Psychoneuroimmunology (PNI)—the interactions among the mind, nervous system, and immune system—is a new discipline that has emerged only in the last fifty years. Even more recent, but no less important, have been the many advances in and applications of psychology to PNI, the contributions of which are essential to the vitality of this rapidly growing field.

The Oxford Handbook of Psychoneuroimmunology comprises perspectives on the state-of-the-art applications of psychological theory to PNI. Chapters in the volume present the multiple ranges of analysis in psychoneuroimmunology, including: genes within cells, cells within organs, organs within individuals, and individuals within both social groups and larger social structures. Furthermore, chapters address the effects of psychological factors on markers of chronic, low-grade, systemic inflammation, which can indicate a risk of such disorders as atherosclerosis, Alzheimer's disease, frailty, and some cancers. The volume provides specific applications of psychoneuroimmunological models to fatigue, cancer, neuroinflammation, and pain, along with a review of how psychotherapeutic approaches, when integrated with psychoneuroimmunological knowledge, can mitigate adverse health outcomes.

This *Oxford Handbook* samples from the best and most sophisticated applications of psychology to PNI, encompassing perspectives from affective science, development, behavioral neuroscience, and clinical psychology.

The Oxford Handbook of
Psychoneuroimmunology

OXFORD LIBRARY OF PSYCHOLOGY

Editor in Chief PETER E. NATHAN

The Oxford Handbook of Psychoneuroimmunology

Edited by

Suzanne C. Segerstrom

UNIVERSITY PRESS

OXFORD
UNIVERSITY PRESS

Oxford University Press, Inc., publishes works that further
Oxford University's objective of excellence
in research, scholarship, and education.

Oxford   New York
Auckland   Cape Town   Dar es Salaam   Hong Kong   Karachi
Kuala Lumpur   Madrid   Melbourne   Mexico City   Nairobi
New Delhi   Shanghai   Taipei   Toronto

With offices in
Argentina   Austria   Brazil   Chile   Czech Republic   France   Greece
Guatemala   Hungary   Italy   Japan   Poland   Portugal   Singapore
South Korea   Switzerland   Thailand   Turkey   Ukraine   Vietnam

Published by Oxford University Press, Inc.
198 Madison Avenue, New York, New York 10016
www.oup.com

Oxford is a registered trademark of Oxford University Press

Library of Congress Cataloging-in-Publication Data
The Oxford handbook of psychoneuroimmunology / edited by Suzanne C. Segerstrom.
    p. cm.
  ISBN 978-0-19-539439-9
  1. Psychoneuroimmunology.   I. Segerstrom, Suzanne C.
  QP356.47.O94 2012
  612.8'043—dc23
  2011052872

9 8 7 6 5 4 3 2 1
Printed in the United States of America
on acid-free paper

SHORT CONTENTS

OXFORD LIBRARY OF PSYCHOLOGY

The *Oxford Library of Psychology*, a landmark series of handbooks, is published by Oxford University Press, one of the world's oldest and most highly respected publishers, with a tradition of publishing significant books in psychology. The ambitious goal of the *Oxford Library of Psychology* is nothing less than to span a vibrant, wide-ranging field and, in so doing, to fill a clear market need.

Encompassing a comprehensive set of handbooks, organized hierarchically, the *Library* incorporates volumes at different levels, each designed to meet a distinct need. At one level are a set of handbooks designed broadly to survey the major subfields of psychology; at another are numerous handbooks that cover important current focal research and scholarly areas of psychology in depth and detail. Planned as a reflection of the dynamism of psychology, the *Library* will grow and expand as psychology itself develops, thereby highlighting significant new research that will impact on the field. Adding to its accessibility and ease of use, the *Library* will be published in print and, later on, electronically.

The *Library* surveys psychology's principal subfields with a set of handbooks that capture the current status and future prospects of those major subdisciplines. This initial set includes handbooks of social and personality psychology, clinical psychology, counseling psychology, school psychology, educational psychology, industrial and organizational psychology, cognitive psychology, cognitive neuroscience, methods and measurements, history, neuropsychology, personality assessment, developmental psychology, and more. Each handbook undertakes to review one of psychology's major subdisciplines with breadth, comprehensiveness, and exemplary scholarship. In addition to these broadly conceived volumes, the *Library* also includes a large number of handbooks designed to explore in depth more specialized areas of scholarship and research, such as stress, health and coping, anxiety and related disorders, cognitive development, or child and adolescent assessment. In contrast to the broad coverage of the subfield handbooks, each of these latter volumes focuses on an especially productive, more highly focused line of scholarship and research. Whether at the broadest or most specific level, however, all of the *Library* handbooks offer synthetic coverage that reviews and evaluates the relevant past and present research and anticipates research in the future. Each handbook in the *Library* includes introductory and concluding chapters written by its editor to provide a road map to the handbook's table of contents and to offer informed anticipations of significant future developments in that field.

An undertaking of this scope calls for handbook editors and chapter authors who are established scholars in the areas about which they write. Many of the nation's and world's most productive and best-respected psychologists have agreed to edit *Library* handbooks or write authoritative chapters in their areas of expertise.

For whom has the *Oxford Library of Psychology* been written? Because of its breadth, depth, and accessibility, the *Library* serves a diverse audience, including graduate students in psychology and their faculty mentors, scholars, researchers, and practitioners in psychology and related fields. Each will find in the *Library* the information they seek on the subfield or focal area of psychology in which they work or are interested.

Befitting its commitment to accessibility, each handbook includes a comprehensive index, as well as extensive references to help guide research. Because the *Library* was designed from its inception as an online as well as a print resource, its structure and contents will be readily and rationally searchable online. Further, once the *Library* is released online, the handbooks will be regularly and thoroughly updated.

In summary, the *Oxford Library of Psychology* will grow organically to provide a thoroughly informed perspective on the field of psychology, one that reflects both psychology's dynamism and its increasing interdisciplinarity. Once published electronically, the *Library* is also destined to become a uniquely valuable interactive tool, with extended search and browsing capabilities. As you begin to consult this handbook, we sincerely hope you will share our enthusiasm for the more than 500-year tradition of Oxford University Press for excellence, innovation, and quality, as exemplified by the *Oxford Library of Psychology.*

Peter E. Nathan
Editor-in-Chief
Oxford Library of Psychology

ABOUT THE EDITOR

Suzanne C. Segerstrom

Suzanne C. Segerstrom is a Professor of Psychology at the University of Kentucky. Her research focuses on how psychological and behavioral factors such as personality, self-control, and stress affect well-being and health, especially the immune system. She has received awards for her work from the American Psychological Association, the Psychoneuroimmunology Research Society, and the National Institutes of Health.

CONTRIBUTORS

Shelley A. Adamo
Department of Psychology and
Neuroscience
Dalhousie University
Halifax, Nova Scotia, Canada

Michael H. Antoni
Department of Psychology
University of Miami
Coral Gables, FL

Arnaud Aubert
Department of Psychology
University of Tours
Tours, France

Wendy Birmingham
Department of Psychology and Health
Psychology Program
University of Utah
Salt Lake City, UT

Lora Black
Department of Psychology
University of Kansas
Lawrence, KS

Roger J. Booth
School of Medical Sciences
The University of Auckland
Auckland, New Zealand

Julienne Bower
Departments of Psychology, Psychiatry, and
Biobehavioral Sciences
Cousins Center of
Psychoneuroimmunology
University of California, Los Angeles
Los Angeles, CA

Anibal Garza Carbajal
Laboratory of Neuroimmunology and
Developmental Origins of Disease
University Medical Center Utrecht
Utrecht, The Netherlands

McKenzie Carlisle
Department of Psychology and Health
Psychology Program
University of Utah
Salt Lake City, UT

Sonia A. Cavigelli
Department of Biobehavioral Health
Pennsylvania State University
State College, PA

Christopher L. Coe
Department of Psychology
University of Wisconsin
Madison, WI

Sheldon Cohen
Department of Psychology
Carnegie Mellon University
Pittsburgh, PA

Steven W. Cole
Department of Medicine
Division of Hematology-Oncology
UCLA School of Medicine
Los Angeles, CA

Erin S. Costanzo
Department of Psychiatry
University of Wisconsin-Madison
Madison, WI

Mary E. Coussons-Read
Department of Psychology
The University of Colorado Denver
Denver, CO

Crista N. Crittenden
Department of Psychology
Carnegie Mellon University
Pittsburgh, PA

Sally S. Dickerson
Department of Psychology & Social Behavior
University of California, Irvine
Irvine, CA

Rita B. Effros
Department of Pathology & Laboratory
Medicine and UCLA AIDS Institute
David Geffen School of Medicine
UCLA Molecular Biology Institute
Los Angeles, CA

Elliot M. Friedman
Department of Human Development
and Family Studies
Purdue University
West Lafayette, IN

Cobi J. Heijnen
Laboratory of Neuroimmunology and
Developmental Origins of Disease
University Medical Center Utrecht
Utrecht, The Netherlands

Michael R. Irwin
Department of Psychiatry and
Biobehavioral Sciences
Cousins Center of Psychoneuroimmunology
University of California, Los Angeles
Los Angeles, CA

Shamini Jain
Samueli Institute
Department of Psychiatry & Behavioral
Medicine
University of California, San Diego
La Jolla, CA

Denise Janicki-Deverts
Department of Psychology
Carnegie Mellon University
Pittsburgh, PA

Heidi S. Kane
Department of Psychology
University of California, Los Angeles
Los Angeles, CA

Annemieke Kavelaars
Department of Pathology
School of Medicine and Department of
Animal Sciences
School of Agricultural and Environmental
Sciences (ACES)
University of Illinois
Urbana-Champaign, IL
Laboratory of Neuroimmunology and
Developmental Origins of Disease
University Medical Center Utrecht
Utrecht, The Netherlands

Gabriele R. Lubach
Harlow Center for Biological Psychology
University of Wisconsin-Madison
Madison, WI

Susan K. Lutgendorf
Departments of Psychology, Obstetrics and
Gynecology, and Urology
Holden Comprehensive Cancer Center
University of Iowa
Iowa City, IA

Kerry C. Michael
Department of Psychiatry
University of Maryland School of
Medicine
Baltimore, MD

Randy J. Nelson
Department of Neuroscience
The Ohio State University
Medical Center
Columbus, OH

Sarah D. Pressman
Department of Psychology
University of Kansas
Lawrence, KS

Theodore F. Robles
Department of Psychology
University of California, Los Angeles
Los Angeles, CA

Suzanne C. Segerstrom
Department of Psychology
University of Kentucky
Lexington, KY

Gregory T. Smith
Department of Psychology
University of Kentucky
Lexington, KY

Rodlescia S. Sneed
Department of Psychology
Carnegie Mellon University
Pittsburgh, PA

Anil K. Sood
Departments of Gynecologic Oncology
and Cancer Biology
Center for RNA Interference and
Non-Coding RNA
M.D. Anderson Cancer Center
University of Texas
Houston, TX

Andrew Steptoe
Department of Epidemiology and Public
Health
University College London
London, UK

Edward C. Suarez
Department of Psychiatry and Behavioral
Sciences
Duke University School of Medicine
Durham, NC

Bert N. Uchino
Department of Psychology and Health
Psychology Program
University of Utah
Salt Lake City, UT

Allison A. Vaughn
Department of Psychology
San Diego State University
San Diego, CA

Zachary M. Weil
Department of Neuroscience
The Ohio State University Medical Center
Columbus, OH

CONTENTS

PREFACE

Suzanne C. Segerstrom

Abstract

The present volume demonstrates how advances in psychological science can contribute to advancing knowledge in psychoneuroimmunology. The traditional focus on stress can be seen in several chapters, but this focus is also modernized in chapters dealing with specific stressful conditions, emotional reactions, and individual differences. The chapters also reveal an expansion of the levels of analysis from molecules to societies. The importance of the immune system for health at the beginning and end of life is reflected in chapters examining psychoneuroimmunological effects from pregnancy through infancy and in the latter decades of life. The chapters in this volume illustrate the best of PNI: cutting-edge models of how the outer and inner worlds interact with each other, and the complexity of both of those worlds.

Key Words: psychoneuroimmunology, stress, development, inflammation

Psychoneuroimmunology (PNI)—the interactions among the mind, nervous system, and immune system—is a fairly new discipline, with many of the earliest, seminal papers having been published less than 50 years ago (e.g., Solomon & Moos, 1964; Ader & Cohen, 1975). However, advances in anatomy and immunology have quickly moved the field along, and it is now widely accepted that the immune system is responsive to many of the messengers employed by the nervous system, and vice versa. This is, of course, a volume in the Oxford Library of Psychology. Therefore, the aim of the present volume is to emphasize recent advances and applications of psychology as they have influenced psychoneuroimmunology. There are six broad sections of chapters that make up the volume. The sections are: Development; Emotion; Personality and Individual Differences; Social Relationships; Ecological Approaches; and Clinical Methods and Models. From these sections, four broad themes emerge: changes in how PNI science approaches stress; expanding the number of levels of analysis; extending PNI along the life course; and a focus on inflammation.

Stress

The first theme addresses a question that may cross the reader's mind when reading the table of contents: Where is the chapter on stress? Stress is one of the earliest and most productive constructs in PNI, and I and many other budding psychoneuroimmunologists were inspired by early studies demonstrating immunological correlates of academic stress, community trauma, caregiving, bereavement, and other stressful events (Irwin, Daniels, Smith, Bloom, & Weiner, 1987; Kiecolt-Glaser, Garner, et al., 1984; Kiecolt-Glaser, Glaser, et al., 1987; McKinnon, Weisse, Reynolds, Bowles, & Baum, 1989). Stress is still a productive construct in PNI, but consistent with advances in how psychologists think about stressful events, it has become more contextualized. For example, it has been some time since Finlay-Jones and Brown (1981) demonstrated the important distinction between threat and loss as they pertain to mental health, and these distinctions may also affect immunological correlates of these different kinds of stressors. Stress can also be productively characterized by its length when considering immunological correlates (Segerstrom & Miller, 2004).

However, the construct of stress was already under criticism before PNI became a discipline. Roberts (1950) famously wrote that "stress, in addition to being itself and the result of itself, is also the cause of itself" (p. 105), having pointed out that the term applies to what organisms respond to, the responses themselves, and the condition caused by these responses. In this volume, we find a more refined view of stress that focuses on specific conditions, such as lack of social status or belonging that may affect the individual (Robles and Kane, chapter 11; Uchino, Vaughn, Carlisle, & Birmingham, chapter 12; Steptoe, chapter 13; and Cole, chapter 14, this volume); on particular emotions, such as shame, that may mediate between external circumstances and immunological responses (e.g., Dickerson, chapter 5, this volume); and on the way that multimodel interventions can address the stress associated with immunologically mediated diseases such as cancer and HIV (Antoni, chapter 21, this volume).

In a related vein, we also find work that recognizes that stress—if such a construct can be pinned down—is an individual phenomenon. A group of people may experience the same event at the same time, but their individual constructions of that event may differ greatly, and these individual differences can drive differences in the immunological sequelae of the event. For example, in a cohort of first-year law students taking the same courses on the same schedule at the same law school, there were large and idiosyncratic differences between and within students in how they appraised their academic futures, and changes in these appraisals were related to changes in cell-mediated immunity (Segerstrom & Sephton, 2010). Personality psychology, having taken a hit in the late 1960s with an influential publication that threw the existence of traits into doubt (Mischel, 1968), has reemerged as an important discipline in psychology in part by work reestablishing the existence and importance of individual differences, and one section of this volume reviews how traits in both humans and nonhuman animals may influence immunity (Michael and Cavigelli, chapter 8; Cohen, Janicki-Deverts, Crittenden, and Sneed, chapter 9; Suarez, chapter 10; this volume).

Of course, traits are not the only individual differences of importance. The past two decades have also seen a rise in affective science: the study of the nature, structure, regulation, and physiology of emotion and mood. Affective science reintroduced the "hot" brain back into the "cool" climate created by the cognitive revolution of the 1960s and the rise of social cognition in the 1970s and 1980s. It also re-ignited a useful debate about whether emotions should be considered distinct from each other or whether they could be usefully arrayed along a smaller number of dimensions. One clear result of this debate that is reflected in this volume is that positive affect is not just the absence of negative affect but may be a separate, orthogonal dimension of experience from negative affect, with its own biological correlates (see Friedman, chapter 3; Pressman and Black, chapter 6, this volume) and that emotion regulation is an important area of study in its own right (Booth, chapter 7, this volume).

Levels of analysis

The study of individual differences interpolates the study of the person between the shared environment and the cell, and this observation provides a segue to the second theme: levels of analysis. In fact, rather than being limited to the more established study of people within groups, organs within people, and cells within organs, the chapters in this volume analyze nearly the whole hierarchy of living systems, from genes and molecules to large social structures (e.g., Cole, chapter 14, this volume). In fact, one section of this volume deals directly with how high-level organization, ecology, coordinates the low-level organizations—organs, cells, and molecules—to align the organism best with the demands of its environment (Adamo, chapter 15; Weil and Nelson, chapter 16; Aubert, chapter 17; this volume). This section on *ecological approaches to psychoneuroimmunology* also provides an alternative perspective on stress—in some cases, the immunological sequelae of stress may appear maladaptive, but in fact may be secondary to adaptive shifts in the energetic priorities of the organism. This perspective has mainly been applied to animal models of energy, stress, and immunity, as reflected in these chapters, but there is clear relevance to human models as well (Segerstrom, 2010; Straub, Cutolo, Buttgereit, & Pongratz, 2010).

The life course

In addition to expanding the dimensions of PNI along levels of analysis, recent work has also been expanding along the life course, the third theme. In the lifespan development section of this volume, authors make the case that the very earliest and latest stages of life are critical for PNI effects, whether those effects relate to pregnancy outcomes, fetal programming, or protection against the deleterious effects of aging on immunity (Cousson-Read, chapter 1; Coe, chapter 2; Friedman, chapter 3; Effros, chapter 4; this volume). In fact, death rates in developed countries such as the United States are curvilinear, with death rates highest under 1 year of age and remaining lower thereafter until age 55 (Centers for Disease Control, 2010a). This U-shaped pattern is also seen in the death rates due to specific infectious causes, including septicemia, meningitis, influenza, and pneumonia (Centers for Disease Control, 2010b), indicating the importance of prenatal and early influences on the developing immune system as well as of immune senescence.

Inflammation

Of course, clinically relevant situations arise all through the lifespan, and even immunological changes present in midlife can increase risk for disease in later life. One final theme that has emerged in the past decade in PNI and is to be found in abundance in this volume is a focus on inflammation. Inflammation contributes to a number of pathologies that develop both acutely and across the lifespan. For example, atherosclerosis is now commonly considered an inflammatory disease (Ross, 1999), and with signs of the disease beginning to develop in late childhood and adolescence (McGill et al., 2000), it is also a lifespan disease. Inflammation increases with age (Friedman, chapter 3; Effros, chapter 4; this volume), is critical to pathologies such as arthritis, autoimmune disease, and neuroinflammation (Kavelaars, Garza Carbajal, and Heijnen, chapter 20, this volume), and also contributes to poorer outcomes in cancer (Lutgendorf, Costanzo, and Sood, chapter 19, this volume). In addition to its effects on peripheral pathologies, inflammation also acts on the brain to affect psychological states, including motivation (Aubert, chapter 17, this volume) and fatigue (Jain, Bower, and Irwin, chapter 18, this volume).

The chapters in this volume illustrate the best of PNI: cutting-edge models of how the outer and inner worlds interact with each other, and the amazing complexity of both of those worlds.

References

Ader, R., & Cohen, N. (1975). Behaviorally conditioned immunosuppression. *Psychosomatic Medicine, 37,* 333–340.

Centers for Disease Control (2010a). GMWK23R: Death rates by 10-year age groups: United States and each state, 1999–2007. Retrieved from http://www.cdc.gov/nchs/data/dvs/MortFinal2007_Worktable23r.pdf, June 25, 2010.

Centers for Disease Control (2010b). GMWK210R: Death rates for 113 selected causes, by 5-year age groups, race, and sex: United States, 1999–2007. Retrieved from http://www.cdc.gov/nchs/data/dvs/MortFinal2007_WorkTable210R.pdf, June 25, 2010.

Finlay-Jones, R., & Brown, G. W. (1981). Types of stressful life event and the onset of anxiety and depressive disorders. *Psychological Medicine, 11,* 803–815.

Irwin, M., Daniels, M., Smith, T. L., Bloom, E., & Weiner, H. (1987). Impaired natural killer cell activity during bereavement. *Brain, Behavior and Immunity, 1,* 98–104.

Kiecolt-Glaser, J. K., Garner, W., Speicher, C., Penn, G. M., Holliday, J., & Glaser, R. (1984). Psychosocial modifiers of immunocompetence in medical students. *Psychosomatic Medicine, 46,* 7–14.

Kiecolt-Glaser, J. K., Glaser, R., Shuttleworth, E. C., Dyer, C. S., Ogrocki, P. & Speicher, C. E. (1987). Chronic stress and immunity in family caregivers of Alzheimer's disease victims. *Psychosomatic Medicine, 49,* 523–535.

McGill, H. C., McMahan, A., Herderick, E. E., Malcom, G. T., Tracy, R. E., Strong, J. P., & the Pathological Determinants of Atherosclerosis in Youth (PDAY) Research Group (2000). Origin of atherosclerosis in childhood and adolescence. *American Journal of Clinical Nutrition, 72,* 1307s–1315s.

McKinnon, W., Weisse, C. S., Reynolds, C. P., Bowles, C. A., & Baum, A. (1989). Chronic stress, leukocyte subpopulations, and humoral response to latent viruses. *Health Psychology, 8,* 389–402.

Mischel, W. (1968). *Personality and assessment.* New York: Wiley.

Roberts, F. (1950). Stress and the general adaptation syndrome. *British Medical Journal, 2,* 104–105.

Ross, R. (1999). Atherosclerosis—an inflammatory disease. *New England Journal of Medicine, 340,* 115–126.

Segerstrom, S. C. (2010). Resources, stress, and immunity: An ecological perspective on human psychoneuroimmunology. *Annals of Behavioral Medicine, 40,* 114–125.

Segerstrom, S. C., & Miller, G. E. (2004). Psychological stress and the human immune system: A meta-analytic study of 30 years of inquiry. *Psychological Bulletin, 130,* 601–630.

Segerstrom, S. C., & Sephton, S. E. (2010). Optimistic expectancies and cell-mediated immunity: The role of positive affect. *Psychological Science, 21,* 448–455.

Solomon, G. F., & Moos, R. H. (1964). Emotions, immunity, and disease: A speculative theoretical integration. *Archives of General Psychiatry, 11,* 657–674.

Straub, R. H., Cutolo, M., Buttgereit, F. & Pongratz, G. (2010). Energy regulation and neuroendocrine–immune control in chronic inflammatory diseases. *Journal of Internal Medicine, 267,* 543–560.

PART 1

Development

Stress and Immunity in Pregnancy

Mary E. Coussons-Read

Abstract

The last decade has seen a dramatic increase in research on the effects of environment and behavior on pregnancy and infant development. A key aspect of these efforts has been to examine how prenatal stress affects pregnancy and maternal and child health and to identify candidate mechanisms for these effects. This chapter describes research addressing how prenatal stress can alter the course of pregnancy and affect infant development and the potential role of neural-immune interactions in mediating these effects. Background research in psychoneuroimmunology, discussion of the role of the immune and endocrine systems in normal and complicated pregnancy, and foundational and ongoing research on how neural-immune interactions are involved in stress-related pregnancy outcomes are presented. The chapter concludes by identifying key future directions and ongoing challenges for research in this field with an eye toward affecting clinical practice.

Key Words: pregnancy, stress, cytokines, inflammatory markers, prematurity, infant outcome, HPA axis

Introduction

The prenatal period is a critical time for all aspects of infant development, and events that affect these processes during pregnancy may have long-lasting negative consequences for infant and child health. Demonstrations of these relationships are provided by studies showing that prenatal events can significantly alter pregnancy outcome and infant well-being with effects ranging from mild to severe perturbations of developmental trajectories to mortality. For example, maternal drug use during pregnancy has been shown to impair a range of aspects of neural, cognitive, and behavioral outcomes with effects that last well into adolescence and adulthood (Curry, 1998). Maternal nutritional status, such as inadequate intake of folic acid, can predispose women to having infants with neural-tube defects (Centers for Disease Control, 2010). More recently, maternal stress has been identified as

a factor that has a potentially important influence on fetal development, and there is growing evidence that psychosocial, cultural, and environmental stressors experienced during gestation can be detrimental to pregnancy outcome and infant physical and mental well-being. Several recent studies have suggested that even milder stresses can affect developmental outcome (Wadhwa et al., 2001; Copper et al., 1996). Many of these studies have focused on how stress impacts birth weight and gestational age, showing that prenatal stress can increase prematurity and the incidence of low birth weight for gestational age (Wadhwa, Sandman, Porto, Dunkel-Schetter, & Garite, 1993; Orr et al., 1996). A few studies that have explored how maternal stress may be associated with complications during pregnancy such as preeclampsia and gestational diabetes have suggested that stress may contribute to the development of pregnancy-related hypertension and frank preeclampsia, and that stress may complicate the potential effects of gestational diabetes (Knackstedt, Hamelmann, & Arck, 2005; Daniells et al., 2003). On the whole, these studies indicate that stress experiences during pregnancy increase the probability of poor outcomes and underscore the importance of understanding these relationships to support healthy mothers and babies. Among the potential shortcomings of many of the aforementioned studies is the fact that they involved retrospective data collection and did not address the pathways that underlie the observed relationships. Ongoing research is focused on clarifying how and when prenatal stress affects pregnancy and the mechanisms of these effects from a psychoneuroimmunology standpoint. This current work extends previous studies of the correlations of stress with poor outcome to explore the pathways that lead from stress exposure to prematurity, preeclampsia, low birth weight, and other suboptimal pregnancy outcomes.

The foundation for this growing area of research is provided by many psychoneuroimmunology studies that show that psychosocial stress alters immune function in nonpregnant individuals. As reviewed elsewhere in this volume, numerous researchers have demonstrated that stressful experiences not only alter cellular immune function in humans but also have a meaningful impact on the health of nonpregnant adults (Kemeny & Gruenewald, 1999; Kemeny & Laudenslager, 1999). Among the findings in this area are studies showing that short-term psychological stress exacerbates symptoms of the common cold and influenza A infection in humans and alters cytokine production in response to respiratory infection Cohen (Cohen, Doyle, & Skoner, 1999). Others have show that the stress of preparing for and taking examinations significantly reduces in vitro natural killer (NK) cell activity and lymphocyte proliferation, exacerbates illness, and slows wound healing, showing that these changes are biologically important for health (Marucha, Kiecolt-Glaser, & Favagehi, 1998; Kiecolt-Glaser, Page, Marucha, MacCallum, & Glaser, 1998; Glaser et al., 1999). Additional work has shown that chronic stress in particular has marked effects on reducing immune function in humans. For example, the persistent social stress of loneliness increases levels of circulating antibodies to herpes virus, indicating alteration of immune function, and the chronic stress of caring for a spouse or relative with Alzheimer's disease reduces NK-cell activity and increases the frequency and duration of illness (Kiecolt-Glaser & Glaser, 1992; Yang & Glaser, 2000). Other typically long-lasting stress experiences including lack of marital satisfaction, divorce, and bereavement have similar negative effects on immunity and health, further emphasizing the role of psychological and social factors in maintaining physical health (Kiecolt-Glaser et al., 1997; Kiecolt-Glaser & Glaser, 1992).

The strength of psychoneuroimmunology-based research showing the impact of stress on immunity in nonpregnant humans together with evidence that stressful experiences during pregnancy can negatively influence gestation and infant health has fueled a significant amount of research on the psychoneuroimmunology of pregnancy. Investigators have hypothesized that chemicals released during the stress response and during activation of the immune system may be responsible for some of these effects, and recent work, described later in this chapter, confirms that this is the case (Cannon, 1998; Gennaro & Fehder, 1996; Livingston, Otado, & Warren, 2003). Work in this area has been focused on first, better characterizing how prenatal stress can change the course of pregnancy and development, second, understanding the state of the immune and endocrine systems in uncomplicated pregnancy and birth, and finally, examining the degree to which stress-related changes in immune and endocrine function are related to perturbations in the normal course of gestation and infant development. By and large, this body of research has supported a role for neural-immune interactions in the effects of stress on pregnancy. Learning more about the psychoneuroimmunology of pregnancy will advance our understanding of the relationships between brain, behavior, and immunity as a whole. This chapter provides a review of our current state of knowledge of the psychoneuroimmunology of pregnancy and how neural-immune interactions play a role in healthy and challenged pregnancies, and the implications of these relationships for clinical practice and ongoing research.

Early Studies

Many of the first demonstrations that stress experienced by mothers during pregnancy can derail the course of normal prenatal development were anecdotal and largely retrospective. Nevertheless, these studies were instrumental in laying the foundation for more recent prospective studies of how and when prenatal stress affects pregnancy. Although a few of these initial studies showed minimal effects of prenatal stress on pregnancy (Milad, Klock, Moses, & Chatterton, 1998), the majority found that stress experiences throughout pregnancy can have a negative impact on infant outcome. Typically, these studies were conducted in groups of women who presented with a pregnancy complication such as preterm labor or preeclampsia, who were then asked to recount stress experiences in the past. Among the critical studies that initially established these connections are findings by Carmichael and Shaw (Carmichael & Shaw, 2000) who noted that significant stress around conception, for example, death of a loved one or divorce, resulted in greater chances of delivering an infant with conotruncal heart defects, neural-tube defects, and isolated cleft lip. Glynn et al. (Glynn, Wadhwa, Dunkel-Schetter, Chicz-DeMet, & Sandman, 2001) found that trauma resulting from an earthquake had a greater negative effect on gestational length if experienced early in pregnancy. Although these and other studies were focused on the effects of major stressors, many women experience less severe stress, either periodically or consistently, through their pregnancies. Several studies addressed this fact by asking women to report other types of stress across their pregnancies, asking for self-report of daily hassles, life events, and stresses related to relationships and work/job stress. Consistent with studies of large magnitude stress, modest and mild stressors have also been shown to be related to low birth weight as well as maternal psychological status during pregnancy (DiPietro, Ghera, Costigan, & Hawkins, 2004; Schempf, Strobino, & O'Campo, 2009).

Collectively, these studies do clearly illustrate that stress during pregnancy may not be a benign event, and potentially can have a significant impact on outcomes for mothers and babies. The implications of these studies are important: 70% of infant perinatal deaths in the United States are related to low birth weight (LBW), preterm delivery, and restricted fetal growth, all of which are more likely to occur in women who experience stress during gestation. This work has generally shown that both major and minor stressors are associated with premature delivery, prolonged labor, and LBW. Complications such as these can affect up to half of pregnancies in healthy adult women (Orr et al., 1996; Carmichael & Shaw, 2000; Peacock, Bland, & Anderson, 1995). Interestingly, high levels of social support do not necessarily insulate women against these effects. Studies suggest that physiological events related to the stress may underlie these untoward effects observed, emphasizing the need for early identification of at-risk women (Williamson, LeFevre, & Hector, 1989). A limitation of many of these earlier studies is that they were retrospective

and their ability to establish which stresses were directly tied to the outcomes observed or the temporal relationship of these effects was limited. As will be discussed later in this chapter, more recent studies have attempted to prospectively assess the effects of prenatal stress on pregnancy outcome and infant development, and they have begun to assess the possible mechanisms of these changes.

Defining and Measuring the Effects of Prenatal Stress

Developing a solid understanding of research on the effects of stress on pregnancy requires being cognizant of the ways in which researchers choose to operationalize and measure stress. Stress is described by psychoneuroimmunology researchers in a variety of ways. Looking for common aspects of how *stress* is defined is important for assessing the current state of our knowledge as well as for framing the overall direction of research in this area. Typically, definitions of stress include events, situations, emotions, and interactions that are perceived as negatively affecting the well-being of the individual or that cause responses perceived as harmful (Dantzer, 1989; Orr, James, & Casper, 1992; Maes et al., 1998). A key feature of this conceptualization of stress is the distinction between the events themselves and how they are perceived. In other words, the same event may be stressful for one individual and may not be perceived as being stressful for another (Kemeny & Laudenslager, 1999). The role of individual differences in the impact of stress on pregnancy remains a fundamental point of challenge for research and provides an essential focus for future research. Current research on how pregnancy is affected by stress, however, has attempted to capture the general concept of stress as described earlier, with particular focus on psychosocial stressors (Coussons-Read, Okun, & Nettles, 2007; Gennaro & Fehder, 1996; Wadhwa et al., 2001; Ruiz & Fullerton, 1999). The concept of a psychosocial stressor encompasses life experiences, including changes in personal life, job status, housing, domestic violence, and family makeup, which require adaptive coping behavior on the part of the affected individual (Yali & Lobel, 1999; Orr et al., 1992). Maternal stress experiences during pregnancy can range from severe trauma to moderate life-event changes to low experience of daily hassles. Research regarding the effects of maternal stress on pregnancy outcome have included a range of definitions of stressors and stress, but there is quite good consistency in these studies supporting the idea that prenatal stress experienced by mothers can have adverse effects on pregnancy and infant health.

It is important to note that, although some investigators use established clinical tools to assess the effects of stress on pregnancy, others have created their own tools to assess stress in a clinical setting (Orr et al., 1992; DiPietro et al., 2004; Coussons-Read, Okun, Schmitt, & Giese, 2005). This reflects some of the peculiarities of measuring stress during pregnancy, such as, in some cases, the need to incorporate stress assessments into already time-pressured prenatal care visits and the desire to capture some of the alterations in stress perception and priorities that may occur when women are pregnant (Coussons-Read et al., 2007; Coussons-Read et al., 2005; Orr et al., 1992; Ruiz & Avant, 2005). One assessment tool that acknowledges that there are pregnancy-specific aspects of stress that need to be measured across pregnancy is the NUPDQ (Prenatal Distress Questionnaire) assessment used by Lobel and colleagues (Hamilton & Lobel, 2008; Lobel, DeVincent, Kaminer, & Meyer, 2000). This approach is important as it adds an important dimension to research in this area because the NUPDQ effectively taps into the fact that, although "typical" stressors affect women during pregnancy, there are pregnancy-specific stressors that can create maternal distress. These pregnancy-specific stressors, such as worry about prenatal screenings and concerns about infant health and development, may change across the trimesters of pregnancy, and the NUPDQ accounts for this. This approach captures the reality that pregnancy has unique characteristics that may alter (a) perceptions of stress by women, (b) what is stressful to women and when, and/or (c) how women respond to stress. Studies using the NUPDQ have shown that pregnancy-specific distress is associated with increased occurrence of maternal anxiety during pregnancy as well as higher rates of unplanned cesarean sections (Saunders, Lobel, Veloso, & Meyer, 2006; Lobel et al., 2008). The addition of these pregnancy-specific measures to more traditional definitions of stress is helping to create a more complete picture of the dimensions of stress that can affect pregnancy.

Possible Mechanisms for the Effects of Stress on Fetal Development

A key question posed by researchers in this area is the degree to which prenatal stress exposures affect infant and child development. A growing body of work is demonstrating that maternal stress during pregnancy can have persistent effects on infant behavioral, physiological, and immunological development. Animal-based studies indicate that brain development, specifically that of the hippocampal system, which is heavily involved in learning and memory, is adversely affected by prenatal stress and stress hormones during gestation (Mandyam, Crawford, Eisch, Rivier, & Richardson, 2008; Short et al., 2010). Similar effects have been demonstrated in human populations, noting not only changes in brain development, but function as well (Lou et al., 1994; Buss, Davis, Muftuler, Head, & Sandman, 2010). Other animal studies show that prenatal stress affects the development of anxiety behavior and acoustic startle responses creating effects that last through adulthood (Kjaer, Wegener, Rosenberg, Lund, & Hougaard, 2010; Kapoor, Kostaki, Janus, & Matthews, 2009). The mechanism of these effects is likely to involve passage of stress hormones from the mother to the infant. Prenatal stress induces the release of glucocorticoids in the mother, which enter the fetal circulation where they gain access to the developing nervous system (Field & Diego, 2008; Kleinhaus et al., 2010). Interestingly, neurons in the developing hippocampus express high numbers of glucocorticoid receptors, and appear to be especially sensitive to the effects of stress in both infant and adult animals (Mandyam et al., 2008; Jia et al., 2010). It has been hypothesized that increases in stress hormones in the fetus induced by maternal stress alter hippocampal development by binding to these receptors and either have a neurotoxic effect or disrupt development in other ways (Jia et al., 2010; Weinstock, 2005; Fukumoto et al., 2009). Prenatal stress-related changes in the development of the hippocampal system have been tied to persistent impairments in learning and memory across the life span in animal models.

Effects of Stress on the Developing Immune System

Exposure to stress hormones in the prenatal environment also appears to have lasting effects on the function of the immune system. This has been demonstrated in a number of animal studies that have examined the effects of prenatal administration of exogenous glucocorticoids to rats. These studies showed that prenatal administration of dexamethasone (DEX) reduced cell numbers in the thymus and spleen and altered the developing HPA axis in a manner that predisposed rats to being stress hyperresponsive later in life (Ruiz & Avant, 2005; Bakker et al., 1995). The importance of these connections is emphasized by work in nonhuman primates showing that maternal prenatal stress reduces the ability of the immune system of offspring to respond to immune challenges. For example, Coe et al. demonstrated that rhesus monkeys whose mothers were chronically stressed during pregnancy had lower proliferation of immune cells in response to a challenge relative to nonstressed offspring, suggesting an impaired ability of the immune system to adequately respond when necessary (Coe, Lubach, & Karaszewski, 1999). Although not as numerous, human studies of the effects of prenatal stress on immune function in offspring are consistent with the animal studies, showing persistent and functionally relevant changes in immune function in the offspring of stressed mothers. For example, experiences of prenatal stress have been associated with increased occurrence of allergy and asthma, reduced response to infection, and lowered immunity at birth (Ruiz & Avant, 2005; Wright et al., 2010). Others have demonstrated that maternal stress during gestation can have lasting effects on immunity into adulthood. For example, Entringer and colleagues found that the lymphocytes of adult women whose mothers experienced a major negative event during pregnancy showed alerted production of cytokines in vitro (Entringer et al., 2008).

Psychosocial Stressors and the Effect of Minority Status

A final facet of the research on the effects of stress during pregnancy on infant outcome is the fact that there continues to be a significant degree of racial disparity in both the frequency of negative pregnancy outcomes and in the impact of stress on pregnancies in minority women. For example, the rates of occurrence of LBW, premature labor and delivery, and small-for-gestational-age infants are significantly higher in nonwhite minority women (Giscombe & Lobel, 2005). The rate of infant mortality and LBW is nearly 2.5 times higher among African American woman than among Caucasians (Copper, Goldenberg, DuBard, & Davis, 1994; Livingston et al., 2003). Although Hispanic women as a whole have been reported to have rates of LBW similar to those of whites (Copper et al., 1994), women of Puerto Rican descent and highly acculturated Hispanic women have significantly higher rates of LBW, pregnancy complications, and poor infant outcomes than their Caucasian counterparts (Tumiel, Buck, Zayas, & Jaen, 1998). Stress, lack of social support, and other psychosocial factors appear to be critical in the disparities in pregnancy outcome observed between minority and

nonminority women. For example, although stress exposure during pregnancy is generally related to poorer outcomes regardless of racial or ethnic group, the negative effects of stress appear to be more severe for African American women than for Caucasians. In a study of LBW in urban populations, although many prenatal behaviors such as smoking and hypertension in pregnancy were risk factors for LBW for both Caucasian and African American women, exposure to stress was only predictive of LBW for African American women (Livingston et al., 2003; Leff et al., 1992). Others have shown that nonwhite women experience more adverse birth outcomes associated with stress and low social support than white women, further suggesting that the combination of being a member of a minority group and psychosocial challenges may be especially perilous for pregnancy success (Mckee, Cunningham, Jankowski, & Zayas, 2001). For Hispanics, for instance, birth outcomes deteriorate as the number of years for which they have lived in America increases, implying that attempting to adapt to a new culture may be a chronic stressor (Luecken, Purdom, & Howe, 2009; Tumiel et al., 1998; Reichman & Kenney, 1998). These findings emphasize that the concept of stress is multifaceted and an individual's experiences of stress during pregnancy are influenced not only by the "stressors" themselves as described earlier, but also by the cultural, social, and environmental context in which the stressors occur. Clearly, a real challenge for research on the psychoneuroimmunology of pregnancy is considering and assessing the social, psychological, cultural, and environmental complexities that create stress for women during pregnancy.

The Pregnant Immune and Endocrine Systems

Although more researchers are exploring the question, to date, few studies have directly addressed whether there is an association between psychological or environmental stress, neural-immune factors, and pregnancy outcome. One explanation for the relative paucity of work on this topic is the view that pregnancy itself is, by necessity, an immunocompromised state full of changes in other physiological systems (Colbern & Main, 1991; Daunter, 1992). It has been argued that due to the changes in immune and endocrine function that occur in pregnancy, assessing the effects of stress on these systems is difficult. Although it is true that successful pregnancy is characterized by a host of adjustments in the endocrine, immune, and nervous systems, given that pregnancy is a normal physiological state for women, it is important to work to tease apart these complexities when possible to understand how stress may perturb normal pregnancies and threaten maternal and child health.

Normal pregnancy has been suggested to be a balance of aspects of the immune, endocrine, and nervous systems that delicately shifts through the course of pregnancy to support maternal well-being and prenatal development (Daunter, 1992; Arck, 2001). There are significant alterations in maternal physiology that together support a healthy pregnancy. Key in this conceptualization of a balance among these systems is the fact that the collective changes in them that are necessary for successful outcome create an interdependence that can be perturbed by stress or other influences. In other words, changes in endocrine system function induced by stress can affect aspects of both the immune and nervous systems, potentially disrupting the balance that supports normal pregnancy. Similarly, strengthening or supporting one or more of these systems may help to ensure that the necessary functional shifts in and among these three systems are maintained to encourage maternal and infant well-being.

The maternal immune system undergoes substantial changes during the course of pregnancy, and these changes reflect the evolving needs of the mother and infant. The immune system has been described as shifting toward a more anti-inflammatory profile than normal during pregnancy out of necessity (Daunter, 1992; Colbern & Main, 1991). The presence of paternal antigens in the fetus could be detected as an immunologic challenge by maternal physiology, and the pregnant woman's immune system must be altered from its normal state to avoid rejection of the conceptus (Gennaro & Fehder, 1996; Hill & Choi, 2000). Modifications made by the maternal immune system during pregnancy to avoid this include separation of maternal and fetal circulation, protection of the uterus as an immunologically privileged location during gestation, and changes in maternal lymphocyte function and subsets (Gennaro & Fehder, 1996). One hypothesis about how the mother's immune system avoids rejecting the baby is that maternal immunity switches to favor a Th 2-type immune response over a Th 1-type immune response, especially early in pregnancy (Saito et al., 1999; Saito, 2000; Vassiliadis, Ranella, Papadimitriou, Makrygiannakis, & Athanassikis, 1998). Th-1 and Th-2 type responses are two arms of the human immune response that serve different but complementary roles. The Th 1-type response

system provides immediate defense against invading pathogens and antigens, and the Th 2-type system mediates formation and maintenance of antibody responses (Elenkov, 1999). Both types of processes are involved in responses to pathogens, with either the Th 1- or Th 2-type response dominating in certain situations. A shift away from Th 1 responsiveness in early pregnancy is supported by observed reductions in maternal NK cell number and activity (Opsahl, Hansen, Klein, & Cunningham, 1994), lymphocyte proliferation (Matthiesen, Berg, Ernerudh, & Hakansson, 1996) (Fiddes et al., 1986), and decreases in Th 1-type cytokines (Pope, 1990). Reduced maternal immunity in pregnancy is further reflected in epidemiological data indicating increased severity and duration of viral and fungal infections and decreased intensity of autoimmune diseases such as systemic lupus erythematosis and rheumatoid arthritis during pregnancy (Zauner, Rother, & Schollmeyer, 1995; Pope, Yoshinoya, Rutstein, & Persellin, 1983). These adjustments of the maternal immune system do not rule out the possibility that stress-induced immunosuppression could magnify these pregnancy-related changes and reduce the success of pregnancy by increasing the likelihood of infection. Moreover, the necessity of reducing Th 1 and more inflammatory responses during pregnancy to support normal gestation suggests that stress-related increases of cytokines and other aspects of the inflammatory response may set the stage for disruption of the normal balance of pregnancy.

Cytokines produced by cells of the immune system are involved in maintenance of pregnancy as well as in the onset of normal labor and delivery. One primary way cytokines are classified is based on whether they are produced by cells involved in the Th 1- or Th 2-type human immune response (Roitt, 1991). The importance of shifting to favor aspects of a Th 2-type immune response in normal pregnancy described earlier suggests that cytokines associated with progression of Th 1 and Th 2 immune responses may be involved in various aspects of pregnancy progression. The possibility that successful pregnancy may be mediated in part by cytokines is supported by studies in which circulating cytokines at various points in gestation are correlated with aspects of pregnancy success. For example, a possible role of Th 1- type immune responsiveness in early miscarriage is suggested by the finding that levels of the Th 1 cytokine interferon gamma (IFN-γ) are significantly elevated in women who have recurrent miscarriages compared to women with normal pregnancies (Piccinni, 2007; Piccinni, Maggi, & Romagnani, 2000). Other studies support a shift away from Th 1 responses during pregnancy, showing reduced IFN-γ and IL-2, both Th 1 cytokines, in women with normal pregnancies (Kruse et al., 2000; Piccinni, Scaletti, Maggi, & Romagnani, 2000). These studies suggest that, indeed, shifting the immune system toward a Th 2-type response may be beneficial in pregnancy, and that increased levels of Th 1-type cytokines may be detrimental.

Another cytokine-related distinction that is critical in understanding the impact of immune activation on pregnancy is that some cytokines help to generate an inflammatory (pro-inflammatory cytokines) response, whereas others reduce such responses (anti-inflammatory cytokines). This distinction is in addition to Th 1 and Th 2 classification and is based on whether a cytokine drives or suppresses the inflammatory process. Inflammation is a fundamental aspect of the immune response in which activated cells attack and disable invading pathogens. Infection or injury reliably initiates an inflammatory response, and although this response is adaptive and effective in eliminating infection, it can be damaging if misdirected or prolonged (Roitt, 1991). Pro-inflammatory cytokines relevant to pregnancy include interleukin 1-β (IL-1β), interleukin 8 (IL-8), tumor necrosis factor alpha (TNF-α), and interleukin-6 (IL-6). As mentioned earlier, stress induces production of pro-inflammatory cytokines that are also produced as part of infection. These cytokines are involved in the ripening of the cervix before delivery, and elevated levels of IL-6, IL-8, and TNF-α are associated with premature labor and delivery (Zhang, Wang, Zhao, & Kang, 2000).

Shifting the maternal immune system away from the Th 1 response toward the Th 2 response and the concomitant changes in the cytokines produced by this switch also affect the pregnant mother's health in other ways. The significance of these changes is best cast in terms of the impact of maternal infection on labor and birth outcome. Both systemic and intrauterine infections contribute to premature labor and delivery (Gibbs, Romero, Hillier, Eschenbach, & Sweet, 1992; Gomez et al., 1995; Wadhwa et al., 2001). For example, although antibiotic treatment has significantly reduced pneumonia-related deaths, pneumonia still drastically increases the incidence of preterm delivery in pregnant women. Other untreated infections, such as malaria and typhoid fever, predispose women to preterm labor and delivery (Gomez et al., 1995; Santhanam et al., 1991).

Moreover, undetected intrauterine infections and urinary tract infections are not uncommon in pregnancy, and they have been shown to contribute to preterm labor (McGregor, French, Lawellin, & Todd, 2000; Wadhwa et al., 2001). Studies have shown that high levels of TNF-α, which is released in response to viral and bacterial infections, are associated with premature labor. Administration of TNF-α to animals also produces preterm labor (McGregor et al., 2000; Romero, Sirtori et al., 1989; Park, Park, Lockwood, & Norwitz, 2005). Similarly, administration of IL1-β induces premature labor and delivery in laboratory animals, and it is significantly elevated in the amniotic fluid of women with intramniotic infections who deliver prematurely (Romero, Sirtori, et al., 1989; Romero, Mazor et al., 1989; Romero, Brody et al., 1989). Interestingly, these cytokines are also elevated in nonpregnant laboratory animals and humans following stress (Persoons, Schornagel, Breve, Berkenbosch, & Kraal, 1995). Not only is there evidence, therefore, that infection-related increases in pro-inflammatory cytokine production may alter pregnancy outcome, but data also suggest that stress-induced changes in these mediators may affect the timing of parturition.

Effects of Maternal Stress during Pregnancy

Alterations and activity in the systems that respond to stress are also critical players in pregnancy outcome. Maternal endocrine and sympathetic nervous system responses to stress, not surprisingly, have the potential to impact fetal physiology and development, and research shows that activation of aspects of these responses may affect the course of pregnancy. The physiological stress response is activated when an individual consciously or unconsciously perceives a physical or psychological stimulus as a threat to their well-being. Components of this response include increased sympathetic arousal, heart rate, and increases in cortisol and catecholamines that have antigrowth, antireproductive, anti-inflammatory and immunosuppressive effects (Chrousos, 1999; Kalantaridou, Makrigiannakis, Mastorakos, & Chrousos, 2003). Perception of a stressor results in activation of the sympathetic nervous system (SNS). A primary component of the fight-or-flight response is an increase in the release of the neurotransmitters norepinephrine (NE) and epinephrine (E). Activation of the hypothalamo-pituitary-adrenal (HPA) axis is essential to this response, and recognition of a psychological or physical stressor induces the release of corticotropin-releasing hormone (CRH) in the hypothalamus. CRH stimulates the anterior pituitary gland to release adrenocorticotropin hormone (ACTH), which, in turn, stimulates cortisol release from the adrenal cortex (Ruiz & Avant, 2005; Field & Diego, 2008). This concert of neurochemical changes temporarily directs energy toward dealing with the stressful situation and away from other bodily functions including reproduction, immune function, and digestion, to name a few. At the conclusion of short-term stress, these changes are no longer needed, and the body quickly returns to homeostasis. Chronic stress, however, prolongs activation of these systems in a manner that has clearly detrimental effects for health, cardiovascular function, metabolism, and immunity (Rabin, 1999).

Activation of this stress response affects pregnancy, and women who encounter psychosocial stress during pregnancy have higher levels of ACTH, CRH, and cortisol than nonstressed pregnant women (Wadhwa et al., 1993; McLean & Smith, 2001) Women experiencing preterm labor and delivery have significantly higher levels of plasma cortisol and CRH prior to onset of labor than women who deliver normally (Pearce et al., 2010; Field & Diego, 2008).

A major component of the response to stress is release of CRH in the hypothalamus, which regulates the peripheral activities of the HPA axis. The placenta also produces CRH, which increases exponentially over gestation (Wadhwa, 2005). Considerable interest has focused on the role of stress-related CRH production in modulation of labor and delivery, because CRH may act as a signal for normal labor, and if stress-related, it may induce premature labor (Kalantaridou et al., 2003; Stamatelou, Deligeoroglou, Farmakides, & Creatsas, 2009). Studies indicate that maternal stress appears to increase CRH levels, and given the role that CRH plays in regulation of parturition, it may be that stress-related increases in it may contribute to premature labor (Wadhwa, 2005).

Other aspects of the stress response appear to be involved in the effects of stress on immunity. There is significant evidence that NE, cortisol, and ACTH are potent immunosuppressors, and some studies suggest that these neurochemicals act to directly suppress immune status (Kimura K. et al., 2000; Wiegers, Croiset, Reul, Holsboer, & de Kloet, 1993). Stressed animals and humans have elevated levels of cortisol, CRH, and ACTH, which correlate with suppressed measures of immune function including NK activity, lymphocyte proliferation, and cytokine production (DeKeyser, Leker, & Weidenfeld, 2000; Rook, 1999; Dunn, 1993). Recent evidence shows that the immune system and the endocrine system talk to each other and can regulate each other's functions. For example, the body perceives infection and immune system activation as stressors, and stress-related hormones are increased in response to these events just as they are to a psychological stressor. Activation of the immune system by antigens activates the HPA axis and results in increases in CRH and corticosterone and cortisol, which, in turn, can suppress immune function if not appropriately controlled (Lacey et al., 2000; Dunn, 1993; Elenkov & Chrousos, 1999). This connection is further solidified by studies showing that addition of very small amounts of cortisol or NE to cell cultures dramatically inhibits lymphocyte proliferation and cytokine production, supporting the suggestion that these substances directly alter immune cell function (Schwarze & Bartmann, 1994; Wiegers et al., 1993; Cardinal, Pretorius, & Ungerer, 2010). These studies emphasize the interactive nature of immune and endocrine regulation and suggest multiple pathways through which psychosocial stress and infection might alter homeostasis in nonpregnant adults. Given the strength of the literature supporting an impact of stress on immune function and health, it is logical to see if these relationships apply to pregnancy, a time in which not only the mother's but also her baby's health depends on the function and integrity of maternal physiology and immunity.

Neural-Immune Interactions in Pregnancy

The above findings have helped to create a working hypothesis that drives a substantial amount of research on how stress affects pregnancy. Several investigators have hypothesized that psychological and social stressors encountered by mothers during pregnancy affect pregnancy outcome by altering immune function via neurochemicals that are released as part of the physiological response to stress (Coussons-Read, 2003; Ruiz & Avant, 2005; Pearce et al., 2010; Knackstedt et al., 2005). There are several possible pathways for these effects. Prenatal stress might directly increase the production of pro-inflammatory and Th1 cytokines by immune cells, perhaps via the endocrine system, or stress might increase susceptibility to infections that, in turn, induce cytokine production. A growing body of research supports these connections and suggests that, indeed, stress-related changes in immune function and cytokine production may play a role in the effects of stress on poor pregnancy outcome.

Several studies have successfully established that stress experiences during pregnancy can alter maternal immune function and cytokine balance, and that these changes appear to be associated with increased occurrence of pregnancy complications and suboptimal outcome. Although there are limitations to research using pregnant women and these studies have a difficult time establishing causal relationships between stress, changes in immune and endocrine function, and pregnancy outcome, they are paving the way for future work that can help complete the picture of how stress-related neural-immune interactions affect pregnancy.

A key feature of more recent work in this area is that researchers have been able to extend earlier work based on prospective assessments of stress to create longitudinal and prospective studies examining how stress experiences across pregnancy affect endocrine and immune function and, in turn, alter pregnancy outcomes. An exciting aspect of these studies is that many of them have assessed stress, biomarkers, and outcome in larger cohorts of women and have done so throughout and, in some cases, after pregnancy. Currently published data from these studies indicates two things: (a) that prenatal stress and associated alterations in production of stress-related hormones are related to poor pregnancy outcome, and (b) that prenatal stress and associated alterations in cytokine balance and production are related to poor pregnancy outcome. These relationships are becoming well established. Current work is now turning toward connecting these bodies of work to test the hypothesis that stress alters immune function and cytokine balance via the SNS and/or HPA axis aspects of the stress response, and these changes, in turn, affect pregnancy outcome. Clearly, another aspect of this research is that the immune and endocrine systems appear to modulate each other in a bidirectional fashion (Rabin, Cohen, Ganguli, Lysle, & Cunnick, 1989), and as such, it will also be important to examine how this relationship relates to pregnancy outcome.

A primary finding that supports work in this area is that, indeed, maternal stress experiences and perceptions do result in strong activation of the stress response (Buss et al., 2009; Pluess, Bolten, Pirke, & Hellhammer, 2010). This is an important piece of information, as it confirms that maternal stress responses are altered during pregnancy (Slattery & Neumann, 2008; Russell, Douglas, & Brunton, 2008), and they may be of sufficient magnitude that they could have the potential to modulate other aspects of maternal health. Within this context,

several studies have connected stress-related changes in HPA axis activity and stress responsiveness with shorter gestational length, higher probability of preterm labor and delivery, and LBW. For example, studies of women in the second trimester of pregnancy indicate that women who had higher levels of cortisol at that time had a substantially higher probability of exhibiting preterm labor (Field & Diego, 2008). Others have shown that women who experience stress and have higher levels of stress-related hormones as a result are more likely to have infants with LBW (Field & Diego, 2008; Diego et al., 2006). Still others have reported that maternal stress experiences and the resulting activation of the HPA axis are related to both preterm labor as well as lasting effects on infant development that result from prematurity (Wadhwa, 2005). Stress hormones have also been tied to the development of pregnancy complications such as preeclampsia and gestational diabetes, further suggesting that there may be direct effects of stress on pregnancy outcome and indicating that, at a minimum, stress experiences impact the severity of pregnancy-related complications (Shamsi et al., 2010; Roberts & Lain, 2002).

Other studies have established that stress experiences alter cytokine balance and production in a manner that predisposes women to poor pregnancy outcomes. The bulk of these studies have relied on serum or plasma assessments of circulating cytokines across pregnancy, with a smaller number looking at production of these substances by immune cells in vitro (Coussons-Read et al., 2007; Coussons-Read et al., 2005; Ruiz & Avant, 2005; Ruiz, Fullerton, & Dudley, 2003). Clearly, these two approaches provide different levels of information, with the former indicating global levels of cytokines produced by the placenta, the maternal immune system, and adipose tissue, and the latter isolating the effects of stress on the ability of stimulated lymphocytes to produce cytokines. A consistent finding from these studies is that psychosocial stress is associated with elevations in circulating levels of pro-inflammatory cytokines that have been associated with poor outcome, including TNF-α and IL-6 (Ruiz & Avant, 2005; Pearce et al., 2010; Coussons-Read, 2003; Coussons-Read et al., 2005). Other work has indicated that such stress increases production of pro-inflammatory cytokines in cultured lymphocytes, indicating that, although other sources of cytokines contribute to measures of circulating levels of these substances, the ability of immune cells to produce these mediators is affected by stress (Coussons-Read et al., 2007; Pearce et al., 2010). Together, these types of studies have established that prenatal stress does perturb the critical balance of immune responsiveness described previously in this chapter, and that these changes appear to map onto the occurrence of preterm labor, LBW, infant complications, and other complications of pregnancy. Importantly, ongoing research is connecting these stress-related changes in pro-inflammatory cytokines to poor pregnancy outcomes including prematurity, higher frequency of pregnancy complications (Coussons-Read, in press). This connection is essential for linking stress-related changes in immune mediators to meaningful outcomes for mothers and infants.

Conclusions and Future Directions

The implications of this body of research reach far beyond labor and delivery into infancy and early childhood. There is significant evidence that prenatal stress can have a negative impact on infant behavioral and cognitive development. For example, infants from stressed pregnancies are harder to soothe and have been characterized as being more temperamental than infants from pregnancies in which the mothers did not report significant stress (Field & Diego, 2008; Martin, Noyes, & Wisenbaker, 1999). Stressful pregnancies are also related to slower cognitive development, and have been correlated with slower infant growth and development in animals and humans (Sandman, Wadhwa, Chicz-DeMet, Dunkel-Schetter, & Porto, 1997; Swolin-Eide, Nilsson, Holmang, & Ohlsson, 2004; Romo, Carceller, & Tobajas, 2009). Animal and human studies have also shown that infants of stressed pregnancies have poorer immune function and are more likely to contract childhood illnesses (Coe & Lubach, 2000; Narendran, Visscher, Abril, Hendrix, & Hoath, 2010; Ruiz & Avant, 2005). These studies implicate prenatal maternal immune system dysfunction resulting from stress in these effects, but human studies have yet to clearly confirm this relationship. Understanding the mechanisms through which prenatal stress affects maternal and infant health may provide clues for how to ameliorate some of these postnatal effects. It is hoped that such studies will eventually provide a basis for providing patients with the psychological and behavioral tools with which they can learn to manage stress in the prenatal period.

Although clearly, research aimed at understanding the impact of stress on pregnancy and infant outcome has already provided important clues

about when and how prenatal stress affects gestation, a great deal of work remains to be done. Some of the challenges facing researchers in this area are common to those faced by researchers in other areas of psychoneuroimmunology, but others are unique. Four major areas for future growth of research in this field are identified and discussed below. Rapidly advancing research in psychoneuroimmunology and in the study of stress and pregnancy suggests that these major goals are within reach.

The first major challenge facing researchers in this area is the need to connect the two bodies of work described in the previous section of this chapter. In other words, at this point, we know that prenatal stress induces changes in endocrine function and that these changes are related to poor outcome. Prenatal stress induces changes in cytokine balance and production, and these changes are related to poor outcome. Now, it is necessary to connect stress-related immune and endocrine changes to each other and then to pregnancy outcome. Given our current state of understanding of the connections between stress, endocrine and immune function, and health outcomes in nonpregnant populations (Dantzer, 1989; Graham, Christian, & Kiecolt-Glaser, 2006; Malarkey, Glaser, Kiecolt-Glaser, & Marucha, 2001), it is likely that additional research will be able to establish these pathways in pregnancy. Such demonstrations will provide more detailed analysis of the biological pathways connecting stress to pregnancy outcome.

The second major challenge is a common one for research in psychoneuroimmunology. If the goal of studying how stress affects pregnancy is to identify at-risk pregnancies and develop therapeutic strategies for supporting pregnant women, it is essential that researchers in this area be able to generalize a specific finding to a larger population or clinical situation. Although studies indicate that prenatal stress and inadequate social support increase levels of circulating pro-inflammatory cytokines, it is unclear what, if any, direct relevance for outcome is related to this finding (Coussons-Read et al., 2005). Although authors of these studies show that such increases in cytokines in the maternal circulation are related to an increased risk of complications, this connection is indirect (Coussons-Read et al., 2007; Pearce et al., 2010). Moreover, although such studies show that "an increase" in these measures occurs, the magnitude of change necessary to observe an increase in pregnancy complications is unknown. A key goal of future research in the effects of stress on pregnancy is to determine the degree to which alterations in immune function and biomarkers associated with prenatal stress are truly predictive of poor obstetrical outcome. Our current understanding of what stress does to pregnancy does suggest that clinically meaningful changes in outcome occur when stress is experienced prenatally, but few studies have prospectively assessed this relationship and tied stress-related changes in immune function to outcome. For example, although studies have shown that bereavement experienced by mothers in pregnancy is associated with increased occurrence of LBW (Khashan et al., 2008), we do not currently understand the timing, duration, and severity of bereavement or what changes in biomarkers are necessary to result in a clinically relevant outcome. Although difficult to do, such investigations are necessary if a goal of research in this area is to develop screening tools and, eventually, interventions that clinicians can use to identify and support women who are at risk for a stress-related pregnancy outcome. Future studies will be able to prospectively assess the magnitude and timing of stress experiences and the biological changes that are associated with them and be able to relate them to changes in pregnancy and birth outcome.

The third major area of focus for research addressing how stress affects pregnancy is developing effective and affordable screening tools that will allow clinical personnel to identify women whose pregnancies are at risk for stress-related poor outcomes. Of course, being able to do this requires success in the first area of focus mentioned earlier; until the importance of stress and stress-related changes in biological mediators for clinical outcome has been established, development of screening tools is impossible. However, once this information is available, it will be essential to translate these research findings into useable and reliable tools that can be used to assess stress-related risk across pregnancy. Depending on what is learned about the strongest predictors of stress-related poor pregnancy outcome, these tools may take the form of interviews or paper-and-pencil assessments, assessment of biomarkers in blood and/or saliva, or a combination of these. The key to accomplishing this task will be to create screening tools that can be completed quickly and inexpensively that can be deployed and used in large patient populations. Partnerships between research teams and clinicians will be necessary to develop and test possible screening options that meet the aforementioned goals and reliably identify at-risk women. The primary challenge associated with these partnerships will be translating research findings and methods into simple, repeatable, processes and tests that provide reliable data while meeting the financial and clinical goals of practitioners.

The final, and perhaps ultimate, goal of research on stress and pregnancy is to develop interventions that help at-risk women deal with stress effectively during pregnancy and support them in having healthy babies. Several investigators are already working in this area to develop stress-reduction interventions that may be effective in improving outcome. For example, the impact of interventions such as relaxation training and yoga have been examined as possible ways of improving birth outcome, and they indicate that, indeed, such practices reduce the need for assisted births and can support healthy pregnancies overall (Beddoe & Lee, 2008; Beddoe, Paul Yang, Kennedy, Weiss, & Lee, 2009; Narendran, Nagarathna, Gunasheela, & Nagendra, 2005). These findings are encouraging, but they were not focused on reducing stress per se. Eventually, research on the impact of stress on pregnancy outcome will be able to address whether such interventions are helpful in reducing maternal stress, positively impacting neural-immune interactions during pregnancy, and ultimately, improving outcome for mothers and their offspring. Progression from our current state of knowledge to the application of reliable screening and interventions for mothers who may be prone to prenatal stress will take time, but the foundation for achieving these goals is already in place.

Related Chapters

For more information on concepts introduced in this chapter, see also Coe, this volume.

References

Arck, P. C. (2001). Stress and pregnancy loss: Role of immune mediators, hormones and neurotransmitters. *American Journal of Reproductive Immunology, 46,* 117–123.

Bakker, J. M., Schmidt, E. D., Kroes, H., Kavelaars, A., Heijnen, C. J., Tilders, F. J. et al. (1995). Effects of short-term dexamethasone treatment during pregnancy on the development of the immune system and the hypothalamo-pituitary adrenal axis in the rat. *Journal of Neuroimmunology, 63,* 183–191.

Beddoe, A. E., & Lee, K. A. (2008). Mind-body interventions during pregnancy. *Journal of Obstetrics, Gynecology, and Neonatal Nursing, 37,* 165–175.

Beddoe, A. E., Paul Yang, C. P., Kennedy, H. P., Weiss, S. J., & Lee, K. A. (2009). The effects of mindfulness-based yoga during pregnancy on maternal psychological and physical distress. *Journal of Obstetric, Gynecological, and Neonatal Nursing, 38,* 310–319.

Buss, C., Davis, E. P., Muftuler, L. T., Head, K., & Sandman, C. A. (2010). High pregnancy anxiety during mid-gestation is associated with decreased gray matter density in 6–9-year-old children. *Psychoneuroendocrinology,35,* 141–153.

Buss, C., Entringer, S., Reyes, J. F., Chicz-DeMet, A., Sandman, C. A., Waffarn, F. et al. (2009). The maternal cortisol awakening response in human pregnancy is associated with the length of gestation. *American Journal of Obstetrics and Gynecology, 201,* 398.

Cannon, J. G. (1998). Adaptive interactions between cytokines and the hypothalamic-pituitary-gonadal axis. *Annals of the New York Academy of Science, 29,* 234–242.

Cardinal, J., Pretorius, C. J., & Ungerer, J. P. J. (2010). Biological and diurnal variation in glucocorticoid sensitivity detected with a sensitive in vitro dexamethasone suppression of cytokine production assay. *Journal of Clinical Endocrinology and Metabolism, 95,* 3657–3663.

Carmichael, S. L., & Shaw, G. M. (2000). Maternal life event stress and congenital anomalies. *Epidemiology, 11,* 30–35.

CDC Grand Rounds: additional opportunities to prevent neural tube defects with folic acid fortification (2010). *Morbidity and Mortality Weekly Report, 59,* 980–984.

Chrousos, G. P. (1999). Reproductive placental corticotropin-releasing hormone and its clinical implications. *American Journal of Obstetrics and Gynecology, 180,* S249–S250.

Coe, C. L., & Lubach, G. R. (2000). Prenatal influences on neuroimmune set points in infancy. *Annals of New York Academy of Science, 917,* 468–477.

Coe, C. L., Lubach, G. R., & Karaszewski, J. W. (1999). Prenatal stress and immune recognition of self and nonself in the primate neonate. *Biology of the Neonate, 76,* 301–310.

Cohen, S., Doyle, W. J., & Skoner, D. P. (1999). Psychological stress, cytokine production, and severity of upper respiratory illness. *Psychosomatic Medicine, 61,* 175–180.

Colbern, G. T., & Main, E. K. (1991). Immunology of the Maternal-Placental Interface in Normal-Pregnancy. *Seminars in Perinatology, 15,* 196–205.

Copper, R. L., Goldenberg, R. L., Das, A., Elder, N., Swain, M., Norman, G., et al. (1996). The preterm prediction study: Maternal stress is associated with spontaneous preterm birth at less than thirty-five weeks' gestation. *American Journal of Obstetrics and Gynecology, 175,* 1286–1292.

Copper, R. L., Goldenberg, R. L., DuBard, M. B., & Davis, R. O. (1994). Risk factors for fetal death in white, black, and Hispanic women. Collaborative Group on Preterm Birth Prevention. *Obstetrics and Gynecology, 84,* 490–495.

Coussons-Read, M. E. (2003). Neural-immune consequences of environmental and psychological stress in pregnancy. In S. G. Pandalai (Ed.), *Recent progress in life sciences* (pp. 113–130). Kerala, India: Research Signpost.

Coussons-Read, M. E., Lobel, M., Carey J. C., Kreither, M. O., D'Anna, K., Argys L., Ross, R. G., Brandt, C., Cole, S. Occurrence of preterm delivery is linked to pregnancy-specific distress and elevated inflammatory markers across gestation. *Brain, Behavior and Immunity.* In press.

Coussons-Read, M. E., Okun, M. L., & Nettles, C. D. (2007). Psychosocial stress increases inflammatory markers and alters cytokine production across pregnancy. *Brain, Behavior, and Immunity, 21,* 343–350.

Coussons-Read, M. E., Okun, M. L., Schmitt, M. P., & Giese, S. (2005). Prenatal stress alters cytokine levels in a manner that may endanger human pregnancy. *Psychosomatic Medicine, 67,* 625–631.

Curry, M. A. (1998). The interrelationships between abuse, substance use, and psychosocial stress during pregnancy. *Journal of Obstetric, Gynecologic, and Neonatal Nursing, 27,* 692–698.

Daniells, S., Grenyer, B. F. S., Davis, W. S., Coleman, K. J., Burgess, J. A., & Moses, R. G. (2003). Gestational diabetes mellitus: Is a diagnosis associated with an increase in maternal anxiety and stress in the short and intermediate term? *Diabetes Care, 26,* 385–389.

Dantzer, R. (1989). Stress and immunity: an integrated view of relationships between the brain and the immune system. *Life Sciences, 44,* 1995–2008.

Daunter, B. (1992). Immunology of pregnancy—Towards a unifying hypothesis. *European Journal of Obstetrics Gynecology and Reproductive Biology, 43,* 81–95.

DeKeyser, F. G., Leker, R. R., & Weidenfeld, J. (2000). Activation of the adrenocortical axis by surgical stress: involvement of central norepinephrine and interleukin-1. *Neuroimmunomodulation, 7,* 182–188.

Diego, M. A., Jones, N. A., Field, T., Hernandez-Reif, M., Schanberg, S., Kuhn, C. et al. (2006). Maternal psychological distress, prenatal cortisol, and fetal weight. *Psychosomatic Medicine, 68,* 747–753.

DiPietro, J. A., Ghera, M. M., Costigan, K., & Hawkins, M. (2004). Measuring the ups and downs of pregnancy stress. *Journal of Psychosomatic Obstetrics and Gynaecology, 25,* 189–201.

Dunn A. J. (1993). Infection as a stressor: a cytokine-mediated activation of the hypothalam-pituitary-adrenal axis? *Ciba Foundation Symposium, 172,* discussion 239–242.

Elenkov I. J., & Chrousos G. P. (1999). Stress hormones, Th1/Th2 patterns, pro/anti-inflammatory cytokines and susceptibility to disease. *Trends in Endocrinology and Metabolism, 10,* 359–368.

Entringer, S., Kumsta, R., Nelson, E. L., Hellhammer, D. H., Wadhwa, P. D., & Wust, S. (2008). Influence of prenatal psychosocial stress on cytokine production in adult women. *Developmental Psychobiology, 50,* 579–587.

Fiddes, T. M., Oreilly, D. B., Cetrulo, C. L., Miller, W., Rudders, R., Osband, M. et al. (1986). Phenotypic and functional-evaluation of suppressor cells in normal-pregnancy and in chronic aborters. *Cellular Immunology, 97,* 407–418.

Field, T., & Diego, M. (2008). Cortisol: The culprit prenatal stress variable. *International Journal of Neuroscience, 118,* 1181.

Fukumoto, K., Morita, T., Mayanagi, T., Tanokashira, D., Yoshida, T., Sakai, A. et al. (2009). Detrimental effects of glucocorticoids on neuronal migration during brain development. *Molecular Psychiatry, 14,* 1119–1131.

Gennaro, S., & Fehder, W. P. (1996). Stress, immune function, and relationship to pregnancy outcome. *Nursing Clinics of North America, 31,* 293–302.

Gibbs, R. S., Romero, R., Hillier, S. L., Eschenbach, D. A., & Sweet, R. L. (1992). A review of premature birth and subclinical infection. *American Journal of Obstetrics and Gynecology, 166,* 1515–1528.

Giscombe, C. L., & Lobel, M. (2005). Explaining disproportionately high rates of adverse birth outcomes among African Americans: The impact of stress, racism, and related factors in pregnancy. *Psychological Bulletin, 131,* 662–683.

Glaser, R., Kiecolt-Glaser, J. K., Marucha, P. T., MacCallum, R. C., Laskowski, B. F., & Malarkey, W. B. (1999). Stress-related changes in proinflammatory cytokine production in wounds. *Archives of General Psychiatry, 56,* 450–456.

Glynn, L. M., Wadhwa, P. D., Dunkel-Schetter, C., Chicz-DeMet, A., & Sandman, C. (2001). When stress happens matters: Effects of earthquake timing on stress responsivity in pregnancy. *American Journal of Obstetrics and Gynecology, 184,* 637–642.

Gomez, R., Ghezzi, F., Romero, R., Munoz, H., Tolosa, J. E., & Rojas, I. (1995). Premature labor and intra-amniotic infection. Clinical aspects and role of the cytokines in diagnosis and pathophysiology. *Clinics in Perinatology, 22,* 281–342.

Graham, J. E., Christian, L. M., & Kiecolt-Glaser, J. K. (2006). Stress, age, and immune function: Toward a life span approach. *29,* 389–400.

Hamilton, J. G., & Lobel, M. (2008). Types, patterns, and predictors of coping with stress during pregnancy: Examination of the Revised Prenatal Coping Inventory in a diverse sample. *Journal of Psychosomatic Obstetrics and Gynaecology, 29,* 97–104.

Hill, J. A., & Choi, B. C. (2000). Maternal immunological aspects of pregnancy success and failure. *Journal of Reproductive Fertility., 55,* 91–97.

Jia, N., Yang, K., Sun, Q., Cai, Q., Li, H., Cheng, D., et al. (2010). Prenatal stress causes dendritic atrophy of pyramidal neurons in hippocampal CA3 region by glutamate in offspring rats. *Developmental Neurobiology, 70,* 114–125.

Kalantaridou, S. N., Makrigiannakis, A., Mastorakos, G., & Chrousos, G. P. (2003). Roles of reproductive corticotropin-releasing hormone. *Annals of New York Academy of Science, 997,* 129–135.

Kapoor, A., Kostaki, A., Janus, C., & Matthews, S. G. (2009). The effects of prenatal stress on learning in adult offspring is dependent on the timing of the stressor. *Behavioral Brain Research, 197,* 144–149.

Kemeny, M. E., & Gruenewald, T. L. (1999). Psychoneuroimmunology update. *Semin Gastrointestinal Disease, 10,* 20–29.

Kemeny, M. E., & Laudenslager, M. L. (1999). Introduction beyond stress: the role of individual difference factors in psychoneuroimmunology. *Brain, Behavior, and Immunity,, 13,* 73–75.

Khashan, A. S., McNamee, R., Abel, K. M., Pedersen, M. G., Webb, R. T., Kenny, L. C. et al. (2008). Reduced infant birthweight consequent upon maternal exposure to severe life events. *Psychosomatic Medicine, 70,* 688–694.

Kiecolt-Glaser, J. K., & Glaser, R. (1992). Psychoneuroimmunology: Can psychological interventions modulate immunity? *Journal of Consulting and Clinical Psychology, 60,* 569–575.

Kiecolt-Glaser, J. K., Glaser, R., Cacioppo, J. T., MacCallum, R. C., Snydersmith, M., Kim, C., et al. (1997). Marital conflict in older adults: Endocrinological and immunological correlates. *Psychosomatic Medicine, 59,* 339–349.

Kiecolt-Glaser, J. K., Page, G. G., Marucha, P. T., MacCallum, R. C., & Glaser, R. (1998). Psychological influences on surgical recovery. Perspectives from psychoneuroimmunology. *American Psychologist, 53,* 1209–1218.

Kimura, K., Kitamura, H., Makondo, K., Okita, K., Kawasaki, M., & Saito, M. (2000). Norepinephrine stimulates interleukin-6 mRNA expression in primary cultured rat hepatocytes. *Journal of Biochemistry.(Tokyo)., 127,* 205–209.

Kjaer, S. L., Wegener, G., Rosenberg, R., Lund, S. P., & Hougaard, K. S. (2010). Prenatal and adult stress interplay—behavioral implications. *Brain Research, 1320,* 106–113.

Kleinhaus, K., Steinfeld, S., Balaban, J., Goodman, L., Craft, T. S., Malaspina, D., et al. (2010). Effects of excessive glucocorticoid receptor stimulation during early gestation on psychomotor and social behavior in the rat. *Developmental Psychobiology, 52,* 121–132.

Knackstedt, M. K., Hamelmann, E., & Arck, P. C. (2005). Mothers in stress: Consequences for the offspring. *American Journal of Reproductive Immunology, 54,* 63–69.

Kruse, N., Greif, M., Moriabadi, N. F., Marx, L., Toyka, K. V., & Rieckmann, P. (2000). Variations in cytokine mRNA expression during normal human pregnancy. *Clinical Experimental Immunology, 119,* 317–322.

Lacey, K., Zaharia, M. D., Griffiths, J., Ravindran, A. V., Merali, Z., & Anisman, H. (2000). A prospective study of neuroendocrine and immune alterations associated with the stress of an oral academic examination amonug graduate students. *Psychoneuroendocrinology, 25,* 339–356.

Leff, M., Orleans, M., Haverkamp, A. D., Baron, A. E., Alderman, B. W., & Freedman, W. L. (1992). The association of maternal low birthweight and infant low birthweight in a racially mixed population. *Paediatrics, Perinatology, and Epidemiology, 6,* 51–61.

Livingston, I. L., Otado, J. A., & Warren, C. (2003). Stress, adverse pregnancy outcomes, and African-American females. *Journal of the National Medical Association, 95,* 1103–1109.

Lobel, M., Cannella, D. L., Graham, J. E., DeVincent, C., Schneider, J., & Meyer, B. A. (2008). Pregnancy-specific stress, prenatal health behaviors, and birth outcomes. *Health Psychology, 27,* 604–615.

Lobel, M., DeVincent, C. J., Kaminer, A., & Meyer, B. A. (2000). The impact of prenatal maternal stress and optimistic disposition on birth outcomes in medically high-risk women. *Health Psychology, 19,* 544–553.

Lou, H. H., Hansen, D., Nordentoft, M., Pryds, O., Jensen, F., Nim, J., et al. (1994). Prenatal stressors of human life affect fetal brain development. *Developmental Medicine and Child Neurology, 36,* 826–832.

Luecken, L. J., Purdom, C. L., & Howe, R. (2009). Prenatal care initiation in low-income Hispanic women: Risk and protective factors. *American Journal of Health Behavior, 33,* 264–275.

Maes, M., Song, C., Lin, A., de Jongh, R., Van Gastel, A., Kenis, G. et al. (1998). The effects of psychological stress on humans: Increased production of pro-inflammatory cytokines and Th1-like response in stress-induced anxiety. *Cytokine, 10,* 313–318.

Malarkey, W. B., Glaser, R., Kiecolt-Glaser, J. K., & Marucha, P. T. (2001). Behavior: The endocrine-immune interface and health outcomes. *Advances in Psychosomatic Medicine, 22,* 104–115.

Mandyam, C. D., Crawford, E. F., Eisch, A. J., Rivier, C. L., & Richardson, H. N. (2008). Stress experienced in utero reduces sexual dichotomies in neurogenesis, microenvironment, and cell death in the adult rat hippocampus. *Developmental Neurobiology, 68,* 575–589.

Martin, R. P., Noyes, J., & Wisenbaker, J. M. (1999). Prediction of early childhood negative emotionality and inhibition from maternal distress during pregnancy. *Merrill-Palmer Quarterly, 45,* 370–391.

Marucha, P. T., Kiecolt-Glaser, J. K., & Favagehi, M. (1998). Mucosal wound healing is impaired by examination stress. *Psychosomatic Medicine, 60,* 362–365.

Matthiesen, L., Berg, G., Ernerudh, J., & Hakansson, L. (1996). Lymphocyte subsets and mitogen stimulation of blood lymphocytes in normal pregnancy. *American Journal of Reproductive Immunology, 35,* 70–79.

McGregor, J. A., French, J. I., Lawellin, D., & Todd, J. K. (2000). Preterm birth and infection: Pathogenic possibilities. *American Journal of Reproductive Immunology and Microbiology, 16,* 123–132.

Mckee, M. D., Cunningham, M., Jankowski, K. R., & Zayas, L. (2001). Health-related functional status in pregnancy: Relationship to depression and social support in a multiethnic population. *Obstetrics and Gynecology, 97,* 988–993.

McLean, M., & Smith, R. (2001). Corticotrophin-releasing hormone and human parturition. *Reproduction, 121,* 493–501.

Milad, M. P., Klock, S. C., Moses, S., & Chatterton, R. (1998). Stress and anxiety do not result in pregnancy wastage. *Human Reproduction, 13,* 2296–2300.

Narendran, S., Nagarathna, R., Gunasheela, S., & Nagendra, H. R. (2005). Efficacy of yoga in pregnant women with abnormal Doppler study of umbilical and uterine arteries. *Journal of the Indian Medical Association, 103,* 12–17.

Narendran, V., Visscher, M. O., Abril, I., Hendrix, S. W., & Hoath, S. B. (2010). Biomarkers of epidermal innate immunity in premature and full-term infants. *Pediatric Research, 67,* 382–386.

Opsahl, M., Hansen, K., Klein, T., & Cunningham, D. (1994). Natural-Killer-Cell Activity in Early Human-Pregnancy. *Gynecologic and Obstetric Investigation, 37,* 226–228.

Orr, S. T., James, S. A., & Casper, R. (1992). Psychosocial stressors and low birthweight: development of a questionnaire. *Developmental and Behavioral Pediatrics, 13,* 343–347.

Orr, S. T., James, S. A., Miller, C. A., Barakat, B., Daikoku, N., Pupkin, M., et al. (1996). Psychosocial stressors and low birthweight in an urban population. *American Journal od Preventive Medicine, 12,* 459–466.

Park, J. S., Park, C. W., Lockwood, C. J., & Norwitz, E. R. (2005). Role of cytokines in preterm labor and birth. *Minerva Ginecologica, 57,* 349–366.

Peacock, J. L., Bland, J. M., & Anderson, H. R. (1995). Preterm delivery: effects of ·socioeconomic factors, psychological stress, smoking, alcohol, and caffeine. *British Medical Journal, 311,* 531–535.

Pearce, B. D., Grove, J., Bonney, E. A., Bliwise, N., Dudley, D. J., Schendel, D. E., et al. (2010). Interrelationship of cytokines, hypothalamic-pituitary-adrenal axis hormones, and psychosocial variables in the prediction of preterm birth. *Gynecologic and Obstetric Investigation, 70,* 40–46.

Persoons, J. H. A., Schornagel, K., Breve, J., Berkenbosch, F., & Kraal, G. (1995). Acute stress affects cytokines and nitric oxide production by aveolar macrophages differently. *American Journal of Respiratory and Critical Care Medicine, 152,* 619–624.

Piccinni, M. P. (2007). T cells in normal pregnancy and recurrent pregnancy loss. *Reproductive Biomedicine Online, 14 Spec No 1,* 95–99.

Piccinni, M. P., Maggi, E., & Romagnani, S. (2000). Role of hormone-controlled T cell cytokines in the maintenance of pregnancy. *Biochemical Social Transactions, 28,* 212–215.

Piccinni, M. P., Scaletti, C., Maggi, E., & Romagnani, S. (2000). Role of hormone-controlled Th1- and Th2-type cytokines in successful pregnancy. *Journal of Neuroimmunology, 109,* 30–33.

Pluess, M., Bolten, M., Pirke, K. M., & Hellhammer, D. (2010). Maternal trait anxiety, emotional distress, and salivary cortisol in pregnancy. *Biological Psychology, 83,* 169–175.

Pope, R. M. (1990). Immunoregulatory mechanisms present in the maternal circulation during pregnancy. *Baillieres Clinical Rheumatology, 4,* 33–52.

Pope, R. M., Yoshinoya, S., Rutstein, J., & Persellin, R. H. (1983). Effect of pregnancy on immune-complexes and rheumatoid factors in patients with rheumatoid-arthritis. *American Journal of Medicine, 74,* 973–979.

Rabin, B. (1999) *Stress, immune function and health: The connection.* New York, NY: Wiley Liss.

Rabin, B., Cohen, S., Ganguli, R., Lysle, D., & Cunnick, J. (1989). Bidirectional interaction between the central nervous system and the immune system. *Critical Revue Immunology, 9,* 279–312.

Reichman, N. E., & Kenney, G. M. (1998). Prenatal care, birth outcomes and newborn hospitalization costs: Patterns among Hispanics in New Jersey. *Family Planning Perspectives, 30,* 182–187.

Roberts, J. M., & Lain, K. Y. (2002). Recent insights into the pathogenesis of pre-eclampsia. *Placenta, 23,* 359–372.

Roitt, I. (1991). *Essntial immunology.* Oxford, England: Blackwell Scientific.

Romero, R., Brody, D. T., Oyarzun, E., Mazor, M., Wu, Y. K., Hobbins, J. C. et al. (1989). Infection and labor. III. Interleukin-1: A signal for the onset of parturition. *American Journal of Obstetrics and Gynecology, 160,* 1117–1123.

Romero, R., Mazor, M., Wu, Y. K., Avila, C., Oyarzun, E., & Mitchell, M. D. (1989). Bacterial endotoxin and tumor necrosis factor stimulate prostaglandin production by human decidua. *Prostaglandins Leukotrienes and Essential Fatty Acids., 37,* 183–186.

Romero, R., Sirtori, M., Oyarzun, E., Avila, C., Mazor, M., Callahan, R. et al. (1989). Infection and labor. V. Prevalence, microbiology, and clinical significance of intraamniotic infection in women with preterm labor and intact membranes. *American Journal of Obstetrics and Gynecology., 161,* 817–824.

Romo, A., Carceller, R., & Tobajas, J. (2009). Intrauterine growth retardation (IUGR): epidemiology and etiology. *Pediatric Endocrinology Review, 6 Suppl 3,* 332–336.

Rook, G. A. (1999). Glucocorticoids and immune function. *Bailliere's Clinical Endocrinology and Metabolism, 13,* 567–581.

Ruiz, R. J., & Avant, K. C. (2005). Effects of maternal prenatal stress on infant outcomes: a synthesis of the literature. *28,* 345–355.

Ruiz, R. J., & Fullerton, J. T. (1999). The measurement of stress in pregnancy. *Nursing and Health Science, 1,* 19–25.

Ruiz, R. J., Fullerton, J., & Dudley, D. J. (2003). The interrelationship of maternal stress, endocrine factors and inflammation on gestational length. *Obstetrics and Gynecology Survey, 58,* 415–428.

Russell, J. A., Douglas, A. J., & Brunton, P. J. (2008). Reduced hypothalamo-pituitary-adrenal axis stress responses in late pregnancy: Central opioid inhibition and noradrenergic mechanisms. *Annals of the New York Academy of Sciences, 1148,* 428–438.

Saito, S. (2000). Cytokine network at the feto-maternal interface. *Journal of Reproductive Immunology, 47,* 87–103.

Saito, S., Sakai, M., Masaki, Y., Tanebe, K., Tsuda, H., & Shimata, T. (1999). Quantitative analysis of peripheral blood Th0, Th1, Th2 and the Th1:Th2 cell ratio during normal human pregnancy and preeclampsia. *Clinical Experimental Immunology, 117,* 550–555.

Sandman, C. A., Wadhwa, P. D., Chicz-DeMet, A., Dunkel-Schetter, C., & Porto, M. (1997). Maternal stress, HPA activity, and fetal/infant outcome. *Annals of the New York Academy of Science, 814,* 266–275.

Santhanam, U., Avila, C., Romero, R., Viguet, H., Ida, N., Sakurai, S., et al. (1991). Cytokines in normal and abnormal Parturition: elevated amniotic fluid interleukin-6 levels in women with premature rupture of membranes associated with intrauterine infection. *Cytokine, 3,* 155–163.

Saunders, T. A., Lobel, M., Veloso, C., & Meyer, B. A. (2006). Prenatal maternal stress is associated with delivery analgesia and unplanned cesareans. *Journal of Psychosomatic Obstetrics and Gynaecology, 27,* 141–146.

Schempf, A., Strobino, D., & O'Campo, P. (2009). Neighborhood effects on birthweight: An exploration of psychosocial and behavioral pathways in Baltimore, 1995–1996. *Social Science and Medicine, 68,* 100–110.

Schwarze, J., & Bartmann, P. (1994). Influence of dexamethasone on lymphocyte proliferation in whole blood cultures of neonates. *Biology of the Neonate, 65,* 295–301.

Shamsi, U., Hatcher, J., Shamsi, A., Zuberi, N., Qadri, Z., & Saleem, S. (2010). A multicentre matched case control study of risk factors for preeclampsia in healthy women in Pakistan. *BioMed Central Womens Health, 10,* 14.

Short, S. J., Lubach, G. R., Karasin, A. I., Olsen, C. W., Styner, M., Knickmeyer, R. C. et al. (2010). Maternal influenza infection during pregnancy impacts postnatal brain development in the rhesus monkey. *Biological Psychiatry, 67,* 965–973.

Slattery, D. A., & Neumann, I. D. (2008). No stress please! Mechanisms of stress hyporesponsiveness of the maternal brain. *Journal of Physiology, 586,* 377–385.

Stamatelou, F., Deligeoroglou, E., Farmakides, G., & Creatsas, G. (2009). Abnormal progesterone and corticotropin releasing hormone levels are associated with preterm labour. *Annals of the Academy of Medicine, Singapore, 38,* 1011–1016.

Swolin-Eide, D., Nilsson, C., Holmang, A., & Ohlsson, C. (2004). Prenatal exposure to IL-1beta results in disturbed skeletal growth in adult rat offspring. *Pediatric Research, 55,* 598–603.

Tumiel, L. M., Buck, G. M., Zayas, L. E., & Jaen, C. R. (1998). Unmasking adverse birth outcomes among Hispanic subgroups. *Ethnicity and Disease, 8,* 209–217.

Vassiliadis, S., Ranella, A., Papadimitriou, L., Makrygiannakis, A., & Athanassikis, I. (1998). Serum levels of pro- and anti-inflammatory cytokines in non-pregnant women, during pregnancy, labour and abortion. *Mediators of Inflammation, 7,* 69–72.

Wadhwa, P. D. (2005). Psychoneuroendocrine processes in human pregnancy influence fetal development and health. *Psychoneuroendocrinology, 30,* 724–743.

Wadhwa, P. D., Culhane, J. F., Rauh, V., Barve, S. S., Hogan, V., Sandman, C. A., et al. (2001). Stress, infection and preterm birth: a biobehavioural perspective. *Paediatr Perinatal Epidemiology, 15 Suppl 2,* 17–29.

Wadhwa, P. D., Sandman, C. A., Porto, M., Dunkel-Schetter, C., & Garite, T. J. (1993). The association between prenatal stress and infant birth weight and gestational age at birth: a prospective investigation. *American Journal of Obstetrics and Gynecology, 169,* 858–865.

Weinstock, M. (2005). The potential influence of maternal stress hormones on development and mental health of the offspring. *Brain, Behavior and Immunity, 19,* 296–308.

Wiegers, G. J., Croiset, G., Reul, J. M., Holsboer, F., & de Kloet, E. R. (1993). Differential effects of corticosteroids on rat peripheral blood T lymphocyte mitogenesis in vivo and in vitro. *American Journal of Physiology, 265,* E825–E830.

Williamson, H. A., LeFevre, M., & Hector, M. (1989). Association between life stress and serious perinatal complications. *Journal of Family Practice, 29,* 489–494.

Wright, R. J., Visness, C. M., Calatroni, A., Grayson, M. H., Gold, D. R., Sandel, M. T. et al. (2010). Prenatal maternal stress and cord blood innate and adaptive cytokine responses in an inner-city cohort. *American Journal of Respiratory and Critical Care Medicine, 182,* 25–33.

Yali, A. M., & Lobel, M. (1999). Coping and distress in pregnancy: an investigation of medically high risk women. *Journal of Psychosomatic Obstetrics and Gynaecology, 20,* 39–52.

Yang, E. V., & Glaser, R. (2000). Stress-induced immunomodulation: impact on immune defenses against infectous disease. *Biomedicine and Pharmacotherapy, 54,* 245–250.

Zauner, I., Rother, E., & Schollmeyer, P. (1995). Systemic lupus erythematosus and pregnancy. *Nieren-und Hochdruckkrankheiten, 24,* 683–685.

Zhang, W., Wang, L., Zhao, Y., & Kang, J. (2000). Changes in cytokine (IL-8, IL-6 and TNF-alpha) levels in the amniotic fluid and maternal serum in patients with premature rupture of the membranes. *Chung Hua I.Hsueh Tsa Chih (Taipei)., 63,* 311–315.

2

The Logic of Developmental Psychoneuroimmunology

Christopher L. Coe *and* Gabriele R. Lubach

Abstract

Research on young animals and children has demonstrated that the prenatal and early rearing environments can leave an indelible mark on the immature immune system. During normal development, these environmental influences can have beneficial consequences including the promotion of immune tolerance during pregnancy, help in the programming of regulatory set points in the fetus, and prime immune responses during childhood. Thus, this aspect of immunity in the young host can be viewed as a "learning system," very amenable to change, and often in a favorable manner. However, this same flexibility may result in a vulnerability to physical and psychological insults, including to a poor diet, pathogen exposure, or parental loss and maltreatment. The take- home message of developmental psychoneuroimmunology (PNI) is that the environmental context can promote resilience and immune vigor, as well as be the reason for lacunae and impairments that persist into adulthood, accounting for individual differences in morbidity and longevity.

Key Words: pregnancy, placenta, fetus, prenatal, rearing, weaning cytokines, thymus, tolerance, microbiota, passive immunity, antibody, autoimmune cortisol, antenatal corticosteroids, allergies, asthma

Saepe ne utile quidem est scire quid futurum sit.
(*Often it is not even advantageous to know what will be*)
—Cicero

Introduction

Infant animals and the human neonate are confronted with an important strategic decision to make with respect to their stage of immune maturation at birth. One option is emerge into the world with a largely formed and competent immune system, but any advantage gained will be at the expense of flexibility. Alternatively, infants can risk first encountering the external world with immature immune responses, and thereby garner the benefits of a more adaptable system that can be shaped and further refined by the postnatal rearing environment.

The consequences of making the wrong choice and an ineffective immune defense may be dire. Even today in many nonindustrialized countries, infant mortality due to respiratory and diarrhea-causing infections exceeds 5–10% of births, if they don't receive adequate nutrition and have access to appropriate medical care and antibiotic treatments (Lawoyin, 2001).

Given what must have been very strong selective pressure on this aspect of immunity over the course of evolution, the infants of most mammalian species appear to have struck a compromise. Many aspects of innate immunity are well established by birth, which affords reasonable protection against bacterial infections, whereas the complex cellular components of adaptive immunity typically mature postpartum. Thus, the latter can be more readily influenced by unique antigenic exposures and pathogens in the rearing environment and by other experiential factors. It is this plasticity that provides empirical support for our chapter title and the logic behind the juxtaposition of the two terms—*developmental* and *psychoneuroimmunology.*

The young infant's immune system should be viewed as a "learning system," almost to the same degree as the developing brain (Hodgson & Coe, 2006). Lymphocyte responses, including antibody production and T cell memory, need to be primed by infections and other antigenic stimuli in the environment. The pace of immune maturation and the ultimate competence of an individual's immune reactions will be affected, not only by these repeated exposures to infectious pathogens, but also by nonantigenic factors, including nutrients in the diet and the quality of parental care. Using nonhuman primate models, our laboratory has spent many years investigating this malleable aspect of immune responses in infants in order to assess how different prenatal and rearing conditions foster or undermine immunity. Select examples from these primate studies are discussed to illustrate some important issues to consider if interested in how early life events alter fetal and infant immune responses.

We, and others, are still in the process of discovering the extent to which psychological processes, such as a stressful experience by the mother or infant, can affect immunity, both acutely and for the long-term into adulthood (Nielsen, Hansen, Simonsen, & Hviid, 2011). As highlighted in this overview, a mother also contributes directly to her infant's protective shield through the provision of antibody and other proteins across the placenta and in breast milk, enabling another flexible process termed *passive immunity.* Beyond providing substantial amounts of antibody against the viruses and bacteria to which she had been exposed in her own lifetime, the mother also bestows some beneficial microbiota from her gut and reproductive tract into and on the previously sterile neonate.

It is of historical interest that developmental studies of this type played a seminal role in the early days of PNI, serving to validate the core belief that psychological factors can change immune responses in a biologically and clinically meaningful manner (Ader, 1983; Solomon, Levine, & Kraft, 1968). For example, pioneering papers on rats and mice documented how early weaning from the mother, or even brief separations from the nest, could lessen their ability to contain a cancerous growth when small tumors were later transplanted into them as adults (Ader & Friedman, 1965). More recently, it has been shown that similar manipulations of rearing conditions can either increase or decrease allergen responses when rats are subsequently sensitized to ovalbumin as adults (Kruschinski et al., 2008). Today, we also know how important the early rearing environment is for humans. It has been found that an impoverished childhood or experiences of familial maltreatment can predispose an individual toward a more pro-inflammatory physiology in adulthood (Chen, Chim, Strunk, & Miller, 2007; Danese, Pariante, Caspi, Taylor, & Poulton, 2007). Moreover, adolescents raised in abusive families appear to have reduced immune control over the latent virus, Herpes simplex (HSV), resulting in the maintenance of higher titers of HSV-specific antibody in their saliva (Shirtcliff, Coe, & Pollak, 2009).

It is equally important to appreciate that many significant immune events have already taken place before birth. In fact, pregnancy could not even be initiated if the implanting blastocyst did not modulate the immune state of the female's reproductive tract. As pregnancy progresses, the fetus induces additional changes in the mother's systemic immune responses in order to prevent rejection, which would otherwise result because of her reaction to paternal antigens on fetal cells. Moreover, within the fetal compartment, the antecedents of lymphoid tissue appear very early in gestation, and both the spleen and thymus are quite developed by birth. This chapter is intended to serve as a brief primer for the reader interested in this remarkable developmental journey, which begins at the moment of implantation and continues onward into the postpartum period. After the infant's birth, we also see the myriad influences of the rearing environment on the immune system. An appreciation of how extensively the environment can affect a young infant's immune competence helps one to understand the now classic papers that first conveyed the potential importance of developmental PNI for pediatric medicine. Those prescient studies showed how the frequency and severity of upper respiratory infections in infants and young children could be affected by the home environment and level of familial discord (Boyce et al., 1977; Meyer & Haggerty, 1962). The observations continue to be relevant to research today on allergies and asthma. Many nonimmune factors, such as the mother's parity, gestation length, and even the amount of violence occurring in a poor neighborhood, can influence the likelihood that a pregnant woman gives birth to an infant with high levels of IgE and a particular cytokine bias that makes her child more prone to atopic disease (Chen, Miller, Kobor, & Cole, 2010; Wright et al., 2010; Karmaus, Arshad, Sadeghnejad, & Twiselton, 2004; Pekkanen, Xu, & Jarevelin, 2001).

Although most of the immune alterations induced by environmental provocations in a fetus or young infant are transient, others can be long lasting (Lowe, Luheshi, & Williams, 2008). In the case of teratogenic exposures to high levels of alcohol during pregnancy, for example, the effects on the developing immune system may be debilitating, resulting in a partial and even complete involution of the fetal thymus and other immune impairments (Amman, Wara, Cowan, Barrett, & Stiehm 1982; Ahluwalia et al., 2000; Ewald & Walden, 1988). Other prenatal processes exert more subtle changes, but with equally important consequences. Not all result in negative outcomes. For example, there are a number of beneficial influences on the immature immune system that take place *in utero*, which are sometimes described as a type of "*fetal programming*" (Bateson et al., 2004).

Some immunomodulation is required to induce a cellular tolerance for maternal and self-antigens, which is critical to fetal survival (Mold et al., 2008). If the thymus does not select against those types of thymocytes, autoimmune reactions will occur, a correction accomplished by cell deletion, largely through a self-imposed cell death (apoptosis and autophagy). Conversely, when some food proteins or environmental pollutants cross the placenta, they may bias the infant's reactions toward an atopy-prone profile by the time of birth (Liobichler, Pichler, & Gestmayr, 2002). Both high IgE and certain cytokines (high IL-5, low IFN and IL-12) in cord blood indicate that the stage has been set for the later emergence of allergic disease during childhood (Fergusson, Crane, Beaseley, & Horwood, 1997; Jones, Holloway, & Warner, 2000). We have a lot more to learn about how environmental and maternal factors predispose for a resilient and healthy trajectory or divert the infant toward a more vulnerable and illness-prone course.

Modulation of Maternal Immunity and the Miracle of Implantation

The immune dialogue between a fetus and the mother begins almost immediately, and then remains vital to the wellbeing and ultimate success of pregnancy. One of the first immune-related tasks for the implanting blastocyst—barely a week after conception when not much more than 100 cells— is to manipulate maternal leukocytes in the uterine endometrium (Figure 2.1). These NK-like cells and monocytic cells, normally present in the reproductive tract to protect against bacterial pathogens, are now recruited to help engulf the front edge of what will become the placenta. Next, the maternal leukocytes must be inhibited from rejecting trophoblast and fetal cells bearing paternal antigens (Nijagal et al., 2011). Many elegant studies in the field of reproductive immunology have demonstrated how this intricate signaling from the fetus is instrumental for changing the immune status of the endometrium in a manner conducive to implantation (Foglia, Ippolito, Stallings, Zelig, & Napolitano, 2010; Faeleabas et al., 1999).

At this stage, any disruptive or infectious factor that stimulates a strong IL-2 dominant reaction can result in miscarriage. In contrast, to initiate a successful pregnancy, rising progesterone levels induced by the trophoblasts' release of chorionic gonadotrophin (HCG) help to dampen down an excessive response by the NK-like cells in the uterus. In addition, maternal monocytic cells are recruited to inhibit the response of her gamma-delta cells, and are also employed to initiate angiogenesis, creating the blood supply that will be life sustaining for the fetus. By Day 12 postconception, the maternal capillaries are penetrated; by 3–4 weeks, the maternal monocytes/macrophages will have assisted in sculpting the blood vessels that support the growing placenta.

Given the specificity and essential timing of these cellular events, it is perhaps not surprising that a number of gynecological conditions that affect maternal immunity, including bacterial vaginosis and endometriosis, are often associated with infertility (Culhane, Rauh, & Farley-McCollum, 2001; McGregor et al., 1995). Both bacterial infections and inflammation change the cytokine milieu of the reproductive tract. When modeling these conditions in female monkeys, we found that endometriosis resulted in the increased release of IL-6. Similarly when there is bacterial overgrowth in a female monkey's reproductive tract, elevated levels of inflammatory cytokines, including IL-1ß, IL-6, and IL-8, are present in her vaginal secretions. Because psychological factors, including stress, have been shown to undermine the effectiveness of microbial defense on tissue surfaces, including in the gut and

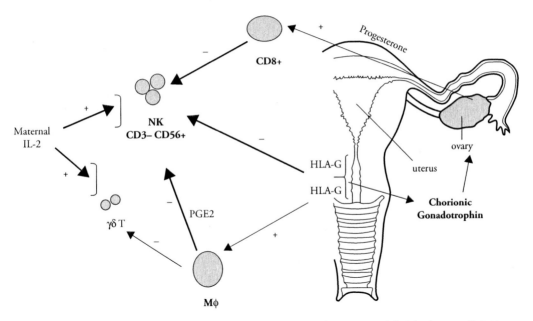

Figure 2.1 Immune processes play a significant role even at the earliest stages of embryonic and fetal development. To initiate a successful pregnancy, the implanting blastocyst and trophoblast cells (which will form the placenta) must induce immune alterations in the uterus. Inflammatory and psychological factors associated with infertility may act through these cellular pathways in the maternal endometrium.

oral cavity, it is likely that these types of inflammatory and bacterial processes in the reproductive tract provide one explanation for the associations found between stressful life events, emotional distress, and infertility.

Fetal Modulation of Maternal Immunity Throughout Pregnancy

Equally important fetal influences on maternal immunity continue to be evident throughout the course of pregnancy. By midgestation they broaden to include significant effects on the mother's systemic immunity. Proteins and hormones of fetal and placental origin act in concert to gradually shift her immune balance away from cellular responses that might result in fetal rejection and toward a greater reliance on other responses more typically associated with humoral defense (Figure 2.2). This change in maternal immunity is evinced both by changes in the circulating levels of several cytokines and the ways in which a gravid female's mononuclear cells (MNC) respond when stimulated in culture. In fact, one sensitive diagnostic predictor of a pregnancy going awry, and destined not to reach normal term, is when pro-inflammatory cytokines, such as TNF-alpha, rise in the blood stream during the third trimester rather than decline. Evidence that there are physiological processes that should normally induce a tonic inhibition of TNF-alpha

in vivo can be obtained by stimulating the cells of pregnant women in vitro with lipopolysaccharide (LPS) (Rigo, Szelenyi, Selmeczy, Papp, & Vizi, 2004). Then, the stimulated cells from women in the third trimester—free of the endogenous suppressive factors—actually show augmented TNF-alpha release as compared to what occurs with cells from a nonpregnant woman.

The disparate finding of low TNF levels in vivo and augmented cellular release following in vitro stimulation takes on a special meaning when one thinks about bacterial and viral infections during pregnancy. Infections induce changes in the inflammatory and immune status of the mother and thereby can potentially harm the developing fetus (Adinolfi, 1993). The list of pathogens of concern includes those known to be teratogenic if they cross the placenta (e.g., Toxoplasma, Syphilus, Cytomegalovirus, Rubella), as well as others that can be harmful indirectly through their effects on placental functioning or via increased transmission of cytokines into the amniotic fluid or fetal blood (Barry et al., 2006; Berrebi et al., 2010; Revello & Gerna, 2002; Yolken, & Torrey, 1997). To mimic the inflammatory response that occurs following an infection during pregnancy, many animal studies have employed endotoxin or Poly I:C as the challenge to recreate the physiology seen after a bacterial or viral infection, respectively (de Miranda

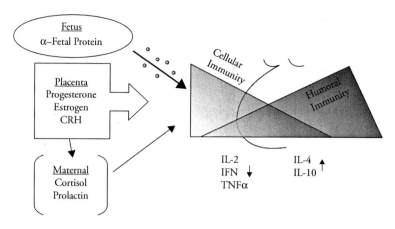

Figure 2.2 The fetus and placenta continue to modulate the immune status of the mother throughout pregnancy in order to prevent rejection. Pro-inflammatory cytokine increases induced by infections or stressful life events in late gestation can result in premature delivery or adverse effects on fetal brain development.

et al., 2010). If high enough doses are administered, both LPS and Poly I:C will cause miscarriages and fetal loss, but even at lower concentrations and when given acutely, they have been found to result in fetal brain damage in rodents, sheep, and primates. Certainly, that is the case if the full-blown physiology of sepsis is induced, which drastically alters blood flow to the uterus and placenta (i.e., causing placental ischemia and insufficiency), inducing hypoxia in the fetal compartment, and sometimes irreversibly damaging the placenta (Kobayashi, Miwa, & Yasui, 2011; Ross, 2010). In the clinical setting, we know that bacterial infections of placental tissues are one of the major causes of premature birth and intra-uterine growth retardation. Moreover, pathological conditions involving inflammation of the amnion and chorion (i.e., chorioamnionitis) are frequently associated with damage to the developing white matter in the fetal brain (Rees, Harding, & Walker, 2008; Saito et al., 2009; Martinez et al., 1998). These types of infections are a major risk factor for cerebral palsy, even when the pregnancy goes to full-term (Damman, & Leviton, 2000; Yoon, Park, & Chaiworapongsa, 2003).

Most of us are inclined to think primarily about the physiology of more affluent women gestating in the hygienic conditions of the modern industrialized world (Lui & Murphy, 2003). However, it is equally important to appreciate that a very high % of pregnant women throughout the world still have babies while infested with worms and parasites, including malaria (Elliott et al., 2005). In some rural regions of Africa, those types of chronic infestations may impact up to 60% of pregnancies (Webb et al. 2011). When we stop to reflect

on how psychosocial processes affect maternal and fetal well-being, we also have to consider the reproductive health of these women who must contend simultaneously with additional immune compromises caused by undernutrition or the chronic anemia associated with a high parasite load (Muhangi et al., 2007; Schwarz et al., 2008).

So far, this section has highlighted maternal infection as the provocation, but there are many reasons to believe that psychological processes can also perturb the immunity of pregnancy and undermine infant well-being through an influence on how a woman responds to the pathogen or even by altering the control over her own endogenous bacteria. For example, stressful psychological events can influence the prevalence of bacterial vaginosis (BV), and worsen the severity of those symptoms during pregnancy for the women who conceived with this gynecological condition (Hiller et al., 1995). The resulting increase in the release of pro-inflammatory cytokines within the reproductive tract has been hypothesized to be one of the pathways accounting for an increase in premature births after stressful pregnancies. If the increased cytokine activity in the mother's reproductive tract then induces a further release of cytokines by the placenta or from fetal leukocytes, there may be cascading effects on the maturing fetal nervous system (De Miranda et al., 2010).

Because the blood-brain-barrier is not yet fully established before birth, nor is it as impervious in most immature animals, cytokines circulating in the bloodstream can more readily gain access to the immature central nervous system (Dammann & Leviton, 1997; Martinez et al., 1998). The results are neuronal damage and deleterious effects on sensitive accessory cells, such as the oligodendrocytes that generate myelin. This type of developmental disturbance is probably a major factor accounting for many neurodevelopmental disorders (e.g., prenatal infection results in a heightened risk for autism) (Braunschweig et al., 2009). In murine models of prenatal infection, the transfer of maternal IL-6 across the placenta has plausibly been implicated as the cytokine mechanism undermining fetal brain development (Shi, Fatemi, Sidwell, & Patterson, 2003). Confirmatory evidence was generated by showing that fewer adverse effects occurred when the same viral infections were conducted in a knockout strain of mouse that could not produce IL-6 (Hsiao & Patterson, 2011; Patterson, 2011; Shi, Tu, & Patterson, 2005).

Many different bacterial and viral pathogens can adversely affect a fetus even when they do not cross the placenta. Influenza viruses are a primary viral vector of concern, at least when more virulent strains circulate in worldwide pandemics (e.g., 1918, 1957, 1968) (Harris, 1919; Irving et al., 2000). In both animal and human studies, influenza infection has been shown to be able to undermine the normal course of fetal brain development (Brown, 2006; Fatemi et al., 2008; Mednick, Machon, Huttunen, & Bonnet, 1988). Our laboratory investigated the effects of maternal infection with a H3N2 strain (A/Sydney/5/97) in pregnant monkeys (Short et al., 2010). To evaluate brain development, we used magnetic resonance imaging (MRI) to scan the offspring from flu-exposed and control pregnancies when they were approximately one year of age. Persistent effects on the maturation of gray matter and white matter were evident in several cortical regions, with the largest deficits in the parietal lobe. When pregnant women have the flu, they are also more prone to progress to secondary bacterial infections and pneumonia, which is another possible cause of adverse effects on the fetus, especially if the disease course is longer, more feverish, and symptomatic (Hartert et al., 2003). It is this public-health concern that motivates the Center for Disease Control (CDC) to recommend immunization against the seasonal influenza viruses when women are planning to get pregnant as well as to endorse vaccination during the first trimester to provide protection across the remainder of pregnancy (Mak, Mangtani, Leese, Watson, & Pfeifer, 2008).

We still have a lot more to learn about how psychological factors influence the normal immune changes associated with pregnancy, as well as a gravid female's responses to infection. Several studies have suggested that stressful events by themselves may change cytokine levels in systematic circulation, increasing the pro-inflammatory bias of late gestation, which would not be advantageous to the developing fetus. It is also reasonable to hypothesize that any psychosocial process or environmental event capable of immunosuppressive actions in the nonpregnant host will undermine immune defense in pregnant women, putting the fetus at greater jeopardy during infections. Sadly, it is known that domestic violence, including spousal abuse of pregnant women, is far too common worldwide (Cokkinides, Coker, Sanderson, Addy, & Bethea, 1999; Gazmararian et al., 1996; Petersen et al. 1997). Although known to increase the risk of premature delivery and low birth weight (LBW) infants, so far the extant research has not sought to establish an immune-mediated explanation for the increased gestational and delivery complications associated with interpersonal violence (Newberger et al., 1992). Similarly, a number of reports have documented that there is a rise in adverse pregnancy outcomes following calamitous environmental events, including earthquakes and societal turmoil, but none have yet specifically implicated immune processes as the main causal agent (Berkowitz et al., 2003; Engel, Berkowitz, Wolff, & Yehuda, 2005; Glynn, Wadhwa, Dunkel-Schetter, & Sandman, 2001).

Nevertheless, it is probably not coincidental that some of the effects on fetal development seen after stressful psychological events appear to be superficially similar to those elicited by the physiological insults of infection and inflammation, at least in animal models (Fortier, Luheshi, & Boksa, 2007; Singer et al., 2009). In both instances, there is often a slowing of fetal growth and lower birth weights at delivery (Byrne, Agerbo, Benndese, Eaton, & Mortensen, 2007). Moreover, in both rodent and primate models of prenatal stress, the offspring frequently exhibit behavioral and brain phenotypes that look a lot like those seen after maternal infections (Hao et al., 2010). The infants from both types of perturbed pregnancies tend to be emotionally reactive, have impaired learning ability, and are less competent in their social skills and reproductive efficiency as adults (Weinstock, 1997). Despite the disparate nature of the psychological and physical provocations during the prenatal period, the similarities in outcomes may reflect common mediating pathways at the level of the placenta (e.g., altered blood flow) or an equivalence induced by the finite number of possible downstream actions on a vulnerable fetus (Welberg, & Seckl, 2001). Both psychological disturbance and immune challenges during pregnancy can result in lasting effects on the offspring's monoamine neurotransmitter systems, especially on the dopaminergic and serotonergic pathways. Moreover, comparable decreases have been found in the size and structural integrity of a number of vulnerable brain regions (e.g., hippocampus and cerebellum), as well as similar changes in the regulation of stress-related neuroendocrine physiology (e.g., on the regulatory set points for hormones from the hypothalamic-pituitary-adrenal axis) (Koehl et al., 1999).

How physical and psychological stressors impact pregnancy physiology and fetal development could easily take up the rest of the chapter because of the many complex issues associated with this topic (Lemaire, Koehl, Le Moal, & Abrous, 2000). One should really consider the many different types of stress, which include the physical demands of work and intense exercise in humans, as well as the emotional distress caused by problematic personal relationships, and the adversity of poverty. In addition, protective factors should be taken into account, including those that contribute to the variation in how pregnant women respond to challenge and illness. Even following environmental disasters and political upheaval that increase the chance of a bad pregnancy outcome, most women do not end up with a foreshortened gestation or an infant born small-for-gestational age. Fortunately, there is also a lot of psychological and biological resiliency both in the mothers and through the protection afforded by the utero-placental barrier. We still have a lot to learn about the factors that account for variation in host vulnerability, which include age, parity, race, and socioeconomic status of the mother. Within the obstetrical and gynecological literatures, there is also interest in genetic risk factors, such as the single nucleotide polymorphisms (SNPs) for IL-6 and TNF, that mediate individual differences in inflammatory responses during pregnancy (Menon et al., 2006). The good news, though, is that delivery and pediatric outcomes today are a far cry from a century ago, when the infant mortality rate in the United States was nearly 10% by one year of age (Centers for Disease Control and Prevention, 2000).

The Evo-Devo Importance of Fetal Immunology

Over a decade ago, researchers began to appreciate that many programming events within cells were already occurring during the earliest stages of embryogenesis. Even as the genetic plan is first starting to unfold, the environment can exert some lasting effects on the infant's phenotype. These findings galvanized a whole field of study that is sometimes called "evo-devo" (Goodman & Coughlin, 2000). Collectively, the research indicates that evolutionary processes and natural selection can act on and through these early influences on embryonic and fetal development. Recent reports on epigenetic changes document how uterine conditions, maternal diet, and the external environment leave permanent marks on the regulation of gene expression and protein transcription (via effects on DNA methylation and histone modifications). There are even effects passed on in an intergenerational manner through persistent alterations in the uterine biology of female offspring (i.e, down matrilines from mother-to-daughter). Some programming of this type also takes place in the immune progenitor cells as the fetal lymphoid tissue is first being created and then later as fetal lymphocytes respond to the antigenic stimuli coming across the placenta from the outside world.

The progenitor cells for the fetal immune system appear early, soon after conception and are found in the yolk sac and the tissue that will become the kidneys and gonads (the par-aortic splanchnopeura/aorta/gonad mesonephros; Yokota et al., 2003). Initially, the fetal liver is an important site for lymphopoiesis and cell differentiation, including the B and NK cell precursors, before the action switches to the bone marrow and spleen. In the human fetus, by two months after conception, lymphocytes in the blood stream can be stimulated to proliferate with mitogen. In addition, the fetal thymus has been forming since Week 6 of gestational age (ga), derived from the third and fourth pharyngeal pouch. As early as Week 8–10 ga, the thymus becomes populated by hematopoietic cells from the liver and bone marrow. In the rodent fetus, the equivalent thymic events also occur by midgestation (by Day 11), although the murine thymus does not progress as far by the time of birth as found in monkey and human infants (De Leon-Luis et al., 2009).

There is not a large literature on how psychological factors affect these important aspects of immune maturation in the fetus, but it is known that they are extremely responsive to maternal and fetal illness, drug exposures including antenatal corticosteroid treatments, and other hormonal and environmental stimuli (Igarashi, Kouro, Yokota, Comp, & Kincade, 2001; Coe & Lubach, 2005).

Many clinical reports have documented that the fetal thymus can shrink dramatically in size and its lymphoid medullary section will become involuted following illness or glucocorticoid treatment (De Felice et al., 1999; Di Naro et al., 2006; Fletcher, Masson, Lisbona, Riggs, & Papageorgiou, 1979; Toti et al., 2000). By midgestation and throughout the latter part of pregnancy, it is also possible to detect activated CD4+ T (Treg) cells in samples of fetal blood (Devereux, Seaton, & Barker, 2001; Warner, Jones, Jones, & Warner, 2000). Some of these cells are likely responding to the small molecular weight (<500 Da) proteins from maternal food crossing the placenta (Liobichler et al., 2002). The proteins include ovalbumin and ß-lactoglobulin, derived from egg and cow's milk, respectively, and even cat dander bound to maternal antibody (Casas & Brjorksten, 2001). In addition, it is known that there is some prenatal exposure to plant and tree pollens based on the seasonal variation one sees in how MNC from neonates react to these allergens when they are tested as in vitro stimulants in cell cultures from cord blood (Piccinni et al., 1993; Van Duren Schmidt et al., 1997)

The fetal stage is also a time when there must be a strong selection against autoreactive T cells that might respond to self-antigens. In a study with rhesus monkeys, we determined whether one could alter this aspect of fetal immunity by repeatedly activating the mother's cortisol levels or subjecting her to a period of psychological disturbance during pregnancy. When the infant monkeys from the disturbed pregnancies were born, we indexed tolerance for self- and maternal antigens by setting up mixed lymphocyte cultures, combining the neonates' mononuclear cells (MNC) with either their own mitomycin C-treated cells (autologous) or stimulator cells from their mother, father, and an unrelated animal (allogeneic) (Coe, Lubach, Karaszewski, & Ershler, 1996). The normal MNC from previously undisturbed infants readily discerned the different stimulators, responding least to their own and the mother's cells, and proliferating more in the presence of the father's and an unrelated animal's lymphocytes. In contrast, the MNC from prenatally disturbed infants did not distinguish the source of the donor's cells as clearly if in late gestation we had (a) exposed to gravid female to several weeks of daily stress, (b) treated her for two days with Dexamethasone, or (c) administered ACTH to her in order to stimulate high cortisol levels each day for two weeks. We also investigated the effects of an equivalent period of psychological disturbance conducted for the same length of time earlier in pregnancy (for 6 weeks of the 24-week pregnancy). In contrast, those infants from this early-gestational-stress condition (Days 50–92 postconception) actually had hyper-responsive MNC at birth, which proliferated excessively in the presence of the allogenic stimulator cells. One can imagine that both an overresponsive immune system as well as a deficient immune capacity to recognize "*other*" could potentially have health ramifications for a young infant.

Maternal Benevolence: Intergenerational Transfer of Passive Immunity

Although it is essential for the immune system to distinguish "self" from "other," the young infant must also be able to temper overwhelming responses to the simultaneous barrage of diverse environmental stimuli. Several processes work in concert to foster that moderation, including the fact that most mammalian young receive some immunological assistance from the mother in the form of transferred antibody. We spent a number of years investigating how maternal antibody is provided to the primate infant because it is known that the placenta and this antibody transfer process varies a lot across species (Wildman et al., 2006). In many species, including farm animals, rats. and mice, the mother's antibody, both of the IgG and IgA class, is mostly provided postnatally in breast milk. However, for that maternal IgG to be of functional value, the infant's gut must be permissive to the translocation of antibody into the bloodstream. Monkeys and humans have evolved a different approach because maternal IgG will not cross the infant's intestine (Figure 2.3). As an alternative strategy, antibody of the G class is transferred across the placenta before birth. Then, sIgA comes later in breast milk to provide a protective coating of the mucosal surfaces of the oral cavity and gut. However, it is the prenatal IgG transfer that confers a neutralizing protection against bacteria and viruses encountered previously by the mother. That IgG enables the infant to temporarily evade many diseases and to not rely as much on its own antibody for the first 3–6 months after birth.

In a comparative survey of five species representing the different primate taxa, we discovered that the more ancestral prosimians (the galago) still do provide IgG after birth like most rodents, but that rhesus monkeys and chimpanzee transfer IgG before birth, more like humans (Coe, Lubach & Izard, 1994). This evolutionary change in the timing coincided with the emergence of a receptor for

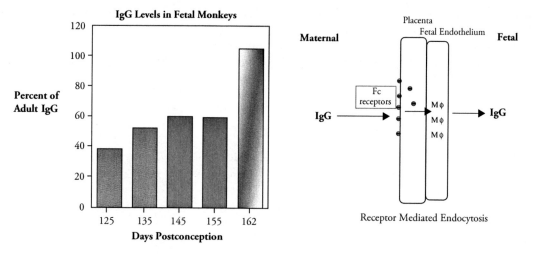

Figure 2.3 Mothers promote the immune defenses of their offspring in many ways, including through the provision of antibody. In monkeys and humans, IgG is transferred more actively at the end of pregnancy via receptors on the placenta, whereas the maternal antibody in breast milk is comprised primarily of the sIgA class. Infants born premature will thus have less maternal antibody and a foreshortened period of protection from these beneficial sources of passive immunity.

IgG on the placenta, which can pull maternal antibody across to the fetal compartment (via receptor-mediated endocytosis). In a follow-up experiment, blood samples from fetal monkeys were also analyzed for antibody— from midgestation to term— revealing that the largest bolus of maternal antibody is transferred during the final two weeks of pregnancy (Figure 2.3). Thus, any infant monkey born premature will be deprived of its normal allotment of maternal antibody, a loss also evident in premature human infants. The postnatal consequence of low IgG is that there will be a quicker depletion of maternal antibody from circulation over the next few months, reducing the duration of the protection provided by this mediator of passive immunity. An infant will then be compelled to more actively generate its own antibody at a younger age. From the pediatric care perspective, such an infant would also be more prone to an earlier respiratory or ear infection, perhaps as soon as 2–3 months postpartum (Alho, Koivu, Hartikainen-Sorri, Sorri & Rantakallio, 1990a, b).

In two studies germane to the topic of developmental PNI, we investigated whether maternal disturbance during pregnancy could interfere with this prenatal transfer of antibody. In the rhesus monkey, which transfers maternal antibody very actively at the end of pregnancy, the amount of IgG acquired by the neonate proved to be resistant to both six weeks of maternal stress during pregnancy and to antenatal Dexamethasone treatments (even though we did find that mother's own IgG levels

did actually decrease (Coe, Kemnitz, & Schneider, 1993). However, when similar effects of maternal stress were examined in another monkey species, the squirrel monkey, with a placenta that does not transfer maternal antibody as affirmatively, gestational stress did affect the amount of IgG present in the neonate. A squirrel monkey infant is born with only 40% of adult IgG. The antibody levels found at birth could be affected by subjecting the gravid female to the stress of two housing relocations into different social groups during pregnancy (Coe & Crispen, 2000).

Nature knows no pause in progress and development,
and attaches her curse on all inaction
J. W. von Goethe (1749–1832)

Other Unique Aspects of Neonatal Immunity

The neonatal stage provides many other unique opportunities to investigate the influence of the prenatal and early rearing environment on the emergence of immune competence. Because so many immune responses are still immature, one can readily discern deficiencies or track the slower progression toward a more mature adult-like immunity (Table 2.1). For example, antigen-presenting cells in the neonate don't recruit lymphocytes as well, and, thus, proliferative and antibody responses are smaller and immature (Schibler, Liechty, White, Rothstein, & Christensen, 1992). The neonate's lymphocytes are also more sensitive to the actions

Table 2.1 Characteristic features of neonatal immunity. At birth, lymphocyte responses are usually less robust than in adults, although inducible following infection and during sepsis

Passive immunity from mother (in primates: placental IgG & sIgA in breast milk).

Innate immune responses functional before birth (e.g., complement activity).

Reduced ability of antigen-presenting cells to stimulate lymphocytes.

Th2-dominant reactions at birth (with atopy prone: less IFN and IL-12, more IL-5).

Unique CD4+ T cell suppression (neonatal type of Treg).

Smaller lymphocyte proliferative and cytokine responses.

Greater sensitivity of lymphocytes to glucocorticoids in neonates.

Smaller antibody responses (usually mount primary responses: more IgM > IgG).

Gradually increasing cytolytic responses with age.

Protective gut microbiota established after birth (e.g., Lactobacilli, Bifidobacteria).

of certain hormones, such as corticosteroids, than are adult cells (Kavelaars et al., 1996). In addition, there are some distinctive cell types in the young infant, including a CD4+ T subpopulation that has a suppressive action on other lymphocytes for the first few months of life.

Traditionally, the activity of this suppressor T cell was evaluated by assessing how the infant's MNC would inhibit the lymphocytes from a "donor" when cultured together. That approach was the one we used to track developmental changes in this suppressive function, in addition to determining if this tonic inhibition might be affected by prior maternal disturbances during the prenatal period (Coe, Lubach, & Karaszewski, 1999). As can be seen in Figure 2.4, the MNC of infant monkeys generated from a normal pregnancy did inhibit how the lymphocytes of an adult animal responded to the mitogen Con A, decreasing proliferation by more than 20%. In contrast, when infants from disturbed pregnancies were assessed—in this particular study after the mothers had their cortisol levels elevated for two weeks by daily injections of ACTH—less inhibition was evident (Coe et al., 1996). At both 2 and 6 weeks of age, the inhibition induced by

their MNC was relatively ineffective, nearly 50% below that of normal infants. We didn't follow-up to determine the actual cause for this defective suppressor activity, but today one might look for a lower number of regulatory T cells in the infants from disturbed pregnancies.

Many Pathways to Altered Immunity and Health in the Young Infant

The availability of maternal antibody provides considerable protection for the neonate, and young infants can respond effectively to many infectious agents, but it is not enough to confer blanket coverage against all pathogens. Young animals and children are especially vulnerable to intestinal disease, and diarrhea-causing enteric pathogens remain a major cause of morbidity and mortality worldwide. To explore this potential vulnerability, we investigated how the gut becomes populated with the beneficial microbiota, and if those bacterial species afford some protection against pathogenic bacteria. While in the sterile womb, an infant's gut should be largely free of bacteria, but even during the birthing process, it begins to encounter and ingest some bacteria from the parturient female. Within a few days, millions of bacteria will have colonized the gut, ultimately reaching almost 10^{14} bacteria, comprised of more than 500 species. We examined developmental changes in two beneficial species, Lactobacilli

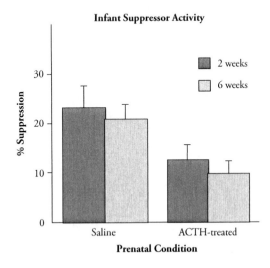

Figure 2.4 Immune responses of neonates to environmental antigens and pathogens are constrained for many reasons, including by a unique CD4+ cell with suppressive actions. This distinctive tempering of immune reactivity was significantly reduced in infant monkeys at 2 and 6 weeks of age if born to females administered ACTH for 2 weeks or if they had been psychologically stressed during late gestation.

and Bifidobacteria across the first 6 months of life, comparing infant monkeys from undisturbed and stressed pregnancies (Bailey, Lubach, & Coe, 2004). Lower concentrations of Lactobacilli and Bifidobacteria were evident in the ones born from disturbed pregnancy conditions. These infants were also more vulnerable to opportunistic infections with diarrhea-causing bacteria, such as Shigella and Campylobacter. In a further extension of this research on the gut microbiome, we determined that the gut Lactobacilli were also responsive to an acute episode of stress. In this case, one relevant to animal husbandry, when the infant monkeys were being weaned from the mother at 6–8 months of age (Bailey & Coe, 1999). Significant decrements in the concentrations of the gut Lactobacilli were evident by the third day after we had re-housed the monkeys away from the mother. The decreases occurred even when they were weaned into small social groups with other young monkeys (in fact, that housing condition increased the likelihood of contagion of diarrhea-causing bacteria among the group-living weanlings).

This impact of a stressful social event on the gut bacteria concurred with a much larger series of studies that our laboratory and others had conducted to directly examine how similar psychological disturbances could affect an infant's immune responses (Table 2.2). During the 1980s and 1990s, many papers were published on the immune changes seen in separated infant monkeys. Disturbances of the mother-infant relationship proved to be

a potent challenge that significantly compromised immune competence. Many aspects of innate and adaptive immunity were perturbed for several days to a few weeks. Lymphocyte proliferation and cytolytic activity becomes markedly decreased, and the capacity to generate an antibody response is reduced (Laudenslager, Reite, & Harbeck, 1982). However, in keeping with what we now know about the bidirectional effects of stress on immunity in humans, not all of the alterations were in a negative direction. Lymphocyte functions become inhibited, but other components of the immune armamentarium are activated in the separated infant monkey. Specifically, there is an activation of innate immunity, including increased complement activity and superoxide release by neutrophils and monocytes (Coe, Rosenberg, & Levine, 1988). Perhaps not coincidentally, during this period of heightened arousal, there is also an enhancement of inflammatory responses, including larger cutaneous hypersensitivity reactions (e.g, more swelling and erythema in the stressed infant when doing a 'recall' test with dinitrochlorobenzene).

Prolonged Immune Alterations Induced by Abnormal Rearing Environments

Notwithstanding the relatively large magnitude of these immune changes in a socially separated monkey, they tend to resolve within a few weeks. One month later, their immune responses typically look close to normal. The rapidity of this recovery suggested to us that the immune system of an older infant is sufficiently mature to have established regulatory set points, enabling a restoration of leukocyte numbers and functions back to the prior healthy level quite quickly. Typically, those experiments were conducted when the young monkeys were between 6–18 months of age, at a stage when they are no longer nursing and are behaviorally independent.

In marked contrast to the transient alterations, very different outcomes were found when the rearing environment was disrupted at a younger age. Almost two decades ago, we evaluated the immune responses of infant monkeys raised by humans in a nursery setting rather than by the biological mother (Lubach, Coe, & Ershler, 1995). Despite the provision of adequate food, benevolent care, and pristine sanitation, we found that there were persistent alterations in several immune responses, including a skewing of the numbers of CD4+ and CD8+ cells in circulation (Figure 2.5). Moreover, when the MNCs of the nursery-reared monkeys were

Table 2.2 Immune alterations seen in young monkeys following separation and weaning from the mother, or in juvenile animals after relocation away from other social companions

Decreased	Increased
Lymphocytopenia	Total WBC
CD4/CD8 ratio	Neutrophilia
Thymic hormones (thymosin)	Neutrophil and monocyte superoxide release
Lymphocyte proliferation	Complement activity; Acute phase response
Cytolytic killing	Other inflammatory mediators
Antibody responses	Cutaneous hypersensitivity reactions

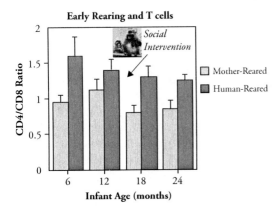

Figure 2.5 Maternal care influences many immune responses in monkeys. When raised by humans in a nursery setting, infant immunity was altered for the first 2 years of life. T cell subsets in circulation and lymphocyte proliferative activity were abnormal, and the differences persisted after an intervention was initiated at 12 months of age. Providing an aged monkey and other yearling monkeys as social companions improved behavioral responses, but did not correct the skewed CD4/CD8 ratio.

stimulated in culture with mitogens, the proliferative responses were markedly exaggerated above normal levels. These differences between mother-reared and nursery-reared monkeys persisted through the second year of life. Further, they were not readily amenable to restoration, even if the infants were transferred as yearlings into social groups with a supportive adult animal. Other research groups have documented that many brain and immune processes remain affected all the way into old age if monkeys have not been mother-reared.

Concluding Thoughts on Priming, Programming, and Disturbed Immunity in the Young Host

The conclusions from our research on nonhuman primates concur with a much larger literature on children and rodent models, which collectively confirms that prenatal and early rearing conditions exert many significant effects on immune responses and health (Barker, 1998; Bilbo, 2010; Coe & Lubach, 2008; LaPlante, Brunet, Schmitz, Ciampi, & King, 2008; Schaub et al., 2009; von Mutius & Vercelli, 2010). As we have emphasized, some environmental modulation of immunity is normal and must occur in both the gravid female and fetus. Lymphoid cells and tissue develop early in gestation, and they are almost immediately exposed to antigenic stimulation from across the placenta, including from food proteins and the external world. The infant's immune responses, both before and after birth, are also be affected by the nutritional status of the mother (Coe, Lubach, & Shirtcliff, 2007). In addition, the placenta is permissive to the bidirectional transfer of some maternal and fetal cells (Bianchi, Zickwolf, Weil, Sylvester, & DeMaria, 1996). Thus, it is reasonable to describe this priming as essential for the normal maturation of the immune system, and the programming aspects are critical for the establishment of immune tolerance, without which the mother's immune system would react against fetal tissues (Singer et al., 2009). However, the same responsiveness can simultaneously create the potential for some vulnerability (Goines, & van de Water, 2010; Kaiser, & Sachser, 2009).

In general, the uterus and placenta provide an effective barrier against viral and bacterial pathogens, but if they reach the fetal compartment, there can be adverse consequences (Arad & Ergaz, 2004). Even in the absence of direct infection of the placenta, amniotic fluids or fetus, increased cytokine activity can impair placental functioning. If the cytokine elevations also occur in the fetal compartment, then there may be deleterious effects on brain development because the blood-brain-brain is still immature and porous. In addition, the fetal thymus is known to be very sensitive to infections, hormones, and physical insults during pregnancy (Rosen, Lee, Cuttitta, Rafiqi, Degan et al., 2006). Much more needs to be learned about the recovery process after a transient thymic involution or loss of thymocytes during the fetal period in order to appreciate whether there are possible long-term consequences (Morrissey, Charrier, Alpert, & Bressler, 1988). In the primate infant, the thymus is relatively larger than it will ever be again for the rest of the life span. After birth, it begins a slow, progressive decline in size, but the factors that guide this age-related trajectory have not been studied.

It is known that there are many ramifications of a premature birth, which is one of the more common adverse events of concern following psychologically or physically challenged pregnancies (Boyd et al., 2009; Reynolds et al., 2001). Even today in the United States, the occurrence of premature births and LBW infants is far too common, still occurring in >12% of pregnancies, with more than 8% born less than 2,500 g (David & Collins, 1997; Martin et al., 2009). Maternal illness and infection of placental tissues are major causes of this negative outcome, with ischemia and placental insufficiency being contributing culprits (Yager & Ashwal, 2009). The degree of risk posed by psychological factors remains more difficult to specify, in part because the magnitude of the effect size varies across epidemiological studies (Wadhwa, Sandman, Porto, Dunkel-Schetter, & Garite, 1993). The inconsistency reflects the wide diversity of the events that have been investigated: ranging from hurricanes to earthquakes, societal catastrophes to the effects of inter-personal violence (Yehuda et al., 2005). There is a pressing need to better identify and understand the many mediating pathways for the increases in bad obstetrical outcomes, which also include a disruption of hormone activity (Murphy, Smith, Giles, & Clifton, 2006; Seckl, 1997; Wadhwa, Sandman, Chicz-DeMet, & Porto, 1997; Wadhwa et al., 2004; Wintour et al., 2003). Of relevance to our field of PNI is whether a dysregulation of maternal and fetal immunity is also a major mediator of these pregnancy and delivery complications after threatening and arousing psychosocial events.

Clearly, female animals and pregnant women have been birthing babies under both good and bad conditions for millennia (Guyer, Freedman, Strobino, Edward, & Sondik, 2000). Thus, there must be a remarkable resiliency as well (Kajantie et al., 2003). In basic science and clinical research, we tend to focus on those factors that derail normal processes and undermine health (Hedegaard, Henriksen, Secher, Hatch, & Sabroe, 1996). However, one could just as easily highlight the ample protection, including the maternal gift of passive immunity, which protects the young infant via the provision of antibody for first 3–6 months after birth. We found this process to be relatively resistant to disruption in the rhesus monkey, except in the case of premature birth. It is also true that the components of innate immunity are well established by birth and, if needed, can be mounted vigorously by the neonate. We did not mention previously that we found the complement system of the fetal rhesus monkey to be quite mature by late gestation, already functional two months before term (Coe et al., 1993). Similarly, when provoked by bacterial infection, the premature and newborn human infant can generate strong cytokine responses, even if their IL-6 levels do not quite reach adult levels (Doellner, Arntzen, Haereid, Aag, & Austgulen, 1998; Messer et al., 1996). After birth, breast-feeding provides many nutrient factors and other proteins that promote the infant's immune competence, including by nurturing a gut microbiome that is more protective against enteric pathogens (Dewey, Jeinig, & Nommsen-Rivers, 1995).

For those interested in PNI, the neonatal and infancy periods provide many opportunities for discovering the potent influences of the environment,

and of stress and hormones, on immune responses. Research on young animals—including the studies on rodent pups, infant primates, and domesticated farm animals—has demonstrated that disturbed early rearing conditions can cause both transient and persistent effects on immunity (Tuchscherer, Kanitz, Oteen, & Tuchscherer, 2002). When the perturbations occur in older infants and juveniles, the stress-related immune alterations in the monkey tend to last a few days to several weeks, followed by a return to the prior level of immune competence (Laudenslager, Berger, Boccia, & Reite, 1996). However, when maternal care is disturbed closer to birth, then some aspects of immunity can be permanently derailed. We briefly described some of our immune findings on infant monkeys reared in a nursery setting. The results raise a serious concern about the possibility of long-term physical health consequences in institutionalized children raised in orphanage settings, beyond the devastating effects on behavioral and emotional well-being that we know about. Nearly two decades ago we examined the immune status of toddlers in Romanian orphanages and found that many had already been infected with Herpes simplex at a very young age. Moreover, they did not appear to be containing the virus in a quiescent state, with high salivary levels of HSV-sIgA indicative of viral shedding. Similarly, in a more recent study of Herpes control in adolescents adopted from many parts of the world, it appeared that an impairment in viral control was still evident at an older age, even while living in benevolent family settings (Shirtcliff et al., 2009).

The research in both animals and humans speaks to the enduring importance of parenting and the early rearing environment for establishing the supportive physical and psychological foundations upon which good health is based. Among the offspring of most mammalian species, there is a "biological expectancy" of a nurturing parent as an essential feature of the postnatal world. In addition, there is extensive research demonstrating that the normal maturation of the brain can be affected by the quality of parental care. Developmental PNI research indicates there are also strong influences on the immune system. It concurs with what we have learned about the immune sequelae of raising young animals in the hygienic realm of a gnotobiotic laboratory. In that setting, without appropriate priming and stimulation, the immune system cannot develop normally (Yazdanbakhsh, van den Biggelaar, & Maizels, 2001). The psychosocial context also has tangible effects: it provides stimulation and positive resources, while serving as a buffer against stressful perturbations. When we discuss the public health implications of a national policy in the United States, such as "No Child Left Behind," the message is clear: Begin early by ensuring high-quality prenatal care for all pregnant women and follow up this societal commitment with adequate support for new parents by making early childhood programs available and accessible. Follow the 13th century proverb that "prevention is worth a pound of cure." That is also the logical conclusion of the extant research on developmental PNI.

Future Directions

1. How can we best distinguish between nonspecific effects (e.g., explained by a general influence on placental functioning) from more specific actions of particular mediators (e.g., hormone or cytokine pathways)?

2. Most research has focused on negative factors and outcomes. What are the primary psychosocial factors that account for maternal resilience and successful pregnancies, especially in the face of adversity?

3. How can we determine when a perturbation or transient disruption should be viewed as a programming event that permanently alters regulatory set points later in life?

4. The premature infant encounters the world at a very different stage of immune maturation than does the full-term infant. Given the high incidence of premature birth in humans, what are the long-term ramifications for immunity and overall health?

5. Newborn infants in our modern society encounter a very different world than that of our ancestors. What are the immune and health consequences of this more hygienic setting, which may at the same time include a number of novel industrial toxicants and pollutants?

6. The mammalian infant, including its immune system, is born with a "biological expectation" of a prolonged period of nursing. What are the ramifications for the maturation of immunity of a foreshortened period of breastfeeding or the decision to bottle-feed exclusively?

7. Sadly, some children do have early experiences with separation and loss. What are the short- and long-term immune and health effects of these events, and how can the adverse outcomes be minimized?

8. There is increasing evidence for intergenerational effects. How much is explained by epigenetic changes in gene regulation and mother-to-daughter changes in the physiology of pregnancy?

9. Prenatal and early rearing conditions certainly affect the development of infant animals. What are the ramifications for veterinary medicine and agricultural practices? What are the optimal husbandry procedures for the breeding and rearing of laboratory rats and mice if we want to standardize these conditions?

10. Given that pregnancy conditions and infant well-being are so important for developmental and population health, what are the policy implications for industrialized countries as well as for the poorer regions of the world?

Acknowledgments

CLC is currently supported in part by grants from the National Institutes of Health, which sponsored the research on nonhuman primates, including several projects on the neural and developmental effects of maternal infection during pregnancy and iron deficiency anemia (AI067518, HD39386, HD057064).

References

Ader, R. (1983). Developmental psychoneurimmunology. *Developmental Psychobiology, 16,* 251–267.

Ader, R., & Friedman, S. G. (1965). Social factors affecting emotionality and resistance to disease in animals. V. Early separation from the mother and response to transplanted tumor in the rat. *Psychosomatic Medicine, 27,* 119–122.

Adinolfi, M. (1993). Infectious diseases in pregnancy, cytokines and neurological impairment: A hypothesis. *Developmental Medicine and Child Neurology, 35,* 549–553.

Ahluwalia, B., Wesley, B., Adyiga, O., Smith, D. M., Da-Silva A., & Rajguru, S. (2000). Alcohol modulates cytokine secretion and synthesis in human fetus, an in vivo and in vitro study. *Alcohol, 21(3),* 207–213.

Alho O-P., Koivu, M., Hartikainen-Sorri, M., Sorri, M., & Rantakallio, P. (1990a). Is a child's history of acute otitis media and respiratory infection already determined in the antenatal and perinatal period? *International Journal of Pediatric Otorhinolaryngology, 19(2),* 129–137.

Alho, O-P., Koivu, M., Sorri, M., & Rantakallio P. (1990b). Risk factors for recurrent acute otitis media and respiratory infection in infancy. *International Journal of Pediatric Otorhinolaryngology, 19(2),* 151–161.

Amman, A. J., Wara, D. W., Cowan, M. J., Barrett, D. J., & Stiehm, E. R. (1982). The DiGeorge syndrome and the fetal alcohol syndrome. *American Journal of Diseases of Children, 136,* 906–908.

Arad, I., & Ergaz, Z. (2004). The fetal inflammatory response syndrome and associated infant morbidity. *Israel Medical Association Journal, 6,* 766–769.

Bailey, M. T., & Coe, C. L. (1999). Maternal separation disrupts indigenous microflora of infant monkeys. *Developmental Psychobiology, 35(2),* 146–155.

Bailey, M. T., Lubach, G. R., & Coe, C. L. (2004). Prenatal conditions alter the bacterial colonization of the gut in the infant monkey. *Journal of Pediatric and Clinical Gastroenterology, 38,* 414–421.

Barker, D. J. P. (1998). In utero programming of chronic disease. *Clinical Science, 95,* 115–128.

Barry P. A., Lockridge, K. M., Salamat, S., Tinling, S. P., Yue, Y., Zhou, S. S., Gospe, S. M., Britt, W. J., & Tarantal, A. F. (2006). Nonhuman primate models of intrauterine cytomegalovirus infection. *Institute for Laboratory Animal Research Journal, 47(1),* 49–64.

Bateson, P., Barker, D. J. P., Clutton-Brock, T., Deb, D., D'Udine, B., Foley, R. A., et al. (2004). Developmental plasticity and human health. *Nature, 430,* 419–421.

Berkowitz, G. S., Wolff, M. S., Janevic, T. M., Holzman, I. R., Yehuda, R., & Landrigan, P. J. (2003). The World Trade Center disaster and intrauterine growth restriction. *Journal of the American Medical Association, 290,* 595–596.

Berrebi, A. B., Assouline, C., Bessieres, M-H, Lathiere, M., Cassling, S., Minville, V., et al. (2010). Long-term outcome of children with congenital toxoplasmosis. *American Journal of Obstetrics and Gynecology 203(6),* 552.e1–552.e6.

Bianchi, D. W., Zickwolf, G. K., Weil, G. J., Sylvester, S., & DeMaria, M. A. (1996). Male fetal progenitor cells persist in maternal blood for as long as 27 years postpartum. *Proceedings of the National Academy of Science, 93(2),* 705–708.

Bilbo, S. D. (2010). Early-life infection is a vulnerability factor for aging-related immune changes and cognitive decline. *Neurobiology of Learning and Memory, 94(1),* 57–64.

Boyce, W. T., Jensen, E. W., Cassel, J. C., Collier, A. M., Smith, A. N., & Ramey, C. T., (1977). Influence of life events and family routines on childhood respiratory tract illness. *Pediatrics, 60,* 609–615.

Boyd, H. A., Pouslen, G., Wohlfahrt, J., Murray, J. C., Feenstra, B., Melbye, M. (2009). Maternal contributions to preterm delivery. *American Journal of Epidemiology, 170(11),* 1358–1364.

Braunschweig, D., Ashwood, P., Krakowiak, P., Hertz-Picciotto, I., Hansen, R., Croen, L, et al. (2009). Autism: maternally derived antibodies specific for fetal brain proteins. *Neurotoxicology, 29(2),* 226–231.

Brown, A. S. (2006). Prenatal infection as a risk factor for schizophrenia. *Schizophrenia Bulletin, 32,* 200–202.

Byrne, M., Agerbo, E., Benndese, B., Eaton, W., & Mortensen, P. (2007). Obstetric conditions and risk of first admission with schizophrenia: A Danish national register based study. *Schizophrenia Research, 97,* 51–59

Casas, R., & Brjorksten, B. (2001). Detection of Fel d-1-immunoglobulin G complexes in cord blood and sera from allergic and nonallergic mothers. *Pediatric Allergy and Immunology, 12(2),* 59–64.

Centers for Disease Control and Prevention (2000). Racial and ethnic differences in infant mortality rates—60 largest US cities, 1995–1998. *Morbidity and Mortality Weekly Report (MMWR), 51,* 329–343.

Chen, E. Chim, L. S., Strunk, R. C., & Miller, G. (2007). The role of the social environment in children and adolescents with asthma. *American Journal of Respiratory and Critical Care Medicine, 176,* 644–649.

Chen, E., Miller, G. E., Kobor, M. S., & Cole S. W. (2010). Maternal warmth buffers the effects of low early-life socioeconomic status on pro-inflammatory signaling in adulthood. *Molecular Psychiatry, 16,* 729–737.

Coe, C. L., & Crispen, H. (2000). Social stress in pregnant monkeys differentially affects placental transfer of maternal antibody to male and female infants. *Health Psychology, 19(6),* 554–559.

Coe, C. L., Kemnitz, J. W., & Schneider, M. L. (1993). Vulnerability of placental antibody transfer and fetal complement synthesis to disturbance of the pregnant monkey. *Journal of Medical Primatology, 22(5),* 294–300.

Coe, C. L., & Lubach, G. R. (2005). Developmental consequences of antenatal dexamethasone treatment in nonhuman primates. *Neuroscience and BioBehavioral Reviews, 29(2),* 227–235.

Coe, C. L., & Lubach, G. R. (2008). Fetal programming: Prenatal origins of health and illness. *Current Directions in Psychological Science, 17(1),* 36–41.

Coe, C. L., Lubach, G. R. & Izard, K. M. (1994). Progressive improvement in the transfer of maternal antibody across the Order Primates. *American Journal of Primatology, 32(1),* 51–55.

Coe, C. L., Lubach, G. R., & Karaszewski, J. (1999). Prenatal stress and immune recognition of self and nonself in the primate neonate. *Biology of the Neonate 76(5),* 301–310.

Coe, C. L., Lubach, G. R., Karaszewski, J. W., & Ershler, W. B. (1996). Prenatal endocrine activation alters postnatal cellular immunity in infant monkeys. *Brain, Behavior and Immunity, 10,* 221–234.

Coe, C. L., Lubach, G. R., & Shirtcliff, E. (2007). Maternal stress during pregnancy increases risk for iron deficient infants impacting innate immunity. *Pediatric Research, 61(5),* 520–524.

Coe, C. L., Rosenberg, L. T., & Levine, S. (1988). Effect of maternal separation on the complement system and antibody responses in infant primates. *International Journal of Neuroscience, 40,* 289–302.

Cokkinides, V. E., Coker, A. L., Sanderson, M., Addy, C., & Bethea, L. (1999). Physical violence during pregnancy: Maternal complications and birth outcomes. *Obstetrics and Gynecology, 93,* 661–666.

Culhane, J. F., Rauh, V., & Farley-McCollum, K. (2001). Maternal stress is associated with bacterial vaginosis in human pregnancy. *Maternal and Child Health Journal, 5,* 127–134.

Dammann, O., & Leviton, A. (1997). Maternal intrauterine infection, cytokines and brain damage in the preterm newborn. *Pediatric Research, 42,* 1–8.

Damman, O., & Leviton, A. (2000). Role of the fetus in perinatal infection and neonatal brain damage. *Current Opinions in Pediatrics, 12,* 99–104.

Danese, A., Pariante, C. M., Caspi, A., Taylor, A., & Poulton, R. (2007). Childhood maltreatment predicts adult inflammation in a life-course study. *Proceedings of the National Academy of Sciences, 104(4),* 1319–1324.

David, R., & Collins, J. (1997). Differing birth weight among infants of US-born blacks, African-born blacks, and US-born whites. *New England Journal of Medicine, 337,* 1209–1219.

De Felice, C., Toti, P., Santopietro, R., Stumpo, M., Pecciarini, L., & Bagnoli, F. (1999). Small thymus in very low birth weight infants born to mothers with subclinical chorioamnionitis. *Journal of Pediatrics, 135,* 384–386.

De Leon-Luis, J., Gamez, F., Pintado, P., Antolin, E., Perez, R., Ortiz-Quintana, L., et al. (2009). Sonographic measurements of the thymus in male and female fetuses. *Journal of Ultrasound Medicine, 28,* 43–48.

De Miranda, J., Yaddanapudi, K., Hornig, M., Villar, G., Serge, R., & Lipkin, W. I. (2010). Induction of toll-like receptor 3-mediated immunity during gestation inhibits cortical neurogenesis and causes behavioral disturbances. *mBio 1*(4), e00176–10. doi:10.1128/mBio.00176–10.

Devereux, G., Seaton, A., & Barker, R. N. (2001). In utero priming of allergen specific helper T cells. *Clinical and Experimental Allergy, 31*(11), 1686–1695.

Dewey, K. G., Jeinig, J., & Nommsen-Rivers, L. A. (1995). Differences in morbidity between breast-fed and formula-fed infants. *Journal of Pediatrics, 126,* 696–702.

Di Naro, E., Cromi, A., Ghezzi, F., Raio, L, Uccella, S., D'Addario, V., et al. (2006). Fetal thymic involution: a sonographic marker of the fetal inflammatory response syndrome. *American Journal of Obstetrics and Gynecology, 194,* 153–159.

Doellner, H., Arntzen, K. J., Haereid, P. E., Aag, S., & Austgulen, R. (1998). Interleukin-6 concentrations in neonates evaluated for sepsis. *Journal of Pediatrics, 132,* 295–299.

Elliott, A. M., Mpairwe, H., Quigley, M. A., Nampijja, M., Muhangi, L., Oweka-Onyee, J., et al. (2005). Helminth infection during pregnancy and development of infantile eczema. *Journal of the American Medical Association, 294*(16), 2032–2034.

Engel, S. M., Berkowitz, G. S., Wolff, M., & Yehuda, Y. (2005). Psychological trauma associated with World Trade Center attacks and its effects on pregnancy outcome. *Paediatrics Perinatalogy and Epidemiology, 19*(5), 334–341.

Ewald, S. J., & Walden, S. M. (1988). Flow cytometric and histological analysis of mouse thymus in fetal alcohol syndrome. *Journal of Leukocyte Biology, 44,* 434–44.

Faeleabas, A. T., Kim, J. J., Srinivasan, S., Donnelly, K. M., Brudney, A., & Jaffe, R. C. (1999). Implantation in the baboon: Endometrial responses. *Seminars in Reproductive Endocrinology, 17*(3), 257–265.

Fatemi, S. H., Reutiman, T. J., Folsom, T. D., Huang, H., Oishi, K., Mori S., et al. (2008). Maternal infection leads to abnormal gene regulation and brain atrophy in mouse offspring. *Schizophrenia Research, 99*(1), 56–70.

Fergusson, D. M., Crane, J., Beaseley, R., & Horwood, L. J. (1997). Perinatal factors and atopic disease in childhood. *Clinical Experimental Allergy, 27,* 1394–1401.

Fletcher, B. D., Masson, M., Lisbona, A., Riggs, T., & Papageorgiou, A. N. (1979). Thymic response to endogenous and exogenous steroids in premature newborn infants. *Journal of Pediatrics, 95,* 111–114.

Foglia, L. M., Ippolito, D. L., Stallings, J. D., Zelig, C. M., & Napolitano, P. G. (2010). Intramuscular 17alpha-hydroxyprogesterone caproate administration attenuates immunoresponsiveness of maternal peripheral mononuclear cells. *American Journal of Obstetrics and Gynecology 203*(6), 561.e1.–5.

Fortier, M-E., Luheshi, G. N., & Boksa, P. (2007). Effects of prenatal infection on PPI in rat depend upon nature of the infectious agent and stage of pregnancy. *Behavioral Brain Research, 181*(2), 270–277.

Gazmararian, J. A., Lazorick, S., Spitz, A. M., Ballard, T. J., Saltzman, L. E., & Marks, J. S. (1996). Prevalence of violence against pregnant women. *Journal of the American Medical Association, 275,* 1915–1920.

Glynn, L. M., Wadhwa, P. D., Dunkel-Schetter, C., & Sandman, C. A. (2001). When stress happens matters: The effects of earthquake timing on stress responsivity in pregnancy. *American Journal of Obstetrics and Gynecology, 184*(4), 637–642.

Goines, P., & van de Water, J. (2010). The immune system's role in the biology of autism. *Current Opinions in Neurology, 23,* 111–117.

Goodman, C. S., & Coughlin, B. C., (2000). The evolution of evo-devo biology. *Proceedings of the National Academy of Sciences, 97*(9), 4424–4425.

Guyer, B., Freedman, M. A., Strobino, D., & Edward, J., Sondik, E. J. (2000). Annual summary of vital statistics: Trends in the health of Americans during the 20th century. *Pediatrics, 106,* 1307–1317.

Hao, X-Q., Zhang, H-G, Li, S-H, Jia, Y., Liu, Y., Zhou, J-Z., et al. (2010). Prenatal exposure to inflammation induced by zymosan results in activation of intrarenal renin-angiotensin system in adult offspring rats. *Inflammation, 33*(6), 408–414.

Harris, J. W. (1919). Influenza occurring in pregnant women. A statistical study of 1350 cases. *Journal of the American Medical Association, 72*(14), 978–980.

Hartert, T. V., Neuzil, K. M., Shintani, A. K., Mitchel, E. F., Snowden, M. S., Wood, L. B., et al. (2003). Maternal morbidity and perinatal outcomes among pregnant women with respiratory hospitalizations during influenza season. *American Journal of Obstetrics and Gynecology 189*(6), 1705–1712.

Hedegaard, M., Henriksen, T. B., Secher, N. J., Hatch, M. C., & Sabroe, S. (1996). Do stressful life events affect duration of gestation and risk of preterm delivery? *Epidemiology, 7*(4), 339–345.

Hiller, S. L., Nugent, R. P., Eschebach, D. A., Krohn, M. A., Gibbs, R. S., Martin, D. H., et al. (1995). Association between bacterial vaginosis and preterm delivery of low-birth weight infants. *New England Journal of Medicine, 333,* 1737–1742.

Hodgson, D. M., & Coe, C. L. (2006). *Perinatal programming: Early life determinants of adult health and disease.* Abingdon, England: Taylor & Francis,

Hsiao, E. Y., & Patterson, P. H. (2011). Activation of the maternal immune system induces endocrine changes in the placenta via IL-6. *Brain, Behavior, & Immunity, 25*(4), 604–615.

Igarashi, H., Kouro, T., Yokota, T., Comp, P. C., & Kincade, P. W. (2001). Age and stage dependency of estrogen receptor expression by lymphocyte precursors, *Proceedings of the National Academy Science, 98,* 15131–1513.

Irving, W. L., James, D. K., Stephenson, T., Laing, P., Jameson, C., Oxford, J. S., et al. (2000). Influenza virus infection in second and third trimesters of pregnancy: A clinical and seroepidemiological study. *British Journal of Obstetrics and Gynecology, 107,* 1282–1289.

Jones, C. A., Holloway, J. A., & Warner, J. O. (2000). Does atopic disease start in foetal life? *Allergy, 55,* 2–10.

Kaiser, S., & Sachser, N. (2009). Effects of prenatal social stress on offspring development: Pathology or adaptation. *Currents Directions in Psychological Science, 18*(2), 118–121.

Kajantie, E., Dunkel, L., Turpeinen, U., Stenman, U-H., Wood, P. J., Nuutila, M., et al. (2003). Placental 11ß- hydroxysteroid dehydrogenase-2 and fetal cortisol/cortisone shuttle in small preterm infants. *Journal of Clinical Endocrinology and Metabolism, 88,* 493–500.

Karmaus, W., Arshad, S. H., Sadeghnejad, A., & Twiselton, R. (2004). Does maternal IgE decrease with increasing order of live offspring? *Clinical and Experimental Allergy, 43,* 853–859.

Kavelaars, A., Cats, B., Visser, G. H. A., Zegers, B. J. M., Bakker, J. M., van Rees E. P., et al. (1996). Ontogeny of the response of human peripheral blood T cells to glucocorticoids. *Brain, Behavior and Immunity, 10,* 288–297.

Kobayashi, K., Miwa, H., & Yasui, M. (2011). Inflammatory mediators weaken the amniotic member barrier through disruption of tight junctions. *Journal of Physiology, 588(24),* 4859–4869.

Koehl, M., Darnaudery, M., Dulluc, J., Van Reeth, O., Le Moal, M., & Maccari S. (1999). Prenatal stress alters circadian activity of hypothalamo-pituitary-adrenal axis and hippocampal corticosteroid receptors in adult rats of both gender. *Journal of Neurobiology, 40(3),* 302–315.

Kruschinski, C., Skripuletz, T., Bedoui, S., Raber, K., Straub, R. H., Hoffman, T., et al. (2008). Postnatal life events affect the severity of asthmatic airway inflammation in the adult rat. *Journal of Immunology, 180,* 3919–3925.

LaPlante, D., Brunet, A., Schmitz, N., Ciampi, A., & King, S. (2008). Project Ice Storm: Prenatal maternal stress affects cognitive and linguistic functioning in 5½ -year old children. *Journal of the American Academy of Child and Adolescent Psychiatry, 47(9),* 1063–1072.

Laudenslager, M. L., Berger, C. L., Boccia, M. L., & Reite, M. L. (1996). Natural cytotoxicity toward K562 cells by macaque lymphocytes form infancy through puberty: Effects of early social challenge. *Brain, Behavior and Immunity, 10,* 275–287.

Laudenslager, M. L., Reite, M. R., & Harbeck, R. J. (1982). Suppressed immune response in infant monkeys associated with maternal separation. *Behavioral and Neural Biology, 36,* 40–48.

Lawoyin, T. O. (2001). Risk factors for infant mortality in a rural community in Nigeria *Journal of Royal Society for the Promotion of Health, 121,* 114–118.

Lemaire, V., Koehl, M., Le Moal, M., & Abrous, D. N. (2000). Prenatal stress produces learning deficits associated with an inhibition of neurogenesis in the hippocampus. *Proceedings of the National Academy of Science, 97(20),* 11032–11037.

Liobichler, C., Pichler, J., & Gestmayr, M. (2002). Materno-fetal passage of nutritive and inhalant allergens across placentas of term and preterm deliveries perfused in vitro *Clinical and Experimental Allergy, 32,* 1546–1551.

Lowe, G. C., Luheshi, G. N., & Williams, S. (2008). Maternal infection and fever during late gestation are associated with altered synaptic transmission in the hippocampus of juvenile offspring rats. *American Journal of Physiology- Regulatory, Integrative and Comparative Physiology, 295,* R1563–R1571.

Lubach, G. R., Coe, C. L., & Ershler, W. B. (1995). Effects of the early rearing environment on immune responses of infant rhesus monkeys. *Brain, Behavior and Immunity 9,* 31–46

Lui, A. H., & Murphy, J. R. (2003). Hygiene hypothesis: fact or fiction? *Journal of Allergy and Clinical Immunology, 111,* 471–478.

Mak, T. K., Mangtani, P., Leese, J., Watson, J. M., & Pfeifer, D. (2008). Influenza vaccination in pregnancy: current evidence and selected national policies. *Lancet Infectious Diseases, 8,* 44–52.

Martin, J. A., Hamilton, B. E., Sutton, P. D., Ventura, S. J., Menacker, F., Kimeyer, S., & et al. (2009). Births: Final data for 2006. *National Vital Statistics Report, 57(7),* 3–104.

Martinez, E., Figueroa, R., Garry, D., Visintainer, P., Patel, K., Verma, U., et al. (1998). Elevated amniotic fluid interleukin-6 as a predictor of neonatal periventricular leukomalacia and intraventricular hemorrhage. *Journal of Maternal and Fetal Investigation, 8,* 101–107.

McGregor, J. A., French, J. I., Parker, R., Draper, D., Patterson, E., Jones, W., et al. (1995). Prevention of premature birth by screening and treatment for common genital tract infections: Results of a prospective controlled evaluation. *American Journal of Obstetrics and Gynecology, 173,* 157–167.

Mednick, S. A., Machon, R. A., Huttunen, M. O. & Bonnet, D. (1988). Adult schizophrenia following prenatal exposure to an influenza epidemic. *Archives of General Psychiatry, 45,* 189–192.

Menon, R., Merialdi, M., Betran, A. P., Dolan, S., Jiang, L., Fortunato, S. J., et al. (2006). Analysis of association between maternal tumor necrosis factor-alpha promoter polymorphism (-308), tumor necrosis factor concentration and preterm birth. *American Journal of Obstetrics and Gynecology, 195,* 1240–1248.

Messer, J., Eyer, D., Donato L., Gallati, H., Matis, J., & Simeoni. U. (1996). Evaluation of interleukin-6 and soluble receptors for tumor necrosis factor for early diagnosis of neonatal infection. *Journal of Pediatrics, 129(4),* 574–580.

Meyer, R. J., & Haggerty, R. J. (1962). Streptococcal infections in families. Factors altering individual susceptibility. *Pediatrics, 29,* 539–549.

Mold, J. E., Michaelsson, J., Burt, T. D., Muench, M. O., Beckerman, K. P., Busch, M. P., et al. (2008). Maternal alloantigens promote the development of tolerogenic fetal regulatory T cells in utero. *Science, 322(5907),* 1562–1565.

Morrissey, P. J., Charrier, K., Alpert, A., & Bressler, L. (1988). In vivo administration of IL-1 induces thymic hypoplasia and increased levels of serum corticosterone. *Journal of Immunology, 141,* 1456–1463.

Muhangi, L., Woodburn, P., Omara, M., Omoding, N., Kizito, D., Mpairwe, H., et al. (2007). Associations between mild-to-moderate anaemia in pregnancy and helminth, malaria and HIV infection in Entebbe, Uganda. *Transactions of the Royal Society of Tropical Medicine and Hygiene, 101(9),* 899–907.

Murphy, V. E., Smith, R., Giles, W. B., & Clifton, V. L. (2006). Endocrine regulation of human fetal growth: The role of the mother, placenta, and fetus. *Endocrine Reviews, 27,* 141–169.

Newberger, E. H., Barkan, S. E., Lieberman, E. S., McCormick, M. C., Yllo, K., Gary, L T., et al. (1992). Abuse of pregnant women and adverse birth outcome: Current knowledge and implications for practice. *Journal of the American Medical Association, 267(17),* 2370–2372.

Nielsen, N. M., Hansen, A. V., Simonsen, J., & Hviid, A. (2011). Prenatal stress and risk of infectious diseases in offspring. *American Journal of Epidemiology,* doi: 10.1093/aje/kwq492

Nijagal, A., Wegorzewska, M., Jarvis, E., Le, T., Tang, Q., & MacKenzie, T. C. (2011). Maternal T cells limit engraftment after in utero hematopoietc cell transplantation in mice. *Journal of Clinical Investigation,* doi:10.1172/JC144907.

Patterson, P. H. (2011). Modeling autistic features in animals. *Pediatric Research, 69(5),* 34R–40R.

Pekkanen, J., Xu, B., & Jarevelin, M-R. (2001). Gestational age and occurrence of atopy at age 31—a prospective birth cohort study in Finland. *Clinical and Experimental Allergy, 31,* 95–102.

Petersen, R., Gazmararian, J. A., Spitz, A. M., Rowley, D. L., Goodwin, M. M., Saltzman, L. E., et al. (1997). Violence and adverse pregnancy outcomes: a review of the literature and directions for future research *American Journal of Preventive Medicine, 13(5),* 366–373.

Piccinni, M. P., Mecacci, F., Sampognaro, S., Manetti, R., Parronchi, P., Maggi, E., et al. (1993). Aeroallergen sensitization can occur during fetal life. *International Archives of Allergy and Immunology, 102(3)*, 301–303.

Rees, S., Harding, R., & Walker, D. (2008). An adverse intrauterine environment: implications for injury and altered development of the brain. *International Journal of Developmental Neuroscience, 26*(1), 3–11.

Revello, M. G., & Gerna, G. (2002). Diagnosis and management of human cytomegalovirus infection in the mother, fetus, and newborn infant. *Clinical Microbiology Reviews, 15*, 680–715

Reynolds, R. M., Walker, B. R., Syddall, H. E., Andrew, R., Wood, P. J., Whorwood, C. B., et al. (2001). Altered control of cortisol secretion in adult men with low birth weight and cardiovascular risk factors. *Journal of Clinical Endocrinology and Metabolism, 86*, 245–250.

Rigo, J. J. R., Szelenyi, J., Selmeczy, Z., Papp, Z, & Vizi, E. S. (2004). Endotoxin-induced TNF production changes inversely to its plasma level during pregnancy. *European Journal of Obstetrics and Gynecology, 114*(2), 236–238.

Rosen, D., Lee, J-H, Cuttitta, F., Rafiqi, F., Degan, S., & Sunday, M. E. (2006). Accelerated thymic maturation and autoreactive T cells in bronchopulmonary dysplasia. *American Journal of Respiratory and Critical Care Medicine, 174*, 75–83.

Ross, M. G. (2010). Inflammatory mediators weaken the amniotic membrane barrier through disruption of tight junctions. *Journal of Physiology, 589*(1), 5.

Saito, M., Matsuda, T., Okuyama, K., Kobayashi, Y., Kitanishi, R., Hanita, T., et al. (2009) Effect of intrauterine inflammation on fetal cerebral hemodynamics and white-matter injury in chronically instrumented fetal sheep. *American Journal of Obstetrics and Gynecology, 200*, 663.e1–664.e11.

Schaub, B., Liu, J., Höppler, S., Schleich, I, Huehn, J., Olek, S., et al. (2009). Maternal farm exposure modulates neonatal immune mechanisms through regulatory T cells. *Journal of Allergy and Clinical Immunology, 123*, 774–782.

Schibler, K. R., Liechty, K. W., White, W. L., Rothstein, G., & Christensen, R. D. (1992). Defective production of interleukin-6 by monocytes: A possible mechanism underlying several host defense deficiencies of neonates. *Pediatric Research, 31*, 18–21.

Shirtcliff, E. A., Coe, C. L., & Pollak, S. D. (2009). Early childhood stress is associated with elevated antibody levels to Herpes simplex virus type 1. *Proceedings National Academy Sciences, 106*(8), 2963–2967.

Schwarz, N. G., Adegnika, A. A., Breitling, L. P., Gabor, J., Agnandji, S. T., Newman, R. D., et al. (2008). Placental malaria increases malaria risk in the first 30 months of life. *Clinical and Infectious Diseases, 47*, 1017–1025.

Seckl, J. R. (1997). Glucocorticoids, feto-placental 11 beta-hydroxysteroid dehydrogenase type 2, and the early life origins of adult disease. *Steroids, 62*(1), 89–94.

Shi, L., Fatemi, S. H., Sidwell, R. W., & Patterson, P. H. (2003). Maternal influenza infection causes marked behavioral and pharmacological changes in the offspring. *Journal Neuroscience, 23*(1), 297–302.

Shi, L., Tu, N., & Patterson, P. H. (2005). Maternal influenza infection is likely to alter fetal development indirectly. *International Journal of Developmental Neuroscience, 23*, 299–305.

Short, S. J., Lubach, G. R., Karasin, A. I., Olsen, C. W., Styner, M., Knickmeyer, R. C., et al. (2010). Maternal influenza infection during pregnancy impacts postnatal brain development in the rhesus monkey. *Biological Psychiatry, 67*, 965–973.

Singer, H. S., Morris C., Gause, C., Pollard, M., Zimmerman, A. W., & Pletnikov, M. (2009). Prenatal exposure to antibodies from mothers of children with autism produces neurobehavioral alterations: A pregnant dam mouse model. *Journal of Neuroimmunology, 211*(1), 39–48.

Solomon, G. F., Levine, S., & Kraft, J. K. (1968). Early experience and immunity. *Nature 220*, 821–822.

Toti, P., De Felice, C., Stumpo, M., Schürfeld, K., Di Leo, L., Vatti, R., et al. (2000). Acute thymic involution in fetuses and neonates with chorioamnionitis. *Human Pathology, 31*, 1121–1128.

Tuchscherer, M., Kanitz, E., Oteen, W., & Tuchscherer, A. (2002). Effects of prenatal stress on cellular and humoral immune responses in neonatal pigs. *Veterinary Immunology and Immunopathology, 86*(3–4), 195–203.

Van Duren Schmidt K., Pichler J., Ebner C., Bartmann P., Forster E., Radvan U., et al. (1997). Prenatal contact with inhalant allergens. *Pediatric Research, 41*, 128–131.

von Mutius, E., & Vercelli, D. (2010). Farm living: Effects on childhood asthma and allergy, *Nature Reviews Immunology, 10*, 861–868.

Wadhwa, P. D., Sandman, C. A., Chicz-DeMet, A., & Porto, M. (1997). Placental CRH modulates maternal pituitary-adrenal function in human pregnancy. *Annals of the New York Academy of Sciences, 814*, 276–281.

Wadhwa, P. D., Sandman, C. A., Porto, M., Dunkel-Schetter, C., & Garite, T. J. (1993). The association between prenatal stress and infant birthweight and gestational age at birth: A prospective investigation. *American Journal of Obstetrics and Gynecology, 169*, 858–65.

Wadhwa, P. D., Garite, T. J., Porto, M., Chicz-DeMet, A., Dunkel-Schetter, C., & Sandman, C. A. (2004). Corticotropin-releasing hormone (CRH), preterm birth and fetal growth restriction: A prospective investigation. *American Journal of Obstetrics and Gynecology, 191*, 1063–1069.

Warner, J. A., Jones, C. A., Jones, A. C., & Warner, J. O. (2000). Prenatal origins of allergic disease. *Journal of Allergy and Clinical Immunology, 105*, 5493–5496.

Webb, E. L., Mawa, P. A., Ndibazza, J., Kizito, D, Namatovu, A, Kyosiimire-Lugemwa, J., et al. (2011). Effect of single-dose antihelmintic treatment during pregnancy on an infant's response to immunisation and on susceptibility to infectious diseases in infancy: a randomised, double-blind, placebo-controlled trial. *Lancet, 377*(9759), 52–62.

Weinstock, M. (1997). Does prenatal stress impair coping and regulation of hypothalamic-pituitary-adrenal axis? *Neuroscience and Biobehavioral Reviews, 21*(1), 1–10.

Welberg, L. A., & Seckl, J. R. (2001). Prenatal stress, glucocorticoids and the programming of the brain. *Journal of Neuroendocrinology, 13*, 113–128.

Wildman, D. E., Chen, C., Erez, O., Grossman, L. I., Goodman, M., & Romero, R. (2006). Evolution of the mammalian placenta revealed by phylogenetic analysis. *Proceedings of the National Academy of Science, 103*(6), 3203–3208.

Wintour, E. M., Johnson, K., Koukoulas, I., Moritz, K., Tersteeg, M., & Dodic, M. (2003). Programming the cardiovascular system, kidney and the brain: A review. *Placenta, 27*(Suppl. A), 65–71.

Wright, R. J., Visness, C. M., Calatroni, A., Grayson, M. H., Gold, D. R., Sandel, M. T., et al. (2010). Prenatal maternal stress and cord blood innate and adaptive cytkine responses in an inner-city cohort. *American Journal of Respiratory and Critical Care Medicine, 182,* 25–33.

Yager, J. Y., & Ashwal, S. (2009). Animal models of perinatal hypoxic-ischemic brain damage. *Pediatric Neurology, 40(3),* 156–167.

Yazdanbakhsh, M, van den Biggelaar, A., & Maizels, R. M. (2001). Th2 responses without atopy: immunoregulation in chronic helminth infections and reduced allergic disease. *Trends in Immunology, 22,* 372–377.

Yehuda, R., Engel, S. M., Brand, S. R., Seckl, J., Marcus, S. M., & Berkowitz, G. S. (2005). Transgenerational effects of post-traumatic stress disorder in babies of mothers exposed to the World Trade Center attacks during pregnancy. *Journal of Clinical and Endocrine Metabolism, 90,* 4115–4118.

Yokota, T, Kouro, T, Hirose, J., Igarashi, H., Garrett, K. P., Gregory, S. C., et al. (2003). Unique properties of lymphoid progenitors identified according to RAG1 gene expression. *Immunity, 19*(3), 365–365.

Yolken, R. H., & Torrey, E. F. (1997). Viruses as etiologic agents of schizophrenia. In: A. E. Henneberg, W. P., Kaschka. (Eds,), Immunological alterations in psychiatric diseases. *Advances in Biological Psychiatry, 18,* 1–12.

Yoon, H., Park, C-W., & Chaiworapongsa, T. (2003). Intrauterine infection and the development of cerebral palsy. *British Journal of Obstetrics and Gynecology, 110* (Supplement 20), 124–127.

Well-Being, Aging, and Immunity

Elliot M. Friedman

Abstract

Aging is associated with progressive declines in multiple aspects of immune function and with corresponding increases in vulnerability to immune-related disease. At the same time, older adults consistently report that they are happier and more satisfied with their lives than adults in middle or early adulthood. There is also growing evidence that well-being is not merely the absence of stress and depression, and that it makes unique contributions to health and longevity, particularly in later life. This chapter examines the intersection of these age-related phenomena. With a particular emphasis on two different aspects of well-being—hedonic and eudaimonic—we consider the extent to which greater well-being is associated with healthier profiles of integrated immune responses, functions of specific immune cell types, and molecular aspects of immune regulation. Physiological and behavioral mechanisms that may underlie these associations, as well as the potential to improve well-being in later life, are also considered.

Key Words: hedonic well-being, eudaimonic well-being, psychological resources, purpose in life, social well-being, well-being therapy, immunosenescence

Introduction

Late life is a time of increased risk of morbidity and mortality from a range of disorders that involve the immune system, including infectious illness, autoimmunity, and cancer. Influenza and pneumonia together, for example, are the sixth leading cause of death in adults 65 years or older (Heron, 2007), and 90% of influenza-related deaths occur in this age group (Thompson, Shay, Weintraub, Brammer, Cox et al., 2003). This increased disease vulnerability in older adults is the product of age-related changes in multiple aspects of immune function, known as immunosenescence. As life expectancy in the United States has increased dramatically over the course of the last century (Arias, Rostron & Tejada-Vera, 2010) and is expected to continue to rise, finding ways to reduce illness vulnerability and burden in late life has become a priority among

health researchers. Appropriately, many of the proposed strategies involve acting at the biological level to stimulate production of new T cells, slow the rate of cellular aging, or develop novel vaccines or vaccine administration regimens (McElhaney & Effros, 2009). However, decades of psychoneuroimmunology (PNI) research have demonstrated the value of a biopsychosocial approach that considers the direct and interactive influences of social and psychological factors to better or worsen profiles of biological functioning and health outcomes. The aim of this chapter is to apply this biopsychosocial perspective to the issue of immunity in later life, and to focus specifically on the potential salutary effects of positive psychological functioning.

This chapter represents the meeting point of two companion pieces in this volume, one on stress and immunological aging (Effros, Chapter 4) and the other on positive affect and immunity (Pressman & Black, Chapter 6). My goal is to complement and extend the conceptual foci of these chapters by borrowing a key concept from each. The chapter on stress and aging centers on the concept of variability in age-related immunological change. That is, although immunological aging is a normative biological process, there are psychosocial factors like stress that can accelerate the rate at which those changes occur, leading to greater impairments of immune function and vulnerability to illness at younger ages. This chapter borrows the concept of variability in age-related changes in immune function, but directs the analytical lens toward the upper end of that distribution by considering the extent to which positive psychosocial factors, like subjective well-being, may be linked to the preservation of or improvements in immune function and resistance to disease in late life. The chapter on positive affect centers on the concept of independence of positive and negative aspects of psychological functioning in their links to immune function. That is, the absence of psychological stress or negative affect is not the same thing either psychologically or biologically as the presence of positive affect and well-being (more on this later).

A consideration of well-being and immunity in the context of aging also adds an interesting wrinkle to most theoretical perspectives and empirical research on positive psychological functioning and immunity. Although there is increasing evidence of direct associations between positive psychological functioning and immunity, a principal mechanism through which positive functioning is thought to contribute to health is by buffering the negative effects of life challenges. Fredrickson's (2001) "broaden-and-build" theory, for example, suggests that positive emotions serve to increase physical and psychosocial resources that can be drawn upon in the face of challenge. Tests of this theory have shown that experiences of positive emotions engender greater psychological and physiological resilience that promote more rapid recovery from both laboratory and naturalistic stressors (Fredrickson, Tugade, Waugh, & Larkin, 2003; Tugade & Fredrickson, 2004; Cohn, Fredrickson, Brown, Mikels, & Conway, 2009). Theoretical formulations of the benefits of positive psychological functioning cite maintenance of or a quick return to a steady and optimal baseline state of immune function. In later life, however, the norm is not a steady baseline state but rather decline in physiological functioning. In the context of this chapter, the specific aspect of biological decline that is of interest

is immunosenescence. The wrinkle then is that the baseline for biological functioning in older adults is a moving target, and the effects of positive psychological functioning are hypothesized to be seen in the form of departures from that baseline in the direction of better functioning and slower decline.

To return to a point raised earlier, a focus on the positive naturally raises the question of how it is distinct from the negative. There is already long history within PNI of studies focused on negative psychosocial experiences and the immune system in late life. Indeed, some of the earliest research on stress and immune function in human beings documented impaired lymphocyte proliferative responses in middle-aged and older adults who were bereaved through the death of a spouse (Bartrop, Luckhurst, Lazarus, Kiloh, & Penny, 1977; Schleifer, Keller, Camerino, Thornton, & Stein, 1983). Later studies linked the chronic stress of caring for a spouse with progressive dementia to significant impairments in multiple aspects of cellular immune function along with increased susceptibility to infectious illness and higher circulating levels of pro-inflammatory cytokines (Kiecolt-Glaser, Glaser, Shuttleworth, Dyer, Ogrocki et al., 1987; Kiecolt-Glaser, Glaser, Gravenstein, Malarkey, & Sheridan, 1996; Kiecolt-Glaser, Preacher, MacCallum, Atkinson, Malarkey et al., 2003). These studies were seminal contributions to what is now a voluminous literature on the impact of adverse psychosocial experiences on host resistance to infection as well as the underlying mechanisms responsible for the effects (Ader, 2007). These studies also helped to highlight the potential contribution of psychosocial processes to age-related changes in immune function, particularly those that put aging adults at increased risk of disease.

Given this rich history of PNI research, a focus on the positive supposes (a) that positive psychological functioning, or well-being, is not merely at the opposite end of a continuum from negative psychological functioning, or ill-being, but, rather, is sufficiently distinct conceptually and empirically to warrant specific interest; and (b) that there are unique gains in immune function and health from increases in well-being that go beyond what is gained from the absence of ill-being. Increasingly, there is support for both these propositions. First, well-being and ill-being are considered to be constructs that are related but distinct, and although the two are typically inversely correlated, the correlation is rarely perfect or even strong (Diener, 1984). Importantly, there is both a theoretical foundation for and empirical evidence of the possibility of experiencing positive and negative emotions at the same time over the same event (Cacioppo & Berntson, 1994; Larsen, McGraw, & Cacioppo, 2001; Norris, Gollan, Berntson, & Cacioppo, 2010), and neuroscience research has shown that positive emotions (associated with a tendency to approach and explore the environment) and negative emotions (associated with a tendency to withdraw from the environment) involve different regions of the brain (Cacioppo & Berntson, 1999). One recent study showed, for example, that greater well-being, but not negative affect, was associated with relatively greater activity in left frontal regions of the brain (Urry, Nitschke, Dolski, Jackson, Dalton et al., 2004). Clinical studies suggest a continuum for mental health ranging from languishing on the negative end to psychological flourishing on the positive end, and there are significant improvements in mental health between those who are moderately mentally healthy (i.e., lacking any mental illness) and those who are flourishing (Keyes, 2002). Finally, two recent literature reviews have shown that higher levels of well-being predict better health and reduced mortality (Chida & Steptoe, 2008; Pressman & Cohen, 2005), and studies that have accounted for ill-being typically find residual associations between well-being and multiple indices of health and immune function. In sum, well-being and ill-being are related but distinct constructs, and there appear to be unique gains in health associated specifically with gains in positive psychological functioning. These conclusions provide a strong justification for examining the unique ways in which positive psychological functioning may be linked to immunity in older adults.

What follows is organized into five parts. We begin with a brief overview of age-related changes in the immune system followed by a consideration of two major perspectives on well-being—hedonic and eudaimonic—that have distinct historical roots, methodological approaches, and implications for intervening to improve well-being. The third section reviews links between well-being and immune function in middle and later life, and the fourth briefly details behavioral and physiological mechanisms that may underlie associations of positive functioning and immunity in older adults. A concluding section then considers future directions for research into the potential for improving well-being and health in later life.

Aging and Immunity

The immune system can be broadly classified into the innate and adaptive branches. The innate immune system represents the first line of defense against pathogens, and it consists of multiple cell types, including monocytes/macrophages, dendritic cells, and natural killer (NK) cells that respond to infectious agents in a largely nonspecific way. The adaptive immune system consists of T and B lymphocytes that are genetically programmed to respond to specific pathogens, and a hallmark feature of adaptive immunity is memory for pathogens that were previously encountered (Goldsby, Kindt, & Osborne, 2006). Optimal immune responses to infection with a bacterial or viral pathogen typically involve cooperation between the innate and adaptive branches, with cells from the innate branch presenting the infectious agent to T and B cells and stimulating them to respond. With age, the ability to respond to infectious agents, particularly ones the individual has not previously encountered, becomes seriously compromised, a consequence of marked changes in the numbers and distribution of specific types of immunocompetent cells, the most profound of which occur within the T cell population.

An ability to mount a robust response to a large range of pathogens upon initial infection depends on the presence of naïve T cells, cells that have emerged from the thymus gland but have not yet encountered their cognate antigen (for which they were specifically programmed). With age, the number of naïve T cells declines and the number of memory T cells increases, and the repertoire of T cells consequently becomes less diverse and less able to mount an effective response to pathogens that are unfamiliar (Agarwal & Busse, 2010; Pfister & Savino, 2008; Weiskopf, Weinberger, & Grubeck-Loebenstein, 2009). Loss of T cell diversity is partially related to one of the hallmarks of immunosenescence: the age-related involution of the thymus gland (Weiskopf et al., 2009). The thymus begins to shrink early in life, and the compartments in which T cells mature are gradually replaced with fat; this process is largely complete by age 40–50. An additional influence on T cell senescence that is receiving more attention recently is chronic exposure to infectious agents, particularly cytomegalovirus (McElhaney & Effros, 2009; Pawelec, Derhovanessian, Larbi, Strindhall, & Wikby, 2009), a herpes virus that remains persistent in the body after initial infection. Prevalence of infection with cytomegalovirus (CMV) in the United States, for example, is 60% in the total population and over 90% in adults 80 years of age or older (Staras, Dollard, Radford, Flanders, Pass et al., 2006). In older adults who are seropositive for CMV, almost

25% of the CD8+ T cell pool is specific for CMV (Khan, Shariff, Cobbold, Bruton, Ainsworth et al., 2002). Latent viruses like CMV are typically contained by immunological surveillance, but under conditions in which the immune system is compromised, such as stress or aging, CMV infection can re-occur leading to a full secondary immune response coordinated by memory T cells. Persistent CMV infection may thus accelerate the loss of T cell diversity with age, thereby increasing vulnerability to novel infections in older adults (Pawelec et al., 2009; Weiskopf et al., 2009).

As with T cells, although the absolute number of B cells typically do not change with age, the distribution of B cell types is altered. There are declines in the number of naïve B cells and increases in the number of memory B cells leading to reductions in B cell diversity. Moreover, B cells are significantly less responsive to stimulation from antigen-presenting cells, in part due to reduced expression of cell surface molecules that facilitate communication with innate immune cells. One result of these changes is a dramatically reduced ability to respond to vaccines. Fewer than half of adults over 65 years of age generate protective levels of antibodies after vaccination against various antigens, including influenza, hepatitis B, or pneumococcal bacteria (Agarwal & Busse, 2010). The number of B cells that are reactive against host tissues also increases with age, a potential source of greater prevalence of autoimmune conditions among older adults (Weiskopf et al., 2009).

Although many aspects of adaptive immunity become impaired with age, the innate immune system tends to be better preserved (Weiskopf et al., 2009). Nevertheless, there are declines in the functional capacities of neutrophils, macrophages, dendritic cells, and natural killer (NK) cells. NK cells are involved in host defense against infectious illness and tumor development (Goldsby et al., 2006). Although the numbers of NK cells do not show significant declines with age, they do become less responsive to stimulation with cytokines such as interferon-γ and interleukin-2 (Weiskopf et al., 2009; Agarwal & Busse, 2010). There is also growing interest in declines in NK receptors as a mechanism for reduced NK activity and increased risk of infectious disease and cancer with aging (Almeida-Oliveira, Smith-Carvalho, Porto, Cardoso-Oliveira, Ribeiro Ados et al., 2011; Mocchegiani & Malavolta, 2004; Raulet & Guerra, 2009). Phagocytic cells, like macophages, show declines in their expression of cell surface molecules

that are involved in the recognition of pathogens, less ability to ingest or kill bacteria, and reductions in stimulated production of pro-inflammatory cytokines (Panda, Arjona et al., 2009; Weiskopf et al., 2009; Agarwal & Busse, 2010).

At the molecular level, immunosenescence is associated with a shortening of the length of telomeres, repetitive sequences of nucleic acids that represent the "tips" of chromosomes. As cells replicate, telomeres shorten, and when they become sufficiently short the cell cycle is arrested, a phenomenon known as replicative senescence (Effros, 2009). The enzyme telomerase extends telomere length, thereby extending the replicative life of the cell (Effros, 2009). Telomere shortening and declining levels of telomerase are regarded as markers of cellular aging and immunosenescence (Kaszubowska, 2008; Effros, 2009; Simpson and Guy, 2010).

Collectively, these widespread changes in immune function with age render older adults significantly more vulnerable to infection by new or latent pathogens, cancer, and autoimmune conditions. A growing literature on chronic stress has shown that stress can exacerbate the effects of age on immune function, and stress may accelerate immunosenescence in aging adults, beginning early in the life span (Bauer, 2008; Gouin, Hantsoo, & Kiecolt-Glaser, 2008; Graham, Christian, & Kiecolt-Glaser, 2006). In other words, this normative process of biological change is sensitive to the influence of psychosocial experience. The remainder of this chapter is devoted to a consideration of whether positive aspects of psychological functioning may have salubrious effects on the biological aging of the immune system.

Hedonic and Eudaimonic Well-Being: A Definition of Terms

There is general agreement among scholars that well-being denotes optimal psychological functioning, but there is less agreement on what aspects of human experience and psychological functioning one should measure in assessing well-being. The two most prominent views of human well-being are the hedonic and eudaimonic approaches, both rooted in notions of what it means to lead a "good life" that date back to Ancient Greece. The third century BC philosopher Aristippus of Cyrene believed that the satisfaction of needs and the consequent experiences of pleasure were the sole source of good (in the ethical sense of the word) (Waterman, 1993). The modern version of the hedonic view centers on experiences of emotion, and well-being is achieved when the preponderance of emotional experiences is positive rather than negative (Diener, 1984; Ryan and Deci, 2001). Interestingly, the frequency of positive emotions tends to be more strongly associated with well-being than the intensity of any single positive emotional experience (Diener, 1984). One of the more widely used constructs that is consistent with the hedonic approach is subjective well-being (SWB), which consists of the presence of positive emotions, an absence of negative emotions, and satisfaction with life (Diener, 1984). SWB is operationalized in various ways, including the Positive and Negative Affect Scale (PANAS) (Watson, Clark, & Tellegen, 1988), the Mood and Anxiety Symptom Questionnaire (MASQ) (Watson, Weber, Assenheimer, Clark, Strauss et al., 1995), and the Satisfaction with Life scale (Diener, Emmons, Larsen, & Griffin, 1985). There are also a number of different methodological approaches to the assessment of hedonic well-being. Scales such as the PANAS or the MASQ, for example, often ask respondents to recall how frequently they experienced a list of emotional states over a recent span of time, such as a week. These scales can also be used to assess current affect. Some studies use semistructured interviews to reconstruct each day's experiences and peoples' emotional reactions to them (Almeida, Wethington, & Kessler, 2002). Finally, ecological momentary assessment methods repeatedly collect information on emotional status in real time and in real-life settings over the course of one or multiple days (Shiffman, Stone, & Hufford, 2008).

The principal alternative to the hedonic view is the eudaimonic perspective. Whereas Aristippus embraced the hedonic gratification of physical pleasure, Aristotle rejected this view as "vulgar" and, instead, championed the pursuit of personal excellence (Ryan & Deci, 2001; Waterman, 1993;). Underlying the eudaimonic view is that notion that each individual possesses a daimon or "true self," and the greatest sense of fulfillment one can experience is when one is fully and holistically engaged in pursuits that are aligned with one's deepest held values (Ryan & Deci, 2001; Waterman, 1993). Waterman (1993) describes the experience of eudaimonia as "a feeling of being intensely alive...an impression that this is what the person was meant to do, and...a feeling that this is who one really is" (p. 679). A useful contrast between hedonic and eudaimonic perspectives is that, although the pursuit of valued personal objectives is likely to engender feelings of happiness (hedonic well-being) and fulfillment (eudaimonic well-being), there are many

needs and desires whose satisfaction will increase hedonic well-being without improving eudaimonic well-being (Ryan & Deci, 2001; Waterman, 1993). Eudaimonic well-being has been conceptualized in different ways. Self-Determination Theory (Ryan & Deci, 2000) cites the meeting of basic needs for autonomy, competence, and relatedness as fundamental to eudaimonic well-being. Ryff (1989) built on a number of social and developmental theories to construct the Psychological Well-Being (PWB) scales that assess six domains of eudaimonic well-being: autonomy, environmental mastery, personal growth, positive relations with others, purpose in life, and self-acceptance. The PWB scales ask respondents to agree or disagree with a set of statements probing the different domains of well-being.

One phenomenon that makes well-being a particularly interesting topic for gerontology research is the so-called "paradox" of aging. That is, although advancing age is generally associated with physical and cognitive decline, well-being is consistently found to be higher in late life than among young or middle-aged adults, and this is true for both hedonic and eudaimonic aspects of well-being (George, 2010). Declines in health certainly are a primary threat to subjective well-being in older adults, and health problems are linked to significantly lower levels of positive affect and life satisfaction and higher levels of depression and depressive symptoms in both cross-sectional and longitudinal analyses (Gerstorf, Ram, Mayrez, Hidajat, Lindenberger et al., 2010; Kunzmann, Little, & Smith, 2000; Mroczek & Spiro, 2005; Strawbridge, Wallhagen, & Cohen, 2002). Health-related declines in well-being are particularly steep for those nearing the end of life (Mroczek & Spiro, 2005; Gerstorf et al., 2010). Nevertheless, mean levels of subjective well-being remain relatively high among adults even in the context of poor health.

A parallel literature on subjective appraisals of successful aging offers similar perspectives. The absence of physical disease or disability is a common criterion for successful aging (Depp and Jeste, 2006; Rowe & Kahn, 1987;). According to a recent report from the 1998 Medical Expenditures Panel Survey, however, almost 50% of women and 40% of men in the United States have at least one chronic medical condition and over 20% of adults have two or more. Among those 65 years old or older, 62% have two or more conditions (Anderson and Horvath, 2004), a number that is projected to increase substantially in coming years (Vogeli, Shields, Lee, Gibson, Marder et al., 2007). Living with medical co-morbidity has thus become the norm for older adults. Indeed, fewer than 19% of participants aged 65–99 years from the Alameda County Study (Strawbridge et al., 2002) and fewer than 12% of respondents over the age of 65 from the Health and Retirement Study (McLaughlin, Connell, Heeringa, Li, & Roberts, 2010) met the criteria for successful aging formulated by Rowe and Kahn, largely because of disease and/or physical impairments.

These numbers stand in stark contrast to older adults' views of their own aging. In one study of approximately 200 community-dwelling adults over the age of 60 in southern California, only 15% were free of physical illness, but 92% of the sample considered themselves to be aging successfully (Montross, Depp, Daly, Reichstadt, Golshan et al., 2006). Similarly, among the older adults from the Alameda County Study, half (50.3%) agreed with the statement "I am aging successfully (or aging well)" in spite of the presence of chronic disease conditions (Strawbridge et al., 2002). When asked what they consider to be important elements of successful aging, older adults volunteer themes such as self-acceptance and contentment with one's life along with continuing to pursue interests, to engage in social interactions, and to grow personally (Reichstadt, Sengupta, Depp, Palinkas, & Jeste, 2010), all of which bear a strong resemblance to the elements of eudaimonic well-being.

These observations collectively underscore the point that well-being in late life is not merely a proxy for physical health; high levels of well-being are consistently found in older adults with chronic health problems, some of them severe. Even among centenarians, the oldest old, most have chronic health conditions and yet continue to lead engaged independent lives (Poon, Clayton, Clayton, Messner, Noble et al., 1992). Good quality of life at older ages is, thus, less likely to involve the avoidance of disease than successful adaptation to age-related physical decline and disease. Importantly, recent prospective studies suggest that those who are able to maintain high levels of well-being in late life also enjoy fewer disabilities and greater longevity (Boyle, Barnes, Buchman, & Bennett, 2009; Boyle, Buchman, Barnes, & Bennett, 2010a,b).

Well-being and Immune Function— Preliminary Considerations

For conceptual clarity, our discussion of links between well-being and immunity in later life is divided into three subsections organized by type of well-being: hedonic well-being and affective style,

eudaimonic and social well-being, and psychological resources. The first includes literature on both experiences of positive affect and the stable tendency to respond positively to external events. Social well-being is combined with eudaimonic well-being because constructs such as social support and quality of social relationships share considerable conceptual space with specific domains of eudaimonic well-being; other aspects of social relationships (e.g., instrumental social support, size of social networks), however, are conceptually distinct and are excluded (and evidence for links between these specific aspects of social relationships and immune function in older adults is weaker anyway). The third subsection, psychological resources, includes a range of psychological constructs that appear in the PNI literature—sense of coherence, optimism, benefit finding, spirituality—and are theorized to provide a buffer against adverse experiences. These will be considered separately, although, as we will see, there is conceptual overlap between some of these constructs and eudaimonic well-being in particular.

The literature review that follows includes studies of middle-aged as well as older adults, the reason being that many aspects of immunosenescence—involution of the thymus, telomere shortening, loss of T cell diversity—are long-term processes that begin in young and middle adulthood. Consideration of associations between well-being and immunity in midlife thus has implications for immune function in older adults. Because these are biological processes with long trajectories of change, the most compelling and useful assessment of life-course changes in immune function would clearly be a study of the same individuals from conception to death. However, longitudinal studies that cover much shorter spans of time, let alone an entire life-course, are rare and typically very expensive. It is, therefore, unlikely that we will ever have access to a life's worth of data on the same individuals. Nonetheless, examination of interindividual variability within the same age cohort can accomplish some of what would be gained from longitudinal data. That is, we can ask the question: why might two people of the same age have very different biological profiles? From the perspective of PNI, we are interested in the current psychosocial correlates and past psychosocial experiences that may contribute to interindividual differences in immune function in late life. Nevertheless, although these kinds of analyses can illuminate important associations, they are vulnerable to the possibility that factors that were not assessed are the most relevant to differences between individuals. This is where we turn to short-term studies of the immunological impact of *intra*individual changes in well-being that occur naturally over time or as a result of interventions designed to reduce ill-being and improve well-being. Because all measurements are within the same individuals, such analyses essentially hold unobserved variables constant, and they provide additional evidence of links between changes in well-being and changes in immune function. These different types of studies—interindividual differences versus intraindividual change—will be noted in the discussion that follows.

HEDONIC WELL-BEING AND AFFECTIVE STYLE

As mentioned at the outset, infectious illness is a significant cause of mortality in older adults. For this reason, psychosocial moderation of vulnerability to infection is a topic with considerable relevance for health in late life. A series of studies, led by psychologist Sheldon Cohen, has examined the associations of positive and negative emotional style and infection after experimental exposure to viruses. As the details of these studies are provided in an accompanying chapter (Pressman & Black, Chapter 6), this section will provide only a brief overview of pertinent research.

In one study, young and middle-aged men and women were presented with a list of adjectives describing emotional states and asked how accurately each adjective described how they had felt that day. They were then exposed to a rhinovirus, and incidence of infection and severity of symptoms in those infected were assessed. The results showed that among those infected, greater positive emotional style was associated with reduced signs and symptoms of illness, and this relationship was dose-related (that is, the greater the positive emotional style, the less severe the illness). There was no such association for negative emotional style, and the relationship with positive emotional style was independent of negative emotional style (Cohen, Doyle, Turner, Alper, & Skoner, 2003). A second study examined social and cognitive variables (e.g., optimism) as potential alternative explanations of the association of positive emotional style and illness susceptibility, and the results showed unique effects of positive emotional style (Cohen, Alper, Doyle, Treanor, & Turner, 2006). A third study of immunological mechanisms linking positive emotional style with respiratory illness showed that IL-6 was inversely associated with positive emotional style and that IL-6 levels explained a significant portion of the association of positive emotional style and

illness severity (Doyle, Gentile, & Cohen, 2006). Collectively, these studies suggest that positive emotional style is linked to greater resistance to viral infection in ways that are independent of (and possibly stronger than) negative emotional style. They also highlight a plausible biological mechanism—the pro-inflammatory cytokine IL-6—through which emotional style may act.

A parallel literature has used a vaccine model to probe the relationship between psychosocial factors and immunological processes related to infection in older adults. Although vaccination against influenza prevents infection in 70–90% of young adults, it only protects 30–40% of older adults (Hannoun, Megas, & Piercy, 2004). There is, thus, growing interest in identifying factors that undermine or increase the efficacy of vaccines, and psychosocial influences have been of some interest. On the negative side, chronic stress associated with caring for a spouse with progressive dementia has been linked to impaired responses to vaccination. In one study, only 38% of older caregivers mounted a significant response (defined as a fourfold increases in virus-specific antibodies) to administration of a trivalent influenza vaccine. In contrast, 66% of matched controls mounted a significant response. Caregivers also exhibited significantly smaller increases in IL-1β and IL-2 in response to vaccination compared to the controls (Kiecolt-Glaser et al., 1996). A larger study of spousal caregivers and matched controls found that, in response to vaccination, only 16% of caregivers compared to 39% of controls mounted a significant antibody response to one of three strains of influenza virus. Caregiver status was also associated with higher levels of daily salivary cortisol, and cortisol levels were modestly and negatively correlated with antibody responses (Vedhara, Cox, Wilcox, Perks, Hunt et al., 1999). Responses to a vaccination with pneumococcal pneumonia showed similar results. Caregivers had significantly lower specific antibody titers than controls; they also showed modest declines in antibody titers over a 6-month follow-up period that were not evident in the control group. Interestingly, caregivers reported significantly less social support than the control group (Glaser, Sheridan, Malarkey, MacCallum, & Kiecolt-Glaser, 2000). Even in the absence of a significant stressor like caring for a chronically ill spouse, reports of greater anger and fatigue in older adults have been linked to lower production of cytokines in cells stimulated with either live virus or vaccine (Costanzo, Lutgendorf, Kohut, Nisly, Rozeboom et al., 2004). Generally, then, ill-being in older adults appears to contribute to impaired immune responses to vaccination.

In contrast, although limited in number, there are studies suggesting that positive psychological functioning may contribute to preserved or improved vaccine responses in older adults. One study of healthy women 57–60 years old, for example, examined links between vaccine responses and brain electrical activity associated with emotion regulation. The results showed that antibody responses to a trivalent influenza vaccine were most robust six months after vaccination in women who exhibited a more positive affective style under resting conditions and a less negative emotional response to recalling an intensely negative event in their lives (Rosenkranz, Jackson, Dalton, Dolski, Ryff et al., 2003).

Whereas vaccine studies probe the links between psychosocial strengths and integrated immune responses, other research examines specific aspects of immune function and how they are associated with well-being. One recent study, for example, focused on the relationship between positive and negative affect on the one hand and innate immune function on the other. Whole-blood samples from 146 community-dwelling middle-aged adults were stimulated in culture with lipopolysaccharide (LPS), and production of both pro- and anti-inflammatory cytokines was measured. Trait positive and negative affect was assessed using the PANAS. The results showed that greater positive affect was associated with lower stimulated levels of IL-6 and IL-10; negative affect was unrelated to any of the cytokines assessed (Prather, Marsland, Muldoon, & Manuck, 2007). These observations paralleled results from an earlier study in which positive affect predicted lower levels of IL-6 in adults infected with rhinovirus (Doyle et al., 2006) and suggest that greater well-being may help to moderate inflammatory responses by innate immune cells when they encounter pathogens, thereby reducing symptoms.

Cancer has long served as a model for PNI research, and over the past few decades, evidence has accumulated showing that psychosocial factors, such as chronic stress or lack of social support, may contribute to the disease development and progression (Antoni, Lutgendorf, Cole, Dhabhar, Sephton et al., 2006). The role of positive psychological functioning in improved outlook for cancer patients is less well examined, although there is growing evidence that psychosocial interventions improve quality of life (Aspinwall & Tedeschi, 2010). Whether these interventions also improve health outcomes is

presently a matter of controversy (Stefanek, Palmer, Thombs, & Coyne, 2009; Aspinwall & Tedeschi, 2010; Coyne, Tennen, & Ranchor, 2010). In contrast, there is a growing literature focused on well-being and immune processes that may be relevant to cancer. Natural killer cells, for example, provide immune surveillance for virally infected and cancerous cells (Antoni et al., 2006) and are implicated in cancer processes in both human and animal models (Zamai, Ponti, Mirandola, Gobbi, Papa et al., 2007). In a sample of 134 women with early and midstage breast cancer who had already undergone surgery but not yet begun adjuvant therapy, positive affect predicted greater in vitro stimulated production of the Th1 cytokines IL-12 and IFN-γ, both of which affect NK cell activity (Blomberg, Alvarez Diaz, Romero, Lechner et al., 2009).

Finally, chronically elevated levels of pro-inflammatory cytokines in the blood are associated cross-sectionally with poor health and prospectively with increased risk of morbidity and mortality from a range of chronic disease conditions (Abraham, Campbell, Cheema, Gluckmen, Blumenthal et al., 2007; Aggarwal & Gehlot, 2009; Blake & Ridker, 2003; Leitch, Chakrabarti, Crozier, McKee, Anderson, et al., 2007). Moreover, pro-inflammatory cytokines tend to increase with age and are implicated in the process of immunosenescence (Franceschi, Capri, Monti, Giunta, Olivieri et al., 2007). Although links between ill-being and higher levels of inflammation are well-documented (Hansel, Hong, Camara, & von Kanel, 2010; Howren, Lamkin, & Suls, 2009;), there is growing evidence of an association between well-being and lower levels of inflammatory proteins in the blood. Much of this newer evidence comes from large epidemiological studies. In one study involving over 2,800 participants from Whitehall II, a survey of health in British civil servants, positive affect was assessed using ecological momentary assessments aggregated across the day. IL-6 and CRP were measured from blood obtained during a clinic visit. The results showed that, in women but not in men, having higher levels of positive affect was associated with lower levels of both IL-6 and CRP. In the same vein, having low levels of positive affect was associated with greater likelihood of having clinically elevated levels of CRP (>3 mg/L; Steptoe, O'Donnell, Badrick, Kumari, & Marmot, 2008). In a smaller sample of 216 men and women from the Whitehall II study, greater positive affect, again measured using ecological momentary assessment, predicted reduced fibrinogen responses to laboratory mental stress, although positive affect was not associated with baseline levels of fibrinogen (Steptoe, Wardle, & Marmot, 2005).

Where chronic elevations of inflammatory proteins in the blood are linked to adverse health outcomes, acute elevations may have a different meaning. A recent paper examined the role of positive affect in pro-inflammatory responses to radiation therapy in cancer patients, a situation in which inflammation may serve a beneficial role in helping promote tissue recovery after radiotherapy sessions. Serum levels of IL-1β and IL-6 were measured in 50 middle-aged men and women newly diagnosed with either prostate or breast cancer as they went through a 6–8-week course of radiation, and positive affect was assessed using four positive items from the CES-D depression scale. The results showed that higher levels of positive affect were associated with greater increases in both cytokines from pretreatment assessments to measurements made during the course of radiation. Both cytokines returned to pretreatment levels by two months after treatment stopped, indicating an acute, treatment-related increase (Sepah & Bower, 2009). These results suggest some contextual specificity for the relationship between positive affect and inflammation. For example, increased inflammation that is acute and associated with localized infection or tissue damage may be indicative of optimal immune function, whereas chronically elevated systemic levels of the same cytokines may be linked to pathology (Lutgendorf, 2009). Current evidence suggests that positive psychological functioning is associated with both greater acute inflammatory responses and lower chronic levels of the same proteins.

EUDAIMONIC AND SOCIAL WELL-BEING

Although eudaimonic well-being has been operationalized in different ways, a central element of the eudaimonic tradition is investment in activities and relationships that are personally meaningful. Two constructs that reflect this fundamental characteristic and have been linked to health outcomes are purpose in life and social relationships. Individuals who score high in purpose in life believe that their activities have meaning, and they make plans for the future that they work to achieve. As assessed using one of Ryff's Psychological Well-Being (PWB) scales, self-rated purpose in life tends to rise through midlife and then to decline in older adults (Ryff, 1989; Ryff &Keyes, 1995), although some studies suggest that there is greater between-person variance in purpose in life than there is within-person change over time

(Springer, Pudrovska, & Hauser, 2011). Higher ratings of purpose in life in large population-based studies of older adults have been linked to a range of positive late-life health outcomes, including lower rates of mortality (Boyle et al., 2009; Koizumi, Ito, Kaneko, & Motohashi, 2008; Krause, 2009), disability (Boyle et al., 2010b), and cognitive impairments (Boyle et al., 2010a). Similarly, there is a large independent literature on links between social relationships and better health (Berkman, Glass, Brissette, & Seeman, 2000; Cohen, 2004; Uchino, 2006; House, Landis, & Umberson, 1988; Kiecolt-Glaser, Gouin, & Hantsoo, 2010). In contrast to purpose in life, though, ratings of social well-being, as assessed by the Ryff's positive relations with others PWB scale, tend to remain high in older adults or even increase (Ryff & Keyes, 1995). This latter observation is consistent with older adults' well-documented preferences for and active selection of the most emotionally satisfying social relationships (Lang & Carstensen, 2002; Scheibe and Carstensen, 2010). Moreover, older adults consistently nominate high-quality social relationships as central to living well in later life (Reichstadt et al., 2010).

Research linking purpose in life and immune function is in its infancy. In our own work, for example, we found that greater purpose in life predicted lower levels of soluble IL-6 receptors, a marker of inflammation, in a sample of older community-dwelling women (Friedman, Hayney, Love, Singer, & Ryff, 2007). Of particular relevance to the current chapter is more recent research examining links between well-being and inflammation in the context of age-related disease conditions. The Survey of Mid-Life in the United States (MIDUS) is a national, longitudinal, population-based study of men and women aged 25–75 at the initial wave of data collection (Brim, Ryff, & Kessler, 2004). MIDUS combines survey assessments with clinical measurement of biological processes related to health and experimental protocols focused on the regulation of physiological and neurological systems related to health and well-being. In a recent study, we found that greater burden of medical co-morbidities in over 1,200 MIDUS participants was associated with higher levels of IL-6 and C-reactive protein (CRP), but higher levels of purpose in life were protective. The association of disease burden and inflammation was significantly weaker in those with higher scores on purpose in life (Friedman & Ryff, 2012). For adults with five chronic conditions, for example, the difference in IL-6 between those in the top tertile of purpose in life and those in the bottom tertile was the equivalent to a difference of 10 years of age.

There is a more substantial literature linking social well-being and immune function in older adults. One study of 184 community-dwelling men and women all over 65 years of age showed that antibody responses to vaccination with two different virus strains was higher in married individuals compared to those who were not (most of whom were widowed); those who reported being happily married also had better antibody responses than those who were unhappily married or not married (Phillips, Carroll, Burns, Ring, Macleod et al., 2006). The Wisconsin Longitudinal Study (WLS) enrolled over 10,000 Wisconsin high school seniors in 1957 and has conducted multiple follow-up waves of data collection since that time. In one study, a sample of 18 WLS participants received the 1998–1999 trivalent flu vaccine. Blood samples were then obtained at various times after vaccination, cells were stimulated in vitro with each of the virus strains, and production of IFN-γ and IL-10 was measured. Participants also completed questionnaires to assess psychological well-being and quality of social relationships. The results showed that greater well-being and better relationship quality, both independently and collectively, predicted higher virus-stimulated levels of IFN-γ and IL-10 (Hayney, Love, Buck, Ryff, Singer et al., 2003). One study of nursing home residents living in upstate New York found that greater social support was associated with lower levels of virus-specific antibodies even before study participants received the vaccinations. The authors surmise that greater social support may slow the loss of protection from prior vaccination (Moynihan, Larson, Treanor, Duberstein, Power et al., 2004).

The tumoricidal cytokine TNF-α was the focus of a prospective study of 44 middle-aged women with recently diagnosed breast cancer. Whole-blood samples were stimulated in culture with LPS to produce TNF-α. Frequency of engaging in social activities and satisfaction with relationship partners were assessed. The results showed that, in those women who increased the frequency of their social activities over the course of the 12-month follow-up period, stimulated TNF-α production was higher compared to women who decreased their activities. Increases in satisfaction with partners also predicted greater TNF-α production. These results suggest that naturalistic improvements in social engagement and well-being are associated with better cancer-relevant aspects of immune function in the context of cancer (Marucha, Crespin, Shelby, & Andersen, 2005).

Social well-being is also linked to age-related inflammation. We examined circulating levels of inflammatory proteins in two independent samples, and we found that IL-6 concentrations were lower in older adults who reported higher levels of eudaimonic well-being, particularly related to social relationships (Friedman et al., 2007; Friedman, Love, Singer, & Ryff, 2008). A recent review finds broad support for links between social relationships and inflammation (Kiecolt-Glaser et al., 2010). We have also found support for the possibility that social well-being may moderate the extent to which other factors are associated with higher levels of inflammation. In a sample of older women, for example, we found that although poor sleep (measured both objectively and subjectively) and low levels of social well-being both predicted higher levels of IL-6, women with poor sleep who also reported strong social ties had IL-6 levels that were similar to those who slept well. The only women with relatively higher levels of IL-6 were those with both poor sleep and low levels of social well-being (Friedman, Hayney, Love, Urry, Rosenkranz et al., 2005). A separate analysis examined links between socioeconomic status (SES) and inflammation and potential moderation by well-being. Low SES, whether assessed using income, educational attainment, or occupational status, is linked to higher circulating levels of inflammatory proteins in large epidemiological studies (Alley, Seeman, Ki, Karlamangla, Hu et al., 2006; Friedman & Herd, 2010; Gruenewald, Cohen, Matthews, Tracy, & Seeman, 2009; Jousilahti, Salomaa, Rasi, Vahtera, & Palosuo, 2003; Loucks, Pilote et al., 2010; Owen, Poulton, Hay, Mohamed-Ali, & Steptoe, 2003; Ranjit, Diez-Roux, Shea, Cushman, Ni, et al., 2007). We examined the association of education and inflammation in the MIDUS study, and we found that although low educational attainment predicted higher levels of IL-6 across the sample, levels of IL-6 were significantly lower in respondents who had high scores on measures of both eudaimonic and hedonic well-being; this was particularly true among the least educated (Morozink, Friedman, Coe & Ryff, 2010). Finally, like purpose in life, higher ratings of social well-being in older adults with multiple chronic medical conditions predicted lower levels of IL-6 and CRP compared to adults with the same disease burden but lower well-being scores (Friedman & Ryff, 2012).

Several recent studies have shown that social relationships are linked to markers of immunosenescence at the molecular level, particularly genes involved in the regulation of immune responses and molecular aspects of cellular aging. Social isolation, for example, has been associated with elevated circulating levels of inflammatory proteins (Ford, Loucks, & Berkman, 2006; Loucks, Berkman, Gruenewald, & Seeman, 2005; 2006), and loneliness is associated with increased blood levels of inflammatory proteins after an acute laboratory stressor (Steptoe, Owen, Kunz-Ebrecht, & Brydon, 2004). There is new evidence that people who are socially isolated or lonely show patterns of gene expression that favor increased production of pro-inflammatory cytokines (Cole, 2009). These changes are found in circulating leukocytes generally (Cole, Hawkley, Arevaio, Sunug, Rose et al. 2007) and antigen-presenting cells, such as monocytes and dendritic cells, specifically (Cole, Hawkley, Arevaio, & Cacioppo, 2011). Because these cells are among the most evolutionarily ancient cells in the immune system, these latter results suggest a significant adaptive function for social modification of gene expression related to inflammation (Cole et al., 2011). It will be important for studies of gene regulation to extend the scope of analyses to positive aspects of social relationships and to psychological well-being more generally.

PSYCHOLOGICAL RESOURCES

This section considers psychological constructs that, although not explicitly linked to hedonic or eudaimonic well-being, are considered aspects of positive psychological functioning. Nonetheless, there is some conceptual overlap between some psychological resources and eudaimonic well-being in particular.

Sense of coherence (SOC) describes a traitlike orientation toward the world as being understandable, manageable, and meaningful (Antonovsky, 1987), and the SOC scale has been widely used in studies focused on how people adapt to challenging situations and stay healthy (Antonovsky, 1993; Eriksson & Lindstrom, 2005). There is some conceptual overlap between SOC and the environmental mastery domain of Ryff's PWB scales, for example, as well as competence, one of the three basic needs that make up self-determination theory (Ryan & Deci, 2001). One study examined the links between SOC and immune function in 30 older adults anticipating a late-life stressor—voluntary relocation to an independent apartment within a larger living facility—and 28 controls who were not planning to relocate. Psychosocial measures and blood samples were obtained one month before each individual's move. As predicted, adults anticipating a relocation experienced decreases in positive mood, more intrusive thoughts, and lower NK activity compared to nonmovers. Importantly, however, SOC moderated the association of moving and NK activity. Higher scores on the SOC scale predicted greater NK activity among relocating adults—at the highest levels of SOC, NK activity was indistinguishable from activity among nonmovers. NK activity did not vary significantly with SOC among the nonmovers (Lutgendorf, Vitaliano, Buckwalter, Reimer, Hong et al., 1999). SOC may, thus, be an important resource for older adults in coping with stressors and may be protective against the potential immunosuppressive effects of late life challenge.

Another construct that is related to eudaimonic well-being is the ability to find positive meaning in the context of adversity through engagement in cognitive processing (Taylor, 1983). Measures of benefit finding or discovery of meaning attempt to capture the extent to which adversities can lead to shifts in values and perspectives and to greater appreciation of existing resources, such as social relationships, and increased commitment to the pursuit of cherished goals. The extent to which such cognitive processing is linked to better health outcomes has been the focus of a number of research efforts. In one study of 40 middle-aged HIV-positive men who had recently lost a close friend or partner because of AIDS, CD4+ cells showed significant declines over the course of a two- to three-year follow-up period. However, in men who engaged in more cognitive processing and thereby found positive meaning in their experiences, CD4+ levels were largely preserved (Bower, Kemeny, Taylor, & Fahey, 2003).

Optimism is the expectation of positive future outcomes, and it can be measured either as a general characteristic (e.g., trait optimism) or in relation to a specific life pursuit. Trait optimism has been linked to multiple aspects of immune function in older adults. Cytokine responses to stimulation with live virus or vaccine in culture, for example, were higher in older adults who reported higher levels of optimism and greater vigor (Costanzo et al., 2004). In one cross-sectional study of 54 middle-aged women newly diagnosed with breast cancer, postoperative stress was associated with significantly lower levels of NK cytotoxicity. However, in women with higher levels of trait optimism, the association between stress and NK activity was significantly weaker, suggesting a buffering effect of optimism (Von Ah, Kang, & Carpenter, 2007).

The Multi-Ethnic Study of Atherosclerosis (MESA) is a large multisite longitudinal survey of risk factors for atherosclerosis involving men and women between 45 and 84 years of age. One recent report using data from over 6,800 MESA participants showed that higher scores on the Life Orientation Test, a measure of dispositional optimism, was associated with lower circulating levels of IL-6 and fibrinogen. Additional analyses suggested that gradients in pessimism were more robustly linked to inflammatory markers than gradients in optimism (Roy, Diez-Roux, Seeman, Ranjit, Shea et al., 2010).

Differences in optimism and pessimism were also at the heart of one of the few studies of positive psychological functioning and telomeres. Interest in links between psychosocial factors and telomere length has been driven in large measure by a landmark study by Epel and colleagues (2004) that examined telomere length and telomerase activity in a sample of healthy women, some of whom were caring for a child with some form of chronic illness. The results showed that, among the caregivers, both length of time caregiving and perceived stress of caregiving were associated with shorter telomeres and reduced telomerase activity (Epel, Blackburn, Lin, Dhabhar, Adler et al., 2004). A recent study extended this line of research to trait optimism and pessimism in a sample of healthy postmenopausal women aged 50–80 years. The results showed that higher levels of pessimism were significantly associated with shorter telomeres; telomere length was not associated with optimism (O'Donovan, Lin, Dhabhar, Wolkowitz, Tillie et al., 2009).

There is growing interest in the potential benefits of spirituality in the context of chronic illness. A recent cross-sectional study examined the association of spiritual well-being and CD4+ cell counts using data for 129 HIV-positive, mostly African American women, culled from two studies of behavioral interventions in HIV patients. Higher levels of spiritual well-being predicted lower levels of depression in the women as well as higher counts and percentages of CD4+ cells, associations that were robust after adjustment for demographic characteristics, HIV viral load, and HIV medication adherence (Dalmida, Holstad, Diiorio, & Laderman, 2009). A recent review focused on positive psychosocial influences in the context of HIV concluded that although the research is in its infancy, initial results are promising, and the benefits of well-being may be particularly helpful in the latter stages of the disease (Ironson & Hayward, 2008).

In some instances, researchers examine links between multiple psychological resources and immune function. For example, a sample of 773 HIV-positive women, 18–55 years old, was recruited from clinics in four large US cities and followed prospectively for 5 years. With multiple aspects of disease status controlled, including viral load, symptoms, antiretroviral therapy, and treatments for opportunistic infections, psychological resources, such as positive affect, positive expectations for disease progression, sense of control, and positive life changes attributed to living with HIV infection, were associated with reduced risk of mortality. Women with three or more of the measured resources were more than 50% less likely to die during the 5-year follow-up than women with none; this difference was even greater for women who started the study with fewer than 200 CD4+ cells, the traditional threshold for progression to AIDS. Women with no psychological resources also showed a steeper decline in CD4+ cells over the course of the study compared to those with two or more resources. These results suggest a protective effect of positive psychological functioning on progression of HIV and AIDS that is independent of the traditional biomedical benchmarks (Ickovics, Milan, Boland, Schoenbaum, Schuman et al., 2006).

INTERVENTIONS

Collectively, the foregoing studies suggest that, at the levels of integrated immune responses, cell numbers and activity, circulating levels of inflammatory proteins, and molecular correlates of immunity, well-being predicts better immune function in aging adults; in many cases this association is independent of ill-being, as predicted from theoretical perspectives on well-being and emotion. These associations are seen in healthy adults and in clinical samples alike. Although these studies constitute suggestive evidence that well-being may promote immune function, stronger evidence would involve prospective analyses examining improvements in immunity—or preservation of immune function at a time of normative decline—within the same individual that are associated with increases in or maintenance of high levels of well-being. Research along these lines is the focus of this final subsection.

I am aware of only one study that has examined the impact of a well-being-based psychosocial intervention on an integrated immune response to vaccination. The focus was the effects of meditation training on brain electrical activity associated with emotion regulation and immune responses to vaccination in a sample of 48 young adults (mean age of 25 years). Participants were randomly assigned to either a wait-list control condition ($n = 16$) or to a group that participated in an 8-week program of mindfulness-based stress reduction (MBSR) of the type pioneered by Jon Kabat-Zinn (Kabat-Zinn, Lipworth, & Burney, 1985) who also delivered this intervention and was a co-author on the study. The protocol consisted of a weekly training class lasting 2.5–3 hours, a 7-hour retreat in week six of the intervention, and home-based meditation for 1 hour a day, 6 days a week. Electroencephalographic (EEG) activity was recorded before, immediately after, and 4 months after the intervention, and patterns of electrical activity associated with positive emotion were assessed. Blood samples were also obtained before and 8–9 weeks after administration of an influenza vaccine; vaccines were administered at the end of the 8-week intervention. The results showed that, compared to the wait-list controls, MBSR participants showed significant increases in EEG patterns associated with positive emotion (specifically, relatively more left-frontal activity) as well as higher influenza-specific antibody titers. Importantly, increases in left-frontal EEG activity in the MBSR group were positively correlated with antibody titers. That is, the greater the increases in positive emotion over the course of the intervention, the better the production of antibodies (Davidson, Kabat-Zinn, Schumacher, Rosenkrantz, Muller, et al., 2003).

Interventions in older adults are more likely to involve behavior change, such as increasing physical activity, and these have shown considerable promise in improving immune function (Kohut & Senchina, 2004). In one study, 14 adults 64 years old or older were assigned to a 10-month program of moderate aerobic activity 3 times per week. They were given trivalent influenza vaccines before and after the exercise program. Compared to the control group, the exercisers showed a significant improvement in their antibody responses as a result of exercising, particularly for virus strains that were repeated in the second vaccination (Kohut, Arntson, Lee, Rozeboom, Yoon et al., 2004). A recent large randomized trial in 160 sedentary older adults 60–83 years old yielded similar results. Among study participants who engaged in moderate cardiovascular exercise 3 times a week for 10 months, 43–55% generated protective levels of antibodies after influenza vaccination compared to 21–39% of participants who were assigned to flexibility training (Woods, Keylock, Lowder, Vieira, Zelkovich et al., 2009). Even gentle movement may have immunological benefits. Tai Chi practice, for

example, has been shown to improve both physical and psychological well-being (Wang, Bannuru, Ramel, Kupelnick, Scott et al., 2010). In one recent study, 41 older adults in their mid to late 70s were assigned to a control condition or to a group that practiced Tai Chi and Qigong for an hour 3 times a week for 5 months. All participants were then vaccinated with a trivalent vaccine. The Tai Chi/Qigong group had significantly greater antibody responses to 2 of the 3 virus strains compared to the control group.

I mention exercise interventions because the improvements in immunity may flow in part from improvements in well-being. In one study, a sample of 28 community-dwelling adults in their 60s and 70s were given a trivalent influenza vaccine and then randomly assigned to a control group or a treatment group that participated in supervised moderate aerobic exercise 3 times a week for 10 months. Serum levels of antibodies to the vaccine and virus-specific IFN-γ were measured along with depression and sense of coherence. As expected, exercising older adults had higher levels of both antibodies and IFN-γ. Also, as predicted, participation in the exercise treatment was associated with declines in depression ratings and increases in sense of coherence. Tests of mediation showed that although the antibody responses to exercise did not depend on improvement in subjective well-being, the increases in IFN-γ did in part (Kohut, Lee, Martin, Arnston, Russell et al., 2005). Exercise is, thus, likely to have myriad benefits for mental and physical health, and some of the improvements in immune function may rely on improvements in well-being.

There is a larger literature on the relationships between psychosocial interventions and changes in discrete aspects of immune function, and most of these have involved clinical samples in which the primary goals are to reduce distress associated with the disease diagnosis and maximize adherence to treatment regimens that are often physiologically and mentally taxing. Breast cancer, for example, has been the focus of considerable research, in part because of early studies suggesting a role for psychosocial factors in disease progression and survival (Levy, Herberman, Lippman, D'Angelo, & Lee, 1991; Spiegel, Bloom, Kraemer, & Gottheil, 1989;). Ongoing research efforts are attempting to bolster immunological processes related to cancer by way of modulating psychological well-being. In what has become a standard design for much research in this area, one study enrolled 227 women who had been diagnosed with breast cancer and had received surgery but who had not yet begun adjuvant therapy. After assessment of a range of psychosocial factors and blood draws for the assessment of in vitro T cell proliferation responses, the women were randomly assigned to a control condition or to an intervention condition designed to reduce stress, and to improve mood, health behaviors, and adherence to treatment. The intervention group met weekly for 4 months. Compared to the controls, women who participated in the intervention had significantly reduced distress, improved health behavior (particularly less smoking), and greater perceived social support. T cell proliferation responses showed significant declines in the control group across the 4-month period, but these responses were preserved in the intervention condition (Andersen, Farrar, Goldern-Kreutz, Glaser, Emery, Crespin, 2004). A follow-up study showed that women who completed the intervention had better global health ratings and fewer illness symptoms than those in the control condition, and these group differences were related to the psychosocial factors that were improved in the intervention group (Andersen, Farrar, Goldern-Kreutz, Emery, Glaser et al., 2007).

Positive psychological functioning in the context of disease may represent a mechanism for immune-enhancing effects of psychosocial interventions. For example, as noted earlier, finding meaning in the context of adversity was linked to preservation of CD4+ cell counts in HIV-infected men (Bower et al., 2003). Antoni, Lehman, Kilbourn, Boyers, Cukver et al (2001) developed a cognitive-behavioral stress management (CBSM) intervention for women with early-stage breast cancer. The intervention consisted of 10 weekly sessions lasting 2 hours each time that combined cognitive restructuring and coping-skills development with relaxation techniques (meditation, progressive muscle relaxation) and opportunities for emotional expression. In the initial study, women were randomly assigned to the intervention or to a control condition consisting of a 1-hour stress- management seminar. The results showed that the intervention significantly increased benefit finding (Antoni et al., 2001). To determine whether the CBSM intervention would improve immune function in women with breast cancer, McGregor and colleagues (2004) examined T cell proliferation responses in the same sample. The results showed that proliferation responses were significantly higher in the CBSM group compared to the control condition. Moreover, increases in benefit finding over the course of a 3-month follow-up

were significantly associated with larger proliferation responses, and this was true for women in both the CBSM and control conditions alike. A later study involving CBSM in a new cohort of women with breast cancer extended these assessments to stimulated production of T cell cytokines, and the results showed that compared to the control group, women in the CBSM group had greater production of IFN-γ and IL-2 at the 6-month follow-up, although these group differences in immune function were not related to differences in psychosocial factors (Antoni, Lechner, Diaz, Vargas, Holley, et al., 2009).

A number of studies have examined the effects of meditation on psychosocial and immune measures in cancer patients. In one preliminary study of women and men with breast and prostate cancer, respectively, counts of immune cells, stimulated production of cytokines, quality of life, and stress were measured before and after an 8-week MBSR intervention that included weekly 90-minute meditation sessions, a 3-hour weekend retreat, and daily home-based guided meditation. The results showed improvements in quality of life, declines in stress, and declines in monocyte counts and stimulated pro-inflammatory cytokine production; many of these changes lasted a full year after the intervention (Carlson, Speca, Faris, & Patel, 2007). A separate study of women with breast cancer included a usual care control condition in addition to an 8-week MBSR protocol. There were 4 assessments each separated by a month beginning before the start of the intervention and continuing until 1 month after its conclusion. Compared to the control group, women who completed the MBSR showed significant increases in quality of life and coping effectiveness, gains in NK activity, and declines in stimulated production of IL-4, IL-6, and IL-10, although links between psychosocial and immunological improvements were not reported. By the time of the final assessment, many of the immune measures in the MBSR group had levels comparable to age-matched women who were cancer-free (Witek-Janusek, Albuquerque, Chroniak, Durazo-Arvizu, & Mathews, 2008). Finally, a recent study examined changes in quality of life, physical symptoms, and physical and mental well-being components of the SF-36, a measure that is widely used in clinical settings (Ware & Sherbourne, 1992; McHorney, Ware, Lu, & Sherbourne, 1994), as well as changes in NK activity and circulating levels of CRP over the course of an 8-week MBSR intervention. The sample was 24 men and women already enrolled in an MBSR program at a university medical center. Pre and post comparisons showed significant declines in distress and improvements in multiple aspects of physical and mental well-being as well as increases in NK activity. Importantly, regression analyses showed that improvements in the mental component score from the SF-36 predicted better postintervention NK activity, and greater improvements in well-being were associated with greater prepost gains in NK activity (Fang, Reibel, Longacre, Rosenzweig, Campbell et al., 2010).

Very few studies to date have examined the impact of psychosocial interventions on molecular processes related to immunosenescence, but one recent study documented changes in telomerase activity associated with meditation. Sixty young and middle-aged men and women were randomly assigned to participate in a 3-month meditation retreat or to a wait-list control group. Results showed that the retreat group had significantly greater increases in mindfulness, purpose in life, and perceived control and decreases in neuroticism compared to the control group. They also had significantly higher levels of telomerase activity, although there were no baseline assessments to determine changes in telomerase from before the retreat, and correlational analyses showed that changes in purpose in life, perceived control, and neuroticism were linearly associated with telomerase activity. Importantly, meditational analyses showed that these improvements in well-being explained the group differences in telomerase, supporting a role for well-being in the regulation of telomerase activity (Jacobs, Epel, Lin, Blackburn, Wolkowitz et al., 2011).

Well-being and Immunity: Candidate Mechanisms

Research on the mechanisms by which positive psychological functioning is linked to better health generally and better immune function specifically is in its infancy, and it is likely that there are multiple pathways. For illustrative purposes, this section will focus on two broad categories that are likely to play a role: physiological regulatory systems and health behaviors.

Candidate physiological systems are principally those that are implicated in linking negative psychological experiences, like chronic stress and depression, to impaired immune function and accelerated immunosenescence, most notably the hypothalamic-pituitary-adrenal (HPA) axis and the sympathetic branch of the autonomic nervous system. The HPA axis regulates the synthesis and release of cortisol from the adrenal gland. Cortisol is considered a stress hormone, as it is released under conditions of physical or psychological challenge, but it also has a marked diurnal rhythm, rising to its peak in human beings within 30 minutes of awakening and falling to its nadir in the evening. Generally, a steeper decline in cortisol from its peak or from levels at awakening to its evening nadir is associated with better health outcomes (Kumari, Shipley, Stafford, & Kivimaki, 2011; Sephton, Sapolsky, Kraemer, & Spiegel, 2000). Cortisol is involved in the physiological regulation of immune function, but prolonged exposure to high levels of cortisol, usually associated with chronic stress, has been associated with multiple aspects of immunosenescence, including thymic involution, impaired cellular immune function, inflammation, and shortened telomeres (Bauer, 2008). There are also normative changes in cortisol regulation that occur with age. Older adults' responses to stressors are typically larger than those in younger men and women (Otte, Hart, Neylan, Marmar, Yaffe et al., 2005). There is also evidence that diurnal patterns of cortisol decline may be blunted in older adults (Deuschle, Gotthardt, Schweiger, Weber, Korner, et al., 1997; Heaney, Phillips, & Carroll, 2010), but this age difference is not observed in other studies (Bauer, 2005). The sympathetic nervous system (SNS) is also involved in both the physiological regulation of immune function under optimal conditions (Felten, Felten, Bellinger, Carlson, Ackerman et al., 1987) and in impaired immune function in the context of chronic stress and clinical depression (Friedman and Irwin, 1995; Irwin, 2002). Research in animal models has shown marked changes in sympathetic regulation of immune function with age (ThyagaRajan, Madden, Teruya, Stevens, Felten et al., 2011) suggesting a role for the SNS in immunosenescence. Age-related changes in both HPA and SNS regulation may underlie observations that stressors can have a more marked effect on immune function in older adults than in the young (Graham et al., 2006).

There is growing evidence that positive psychological functioning is linked to improved regulation of HPA and SNS activity under resting conditions and in response to both laboratory-based and naturalistic stressors (see Dockray & Steptoe, 2010 for review). Research involving older adults specifically is less common, however. One recent study enrolled 33 men and women with an average age of 74 years and monitored blood pressure for 60 days while the participants used diaries to record daily emotional experiences. The results showed that extended periods of positive emotion, usually the product of social connectedness, predicted lower blood pressure and more rapid recovery from negative psychological experiences (Ong & Allaire, 2005). Analysis of data from a sample of 135 women over age 75 living independently in the community found that several dimensions of eudaimonic well-being were associated with steeper cortisol slopes across the day (Ryff, Dienberg Love, Urry, Muller, Rosenkranz et al., 2006). Another study used data on middle-aged and older adults from MIDUS to examine the impact of spousal loss on cortisol regulation. The results showed that bereavement resulted in blunted rises in cortisol in the morning and a flattened rate of decline across the day. Importantly, though, the effect of bereavement on diurnal slope patterns, but not morning cortisol rise, was mediated by positive emotion. That is, the greater the deficits in positive emotion after spousal loss, the larger the impact of bereavement on cortisol decline across the day (Ong, Fuller-Rowell, Bonanno, & Almeida, 2011). Collectively, these results suggest that positive psychological functioning may promote better regulation of physiological systems related to health and immunity and may exert a protective effect on the physiological response to a negative life event. The lack of a mediating effect for cortisol rise in the morning in the preceding study also suggests some specificity in the relationship between positive psychological functioning and biological processes. The extent to which these physiological pathways mediate links between well-being and immune function in older adults remains to be determined.

It is also possible that positive aspects of psychological functioning may be linked to the immune system by alternative physiological pathways (Bower & Segerstrom. 2004), one intriguing possibility being growth factors (Dorshkind, Montecino-Rodriguez, & Signer, 2009). Growth hormone and insulin-like growth factor-1 (IGF-1), for example, have long been known to be sensitive to psychological stress (Tsigos & Chrousos, 2002), and growth factors are important regulators of immune function (Kelley, Weigent, & Kooijman, 2007). The decline in growth factor activity across the life span has been implicated in the process of immunosenescence, particularly the involution of the thymus, and recent research suggests that therapeutic administration of growth factors may improve thymic function (Dorshkind et al., 2009). Although links between well-being and growth factors have not been established, the past research on the negative effects of stress and more recent research linking higher urinary levels of growth hormone to better self-rated physical health and lower stress (Epel, Adler, Ickovics, & McEwen, 1999) indicate that growth factors should be considered another candidate pathway through which psychological well-being may be linked to late-life immunity.

A second general pathway by which well-being may promote better immune function in late life involves health behavior. There are myriad behaviors that have the potential to affect immunity—smoking, alcohol consumption, diet—but two that seem to have particular salience for considerations of aging are physical activity and sleep. Older adults are significantly less active than younger men and women, a function of declines in energy (Schrack, Simonsick, & Ferrucci, 2010) and increases in functional limitations (Motl & McAuley, 2010). As noted earlier, adopting or maintaining a regular routine of physical activity is linked to marked improvements in immune function and resistance to infectious illness (Senchina & Kohut, 2007), and engaging in physical activity in late life may depend in part on psychosocial factors like social support. Results from the MacArthur Studies of Successful Aging showed, for example, that strong social relationships were associated with higher levels of physical activity (Seeman, Berkman, Charpentier, Blazer, Albert et al., 1995). Among middle-aged adults, social support predicted higher levels of physical activity, and physical activity mediated the relationship between social support and reductions in cardiovascular disease (Fischer Aggarwal, Liao, & Mosca, 2008), Because positive affect has been shown to promote the building and strengthening of social relationships (Fredrickson, 2001; Steptoe, O'Donnell, Marmot, & Wardle, 2008a), social support may be an important mechanism by which positive psychological functioning can lead to increases in physical activity and thereby to improvements in immune function in late life.

Sleep is often reduced or disrupted in late life, and poor sleep and sleepiness are common complaints among older adults (Ohayon, 2002; Ohayon, Carskadon, Guilleminault, & Vitiello, 2004; Van Cauter, Leproult, & Plat, 2000). There is a large literature linking experimental and naturalistic sleep loss to impairments in immune function (Bollinger, Bollinger, Oster, & Solbach, 2010; O'Connor & Irwin, 2010) and an equally large literature linking psychosocial factors, almost exclusively negative, to poorer sleep. Both clinical and subclinical levels of depression, for example, are associated with poorer sleep (Benca & Peterson, 2008; Paudel, Taylor, Diem, Stone, Ancoli-Israel et al., 2008), and the association of depression and sleep may be particularly strong in the elderly (Buysse, 2004). Three recent studies focused specifically on the links between positive psychological functioning and sleep in middle aged and older adults. Over 700 participants from the Whitehall II cohort between 58 and 72 years of age completed questionnaire assessments of sleep problems and eudaimonic well-being, and positive affect was measured using ecological sampling across a single day. The results showed that higher levels of both hedonic and eudaimonic well-being predicted fewer sleep problems, and this was true after adjustments for multiple covariates, including negative affect. Moreover, consistent with the theoretical distinctions noted earlier in this chapter, hedonic and eudamonic well-being were weakly correlated, and eudaimonic well-being was more strongly associated with better sleep than hedonic assessments (Steptoe, O'Donnell, Marmot, & Wardle, 2008b). A second study examined well-being and sleep, measured subjectively and objectively, in the MIDUS study. In addition to completing questionnaire assessments of hedonic and eudaimonic well-being, a subsample of MIDUS participants ($N = 1,229$) underwent an overnight clinic stay where they completed the Pittsburgh Sleep Quality Index (PSQI) (Buysse, Reynolds, Monk, Berman, & Kupfer, 1989; Buysse, Reynolds, Monk, Hoch, Yeager, et al., 1991). Some of these participants ($N = 440$) also wore actigraphic watches for seven consecutive days after leaving the clinic. The results showed that higher levels of purpose in life and social well-being were associated with better subjective assessments of sleep quality (using the PSQI) and with better sleep quality as assessed by actigraphy. These associations were robust after adjustments for potential demographic and health confounds; they also remained after adjustments for positive and negative affect, underscoring the independence of eudaimonic and hedonic domains of well-being (Friedman, 2011).

A broader literature on social relationships also provides suggestive evidence linking social well-being specifically with better sleep. Marriage, for example, predicts better sleep than divorced or single status (Hale, 2005; Krueger & Friedman, 2009). Moreover, loneliness, the emotional manifestation of social isolation, predicts poorer objectively measured sleep quality in both young and old individuals (Cacioppo, Hawkley, Berntson, Ernst, Gibbs et al., 2002; Cacioppo, Hawkley, Crawford, Ernst, Burleson et al., 2002; Pressman, Cohen, Miller, Barkin, Rabin et al., 2005). The quality of social relationships matters as well. Among married women, those who are satisfied with their marriages have fewer sleep complaints that those who are less satisfied (Troxel, Buysse, Hall, & Matthews, 2009). Among Japanese civil servants, those lacking someone to confide in when distressed reported more difficulty initiating and maintaining sleep and more daytime fatigue (Murata, Yatsuya, Tamakoshi, Otsuka, & Wada, 2007). Disturbed sleep was associated with low social support in a sample of Swedish women, and sleep mediated the link between low social support and myocardial infarction (Nordin, Knutsson, & Sundbom, 2008).

There are likely to be multiple pathways linking positive psychological functioning and immune function, but it is notable that some of the best described physiological and behavioral regulators of immune function are sensitive to the well-being of the individual, and the links between well-being and these candidate-mediating pathways appears to be independent of the well-documented associations with negative functioning. Thus, they provide potential routes by which positive psychological functioning may be linked to immune function in older adults. It is important to note that this list of candidates is far from complete. Moreover, there are almost certain to be multiple ways of arriving at healthy profiles of immune function in later life—unique combinations of factors that both undermine and promote better immunity—and it will be important to be mindful of the strong likelihood of complex interactions among behavioral and physiological processes in predicting immune function and vulnerability to disease in the elderly.

Promoting Well-being

This chapter has emphasized the potential immunological benefits associated with positive psychosocial factors. Given this emphasis, a fundamental question is whether psychosocial strengths can be cultivated. To the extent that protective resources can be promoted, they could potentially be made available to older adults. Fortunately, work in interventions for treatment of psychological disorders suggests this is possible. Specifically, "well-being therapy" (WBT), developed by Fava and colleagues, has helped to prevent relapse among individuals suffering from mood and anxiety disorders (Fava, 1999; Fava, Rafanelli, Cazzaro, Conti, & Grandi, 1998). The intervention, provided in combination with cognitive behavioral therapy (CBT), was initially effective in preventing relapse of major depression over a two-year period (Fava, Rafanelli, Grandi, Conti, & Belluardo, 1998). Subsequent work showed that these effects persisted over six years (Fava, Ruini, Rafanelli, Finos, Conti et al., 2004). Other related studies showed the effectiveness of the CBT WBT combination in treating generalized anxiety disorder (Fava, Ruini, Rafanelli, Finos, Salmaso et al., 2005).

What is well-being therapy? Fava and Ruini (2003) describe the key components of the intervention, which is based on Ryff's (1989) multidimensional model of psychological well-being. It is a short-term (8-week) therapeutic strategy involving the use of structured diaries kept by patients, combined with interaction with the therapist about diary entries, the overarching goal being to improve participants' experiences of well-being. Clients are required to record positive experiences from their daily lives, however fleeting. The focus in therapy sessions is, then, on helping clients sustain such experiences, rather than on prematurely interrupting them by maladaptive cognitions. The fundamental idea behind the therapy is that recovery from mood and anxiety disorders requires the capacity to experience well-being (Fava, Ruini, & Belaise, 2007). That is, eliminating the symptoms of psychological distress is, in and of itself, insufficient to achieve full recovery; the client must also be able to participate in positive psychological functioning.

Because well-being therapy has been shown to be effective in preventing relapse of psychological disorders, it is now being adapted for use in preventive contexts as well. Ruini, Belaise, Brombin, Caffo, & Fava (2006) developed an intervention protocol, derived from well-being therapy, for students in school settings. Pilot research showed that the intervention resulted in a reduction in psychological symptoms and an increase in psychological well-being. Interventions designed to instill and enhance experiences of well-being among the elderly may also constitute promising future directions in promoting successful aging. That is, because research shows that well-being constitutes an important moderator of later life morbidity and mortality, and because clinical findings show that the promotion of well-being helps prevent relapse of psychological disorders, there is notable promise for interventions designed to nurture psychological well-being among the elderly. The existing evidence showing (a) interindividual differences in well-being associated with corresponding differences in multiple aspects of host defense and immune function in later life, and

(b) changes in well-being during the course of interventions associated with improvements in or preservation of immune processes support the possibility that the promotion of well-being in older adults may have the potential to improve immunological outcomes in this vulnerable population.

Summary and future directions

The twin objectives of this chapter were to highlight the variability in health outcomes that are evident in older adults and to examine the extent to which positive psychological functioning may make unique contributions to that variability. Because immunosenescence is a dynamic normative biological process, the question becomes whether and how positive psychosocial factors can delay, slow, or stall age-related declines in multiple aspects of immune function. Two different historical approaches to the well-being—hedonic and eudaimonic—were discussed, and, although most studies of well-being have not examined the empirical independence of these conceptually different traditions, there is evidence that they may be differentially related to some aspects of biological functioning generally and immune function specifically. Ultimately, though, the goal should not be to treat these different types of well-being as competitors. Rather, they are both theorized to make important contributions to immunological aging, and, to the extent that well-being is involved, achievement of health in later life is likely to involve combinations of features from both traditions. These formulations of well-being were then used as lenses on a broad scope of research studies examining links between immune function and both interindividual differences in positive psychological factors and changes in well-being as a function of interventions. In most cases, positive functioning is associated with better profiles of and improvements in immune function. Finally, the recurrent emphasis on the positive side of the psychosocial ledger led to an important question: namely, are these factors modifiable? Can they be promoted? We briefly reviewed recent intervention strategies to treat individuals with mood and anxiety disorders using WBT. Because these strategies have been shown to be effective in preventing relapse, they are now used in educational contexts with children in the hope of engendering skills that nurture and sustain experiences of well-being and that will last into adulthood and later life. The underlying assumption, which rests at the core of the WBT approach, is that seeking, savoring, and sustaining well-being offers benefits, not only for how one feels subjectively, but also for healthy regulation of underlying biological systems.

It is worth noting that research into the immunological correlates of positive psychological functioning is in its infancy, and rigorous work along many lines will be required to move the field forward. For the same reason, it is an exciting time for this area of research, because evidence that well-being has unique associations with multiple health outcomes continues to accumulate. Below are suggestions for a number of directions future research in this area could take:

- How much overlap exists among different domains of well-being in their associations with immune function in older adults? To what extent are their associations with immunity distinct from one another? Answers to these questions are interesting from a basic science perspective as they will guide identification of important psychological, behavioral, and biological mediating pathways. Differential associations are particularly valuable, because they can inform targeted hypotheses related to specific aspects of well-being and specific pathways. Such answers will also provide a foundation for interventions to improve well-being in older adults. Unique links between hedonic well-being and immunity, for example, might point toward interventions to improve mood, and unique links between eudaimonic well-being and immunity could inform broader policies to increase opportunities for community involvement for older adults.

- A related question relates to whether different kinds of well-being assessments may be related to different aspects of immune function. Multiple methods for the evaluation of well-being are currently in use, and it is likely that each provides a unique snapshot of psychological functioning that may be linked to biological processes in different but no-less-meaningful ways. Momentary assessments of emotion, for example, may be more tightly linked to daily fluctuations in immune processes, for example, than to long-term trajectories of immune function; the reverse may be true of more stable aspects of well-being.

- For which people is well-being most strongly predictive of better immune function? Some of the research reviewed here, for example, suggests that variation in well-being may make the most difference in those who are at some disadvantage (e.g., low social position). Better understanding of who stands to gain the most from improvements in well-being would help in targeting effective interventions.

- To what extent is immunity in later life a product of psychosocial processes accumulating across the life course? To what degree can later life well-being compensate for or reverse the effects of earlier adversity? Immunosenescence is a long-term process that begins in early adulthood. How much of a difference in late-life immune function can well-being in older adults make? Research in cognitive aging shows, for example, that well-being reduces the risk of dementia (Boyle et al., 2010a), and that cognitive function can be preserved even in the context of substantial neuropathology that is typically related to dementia (Snowdon, 1997). Well-being may thus contribute to cognitive resources that preserve cognitive function even in the face of age-related biological decline. Whether the same is true for well-being and immune function remains to be determined.

- Can interventions that promote well-being in older adults lead to improvements in resistance to illness? As is the case for much PNI research, changes in immune function associated with psychosocial processes do not necessarily translate into improvements in health. To date, well-being-based interventions documenting changes in clinically meaningful health outcomes are limited. Future studies must also include greater experimental rigor (e.g., random assignment to conditions) in order to produce the most cogent results.

There are likely to be multiple routes to good health in later life, many of which will involve complex interactions occurring across the life course. It is increasingly possible to address these complex issues in multiple ways, ranging from carefully controlled experimental protocols to large epidemiological datasets in which one can observe heterogeneity in immune function within the population and link it to myriad demographic, psychosocial, and biological processes. The results of these efforts are likely to point to novel approaches to promoting health and well-being in later life.

Related Chapters

For more information on concepts introduced in this chapter, see also Effros; Pressman; and Cole, this volume.

References

Abraham, J., Campbell, C. Y., Cheema, A., Gluckmen, T. J. Blumenthal, R. S., & Danyi, P. (2007). C-reactive protein in cardiovascular risk assessment: a review of the evidence. *Journal of the CardioMetabolic Syndrome, 2*(2), 119–123.

Ader, R. (Ed.). (2007). *Psychoneuroimmunology*. San Diego, CA: Academic Press.

Agarwal, S., & Busse, P. J. (2010). Innate and adaptive immunosenescence. *Annals of Allergy, Asthma & Immunology 104*(3), 183–190.

Aggarwal, B. B., & Gehlot, P. (2009). Inflammation and cancer: how friendly is the relationship for cancer patients? *Current Opinions in Pharmacology, 9*(4), 351–369.

Alley, D. E., Seeman, T. E., Ki, K. J., Karlamangla, A., Hu, P., & Crimmins, E. M. (2006). Socioeconomic status and C-reactive protein levels in the US population: NHANES IV. *Brain, Behavior and Immunity, 20*(5), 498–504.

Almeida, D. M., Wethington, E., & Kessler, R. C. (2002). The daily inventory of stressful events: an interview-based approach for measuring daily stressors. *Assessment 9*(1), 41–55.

Almeida-Oliveira, A., Smith-Carvalho, M., Porto, L. C., Cardoso-Oliveira, J., Ribeiro Ados, S., Falcao, R. R., et al. (2011). Age-related changes in natural killer cell receptors from childhood through old age. *Human Immunology 72*(4), 319–329.

Andersen, B. L., Farrar, W. B., Goldern-Kreutz, D. M., Glaser, R., Emery, C. F., Crespin, T. R., et al. (2004). Psychological, behavioral, and immune changes after a psychological intervention: A clinical trial. *Journal of Clinical Oncology, 22*(17), 3570–3580.

Andersen, B. L., Farrar, W. B., Goldern-Kreutz, D. M., Emery, C. F., Glaser, R., Crespin, T. R., et al. (2007). Distress reduction from a psychological intervention contributes to improved health for cancer patients. *Brain, Behavior and Immunity, 21*(7), 953–961.

Anderson, G., & Horvath, J. (2004). The growing burden of chronic disease in America. *Public Health Report, 119*(3), 263–270.

Antoni, M. H., Lechner, S., Diaz, A., Vargas, S., Holley, G., Phillips, K., et al. (2009). Cognitive behavioral stress management effects on psychosocial and physiological adaptation in women undergoing treatment for breast cancer. *Brain, Behavior and Immunity, 23*(5), 580–591.

Antoni, M. H., Lehman, J. M., Kilbourn, K. M., Boyers, A. E., Cukver, J. L., Alferi, S. M., et al. (2001). Cognitive-behavioral stress management intervention decreases the prevalence of depression and enhances benefit finding among women under treatment for early-stage breast cancer. *Health Psychology, 20*(1), 20–32.

Antoni, M. H., Lutgendorf, S. K., Cole, S. W., Dhabhar, F. S., Sephton, S. E., McDonald, P. G., et al. (2006). The influence of bio-behavioural factors on tumour biology: Pathways and mechanisms. *Nature Reviews Cancer, 6*(3), 240–248.

Antonovsky, A. (1987). Unraveling the mystery of health: How people manage stress and stay well. San Francisco: Josey-Bass.

Antonovsky, A. (1993). The structure and properties of the sense of coherence scale. *Social Science Mediciine, 36*(6), 725–733.

Arias, E., Rostron, B. L., & Tejada-Vera, B. (2010). United States life tables, 2005. *National Vital Statistics Report, 58*(10), 1–132.

Aspinwall, L. G., & Tedeschi, R. G. (2010). The value of positive psychology for health psychology: Progress and pitfalls in examining the relation of positive phenomena to health. *Annals of Behavioral Medicine, 39*(1), 4–15.

Bartrop, R. W., Luckhurst, E., Lazarus, L., Kiloh, L. G., & Penny, R. (1977). Depressed lymphocyte function after bereavement. *Lancet, 1*(8016), 834–836.

Bauer, M. E. (2005). Stress, glucocorticoids and ageing of the immune system. *Stress 8*(1), 69–83.

Bauer, M. E. (2008). Chronic stress and immunosenescence: a review. *Neuroimmunomodulation, 15*(4–6), 241–250.

Benca, R. M., & Peterson, M. J. (2008). Insomnia and depression. *Sleep Med 9 Suppl 1*, S3–9.

Berkman, L. F., Glass, T., Brissette, I., Seeman, T. E. (2000). From social integration to health: Durkheim in the new millennium. *Social Science Medicine, 51*(6), 843–857.

Blake, G. J., & Ridker, P. M. (2003). C-reactive protein and other inflammatory risk markers in acute coronary syndromes. *Journal of the American College of Cardiology, 41*(4 Suppl S), 37S–42S.

Blomberg, B. B., Alvarez, J. P., Diaz, A., Romero, M. G., Lechner, S. C., Carver, C. S., et al. (2009). Psychosocial adaptation and cellular immunity in breast cancer patients in the weeks after surgery: An exploratory study. *Journal of Psychosomatic Research, 67*(5), 369–376.

Bollinger, T., Bollinger, A., Oster, H., & Solbach, W. (2010). Sleep, immunity, and circadian clocks: a mechanistic model. *Gerontology, 56*(6), 574–580.

Bower, J. E., Kemeny, M. E., Taylor, S. E., & Fahey, J. L. (2003). Finding positive meaning and its association with natural killer cell cytotoxicity among participants in a bereavement-related disclosure intervention. *Annals of Behavioral Medicine, 25*(2), 146–155.

Bower, J. E., & Segerstrom, S. C. (2004). Stress management, finding benefit, and immune function: positive mechanisms for intervention effects on physiology. *Journal of Psychosomatic Research, 56*(1), 9–11.

Boyle, P. A., Barnes, L. L., Buchman, A. S., & Bennett, D. A. (2009). Purpose in life is associated with mortality among community-dwelling older persons. *Psychosomatic Medicine, 71*(5), 574–579.

Boyle, P. A., Buchman, A. S., Barnes, L. L., & Bennett, D. A. (2010a). Effect of a purpose in life on risk of incident Alzheimer disease and mild cognitive impairment in community-dwelling older persons. *Archives of General Psychiatry, 67*(3), 304–310.

Boyle, P. A., Buchman, A. S., Barnes, L. L., & Bennett, D. A. (2010b). Purpose in life is associated with a reduced risk of incident disability among community-dwelling older persons. *American Journal of Geriatric Psychiatry, 18*(12), 1093–1102.

Brim, O. G., Ryff, C. D., & Kessler, R. C., Eds. (2004). *How healthy are we? A national study of well-being at midlife*. The John D. and Catherine T. MacArthur Foundation Series on Mental Health and Human Development. Chicago: Chicago University Press.

Buysse, D. J. (2004). Insomnia, depression and aging. Assessing sleep and mood interactions in older adults. *Geriatrics, 59*(2), 47–51; quiz 52.

Buysse, D. J., Reynolds, C. F., III, Monk, T. H., Berman, S. R., & Kupfer, D. J. (1989). The Pittsburgh Sleep Quality Index: a new instrument for psychiatric practice and research. *Psychiatry Research, 28*(2), 193–213.

Buysse, D. J., Reynolds, C. F., III, Monk, T. H., Hoch, C. C., Yeager, A. L., Kupfer, D. J. (1991). Quantification of subjective sleep quality in healthy elderly men and women using the Pittsburgh Sleep Quality Index (PSQI). *Sleep 14*(4), 331–338.

Caccioppo, J. T., & Berntson, G. G. (1994). Relationship between attitudes and evaluative space: a critical review with emphasis on the separability of positive and negative substrates. *Psychological Bulletin 115*(3), 401–423.

Cacioppo, J. T., & Berntson, G. G. (1999). The affect system: architecture and operating characteristics. *Current Directions in Psychological Science, 8*(5), 133–137.

Cacioppo, J. T., Hawkley, L. C., Berntson, G. G., Ernst, J. M., Gibbs, A. C., Stickgold, R., et al. (2002a). Do lonely days invade the nights? Potential social modulation of sleep efficiency. *Psychological Science, 13*(4), 384–387.

Cacioppo, J. T., Hawkley, L. C., Crawford, L. E., Ernst, J. M., Burleson, M. H., Kowalewski, R. B., et al. (2002). Loneliness and health: potential mechanisms. *Psychosomatic Medicine, 64*(3), 407–417.

Carlson, L. E., Speca, M., Faris, P., & Patel, K. D. (2007). One year pre-post intervention follow-up of psychological, immune, endocrine and blood pressure outcomes of mindfulness-based stress reduction (MBSR) in breast and prostate cancer outpatients. *Brain, Behavior and Immunity, 21*(8), 1038–1049.

Chida, Y., & Steptoe, A. (2008). Positive psychological well-being and mortality: A quantitative review of prospective observational studies. *Psychosomatic Medicine, 70*(7), 741–756.

Cohen, S. (2004). Social relationships and health. *American Psychologist, 59*(8), 676–684.

Cohen, S., Alper, C. M., Doyle, W. J., Treanor, J. J., & Turner, R. B. (2006). Positive emotional style predicts resistance to illness after experimental exposure to rhinovirus or influenza a virus. *Psychosomatic Medicine, 68*(6), 809–815.

Cohen, S., Doyle, W. J., Turner, R. B., Alper, C. M., & Skoner, D. P. (2003). Emotional style and susceptibility to the common cold. *Psychosomatic Medicine, 65*(4), 652–657.

Cohn, M. A., Fredrickson, B. L., Brown, S. L., Mikels, J. A., & Conway, A. M. (2009). Happiness unpacked: Positive emotions increase life satisfaction by building resilience. *Emotion, 9*(3), 361–368.

Cole, S. W. (2009). Social regulation of human gene expression. *Current Directions in Psychological Science, 18*(3), 132–137.

Cole, S. W., Hawkley, L. C., Arevaio, J. M., Sunug, C. Y., Rose, R. M., & Cacioppo, J. T. (2007). "Social regulation of gene expression in human leukocytes." *Genome Biology, 8*(9), R189.

Cole, S. W., Hawkley, L. C., Arevaio, J. M., Cacioppo, J. T. (2011). Transcript origin analysis identifies antigen-presenting cells as primary targets of socially regulated gene expression in leukocytes. *Proceedings of the National Academy of Science USA, 108*(7), 3080–3085.

Costanzo, E. S., Lutgendorf, S. K., Kohut, M. L., Nisly, N., Rozeboom, K., Spooner, S., et al. (2004). Mood and cytokine response to influenza virus in older adults. *Journals of Gerontology Series A: Biological Science and Medical Science, 59*(12), 1328–1333.

Coyne, J. C., Tennen, H., & Ranchor, A. V. (2010). Positive psychology in cancer care: a story line resistant to evidence. *Annals of Behavioral Medicine, 39*(1), 35–42.

Dalmida, S., Holstad, M., Diiorio, C., & Laderman, G. (2009). Spiritual well-being, depressive symptoms, and immune status among women living with HIV/AIDS. *Womens Health 49*(2–3), 119–143.

Davidson, R. J., Kabat-Zinn, J., Schumacher, J., Rosenkrantz, M., Muller, D., Santorelli, S. F., et al. (2003). Alterations in brain and immune function produced by mindfulness meditation. *Psychosomatic Medicine, 65*(4), 564–570.

Depp, C. A., & Jeste D. V. (2006). Definitions and predictors of successful aging: a comprehensive review of larger quantitative studies. *American Journal of Geriatric Psychiatry, 14*(1), 6–20.

Deuschle, M., Gotthardt, U., Schweiger, U., Weber, B., Korner, A., Schmider, J., et al. (1997). With aging in humans the activity of the hypothalamus-pituitary-adrenal system increases and its diurnal amplitude flattens. *Life Science, 61*(22), 2239–2246.

Diener, E. (1984). Subjective well-being. *Psychological Bulletin, 95*(3): 542–575.

Diener, E., Emmons, R. A., Larsen, R. J., & Griffin, S. (1985). The Satisfaction With Life Scale. *Journal of Personality Assessment, 49*(1), 71–75.

Dockray, S., & Steptoe, A. (2010). Positive affect and psychobiological processes. *Neuroscience and Biobehavioral Review, 35*(1), 69–75.

Dorshkind, K., Montecino-Rodriguez, E., & Signer, R. A. (2009). The ageing immune system: Is it ever too old to become young again? *National Review of Immunology, 9*(1), 57–62.

Doyle, W. J., Gentile, D. A., & Cohen, S. (2006). Emotional style, nasal cytokines, and illness expression after experimental rhinovirus exposure. *Brain, Behavior, and Immunity, 20*(2), 175–181.

Effros, R. B. (2009). Kleemeier Award Lecture 2008. The canary in the coal mine: telomeres and human healthspan. *The Journals of Gerontology Series A: Biological Sciences and Medical Sciences 64A*(5), 511–515.

Epel, E., Adler, N., Ickovics, J., & McEwen, B. (1999). Social status, anabolic activity, and fat distribution. *Annals of the New York Academy of Science 896:* 424–426.

Epel, E. S., Blackburn, E. H., Lin, J., Dhabhar, F. S., Adler, N. E., Morrow, J. D., et al. (2004). Accelerated telomere shortening in response to life stress. *Proceedings of the National Academy of Science USA, 101*(49), 17312–17315.

Eriksson, M., & Lindstrom, B. (2005). Validity of Antonovsky's sense of coherence scale: a systematic review. *Journal of Epidemiology and Community Health, 59*(6), 460–466.

Fang, C. Y., Reibel, D. K., Longacre, M. L., Rosenzweig, S., Campbell, D. E., & Douglas, S. D. (2010). Enhanced psychosocial well-being following participation in a mindfulness-based stress reduction program is associated with increased natural killer cell activity. *Journal of Alternative and Complementary Medicine, 16*(5), 531–538.

Fava, G. A. (1999). Well-being therapy: Conceptual and technical issues. *Psychotherapy and Psychosomatics, 68*(4), 171–179.

Fava, G. A., Rafanelli, C., Cazzaro, M., Conti, S., & Grandi, S. (1998). Well-being therapy. A novel psychotherapeutic approach for residual symptoms of affective disorders. *Psychological Medicine, 28*(2), 475–480.

Fava, G. A., Rafanelli, C., Grandi, S., Conti, S., & Belluardo, P. (1998). Prevention of recurrent depression with cognitive behavioral therapy. *Archives of General Psychiatry, 55*, 816–821.

Fava, G. A., & Ruini, C. (2003). Development and characteristics of a well-being enhancing psychotherapeutic strategy: Well-being therapy. *Journal of Behavior Therapy and Experimental Psychiatry, 34*(1), 45–63.

Fava, G. A., Ruini, C., Rafanelli, C., Finos, L., Conti, S., & Grandi, S. (2004). Six-year outcome of cognitive behavior therapy for prevention of recurrent depression. *American Journal of Psychiatry, 161*(10), 1872–1876.

Fava, G. A., Ruini, C., Rafanelli, C., Finos, L., Salmaso, L., Mangelli, L., et al. (2005). Well-being therapy of Generalized

Anxiety Disorder. *Psychotherapy and Psychosomatics, 74*(1), 26–30.

Fava, G. A., Ruini, C., & Belaise, C. (2007). The concept of recovery in major depression. *Psychological Medicine, 37*(3), 307–317.

Felten, D. L., Felten, S. Y., Bellinger, D. L., Carlson, S. L., Ackerman, K. D., Madden, K. S., et al. (1987). Noradrenergic sympathetic neural interactions with the immune system: structure and function. *Immunology Review, 100,* 225–260.

Fischer Aggarwal, B. A., Liao, M., & Mosca, L. (2008). Physical activity as a potential mechanism through which social support may reduce cardiovascular disease risk. *Journal of Cardiovascular Nursing, 23*(2), 90–96.

Ford, E. S., Loucks, E. B., & Berkman, L. F. (2006). Social integration and concentrations of C-reactive protein among US adults. *Annals of Epidemiology, 16*(2), 78–84.

Franceschi, C., Capri, M., Monti, D., Giunta, S., Olivieri, F., Sevini, F., et al. (2007). Inflammaging and anti-inflammaging: A systemic perspective on aging and longevity emerged from studies in humans. *Mechanisms of Ageing and Development, 128*(1), 92–105.

Fredrickson, B. L. (2001). The role of positive emotions in positive psychology. The broaden-and-build theory of positive emotions. *American Psychologist, 56*(3), 218–226.

Fredrickson, B. L., Tugade, M. M., Waugh, C. E., & Larkin, G. R. (2003). What good are positive emotions in crises? A prospective study of resilience and emotions following the terrorist attacks on the United States on September 11th, 2001. *Journals of Personality and Social Psychology, 84*(2), 365–376.

Friedman, E. M. (2011). Sleep quality, social well-being, gender, and inflammation: an integrative analysis in a national sample. *Annals of the New York Academy of Sciences, 1231,* 23–34.

Friedman, E. M., Hayney, M. S., Love, G. D., Urry, H. L., Rosenkranz, M. A., Davidson, R. J., et al. (2005). Social relationships, sleep quality, and interleukin-6 in aging women. *Proceedings of the National Academy of Science USA, 102*(51), 18757–18762.

Friedman, E. M., Hayney, M., Love, G. D., Singer, B. H., & Ryff, C. D. (2007). Plasma interleukin-6 and soluble IL-6 receptors are associated with psychological well-being in aging women. *Health Psychology, 26*(3), 305–313.

Friedman, E. M., & P. Herd (2010). Income, education, and inflammation: differential associations in a national probability sample (The MIDUS study). *Psychosomatic Medicine, 72*(3), 290–300.

Friedman, E., Love, G., Singer, B. H., & Ryff, C. D. (2008). Social well-being predicts reduced inflammation in aging women. *Gerontologist, 48*(Special Issue III), 291.

Friedman, E. M., & Irwin, M. R. (1995). A role for CRH and the sympathetic nervous system in stress-induced immunosuppression. *Annals of the New York Academy of Science, 771,* 396–418.

Friedman, E., & Ryff, C. D. (2012). Living well with medical comorbidities: A biopsychosocial perspective. *Journals of Gerontology, Series B, Psychological and Social Sciences.* Published online, February 29, 2012.

George, L. K. (2010). Still happy after all these years: research frontiers on subjective well-being in later life. *Journal of Gerontology Series B: Psychological Sciences and Social Sciences, 65B*(3), 331–339.

Gerstorf, D., Ram, N., Mayrez, G., Hidajat, M., Lindenberger, U., Wagner, G. G., et al. (2010). Late-life decline in well-being across adulthood in Germany, the United Kingdom, and the United States: Something is seriously wrong at the end of life. *Psychology of Aging, 25*(2): 477–485.

Glaser, R., Sheridan, J., Malarkey, W. B., MacCallum, R. C., & Kiecolt-Glaser, J. K. (2000). Chronic stress modulates the immune response to a pneumococcal pneumonia vaccine. *Psychosomatic Medicine, 62*(6): 804–807.

Goldsby, R. A., Kindt, T. J., & Osborne, B. A. (2006). *Kuby Immunology.* New York: W.H. Freeman.

Gouin, J. P., Hantsoo, L., & Kiecolt-Glaser, J. K. (2008). Immune dysregulation and chronic stress among older adults: a review. *Neuroimmunomodulation, 15*(4–6), 251–259.

Graham, J. E., Christian, L. M., & Kiecolt-Glaser, J. K. (2006). Stress, age, and immune function: toward a life span approach. *Journal of Behavioral Medicine, 29*(4), 389–400.

Gruenewald, T. L., Cohen, S., Matthews, K. A., Tracy, R., & Seeman, T. E. (2009). Association of socioeconomic status with inflammation markers in black and white men and women in the Coronary Artery Risk Development in Young Adults (CARDIA) study. *Social Science Medicine, 69,* 451–459.

Hale, L. (2005). Who has time to sleep? *Journal of Public Health, 27*(2), 205–211.

Hannoun, C., Megas, F., & Piercy, J. (2004). Immunogenicity and protective efficacy of influenza vaccination. *Virus Research, 103*(1–2): 133–138.

Hansel, A., Hong, S., Camara, R. J., & von Kanel, R. (2010). Inflammation as a psychophysiological biomarker in chronic psychosocial stress. *Neuroscience and Biobehavioral Reviews, 35*(1), 115–121.

Hayney, M. S., Love, G. D., Buck, J. M., Ryff, C. D., Singer, B. H., & Muller, D. (2003). The association between psychological factors and vaccine-induced cytokine production. *Vaccine, 21,* 2428–2432.

Heaney, J. L., Phillips, A. C. & Carroll, D. (2010). Ageing, depression, anxiety, social support and the diurnal rhythm and awakening response of salivary cortisol. *International Journal of Psychophysiology, 78*(3): 201–208.

Heron, M. (2007). Deaths: Leading causes for 2004. *National Vital Statistics Report, 56*(5), 1–95.

House, J. S., Landis, K. R., & Umberson, D. (1988). Social relationships and health. *Science, 241*(4865), 540–545.

Howren, M. B., Lamkin, D. M., & Suls, J. (2009). Associations of depression with C-reactive protein, IL-1, and IL-6: a meta-analysis. *Psychosomatic Medicine, 71*(2), 171–186.

Ickovics, J. R., Milan, S., Boland, R. Schoenbaum, E., Schuman, P., & Vlahov, D. (2006). Psychological resources protect health: 5-year survival and immune function among HIV-infected women from four US cities. *AIDS, 20*(14), 1851–1860.

Ironson, G., & Hayward, H. (2008). Do positive psychosocial factors predict disease progression in HIV-1? A review of the evidence. *Psychosomatic Medicone, 70*(5), 546–554.

Irwin, M. (2002). Psychoneuroimmunology of depression: Clinical implications. *Brain, Behavior and Immunity, 16*(1) 1–16.

Jacobs, T. L., Epel, E. S., Lin, J., Blackburn, E. H., Wolkowitz, O. M., Bridwell, D. A., et al. (2011). Intensive meditation training, immune cell telomerase activity, and psychological mediators. *Psychoneuroendocrinology, 36*(5), 664–681.

Jousilahti, P., Salomaa, V., Rasi, V., Vahtera, E., & Palosuo, T. (2003). Association of markers of systemic inflammation, C reactive protein, serum amyloid A, and fibrinogen, with socioeconomic status. *Journal of Epidemiology and Community Health, 57*(9), 730–733.

Kabat-Zinn, J., Lipworth, L., & Burney, R. (1985). The clinical use of mindfulness meditation for the self-regulation of chronic pain. *Journal of Behavioral Medicine, 8*(2), 163–190.

Kaszubowska, L. (2008). Telomere shortening and ageing of the immune system. *Journal of Physiological Pharmacology, 59 Suppl 9*, 169–186.

Kelley, K. W., Weigent, D. A., & Kooijman, R. (2007). Protein hormones and immunity. *Brain, Behavior and Immunity, 21*(4), 384–392.

Keyes, C. L. (2002). The mental health continuum: From languishing to flourishing in life. *Journal of Health and Social Behavior, 43*(2), 207–222.

Khan, N., Shariff, N., Cobbold, M., Bruton, R., Ainsworth, J. A., Sinclair, A. J., et al. (2002). Cytomegalovirus seropositivity drives the CD8 T cell repertoire toward greater clonality in healthy elderly individuals. *Journal of Immunology, 169*(4), 1984–1992.

Kiecolt-Glaser, J. K., Glaser, R., Shuttleworth, E. C., Dyer, C. S., Ogrocki, P., & Speicher, C. E. (1987). Chronic stress and immunity in family caregivers of Alzheimer's disease victims. *Psychosomatic Medicine, 49*(5): 523–535.

Kiecolt-Glaser, J. K., Glaser, R., Gravenstein, S., Malarkey, W. B., & Sheridan, J. F. (1996). Chronic stress alters the immune response to influenza virus vaccine in older adults. *Proceedings of the National Academy of Science USA, 93*, 3042–3047.

Kiecolt-Glaser, J. K., Gouin, J. P., & Hantsoo, L. (2010). Close relationships, inflammation, and health. *Neuroscience and Biobehavioral Reviews, 35*(1), 33–38.

Kiecolt-Glaser, J. K., Preacher, K. J., MacCallum, R. C., Atkinson, C., Malarkey, W. B., & Glaser, R. (2003). Chronic stress and age-related increases in the proinflammatory cytokine IL-6. *Proceedings of the National Academy of Science USA, 100*(15), 9090–9095.

Kohut, M. L., Arntson, B. A., Lee, W., Rozeboom, K., Yoon, K. J., Cunnick, J. E., et al. (2004). Moderate exercise improves antibody response to influenza immunization in older adults. *Vaccine, 22*(17–18), 2298–2306.

Kohut, M. L., Lee, W., Martin, A., Arnston, B., Russell, D. W., Ekkekakis, P., et al. (2005). The exercise-induced enhancement of influenza immunity is mediated in part by improvements in psychosocial factors in older adults. *Brain, Behavior and Immunity, 19*(4): 357–366.

Kohut, M. L., & Senchina, D. S. (2004). Reversing age-associated immunosenescence via exercise. *Exercise Immunology Review, 10*, 6–41.

Koizumi, M., Ito, H., Kaneko, Y., & Motohashi, Y. (2008). Effect of having a sense of purpose in life on the risk of death from cardiovascular diseases. *Journal of Epidemiology, 18*(5), 191–196.

Krause, N. (2009). Meaning in life and mortality." *Journals of Gerontology Series B: Psychological Sciences and Social Sciences, 64*(4): 517–527.

Krueger, P. M., & Friedman, E. M. (2009). Sleep duration in the United States: a cross-sectional population-based study. *American J ournal of Epidemiology, 169*(9), 1052–1063.

Kumari, M., Shipley, M., Stafford, M., & Kivimaki, M. (2011). Association of diurnal patterns in salivary cortisol with all-cause and cardiovascular mortality: Findings from the Whitehall II Study. *Journal of Clinical Endocrinology and Metabolism, 96*(5), 1478–1485.

Kunzmann, U., Little, T. D., & Smith, J. (2000). Is age-related stability of subjective well-being a paradox? Cross-sectional and longitudinal evidence from the Berlin Aging Study. *Psychology and Aging, 15*(3), 511–526.

Lang, F. R., & Carstensen, L. L. (2002). Time counts: future time perspective, goals, and social relationships. *Psychology and Aging 17*(1), 125–139.

Larsen, J. T., McGraw, A. P., & Cacioppo, J. T. (2001). Can people feel happy and sad at the same time? *Journal of Personality and Social Psychology, 81*(4), 684–696.

Leitch, E. F., Chakrabarti, M., Crozier, J. E., McKee, R. F., Anderson, J. H., Horgan, P. G., et al. (2007). Comparison of the prognostic value of selected markers of the systemic inflammatory response in patients with colorectal cancer. *British Journal of Cancer, 97*(9), 1266–1270.

Levy, S. M., Herberman, R. B., Lippman, M., D'Angelo, T., & Lee, J. (1991). Immunological and psychosocial predictors of disease recurrence in patients with early-stage breast cancer. *Behavioral Medicine, 17*(2), 67–75.

Loucks, E. B., Berkman, L. F., Gruenewald, T. L., & Seeman, T. E. (2005). Social integration is associated with fibrinogen concentration in elderly men. *Psychosomatic Medicine, 67*(3), 353–358.

Loucks, E. B., Berkman, L. F., Gruenewald, T. L., & Seeman, T. E. (2006). Relation of social integration to inflammatory marker concentrations in men and women 70 to 79 years. *American Journal of Cardiology, 97*(7): 1010–1016.

Loucks, E. B., Pilote, L., Lynch, J. W., Richard, H., Almeida, N. D., Benjamin, E. J., et al. (2010). Life course socioeconomic position is associated with inflammatory markers: The Framingham Offspring Study. *Social Science and Medicine, 71*(1), 187–195.

Lutgendorf, S. K. (2009). Positive affect and radiation-induced inflammation: insights into inflammatory regulation? *Brain, Behavior and Immunity, 23*(8), 1066–1067.

Lutgendorf, S. K., Vitaliano, P. P., Buckwalter, K. C., Reimer, T. T., Hong, S. Y., Lubaroff, D. M. (1999). Sense of coherence moderates the relationship between life stress and natural killer cell activity in healthy older adults. *Psychology and Aging, 14*(4), 552–563.

Marucha, P. T., Crespin, T. R., Shelby, R. A., & Andersen, B. L. (2005). TNF-[alpha] levels in cancer patients relate to social variables. *Brain, Behavior, and Immunity, 19*(6), 521–525.

McElhaney, J. E., & Effros, R. B. (2009). Immunosenescence: what does it mean to health outcomes in older adults? *Current Opinions in Immunology, 21*(4), 418–424.

McGregor, B. A., Antoni, M. H., Boyers, A., Alferi, S. M., Blomberg, B. B., & Carver, C. S. (2004). Cognitive-behavioral stress management increases benefit finding and immune function among women with early-stage breast cancer. *Journal of Psychosomatic Research 56*(1), 1–8.

McHorney, C. A., Ware, J. E., Jr., Lu, J. F., & Sherbourne, C. D. (1994). The MOS 36-item Short-Form Health Survey (SF-36): III. Tests of data quality, scaling assumptions, and reliability across diverse patient groups. *Medical Care, 32*(1), 40–66.

McLaughlin, S. J., Connell, C. M., Heeringa, S. G., Li, L. W., & Roberts, J. S. (2010). Successful aging in the United States: prevalence estimates from a national sample of older adults. *Journals of Gerontology Series B: Psychological Sciences and Social Sciences, 65B*(2): 216–226.

Mocchegiani, E., & Malavolta, M. (2004). NK and NKT cell functions in immunosenescence. *Aging Cell 3*(4), 177–184.

Montross, L. P., Depp, C., Daly, J., Reichstadt, J., Golshan, S., Moore, D., et al. (2006). Correlates of self-rated successful aging among community-dwelling older adults. *American Journal of Geriatric Psychiatry, 14*(1), 43–51.

Morozink, J. A., Friedman, E. M., Coe, C. L., & Ryff, C. D. (2010). Socioeconomic and psychosocial predictors of interleukin-6 in the MIDUS national sample. *Health Psychology, 29*(6), 626–635.

Motl, R. W., & McAuley, E. (2010). Physical activity, disability, and quality of life in older adults. *Physical Medicine and Rehabilitation Clinics of North America, 21*(2), 299–308.

Moynihan, J. A., Larson, M. R., Treanor, J., Duberstein, P. R., Power, A., Shore, B., et al. (2004). Psychosocial factors and the response to influenza vaccination in older adults. *Psychosomatic Medicine, 66*(6), 950–953.

Mroczek, D. K., & Spiro, A., III (2005). Change in life satisfaction during adulthood: Findings from the veterans affairs normative aging study. *Journal of Personality and Social Psychology, 88*(1), 189–202.

Murata, C., Yatsuya, H., Tamakoshi, K., Otsuka, R., Wada, K., & Toyoshima, H. (2007). Psychological factors and insomnia among male civil servants in Japan. *Sleep Medicine, 8*(3), 209–214.

Nordin, M., Knutsson, A., & Sundbom, E. (2008). Is disturbed sleep a mediator in the association between social support and myocardial infarction? *Journal of Health Psychology, 13*(1), 55–64.

Norris, C. J., Gollan, J., Berntson, G. G., & Cacioppo, J. T. (2010). The current status of research on the structure of evaluative space. *Biological Psychology, 84*(3), 422–436.

O'Connor, M. F., & Irwin, M. R. (2010). Links between behavioral factors and inflammation. *Clinical Pharmacology and Therapeutics, 87*(4): 479–482.

O'Donovan, A., Lin, J., Dhabhar, F. S., Wolkowitz, O., Tillie, J. M., Blackburn, E., et al. (2009). Pessimism correlates with leukocyte telomere shortness and elevated interleukin-6 in post-menopausal women. *Brain, Behavior and Immunity, 23*(4), 446–449.

Ohayon, M. M. (2002). Epidemiology of insomnia: what we know and what we still need to learn. *Sleep Medicine Reviews, 6*(2): 97–111.

Ohayon, M. M., Carskadon, M. A., Guilleminault, C., & Vitiello, M. V. (2004). Meta-analysis of quantitative sleep parameters from childhood to old age in healthy individuals: developing normative sleep values across the human life span. *Sleep, 27*(7): 1255–1273.

Ong, A. D. & Allaire, J. C. (2005). Cardiovascular intraindividual variability in later life: the influence of social connectedness and positive emotions. *Psychology of Aging, 20*(3), 476–485.

Ong, A. D., Fuller-Rowell, T. E., Bonanno, G. A., & Almeida, D. M. (2011). Spousal loss predicts alterations in diurnal cortisol activity through prospective changes in positive emotion. *Health Psychology, 30*(2): 220–227.

Otte, C., Hart, S., Neylan, T. C., Marmar, C. R., Yaffe, K., & Mohr, D. C. (2005). A meta-analysis of cortisol response to challenge in human aging: importance of gender. *Psychoneuroendocrinology, 30*(1), 80–91.

Owen, N., Poulton, T., Hay, F. C., Mohamed-Ali, V., & Steptoe, A. (2003). Socioeconomic status, C-reactive protein, immune factors, and responses to acute mental stress. *Brain, Behavior and Immunity, 17*(4), 286–295.

Panda, A., Arjona, A., Sapey, E., Bai, F., Fikrig, E., Montgomery, R., et al. (2009). Human innate immunosenescence: causes and consequences for immunity in old age. *Trends in Immunology, 30*(7), 325–333.

Paudel, M. L., Taylor, B. C., Diem, S. J., Stone, K. L., Ancoli-Israel, S., Redline, S., et al. (2008). Association between depressive symptoms and sleep disturbances in community-dwelling older men. *Journal of the American Geriatric Society, 56*(7), 1228–1235.

Pawelec, G., Derhovanessian, E., Larbi, A., Strindhall, J., & Wikby, A. (2009). Cytomegalovirus and human immunosenescence. *Review of Medical Virology, 19*(1), 47–56.

Pfister, G., & Savino, W. (2008). Can the immune system still be efficient in the elderly? An immunological and immunoendocrine therapeutic perspective. *Neuroimmunomodulation, 15*(4–6), 351–364.

Phillips, A. C., Carroll, D., Burns, V. E., Ring, C., Macleod, J., & Drayson, M. (2006). Bereavement and marriage are associated with antibody response to influenza vaccination in the elderly. *Brain, Behavior and Immunity, 20*(3), 279–289.

Poon, L. W., Clayton, G. M., Clayton, G. M., Messner, S., Noble, C. A., & Johnson, M. A. (1992). The Georgia Centenarian Study. *International Journal of Aging and Human Development, 34*(1), 1–17.

Prather, A. A., Marsland, A. L., Muldoon, M. F., & Manuck, S. B. (2007). Positive affective style covaries with stimulated IL-6 and IL-10 production in a middle-aged community sample. *Brain, Behavior, and Immunity, 21*(8), 1033–1037.

Pressman, S. D., & Cohen, S. (2005). Does positive affect influence health? *Psychology Bulletin, 131*(6), 925–971.

Pressman, S. D., Cohen, S., Miller, G. E., Barkin, A., Rabin, B. S., & Treanor, J. J. (2005). Loneliness, social network size, and immune response to influenza vaccination in college freshmen. *Health Psychology, 24*(3), 297–306.

Ranjit, N., Diez-Roux, A. V., Shea, S., Cushman, M., Ni, H., & Seeman, T. (2007). Socioeconomic position, race/ethnicity, and inflammation in the multi-ethnic study of atherosclerosis. *Circulation, 116*(21), 2383–2390.

Raulet, D. H., & Guerra, N. (2009). Oncogenic stress sensed by the immune system: role of natural killer cell receptors. *National Review of Immunology, 9*(8), 568–580.

Reichstadt, J., Sengupta, G., Depp, C. A., Palinkas, L. A., & Jeste, D. V. (2010). Older adults' perspectives on successful aging: qualitative interviews. *American Journal of Geriatric Psychiatry, 18*(7), 567–575.

Rosenkranz, M. A., Jackson, D. C., Dalton, K. M., Dolski, I. Ryff, C. D., Singer, B. H., et al. (2003). Affective style and in vivo immune response: neurobehavioral mechanisms. *Proceedings of the National Academy of Science USA, 100*(19), 11148–11152.

Rowe, J. W., & Kahn, R. L. (1987). Human aging: Usual and successful. *Science, 237*(4811), 143–149.

Roy, B., Diez-Roux, A. V., Seeman, T., Ranjit, N., Shea, S., & Cushman, M. (2010). Association of Optimism and Pessimism With Inflammation and Hemostasis in the Multi-Ethnic Study of Atherosclerosis (MESA). *Psychosomatic Medicine, 72*(2), 134–140.

Ruini, C., Belaise, C., Brombin, C., Caffo, E., & Fava, G. A. (2006). Well-being therapy in school settings: A pilot study. *Psychotherapy and Psychosomatics, 75*(6), 331–336.

Ryan, R. M., & Deci, E. L. (2000). Self-determination theory and the facilitation of intrinsic motivation, social development, and well-being. *American Psychologist, 55*(1), 68–78.

Ryan, R. M., & Deci, E. L. (2001). On happiness and human potentials: A review of research on hedonic and eudaimonic well-being. *Annual Review of Psychology, 52*, 141–166.

Ryff, C. D. (1989). Happiness is everything, or is it?: Explorations on the meaning of psychological well-being. *Journal of Personality and Social Psychology, 57,* 1069–1081.

Ryff, C. D., Dienberg Love, G., Urry, H. L., Muller, D., Rosenkranz, M. A., Friedman, E. M., et al. (2006). Psychological well-being and ill-being: Do they have distinct or mirrored biological correlates? *Psychotherapy and Psychosomatics, 75*(2), 85–95.

Ryff, C. D., & Keyes, C. L. (1995). The structure of psychological well-being revisited. *Journal of Personality and Social Psychology, 69*(4), 719–727.

Scheibe, S., & Carstensen, L. L. (2010). Emotional aging: recent findings and future trends. *Journal of Gerontology Series B: Psychological Sciences and Social Sciences, 65B*(2), 135–144.

Schleifer, S. J., Keller, S. E., Camerino, M., Thornton, J. C., & Stein, M. (1983). Suppression of Lymphocyte Stimulation Following Bereavement. *JAMA: The Journal of the American Medical Association, 250*(3): 374–377.

Schrack, J. A., Simonsick, E. M., & Ferrucci, L. (2010). The energetic pathway to mobility loss: an emerging new framework for longitudinal studies on aging. *Journal of the American Geriatric Society, 58 Suppl 2,* S329–336.

Seeman, T. E., Berkman, L. F., Charpentier, P. A., Blazer, D. G., Albert, M. S., & Tinetti, M. E. (1995). Behavioral and psychosocial predictors of physical performance: MacArthur studies of successful aging. *Journal of Gerontology Series A: Biological Sciences and Medical Sciences, 50*(4): M177–183.

Senchina, D. S., & Kohut, M. L. (2007). Immunological outcomes of exercise in older adults. *Clinical Interventions in Aging, 2*(1): 3–16.

Sepah, S. C., & Bower, J. E. (2009). Positive affect and inflammation during radiation treatment for breast and prostate cancer. *Brain, Behavior and Immunity, 23*(8), 1068–1072.

Sephton, S. E., Sapolsky, R. M., Kraemer, H. C., & Spiegel, D. (2000). Diurnal cortisol rhythm as a predictor of breast cancer survival. *Journal of the National Cancer Institute, 92*(12): 994–1000.

Shiffman, S., Stone, A. A., & Hufford, M. R. (2008). Ecological momentary assessment. *Annual Review of Clinical Psychology, 4,* 1–32.

Simpson, R. J., & Guy, K. (2010). Coupling aging immunity with a sedentary lifestyle: Has the damage already been done? A Mini-Review. *Gerontology, 56*(5), 449–458.

Snowdon, D. A. (1997). Aging and Alzheimer's disease: Lessons from the Nun Study. *Gerontologist, 37*(2), 150–156.

Spiegel, D., Bloom, J. R., Kraemer, H. C., & Gottheil, E. (1989). Effect of psychosocial treatment on survival of patients with metastatic breast cancer. *Lancet, 2*(8668), 888–891.

Springer, K. W., Pudrovska, T., & Hauser, R. M. (2011). Does psychological well-being change with age?: Longitudinal tests of age variations and further exploration of the multidimensionality of Ryff's model of psychological well-being. *Social Science Research, 40*(1), 392–398.

Staras, S. A., Dollard, S. C., Radford, K. W., Flanders, W. D., Pass, R. F., & Cannon, M. J. (2006). Seroprevalence of cytomegalovirus infection in the United States, 1988–1994. *Clinical Infectious Diseases, 43*(9), 1143–1151.

Stefanek, M. E., Palmer, S. C., Thombs, B. D., & Coyne, J. C. (2009). Finding what is not there: Unwarranted claims of an effect of psychosocial intervention on recurrence and survival. *Cancer, 115*(24), 5612–5616.

Steptoe, A., O'Donnell, K., Badrick, E., Kumari, M., & Marmot, M. (2008). Neuroendocrine and inflammatory factors associated with positive affect in healthy men and women: The Whitehall II Study. *American Journal of Epidemiology, 167*(1), 96–102.

Steptoe, A., O'Donnell, K., Marmot, M., & Wardle, J. (2008a). Positive affect and psychosocial processes related to health. *British Journal of Psychology, 99*(Pt 2), 211–227.

Steptoe, A., O'Donnell, K., Marmot, M., & Wardle, J. (2008b). Positive affect, psychological well-being, and good sleep. *Journal of Psychosomatic Research, 64*(4), 409–415.

Steptoe, A., Owen, N., Kunz-Ebrecht, S. R., & Brydon, L. (2004). Loneliness and neuroendocrine, cardiovascular, and inflammatory stress responses in middle-aged men and women. *Psychoneuroendocrinology, 29*(5), 593–611.

Steptoe, A., Wardle, J., & Marmot, M. (2005). Positive affect and health-related neuroendocrine, cardiovascular, and inflammatory processes. *Proceedings of the National Academy of Science USA, 102*(18), 6508–6512.

Strawbridge, W. J., Wallhagen, M. I., & Cohen, R. D. (2002). Successful aging and well-being: self-rated compared with Rowe and Kahn. *Gerontologist, 42*(6), 727–733.

Taylor, S. E. (1983). Adjustment to threatening events: A theory of cognitive adaptation. *American Psychologist., 38*(11), 1161–1173.

Thompson, W. W., Shay, D. K., Weintraub, E., Brammer, L., Cox, N., Anderson, L. J., et al. (2003). Mortality associated with influenza and respiratory syncytial virus in the United States. *Journal of the American Medical Association, 289*(2), 179–186.

ThyagaRajan, S., Madden, K. S., Teruya, B., Stevens, S. Y., Felten, D. L., & Bellinger, D. L. (2011). Age-associated alterations in sympathetic noradrenergic innervation of primary and secondary lymphoid organs in female Fischer 344 rats. *Journal of Neuroimmunology, 233*(1), 54–64.

Troxel, W. M., Buysse, D. J., Hall, M., & Matthews, K. A. (2009). Marital happiness and sleep disturbances in a multiethnic sample of middle-aged women. *Behavioral Sleep Medicine, 7*(1), 2–19.

Tsigos, C., & Chrousos, G. P. (2002). Hypothalamic-pituitary-adrenal axis, neuroendocrine factors and stress. *Journal of Psychosomatic Research, 53*(4), 865–871.

Tugade, M. M., & Fredrickson, B. L. (2004). Resilient individuals use positive emotions to bounce back from negative emotional experiences. *Journal of Personality and Social Psychology, 86*(2), 320–333.

Uchino, B. N. (2006). Social support and health: A review of physiological processes potentially underlying links to disease outcomes. *Journal of Behavioral Medicine, 29*(4), 377–387.

Urry, H. L., Nitschke, J. B., Dolski, I., Jackson, D. C., Dalton, K. M., Mueller, C. J., et al. (2004). Making a life worth living: Neural correlates of well-being. *Psychological Science, 15*(6), 367–372.

Van Cauter, E., Leproult, R., & Plat, L. (2000). Age-related changes in slow wave sleep and REM sleep and relationship with growth hormone and cortisol levels in healthy men. *Journal of the American Medical Association, 284*(7), 861–868.

Vedhara, K., Cox, N. K., Wilcox, G. K., Perks, P., Hunt, M., Anderson, S., et al. (1999). Chronic stress in elderly carers of dementia patients and antibody response to influenza vaccination. *Lancet, 353*(9153), 627–631.

Vogeli, C., Shields, A. E., Lee, T. A., Gibson, T. B., Marder, W. D., Weiss, K. B., et al. (2007). Multiple chronic conditions: Prevalence, health consequences, and implications for quality, care management, and costs. *Journal of General Internal Medicine, 22 Suppl 3,* 391–395.

Von Ah, D., Kang, D. H., & Carpenter, J. S. (2007). Stress, optimism, and social support: Impact on immune responses in breast cancer. *Research in Nursing and Health, 30*(1), 72–83.

Wang, C., Bannuru, R., Ramel, J., Kupelnick, B., Scott, T., & Schmid, C. H. (2010). Tai Chi on psychological well-being: Systematic review and meta-analysis. *BMC Complementary and Alternative Medicine, 10,* 23.

Ware, J. E., Jr., & Sherbourne C. D. (1992). The MOS 36-item short-form health survey (SF-36). I. Conceptual framework and item selection. *Medical Care, 30*(6), 473–483.

Waterman, A. S. (1993). Two conceptions of happiness: contrasts of personal expressiveness (eudaimonia) and hedonic enjoyment. *Journal of Personality and Social Psychology, 64*(4), 678–691.

Watson, D., Clark, L. A., & Tellegen, A. (1988). Development and validation of brief measures of positive and negative affect: The PANAS scales. *Journal of Personality and Social Psychology, 54*(6), 1063–1070.

Watson, D., Weber, K., Assenheimer, J. S., Clark, L. A., Strauss, M. E., & McCormick, R. A. (1995). Testing a tripartite model: I. Evaluating the convergent and discriminant validity of anxiety and depression symptom scales. *J Abnormal Psychology, 104*(1), 3–14.

Weiskopf, D., Weinberger, B., & Grubeck-Loebenstein, B. (2009). The aging of the immune system. *Transplant International, 22*(11), 1041–1050.

Witek-Janusek, L., Albuquerque, K., Chroniak, C., Durazo-Arvizu, R., & Mathews, H. L. (2008). Effect of mindfulness based stress reduction on immune function, quality of life and coping in women newly diagnosed with early stage breast cancer. *Brain, Behavior and Immunity, 22*(6), 969–981.

Woods, J. A., Keylock, K. T., Lowder, K. T., Vieira, V. J., Zelkovich, W., Dumich, S., et al.et al. (2009). Cardiovascular exercise training extends influenza vaccine seroprotection in sedentary older adults: the immune function intervention trial. *Journal of the American Geriatric Society, 57*(12), 2183–2191.

Zamai, L., Ponti, C., Mirandola, P., Gobbi, G., Papa, S., Galeotti, L., et al. (2007). NK cells and cancer. *Journal of Immunology 178*(7), 4011–4016.

Stress and Immune System Aging

Rita B. Effros

Abstract

Aging of the immune system is responsible for increased severity of infections, reduced vaccine responsiveness, and higher cancer incidence in the elderly. These outcomes can be attributed to several types of stress, including latent viral infections, oxidative stress and psychological stress. The major infectious stressors are herpes viruses, which are usually acquired early in life, persist for many decades and drive certain T cells to replicative senescence, a terminal state characterized by reduced immune function, shortened telomeres, and production of pro-inflammatory cytokines. Chronic psychological and oxidative stress are also associated with shortened telomeres and reduced immune function. Given the wide range of deleterious effects associated with telomere shortening and the resultant immune dysfunction and inflammation, research aimed at retarding the process of replicative senescence—for example, by enhancing telomerase in T cells or by life-style and stress-reduction techniques—are promising approaches for enhancing healthspan in older persons.

Key Words: stress, telomere, telomerase, T cells, immune, human, latent infection, aging, HIV/AIDS

Introduction

Human aging is associated with a variety of clinical problems, the most significant ones relating to infections and cancer. For example, in the United States, influenza and pneumonia rank as the fifth leading cause of death in adults aged 65 and older. In addition to actual mortality, morbidity and prolonged periods of illness due to infections are substantially increased with age. With respect to cancer, epidemiological studies show that old age—even more than known harmful lifestyle factors such as smoking—is the greatest risk factor for the development of cancer. One of the major contributory factors to the age-related changes in severity and incidence of infections and cancer is the waning protective function of the immune system.

The complex remodeling of the human immune system with age is due to both intrinsic events, such as the reduction in size and function of the thymus, as well as to environmental factors, including the life-long exposure to various pathogens, and situations associated with psychological stress. The combined influences of these intrinsic and extrinsic factors lead to major alterations in immune function with age, changes that have been implicated in the deleterious effects of pathogens and cancer in the elderly. Ironically, vaccination, which is aimed at manipulating the immune system in ways that would prevent infection or retard cancer progression, is far less effective in the elderly, as well as in persons experiencing psychological stress (McElhaney, Upshaw, Hooton, Lechelt, & Meneilly, 1998; Glaser & Kiecolt-Glaser, 2005). Even immune memory to certain pathogens that is generated early in life declines during aging.

Interestingly, although there is no change in total lymphocyte number with age, the proportional representation of different types of lymphocytes, particularly within the T cell compartment, is dramatically altered. The population of naïve T cells emerging from the thymus progressively declines, and the proportion of various types of memory T cells increases. Within the memory T lymphocyte pool, there is a striking change in the phenotype and function of the so-called CD8, or cytotoxic T lymphocytes, with progressively increasing proportions of cells showing features of replicative senescence.

This chapter will review the effect of prolonged stress on the human immune system, with a focus on telomere/telomerase dynamics in T lymphocytes. The major age-related immune system changes that occur in humans seem to be driven by life-long stress of maintaining control over latent viral infections acquired in childhood, such as cytomegalovirus (CMV) and Epstein-Barr virus (EBV). During periods of psychological stress, these latent viruses can become reactivated and detected in the blood or urine, causing increased "work" by the immune system to suppress the viral re-emergence. Indeed, over many decades, the proportion of memory cells directed at these viruses undergoes a progressive increase, so that by old age, these virus-specific T cells occupy a progressively larger proportion of the total T cell "repertoire." Indeed, in older persons, the greater the number of clonally expanded virus-specific T cells, the less diverse is the remaining T cell antigen recognition repertoire (i.e., the overall range of antigens that the T cells are able to recognize). It remains to be determined if the constriction of the T cell repertoire is the cause or the effect of the large proportions of clonal populations of CD8 T cells. In fact, it is possible that the age-associate constriction of the T cell repertoire is actually due to the progressive decline in production of new, so-called naive T cells by the shrinking thymus. Although the naïve T cell repertoire is, nevertheless, maintained for a few decades after the dwindling of the thymic output, during the seventh decade, the overall repertoire of different antigen recognition units in humans decreases dramatically (Goronzy & Weyand, 2005)

In addition to viral infection and chronic psychological stress, oxidative stress also contributes to generation of senescent T cells. The progressive changes in immune system function and telomere dynamics can provide novel insights into multiple facets of human aging and healthspan, as well as how immunological history, starting in childhood, can have late-life effects on a variety of physiological processes. Following a brief introduction to the immune system, the features of T cell replicative senescence and telomere/telomerase dynamics

will be discussed. The role of senescent T cells in vivo, as well as the complex relationship between the immune system and age-related pathologies will next be reviewed. Finally, recent advances in psychoneuroimmunology, particularly with respect to aging, will be presented, as well as possible therapeutic approaches. The chapter will end with a discussion of several important questions and suggested avenues for future research.

Immune System Basics

The immune system is a complex and highly integrated network of cells and lymphoid organs, consisting of two interacting components that function in coordinated fashion to combat invading organisms. The so-called innate immune system is capable of dealing with certain pathogens in a rapid, albeit, somewhat nonspecific manner. By contrast, the activity of the adaptive immune system takes longer to develop, but has the advantage of exquisite specificity and long-term memory. Indeed, this anamnestic response is the basis for the efficacy of vaccines (Sompayrac, 2008).

The immune system is derived from primitive stem cells in the bone marrow. A significant feature of T and B lymphocytes, the main players in adaptive immunity, is the presence of antigen receptors on the surface of each cell that confer the ability to recognize a specific region of a particular pathogen. These antigen receptors are generated during the complex transition from hematopoietic stem cells to mature lymphocytes by an intricate process of cutting and pasting that leads to random joining of DNA segments from several different gene families (Janeway, Travers, & Walpert, 2001). The outcome of this process is that each lymphocyte, as well as all of its progeny, expresses a unique antigen receptor. If that lymphocyte encounters the appropriate antigen, it will become activated and undergo cell division, with the identical receptor expressed on all the resulting daughter cells. Some lymphocytes never encounter their specific antigen; these cells are called virgin or naïve cells, in contrast to memory cells, which are antigen experienced.

The random nature of the cutting and splicing process by which antigen receptors are generated results in an extremely large repertoire of antigen specificities, estimated to be in the range of 10^{14}. Thus, the immune system is able to respond to an extraordinarily broad range of pathogens. However, precisely because of this large repertoire, the number of lymphocytes that can respond to any single pathogen is extremely small. This feature leads to the requirement for massive cell division and clonal expansion of the few cells whose receptors recognize the invading pathogen, or, in the case of cancer, a tumor-specific antigen.

The main players within the adaptive immune system—the B and T lymphocytes—have distinct functional roles upon encounter with antigen. B cells produce soluble proteins called antibodies, which can neutralize or otherwise inactivate pathogens that are present within the blood. T cells, on the other hand, are unable to recognize "free" antigen, and can only recognize pathogens that have already infected other cells. In the case of a viral infection, for example, the infected cells become decorated with components of the virus, indicating to the immune system that the cell is no longer normal and must be eliminated. Those cytotoxic T cells whose receptors recognize the specific viral antigens on the surface of the infected cell become activated and then undergo massive cell division, migrate into the tissues, where they actually kill infected or otherwise abnormal (i.e., tumor) cells, thereby controlling the infection or the cancer. Once the antigen-specific T cells complete their function, most of the expanded cell population dies by apoptosis, leaving only a few memory cells to handle possible future encounters with the same antigen. Thus, proliferation and the ability to undergo repeated rounds of clonal expansion is a critical feature of effective T lymphocyte function, as will be discussed next.

Telomere Shortening and Other Changes in Chronically Stimulated T Cells

Some T cells never encounter their antigen, and others may have only a single encounter with antigen during the entire life span of the organism. By contrast, T cells whose receptors recognize viruses that establish a persistent infection have the potential for multiple, repeated exposures to antigen over many decades. With each antigen encounter, these virus-specific T cells become activated and undergo cell division. To model this scenario in the laboratory, our group has established a unique long-term culture system, whereby T cells are driven by chronic antigenic stimulation to an end stage of differentiation known as replicative senescence. Thus, the effects of this intrinsic barrier to unlimited cell division can be studied longitudinally as a population of T cells transitions from naïve to memory status, and eventually to senescence.

The basic protocol of our in vitro model of cellular aging is to isolate peripheral blood mononuclear cells from venous blood samples, and to stimulate the cells with either irradiated foreign (allogeneic) tumor cells, with antibodies to the T cell receptor, or with viral antigens (Dagarag, Evazyan, Rao, & Effros, 2004). Irrespective of the mode of stimulation, after a period of 2–3 weeks, the vigorous cell proliferation subsides, and the cells became quiescent. The cycle of stimulation-proliferation-quiescence is repeated multiple times until the culture reaches an irreversible final stage of quiescence that cannot be overcome by further stimulation or by the addition of growth factors (Perillo, Naeim, Walford, & Effros, 1993; Perillo, Walford, Newman, & Effros, 1989). It is important to note that this end stage of replicative senescence does not imply loss of viability. Indeed, with appropriate feeding, senescent cells remain viable and metabolically active for several months (Wang, Lee, & Pandey, 1994; Spaulding, Guo, & Effros, 1999). Moreover, despite the emphasis on replication, the functional, genetic, and phenotypic alterations associated with senescence may be at least as important to the biology of cells as the inability to proliferate (Campisi, 1997).

Arguably, one of the most significant changes associated with T lymphocyte replicative senescence in cell culture is the complete and irreversible loss of expression of the major signaling molecule, CD28 (Effros et al., 1994; Vallejo, Nestel, Schirmer, Weyand, & Goronzy, 1998). This co-stimulatory receptor is involved in a variety of T cell functions, including activation, proliferation, stabilization of cytokine messenger RNA levels, cell trafficking, and glucose metabolism (Shimizu et al., 1992; Holdorf, Kanagawa, & Shaw, 2000; Sansom, 2000; Frauwirth et al., 2002). Thus, a T cell that no longer expresses CD28 is a fundamentally different cell from one that has CD28 on its surface. In parallel with the loss of CD28 expression, CD8 T lymphocytes lose the ability to upregulate the telomere-extending enzyme, telomerase. Although robust telomerase activity is observed in concert with initial activation, by the third and all subsequent rounds of stimulation, CD8 T cells show no detectible telomerase activity (Valenzuela & Effros, 2002). The loss of telomerase activity parallels the loss of CD28 expression, suggesting a possible link between CD28 and upregulation of telomerase. This notion was confirmed in studies in which blocking the binding of CD28 to its receptor led to complete abrogation of telomerase activity.

With the loss of telomerase activity, the T lymphocytes undergo progressive telomere shortening as they continue to divide, ultimately reaching the critically short telomere length of 5–7 kb that has been associated with replicative senescence in a variety of human cell types (Vaziri et al., 1993). The process of telomere shortening can be accelerated in the presence of oxidative stress and the accumulation of reactive oxygen species, due to less efficient repair of certain types of DNA damage in telomeres, as compared to other regions of the chromosome. Oxidative stress, in the form of exposure to oxidized low density lipoproteins (the "bad" cholesterol) also accelerates the process of replicative senescence, and, furthermore enhances the production of several cytokines known to impact bone homeostasis (Graham et al., 2009).

Even in the absence of oxidized lipids, alteration in the pattern of cytokine production is a prominent feature of senescent T cells (Effros, Dagarag, Spaulding, & Man, 2005). Cytokine secretion by T lymphocytes is essential for cell-to-cell communication and efficient immune function. Our research has documented that, as T lymphocytes progress to senescence in cell culture, they produce increasing amounts of two pro-inflammatory cytokines. Specifically, the levels of both TNFα and IL-6 increase progressively as the cells reach senescence (Effros et al., 2005). These two cytokines are often associated with frailty in the elderly (Hubbard, O'Mahony, Savva, Calver, & Woodhouse, 2009), as well as with increased maturation and activation of bone-resorbing osteoclasts (Arron J.R. & Choi, 2000). A second important change in cytokine secretion is the anti-viral cytokine IFNγ, which CD8 T cells secrete in conjunction with their cytotoxic function. With progressive cell divisions in culture, virus-specific CD8 T cells show significantly reduced production and secretion of IFNγ, along with reduced capacity to kill virally infected cells (Dagarag et al., 2004; Dagarag, Ng, Lubong, Effros, & Yang, 2003; Yang et al., 2005). Senescent T cell cultures also produce a significantly blunted heat shock response, indicative of reduced ability to respond to physical stressors (Effros, Zhu, & Walford, 1994).

A final important feature of T cells that reach the end stage of replicative senescence is the inability to initiate a process known as apoptosis, by which T cells can "commit suicide" (Spaulding, Guo, & Effros, 1999). This change in the capacity to initiate timely and efficient programmed cell death is highly relevant to effective immune function in vivo, since elimination of the majority of activated virus-specific CD8 T cells is an essential event once an infection has been resolved and the virus is no longer present in the body (Effros & Pawelec, 1997). However, in the case of latent viral infections, the virus persists, causing ongoing recognition, activation, and proliferation of the T cells that recognize that virus. This extensive cell division will ultimately lead to critically short telomeres and replicative senescence. Once a T cell reaches senescence in vivo, it will persist, due to its apoptosis resistance. The following section will provide evidence that senescent cells do, in fact, accumulate over time in vivo.

Senescent T Cells are Increased during Aging, HIV/AIDS, and Cancer

The permanent loss of CD28 expression in senescent T lymphocyte cultures has been an informative biomarker for determining whether replicative senescence of T cells is actually occurring in vivo. This analysis involves subjecting samples of peripheral blood to a technique known as flow cytometry, whereby the proportion of CD8 T cells that do or do not express CD28 on their surface can be enumerated. Flow cytometry studies have demonstrated that persons age 70–90 have high proportions of CD8 T lymphocytes that lack CD28 surface expression. Indeed, in some elderly persons, more than 50% of the CD8 T lymphocytes within the total peripheral blood T cell pool do not express the CD28 molecule (Effros et al., 1994). Interestingly, younger persons who are chronically infected with HIV have proportions of CD8+CD28- T cells that are similar to those observed in uninfected person decades older. Moreover, the proportion of such cells at an early stage of the disease is predictive of more rapid, versus very slow, subsequent progression to AIDS (Cao, 2009). As with T lymphocyes that reach senescence in culture, CD8+CD28– T lymphocytes isolated from fresh blood samples show minimal proliferative activity, and have shorter telomeres than CD8+CD28+ T cells from the same donor (Effros et al., 1996).

It has been suggested that latent infection with several herpes viruses, which are endemic and persist throughout life in infected individuals, is the main driving force for the generation of senescent CD8 T cells in vivo (Pawelec et al., 2004) Clinical data on bone-marrow and organ-transplant recipients indicate that, under conditions of immunosuppression, cytomegalovirus (CMV) and other latent herpes viruses are often reactivated. These observations suggest that maintaining viral latency requires active participation by the immune system. The constant and prolonged exposure of CD8 T cells to latently infected cells leads to chronic activation and extensive proliferation, ultimately driving virus-specific T cells to senescence (Pawelec et al., 2004). This notion is consistent with the studies on HIV/AIDS discussed above, and with studies on persons infected with Epstein-Barr Virus (EBV). During the acute phase of EBV infection (the first 10 days), telomerase activity is high in the EBV-specific T cells present in the peripheral blood, and telomere length remains stable. However, one year later, when the infection has become latent, telomere shortening is observed in antigen-specific CD8 T lymphocytes (Hathcock, Weng, Merica, Jenkins, & Hodes, 1998; Maini, Soares, Zilch, Akbar, & Beverley, 1999), presumably due to the down regulation of telomerase activity associated with repeated antigen-driven proliferation (Valenzuela & Effros, 2002).

Chronic exposure to viral antigens is not the only mechanism driving CD8 T cell replicative senescence in vivo. Similar antigen-driven proliferation is presumably also responsible for the presence of senescent CD8 T cells in the context of certain forms of cancer. Indeed, T cells with features of senescence have been purified from a large spectrum of human tumors, including lung (Meloni et al., 2006), colorectal (Ye et al., 2006), endometrial (Chang et al., 2010), ovarian (Webb et al., 2010), lymphoma (Urbaniak-Kujda et al., 2009) and breast (Gruber et al., 2008; Schule, Bergkvist, Hakansson, Gustafsson, & Hakansson, 2004), as well as from patients with melanoma and multiple myeloma patients (Ahmadzadeh et al., 2009; Sze et al., 2001), Moreover, in advanced renal carcinoma, higher proportions of CD8 T cells with markers of senescence are predictive of reduced patient survival (Characiejus et al., 2002). Conversely, the maintenance of CD28 expression is associated with improved in vitro expansion capability of CD8 T cells that have been isolated from actual melanoma tumors (Li et al., 2010). The common theme among all these reports of senescent CD8 T cells present in vivo is chronic antigenic stimulation, which leads to extensive proliferation, and finally to the end stage of replicative senescence. Due to the apoptosis resistance of these cells, once generated, they persist.

Role of the Immune System in Health, Disease, and Life Span

The biological significance of T lymphocyte replicative senescence is underscored by the prognostic value of these cells in several longitudinal analyses. In the very old, for example, T lymphocytes with markers of senescence are part of the so-called "immune-risk phenotype," which is predictive of earlier all-cause mortality (Wikby et al., 2002). Another study analyzed telomere length in total peripheral blood mononuclear cells (PBMC) derived from a cohort of 60-year-old persons. That study showed that the shortest telomere size quartile at age 60 was associated with earlier mortality, as compared with those individuals with the longest quartile of telomere length. Moreover, the short-telomere quartile showed a 7–8 fold increased risk of dying from infection, further implicating the immune system in health and life span (Cawthon, Smith, O'Brien, Sivatchenko, & Kerber, 2003).

Recent more extensive analysis of distinct populations of peripheral blood cells has shown that CD8+CD28– T lymphocytes not only exhibit lower telomerase activity, but also have telomere lengths that are shorter than any other T and B cell subset. Importantly, this extensive study on blood samples from 60 individuals shows a significant inverse correlation between the percentage of CD8+CD28– T lymphocytes and overall telomere length of the total PBMC population (Lin et al., 2010.). Thus, the shorter the overall PBMC telomere length, the higher the proportion of senescent CD8 T cells. This observation is significant, because numerous studies have shown associations between overall PBMC telomere length and various diseases (Effros, 2009a), suggesting that the proportions of CD8+CD28- T lymphocytes may be increased in multiple human pathologies, as will be discussed below. It should be emphasized that telomere shortening—like the canary in the coal mine—is not the *cause* of the deleterious effects, but rather, the harbinger of increased health risk (Effros, 2009b).

Telomere length, telomerase activity, and CD28 expression are increasingly being used as biomarkers of disease, immune status, and overall health. The importance of telomerase in lymphocyte function is dramatically illustrated by the multiple immune abnormalities in persons with the autosomal dominant form of dyskeratosis congenita, a disease caused by a mutation in the gene encoding the RNA component of telomerase (Knudson, Kulkarni, Ballas, Bessler, & Goldman, 2005). By contrast, enhanced telomerase activity and increased telomere length in immune cells, due to another type of mutation in a telomerase gene, is associated with the extreme longevity of centenarians (Clowes, Riggs, & Khosla, 2005). For whatever reason, the increased telomerase activity in the immune cells is not associated with increased cancer. Indeed, it is possible that the enhanced immune function may increase tumor immunosurveillance. In terms of age-associated diseases, telomere shortening has been documented in individuals with Alzheimer's disease (Jenkins et al., 2006; Panossian et al., 2002) and Down syndrome (Vaziri et al., 1993), which shows premature neurological and immunological aging. Accelerated telomere shortening also occurs in patients with coronary heart disease (Spyridopoulos et al., 2009), atherosclerosis (Samani, Boultby, Butler, Thompson, & Goodall, 2001), and premature myocardial infarction (Brouilette, Singh, Thompson, Goodall, & Samani, 2003). In addition, insulin resistance and Type 2 diabetes are associated with telomere loss (Demissie et al., 2006; Tentolouris et al., 2007). Finally, as noted earlier, HIV/AIDS is associated with increased proportions of T cells lacking CD28 expression (a marker of senescence) and telomeres that are in the range usually observed in persons decades their senior (Effros et al., 1996).

The underlying mechanisms for the aforementioned associations are being increasingly investigated. One of prominent connections between the immune system and age-related disease is in the field of "osteoimmunology," which is relevant to both immune involvement in rheumatoid arthritis, an autoimmune disease that affects a large number of older persons, and to the normal age-related reduced bone mass that is mediated, at least in part, by T cells. Indeed, there is accumulating evidence indicating that bone biology is directly linked to immune-system activity, and that chronic immune activation is associated with bone loss (Arron & Choi, 2000). The CD8 T cell subset, in particular, has been implicated in both bone resorption activity (Buchinsky et al., 1996; John, Hock, Short, Glasebrook, & Galvin, 1996) and osteoporotic fractures in the elderly (Pietschmann et al., 2001).

One of the central regulators of bone resorption is both expressed on and secreted by activated T cells. This molecule, known as "RANKL" (receptor activator of NFkB ligand) binds to RANK on osteoclasts, inducing these bone-resorbing cells to mature and become activated (Kong, Boyle, & Penninger, 2000). Under normal circumstances, the bone-resorbing activity induced by RANKL is kept in check by IFNγ, a cytokine also produced by the activated T cells (Takayanagi et al., 2000). However, senescent CD8 T lymphocytes show reduced ability to produce IFNγ (Dagarag et al., 2004). Increased RANKL production by T cells is also induced by exposure to oxidized low-density lipids (LDL, the "bad" cholesterol). We have shown that both resting and activated T cells produce high levels of RANKL following a 72-hour exposure to oxidized LDL

versus native LDL. Moreover, in mice that show bone loss due to a high-fat diet, T cells within the bone marrow were shown to stimulate the maturation and activation of osteoclasts, and T cells present in the spleen of these mice show increased transcription of the genes for TNF-alpha and IL-6, cytokines implicated in bone loss (Graham et al., 2010). Thus, the immune system may disrupt bone homeostasis via multiple pathways, and the effects are exacerbated by chronic activation and exposure to oxidized lipids.

The enhanced immune system activity induced by oxidized lipids is also relevant to atherosclerosis. Both osteoporosis and atherosclerosis not only have immune components involved in disease initiation and progression, but these immune factors are subject to dietary modulation, particularly via high levels of LDL, which are then subject to oxidation. Thus, oxidative stress, which enhances inflammation, is a central feature of both of these diseases. Several large population-based studies have shown that diets consisting of higher fat intake are associated with increased levels of C-reactive protein, IL-6, and other markers of inflammation. Moreover, epidemiological analyses have repeatedly shown that patients with lower bone density and osteoporosis have higher lipid levels, more severe coronary atherosclerosis and increased risk of stroke (Barengolts et al., 1998; Laroche et al., 1994; Uyama, Yoshimoto, Yamamoto, & Kawai, 1997). Conversely, lipid-lowering treatments are associated with both reduced coronary vascular calcification (Edwards, Hart, & Spector, 2000) and fewer osteoporotic fractures (Meier, Schlienger, Kraenzlin, Schlegel, & Jick, 2001).

Immune system involvement has also been documented for neurological diseases of aging, such as Alzheimer's disease (AD). Several studies have described differences in immune cell reactivity to amyloid beta between healthy elderly persons and those with AD (Loewenbrueck, Tigno-Aranjuez, Boehm, Lehmann, & Tary-Lehmann, 2008; Trieb, Ransmayr, Sgonc, Lassmann, & Grubeck-Loebenstein, 1996). These differences may explain the massive inflammatory response elicited by a putative therapeutic AD vaccine, which led to the immediate cessation of the clinical trial. It seems that the immune system of persons with AD may already be perturbed in some way, and is, therefore, quite distinct from the immune system of mice that are genetically engineered to express beta amyloid. Indeed, telomere shortening has been reported for T cells (but not B cells or monocytes) from persons with AD, suggesting some sort of alteration in cellular immunity (Panossian et al., 2002).

Psychoneuroimmunology: Mind-Body Connections

As early as 1974, the immunologist, Niels Jerne pointed out the apparent functional similarities between the immune system and the brain (Jerne, 1974). Both are involved with the recognition of "self" versus "non-self." Another parallel is that the immune network can be considered to constitute the identity of the organism at the molecular level, whereas neural networks of the brain represent the physiological "self" of the organism. Moreover, both systems involve innate responses as well as learning and memory acquired via interaction with the environment. Finally, both the brain and the immune system can be considered sensory organs (Zachariae, 2009). Indeed, the immune system is actually the "sixth sense," because it enables the organism to recognize a host of foreign pathogens.

The preceding notions, originally proposed by Jerne, are now widely accepted, and research in the growing interdisciplinary field of psychoneuroimmunology has played a key role in establishing a biological basis for the ancient notion that the mind can play a role in health, disease, and even life span itself. Many of the age-associated immune changes discussed earlier can be exacerbated by emotional stress, and it is now clear that, as with other physiological systems, the immune system is modulated by neural reflexes, and these connections operate in a bidirectional fashion. For example, the so-called inflammatory reflex is comprised of an afferent arm that senses inflammation, and an efferent arm (the cholinergic anti-inflammatory pathway) that functions to inhibit innate immune responses (Rosas-Ballina & Tracey, 2009).

Multiple components of the immune system, including bone marrow, thymus, lymph nodes, and spleen, are innervated by fibers of the autonomic nervous system that utilize a wide range of neurotransmitters (Mignini, Streccioni, & Amenta, 2003). Moreover, the number of nerve endings and their distribution within immune organs undergoes a dynamic process of remodeling based, in part, on immune cell function, and neurotransmitters are involved in the modulation of T cell responses to antigen (Pacheco, Riquelme, & Kalergis, 2010). Thus, it is not surprising that, over the long human life span, the cumulative immunological history can have dramatic effects on the interactions between immune and nervous systems.

There are many excellent reviews covering mind-body interactions (Kiecolt-Glaser, 2009; Gouin, Hantsoo, & Kiecolt-Glaser, 2008; O'Connor & Irwin, 2010). Here, I will focus on research specifically linking stress and immune function in the elderly population. During aging, psychological stress seems to synergize with the effects of replicative senescence. It had previously been reported that reduced antibody titers to influenza vaccination are associated with increased proportions of senescent T cells (Goronzy et al., 2001; Saurwein-Teissl et al., 2002;). A similarly decreased antibody response to flu vaccination has been documented in older caregivers of relatives with dementia (Vedhara et al., 1999). These individuals also show reduced telomerase activity compared to a matched control group. Reduced telomerase activity is also seen in younger caregivers of chronically ill children (Epel et al., 2004). These observations may be explained by the fact that exposure of T cells to cortisol, the major stress hormone, causes a significant suppression of telomerase activity (Choi, Fauce, & Effros, 2008). Diminished telomerase activity leads to accelerated generation of senescent T cells, which, in turn, can suppress immune responses to vaccines and other antigenic encounters.

As mentioned earlier, long term exposure to latent viruses accelerates the generation of senescent T cells. Although these viruses usually remain latent, it is clear that the immune system is intimately involved in the maintenance of latency, because organ transplant patients who are taking immunosuppresive medications to prevent organ rejection often experience re-emergence of latent infections or the development of certain forms of virally induced cancer, such as EBV lymphoma. Re-emergence of latent viral infection in persons with normal immune systems can also occur in situations of psychological stress. For example, physically fit, healthy astronauts show reactivation and viral shedding of CMV during spaceflight (Mehta, Stowe, Feiveson, Tyring, & Pierson, 2000), and there is evidence of subclinical reactivation of the varicella zoster virus (VZV) and Epstein-Barr virus (EBV) in these astraunats as well (Mehta et al., 2004). The stress of spaceflight is also associated with acute changes in dehydroepiandrosterone sulfate (DHEAS) and cortisol, resulting in a pronounced decrease in the DHEAS/cortisol ratio (Stowe, Mehta, Ferrando, Feeback, & Pierson, 2001).

A novel connection between the nervous and immune systems is adenosine, a potent extracellular messenger, which is well-known for its neuromodulatory function. Indeed, recent work in mice has implicated adenosine as the main mediator of acupuncture treatment (Goldman et al., 2010). Interestingly, adenosine also functions as an immunosuppressor. Under normal conditions, the adenosine level in the blood is maintained at concentrations in the 100–300 nM range (Hershfield, 2005). However, under metabolically unfavorable conditions, such as tissue hypoxia and inflammation, a variety of cell types, such as regulatory T cells, mast cells, and neural cells secrete adenosine, which can have severe clinical implications on immune function (Gessi et al., 2007). Adenosine is also present in the microenvironment of tumor cells, possibly contributing to reduced cancer immunosurveillance (MacKenzie, Hoskin, & Blay, 1994).

ADA is the enzyme that converts adenosine to inosine, thereby playing a key role in normal immune function (Gessi et al., 2007). Indeed, a variety of studies have documented some of the negative effects of adenosine on T lymphoctyes, such as suppression of IL-2 production (DosReis, Nobrega, & de Carvalho, 1986) and at high levels, induction of apoptosis (Szondy, 1994). Short term (~36 hrs) exposure of murine T lymphocytes to adenosine alters multiple effector functions (Ohta et al., 2009) and also results in a loss of CD28 expression (Butler et al., 2003). Recent studies have shown that chronic stimulation of T cells in culture leads to a progressive loss of ADA expression and function. Moreover, cells that lack ADA have significantly reduced telomerase activity, and exposure of T cells to adenosine in the absence of ADA accelerates the progression to replicative senescence (Parish et al., 2010).

Preventive/Treatment Strategies

A variety of approaches are addressing possible strategies to enhance immune function and reduce stress, particularly in the elderly. This section will review the results of several types of basic science experiments, as well conclusions from lifestyle studies that aim to enhance healthspan in the elderly.

Biological Approaches

As noted earlier, shorter telomeres and/or reduced telomerase activity of either total PBMC, or various subsets of lymphocytes, are increasingly being documented to correlate with a variety of diseases. Given the intimate relationship of telomerase with replicative senescence dynamics, and the emerging picture of pleiotropic negative effects exerted by senescent CD8 T cells in vivo, many of the approaches to modulate the process have focused on telomerase.

Targeting telomerase is consistent with several recent studies showing that high telomerase activity is associated with several favorable health outcomes. In HIV disease, increased telomerase activity in the virus-specific CD8 T lymphocyte subset is present in persons who have strong control over the infection (i.e., elite controllers) (Lichterfeld et al., 2008). Moreover, many centenarians have a genetic variation in telomerase, leading to increased activity of the enzyme and longer telomeres (Atzmon et al., 2010). Laboratory studies have, therefore, used telomerase-based approaches to retard the process of replicative senescence. Gene transduction of CD8 T cells from HIV-infected persons with the catalytic component of telomerase (hTERT) led to telomere length stabilization and reduced expression of two cell-cycle inhibitors, implicating both of these proteins in the senescence program (Dagarag et al., 2004). Notably, the transduced cultures showed indefinite proliferation, with no signs of change in growth characteristics or karyotypic abnormalities. In terms of protective immune function, the "telomerized" HIV-specific-specific CD8 T cells were able to maintain the production of IFNγ for extended periods, and showed significantly enhanced capacity to inhibit HIV replication.

Telomerase enhancement has also been achieved using nongenetic strategies, which would offer more practical approaches to therapeutic interventions in the elderly. Pharmacologic enhancement of telomerase has the important advantage over gene therapy approaches of allowing control over the dose and timing. We recently showed that short term exposure to a small molecule telomerase activator led to a significant enhancement of telomerase activity in T cells from both healthy and HIV-infected persons. For HIV-specific CD8 T lymphocytes, the increased telomerase activity was accompanied by increased proliferation and, importantly, significant enhancement of a variety of antiviral functions (Fauce et al., 2008).

Several additional categories of nongenetic telomerase-enhancing treatments show preliminary promise in cell culture studies. Inhibition of TNFα in cell cultures of CD8 T lymphocytes allows for increased telomerase activity, prolonged maintenance of CD28 expression, and enhanced proliferation (Parish, Wu, & Effros, 2009). Estrogen or modified "designer" versions of the hormone may also have the desired effect. It is well-established that estrogen is able to enhance telomerase activity in reproductive tissues. The complex formed when estrogen binds to its receptors migrates to the nucleus and regulates the expression of certain genes, including telomerase (Misiti et al., 2000). It has been known for some time that T cells can bind to estrogen via specific estrogen receptors. Thus, we tested whether pre-incubation of T cells to 17β-estradiol prior to activation might augment telomerase activity. Our data suggest that estrogen does, in fact, enhance T cell telomerase activity (Effros et al., 2005).

Another potential modulator of telomerase activity in human T cells is Vitamin D (Chou, Parish, & Effros R.B., 2010), which is actually a hormone that is increasingly being studied for its immune system effects (Adams, Liu, Chun, Modlin, & Hewison, 2007; Liu & Modlin, 2008; Walker & Modlin, 2009). Thus, therapeutic approaches that are based on telomerase modulation would seem to be promising candidates for clinical interventions that are aimed at reversing or retarding the process of replicative senescence in T cells.

Other possible strategies for regenerating/ rejuvenating the immune system are also worth considering. It has been repeatedly observed that a large proportion of senescent CD8 T cells are directed at CMV (Pawelec et al., 2004; Pawelec, Derhovanessian, Larbi, Strindhall, & Wikby, 2009). Therefore, development of a vaccine against this virus might offer a practical preventive approach for eliminating one of the major driving forces for generating senescent CD8 T cells (Pawelec et al., 2004). Alternatively, actual physical removal of senescent cells from the circulation might stimulate both the expansion of more functional (nonsenescent) memory cells and the production of naïve T cells by the thymus. Indeed, it is possible that thymic output may be inhibited during old age, at least in part, by the presence of expanded T cell populations in the periphery.

Life-Style Interventions

Another category of therapeutic approaches relate to lifestyle, which has been repeatedly shown to affect health status and immune function. Indeed, several mechanistic studies have shown how various dietary components can modulate certain inflammatory pathways, including sympathetic activity, oxidative stress, and proinflammatory cytokine secretion (Kiecolt-Glaser, 2010; Wu & Meydani, 2008). The current obesity epidemic is predicted to further exacerbate the inflammatory milieu, leading to metabolic disfunction and

several age-related pathologies (Iyer, Fairlie, Prins, Hammock, & Brown, 2010). Recent behavioral studies have shown that stressful events and depression can have similar pro-inflammatory effects. Moreover, stress can influence food choices and can even enhance maladaptive metabolic responses to unhealthful meals. Diet can also affect mood and the cytokine production patterns (Kiecolt-Glaser, 2010). Ongoing studies are addressing the bi-directional interactions between the vagus nerve, which innervates tissues involved in digestion, with nutrient absorption, metabolism, in signal transduction within the gut that leads to inflammation. These studies will undoubtedly increase our understanding of how stressors, unhealthful diet choices, and negative emotions synergize to enhance inflammation, which plays a key role in chronic disease and life span.

Inflammation can also be modulated by exercise, which is well known to not only enhance immune function, but also to reduce psychological stress. A review covering research performed over a 30-year period concludes that habitual physical activity is associated with a long-term "anti-inflammatory" effect (Kasapis & Thompson, 2005). Consistent with those studies, Tai Chi, a traditional Chinese martial art that incorporates aerobic activity, relaxation, and mediation, has also been shown to improve immune function. This form of exercise is particularly appropriate for use in older people, who often have physical limitations in their ability to tolerate even moderately intensive exercise. A recent 16-week prospective randomized control trial documented that Tai Chi induced an increase in cell-mediated immunity to the varicella zoster virus that was comparable in magnitude to that induced by the varicella vaccine. Moreover, there was an additive effect: Tai Chi, together with vaccine, produced a substantially higher level of immunity than the vaccine alone (Irwin, Olmstead, & Oxman, 2007).

It has been suggested that mindfulness meditation may have salutory effects on health by reducing psychological stress and arousal (Epel, Daubenmier, Moskowitz, Folkman, & Blackburn, 2009). Meditation has also been suggested to affect aging at the cellular level (Epel et al., 2009). Given the role of telomere maintenance in immune cell function, and its association with human longevity and optimal health, interventions that can reduce psychological stress, which has been associated with telomere shortening (Epel et al., 2004; Damjanovic et al., 2007), are predicted to improve health status. Thus, meditative practices may retard

T cell replicative senescence both by decreasing the levels of stress hormones (e.g., cortisol) and oxidative stress, and by increasing certain hormones that protect telomeres. Another example of the biological effect of mindfulness meditation comes from studies on HIV/AIDS, which, as noted earlier, is a model of premature immunological aging (Appay & Rowland-Jones, 2002; Effros, 2009a). In a small randomized controlled trial on stressed HIV-infected adults, meditation was shown to retard the loss of helper (CD4) T cells (Creswell, Myers, Cole, & Irwin, 2009). Since CD4 T cell count is one of the prime biomarkers of disease status, these studies suggest that changes in psychological stress can actually modulate HIV disease pathogenesis. In sum, the field of stress-induced cell aging, although still in its early stage of development, holds great promise to provide novel mechanistic insights into the field of psychoneuroimmunology.

Concluding Remarks

It is clear that multiple factors can function as immune-system stressors. The effects of persistent viral infections on immune function have been fairly well described, particularly with respect to mechanistic pathways involving telomere-based cellular aging. Other immune system stressors, induced by free radicals and oxidative changes are also under extensive investigation. Least understood are the precise pathways by which emotional problems, chronic psychological stress, and mental disorder, such as depression, can affect immune function and health. These issues will become increasingly relevant with the current demographic shift. The immune systems of elderly persons are already substantially altered, due to chronological aging. The added burden of psychological stressors may further compromise immunity and contribute to disease. Thus, the main research challenge with respect to health enhancement of the ever-increasing elderly population will be to translate some of the basic science observations into practical approaches for improving the quality of life of older persons. Some of the lifestyle interventions discussed earlier represent noninvasive, practical approaches that are particularly relevant to older persons.

Future Directions/Unsolved Problems

The field of psychoneuroimmunology has finally become part of mainstream biomedical science. Anecdotal reports of catching colds during final-exam week, or becoming ill during periods of grief are being replaced by complex mechanistic studies that address multiple important issues related to the mind-body connection. Indeed, advances in neuroscience and immunology have established both anatomical and cellular basis for interactions between the nervous and immune systems. However, most of this work has been done on the innate immune system. Thus, one new promising direction will address the following question: What anatomical links exist between the nervous system and cells/organs involved in adaptive immunity?

A second important question regarding the mind/body connection is: What is the role of the immune system in the initiation and progression of dementia and Alzheimer's disease? This issue is becoming increasingly urgent, based on the high risk of developing AD after reaching age 85. The vaccine that prevented AD in a mouse "model" of the disease actually caused massive brain inflammation in some humans with AD, suggesting that the human disease may not be accurately modeled in rodents. Recent studies on T cells from young, young trisomy 21, old, and old AD have clearly demonstrated differences in T cell reactivity to the amyloid-beta protein, which accumulates in AD brains. The cytokine patterns of T cells stimulated with amyloid beta peptides were quite distinct in the different groups—specifically, older persons with AD and persons with trisomy 21 (all of whom develop AD by age 40) showed a switch from the usual Th1 pattern to an IL-10-mediated regulatory pattern (Loewenbrueck et al., 2008). Further research into the early events involved in the disease initiation will be important in enhancing healthspan and quality of life in the very old.

Finally, there are multiple associations between having high proportions of senescent T cells and with poor health outcomes and mortality. Understanding the cellular basis for these epidemiological links will be critical in developing treatment approaches. Do senescent cells act directly to suppress an ongoing immune response, or does their enhanced production of pro-inflammatory cytokines functions indirectly blunt immunity and promote disease? And what are the cellular pathways by which psychological stress exacerbates various diseases of aging? These and other questions will undoubtedly be essential as the field of psychoneuroimmunology matures further and contributes novel insights into health and longevity.

References

Adams, J. S., Liu, P. T., Chun, R., Modlin, R. L., & Hewison, M. (2007). Vitamin D in defense of the human immune response. *Annals of the New York Academy of Sciences, 1117,* 94–105.

Ahmadzadeh, M., Johnson, L. A., Heemskerk, B., Wunderlich, J. R., Dudley, M. E., White, D. E., & Rosenberg, S. A. (2009). Tumor antigen-specific CD8 T cells infiltrating the tumor express high levels of PD-1 and are functionally impaired. *Blood, 114,* 1537–1544.

Appay, V., & Rowland-Jones, S. (2002). Premature ageing of the immune system: The cause of AIDS? *Trends in Immunology, 23,* 580–585.

Arron J. R., & Choi, Y. (2000). Bone versus immune system. *Nature, 408,* 535–536.

Atzmon, G., Cho, M., Cawthon, R. M., Budagov, T., Katz, M., Yang, X.,…Suh, Y. (2010). Evolution in health and medicine Sackler colloquium: Genetic variation in human telomerase is associated with telomere length in Ashkenazi centenarians. *Proceedings of the National Academy of Science U.S.A, 107*(1), 1710–1717.

Barengolts, E. I., Berman, M., Kukreja, S. C., Kouznetsova, T., Lin, C., & Chomka, E. V. (1998). Osteoporosis and coronary atherosclerosis in asymptomatic postmenopausal women. *Calcified Tissue International, 62,* 209–213.

Brouilette, S., Singh, R. K., Thompson, J. R., Goodall, A. H., & Samani, N. J. (2003). White cell telomere length and risk of premature myocardial infarction. *Arteriosclerosis, Thrombosis, Vascular Biology, 23,* 842–846.

Buchinsky, F. J., Ma, Y., Mann, G. N., Rucinski, B., Bryer, H. P., Romero, D. F.,…Epstein, S. (1996). T lymphocytes play a critical role in the development of cyclosporin A-induced osteopenia. *Endocrinology, 137,* 2278–2285.

Butler, J. J., Mader, J. S., Watson, C. L., Zhang, H., Blay, J., & Hoskin, D. W. (2003). Adenosine inhibits activation-induced T cell expression of CD2 and CD28 co-stimulatory molecules: role of interleukin-2 and cyclic AMP signaling pathways. *Journal of Cellular Biochemistry, 89,* 975–991.

Campisi, J. (1997). The biology of replicative senescence. *Europeaan Journal of Cancer, 33,* 703–709.

Cao, W., Jamieson, B. D., Hultin, L. E., Hultin, P. M., Effros, R. B., & Detels, R. (2009). Premature aging of t-cells is associated with faster hiv-1 disease progression. *Journal of Acquired Immunodeficiency Syndrome, 50,* 137–147.

Cawthon, R. M., Smith, K. R., O'Brien, E., Sivatchenko, A., & Kerber, R. A. (2003). Association between telomere length in blood and mortality in people aged 60 years or older. *Lancet, 361,* 393–395.

Chang, W. C., Li, C. H., Huang, S. C., Chang, D. Y., Chou, L. Y., & Sheu, B. C. (2010). Clinical significance of regulatory T cells and CD8+ effector populations in patients with human endometrial carcinoma. *Cancer, 116,* 5777–5788.

Characiejus, D., Pasukoniene, V., Kazlauskaite, N., Valuckas, K. P., Petraitis, T., Mauricas, M., & Den Otter, W. (2002). Predictive value of CD8highCD57+ lymphocyte subset in interferon therapy of patients with renal cell carcinoma. *Anticancer Research, 22,* 3679–3683.

Choi, J., Fauce, S. R., & Effros, R. B. (2008). Reduced telomerase activity in human T lymphocytes exposed to cortisol. *Brain, Behavior, and Immunity, 22,* 600–605.

Chou, J., Parish, S. T., & Effros R. B. (2010). Modulatory effects of inflammatory isoprostanes and vitamin D on telomerase in human T lymphocytes: Impact on bone loss during aging. Inflammation and Aging: Causes and Consequences.39th Annual Meeting of the American Aging Association, 2010, oral presentation.

Clowes, J. A., Riggs, B. L., & Khosla, S. (2005). The role of the immune system in the pathophysiology of osteoporosis. *Immunogical Reviews, 208,* 207–227.

Creswell, J. D., Myers, H. F., Cole, S. W., & Irwin, M. R. (2009). Mindfulness meditation training effects on CD4+ T lymphocytes in HIV-1 infected adults: A small randomized controlled trial. *Brain, Behavior, and Immunity, 23,* 184–188.

Dagarag, M. D., Evazyan, T., Rao, N., & Effros, R. B. (2004). Genetic manipulation of telomerase in HIV-specific CD8+ T cells: Enhanced anti-viral functions accompany the increased proliferative potential and telomere length stabilization. *Journal of Immunology, 173,* 6303–6311.

Dagarag, M. D., Ng, H., Lubong, R., Effros, R. B., & Yang, O. O. (2003). Differential impairment of lytic and cytokine functions in senescent HIV-1-specific cytotoxic T lymphocytes. *Journal of Virology, 77,* 3077–3083.

Damjanovic, A. K., Yang, Y., Glaser, R., Kiecolt-Glaser, J. K., Nguyen, H., Laskowski, B., et al. (2007). Accelerated telomere erosion is associated with a declining immune function of caregivers of Alzheimer's disease patients. *Journal of Immunology, 179,* 4249–4254.

Demissie, S., Levy, D., Benjamin, E. J., Cupples, L. A., Gardner, J. P., Herbert, A., et al. (2006). Insulin resistance, oxidative stress, hypertension, and leukocyte telomere length in men from the Framingham Heart Study. *Aging Cell, 5,* 325–330.

DosReis, G. A., Nobrega, A. F., & de Carvalho, R. P. (1986). Purinergic modulation of T lymphocyte activation: Differential susceptibility of distinct activation steps and correlation with intracellular 3',5'-cyclic adenosine monophosphate accumulation. *Cellular Immunology, 101,* 213–231.

Edwards, C. J., Hart, D. J., & Spector, T. D. (2000). Oral statins and increased bone-mineral density in postmenopausal women. *Lancet, 355,* 2218–2219.

Effros, R. B. (2009a). HIV disease: Model of premature immunological aging. In T.Fulop, C. Franceschi, K. Hirokawa, & G. Pawelec (Eds.), *Handbook on immunosenescence: Basic understanding and clinical applications* (pp. 949–964). Springer Science+Business Media B.V.

Effros, R. B. (2009b). Kleemeier Award lecture 2008. The canary in the coal mine: Telomeres and human healthspan. *Journals of Gerontology Series A: Biological Sciences and Medical Sciences, 64,* 511–515.

Effros, R. B., Allsopp, R., Chiu, C. P., Wang, L., Hirji, K., Harley, C. B., et al. (1996). Shortened telomeres in the expanded CD28-CD8+ subset in HIV disease implicate replicative senescence in HIV pathogenesis. *AIDS/Fast Track, 10,* F17–F22.

Effros, R. B., Boucher, N., Porter, V., Zhu, X., Spaulding, C., Walford, R. L., et al. (1994). Decline in CD28+ T cells in centenarians and in long-term T cell cultures: A possible cause for both in vivo and in vitro immunosenescence. *Experimental Gerontology, 29,* 601–609.

Effros, R. B., Dagarag, M. D., Spaulding, C. C., & Man, J. (2005). The role of CD8 T cell replicative senescence in human aging. *Immunological Reviews, 205,* 147–157.

Effros, R. B., & Pawelec, G. (1997). Replicative senescence of T lymphocytes: Does the Hayflick Limit lead to immune exhaustion? *Immunology Today, 18,* 450–454.

Effros, R. B., Zhu, X., & Walford, R. L. (1994). Stress response of senescent T lymphocytes: Reduced hsp70 is independent of the proliferative block. *Journal of Gerontology, 49,* B65–B70.

Epel, E. S., Blackburn, E. H., Lin, J., Dhabhar, F. S., Adler, N. E., Morrow, J. D., et al. (2004). Accelerated telomere shortening in response to life stress. *Proceedings of the .Nationall. Academy. of Science. U.S.A, 101,* 17312–17315.

Epel, E., Daubenmier, J., Moskowitz, J. T., Folkman, S., & Blackburn, E. (2009). Can meditation slow rate of cellular aging? Cognitive stress, mindfulness, and telomeres. *Annals of the New York Academy of Sciences, 1172,* 34–53.

Fauce, S. R., Jamieson, B. D., Chin, A. C., Mitsuyasu, R. T., Parish, S. T., Ng, H. L., et al. (2008). Telomerase-based pharmacologic enhancement of anitviral function of human CD8+ T lymphocytes. *Journal of Immunology, 181,* 7400–7406.

Frauwirth, K. A., Riley, J. L., Harris, M. H., Parry, R. V., Rathmell, J. C., Plas, D. R. et al. (2002). The CD28 signaling pathway regulates glucose metabolism. *Immunity, 16,* 769–777.

Gessi, S., Varani, K., Merighi, S., Fogli, E., Sacchetto, V., Benini, A. et al. (2007). Adenosine and lymphocyte regulation. *Purinergic Signalling, 3,* 109–116.

Glaser, R., & Kiecolt-Glaser, J. K. (2005). Stress-induced immune dysfunction: Implications for health. *Nature Reviews Immunology., 5,* 243–251.

Goldman, N., Chen, M., Fujita, T., Xu, Q., Peng, W., Liu, W., et al. (2010). Adenosine A1 receptors mediate local antinociceptive effects of acupuncture. *Nature Neuroscience, 13,* 883–888.

Goronzy, J. J., Fulbright, J. W., Crowson, C. S., Poland, G. A., O'Fallon, W. M., & Weyand, C. M. (2001). Value of immunological markers in predicting responsiveness to influenza vaccination in elderly individuals. *Journal of Virology, 75,* 12182–12187.

Goronzy, J. J., & Weyand, C. M. (2005). T cell development and receptor diversity during aging. *Current Opinion in Immunology, 17,* 468–475.

Gouin, J. P., Hantsoo, L., & Kiecolt-Glaser, J. K. (2008). Immune dysregulation and chronic stress among older adults: A review. *Neuroimmunomodulation, 15,* 251–259.

Graham, L. S., Parhami, F., Tintut, Y., Kitchen, C. M., Demer, L. L., & Effros, R. B. (2009). Oxidized lipids enhance RANKL production by T lymphocytes: implications for lipid-induced bone loss. *Clinical Immunology, 133,* 265–275.

Graham, L. S., Tintut, Y., Parhami, F., Kitchen, C. M., Ivanov, Y., Tetradis, S., et al. (2010). Bone density and hyperlipidemia: The T lymphocyte connection. *Journal of Bone and Mineral Research, 11,* 2460–2469.

Gruber, I. V., El Yousfi, S., Durr-Storzer, S., Wallwiener, D., Solomayer, E. F., & Fehm, T. (2008). Down-regulation of CD28, TCR-zeta (zeta) and up-regulation of FAS in peripheral cytotoxic T cells of primary breast cancer patients. *Anticancer Research, 28,* 779–784.

Hathcock, K. S., Weng, N. P., Merica, R., Jenkins, M. K., & Hodes, R. (1998). Antigen-dependent regulation of telomerase activity in murine T cells. *Journal of Immunology, 160,* 5702–5706.

Hershfield, M. S. (2005). New insights into adenosine-receptor-mediated immunosuppression and the role of adenosine in causing the immunodeficiency associated with adenosine deaminase deficiency. *European Journal of Immunology, 35,* 25–30.

Holdorf, A. D., Kanagawa, O., & Shaw, A. S. (2000). CD28 and T cell co-stimulation. *Reviews in Immunogenetics, 2,* 175–184.

Hubbard, R. E., O'Mahony, M. S., Savva, G. M., Calver, B. L., & Woodhouse, K. W. (2009). Inflammation and frailty measures in older people. *Journal of Cellular and Molecular Medicine, 13,* 3103–3109.

Irwin, M. R., Olmstead, R., & Oxman, M. N. (2007). Augmenting immune responses to varicella zoster virus in older adults: A randomized, controlled trial of Tai Chi. *Journal of the American Geriatrics Society, 55,* 511–517.

Iyer, A., Fairlie, D. P., Prins, J. B., Hammock, B. D., & Brown, L. (2010). Inflammatory lipid mediators in adipocyte function and obesity. *Nature Reviews Endocrinology, 6,* 71–82.

Janeway C. A., Jr, Travers, P., & Walpert, M. S. M. (2001). *The immune system in health and disease* (5th ed.). Princeton, NJ: Garland Publishing, Inc..

Jenkins, E. C., Velinov, M. T., Ye, L., Gu, H., Li, S., Jenkins, E. C., Jr. et al. (2006). Telomere shortening in T lymphocytes of older individuals with Down syndrome and dementia. *Neurobiology of Aging, 27,* 941–945.

Jerne, N. K. (1974). Towards a network theory of the immune system. *Annals of Immunology(Paris), 125*(C), 373–389.

John, V., Hock, J. M., Short, L. L., Glasebrook, A. L., & Galvin, R. J. (1996). A role for CD8+ T lymphocytes in osteoclast differentiation in vitro. *Endocrinology, 137,* 2457–2463.

Kasapis, C., & Thompson, P. D. (2005). The effects of physical activity on serum C-reactive protein and inflammatory markers: A systematic review. *Journal of the American College of Cardiology, 45,* 1563–1569.

Kiecolt-Glaser, J. K. (2009). Psychoneuroimmunology psychology's gateway to the biomedical future. *Perspectives on Psychological Science, 4,* 367–369.

Kiecolt-Glaser, J. K. (2010). Stress, food, and inflammation: Psychoneuroimmunology and nutrition at the cutting edge. *Psychosomatic Medicine, 72,* 365–369.

Knudson, M., Kulkarni, S., Ballas, Z. K., Bessler, M., & Goldman, F. (2005). Association of immune abnormalities with telomere shortening in autosomal-dominant dyskeratosis congenita. *Blood, 105,* 682–688.

Kong, Y. Y., Boyle, W. J., & Penninger, J. M. (2000). Osteoprotegerin ligand: A regulator of immune responses and bone physiology. *Immunology Today, 21,* 445–502.

Laroche, M., Pouilles, J. M., Ribot, C., Bendayan, P., Bernard, J., Boccalon, H. et al. (1994). Comparison of the bone mineral content of the lower limbs in men with ischaemic atherosclerotic disease. *Clinical Rheumatology, 13,* 611–614.

Li, Y., Liu, S., Hernandez, J., Vence, L., Hwu, P., & Radvanyi, L. (2010). MART-1—Specific melanoma tumor-infiltrating lymphocytes maintaining CD28 expression have improved survival and expansion capability following antigenic restimulation in vitro. *Journal of Immunology, 184,* 452–465.

Lichterfeld, M., Mou, D., Cung, T. D., Williams, K. L., Waring, M. T., Huang, J., et al. (2008). Telomerase activity of HIV-1-specific CD8+ T cells: Constitutive upregulation in controllers and selective increase by blockade of PD ligand 1 in progressors. *Blood, 112,* 3679–3687.

Lin, J., Epel, E., Cheon, J., Kroenke, C., Sinclair, E., Bigos, M. et al. (2010). Analyses and comparisons of telomerase activity and telomere length in human T and B cells: Insights for epidemiology of telomere maintenance. *Journal of Immunological Methods, 352,* 71–80.

Liu, P. T., & Modlin, R. L. (2008). Human macrophage host defense against Mycobacterium tuberculosis. *Current Opinion In Immunology, 20,* 371–376.

Loewenbrueck, K. F., Tigno-Aranjuez, J. T., Boehm, B. O., Lehmann, P. V., & Tary-Lehmann, M. (2008). Th1 responses to beta-amyloid in young humans convert to regulatory IL-10 responses in Down syndrome and Alzheimer's disease. *Neurobiology of Aging, 10,* 1732–1742.

MacKenzie, W. M., Hoskin, D. W., & Blay, J. (1994). Adenosine inhibits the adhesion of anti-CD3-activated killer lymphocytes to adenocarcinoma cells through an A3 receptor. *Cancer Research, 54,* 3521–3526.

Maini, M. K., Soares, M. V., Zilch, C. F., Akbar, A. N., & Beverley, P. C. (1999). Virus-induced CD8+ T cell clonal expansion is associated with telomerase up-regulation and telomere length preservation: a mechanism for rescue from replicative senescence. *Journal of Immunology, 162,* 4521–4526.

McElhaney, J. E., Upshaw, C. M., Hooton, J. W., Lechelt, K. E., & Meneilly, G. S. (1998). Responses to influenza vaccination in different T cell subsets: A comparison of healthy young and older adults. *Vaccine, 16,* 1742–1747.

Mehta, S. K., Cohrs, R. J., Forghani, B., Zerbe, G., Gilden, D. H., & Pierson, D. L. (2004). Stress-induced subclinical reactivation of varicella zoster virus in astronauts. *Journal of Medical Virology, 72,* 174–179.

Mehta, S. K., Stowe, R. P., Feiveson, A. H., Tyring, S. K., & Pierson, D. L. (2000). Reactivation and shedding of cytomegalovirus in astronauts during spaceflight. *Journal of Infectious Diseases, 182,* 1761–1764.

Meier, C. R., Schlienger, R. G., Kraenzlin, M. E., Schlegel, B., & Jick, H. (2001). Statins and fracture risk. *JAMA, 286,* 669–670.

Meloni, F., Morosini, M., Solari, N., Passadore, I., Nascimbene, C., Novo, M. et al. (2006). Foxp3 expressing CD4+ CD25+ and CD8+CD28- T regulatory cells in the peripheral blood of patients with lung cancer and pleural mesothelioma. *Human Immunology, 67,* 1–12.

Mignini, F., Streccioni, V., & Amenta, F. (2003). Autonomic innervation of immune organs and neuroimmune modulation. *Autonomic and Autacoid Pharmacology, 23,* 1–25.

Misiti, S., Nanni, S., Fontemaggi, G., Cong, Y. S., Wen, J., Hirte, H. W., et al. (2000). Induction of hTERT expression and telomerase activity by estrogens in human ovary epithelium cells. *Molecular and Cellular Biology, 20,* 3764–3771.

O'Connor, M. F., & Irwin, M. R. (2010). Links between behavioral factors and inflammation. *Clinical Pharmacology and Therapeutics, 87,* 479–482.

Ohta, A., Ohta, A., Madasu, M., Kini, R., Subramanian, M., Goel, N., et al. (2009). A2A adenosine receptor may allow expansion of T cells lacking effector functions in extracellular adenosine-rich microenvironments. *Journal of Immunology, 183,* 5487–5493.

Pacheco, R., Riquelme, E., & Kalergis, A. M. (2010). Emerging evidence for the role of neurotransmitters in the modulation of T cell responses to cognate ligands. *Central Nervous System Agents in Medicinal Chemistry, 10,* 65–83.

Panossian, L., Porter, V. R., Valenzuela H. F., Masterman, D., Reback, E., Cummings, J., et al. (2002). Telomere shortening in T cells correlates with Alzheimer's disease status. *Neurobiology of Aging, 24,* 77–84.

Parish, S. T., Kim, S., Sekhon, R. K., Wu, J. E., Kawakatsu, Y., & Effros, R. B. (2010). Adenosine deaminase modulation of telomerase activity and replicative senescence in human CD8 T lymphocytes. *Journal of Immunology, 184,* 2847–2854.

Parish, S. T., Wu, J. E., & Effros, R. B. (2009). Modulation of T lymphocyte replicative senescence via TNF-{alpha} inhibition: role of caspase-3. *Journal of Immunology, 182,* 4237–4243.

Pawelec, G., Akbar, A., Caruso, C., Effros, R. B., Grubeck-Loebenstein, B., & Wikby, A. (2004). Is immunosenescence infectious? *Trends in Immunology, 25,* 406–410.

Pawelec, G., Derhovanessian, E., Larbi, A., Strindhall, J., & Wikby, A. (2009). Cytomegalovirus and human immunosenescence. *Reviews in Medical Virology, 19,* 47–56.

Perillo, N. L., Naeim, F., Walford, R. L., & Effros, R. B. (1993). The in vitro senescence of human lymphocytes: Failure to divide is not associated with a loss of cytolytic activity or memory T cell phenotype. *Mechanisms of Ageing and Development, 67,* 173–185.

Perillo, N. L., Walford, R. L., Newman, M. A., & Effros, R. B. (1989). Human T lymphocytes possess a limited in vitro lifespan. *Experimental Gerontology, 24,* 177–187.

Pietschmann, P., Grisar, J., Thien, R., Willheim, M., Kerschan-Schindl, K., Preisinger, E. et al. (2001). Immune phenotype and intracellular cytokine production of peripheral blood mononuclear cells from postmenopausal patients with osteoporotic fractures. *Experimental Gerontology, 36,* 1749–1759.

Rosas-Ballina, M., & Tracey, K. J. (2009). The neurology of the immune system: Neural reflexes regulate immunity. *Neuron, 64,* 28–32.

Samani, N. J., Boultby, R., Butler, R., Thompson, J. R., & Goodall, A. H. (2001). Telomere shortening in atherosclerosis. *Lancet, 358,* 472–473.

Sansom, D. M. (2000). CD28, CTLA-4 and their ligands: Who does what and to whom? *Immunology, 101,* 169–177.

Saurwein-Teissl, M., Lung, T. L., Marx, F., Gschosser, C., Asch, E., Blasko, I. et al. (2002). Lack of antibody production following immunization in old age: association with CD8(+) CD28(-) T cell clonal expansions and an imbalance in the production of Th1 and Th2 cytokines. *Journal of Immunology, 168,* 5893–5899.

Schule, J. M., Bergkvist, L., Hakansson, L., Gustafsson, B., & Hakansson, A. (2004). CD28 expression in sentinel node biopsies from breast cancer patients in comparison with CD3-zeta chain expression. *Journal of Translational Medicine, 2,* 45.

Shimizu, Y., Van Seventer, G., Ennis, E., Newman, W., Horgan, K., & Shaw, S. (1992). Crosslinking of the T cell-specific accessory moleculesCD7 and CD28 modulates T cell adhesion. *Journal of Experimental Medicine, 175,* 577–582.

Sompayrac, L. (2008). *How the immune system works* (3rd ed.). Malden, MA: Blackwell Publishing , Inc.

Spaulding, C. S., Guo, W., & Effros, R. B. (1999). Resistance to apoptosis in human CD8+ T cells that reach replicative senescence after multiple rounds of antigen-specific proliferation. *Experimental Gerontology, 34,* 633–644.

Spyridopoulos, I., Hoffmann, J., Aicher, A., Brummendorf, T. H., Doerr, H. W., Zeiher, A. M., et al. (2009). Accelerated telomere shortening in leukocyte subpopulations of patients with coronary heart disease: role of cytomegalovirus seropositivity. *Circulation, 120,* 1364–1372.

Stowe, R. P., Mehta, S. K., Ferrando, A. A., Feeback, D. L., & Pierson, D. L. (2001). Immune responses and latent herpesvirus reactivation in spaceflight. *Aviation, Space, and Environmental Medicine, 72,* 884–891.

Sze, D. M., Giesajtis, G., Brown, R. D., Raitakari, M., Gibson, J., Ho, J. et al. (2001). Clonal cytotoxic T cells are expanded in myeloma and reside in the CD8(+)CD57(+)CD28(–) compartment. *Blood, 98*, 2817–2827.

Szondy, Z. (1994). Adenosine stimulates DNA fragmentation in human thymocytes by Ca(2+)-mediated mechanisms. *Biochemical Journal, 304*(3), 877–885.

Takayanagi, H., Ogasawara, K., Hida, S., Chiba, T., Murata, S., Sato, K., et al. (2000). T cell-mediated regulation of osteoclastogenesis by signalling cross-talk between RANKL and IFN-gamma. [Comment In: Nature. 2000 Nov 30;408(6812):535–6 UI: 21003806]. *International Immunology, 408*, 600–605.

Tentolouris, N., Nzietchueng, R., Cattan, V., Poitevin, G., Lacolley, P., Papazafiropoulou, A., et al. (2007). White blood cells telomere length is shorter in males with type 2 diabetes and microalbuminuria. *Diabetes Care, 30*, 2909–2915.

Trieb, K., Ransmayr, G., Sgonc, R., Lassmann, H., & Grubeck-Loebenstein, B. (1996). APP peptides stimulate lymphocyte proliferation in normals, but not in patients with Alzheimer's disease. *Neurobiology of Aging, 17*, 541–547.

Urbaniak-Kujda, D., Kapelko-Slowik, K., Wolowiec, D., Dybko, J., Halon, A., Jazwiec, B. et al. (2009). Increased percentage of CD8+CD28- suppressor lymphocytes in peripheral blood and skin infiltrates correlates with advanced disease in patients with cutaneous T-cell lymphomas. *Postepy higieny i medycyny doswiadczalnej (Online.), 63*, 355–359.

Uyama, O., Yoshimoto, Y., Yamamoto, Y., & Kawai, A. (1997). Bone changes and carotid atherosclerosis in postmenopausal women. *Stroke, 28*, 1730–1732.

Valenzuela, H. F., & Effros, R. B. (2002). Divergent telomerase and CD28 expression patterns in human CD4 and CD8 T cells following repeated encounters with the same antigenic stimulus. *Clinical Immunology, 105*, 117–125.

Vallejo, A. N., Nestel, A. R., Schirmer, M., Weyand, C. M., & Goronzy, J. J. (1998). Aging-related deficiency of CD28 expression in CD4+ T cells is associated with the loss of gene-specific nuclear factor binding activity. *Journal of Biological Chemistry, 273*, 8119–8129.

Vaziri, H., Schachter, F., Uchida, I., Wei, L., Zhu, X., Effros, R. et al. (1993). Loss of telomeric DNA during aging of normal and trisomy 21 human lymphocytes. *American Journal of Human Genetics, 52*, 661–667.

Vedhara, K., Cox, N. K., Wilcock, G. K., Perks, P., Hunt, M., Anderson, S. et al. (1999). Chronic stress in elderly careers of dementia patients and antibody response to influenza vaccination. *Lancet, 353*, 627–631.

Walker, V. P., & Modlin, R. L. (2009). The vitamin D connection to pediatric infections and immune function. *Pediatric Research, 65*, 106R–113R.

Wang, E., Lee, M. J., & Pandey, S. (1994). Control of fibroblast senescence and activation of programmed cell death. *Journal of Cellular Biochemistry, 54*, 432–439.

Webb, J. R., Wick, D. A., Nielsen, J. S., Tran, E., Milne, K., McMurtrie, E., et al. (2010). Profound elevation of CD8+ T cells expressing the intraepithelial lymphocyte marker CD103 (alphaE/beta7 Integrin) in high-grade serous ovarian cancer. *Gynecologic Oncology, 118*, 228–236.

Wikby, A., Johansson, B., Olsson, J., Lofgren, S., Nilsson, B. O., & Ferguson, F. (2002). Expansions of peripheral blood CD8 T lymphocyte subpopulations and an association with cytomegalovirus seropositivity in the elderly: the Swedish NONA immune study. *Experimental Gerontology, 37*, 445–453.

Wu, D., & Meydani, S. N. (2008). Age-associated changes in immune and inflammatory responses: Impact of vitamin E intervention. *Journal of Leukocyte Biology, 84*, 900–914.

Yang, O. O., Lin, H., Dagarag, M., Ng, H. L., Effros, R. B., & Uittenbogaart, C. H. (2005). Decreased perforin and granzyme B expression in senescent HIV-1-specific cytotoxic T lymphocytes. *Virology, 332*, 16–19.

Ye, S. W., Wang, Y., Valmori, D., Ayyoub, M., Han, Y., Xu, X. L., et al. (2006). Ex-vivo analysis of CD8+ T cells infiltrating colorectal tumors identifies a major effector-memory subset with low perforin content. *Journal of Clinical Immunology, 26*, 447–456.

Zachariae, R. (2009). Psychoneuroimmunology: A bio-psycho-social approach to health and disease. *Scandanavian Journal of Psychology, 50*, 645–651.

PART 2

Emotion

Physiological Correlates of Self-Conscious Emotions

Sally S. Dickerson

Abstract

Self-conscious emotions, such as shame and embarrassment, are painful and intense emotions, yet they have been understudied within psychoneuroimmunology. However, several studies have examined the biological correlates of self-conscious emotions, and far more have demonstrated that the social-evaluative stressors, which can induce these emotions, are potent elicitors of physiological reactivity. Self-conscious emotions—and the social contexts that elicit them—can be associated with immunological changes, including increases in pro-inflammatory cytokine activity. These conditions can also lead to increases in cortisol and sympathetic nervous system activity, which have implications for immunological functioning. The self-conscious emotional and physiological changes can occur in concert under social-evaluative threat, leading to correlations between the affective and physiological responses. Future research should continue to examine the specificity of the associations between self-conscious emotions and physiological outcomes, the role of the social context in eliciting these changes, and the health implications of these effects.

Key Words: social-evaluative threat, self-conscious emotion, cortisol, pro-inflammatory cytokine, stress, shame, guilt, cardiovascular reactivity

Self-conscious emotions—such as shame, humiliation, and embarrassment—are considered among the most intense and painful of human emotions. Although research has carefully documented the elicitors and functions of self-conscious emotions as well as their consequences for behavioral and mental health outcomes (e.g., Tracy, Robins & Tangney, 2007), relatively little attention has focused on the physiological correlates of these emotional states. Instead, much of the work documenting associations between emotion and physiology centers on distress, negative affect, or depression; when specific emotions are examined, the focus is often on anger, fear, or other "basic" emotions. However, a growing body of evidence suggests that self-conscious emotions can have physiological correlates, including immunologic, neuroendocrine, and autonomic

parameters. Several studies have now directly examined the biological correlates of self-conscious emotions, and far more have demonstrated that the social-evaluative stressors, which can induce these emotions, are potent elicitors of physiological reactivity. This chapter will review the findings demonstrating that self-conscious emotions—and the social contexts that elicit these emotions—can be associated with immunological changes, as well as shifts in neuroendocrine and autonomic parameters that have implications for immunological functioning.

One theoretical perspective linking self-conscious emotion to physiological parameters is social self-preservation theory (e.g., Dickerson, Gruenewald & Kemeny, 2004; Dickerson, Gruenewald & Kemeny, 2011; Gruenewald, Dickerson, & Kemeny, 2007). This theory proposes that conditions that threaten one's social self—or threaten one's social esteem, status, or acceptance—are capable of triggering psychological and physiological responses. These include increases in self-conscious emotions, such as shame, and increases in different physiological parameters, including cortisol, pro-inflammatory cytokine production and cardiovascular or sympathetic nervous system activity. These changes can occur in concert, leading to correlations between the self-conscious emotional and physiological responses. Although acute social self threats, and the self-conscious emotions engendered, may elicit short-term changes in these physiological parameters, more chronic or enduring forms of social threat could have implications for physiological and health outcomes.

Prototypical threats to the social self include conditions in which an important aspect of the self is or could be negatively judged by others (i.e., social-evaluative threat [SET]; Dickerson & Kemeny, 2004). Many different contexts could induce SET. For example, it could be experienced in performance situations that require displays of valued attributes, such as competence or intelligence, in front of others (e.g., a speech, competition, or interview). Social-evaluative threat could also occur in contexts of potential or explicit rejection, in which one could be judged unworthy of acceptance. The underlying evaluative, rejecting component of these situations could jeopardize or threaten the social self and set into motion these psychobiological changes, with self-conscious emotional and physiological responses elicited in parallel under SET.

Self-Conscious Emotion: Elicitors and Functions

The category of "negative self-conscious emotions" typically includes the similar yet distinct emotions of shame, guilt, and embarrassment. Following Gilbert (1997), we view shame as the prototypical emotion elicited under threats to the social self, although other self-conscious emotions (e.g., embarrassment, humiliation) may often be experienced as well.

Shame is experienced when a core aspect of the self is judged as flawed, inadequate, or inferior (Gilbert, 1997; Tangney, 1995; Tracy & Robins, 2004). It often is associated with a sense of exposure, in which a negative characteristic is revealed before a real or imagined audience (Tangney, 1995). Shame is accompanied by the motivation to disengage or withdraw from the situation (e.g., wanting to "shrink," "disappear" and avoid interpersonal interaction; Tangney, 1995) and is often associated by nonverbal displays denoting submission or appeasement (e.g., head down, gaze avoidance, slumped posture; Gilbert, 1997; Keltner & Buswell, 1996; Tracy, Robins & Schriber, 2009). This could be an adaptive social signal of appeasement, which could serve to reduce conflict and aggression and increase social bonds and cohesion (e.g., Keltner, 1995; Gilbert, 2000).

The self-evaluative nature of shame is often contrasted with the related emotion of guilt. With shame, the self is thought to be the object of negative evaluation; with guilt, the negative evaluation is an aspect of one's behavior (Lewis, 1971; Weiner, 1985). Indeed, empirical studies support that negative characterological self-evaluation is fundamental to shame, and can be differentiated from guilt along this dimension (Niedenthal, Tangney, & Gavanski, 1994; Tangney, Niedenthal, Covert, & Barlow, 1998).

Embarrassment and shame are closely related, as both can be elicited from social transgressions and self-presentational flaws. However, embarrassment is thought to stem from more trivial social transgressions or revealing a flaw that is not central to the self, in comparison to the more serious transgressions or characterological flaws associated with shame (Tangney, Miller, Flicker, & Barlow, 1996; Miller & Tangney, 1994). In response to social self threat, shame and embarrassment are often experienced together, whereas guilt is reported to a lesser extent (e.g., Dickerson, Mycek, & Zaldivar, 2008; Gruenewald, Kemeny, Aziz, & Fahey, 2004).

Social-Evaluative Threat and Self-Conscious Emotion

A rich theoretical and empirical literature documents that self-conscious emotions can be triggered by threats to the social self. For example, Darwin (1871/1899) proposed that shame "relates almost exclusively to the judgment of others" (p. 144) and William James (1890/1950) thought this emotion originated from others' perceptions of an impaired image of the self. This resonates with modern theories that shame and related emotions serve as a marker of a loss of belonging, social status, and acceptance (e.g., Gilbert, 1997; Leary, Tambor, Terdal, & Downs, 1995).

Studies that have experimentally manipulated SET in the laboratory also support the premise that self-conscious emotion is induced by these contexts. Gruenewald and colleagues (2004) randomly assigned participants to complete a speech and computerized math task either alone in a room (non-SET condition) or in front of a two-member audience panel that was stoic throughout the tasks (SET condition). Participants in the SET condition reported greater increases in shame from pre- to posttask than those in the non-SET condition; an effect recently replicated other investigations (e.g., Bosch et al., 2009; Dickerson et al., 2008). Furthermore, several studies have reported that among those in SET conditions, greater levels of shame were observed than other negative emotions, such as distress or anxiety (Dickerson et al., 2008; Gruenewald et al., 2004; Raspopow, Abizaid, Matheson, & Anisman, 2010). Taken together, these findings suggest that self-conscious emotions such as shame can be elicited under SET, and they often can be experienced to a greater degree than other negative emotional states under these conditions.

Physiological Effects of Social Threat and Self-Conscious Emotion

Relatively few studies have directly examined the physiological correlates of self-conscious emotion. However, the physiological concomitants of this class of emotions can be inferred through research on their eliciting conditions—social-evaluative and rejecting contexts.

Research in nonhuman primates and other animals have documented the effects of social threat on physiological parameters. Studies of acute and chronic threats to social status have demonstrated that subordinate, low-ranked animals have higher levels of cortisol and other HPA hormones compared to their more dominant, higher-ranked peers (e.g., Sapolsky, 2005; Shively, Laber-Laird, & Anton, 1997). Additionally, the subordinate animals who display greater levels of submissive behaviors also show the greatest elevations in HPA activation (e.g., Shively et al., 1997). Social subordination or threats to status can elicit increases in autonomic and cardiovascular parameters, including increases in heart rate and the hormones epinephrine and norepinephrine (e.g., Shively, Register, Friedman, Morgan, Thompson, & Lanier, 2005; Stefanski, 2000).

Social threat can also alter immunological functioning, including processes related to inflammation. Following tissue injury or infection, an inflammatory response can be initiated. This process is orchestrated by pro-inflammatory cytokines, including tumor necrosis factor-alpha (TNFα), interleukin-6 (Il-6), and interleukin-1β (Il-1β), which are produced primarily by macrophages and monocytes. Pro-inflammatory cytokines are

chemical communication molecules that can alter the production and movement of different types of immune cells and can induce the signs and symptoms of inflammation.

There is evidence that other threats besides pathogens and injuries can trigger inflammatory responses; a number of studies have shown that threats to social status in nonhuman animals are capable of increasing inflammatory markers. Subordinate or socially defeated animals have shown increases in pro-inflammatory cytokines (e.g., TNF-α, Il-6) and other parameters indicative of inflammation (e.g., increases in granulocytes, nerve growth factor; (e.g., Avitsur, Stark, & Sheridan, 2001; Quan et al., 2001; Stark, Avitsur, Padgett, & Sheridan, 2001; Stark, Avitsur, Hunzeker, Padgett, & Sheridan, 2002).

Taken together, these studies show that social threat in nonhuman animals can elicit inflammatory processes as well as increases in cortisol and autonomic activity. Importantly, in some studies, submissive behavior has correlated with these physiological changes. Submissive behaviors in nonhuman primates and other animals have been proposed as primitive analogues of submission and shame behaviors in humans (e.g., Gilbert, 2000; Keltner, Young, & Buswell, 1997). Therefore, these investigations into the physiological consequences of social threat—and the physiological correlates of submissive behavior more specifically—suggest that shame displays and social threat in humans may be accompanied by similar psychobiological responses.

In the following sections, the literature on the neuroendocrine, autonomic, and immunologic effects of social-evaluative threat are reviewed, accompanied by a discussion of the smaller number of studies that have specifically examined the relationship between self-conscious emotion and these parameters.

Self-Conscious Emotion and Cortisol
Social-Evaluation and Cortisol Reactivity

This is now a great deal of evidence that social-evaluative threat can elicit strong and significant cortisol responses. In a meta-analysis of 208 acute psychological stressor studies (Dickerson & Kemeny, 2004), we found that tasks with social evaluation (e.g., audience present) were associated with much larger cortisol increases than those without this element; in fact, the SET stressors were associated with an effect size of approximately three times the magnitude of those without an evaluative component. This effect was particularly heightened under uncontrollable, social-evaluative tasks; this combination was associated with heightened reactivity and delayed times to recovery compared to those with just one or none of these characteristics.

Other studies have experimentally manipulated SET in the laboratory. Gruenewald and colleagues (2004) had participants deliver a speech and perform a difficult computerized math task in one of two conditions: a social-evaluative condition, in which two panelists were present to evaluate their performance, and a nonsocial evaluative condition, in which the participants were alone in a room. Only the SET condition elicited a significant cortisol response; those completing the identical task in a nonsocial context showed no increases in cortisol. This demonstrates that social-evaluative contexts can elicit robust cortisol responses, particularly when contrasted with otherwise equivalent non-SET conditions. This finding has now been replicated in a number of studies that have manipulated SET utilizing psychosocial laboratory stressors (e.g, Bosch et al., 2009; Dickerson et al., 2008; Het, Rohleder, Schoofs, Kirschbaum, & Wolf, 2009; Taylor et al., 2010) or physical stressors (i.e., cold pressor task; Schwabe, Haddad, & Schachinger, 2008).

The SET/cortisol linkage has also been examined in naturalistic contexts. Rohleder and colleagues (2007) used ballroom-dancing competitions as a naturally occurring model of SET. Cortisol samples were collected from dancers on a practice day and on a competition day, in which their performances were judged by an evaluative panel. The competition day was associated with much more pronounced increases in cortisol compared to the practice day, demonstrating the heightened cortisol response under social-evaluative threat. Furthermore, the more the dancers reported feeling stressed by the judges, the larger their cortisol responses, suggesting that increasing perceptions of social evaluation were associated with increasing cortisol responses.

Other research has examined the effects of rejection on cortisol responses. For example, children who were rejected by peers showed elevated cortisol levels compared to those who were more accepted (Gunnar, Sebanc, Tout, Donzella, & van Dulman, 2003). Studies that have manipulated rejection in the lab (e.g., through ostracism, ignoring) have demonstrated greater increases in cortisol in response to rejecting rather than accepting conditions, however, these effects appear stronger among subsets of participants, such as women (Stroud, Tanofsky-Kraff, Wilfley, & Salovey, 2000), those low on defensiveness (Blackhart, Eckel, & Tice,

2007), those experiencing high levels of peer victimization (Zwolinski, 2008), or those low on self-esteem (Ford & Collins, 2010).

Self-Conscious Emotion and Cortisol

The findings just described demonstrate that shame-inducing experiences of SET can elicit cortisol reactivity. A growing number of studies have tested the specific association between state self-conscious emotion and cortisol responses in this type of an acute social-evaluative context. For example, in the Gruenewald et al. (2004) study, those in the social-evaluative condition reported greater levels of self-conscious emotion and showed greater cortisol responses compared to those in the non-SET condition. In addition, the emotional and physiological responses were correlated; those that showed greater increases in self-conscious emotions also showed the greatest increases in cortisol. Importantly, this was specific to self-conscious emotions; this did not emerge for other negative emotions, such as anxiety. Therefore, the cortisol response was more closely tied to self-conscious emotions than other emotions assessed.

Several studies have now replicated this association between cortisol reactivity and self-conscious emotion. Dickerson et al. (2008) also found that participants in a social-evaluative condition who reported greater increases in self-conscious cognitions and emotions also had greater cortisol responses. Again, there was no relationship between other negative emotions (e.g., fear, sadness) and cortisol reactivity. More recently, another study also found the same association between heightened self-conscious emotions and cortisol responses (Raspopow, Abizaid, Matheson, & Anisman, 2010); although this correlation has not always emerged (Bosch et al., 2009).

Other studies have primed the emotion of shame in order to experimentally test this association between self-conscious emotion and cortisol reactivity. Matheson and Anisman (2009) had participants complete a short-story writing task in which they were to recreate and extend a scenario in their own words; they were randomly assigned to include a list of target words in their story, which were descriptors of either anger (anger prime condition), shame (shame prime condition), or had no affective content (control condition). The participants then experienced a discrimination stressor, in which they were lead to believe that the reason they had received a failing grade on a previous task was due to discrimination from the grader. Those who were primed with shame showed elevated cortisol levels after this discrimination stressor compared to those primed with anger or in the control condition. Interestingly, when participants received failure feedback allegedly based on their performance (rather than discrimination), there was no association with cortisol. This suggests that the stressor may need to have a social component for this self-conscious emotion/cortisol linkage to emerge.

The self-conscious emotion/cortisol association has also been examined in the context of economic decision making. Dunn and colleagues (2010) had participants play a game in which they could choose to donate some of their payment to others. They found that the more money participants chose to keep for themselves, the higher their levels of shame; furthermore, shame predicted postgame cortisol levels. Additional analyses demonstrated that shame mediated the effect of donation amount on cortisol; those who donated less felt higher levels of shame, which in turn was associated with elevated cortisol.

Developmental studies have provided additional evidence for a relationship between self-conscious emotion and cortisol. For example, Lewis and Ramsay (2002) had four-year-old children complete different tasks, and self-conscious emotional expressions were subsequently coded (e.g., body collapsed, gaze downward, withdrawal). Those children who displayed more self-conscious emotion across the session had elevated cortisol levels; this was a large effect, $d = 0.79$. In fact, there was a 127% increase in the likelihood of self-conscious emotional expression for each standard deviation increase in cortisol.

Another study with four-year-old children examined self-conscious emotion and cortisol (Mills, Imm, Walling, & Weiler, 2008). They found that the expression of shame in response to failure in boys predicted greater cortisol reactivity as well as slower recovery. There was also some evidence for emotion specificity in this effect; although both shame and sadness correlated with reactivity, only shame correlated with recovery, and there was no association between cortisol and anger. For girls, it was a more complicated story, but there was evidence that a subset of those showing high levels of shame also showed higher peak cortisol and slower times to recovery.

Taken together, these developmental studies demonstrate an association between self-conscious emotional expression and cortisol among young children. It is important to note that these studies assessed nonverbal self-conscious emotional expression, rather than self-reported emotion, which is often assessed with studies in adult populations. This dovetails nicely with recent evidence that nonverbal submissive, self-conscious displays predict elevations in cortisol in adults (Carney, Cuddy, & Yap, 2010). Participants who were randomly assigned to assumed submissive postures had elevated cortisol relative to participants in a dominant posture condition. This demonstrates that, across children and adults, expressive displays indicative of submission or self-consciousness are associated with elevations in cortisol.

The studies just reviewed all examined the association between self-conscious emotion and cortisol in an acute stressor context. However, many stressors are chronic and ongoing. Preliminary evidence suggests that social stressors—and the self-conscious emotions they elicit—are associated with elevated HPA activity as well. A meta-analysis found that chronic stressors that threatened the social self were associated with higher cortisol levels throughout the day compared to nonsocial chronic stressors (Miller, Chen & Zhou, 2007). Additionally, chronic stressors that were likely to induce shame were associated with higher levels of evening cortisol than those less likely to be associated with this emotion. Therefore, chronic social stressors and those associated with self-conscious emotion were associated with greater HPA activity.

Self-Conscious Emotion and Cortisol: Boundary Conditions
SOCIAL CONTEXT

The social context of the shame experience may be an important factor to consider when examining associations. Indeed, it has been proposed that threats to the social self trigger self-conscious emotion and cortisol reactivity, and that the nature of the threat is central to the elicitation of an emotional and physiological response (e.g., Dickerson et al., 2004). Therefore, shame experienced in a nonsocial context (i.e., in the absence of social-evaluative threat) may not be accompanied by the same biological responses. Consistent with this premise, two studies (Gruenewald et al., 2004; Dickerson et al., 2008) have found correlations between self-conscious emotion and cortisol to emerge only under social-evaluative conditions; there was no relationship between self-conscious emotion and cortisol reactivity in stressor context that was not explicitly evaluative (e.g., alone in a room).

This idea that only self-conscious emotion experienced under SET may be associated with cortisol reactivity is also consistent with several studies that have not found relationships between self-conscious emotion and cortisol. Dickerson and colleagues (Dickerson, Kemeny, Aziz, Kim, & Fahey, 2004) had participants anonymously and confidentially write essays on experiences in which they blamed themselves. Although this did lead to significant increases in shame and guilt, cortisol levels declined across the session, and there was no relationship between cortisol and shame. Danielson, Matheson, & Anisman (2011) found similar results using an essay-writing task in which participants read and wrote essays on abuse or a control topic; no relationship between cortisol and shame (or other negative emotions) emerged. However, the writing tasks in these studies were not explicitly social, and, in fact, they downplayed any evaluative component. Therefore, the social context of the stressor may be an important moderator of the shame/cortisol relationship.

This premise may also in part account for why *trait* shame has not consistently been associated with cortisol (although very few studies have investigated this question). One study failed to find a relationship between shame proneness and cortisol responses (Tops, Boksem, Wester, Lorist, & Meijman, 2006), although this was examined in the context of a nonsocial stressor task. Additionally, Rohleder and colleagues (Rohelder, Chen, Wolf, & Miller, 2008) found that trait shame was not associated with several indices of hypothalamic-pituitary-adrenal (HPA) activity: total cortisol output throughout the day, cortisol slope, or the cortisol awakening response. However, it was not clear whether the participants experienced shame in response to a social threat, which could be an important antecedent for triggering cortisol responses.

Taken together, these findings suggest that the social context may be an important factor to consider when examining the relationship between self-conscious emotion and cortisol. This is consistent with the premise that SET triggers a psychobiological response that includes self-conscious emotion and HPA activity; with the association between self-conscious emotion and cortisol reactivity hinging on the presence of this threat.

INDIVIDUAL DIFFERENCES

Individual differences may also be important moderators of the relationship between self-conscious emotion and cortisol. For example, Gruenewald and colleagues (Gruenewald, Kemeny, & Aziz, 2006) found the relationship between self-conscious emotion and cortisol reactivity emerged only among those reporting high subjective status. Although those lower in status reported equally high levels of self-conscious emotion, they showed dissociations between self-conscious and cortisol responses; despite increases in self-conscious emotion, they did not show increases in cortisol in the context of social-evaluative threat. This suggests that certain individual difference factors may dissociate the affective and physiological responses. Future research, which incorporates individual differences, affective responses, and cortisol reactivity will further delineate these relationships.

Psychiatric disorders may also alter the relationship between self-conscious emotion and cortisol. For example, one study reported that self-conscious emotion correlated with *lower* levels of cortisol among combat veterans with posttraumatic stress disorder (PTSD) (Mason et al., 2001). Specifically, veterans who were undergoing inpatient PTSD treatment had lower levels of 24-hour urinary cortisol when they reported higher levels of shame and guilt. There are several ways to interpret this finding. First, it could be that these relationships are different or altered in the context of a psychiatric diagnosis. Second, PTSD has been associated with hypocortisolism; therefore, it is possible that higher levels of shame could lead to greater dysregulation (e.g., lower levels in this context). Future research that teases apart these complex relationships between chronic stressors, psychiatric disorders, and HPA activity are needed to address these complex questions.

Self-Conscious Emotion and Autonomic Activity
Social-Evaluative Threat and Autonomic Responses

Social-evaluative conditions can strongly increase cardiovascular parameters. Social-evaluative tasks can lead to increases in systolic blood pressure (SBP), diastolic blood pressure (DBP), and heart rate (HR; e.g., Kirschbaum, Pirke, & Hellhammer, 1993). Naturally occurring instances of SET can also elicit increases in cardiovascular activity; when participants reported feeling social evaluation in daily contexts, they showed elevated levels of SBP and DBP compared to times in which they did not feel others were evaluating them (Lehman & Conley, 2010). Other studies have shown that SET can elicit increases in markers of sympathetic activity (e.g., epinephrine, norepinephrine, alpha-amylase; Lovallo & Thomas, 2000; Nater & Rohleder, 2009).

A number of studies have manipulated the social-evaluative nature of the stressor and examined the effects on cardiovascular parameters. This has been accomplished through the presence or absence of social evaluation, emphasizing or de-emphasizing evaluative components, or having confederates display evaluative versus neutral or supportive behavior. Taken together, these studies have found that tasks that are more social-evaluative are associated with greater cardiovascular or sympathetic reactivity when compared to less evaluative conditions (e.g., Christian & Stoney, 2006; Gerin, Pieper, Levy & Pickering, 1992; Gruenewald et al., 2004; Lepore, Allen & Evans, 1993; Sheffield & Carroll, 1994; Smith, Nealey, Kircher, & Limon, 1997). However, this has not been found in all cases (e.g, Dickerson, Gable, Irwin, Aziz, & Kemeny, 2009; Kelsey et al., 2000). Social-evaluative threat may interact with other factors, such as task difficulty, to predict heightened cardiovascular reactivity (Blascovich, Mendes, Hunter, & Salomon, 1999; Wright, Tunstall, Williams, Goodwin, & Harmon-Jones, 1995).

Other research has examined impedance and electrocardiographic assessment when testing the effects of social evaluation on cardiovascular responses. This can help determine whether the increases in cardiovascular activity are due to myocardial (i.e., the heart beating faster) or vascular (i.e., blood vessels constricting) changes. Several studies have demonstrated shortening of pre-ejection period (PEP) in response to performing under social-evaluative versus nonsocial evaluative conditions (e.g., Christian & Stoney, 2006; Kelsey et al., 2000), which may indicate greater myocardial reactivity when social evaluation is present.

One study manipulated SET by randomly assigning participants to deliver speeches in front of audiences of various sizes (no panelists, 1 panelist, or 4 panelists; Bosch et al., 2009). They found greater increases in heart rate and reductions in PEP with increasing audience size, and vagal withdrawal was also greater in audience conditions. Taken together, these studies demonstrate marked cardiovascular and/or sympathetic reactivity under conditions of SET.

Self-Conscious Emotion and Autonomic Activity

There have been several studies that have directly examined the effects of self-conscious emotion on cardiovascular reactivity. Harris (2001) induced embarrassment by having participants sing "The

Star Spangled Banner" in front of a videocamera, and then they watched, with several confederates, the video of themselves singing. In two studies that utilized this paradigm, when participants then publically watched the video, they showed increases in systolic and diastolic blood pressure as well as heart rate. These effects were heightened when participants were told to suppress their emotions while watching their singing video. Furthermore, the increase in heart rate correlated with self-reported increase in embarrassment; no other emotions were associated with the cardiovascular parameters.

Another study also found that embarrassment-inducing tasks (e.g., singing a song and delivering a speech, then watching the videotapes of both performances) lead to increases in heart rate, higher skin conductance levels, and decreases in respiratory sinus arrhythmia (RSA; Hofmann, Moscovitch, & Kim, 2006). Similar patterns of results were found for social anxiety, indicating that there may be overlap in the autonomic correlates of these two emotional states. Another study that utilized similar methodology found increases in heart rate and skin conductance and no change in RSA (Gerlach, Wilhelm, & Roth, 2003). The authors conclude that this is indicative of sympathetic activation, and that parasympathetic activity may play less of a role in the psychophysiology of embarrassment (Gerlach et al., 2003).

Only a handful of studies have specifically focused on the autonomic correlates of shame. Rohleder and colleagues (2008) found that trait shame predicted greater sympathetic activity (salivary alpha amylase) across the day. Herrald and Tomaka (2002) induced shame in participants by having them complete a public speaking task in the presence of social evaluation, which highlighted the participant's inability to live up to expectations. They found increases in heart rate and PEP responses (indicative of sympathetic activation) when compared to a neutral stressor condition. They also found greater increases in total peripheral resistance in this shame-inducing context as well. This pattern of cardiovascular changes, characterized by increases in cardiac reactivity and high vascular resistance is indicative of the "threat" response described by Blascovich and colleagues (e.g., Blascovich & Mendes, 2000).

Taken together, research has demonstrated that self-conscious emotion is often accompanied by broad sympathetic activation and vagal withdrawal (Kreibig, 2010). Very few studies have directly compared the autonomic and/or cardiovascular correlates of self-conscious emotion to other negative emotional states (cf. Herrald & Tomaka, 2002) and so it is difficult to determine whether these effects are unique to self-conscious emotion or whether they overlap with others. Indeed, the patterns of psychophysiological changes seen with self-conscious emotional expression share similarities with anger and anxiety (Kreibig, 2010). Future research is needed to delineate the psychophysiological correlates of self-conscious emotions, and to determine the overlap and divergence with other related emotional states.

Immunologic Correlates of Self-Conscious Emotion
Immunological Effects of SET

Many studies have demonstrated that acute social threat can lead to changes in immunological parameters, including the number and type of cells in circulation and how these cells function. A meta-analytic review found that acute stressors can reliably elicit shifts in immunologic parameters, including increases in natural killer cell and cytotoxic T lymphocyte numbers (Segerstrom & Miller, 2004). Additionally, increases in circulating levels of inflammatory markers, such as Il-6 and Il-1β, have also been observed (Steptoe, Hamer, & Chida, 2007). Acute stressors can also lead to functional changes, including increases in natural killer (NK) cell cytotoxicity (i.e., the ability of NK cells to lyse a target cell) and decreases in lymphocyte proliferation (i.e., the ability of lymphocytes to multiply and divide upon stimulation; Segerstrom & Miller, 2004). Taken together, this suggests that acute stressors can up-regulate nonspecific or natural immunity while down-regulating specific immunity. This pattern of changes is thought to be adaptive under conditions of acute threat, in which injury or exposure to pathogens would require a rapid mobilization of the immune system. It is important to note that these meta-analyses included many different types of stressors, some of which were social-evaluative and others which were not.

We specifically compared the pro-inflammatory response to stressors that varied in their social-evaluative context (Dickerson et al., 2009). This was based evidence from research in nonhuman animals demonstrating that inflammatory parameters can increase in response to social threat (e.g., Avitsur et al., 2001). We randomly assigned healthy women to perform a speech and math stressor either alone in a room (non-SET) or in front of an evaluative audience (SET). Among those in the SET condition, we found increases in the production of TNF-α from

pre- to poststressor, and these increases were maintained throughout a 40 minute recovery period. In contrast, there were no increases in TNF-α among those in the non-SET condition. Participants in both conditions reported that the task was difficult, demanding, and effortful; however, only those performing the in front of an evaluative audience showed increases in this marker of inflammation. Furthermore, we found that those participants who felt the most evaluated during the task showed the largest increases in TNF-α production; no relationship emerged with other task appraisals (e.g., perceptions of effort, task difficulty, or how well they performed). Therefore, the SET condition elicited greater increases in pro-inflammatory activity, and individual differences in perceptions of social evaluation were linked with these changes.

Research has also linked chronic forms of social threat to inflammatory processes. For example, experiencing more interpersonal stressors predicted elevated levels of C-reactive protein, a marker of systemic inflammation (Fuligni et al., 2009). Higher levels of chronic interpersonal stress have also been associated with greater increases over time in stimulated production of the pro-inflammatory cytokine Il-6 (Miller, Rohleder, & Cole, 2009). This study also demonstrated that chronic interpersonal stress predicted greater expression of genes involved in transducing inflammatory signals. This is consistent with research showing that individuals high on loneliness (who may experience chronic threats to social acceptance or belonging) also have increased gene expression related to inflammatory signaling pathways (Cole, 2008). Taken together, this research documents that, like acute social threats, chronic interpersonal threats are linked with an upregulation of inflammatory processes.

Inflammation and Self-Conscious Emotion

Few studies have specifically have examined the immunological correlates of self-conscious emotion. We examined this association by randomly assigning participants to write about a traumatic experience in which they blamed themselves, or to write about a neutral topic (Dickerson, Kemeny, Aziz, Kim, & Fahey, 2004). Those writing about an experience of self-blame increased in their feelings of the self-conscious emotions of shame and guilt from pre- to postwriting, whereas those in the neutral condition showed no changes in self-conscious emotion as a result of the procedures. Those in the self-blame condition showed increases in the soluble receptor for TNF-α, a marker of TNF-α activity, whereas those writing about a neutral topic did not show changes in this parameter. Furthermore, those reporting the greatest increase in shame also showed the greatest increase in TNF-α activity; no relationship emerged between this inflammatory marker and other negative emotions (e.g., guilt, fear, or sadness). This demonstrates that conditions that induce self-conscious emotions can also elicit increases inflammatory activity.

Another study examined the association between trait shame and inflammatory activity. Rohleder and colleagues (2008) had participants complete a measure assessing experiences of shame over the past few months. They found that this measure of trait shame correlated with stimulated Il-6 production, such that the more shame participants felt, the greater their pro-inflammatory response. However, Il-6 production was not associated with trait guilt. Therefore, this study extends previous findings of a relationship between self-conscious emotion and pro-inflammatory cytokine activity to a chronic or trait context.

SET, Inflammation, and Hormonal Interactions

What might be the physiological mechanism leading to exaggerated inflammatory responses in the context of SET? Sympathetic and HPA products can influence macrophage activity as well as cytokine expression and production, and these systems have been proposed as mediators of the stressor/psychological state/cytokine relationship.

Autonomic products could elicit changes in pro-inflammatory cytokine expression and production. Specifically, at physiological doses, the ANS hormones norepinephrine and epinephrine can have direct, stimulatory effects on pro-inflammatory cytokines (DeRijk, Boelen, Tilders, & Berkenbosch, 1994; Norris & Benveniste, 1993). Autonomic activity could also lead to activation of the pro-inflammatory cytokine system through an additional mechanism. The transcription factor nuclear factor κB (NF-κB) can regulate the transcription of genes involved in the inflammatory response, including the expression and production of TNFα and Il-6. Therefore, increases in NF-κB could translate into increases in downstream pro-inflammatory cytokine activation.

Research has demonstrated that NF-κB activity in response to social-evaluative threat in humans (Bierhaus et al., 2003). In a subsequent in vitro study, a dose-dependent relationship was found between physiologically relevant increases in norepinephrine and NF-κB expression (Bierhaus et al., 2003). This suggests the possibility that heightened autonomic activity in response to social-evaluative stressors could be associated with increases in pro-inflammatory cytokine expression and production. Future studies that manipulate social-evaluative threat and/or self-conscious emotion could clarify the mechanism through which increased pro-inflammatory cytokine production may occur.

Research has demonstrated that social threat may influence the relationship between inflammatory processes and cortisol. Under basal conditions, the glucocorticoid hormone cortisol is an anti-inflammatory that can suppress pro-inflammatory cytokine production and other components of the immune system. This relationship may be altered under social threat. Research in nonhuman animal models demonstrates that glucocorticoids are less able to reign in or suppress inflammatory responses after social threat, leading to decreases in glucocorticoid sensitivity (Avistur, Padgett, & Sheridan, 2006). These decreases in glucocorticoid sensitivity may be specific to social threat, because other types of stressors have not resulted in this shift (e.g., physical restraint; Sheridan, Stark, Avitsur, & Padgett, 2000). Studies in humans have also shown that acute social threat can affect glucocorticoid sensitivity (Rohleder, Wolf, & Kirschbaum, 2003).

To test whether glucocorticoid sensitivity is specific to social threat, as demonstrated in the nonhuman animal literature, we manipulated social-evaluative threat in the laboratory (Dickerson, Gable et al., 2009). To test glucocorticoid sensitivity, cortisol was added to wells containing pro-inflammatory cytokine-producing cells, and then the ability of the glucocorticoid to suppress the production of these cytokines was determined. Consistent with hypotheses, women performing a speech and math task in front of an evaluative audience (SET) showed decreases in the suppressive effects of glucocorticoids, compared to those performing the identical task but in a non-SET context (alone in a room). These findings demonstrate that social threat not only can elicit cortisol and pro-inflammatory activity, but it can also affect the regulation of these processes.

Only one study to date has examined the association between shame and glucocorticoid sensitivity. Contrary to hypotheses, they found that higher levels of trait shame predicted increases in glucocorticoid sensitivity (Rohleder et al., 2008). Clearly, more research is needed to tease apart the complex relationships between social threat, self-conscious emotion, and glucocorticoid regulation of the inflammatory response.

Questions and Future Directions

Although there is substantial evidence that the social-evaluative conditions that induce the self-conscious emotions can elicit a range of physiological responses, fewer studies have directly examined the correlates of self-conscious emotions. Studies that incorporate the assessment of self-conscious emotions—as well as other comparative negative emotions—are needed to further clarify their role in the SET-physiological reactivity associations. Despite the small number of studies that have been conducted on the physiological correlates of self-conscious emotion, the emerging findings suggests that this class of emotions is worthy of continuing empirical investigation. These future studies should replicate and extend these findings, and they should address important questions that are raised by this nascent area of research.

One important issue to examine is whether self-conscious emotions mediate the effects of SET on physiological outcomes. Although a growing number of studies have reported correlations between self-conscious emotions and physiological parameters (e.g., cortisol; Dickerson et al., 2008; Gruenewald et al., 2004; Raspopow et al., 2010), these studies have not been able to find evidence of mediation, that is, that the increases in cortisol observed under SET hinges on the experience of self-conscious emotion. There are several reasons that studies may have failed to establish mediation. First, physiological changes observed under SET have their own temporal sequencing; for example, cortisol peaks approximately 20–40 minutes after the onset of a stressor (Dickerson & Kemeny, 2004). Models that test for different time-lagged effects may be more likely to establish potential mediation. Second, most studies only assess self-reported emotion; composites that incorporate nonverbal expressions may provide a more comprehensive marker of self-conscious emotional expression to include in meditational tests. Third, and most importantly, it may be that SET elicits implicit or explicit appraisals of social evaluation, which, in turn, then drive both self-conscious emotion and physiological responses. This would explain the pattern of findings that self-conscious emotion and physiological parameters are correlated, but no mediation is observed. Future research that further delineates the causal ordering of these processes will be important to clarify these complex relationships.

Another question facing this area of research is the specificity of the physiological changes observed when self-conscious emotion is experienced. Very few studies have compared the relationship between physiological parameters and a wide variety of emotional states; incorporating assessment of a fuller range of emotions could help further articulate the conditions under which certain threats trigger certain emotional and physiological responses. A growing number of studies have demonstrated correlations between self-conscious emotion and cortisol responses under social-evaluative conditions, and this association has not emerged with other negative emotions (i.e. fear; Gruenewald et al., 2004; Dickerson et al., 2008). However, other studies have reported correlations between other negative emotions and cortisol reactivity such as anger (Moons, Eisenberger, & Taylor, 2010) or fear (Lerner, Dahl, Hariri, & Taylor, 2007). Simultaneously and comprehensively assessing a variety of physiological systems may uncover physiological "signatures" that could be associated with different emotional states. For example, it may be that self-conscious emotion experienced under social-evaluative conditions may be associated with increases in cortisol, pro-inflammatory cytokine production, and sympathetic activity; this combination of changes may be different for different threats, and for different emotions.

It will also be important to differentiate between the self-conscious emotions and to examine to what degree their physiological correlates are unique or overlapping. There is evidence that shame and guilt are associated with different physiological profiles. Multiple studies have demonstrated that shame—but not guilt—correlates with cortisol and pro-inflammatory cytokine production (e.g., Dickerson, Kemeny et al., 2004; Gruenewald et al., 2004; Rohleder et al., 2008), suggesting that the physiological profiles of these emotions may be distinct. Whether other self-conscious emotional pairings, such as shame and embarrassment, are also associated with different physiological parameters has received less attention. This is likely due, in part, to high correlations between these emotions under social-evaluative conditions (e.g., Dickerson et al., 2008).

Another issue is whether the physiological correlates of self-conscious emotion hinge on the social context. There is evidence for this within cortisol research; shame elicited under SET is associated with cortisol reactivity, whereas more private shame experiences are less closely tied to this physiological parameter. It is less clear how the social context may moderate the effects of self-conscious emotion on other physiological outcomes, such as autonomic or cardiovascular activity. The degree to which the physiology of self-conscious emotions is shaped by the social nature of the threat is important to disentangle in future research.

Taken together, the research on the physiological correlates of self-conscious emotion suggests promising new avenues to explore relationships between stress, emotion, and health. Continuing to elucidate the pathways through which certain social threats may trigger specific emotional and physiological responses could isolate mechanisms through which stressors could lead to disease.

References

Avitsur, R., Padgett, D. A., & Sheridan, J. F. (2006). Social interactions, stress, and immunity. *Neurology Clinics, 24,* 483–491.

Avitsur, R., Stark, J. L., & Sheridan, J. F. (2001). Social stress induces glucocorticoid resistance in subordinate animals. *Hormones and Behavior, 39,* 247–257.

Bierhaus, A., Wolf, J., Andrassy, M., Rohleder, N., Humpert, P. M., Petrov, D., et al. (2003). A mechanism converting psychosocial stress into mononuclear cell activation. *Proceedings of the National Academy of Sciences of the USA, 100,* 1920–1925.

Blackhart, G. C., Eckel, L. A., & Tice, D. M. (2007). Salivary cortisol in response to acute social rejection and acceptance by peers. *Biological Psychology, 75,* 267–276.

Blascovich, J., & Mendes, W. B. (2000). Challenge and threat appraisals: The role of affective cues. In J. P. Forgas (Ed.), *Feeling and thinking: The role of affect in social cognition* (pp. 59–82). New York: Cambridge University Press.

Blascovich, J., Mendes, W. B., Hunter, S. B., & Salomon, K. (1999). Social facilitation as challenge and threat. *Journal of Personality and Social Psychology, 77,* 68–77.

Bosch, J. A., De Gues, E. J. C., Carroll, D., Goedhart, A. D., Anane, L. A., Veldhuizen, et al. (2009). A general enhancement of autonomic and cortisol responses during social evaluative threat. *Psychosomatic Medicine, 71,* 877–885.

Carney, D. R., Cuddy, A. J., & Yap, A. J. (2010). Power posing: Brief nonverbal displays affect neuroendocrine levels and risk tolerance. *Psychological Science, 21,* 1363–1368.

Christian, L. M., & Stoney, C. M. (2006). Social support versus social evaluation: Unique effects on vascular and myocardial response patterns. *Psychosomatic Medicine, 68,* 914–921.

Cole, S. W. (2008). Social regulation of leukocyte homeostasis: The role of glucocorticoid sensitivity. *Brain, Behavior, and Immunity, 22,* 1049–1055.

Danielson, A. M., Matheson, K., & Anisman, H. (2011). Cytokine levels at a single time point following a reminder stimulus among women in abusive dating relationships: Relationship to emotional states. *Psychoneuroendocrinology, 36,* 40–50.

Darwin, C. (1871/1899). *The descent of man* (2nd ed.). London, England: Murray.

DeRijk, R. H., Boelen, H., Tilders, F. J., & Berkenbosch, F. (1994). Induction of plasma interleukin-6 by circulating adrenaline in the rat. *Psychoneuroendocrinology, 19,* 155–163.

Dickerson, S. S., Gable, S. L., Irwin, M. R., Aziz, N., & Kemeny, M. E. (2009). Social-evaluative threat and proinflammatory cytokine regulation: An experimental laboratory investigation. *Psychological Science, 20,* 1237–1244.

Dickerson, S. S., Gruenewald, T. L., & Kemeny, M. E. (2011). Physiological effects of social threat: Implications for health. In J. Cacioppo & J. Decety, (Eds.), *Handbook of Social Neuroscience* (pp. 787–803). New York: Oxford University Press.

Dickerson, S. S., Gruenewald, T. L., & Kemeny, M. E. (2004). When the social self is threatened: Shame, physiology, and health. *Journal of Personality, 72,* 1191–1216.

Dickerson, S. S., & Kemeny, M. E. (2004). Acute stressors and cortisol responses: A theoretical integration and synthesis of laboratory research. *Psychological Bulletin, 130*(3), 355–391.

Dickerson, S. S., Kemeny, M. E., Aziz, N., Kim, K. H., & Fahey, J. L. (2004). Immunological effects of induced shame and guilt. *Psychosomatic Medicine, 66,* 124–131.

Dickerson, S. S., Mycek, P. M., & Zaldivar, F. P. (2008). Negative social evaluation, but not mere social presence, elicits cortisol responses to a laboratory stressor task. *Health Psychology, 27,* 116–121.

Dunn, E. W., Ashton-James, C. E., Hanson, M. D., & Aknin, L. B. (2010). On the costs of self-interested economic behavior: How does stinginess get under the skin? *Journal of Health Psychology, 15,* 627–633.

Ford, M. B., & Collins, N. L. (2010). Self-esteem moderates neuroendocrine and psychological responses to interpersonal rejection. *Journal of Personality and Social Psychology, 98,* 405–419.

Fuligni, A., Telzer, E. H., Bower, J., Cole, S. W., Kiang, L., & Irwin, M. R. (2009). A preliminary study of daily interpersonal stress and c-reactive protein levels among adolescents from Latin American and European Backgrounds. *Psychosomatic Medicine, 71*(3), 329–333.

Gerin, W., Pieper, C., Levy, R., & Pickering, T. G. (1992). Social support in social interaction: A moderator of cardiovascular reactivity. *Psychosomatic Medicine, 54,* 42–58.

Gerlach, A. L., Wilhelm, F. H., & Roth, W. T. (2003). Embarrassment and social phobia: The role of parasympathetic activation. *Anxiety Disorders, 17,* 197–210.

Gilbert, P. (1997). The evolution of social attractiveness and its role in shame, humiliation, guilt, and therapy. *British Journal of Medical Psychology, 70,* 113–147.

Gilbert, P. (2000). Varieties of submissive behavior as forms of social defense: Their evolution and role in depression. In L. Sloman & P. Gilbert (Eds.), *Subordination and defeat: An evolutionary approach to mood disorders and their therapy.* Mahwah, NJ: Erlbaum.

Gruenewald, T. L., Dickerson, S. S., & Kemeny, M. E. (2007). A social function for the self-conscious emotions: Social-self preservation theory. In J. Tracy, R. Robins, & J. Tangney (Eds.), *Self-conscious emotions* (2nd ed., pp. 68–87). New York: Guilford Press.

Gruenewald, T. L., Kemeny, M. E., & Aziz, N. (2006). Subjective social status moderates cortisol responses to social threat. *Brain, Behavior, and Immunity, 20*(4), 410–419.

Gruenewald, T. L., Kemeny, M. E., Aziz, N., & Fahey, J. L. (2004). Acute threat to the social self: Shame, social self-esteem, and cortisol activity. *Psychosomatic Medicine, 66,* 915–924.

Gunnar, M. R., Sebanc, A. M., Tout, K., Donzella, B., & van Dulmen, M. M. H. (2003). Peer rejection, temperament, and cortisol activity in preschoolers. *Developmental Psychobiology, 43,* 346–358.

Harris, C. R. (2001). Cardiovascular responses of embarrassment and effects of emotional suppression in a social setting. *Journal of Personality and Social Psychology, 81,* 886–897.

Herrald, M. M., & Tomaka, J. (2002). Patterns of emotion-specific appraisal, coping, and cardiovascular reactivity during an ongoing emotional episode. *Journal of Personality and Social Psychology, 83,* 434–450.

Het, S., Rohleder, N., Schoofs, D., Kirschbaum, C., & Wolf, O. T. (2009). Neuroendocrine and psychometric evaluation of a placebo version of the "Trier Social Stress Test." *Psychoneuronendocrinology, 34,* 1075–1086.

Hofmann, S. G., Moscovitch, D. A., & Kim, H.-J. (2006). Autonomic correlates of social anxiety and embarrassment in shy and non-shy individuals. *International Journal of Psychophysiology, 61,* 134–142.

James, W. J. (1950). *The principles of psychology Vol. 1.* New York: Dover. Originally published in 1890.

Keltner, D. (1995). Signs of appeasement: Evidence for the distinct displays of embarrassment, amusement, and shame. *Journal of Personality and Social Psychology, 68,* 441–454.

Keltner, D., & Buswell, B. N. (1996). Evidence for the distinctness of embarrassment, shame, and guilt: A study of recalled antecedents and facial expressions of emotion. *Cognition & Emotion, 10,* 155–171.

Kelsey, R. M., Blascovich, J., Leitten, C., Schneider, T. R., Tomaka, J., & Weins, S. (2000). Cardiovascular reactivity and adaptation to recurrent psychological stress: The moderating effects of evaluative observation. *Psychophysiology, 37,* 748–756.

Keltner, D., Young, R. C., & Buswell, B. N. (1997). Appeasement in human emotion, social practice, and personality. *Aggressive Behavior, 23,* 359–374.

Kirschbaum, C., Pirke, K. M., & Hellhammer, D. H. (1993). The "Trier Social Stress Test": A tool for investigating psychobiological responses in a laboratory setting. *Neuropsychobiology, 28,* 76–81.

Kreibig, S. D. (2010). Autonomic nervous system activity in emotion: A review. *Biological Psychology, 84,* 394–421.

Leary, M. R., Tambor, E. S., Terdal, S. K., & Downs, D. L. (1995). Self-esteem as an interpersonal monitor: The sociometer hypothesis. *Journal of Personality and Social Psychology, 68,* 518–530.

Lehman, B. J., & Conley, K. M. (2010). Momentary reports of social-evaluative threat predict ambulatory blood pressure. *Social Psychological and Personality Science, 1,* 51–56.

Lepore, S. J., Allen, K. A., & Evans, G. W. (1993). Social support lowers cardiovascular reactivity to an acute stressor. *Psychosomatic Medicine, 55,* 518–524.

Lerner, J. S., Dahl, R. E., Hariri, A. R., & Taylor, S. E. (2007). Facial expressions of emotion reveal neuroendocrine and cardiovascular stress responses. *Biological Psychiatry, 61,* 253–260.

Lewis, H. B. (1971). *Shame and guilt in neurosis.* New York: International Universities Press.

Lewis, M., & Ramsay, D. (2002). Cortisol response to embarrassment and shame. *Child Development, 73,* 1034–1045.

Lovallo, W. R., & Thomas, T. L. (2000). Stress hormones in psychophysiological research: Emotional, behavioral, and cognitive implications. In J. T. Cacioppo, L. G. Tassinary, & G. G. Bertson (Eds.), *Handbook of psychophysiology* (pp. 342–367). Cambridge, England: Cambridge University Press.

Mason, J. W., Wang, S., Yehuda, R., Riney, S., Charney, D. S., & Southwick, S. M. (2001). Psychogenic lowering of urinary cortisol levels linked to increased emotional numbing and a shame-depressive syndrome in combat-related post-traumatic stress disorder. *Psychosomatic Medicine, 63,* 387–401.

Matheson, K., & Anisman, H. (2009). Anger and shame elicited by discrimination: moderating role of coping on action endorsements and salivary cortisol. *European Journal of Social Psychology, 39,* 163–185.

Miller, G. E., Chen, E., & Zhou, E. (2007). If it goes up, must it come down? Chronic stress and the hypothalamic-pituitary-adrenocortical axis in humans. *Psychological Bulletin, 133,* 25–45.

Miller, G. E., Rohleder, N., & Cole, S. W. (2009). Chronic interpersonal stress predicts activation of pro- and anti-inflammatory signaling pathways 6 months later. *Psychosomatic Medicine, 71,* 57–62.

Miller, R. S., & Tangney, J. P. (1994). Differentiating embarrassment and shame. *Journal of Social and Clinical Psychology, 13*(3), 273–287.

Mills, R. S. L., Imm, G. P., Walling, B. R., & Weiler, H. A. (2008). Cortisol reactivity and regulation associated with shame resonding in early childhood. *Developmental Psychology, 44,* 1369–1380.

Moons, W. G., Eisenberger, N. I., & Taylor, S. E. (2010). Anger and fear responses to stress have different biological profiles. *Brain, Behavior, and Immunity, 24,* 215–219.

Nater, U. M., & Rohleder, N. (2009). Salivary alpha-amylase as a non-invasive biomarker for the sympathetic nervous system: Current state of research. *Psychoneuroendocrinology, 34,* 486–496.

Neidenthal, P. M., Tangney, J. P., & Gavanski, I. (1994). "If only I weren't" versus "if only I hadn't": Distinguishing shame and guilt in counterfactual thinking. *Journal of Personality and Social Psychology, 67,* 585–595.

Norris, J. G., & Benveniste, E. N. (1993). Interleukin-6 production by astrocytes: Induction by the neurotransmitter norephineprhine. *Journal of Neuroimmunology, 45,* 137–145.

Quan, N., Avitsur, R., Stark, J. L., He, L., Shah, M., Caligiuri, M., et al. (2001). Social stress increases the susceptibility to endotoxic shock. *Journal of Neuroimmunology, 115,* 36–45.

Raspopow, K., Abizaid, A., Matheson, K., & Anisman, H. (2010). Psychosocial stressor effects on cortisol and ghrelin in emotional and non-emotional eaters: Influence of anger and shame. *Hormones and Behavior, 58,* 677–684.

Rohleder, N., Beulen, S. E., Chen, E., Wolf, J. M., & Kirschbaum, C. (2007). Stress on the dance floor: The cortisol stress response to social-evaluative threat in competitive ballroom dancers. *Personality and Social Psychology Bulletin, 33,* 69–84.

Rohleder, N., Chen, E., Wolf, J. M., & Miller, G. E. (2008). The psychobiology of trait shame in young women: Extending the social self preservation theory. *Health Psychology, 27,* 523–532.

Rohleder, N., Wolf, J. M., & Kirschbaum, C. Glucocorticoid sensitivity in humans: Interindividual differences and acute stress effects. *Stress, 6*(3), 207–222.

Sapolsky, R. M. (2005). The influence of social hierarchy on primate health. *Science, 308,* 648–652.

Schwabe, L., Haddad, L., & Schachinger, H. (2008). HPA axis activation by a socially evaluated cold-pressor task. *Psychoneuroendocrinology, 33,* 890–895.

Segerstrom, S. C., & Miller, G. E. (2004). Psychological stress and the human immune system: A meta-analytic study of 30 years of inquiry. *Psychological Bulletin, 130,* 601–630.

Sheffield, D., & Carroll, D. (1994). Social support and cardio-vascular reactions to active laboratory stressors. *Psychology & Health, 9,* 305–316.

Sheridan, J. F., Stark, J. L., Avitsur, R., & Padgett, D. A. (2000). Social disruption, immunity, and susceptibility to viral infection. Role of glucocorticoid insensitivity and NGF. *Annals of the New York Academy of Sciences, 917,* 894–905.

Shively, C. A., Laber-Laird, K., Anton, R. F. (1997). Behavior and physiology of social stress and depression in female cynomolgus monkeys. *Biological Psychiatry, 41,* 871–882.

Shively, C. A., Register, T. C., Friedman, D. P., Morgan, T. M., Thompson, J., & Lanier, T. (2005). Social stress-associated depression in adult female cynomolgus monkeys (Macaca fascicularis). *Biological Psychology, 69,* 67–84.

Smith, T. W., Nealey, J. B., Kircher, J. C., & Limon, J. P. (1997). Social determinants of cardiovascular reactivity: Effects of incentive to exert influence and evaluative threat. *Psychophysiology, 34,* 65–73.

Stark, J. L., Avitsur, R., Hunzeker, J., Padgett, D. A., & Sheridan, J. F. (2002). Interleukin-6 and the development of social disruption-induced glucocorticoid resistance. *Journal of Neuroimmunology, 124,* 9–15.

Stark, J., Avitsur, R., Padgett, D. A., & Sheridan, J. F. (2001). Social stress induces glucocorticoid resistance in macrophages. *American Journal of Physiology: Regulatory, Integrative, and Comparative Physiology, 280,* 1799–1805.

Stefanski, V. (2000). Social stress in laboratory rats: Hormonal responses and immune cell distribution. *Psychoneuroendocrinology, 25,* 389–406.

Steptoe, A., Hamer, M., & Chida, Y. (2007). The effects of acute psychological stress on circulating inflammatory factors in humans: A review and meta-analysis. *Brain, Behavior, and Immunity, 21*(7), 901–912.

Stroud, L. R., Tanofsky-Kraff, M., Wilfley, D. E., & Salovey, P. (2000). The Yale Interpersonal Stressor (YIPS): Affective, physiological, and behavioral responses to a novel interpersonal rejection paradigm. *Annals of Behavioral Medicine, 22,* 204–213.

Tangney, J. P. (1995). Recent advances in the empirical study of shame and guilt. *American Behavioral Scientist, 38,* 1132–1145.

Tangney, J. P., Miller, R. S., Flicker, L., & Barlow, D. H. (1996). Are shame, guilt, and embarrassment distinct emotions? *Journal of Personality and Social Psychology, 70,* 1256–1269.

Tangney, J. P., Neidenthal, P. M., Covert, M. V., & Barlow, D. H. (1998). Are shame and guilt related to distinct self-discrepancies? A test of Higgins's (1987) hypotheses. *Journal of Personality and Social Psychology, 73,* 256–268.

Taylor, S. E., Seeman, T. E., Eisenberger, N. I., Kozanian, T. A., Moore, A. N., & Moons, W. G. (2010). Effects of a supportive or unsupportive audience on biological and psychological responses to stress. *Journal of Personality and Social Psychology, 98,* 47–56.

Tops, M., Boksem, M. A. S., Wester, A. E., Lorist, M. M., & Meijman, T. F. (2006). Task engagement and the relationships between the error-related negativity, agreeableness, behavioral shame-proneness and cortisol. *Psychoneuroendocrinology, 31,* 847–858.

Tracy, J. L., & Robins, R. W. (2004). Putting the self into self-conscious emotions: A theoretical model. *Psychological Inquiry, 15*(2), 103–125.

Tracy, J. L., Robins, R. W., & Schriber, R. A. (2009). Development of a FACS-verified set of basic and self-conscious emotion expressions. *Emotion, 9,* 554–559.

Tracy, J. L., Robins, R. W., & Tangney, J. P. (2007). *Self-conscious emotions* (2nd ed.). New York: Guilford Press.

Weiner, B. (1985). An attributional theory of achievement motivation and emotion. *Psychological Review, 92,* 548–573.

Wright, R. A., Tunstall, A. M., Williams, B. J., Goodwin, J. S., & Harmon-Jones, E. (1995). Social evaluation and cardiovascular response: An active coping approach. *Journal of Personality and Social Psychology, 69,* 530–543.

Zwolinski, J. (2008). Biopsychosocial responses to social rejection in targets of relational aggression. *Biological Psychology, 79,* 260–267.

Positive Emotions and Immunity

Sarah D. Pressman *and* Lora L. Black

Abstract

In this section, we examine the evidence tying positive emotions to immune function. Studies reviewed here focus on the *short-term* alterations in immune function that occur as a result of experimentally induced emotions as well as naturally occurring emotional states. We begin by discussing the larger theoretical concerns in this field, such as measurement of positive emotions, independence from related constructs, and the pathways by which positive feelings might lead to alterations in immune outcomes. We follow with a brief review of the literature showing ties between manipulations of positive emotions and immune outcomes, as well as studies tying short term, naturally occurring states to immunity. We conclude that this literature is suggestive in that many studies show immune enhancing benefits of positive emotions. However, a number of studies have methodological concerns making it difficult to determine the true effect sizes and active components of these associations and we, therefore, make a call for further work in this area.

Key Words: positive affect, positive emotion, vigor, calm, happiness, laughter, immunity, immune function, mood induction

Introduction

It has been almost 50 years since it was first postulated that emotions could influence immune system function (Solomon & Moos, 1964). Since then, there has been extensive research into the field with numerous studies showing consistent and robust associations between negative states and traits (e.g., stress, depression, anxiety) and worsened immune system function (see reviews by Herbert & Cohen, 1993a,b; Segerstrom & Miller, 2004). There has, however, been relatively less research focusing on the ties between positive emotional states and immune function with approximately 1/100th the number of studies in this area. Given the growing excitement in the field of positive psychology tied with an upsurge of research linking positive psychological measures to better health outcomes (e.g., Pressman & Cohen, 2005; Rasmussen, Scheier, &

Greenhouse, 2009), it is of the utmost importance to understand the underlying mediators of the positive emotion-health correlation, including the role of the immune system.

What Is Positive Affect?

There is much contention within the field of emotion about how to precisely measure and define positive affect (PA). Although negative affect (NA) has been extensively researched, both as a broad construct and via its negative subcomponents (e.g., shame, depression, hostility), PA has often been neglected in research with the subcomponents not being universally agreed on (for examples see: Ekman, 1992, Watson & Tellegen, 1985; Russell, 1980). A broad definition of PA is that it reflects pleasant engagement with the environment (Clark, Watson, & Leeka, 1989). Adjectives that might be included in PA assessment tools represent feelings of calm and peace (low arousal); happiness and well-being (medium arousal); or excitement, vigor, and even overt laughter (high arousal). Depending on the researcher's preferred model of affect, some of these adjective categories may be excluded or included, and additional categories or adjectives may be added. Frequently these distinctions among adjectives in different scales are ignored, given that the vast majority of studies aggregate the adjectives for a *general* PA measure. However, in the field of psychoneuroimmunology, it may be critical to consider the *types* of PA, given the known autonomic differences of aroused versus relaxed states, and the likely impact that these differences would have on immunity. However, types of PA are rarely highlighted in these studies, and they are frequently ignored, with studies of mild positive induction grouped with those inducing highly arousing laughter states.

Another critical consideration in affect measurement is timing. For example, reflecting on a given moment in time or manipulating PA momentarily would typically be discussed as *state* PA, emotional experience, and in some cases as mood (which may last minutes to days). Once affect is reported as a *general trait* of a person or assessed in terms of how someone feels "on average" or over the last few months, it is considered personality-like trait PA. Long lasting feelings of affect (e.g., being a happy person or being a generally depressed person) have more obvious implications for long-term health because of their known impacts on health behaviors, social relationships, and the likely long-lasting impacts on physiological function (see review by Pressman & Cohen, 2005). However, physiology is clearly responsive to momentary changes in affect, making it critical to understand how variation in these emotional experiences (both natural and induced) impact the immune system. Furthermore, it is these momentary changes that are responsible for the averaged impacts that we see with trait affect measures. This section will focus on the short-term changes in the immune system associated with state and emotional positive affect with allusions to implications for health.

Finally, given the glut of literature on NA, and its ties to immune function and health, it is essential to consider the role that an *absence* of NA plays in the findings of PA with immune function. There is some contention remaining regarding the independence of measures of PA and NA. Some researchers assume that these variables are dependent on one another and represent opposite ends of the same continuum, whereas others believe in their relative independence (e.g., Diener & Emmons, 1984; Watson, 1988). PA and NA are especially likely to be negatively and highly correlated with one another in the short term (e.g., when assessing momentary feelings) (Diener, Larsen, Levine, & Emmons, 1985), which makes it essential to consider whether *both* PA and NA are measured or manipulated. It may be that any finding of PA is simply the absence of NA and vice versa. However, some measures of affect, such as the Positive and Negative Affect Schedule (Watson, Clark, & Tellegen, 1988), are specifically designed to avoid this interdependence, making the utilized affect measure of importance as well.

Why Study Positive Affect and Immunity?

Growing numbers of research studies have now shown that PA is tied to diverse health outcomes ranging from reduced symptom and pain report to enhanced longevity (see reviews by Pressman & Cohen, 2005; Chida & Steptoe, 2008). Most relevant to immunology, PA has been linked to better outcomes for immune relevant diseases like cancer and HIV (Levy, Lee, Bagley, & Lippman, 1988; Moskowitz, 2003), and PA over the course of a few weeks has been tied to reduced incidence of infectious disease when experimentally exposed to a virus (Cohen, Alper, Doyle, Treanor, & Turner, 2006; Cohen, Doyle, Turner, Alper, & Skoner, 2003). Critical to the results of these studies is that PA, not the absence of NA, was responsible for the effects. Given these relevant health outcomes, it seems essential, then, to understand the underlying immune processes that allow these PA-associated benefits to occur, especially in the context of controlled experimental manipulations.

Pathways Connecting PA to Immune Function

When conceptualizing how PA might influence objective health outcomes, changes in health practices (e.g., smoking, exercise), social-relationship formation, and stress responses are frequently called on to explain the plausible mediators allowing PA to "get under the skin" and influence disease and other health outcomes. However, when focusing on short term, transient state levels of PA (e.g., PA induced in the laboratory by watching a humorous movie) we must move away from these broader and slower pathways to a more narrow focus on how the experience of emotion directly translates into physiological changes that might alter the immune system.

Pressman and Cohen (2005) have proposed two models linking trait PA to immune function: a main effect model and a stress-buffering model. In the first case, PA has a direct effect on behavioral and biological mechanisms that influence immune function. In the second model, PA acts as a buffer of behavioral and physiological responses to stress. Direct (fast) pathways include neurological and endocrine mechanisms. PA may directly alter immune function through the activation of neurological and neuroendocrine pathways and the release of hormones and neurotransmitters, such as catecholamines. Here, there is extensive evidence for direct anatomical and functional links between the central nervous and immune systems, as indicated by the sympathetic and parasympathetic innervation of lymphoid organs (Felten & Olschowka, 1987; Livnat, Felten, Carlson, Bellinger, & Felten, 1985) and the presence of receptors on immune cells for a variety of hormones and neurotransmitters that are released in response to emotional stimuli, such as epinephrine and norepinephrine, corticosteroids, and opiates (Rabin, 1999). In support of this pathway, trait and state PA have been associated with lower blood concentrations of epinephrine and norepinephrine (Berk et al., 1989; Codispoti et al., 2003; Cohen et al., 2003), suggesting a dampening of sympathetic nervous system (SNS) activation. Others have suggested that it is the arousal dimension of acute mood states that induces autonomic arousal, with activated positive and negative emotional states resulting in SNS activation (e.g., Futterman, Kemeny, Shapiro, & Fahey, 1994; Knapp et al., 1992; Neumann & Waldstein, 2001). In contrast, less activated positive emotions (e.g., calm) have been associated with decreases in SNS activation and possible activation of the parasympathetic (PNS) branch of the autonomic system (e.g., Bacon et al., 2004), which may play a role in the downregulation of inflammation (Borovikova et al., 2000; Tracey, 2002).

In addition to autonomic pathways, it is widely accepted that psychological factors can regulate immune function by activation of the hypothalamic-pituitary-adrenal (HPA) axis and release of hormones, including cortisol, from the adrenal cortex. A number of studies have demonstrated that both the experimental induction of positive mood states and higher levels of trait PA are associated with lower levels of cortisol (Berk et al., 1989; Buchanan, al'Absi, & Lovallo, 1999; Cohen et al., 2003; Polk, Cohen, Doyle, Skoner, & Kirschbaum, 2005; Smyth et al., 1998; Steptoe, Wardle, & Marmot,

2005) Glucocorticoid receptors are expressed on a variety of immune cells, and ligand binding to these receptors has a number of immune inhibitory effects (e.g., Almawi, Beyhum, Rahme, & Rieder, 1996; Cato & Wade, 1996). Other hormones are also found to increase in response to positive emotions, such as growth hormone (Berk et al., 1989), prolactin (Codispoti et al., 2003), as well as endogenous opioids (Gerra et al., 1996; Gerra et al., 1998), which might also play a role in the regulation of immune function. Oxytocin has been hypothesized to play a role in the PA-immune pathway due to its known cortisol-regulating functions and its ties to positive social interactions (e.g., Taylor et al., 2006); however, to date, this association has not been reported.

Positive affect may also act as a buffer of the immune influences of stressful life events (Pressman & Cohen, 2005). Although there is a substantial literature demonstrating that psychological stress dysregulates immune function, not all individuals display immune changes following stressful life events. Variability among individuals in the magnitude of their immune responses to stress is attributed to their level of perceived stress. A psychological stress response comprised of negative cognitive and emotional states is proposed to be the consequence of perceptions that demands exceed individuals' ability to cope (Lazarus & Folkman, 1984). These stress responses are thought to influence immune function through their effects on neuroendocrine responses and behavior. Momentary PA may act as a buffer of stress responses, acting to reduce negative appraisals of events and to facilitate adaptive coping. As a result, PA may ameliorate stress-related autonomic nervous system (ANS) and HPA activation (Fredrickson, Mancuso, Branigan, & Tugade, 2000; Kraft & Pressman, in press). Beyond transient state PA, dispositional levels of PA may also encourage restorative coping activities such as sleep, exercise, relaxation, social support, and vacation (Pressman et al., 2009; Smith & Baum, 2003). These hypotheses are consistent with Fredrickson's proposal that positive emotions broaden and diversify individuals' thoughts and actions, which enable them to build "enduring personal resources," such as social contacts that can be drawn on when facing environmental threats (Fredrickson, 1998). In addition to buffering the effects of stress, PA may also facilitate faster recovery from stress-related psychological and physiological activation. In support of this possibility, Fredrickson and associates (2000) demonstrated that inducing PA following a stressful stimulus resulted in faster recovery to baseline levels of heart rate and blood pressure.

Conceptual Issues in the Study of PA and Immunity

As mentioned earlier, there are many aspects of PA measurement and manipulation that should be attended to when reviewing the literature on state PA and immune outcomes. First, of course, are the previously discussed critical issues in the general field of emotions and health. This includes a consideration of the types of emotions being induced (high versus low arousal, for example). This raises the question of whether studies on mindfulness and immune change are relevant in the study of PA. Mindfulness is frequently thought of as a neutral state without any type of affective tone (Shapiro, Carlson, Astin, & Freedman, 2006). However, given its known relaxing effects and the assumption that low arousal PA includes similar feelings, these manipulations are not necessarily distinct. That being said, it should not be assumed that changes in immunity tied to mindfulness and relaxation will have overlap with those induced by laughter and other high arousal states such as excitement, because there are likely differences in hormonal and sympathetic or parasympathetic changes in the body.

Also problematic is the distinction between state and trait PA. Even emotion theorists struggle to define the precise moment that a state becomes a trait. In this case, it is also important to consider how immune changes associated with state alterations in mood eventually become engrained into real health differences. Complicating this type of work is the difference between naturally occurring state emotion and what is manipulated in the laboratory. Although we are presumably studying alterations due to day-to-day variation in emotion (e.g., in a daily diary study with multiple immune samples), we know from existing work that these day-to-day variations are highly correlated with trait levels of affect. Most of these studies do not control for existing dispositional changes, making it difficult to know whether immune-associations are due to state alterations in emotion or simply due to the underlying trait differences in emotion and possibly health. Although experimental studies of mood induction can help clear up this problem via randomization to group, it is still possible that trait affect and the underlying health and physiological differences tied to trait PA have an impact. Again, this is rarely considered in this type of work because of the assumption that randomization will mitigate these influences.

In experimental research, the manipulation of emotion is infrequently checked to determine what emotions have changed. The typical study engages in a mood manipulation, and then it tests the immune correlates after the manipulation as compared with resting immune activity. This neglects several interesting questions, such as whether the amount of affective change (e.g., self-reported change in duration, frequency, or intensity) is correlated with the magnitude of the immune change. It also ignores the possibility that the wrong types of emotions were being manipulated, that certain types of emotions are responsible for the effects found (as opposed to general PA), or that there was no emotion change at all. Without manipulation checks, there is uncertainty about the exact pathways that resulted in the immune change found.

Finally, in many of these studies the impact of negative emotion is not assessed, which makes it difficult for the researcher to understand whether these findings are due to a reduction in NA or due to an increase in PA. Although many studies do record emotion changes via self-reported emotion scales, researchers frequently focus only on the positive items of these measures.

Review

Below is a short review on the studies of state affect and immune change. We first review experimental studies on mood induction, focusing on those inducing high-arousal PA (laughter), followed by those that induce more typical PA (joy, happiness), and finally ending with low arousal PA. Next, we consider studies of naturally occurring state PA and their associations with immune outcomes. Again, we focus on studies looking at short-term measures (e.g., in daily diaries or over the course of a day).

Induction Studies

Mood induction studies aim to rouse a certain mood in subjects. A common procedure uses film or stories to elicit specific moods by having the participant watch/listen to a movie or story that is thought to be emotionally stimulating (Westermann, Spies, Stahl, & Hesse, 1996). Although there are a number of criticisms of mood induction procedures, such as the ability to produce the sufficient mood intensity or whether the effect is due to other factors (Westermann et al., 1996), mood induction studies are used frequently in the study of immune change.

High-Arousal PA Induction

The most common measure of immunity in mood induction studies is secretory immunoglobulin A (sIgA) in saliva. This is an important antibody that plays a role in defending against viral and bacterial infection and is often considered a first line of defense. It is popular in this type of research because it is noninvasive, easy to collect, relatively stable, and relevant to functional immunity. Nevertheless, there remains controversy about what specific outcome variable to analyze (e.g., whether to look at total amounts, specific titers, and whether salivary flow rate is assessed) (Stone, Cox, Valdimarsdottir, & Neale, 1987). At least eight studies have examined the association between watching a *humorous* video and increases in sIgA (Dillon, Minchoff, & Baker, 1985; Harrison et al., 2000; Labott, Ahleman, Wolever, & Martin, 1990; Lambert & Lambert, 1995; McClelland & Cheriff, 1997; McCraty, Atkinson, Rein, & Watkins, 1996; Njus, Nitschke, & Bryant, 1996; Perera, Sabin, Nelson, & Lowe, 1998). These were all done in healthy populations, and all but two (Lambert & Lambert, 1995; McCraty et al., 1996) confirmed that the mood induction was successful. Beyond this strength, the majority of the studies also included an emotionally neutral condition to control for diurnal variation in immunity, passage of time, and other contextual factors. In addition to the consensus of these sIgA findings, levels of blood immunoglobulins G, A, and M have also been shown to increase in response to a laughter-inducing film (Berk, Felten, Tan, Bittman, & Westengard, 2001).

Induced high-arousal positive emotions and laughter have also been show to affect a handful of other immunologic parameters. Three studies of healthy adult men and women have examined Natural Killer Cell Cytotoxicity (NKCC), which is another indicator of innate immunity that plays a role in the destruction of virus-infected and tumor cells. These studies show NKCC increases with the induction of humor via video (Bennett, Zeller, Rosenberg, & McCann, 2003; Berk et al., 2001; Takahashi et al., 2001). Moreover, one study shows NKCC and total numbers of NK cells increasing in response to the PA induction (Berk et al., 2001). However, one study found no impact of PA on NKCC or total NK cell numbers (Takahashi et al., 2001). All these types of increases are believed to be markers of increased immune function. Interestingly, in one study, this increase was found to depend on the *overt* display of humor (observer ratings of laughter) by the subjects (Bennett et al.,

2003), whereas, in another, there was no impact due to the magnitude of laughter or pleasantness ratings of the video, which were both measured by self-report (Takahashi et al., 2001). These differences may be due to measurement error, cultural differences in emotional expression behavior, or simply inaccurate self-report as opposed to an observer coding overt laughter. The Berk (2001) study did not report on the effectiveness of the manipulation, and there was no control group, but it is consistent with the other two studies.

More recent attention in the field has turned to relationships between emotions and the concentration of cytokines in circulation. Pro-immune response (or pro-inflammatory) cytokines are related to the proliferation of T and B lymphocytes and are produced by the body during the immune response, whereas anti-immune responses (or anti-inflammatory) cytokines work with cytokine inhibitors and work to regulate the immune system. Commonly measured pro-inflammatory cytokines include interleukin (IL)-2, IL-3, interferon (IFN)-γ, and tumor necrosis factor (TNF)-α, whereas anti-inflammatory cytokines include IL-1, IL-1β, and IL-4. The health significance of circulating peripheral cytokines is difficult to interpret, because it is a regulation of levels in response to a *specific demand* that confers immune efficiency. For example, higher levels of pro-immune response/inflammatory cytokines are associated with disease prevention and treatment (Margolin, 2000), but high levels of TNF-α (a pro-inflammatory cytokine) have been associated with increased disease progression in rheumatoid arthritis (RA) patients (Feldmann, Brennan, & Maini, 1996). In addition, elevated IL-6 has been implicated in the development of heart disease (e.g., Yudkin, Kumari, Humphries, & Mohamed-Ali, 2000). The few studies that have examined cytokine levels in response to positive-mood induction provide some evidence that state PA is associated with increases in IL-2, IL-3, and decreases in TNF-α in healthy populations (Berk et al., 2001; Mittwoch-Jaffe, Shalit, Srendi, & Yehuda, 1995). More relevant are studies examining cytokines in populations with heightened inflammation (and pro-inflammatory cytokines) due to autoimmune disease. One study compared cytokine responses to humor (watching a funny theatrical presentation) in healthy controls versus RA patients and found a decrease in IL-4 and IL-6 in the RA patients, but not the controls, as well as a decrease in TNF-α concentrations for those with controllable RA (Matsuzaki, Nakajima, Ishigami, Tanno & Yoshino, 2006). This finding indicates possible short-term beneficial health benefits (i.e., decreases in pro-inflammatory cytokines) of PA for the RA population, but perhaps not for healthy individuals. Findings are less consistent for IFN-γ, with one study showing mood-related increases (Berk et al., 2001) and another decreases (Yoshino, Fujimori, & Kohda, 1996) for both healthy and RA patients. Taken together, these studies suggest that PA induction *may* increase disease-preventing/anti-inflammatory cytokines while decreasing disease-promoting/pro-inflammatory cytokines.

A single study examined whether induced humor is associated with a more clinically meaningful measure of cellular immune function: allergic hypersensitivity reactions in response to skin prick tests using commercial or dust-mite allergens. In support of a health benefit of state PA, a reduction in allergic response (wheal size) was found in response to the introduction of the allergen (a substance that stimulates an allergic response) when humor was induced by watching a funny film as compared with a control movie (Kimata, 2001).

Midarousal PA Induction

More relevant to naturally occurring PA, are studies of midarousal PA induction, or specifically, manipulations of happiness, joy, and other pleasant states. Although these feelings are likely altered in the humor manipulations described previously, the expectation is that the intensity for happiness manipulations is lower. The typical study might show a pleasant clip with an attractive person or situation and examine the concomitant changes in immune function. For example, Matsunaga et al., (2008) showed subjects a favorite actress, and these participants showed heightened Natural Killer Cell Activity (NKCA) as compared with those viewing a control film (a newscast about past weather not featuring a favorite person).

Although the preceding example is similar to the laughter studies discussed earlier, studies of happiness induction are more likely to also include NA manipulation unlike the humor work that typically only has a control group or no comparison at all. Two small studies by Futterman and colleagues (1994; 1992) examined the impact of positive, neutral, and negative mood inductions as well as the impact of high and low arousal emotions by using actors who are able to easily experience feelings via readings and personal memories. They found that, in general, *all* mood states were associated with increased immune activity (e.g., NKCC and NK cell numbers), and there were more fluctuations present in the aroused

emotions. Two other papers have similarly found no distinction between the immune effects of different emotional valences (Hucklebridge et al., 2000; Njus et al., 1996). In all three studies (Hucklebridge had two separate experiments), when healthy participants were instructed to write about a positive or negative experience (films in one study, personal recollections in the other) or listen to emotionally valenced music, there was no differential effect of PA versus NA on sIgA. Once again, *both* types of emotional manipulations showed increases as compared with baseline. This was true even after doing a manipulation check and when there was a comparison control group for one study (Njus et al., 1996). Thus, although there is consistent evidence for mood-induced increases in total sIgA concentration in activated emotions, including laughter and happiness, it may be the *activation* of the emotion, rather than the valence, that is associated with increased antibody levels. This conclusion is consistent with studies showing an increase in total salivary sIgA levels in response to acute laboratory stress tasks that typically induce negative mood states (e.g., Bristow, Hucklebridge, Clow, & Evans, 1997; Willemsen et al., 1998).

One distinction between valences was found in Futterman et al. (1994) when examining lymphocyte proliferation to phytohaemagglutinin (PHA; a plant mitogen). This is one test of the body's immune function in response to the introduction of a foreign invader. Specifically, higher lymphocyte proliferation is indicative of a higher immune response to the mitogen. Although PA was associated with enhanced response to PHA, the opposite was found for NA. Unfortunately, this was not replicated in a similar study by Knapp and colleagues (1992) who found no impact of PA *or* NA (induced via recall) on PHA stimulation; however, they did find a decrease in white blood cell proliferative response to Concanavalin A (a plant mitogen) with NA only, consistent with the direction of the Futterman finding.

The only study with no impact of midarousal positive emotion was a study by Zachariae and colleagues (2001) who did not find an effect of hypnotically induced positive or negative moods on the immune hypersensitivity response (skin reactions in response to a histamine skin prick that would indicate higher immune activity). Although this might suggest a failure of the hypnosis manipulation, in a previous study conducted by the same group, results showed changes in monocyte chemotaxis (the migration of white blood cells) after a relaxed happiness induction, but no impact resulting from neutral or negative manipulations (Zachariae et al., 1991).

Meditation, Relaxation, and Calm Inductions

The following studies investigated the relationship between low-arousal PA inductions (e.g., meditation, relaxation, and calm) with immune functioning. It is important to note that PA was not directly measured in this work, requiring the reader to make the assumption that feelings like calm and relaxation are likely being altered.

In support of a health benefit of state PA, a reduction in allergic histamine-triggered hypersensitivity response (wheal size) was found when pleasantness and relaxation were induced by hypnotic suggestion (Laidlaw, Booth, & Large, 1996). Although no other immune study examined relaxation hypnosis, studies on calm music (McCraty et al., 1996), progressive muscle relaxation (Pawlow & Jones, 2005), and Integrative Mind-Body Training (IMBT—a form of meditation) (Yaxin, Yi-Yuan, Yinghua, & Posner, 2010) all found increases in sIgA. In addition, IBMT immediately following a stressor was related to a significant sIgA concentration increase, which reveals evidence of stress buffering.

In a similar stress buffering study by Pace and colleagues (2009), compassion meditation (a technique focused on developing kindness and love for others) was examined as a possible reducer of laboratory stress. After six weeks of meditation training, those individuals who practiced regularly were found to have lower IL-6 levels after the stressor as compared with those who did not practice. In addition, participants who reported meditation practice rates above the median showed significantly lower IL-6 levels on average compared with those below the median.

Finally, although beyond the scope of this chapter, it is also important to consider related relaxation activities such as Mindfulness Based Stress Reduction (MBSR), a meditative technique that includes exercises in mindfulness, meditation, and mind-body connection (Carlson, Speca, Patel, & Goodey, 2003; Robinson, Mathews, & Witek-Janusek, 2003). We will not review the literature here because techniques do not specifically discuss low-arousal PA, but it is likely that these studies are inducing feelings of calm and relaxation. Not surprisingly, MBSR has been tied to a range of immune outcomes, such as NKCA enhancement, higher vaccine-related antibody levels, and cytokine alteration (Carlson et al., 2003; Davidson et al., 2003; Robinson et al., 2003; Witek-Janusek et al., 2008), but the psychological mechanisms and the role of PA has been unstudied up to this point.

Conclusions of Induction Studies

In sum, the most consistent findings from studies examining the effects of brief positive mood induction on immune functioning in healthy individuals support PA-related increases in sIgA levels, numbers of immune cells in peripheral circulation, and NK cell activity, which suggests an upregulation of parameters of innate immunity. These findings are consistent with those found in response to acute laboratory stress tasks designed to elicit negative moods, such as speech and mental arithmetic tasks (for review see Segerstrom & Miller, 2004). Similar immune responses to positive and negative mood states suggest that it may be the increase in affective arousal, rather than the positive or negative valence of the emotion, that contributes to immunological variability. To date, the majority of positive mood induction protocols have induced activated positive states, such as humor and excitement. This arousal theory is consistent with evidence that immune changes in response to acute laboratory stress are largely mediated by activation of the SNS (e.g., Manuck, Cohen, Rabin, Muldoon, & Bachen, 1991; Marsland, Bachen, Cohen, & Manuck, 2001), and studies showing that brief stress-related immune responses are blocked by adrenergic receptor inhibition (Bachen et al., 1995). Given the similarity in immune responses to both positive and negative mood induction, it is possible that the arousal dimension of these mood states induces activation of the SNS and an upregulation of innate immunity. It has been proposed that brief increases in innate immune function in response to acute challenge are adaptive, reducing risk of infection and aiding in wound healing (Segerstrom & Miller, 2004).

Inconsistent with the arousal-only hypothesis is the growing evidence that relaxed low-arousal PA inductions are similarly beneficial to immune function (primarily sIgA outcomes). Unfortunately, because many of these studies do not use manipulation checks and neglect to measure low arousal PA, it is unclear whether these changes are due to feelings of calm per se, or whether high-arousal PA is also inadvertently altered by these manipulations (e.g., increased vigor from meditation). Given that low arousal negative emotions are well-known immune modulators (e.g., sadness and depression), it seems unlikely that SNS activity is the only actor in the state affect-immune connection.

Naturally Occurring Mood

Studies investigating state affect and immunity aim to understand the impact of brief and transient mood states that may fluctuate from day to day or even minute to minute. State affect is commonly measured by asking the participant how they feel over specific time points, such as at the *present moment* or over a period of time ranging from today to the past weeks (at which point state begins to transition into trait measures of PA). It is likely that studies looking at naturally occurring mood states are more generalizable to real life settings, because the moods are not artificially induced in a laboratory. As a result, findings may be more reflective of the real world experience of PA, which is frequently less intense than some laboratory manipulations. Typically, these studies use self-report adjective evaluation measures of positive and negative affect such as the Positive and Negative Affect Schedule (PANAS; Watson, Clark, & Tellegen, 1988), the Profile of Mood States (POMS; Usala & Hertzog, 1989), or positive items from an existing measure (e.g., the Center for Epidemiological Studies Depression Scale [CES-D]; Radloff, 1977). These tend to be focused on activated positive emotions, such as vigor and excitement with the PANAS, and also include measures of other types of positive emotions. However, many of these measures also combine low- and high-arousal adjectives. Therefore, we will discuss the following naturalistic studies based on timing as opposed to arousal.

Momentary Positive Emotion (Minute to Day)

Naturalistic studies interested in the immune correlates of daily fluctuations in mood utilize daily diary measures of mood states partnered with immune measures (typically salivary). A well-designed study by Stone, Cox, Valdimarsdottir, Jandorf, and Neale (1987) had volunteers ingest a capsule containing an innocuous novel antigen (rabbit albumin) daily for 10 weeks so that the researchers could determine the *specific* sIgA response to the novel antigen, unlike the previously discussed studies that look at general (nonspecific) levels of this marker (for a discussion on the rationale for this please see Stone, et al., 1987). For the latter 8 weeks of this period, volunteers also completed daily mood diaries and gave daily saliva samples to assess specific sIgA to

the novel antigen. Within subjects analyses revealed that antigen-specific sIgA was higher on days with higher positive mood and lower on days with high negative mood. These results were replicated in a subsequent study that monitored mood and antibody levels over a 12-week period (Stone et al., 1994). Evans et al. (Evans, Bristow, Hucklebridge, & Chow, 1993) examined relationships between daily mood and *non-specific* sIgA over a 2-week measurement period. However, in this case, no associations between positive mood and total sIgA were found. Negative mood was associated with higher total sIgA concentration and secretion rate. It may be that this result diverges because specific markers of immune activity are a better gauge of immune function than general markers. It may also be that higher arousal PA (like that induced by laughter in the lab) is necessary for a general sIgA response. Further naturalistic studies are necessary to aid in better understanding relationships between acute mood states and immune function and disentangling the differential roles of emotional valence and arousal.

Positive Mood (PA from One to Several Weeks)

Other naturalistic research has explored the relationship between longer lasting PA and NKCC. For example, Lutgendorf et al. (2001) found that, in a sample of 58 older adults (65 and up), PA assessed over a one-week period using the POMS was tied to immune function. For example, higher levels of vigor were associated with higher NKCC and lower IgG antibody titers to Epstein Barr virus (EBV) (suggesting more effective immune control of latent EBV). These longer-term PA-related changes of specific IgG may reflect changes in the efficacy of other immune cells (like B and T cells) via their response to the circulating antigen. Valdimarsdottir & Bovbjerg (1997) also found a relationship between PA (averaged over a 2-day period) and NKCC in a population of healthy female volunteers. Interestingly, there was also an interaction between PA and NA scores in predicting NKCC: Those who endorsed both lower levels of PA and the presence of some NA showing lower NKCC than individuals with either higher PA or no negative mood. Thus, it is possible that PA is *protective* for individuals who also experience negative mood traits. In contrast to the preceding two studies, Moss and colleagues (Moss, Moss, & Peterson, 1989) tracked relationships between weekly positive moods and NKCC for 4 weeks during summer vacation among 10 healthy professional students and found no consistent effects of mood on NKCC. These findings are more difficult to interpret as a consequence of a large interindividual variability in NKCC and a small sample size. In addition, interpretation of these results may be misleading as the studies did not control for effector mix when determining NKCC levels (Kiecolt-Glaser & Glaser, 1991).

Also relevant to immune function is healing ability in an experimental wounding paradigm. Although most studies of wound healing focus on the slowing that occurs with stress, a single study has found that PA (as measured over the past week with the PANAS, a high arousal assessment of affect) was tied to faster healing in a skin disruption paradigm in the context of an acute stressor (Robles, Brooks, & Pressman, 2009). Importantly, NA was not associated with healing, and controlling for it experimentally did not eliminate the PA impact.

A few other studies have examined associations between affect and immune responses among individuals with immune-related diseases. For example, Logan et al. (Logan, Lutgendorf, Hartwig, Lilly, & Berberich, 1998) followed 10 individuals with a history of herpes labialis (cold sores) over a 3-month period, recorded daily state measures of PA and NA, and drew blood each week for the determination of numbers of circulating T lymphocytes (a measure of cell-mediated immunity) and NK cells. In the week prior to a cold sore outbreak, individuals who endorsed being more content demonstrated higher numbers of NK cells and cytotoxic T cells (T cells that kill virus-infected cells) than individuals who were discontent. Conversely, individuals who reported low happiness/hopefulness showed lower numbers of cytoxic T cells than those at the other end of the happiness continuum. Similarly, Laidlaw et al. (Laidlaw, Booth, & Large, 1994) found that individuals with allergies, who endorsed higher liveliness on a bipolar continuum from liveliness to listless and more vigor on the POMS, as averaged over a 2-week period, had smaller mean hypersensitivity skin responses to allergens than their more listless and lower vigor counterparts. Because PA and NA were assessed in these studies on a single continuum, it is impossible to know whether one or affect both valences contributed to the reported associations. Finally, Sepah and Bower (2009) examined the association between PA and cytokines (IL-6 and IL-1β) in a population of breast and prostate cancer patients (all over the age of 55). PA over the last week (measured with the positive items from the CESD) was assessed alongside IL-6

and IL-1β serum levels prior to radiation, 4 times during a 6- to 8-week treatment and at 2 follow-up visits after treatment. Results showed that there was no significant correlation between PA and pre- or posttreatment IL-6 or IL-1β levels. However, higher PA was significantly associated with higher IL-1β and IL-6 levels *during* the treatment phase.

Naturalistic Study Conclusions

In sum, available evidence from the few naturalistic studies examining mood across periods ranging from a few days to weeks suggests that PA is associated with markers of immune function, including higher NK cell number and activity, better control of latent EBV, faster wound healing, and increased cytokine responses to live influenza virus and cancer treatment. Of interest are studies linking PA to an increasing number of circulating cytotoxic T cells and NK cells among individuals with herpes, studies showing a reduction in allergic response in individuals with allergies, and a single study indicating better skin healing in those with higher PA when faced with duress. These findings raise the possibility that PA-related changes in immune function have a health benefit.

General Conclusions

This review highlights a general a relationship between better PA and higher immune function in both induction studies, as well as naturally occurring PA studies. Overall, studies show that both high and midarousal PA induction is associated with higher immune function (as measured by sIgA, NKCA, NKCC, and pro- and anti-inflammatory cytokine levels). However, it is often difficult to compare these studies because induced PA may be different than naturally occurring PA. Although many of the studies use various types of humor for PA induction, others induce PA without humor, and the laboratory itself may also be a different type of arousal agent. It is, therefore, possible that these studies are associated with different types of arousal, and are, thus, conceptually different forms of PA. Furthermore, it is unclear the role that PA plays in calm induction studies and whether calm is manipulated at all in mindfulness studies (given that it is rarely measured). This may make it inappropriate to compare these studies to those that specifically induce PA. Overall, studies investigating naturally occurring PA have found an association between PA (with measurement periods ranging from days to weeks) and immune function, where higher levels of PA are generally associated with enhanced immune function. The precise relationship differed depending on the immune parameter of interest, subject sample, and other factors, which suggests a more complex relationship between immune function and naturally occurring PA. Findings are, however, consistent with trait PA studies that reveal immune benefits (also refer Chapter 9) and even animal literature showing that positive temperaments (e.g., calm cows) are associated with higher levels of immune parameters (Burdick, Randel, Carroll, & Welsh Jr, 2011).

Future Directions

Although the studies reviewed in this chapter suggest a relationship between PA and immune function, it is important to note that many of the studies had small samples sizes or inadequate control groups. Many of the studies also lack measurement of NA, making it difficult to separate the effects of PA and NA on immune function. This is especially important given that some studies found that *both* positive and negative mood states were associated with similar immune alterations. These findings suggest it may be the activation rather than the valence that produces immune change. Future studies should assess PA *and* NA to determine the differing effects of these emotions, but this will be difficult because these valences can be highly correlated in momentary assessments. A thoughtful approach about which emotions might be altered and which might be important for a given manipulation is warranted. One final limitation of this work is the frequent failure to conduct a manipulation check for inducing PA or a lack of reported specifics on the check. It is important for future induction studies to separate high and midarousal PA and use the correct manipulation for each one. For example, laughter manipulations are aimed at inducing high arousal PA, whereas the viewing of pleasant video clips may result in midarousal PA. These differences in arousal may produce differing effects on the immune system and thus should be carefully outlined and controlled for. Further, it is essential to select the appropriate measures for assessing the different types of PA. For example, use of the PANAS might not be appropriate for assessing the effects of mindfulness or calm inductions because this measure does not adequately address the low arousal emotions thought to be associated with these manipulations.

In addition to measurement and manipulation checks, it is also important for future studies to investigate the relationship between mindfulness and emotional changes including low-arousal PA.

It is currently unclear whether mindfulness manipulations are actually manipulating calmness or any another emotion. It may be the case that the relaxed state of mindfulness actually produces later vigor raising very different mechanistic pathways.

Finally, it is critical that future studies attempt a more integrated view of the relationship between state PA and immune function. This would include a better understanding of the progression of changes that occur following emotion induction such as brain activity alterations, neurotransmitter release, hormone changes, and the resulting immune function. Although these relations are complex and costly to investigate simultaneously, a multisystems approach will help develop an advanced understanding of exactly how PA influences the immune system. It will also advance the goal of fully understanding when and why happiness might be good for us.

Related Chapters

For more information on concepts introduced in this chapter, see also Suarez; and Cohen, this volume.

References

Almawi, W., Beyhum, H. N., Rahme, A. A., & Rieder, M. (1996). Regulation of cytokine and cytokine receptor expression by glucocorticoids. *Journal of Leukocyte Biology, 60*(5), 563–572.

Bachen, E. A., Manuck, S. B., Cohen, S., Muldoon, M. F., Raible, R., Herbert, T. B., et al. (1995). Adrenergic blockade ameliorates cellular immune responses to mental stress in humans. *Psychosomatic Medicine, 57*(4), 366–372.

Bacon, S. L., Watkins, L. L., Babyak, M., Sherwood, A., Hayano, J., Hinderliter, A. L., et al. (2004). Effects of daily stress on autonomic cardiac control in patients with coronary artery disease. *The American Journal of Cardiology, 93*(10), 1292–1294.

Bennett, M. P., Zeller, J. M., Rosenberg, L., & McCann, J. (2003). The effect of mirthful laughter on stress and natural killer cell activity. *Alternative Therapies in Health and Medicine, 9*(2), 38–45.

Berk, L. S., Felten, D. L., Tan, S. A., Bittman, B. B., & Westengard, J. (2001). Modulation of neuroimmune parameters during the eustress of humor-associated mirthful laughter. *Alternative Therapies in Health and Medicine, 7*(2), 62–76.

Berk, L. S., Tan, S. A., Fry, W. F., Napier, B. J., Lee, J. W., Hubbard, R. W., et al. (1989). Neuroendocrine and stress hormone changes during mirthful laughter. *The American Journal of the Medical Sciences, 298*(6), 390–396.

Borovikova, L. V., Ivanova, S., Zhang, M., Yang, H., Botchkina, G. I., Watkins, L. R., et al. (2000). Vagus nerve stimulation attenuates the systemic inflammatory response to endotoxin. *Nature, 405*(6785), 458–462.

Bristow, M., Hucklebridge, F., Clow, A., & Evans, P. D. (1997). Modulation of secretory immunoglobin A in saliva in relation to an acute episode of stress and arousal. *Journal of Psychophysiology, 11,* 248–255.

Buchanan, T. W., al'Absi, M., & Lovallo, W. R. (1999). Cortisol fluctuates with increases and decreases in negative affect. *Psychoneuroendocrinology, 24,* 227–241.

Burdick, N., Randel, R., Carroll, J., & Welsh, T. Jr. (2011). Interactions between temperament, stress, and immune function in cattle. *Journal of Animal Science, 87,* 3202–3210.

Carlson, L. E., Speca, M., Patel, K. D., & Goodey, E. (2003). Mindfulness-based stress reduction in relation to quality of life, mood, symptoms of stress, and immune parameters in breast and prostate cancer outpatients. *Psychosomatic Medicine, 65*(4), 571–581.

Cato, A. C. B., & Wade, E. (1996). Molecular mechanisms of anti inflammatory action of glucocorticoids. *Bioessays, 18*(5), 371–378.

Chida, Y., & Steptoe, A. (2008). Positive psychological well-being and mortality: A quantitative review of prospective observational studies. *Psychosomatic Medicine, 70*(7), 741–756.

Clark, L. A., Watson, D., & Leeka, J. (1989). Diurnal variation in the positive affects. *Motivation and Emotion, 13*(3), 205–234.

Codispoti, M., Gerra, G., Montebarocci, O., Zaimovic, A., Augusta Raggi, M., & Baldaro, B. (2003). Emotional perception and neuroendocrine changes. *Psychophysiology, 40*(6), 863–868.

Cohen, S., Alper, C. M., Doyle, W. J., Treanor, J. J., & Turner, R. B. (2006). Positive emotional style predicts resistance to illness after experimental exposure to rhinovirus or influenza a virus. *Psychosomatic Medicine, 68*(6), 809–815.

Cohen, S., Doyle, W. J., Turner, R. B., Alper, C. M., & Skoner, D. P. (2003). Emotional style and susceptibility to the common cold. *Psychosomatic Medicine, 65*(4), 652–657.

Davidson, R. J., Kabat-Zinn, J., Schumacher, J., Rosenkranz, M., Muller, D., Santorelli, S. F., et al. (2003). Alterations in brain and immune function produced by mindfulness meditation. *Psychosomatic Medicine, 65*(4), 564–570.

Diener, E., & Emmons, R. A. (1984). The independence of positive and negative affect. *Journal of Personality and Social Psychology, 47*(5), 1105–1117.

Diener, E., Larsen, R. J., Levine, S., & Emmons, R. A. (1985). Intensity and frequency: Dimensions underlying positive and negative affect. *Journal of Personality and Social Psychology, 48*(5), 1253–1265.

Dillon, K. M., Minchoff, B., & Baker, K. H. (1985). Positive emotional states and enhancement of the immune system. *The International Journal of Psychiatry in Medicine, 15,* 13–18.

Ekman, P. (1992). Are there basic emotions? *Psychological Review, 99,* 550–553.

Evans, P., Bristow, M., Hucklebridge, F., & Clow, A. (1993). The relationship between secretory immunity, mood and life-events. *British journal of clinical psychology, 32,* 227–236.

Feldmann, M., Brennan, F. M., & Maini, R. N. (1996). Role of cytokines in rheumatoid arthritis. *Annual Review of Immunology, 14*(1), 397–440.

Felten, S., & Olschowka, J. (1987). Noradrenergic sympathetic innervation of the spleen: II. Tyrosine hydroxylase (TH) positive nerve terminals form synapticlike contacts on lymphocytes in the splenic white pulp. *Journal of Neuroscience Research, 18,* 37–48.

Frazier, T. W., Strauss, M. E., & Steinhauer, S. R. (2004). Respiratory sinus arrhythmia as an index of emotional response in young adults. *Psychophysiology, 41,* 75–83.

Fredrickson, B. L. (1998). What good are positive emotions? *Review of General Psychology, 2*(3), 300–319.

Fredrickson, B. L., Mancuso, R. A., Branigan, C., & Tugade, M. M. (2000). The undoing effect of positive emotions. *Motivation & Emotion, 24*(4), 237–258.

Futterman, A. D., Kemeny, M. E., Shapiro, D., & Fahey, J. L. (1994). Immunological and physiological changes associated with induced positive and negative mood. *Psychosomatic Medicine, 56*(6), 499.

Futterman, A. D., Kemeny, M. E., Shapiro, D., Polonsky, W., & Fahey, J. L. (1992). Immunological variability associated with experimentally-induced positive and negative affective states. *Psychological medicine, 22,* 231–238.

Gerra, G., Fertomani, G., Zaimovic, A., Caccavari, R., Reali, N., Maestri, D., et al. (1996). Neuroendocrine responses to emotional arousal in normal women. *Neuropsychobiology, 33*(4), 173–181.

Gerra, G., Zaimovic, A., Franchini, D., Palladino, M., Giucastro, G., Reali, N., et al. (1998). Neuroendocrine responses of healthy volunteers to techno-music': Relationships with personality traits and emotional state. *International Journal of Psychophysiology, 28,* 99–111.

Harrison, L. K., Carroll, D., Burns, V. E., Corkill, A. R., Harrison, C. M., Ring, C., et al. (2000). Cardiovascular and secretory immunoglobulin A reactions to humorous, exciting, and didactic film presentations. *Biological psychology, 52*(2), 113–126.

Herbert, T. B., & Cohen, S. (1993a). Depression and immunity: A meta-analytic review. *Psychological Bulletin, 113*(3), 472–486.

Herbert, T. B., & Cohen, S. (1993b). Stress and immunity in humans: A meta-analytic review. *Psychosomatic Medicine, 55*(4), 364–379.

Hucklebridge, F., Lambert, S., Clow, A., Warburton, D., Evans, P. D., & Sherwood, N. (2000). Modulation of secretory immunoglobulin A in saliva: Response to manipulation of mood. *Biological psychology, 53,* 25–35.

Kiecolt-Glaser, J. K., & Glaser, R. (1991). Stress and immune function in humans. In R. Ader, D. L. Felten, & N. Cohen (Eds.), *Psychoneuroimmunology* (pp. 849–867). San Diego, CA: Academic Press.

Kimata, H. (2001). Effect of humor on allergen-induced wheal reactions. *JAMA, 285*(6), 738.

Knapp, P. H., Levy, E. M., Giorgi, R. G., Black, P. H., Fox, B. H., & Heeren, T. C. (1992). Short-term immunological effects of induced emotion. *Psychosomatic Medicine, 54*(2), 133–148.

Kraft, T. L., & Pressman, S. D. (in press). Grin and bear it: The influence of manipulated facial expression on the stress response. *Psychological Science.*

Labott, S. M., Ahleman, S., Wolever, M. E., & Martin, R. B. (1990). The physiological and psychological effects of the expression and inhibition of emotion. *Behavioral Medicine, 16*(4), 182–189.

Laidlaw, T. M., Booth, R. J., & Large, R. G. (1994). The variability of Type I hypersensitivity reactions: The importance of mood. *Journal of Psychosomatic Research, 38,* 51–61.

Laidlaw, T. M., Booth, R. J., & Large, R. G. (1996). Reduction in skin reactions to histamine after a hypnotic procedure. *Psychosomatic Medicine, 58*(3), 242–248.

Lambert, R., & Lambert, N. K. (1995). The effects of humor on secretory immunoglobulin A levels in school-aged children. *Pediatric Nursing, 21,* 16–19.

Lazarus, R. S., & Folkman, S. (1984). *Stress, appraisal, and coping.* New York: Springer.

Levy, S. M., Lee, J., Bagley, C., & Lippman, M. (1988). Survival hazards analysis in first recurrent breast cancer patients: Seven-year follow-up. *Psychosomatic Medicine, 50*(5), 520–528.

Livnat, S., Felten, S. Y., Carlson, S. L., Bellinger, D. L., & Felten, D. L. (1985). Involvement of peripheral and central catecholamine systems in neural-immune interactions. *Journal of Neuroimmunology, 10,* 5–30.

Logan, H. L., Lutgendorf, S., Hartwig, A., Lilly, J., & Berberich, S. L. (1998). Immune, stress, and mood markers related to recurrent oral herpes outbreaks. *Oral Surgery, Oral Medicine, Oral Pathology, Oral Radiology, and Endodontology, 86,* 48–54.

Lutgendorf, S. K., Reimer, T. T., Harvey, J. H., Marks, G., Hong, S. Y., Hillis, S. L., et al. (2001). Effects of housing relocation on immunocompetence and psychosocial functioning in older adults. *The Journals of Gerontology Series A: Biological Sciences and Medical Sciences, 56*(2), M97–105.

Manuck, S. B., Cohen, S., Rabin, B. S., Muldoon, M. F., & Bachen, E. A. (1991). Individual differences in cellular immune response to stress. *Psychological Science, 2*(2), 111–115.

Margolin, K. A. (2000). Interleukin-2 in the treatment of renal cancer. *Seminars in Oncology, 27*(2), 194–203.

Marsland, A. L., Bachen, E. A., Cohen, S., & Manuck, S. B. (2001). Stress, immunity, and susceptibility to infectious disease. In A. Baum, T. A. Revenson, & J. E. Singer (Eds.), *Handbook of Health Psychology* (pp. 683–695). Mahwah, NJ: Erlbaum.

Matsunaga, M., Isowa, T., Kimura, K., Miyakoshi, M., Kanayama, N., Murakami, H., et al. (2008). Associations among central nervous, endocrine, and immune activities when positive emotions are elicited by looking at a favorite person. *Brain, Behavior, and Immunity, 22*(3), 408–417.

Matsuzaki, T., Nakajima, A., Ishigami, S., Tanno, M., & Yoshino, S. (2006). Mirthful laughter differentially affects serum pro- and anti-inflammatory cytokine levels depending on the level of disease activity in patients with rheumatoid arthritis. *Rheumatology, 45*(2), 182–186.

McClelland, D. C., & Cheriff, A. D. (1997). The immunoenhancing effects of humor on secretory IgA and resistance to respiratory infections. *Psychology & Health, 12*(3), 329–344.

McCraty, R., Atkinson, M., Rein, G., & Watkins, A. D. (1996). Music enhances the effect of positive emotional states on salivary IgA. *Stress Medicine, 12,* 167–175.

Mittwoch-Jaffe, T., Shalit, F., Srendi, B., & Yehuda, S. (1995). Modification of cytokine secretion following mild emotional stimuli. *Neuroreport, 6,* 789–792.

Moskowitz, J. T. (2003). Positive affect predicts lower risk of AIDS mortality. *Psychosomatic Medicine, 65*(4), 620–626.

Moss, R. B., Moss, H. B., & Peterson, R. (1989). Microstress, mood, and natural killer-cell activity. *Psychosomatics, 30*(3), 279–289.

Neumann, S. A., & Waldstein, S. R. (2001). Similar patterns of cardiovascular response during emotional activation as a function of affective valence and arousal and gender. *Journal of Psychosomatic Research, 50*(5), 245–253.

Njus, D. M., Nitschke, W., & Bryant, F. B. (1996). Positive affect, negative affect, and the moderating effect of writing on sIgA antibody levels. *Psychology & Health, 12,* 135–148.

Pace, T. W. W., Negi, L. T., Adame, D. D., Cole, S. P., Sivilli, T. I., Brown, T. D., et al. (2009). Effect of compassion meditation on neuroendocrine, innate immune and behavioral responses to psychosocial stress. *Psychoneuroendocrinology, 34,* 87–98.

Pawlow, L., & Jones, G. (2005). The impact of abbreviated progressive muscle relaxation on salivary cortisol and salivary immunoglobulin A (sIgA). *Applied Psychophysiology and Biofeedback, 30*(4), 375–387.

Perera, S., Sabin, E., Nelson, P., & Lowe, D. (1998). Increases in salivary lysozyme and IgA concentrations and secretory rates independent of salivary flow rates following viewing of a humorous videotape. *International Journal of Behavioral Medicine, 5*(2), 118–128.

Polk, D. E., Cohen, S., Doyle, W. J., Skoner, D. P., & Kirschbaum, C. (2005). State and trait affect as predictors of salivary cortisol in healthy adults. *Psychoneuroendocrinology, 30*(3), 261–272.

Pressman, S. D., & Cohen, S. (2005). Does positive affect influence health? *Psychological Bulletin, 131*(6), 925–971.

Pressman, S. D., Matthews, K. A., Cohen, S., Martire, L. M., Scheier, M., Baum, A., & Schulz, R. (2009). Association of enjoyable leisure activities with psychological and physical well-being. *Psychosomatic Medicine, 71,* 725–732.

Rabin, B. S. (1999). *Stress, immune function, and health: The connection.* New York: Wiley-Liss.

Radloff, L. S. (1977). The CES-D scale: A self-report depression scale for research in the general population. *Applied Psychological Measurement, 1*(3), 385–401.

Rasmussen, H. N., Scheier, M. F., & Greenhouse, J. B. (2009). Optimism and physical health: A meta-analytic review. *Annals of Behavioral Medicine, 37*(3), 239–256.

Robinson, F. P., Mathews, H. L., & Witek-Janusek, L. (2003). Psycho-endocrine-immune response to mindfulness-based stress reduction in individuals infected with the human immunodeficiency virus: A quasiexperimental study. *Journal of Alternative & Complementary Medicine, 9*(5), 683–694.

Robles, T. F., Brooks, K. P., & Pressman, S. D. (2009). Trait positive affect buffers the effects of acute stress on skin barrier recovery. *Health Psychology, 28*(3), 373.

Russell, J. A. (1980). A circumplex model of affect. *Journal of Personality and Social Psychology, 39*(6), 1161–1178.

Ryff, C. D., Singer, B. H., & Love, G. D. (2004). Positive health: Connecting well-being with biology. *Philosophical Transactions of the Royal Society B: Biological Sciences, 359*(1449), 1383–1394.

Segerstrom, S. C., & Miller, G. E. (2004). Psychological stress and the human immune system: A meta-analytic study of 30 years of inquiry. *Psychological Bulletin, 130*(4), 601–630.

Sepah, S. C., & Bower, J. E. (2009). Positive affect and inflammation during radiation treatment for breast and prostate cancer. *Brain, Behavior, and Immunity, 23*(8), 1068–1072.

Shapiro, S. L., Carlson, L. E., Astin, J. A., & Freedman, B. (2006). Mechanisms of mindfulness. *Journal of clinical psychology, 62*(3), 373–386.

Smith, A. W., & Baum, A. (2003). The influence of psychological factors on restorative function in health and illness. In J. Suls & K. A. Wallston (Eds.), *Social Psychological Foundations of Health and Illness* (pp. 431–457). Malden, MA: Blackwell.

Smyth, J., Ockenfels, M. C., Porter, L., Kirschbaum, C., Hellhammer, D. H., & Stone, A. A. (1998). Stressors and mood measured on a momentary basis are associated with salivary cortisol secretion. *Psychoneuroendocrinology, 23*(4), 353–370.

Solomon, G. F., & Moos, R. (1964). Emotions, immunity, and disease. *Archives of General Psychiatry, 11,* 657–674.

Steptoe, A., Wardle, J., & Marmot, M. (2005). Positive affect and health-related neuroendocrine, cardiovascular, and inflammatory processes. *Proceedings of the National Academy of Sciences of the United States of America, 102*(18), 6508–6512.

Stone, A. A., Cox, D. S., Valdimarsdottir, H., Jandorf, L., & Neale, J. M. (1987). Evidence that secretory IgA antibody is associated with daily mood. *Journal of personality and social psychology, 52*(5), 988–993.

Stone, A. A., Cox, D. S., Valdimarsdottir, H., & Neale, J. M. (1987). Secretory IgA as a measure of immunocompetence. *Journal of Human Stress, 13*(3), 136–140.

Stone, A. A., Neale, J. M., Cox, D. S., Napoli, A., Valdimarsdottir, H., & Kennedy-Moore, E. (1994). Daily events are associated with a secretory immune response to an oral antigen in men. *Health Psychology, 13*(5), 440–446.

Szcepanski, R., Napolitano, M., Feaganes, J. R., Barefoot, J. C., Luecken, L., Swoap, R., et al. (1997). Relation of mood ratings and neurohormonal responses during daily life in employed women. *International Journal of Behavioral Medicine, 4,* 1–16.

Takahashi, K., Iwase, M., Yamashita, K., Tatsumoto, Y., Ue, H., Kuratsune, H., et al. (2001). The elevation of natural killer cell activity induced by laughter in a crossover designed study. *International Journal of Molecular Medicine, 8*(6), 645–650.

Taylor, S. E., Gonzaga, G. C., Klein, L. C., Hu, P., Greendale, G. A., & Seeman, T. E. (2006). Relation of oxytocin to psychological stress responses and hypothalamic-pituitary-adrenocortical axis activity in older women. *Psychosomatic Medicine, 68*(2), 238–245.

Tracey, K. J. (2002). The inflammatory reflex. *Nature, 420*(6917), 853–859.

Usala, P. D., & Hertzog, C. (1989). Measurement of affective states in adults. *Research on Aging, 11*(4), 403–426.

Valdimarsdottir, H. B., & Bovbjerg, D. H. (1997). Positive and negative mood: Association with natural killer cell activity. *Psychology & Health, 12*(3), 319–327.

Watson, D. (1988). The vicissitudes of mood measurement: Effects of varying descriptors, time frames, and response formats on measures of positive and negative affect. *Journal of Personality and Social Psychology, 55,* 128–141.

Watson, D., Clark, L. A., & Tellegen, A. (1988). Development and validation of brief measures of positive and negative affect: The PANAS scales. *Journal of Personality and Social Psychology, 54*(6), 1063–1070.

Watson, D., & Tellegen, A. (1985). Toward a consensual structure of mood. *Psychological Bulletin, 98*(2), 219–235.

Westermann, R., Spies, K., Stahl, G., & Hesse, F. W. (1996). Relative effectiveness and validity of mood induction procedures: A meta-analysis. *European Journal of Social Psychology, 26*(4), 557–580.

Willemsen, G., Ring, C., Carroll, D., Evans, P., Clow, A., & Hucklebridge, F. (1998). Secretory immunoglobulin A and cardiovascular reactions to mental arithmetic and cold pressor. *Psychophysiology, 35*(3), 252–259.

Witek-Janusek, L., Albuquerque, K., Chroniak, K. R., Chroniak, C., Durazo-Arvizu, R., & Mathews, H. L. (2008). Effect of mindfulness based stress reduction on immune function, quality of life and coping in women newly diagnosed with early stage breast cancer. *Brain, Behavior, and Immunity, 22*(6), 969–981.

Yaxin, F., Yi-Yuan, T., Yinghua, M., & Posner, M. I. (2010). Mucosal immunity modulated by integrative meditation in a dose-dependent fashion. *Journal of Alternative & Complementary Medicine, 16*(2), 151–155.

Yoshino, S., Fujimori, J., & Kohda, M. (1996). Effects of mirthful laughter on neuroendocrine and immune systems in patients with rheumatoid arthritis. *The Journal of Rheumatology, 23*(4), 793–794.

Yudkin, J. S., Kumari, M., Humphries, S. E., & Mohamed-Ali, V. (2000). Inflammation, obesity, stress and coronary heart disease: Is interleukin-6 the link? *Atherosclerosis, 148*(2), 209–214.

Zachariae, R., Bjerring, P., Zachariae, C., Arendt Nielsen, L., Nielsen, T., Eldrup, E., et al. (1991). Monocyte chemotactic activity in sera after hypnotically induced emotional states. *Scandinavian Journal of Immunology, 34,* 71–79.

Zachariae, R., Jørgensen, M., Egekvist, H., & Bjerring, P. (2001). Skin reactions to histamine of healthy subjects after hypnotically induced emotions of sadness, anger, and happiness. *Allergy, 56*(8), 734–740.

Emotional Expression and Disclosure

Roger J. Booth

Abstract

Writing or talking about past emotionally laden events in our lives has been found to result in a variety of psychological, social, and physiological changes that often lead to improvements in health for those who participate in the disclosure process in particular ways. This chapter will review the range of effects reported using emotional expression and disclosure as an experimental or therapeutic tool, highlighting illnesses and patient groups for which it has been effective. It will discuss the factors required for effectiveness and consider the likely importance of such psychological theories as disinhibition, cognitive processing, self-regulation, social integration, and exposure as explanations of the process. The findings of several recent meta-analyses will also be summarized. Finally, the neuroimmune changes identified in disclosure research will be considered, and a possible psychoneuroimmune mechanism to explain this intriguing field of research will be presented.

Key Words: autonomic, cognitive processing, cytokines, disclosure, disinhibition, emotion, expression, goals, inflammation, meaning-making, neuroimmune, self-regulation, self/no-self, social integration, trauma, word use

Introduction

As social animals, humans live in a realm of shared activities coordinated through the domain of consensual linguistic coupling involving recurrent gestural and verbal coordinating activities. We express ourselves and make sense of our lives and events in them through the vehicle of these meaningful linguistic behaviors. Moreover, because linguistic activities necessarily require shared understandings of the meanings of the coordinating tokens out of which they are constructed (e.g., words, gestures, body postures, etc.), expressing ourselves in any sort of linguistic domain (e.g., thinking private thoughts, or communicating them to others) always assumes the presence of an observer (listener) or observers, who can include ourselves.

As we live, the structure of our bodies constantly changes to enable us to act in ways that maintain viable relationships with our worlds. When events

happen in our lives, our bodily structure changes to prepare us for actions relevant to those events, and we experience those structural changes as our "emotions"—literally, our bodily dispositions for particular sets of actions. When we reflect upon our emotions and the events associated with them, we generate narratives that we call "feelings," describing the impact of those emotions and events on our experiences of ourselves and, through this process, we construct cognitive representations linking the events and associated emotions. Recalling events in our lives, therefore, always brings forth an associated emotional context to the extent that sometimes we prefer not to remember particular events because we consider the associated emotions are too painful or overwhelming for us.

The value of sharing our thoughts and feelings with sympathetic others has long been recognized as a salutary activity for humans. Following any sort of emotional experience, people generally talk about the experience, and the rate of sharing is often very high and remarkably similar across different cultures (Rimé, Philippot, Boca, & Mesquita, 1992). Most of us expect to feel better after sharing our emotional episodes with others, and in a study with over 1,000 college students, 89% agreed that talking about an emotional experience was relieving (Zech, 1981). Although no significant positive relationship was found between the amount of social sharing after the emotional event and the degree of emotional recovery (Pennebaker, Emmanuelle, & Bernard, 2001), in 1986, Pennebaker and Beall published a study that indicated health benefits from written emotional disclosure (Pennebaker & Beall, 1986). This study triggered a burgeoning interest in the use of emotional expression and emotional disclosure as health-promoting interventions. Because there have been several reviews and meta-analyses of the emotional expression literature (Booth, 2005; Booth & Petrie, 2002; Frattaroli, 2006; Lepore & Smyth, 2002; Pennebaker, Mehl, & Niederhoffer, 2003), this chapter will not review in detail the field as a whole but focus on what has been done in this area that is relevant to psychoneuroimmunology and how we might make sense of it.

The Background of Emotional Disclosure Interventions

Following his initial finding that writing about emotionally traumatic issues compared with writing descriptively about mundane topics resulted in reduced health-center visits over the subsequent 6 months in first-year college students (Pennebaker & Beall, 1986), James Pennebaker and his colleagues explored the use of expressive writing in a variety of laboratory-based experimental studies. In what have now become known as "Pennebaker-type" interventions, volunteers are asked to write about traumatic or upsetting events in their lives and to explore their deepest thoughts and feelings about those events in their writing. Typically, a simple randomized control design is employed in which participants are asked to write anonymously and confidentially for 15–20 minutes every day for 3–4 days about either traumatic experiences in an emotionally expressive way or mundane events in a descriptive way.

Since the initial research, subsequent studies by Pennebaker and colleagues revealed beneficial effects of emotionally expressive writing on grade averages of students (Dalton & Glenwick, 2009; Pennebaker, Colder, & Sharp, 1990), absentee rates in university employees (Francis & Pennebaker,

1992), and re-employment rate following job loss (Spera, Buhrfeind, & Pennebaker, 1994). Others have reported positive cognitive changes (Murray & Segal, 1994), improvements in upper respiratory illness symptoms following a relationship break-up (Lepore & Greenberg, 2002), and reduced depressive symptoms and intrusive thoughts (Lepore, 1997; Schoutrop, Lange, Hanewald, Davidovich, & Salomon, 2002) using emotional writing interventions with student volunteers. Although much research into emotional disclosure has centered on college students, this is not the only group to benefit. The expressive writing paradigm has led to remarkable salutary effects among children, elderly people, college students, homeless people, abuse and trauma victims, prisoners in maximum security, and patients suffering from serious disease (Frattaroli, 2006; Pennebaker et al., 2001; Smyth, 1998).

The positive effects have been reported in different parts of the world including the United States, New Zealand, Australia, Japan, England, and other European countries (Pennebaker et al., 2001). Further, despite a potentially stressful process of emotionally reexperiencing the event during writing, many participants have found that the disclosure process is valuable and meaningful and few participants have reported difficulty dealing with negative emotions evoked by the writing exercise (Pennebaker et al., 2001; Smyth, 1998). In the early studies, writing times and frequencies (20 minutes per day for 4 consecutive days) and a laboratory venue were chosen on purely pragmatic grounds— to enable college students to complete the process within a week—and although much of the research subsequently has used the similar parameters, some has explored other time intervals and locations. The most recent meta-analysis of 146 published and unpublished studies (Frattaroli, 2006) concluded that effect sizes tended to be larger in studies in which participants had at least 3 disclosure sessions lasting at least 15 minutes and with an interval between writing sessions being at least a day. Further, a private setting for disclosure was found to produce the better psychological results and writing at home rather than in a laboratory setting also produced desirable psychological outcomes (Frattaroli, 2006; van Middendorp, Geenen, Sorbi, van Doornen, & Bijlsma, 2009), although most home-based studies have found minimal beneficial effects on physical health (Bower, Kemeny, Taylor, & Fahey, 2003; Broderick, Stone, Smyth, & Kaell, 2004; Kelley, Lumley, & Leisen, 1997; Sheese, Brown, & Graziano, 2004; Stroebe, Stroebe, Schut, Zech, &

van den Bout, 2002; Ullrich & Lutgendorf, 2002; Walker, Nail, & Croyle, 1999).

Short-Term Effects

Many disclosure studies have assessed immediate mood changes using a short questionnaire before and after the writing. Writing about traumatic experiences tends to make people feel transiently unhappy and distressed. In his meta-analysis, Smyth (Smyth, 1998) reported a large effect size (0.84) for immediate increases in distress following writing, although prior to expressive writing, highly distressed participants, such as senior engineers who had been laid off from their jobs (Spera et al., 1994) and college students who presented with multiple physical symptoms (Lumley & Provenzano, 2003) reported immediate mood improvements during the course of the writing. Thus, emotional state after writing may depend on how participants were feeling prior to writing—the better they feel before the task, the worse they feel after and vice versa (Pennebaker et al., 2001). Along with moods, participants have often been asked to record physical sensations after emotional expression (Booth, Petrie, & Pennebaker, 1997; Paez, Velasco, & Gonzalez, 1999; Richards, Beal, Seagal, & Pennebaker, 2000; Sloan & Marx, 2004; Ullrich & Lutgendorf, 2002). In these studies, unpleasantness and physical arousal were present after each writing session but most evident after the first session.

Short-term physiological effects including autonomic nervous system (ANS) effects and endocrine modulation have been found, also. Three studies found a drop in skin conductance levels (SCL) during emotionally expressive writing but not during nonemotional writing (Pennebaker, Barger, & Tiebout, 1989; Pennebaker, Hughes, & O'Heeron, 1987; Petrie, Booth, Pennebaker, Davison, & Thomas, 1995), and greater severity of disclosed trauma was associated with larger drop in SCL (Pennebaker et al., 1989; Pennebaker et al., 1987). Because SCL has been regarded as an indicator of behavioral inhibition (Fowles, 1980) and experimentally induced thought suppression has been found to increase SCL (Wegner, Shortt, Blake, & Page, 1990), Pennebaker suggested that not disclosing or confronting trauma represents ongoing inhibition, whereas emotionally expressive writing reverses the process (Pennebaker et al., 1987; Pennebaker, Kiecolt-Glaser, & Glaser, 1988). Short-term cardiovascular reactivity is also associated with emotional disclosure, with both blood pressure and heart rate generally being found to be more reactive to emotional writing than to descriptive writing (Knapp et al., 1992; Pennebaker & Beall, 1986; Pennebaker et al., 1987; Pennebaker et al., 1988) and the pattern of changes is consistent with motivating and cognitively challenging tasks rather than with fearful experiences (Mendes, Reis, Seery, & Blascovich, 2003). Sloan and Marx (Sloan & Marx, 2004) found increased self-reports of unpleasantness and physical sensations and greater cortisol levels among those who wrote about a traumatic event relative to those who wrote about a trivial topic, but as sessions progressed, the group differences in self-reported affect and cortisol diminished. In contrast, (Dickerson, Gruenewald, & Kemeny, 2004) found no significant difference in cortisol between two writing conditions, although increased negative self-perceptions of guilt and shame were reported by those in the expressive condition, relative to those in the neutral condition.

Emotional expression in a variety of situations has been found to result in short-term changes in several immune variables. For example, expressing or inhibiting emotions while viewing emotionally rich videos has been found to affect salivary IgA (sIgA) concentrations (Labott, Ahleman, Wolever, & Martin, 1990; Martin, Guthrie, & Pitts, 1993), and deliberately expressing emotions affected circulating natural killer (NK) cell and CD8 T percentages (Futterman, Kemeny, Shapiro, & Fahey, 1994; Futterman, Kemeny, Shapiro, Polonsky, & Fahey, 1992). Also, healthy volunteers asked to recall maximally disturbing or maximally pleasurable emotional experiences, displayed significant cardiovascular activation, transient declines in mitogen-induced T lymphocyte proliferation and small changes in NK cell activity (Knapp et al., 1992). Circulating immunological regulatory cytokines concentrations have also been found to be affected by mood changes. For example, increased secretion of cytokines associated with T lymphocyte proliferation (e.g., IL-2) but not those associated with inflammation (e.g., IL-1 and IL-6) was observed in response to mild induced negative emotional changes, whereas the reverse of this (i.e., increased inflammatory cytokines but not T cell proliferative cytokines) occurred following positive mood changes (Mittwoch-Jaffe, Shalit, Srendi, & Yehuda, 1995). "Pennebaker-type" written emotional disclosure studies have also found short-term changes in immunological variables such as circulating lymphocyte counts (Booth et al., 1997; Petrie, Booth, & Pennebaker, 1998; Petrie et al., 1995), lymphocyte responsiveness to mitogens (Knapp et al., 1992; Pennebaker et al., 1988), proinflammatory cytokine activity (Dickerson et al., 2004), and NK cell cytotoxicity (Bower et al., 2003), and some of these may be associated with concomitant cortisol and neuroendocrine changes (Dickerson, Kemeny, Aziz, Kim, & Fahey, 2004; Sloan & Marx, 2004).

Moderators of Emotional Disclosure

In the early studies of students following emotional disclosure, changes in health-center visits and measures associated with psychological well-being, such as anxiety, depression, and stress, were often assessed over subsequent weeks or months (Pennebaker, 2004) and it became apparent that the short-term changes (summarized earlier) were not necessarily related to longer-term effects. Immediate postdisclosure effects are likely to be the result of transient autonomic and cardiovascular activation resulting from the upsetting or "stressful" nature of the disclosure process and bearing little relationships to longer-term disease-relevant changes. Instead, the characteristics of the people doing the emotional writing and the nature of their disclosures are better predictors of beneficial outcomes. For example, analyzing the cognitive and emotional content of the disclosed material has suggested that positive health changes are associated with negative-emotion word use (Pennebaker, Mayne, & Francis, 1997); increased use of positive emotion; cognition- and insight-related words across writing sessions (Pennebaker et al., 1997; Ramírez-Esparza & Pennebaker, 2006); changes in function words, especially pronouns, across writing sessions (Campbell & Pennebaker, 2003); and evidence of finding meaning in the events being described (Bower et al., 2003; Burke & Bradley, 2006; O'Cleirigh et al., 2003). Consistent with these findings, several emotional and personality characteristics have been identified to moderate the effectiveness of emotional disclosure. After reviewing several studies, Stroebe and colleagues (Stroebe, Schut, & Stroebe, 2006) concluded that people with secure attachment styles are less likely to benefit from the disclosure paradigm, because they are normally able to disclose in ways that further the adjustment process in their everyday lives. They suggested that targeting people with insecure attachment styles and providing attachment-style-specific disclosure instructions are likely to increase the power of the manipulation.

People with a tendency to experience negative emotions and to inhibit their expression (sometimes referred to as type D or repressor personality) have elevated levels of soluble markers associated with inflammatory immune responses (TNF-alpha and soluble TNF-alpha receptors) (Conraads et al., 2006). Further, people who have difficulty in recognizing and describing their emotional states (often referred to as alexithymia) have elevated levels of circulating cytokines (IL-1, IL-2 and IL-4) associated with an impaired pro-/anti-inflammatory immune balance (Corcos et al., 2004). E repressive or alexithymic characteristics have been found to attenuate the health benefits of disclosure (Lumley, 2004). Consistent with this, Petrie and colleagues (1998) found that, although emotional writing was associated with postwriting increases in circulating helper T lymphocyte numbers in healthy volunteers, deliberate suppression of thoughts about the written events following writing decreased circulating T lymphocyte numbers. In contrast, allowing appropriate emotions to be expressed in response to events may be salutary. Ishii and colleagues (Ishii, Nagashima, Tanno, Nakajima, & Yoshino, 2003) compared the levels of plasma cortisol and IL-6, the CD4/CD8 ratio, and NK cell activity in peripheral blood between the patients with easily controlled rheumatoid arthritis (RA) and those with difficult-to-control RA before and after a psychological stress session and found that overtly expressing emotions had a greater influence on these blood variables in patients with difficult-to-control RA than in those with easily controlled RA. Moreover, patients who were moved to tears were likely to develop good control of RA over the subsequent year.

Further, in a study in which 61 HIV-seropositive women without AIDS underwent coping interviews to assess HIV-specific emotional support and emotional expression and inhibition, using the percentage of positive/negative emotion words and inhibition words, respectively, a higher percentage of inhibition words was associated with lower CD4 T lymphocyte concentrations (Eisenberger, Kemeny, & Wyatt, 2003). This, also, is consistent with their being a relationship between psychological inhibition and deleterious health outcomes.

Emotional and behavioral volatility in the form of hostility is known to have a significant association with development and progression of arteriosclerosis and heart disease, and this has been linked to immune and inflammatory processes (Everson-Rose & Lewis, 2005; Miller, Freedland, Carney, Stetler, & Banks, 2003). Comparing immune response and psychological factors among 74 patients with heart disease and 64 healthy controls, Ishihara and colleagues (Ishihara, Makita, Imai, Hashimoto, & Nohara, 2003) found that, not only was NK cell activity significantly higher in the heart disease group, but, also, it was significantly elevated by suppression of anger and negative emotions. Christensen and colleagues (1996) explored the effect of cynical hostility on the relationship between emotional expression and NK cell activity further. In a cohort of 43 male college undergraduates classified as high or low on the Cook-Medley Hostility scale and randomly assigned to either a verbal self-disclosure or a nondisclosure discussion condition, they found that, among subjects in the self-disclosure condition, high hostility subjects exhibited a significantly greater increase in NK cell activity than did low hostility subjects. They suggest that this may be the consequence of a more pronounced acute arousal response elicited by the self-disclosure task in the high hostility group.

Austenfeld and colleagues (Austenfeld, Paolo, & Stanton, 2006) compared the effects of writing about emotions versus goals ("best possible self") on psychological and physical health among medical students. They found that, in participants with higher baseline hostility, the emotional writing condition was associated with less hostility at 3 months compared with the goal-writing and control conditions. Further, participants high in trait emotional processing (EP) reported fewer depressive symptoms in the emotional writing condition, whereas those low in EP reported fewer depressive symptoms in the goal-writing condition. A moderating effect on physical health was also identified, such that low-EP participants who wrote about goals had fewer health-care visits at 3 months, whereas high-EP participants who wrote about goals had more visits relative to other conditions (Austenfeld & Stanton, 2008). These results indicate that benefits may accrue when the expressive task is matched to the individual's preferred coping strategy. Cognitive factors, such as attentional bias, are known to influence emotional processing. In a recent study by Vedhara and colleagues (Vedhara et al., 2010), individuals with negative and avoidant attentional bias (i.e., individuals vigilant for and individuals avoidant of negative emotional material, respectively) participated in an emotional disclosure intervention, and then their mood was assessed over the following 8 weeks. Individuals with negative attentional bias showed greater improvements in depression, anger, fatigue, and total mood disturbance than did those with avoidant attentional bias, and the effects were unrelated to alexithymia, adding weight to the

proposition that matching disclosure interventions to personality and coping styles may be required for effectiveness. In summary, the data from several studies indicate that, for people with emotionally focused coping styles, or those who engage with their emotions, or those who are low in cynical hostility, direct emotionally expressive writing may be beneficial, whereas, for those low in emotional coping, or those who avoid engaging with negative emotions, or those who are high in cynical hostility, a more directed or task-oriented form of emotionally expressive writing may be more effective.

Health Effects
Pain

Several studies have investigated whether emotional disclosure interventions can alleviate pain and affect well-being in people suffering from chronic pain. For example, in a study of 48 women with chronic pelvic pain randomized to write for 3 days about stressful consequences of their pain (disclosure) or positive events (control) and assessed 2 months later, although the main effects of writing about the stress of pelvic pain were limited, women with higher baseline ambivalence about emotional expression or negative affect appear to respond more positively to this intervention (Norman, Lumley, Dooley, & Diamond, 2004). More recently, Cepeda and colleagues (2008) randomized 234 patients with cancer pain to one of three groups: a narrative group, in which patients wrote a story about how cancer affected their lives for at least 20 minutes once a week for three weeks; a questionnaire group, in which patients filled out a pain questionnaire; and a control group (weekly routine medical visits). Pain intensity and sense of well-being were similar in all groups before and after treatment, but during the 8 weeks after the intervention, patients whose narratives had high emotional disclosure had significantly less pain and reported higher well-being scores than patients whose narratives were less emotional.

Anger can be a problem for chronic pain sufferers, and, in a study involving 102 outpatients randomly assigned to express their anger constructively or to write about their goals nonemotionally in a letter-writing format on two occasions, participants in the anger-expression group over the subsequent 9 weeks experienced greater improvements in pain control, depressed mood, and pain severity than did the control group, suggesting that anger expression may be helpful for chronic pain sufferers, particularly if it leads to meaning making (Graham, Lobel,

Glass, & Lokshina, 2008). In people with migraine headaches, relaxation training has been found to be more effective at reducing headache frequency and disability relative to written emotional disclosure (D'Souza, Lumley, Kraft, Lumley, D'Souza, & Dooley, 2008), although in a subsequent study, undergraduates with migraine headaches who reported emotion-focused coping benefitted from relaxation training, whereas those who were low in headache-management self-efficacy improved with either relaxation training or emotional expression, suggesting that different coping strategies may affect the outcome of emotional disclosure interventions, at least in some patient groups (Kraft, Lumley, D'Souza, & Dooley, 2008).

Psychosis and Posttraumatic Stress

Written emotional disclosure reduced psychosis-related posttraumatic stress disorder (PTSD) symptoms in a small clinical sample recovering from a first episode of psychosis. Two to three years after their first episode of psychosis, 22 people completed measures of traumatic symptoms, recovery style, insight, anxiety, and depression, and then wrote about the most stressful aspects of their illness or about emotionally neutral topics for 15 minutes on three separate occasions. Five weeks later, those who had written about their psychotic experiences showed less overall severity and avoidance of traumatic symptoms compared with those who hadn't (Bernard, Jackson, & Jones, 2006).

The type of writing instructions also appears to be influential in determining the efficacy of emotional disclosure in posttraumatic stress sufferers. Sloan and colleagues (Sloan, Marx, & Epstein, 2005) studied college undergraduates with a trauma history and at least moderate posttraumatic stress symptoms. They were asked to write about the same traumatic experience, different traumatic experiences, or nontraumatic experiences every day for 3 days, and the results revealed that the group who wrote about the same traumatic experience reported significant reductions in psychological and physical symptoms at follow-up assessments compared with the other groups. Subsequently, investigations by the same researchers highlighted the importance of writing instructions on outcome. They randomly assigned 82 participants to one of three writing conditions that focused on emotional expression, insight, and cognitive assimilation, or to a control condition. Participants assigned to the emotional expression condition reported significant improvements in psychological and physical

health one month later, relative to the other two conditions. In addition, the emotional expression participants relative to those in the other two conditions also displayed significantly greater initial psycho-physiological reactivity and subsequent habituation (Sloan, Marx, Epstein, & Lexington, 2007).

With sexual assault victims, emotional disclosure interventions may benefit the perpetrators more than it does the victims. When psychiatric prison inmates were randomly assigned to one of three conditions (trauma writing, trivial writing, or no-writing control), although participants in the trauma condition reported experiencing more physical symptoms subsequent to the intervention relative to those in the other conditions, they significantly decreased their doctor visits postwriting (Richards et al., 2000). By contrast, in undergraduate women who acknowledged attempted or completed rape, there were no significant symptom reductions (Brown & Heimberg, 2001), nor were psychological or physical health benefits observed in women who reported a history of child sexual abuse (Batten, Follette, Rasmussen Hall, & Palm, 2002) following emotional disclosure. More recently, 74 college women with a history of sexual assault wrote about their most severe victimization or about how they spend their time. One month later, the disclosure group reported greater reductions in negative mood immediately postwriting. However, both groups showed significant reductions in physical complaints, psychological distress, and traumatic stress symptoms, suggesting no added benefit to disclosure of a sexual assault (Kearns, Edwards, Calhoun, & Gidycz, 2010).

Marital Conflict

Marital conflict is a source of emotionally related expression that has been used as a socially meaningful "stressor" in several studies (Kiecolt-Glaser et al., 1993; Dopp et al., 2000; Kiecolt-Glaser et al., 1997; Miller et al., 1999) The physiological effects of displaying anger during conflict differ depending on whether subjects are categorized as high or low in cynical hostility. Recently, Graham and colleagues (2009) assessed whether greater cognitive engagement during a marital conflict discussion, as evidenced by the use of words that suggest thinking and meaning making, would affect pro-inflammatory cytokine increases. They found that, after controlling for demographics, hostility, depressed mood, positive and negative interactions, and marital quality, individuals who used more cognitive-processing words during the conflict discussion showed smaller increases in serum IL-6 and TNF-alpha over 24 hours. They suggested that productive expression and communication patterns may help mitigate the adverse effects of relationship conflict on inflammatory dysregulation.

Rheumatoid Arthritis

The relationship of emotions and emotional disclosure to inflammation and inflammatory processes is relevant to autoimmune diseases such as rheumatoid arthritis (RA) where inappropriately aggressive or inflammatory immune responsiveness toward aspects of bone or joint tissue are evident. Evidence of inflammatory reactivity autoimmune diseases is often associated with blood changes typified by increased pro-inflammatory cytokines such as IL-1, IL-6, TNF-alpha and IFN-gamma, increases in C-reactive protein (CRP), and changes in erythrocyte sedimentation rate (ESR). Many patients with autoimmune diseases such as RA report that their disease activity fluctuates over time and is often worse at times of stress, therefore, the possibility that emotional disclosure interventions might diminish stress-related inflammation or auto-reactivity has been considered. The first research to address this randomly assigned 72 patients with RA either to talk privately about stressful events or to talk about trivial topics for four consecutive days (Kelley et al., 1997). Two weeks later, there were no differences between the groups in any health measures, but at 3 months, the disclosure patients have less affective disturbance and better physical functioning in daily activities. Interestingly, those patients who experienced larger increases in negative affect immediately after emotional disclosure also demonstrated improvements in the condition of their joints.

A subsequent study confirmed the positive effect of emotional disclosure for RA patients and extended it to asthmatic patients as well (Smyth, Stone, Hurewitz, & Kaell, 1999), measuring effectiveness in terms of changes in clinically assessed disease activity in the case of RA and objective lung function in asthma. Although in the 2 weeks following emotionally expressive or trivial writing, patients in the emotional writing group had less positive affect, increased experience of stress and more stressful thoughts, 4 months after writing there were significant improvements in disease activity for both RA and asthma patients in the emotional writing group but no change in patients in the control group, and the effects could not be explained by changes in activities, locations, or social contacts of the patients. Following this, Wetherell and colleagues (2005) conducted an exploratory home-based study (20 minutes a day for 4 days) using 34 RA patients randomly assigned either to a disclosure group in which they wrote or talked about traumatic personal experiences or to a control group in which they wrote or talked about the events of a particular day. As found in the previous studies, the disclosure group demonstrated increases in negative mood and objective markers of disease activity at 1week postintervention, but unlike previous studies, although there were significant trends for the disclosure group to demonstrate minor improvements in mood and stabilization of disease activity, these group differences appeared to be due to deteriorations in the control group rather than to improvements in the disclosure group.

Van Middendorp and colleagues (van Middendorp, & Geenen, 2008) speculated that poor cognitive-emotional processing in RA patients may adversely affect the outcome of emotional disclosure interventions. To test this, they compared alexithymia and emotional and cognitive word use with self-assessed psychological and disease activity outcome in 37 RA patients, and they found that cognitive and positive-emotion word use during disclosure sessions predicted improved psychological well-being but not disease activity after the intervention. By contrast, negative-emotion word use and alexithymia did not significantly predict outcome. Building on this, they then adapted the emotional disclosure intervention for use in home-based settings by stimulating the suggested effective ingredients of cognitive-emotional processing (van Middendorp et al., 2009). Using 68 RA patients randomly assigned to 4 weekly oral emotional-disclosure or time-management sessions, they were neither able to find any effect on psychological well-being or clinical outcome 3 months after the intervention, nor were cortisol or IFN-gamma concentrations differentially affected by the two conditions, although the change of IL-6 nearly reached significance. Another recent randomized, controlled trial of emotional disclosure in 98 RA patients explored whether clinician assistance could enhance the effects. Three conditions—private verbal emotional disclosure, clinician-assisted verbal emotional disclosure, arthritis information—in four, 30-minute laboratory sessions, were compared with a no-treatment control group, and pain, disability, affect, and stress were assessed at intervals up to 15 months postintervention. The results revealed little or no benefit of verbal emotional disclosure about stressful experiences, whether conducted privately or assisted by a clinician (Keefe et al., 2008). Taken together, the studies of emotional disclosure with RA patients have not consistently found beneficial effects, but whether this is a function of the characteristics of the patients or the disease has yet to be determined.

Infection

Human Immunodeficiency Virus (HIV) infects CD4 (helper) T lymphocytes and leads to their immune-mediated destruction resulting ultimately in Acquired Immunodeficiency Syndrome (AIDS). The course of the infectious process and its progression to AIDS is positively correlated with the amount of HIV in the blood (HIV viral load) and negatively correlated with circulating CD4 T lymphocyte concentrations. Both these markers are affected by psychosocial factors. For example, Cole and colleagues (Cole, Kemeny, Taylor, Visscher, & Fahey, 1996) have explored the effects of social isolation on psychoneuroimmune measures, and the results of their work indicates that at least some of the value of emotional expression may be related to a diminution of socially related inhibition. In a study that sought to determine whether HIV infection might progress more rapidly among gay men who conceal their homosexual identity than among those who do not, they found that HIV infection, as assessed by circulating CD4 T lymphocyte changes, advanced in proportion to the degree that participants concealed their homosexual identity. The effect could neither be explained by demographic characteristics, health practices, sexual behavior, or antiretroviral therapy, nor was it attributable to differences in depression, anxiety, social support, or repressive coping style.

Because HIV has readily measurable variables associated with disease progression (circulating HIV viral load and CD4 T lymphocyte concentrations), and because of the potential stigma and social marginalization associated with it, HIV provides an ideal infection in which to study the relationships between emotional disclosure and immune function. Lutgendorf and colleagues (1997) explored the effects of emotional disclosure on the outcome of notification of HIV status in men at risk of AIDS. In the weeks following HIV sero-status notification, avoiding thinking about HIV positivity predicted poorer mitogen-induced T lymphocyte proliferative responses as well as trends toward lower circulating CD4 T lymphocytes. They suggested that increases in avoidant and intrusive thought processing may indicate difficulties in working through the trauma of a confirmed HIV infection, and, thus, their results highlight the importance of cognitively processing stressful or emotional material for immune functioning in HIV-positive individuals. The question of whether a standard "Pennebaker-type" emotional disclosure study would result in health benefits for HIV-positive subjects was investigated in a pilot study by Petrie and colleagues (Petrie, Fontanilla, Thomas, Booth, Pennebaker, 2004). They randomly assigned 37 HIV-positive volunteers to 4 daily sessions of emotionally expressive writing or descriptive writing, and then they compared viral load and CD4 T lymphocyte levels over the subsequent 6 months, controlling for prewriting levels. Relative to the drop in viral load, CD4 T lymphocyte counts increased following the intervention for participants in the emotional-writing condition compared with control writing participants, suggesting that emotionally expressive writing may well have therapeutic benefits in HIV-infected people.

The work of Bower and colleagues (Bower, Kemeny, Taylor, & Fahey, 1998) gives clues to how this benefit might arise. When HIV-sero-positive men who had recently experienced an AIDS-related bereavement participated in structured interviews, these researchers found that men whose interviews showed evidence of engaging in cognitive processing were more likely to find meaning from the loss. Importantly, men who found meaning showed less rapid declines in CD4 T lymphocyte concentrations and lower rates of AIDS-related mortality independent of health status at baseline or health behaviors. The importance of cognitive processing, finding or reconstructing meaning, and working through, rather than simply releasing emotion was reinforced by related studies with HIV-infected volunteers. For example, HIV-positive subjects with the highest circulating CD4 T lymphocyte numbers were those with intermediate levels of expressed emotion and a high capacity for emotional processing (Solano et al., 2002). Another study analyzed the percentage of positive/negative emotion words and inhibition words used in coping interviews to assess HIV-specific emotional support and emotional expression and inhibition, respectively (Eisenberger et al., 2003). After controlling for health behaviors and other variables, a higher percentage of inhibition words was associated with lower CD4 T lymphocyte numbers.

A study of patients living with AIDS examined the relationship between long-term survival and emotional expression and depth processing of trauma (O'Cleirigh et al., 2003). Subjects wrote essays describing their reactions to past traumas and these were scored for emotional expression and evidence of depth processing such as positive cognitive appraisal change, experiential involvement, self-esteem enhancement, and adaptive coping strategies. Participants who had survived at least 4 years past an AIDS-defining symptom were compared with HIV-positive subjects who had comparably low CD4 T lymphocyte numbers but no AIDS symptoms. The long-term survivor group scored significantly higher on emotional expression and depth processing. For women, depth processing was positively related to CD4 T lymphocyte numbers, whereas emotional expression was also significantly related negatively to viral load and positively to CD4 T lymphocyte numbers. Subsequently, the same researchers compared written emotional disclosure and processing of trauma among a relatively rare group of healthy AIDS survivors (low CD4 numbers but asymptomatic for more than 9 months) with a standard HIV-positive comparison group (O'Cleirigh, Ironson, Fletcher, & Schneiderman, 2008). Each group wrote essays describing their reactions to past traumas and these were scored for emotional disclosure/processing. The healthy survivors had higher levels of emotional disclosure and emotional/cognitive processing than did the comparison group, and these psychological factors were also associated with NK cell numbers. All these findings again highlight the importance of cognitive processing rather than just emotional expression of traumatic experiences. Finally, in a more recent study by Rivkin and colleagues (Rivkin, Gustafson, Weingarten, & Chin, 2006), 50 HIV-positive volunteers participated in a structured interview and wrote about either their deepest thoughts and feelings about living with HIV or their activities over the past 24 hours. Salivary beta2-microglobulin concentrations (as an indicator of immune activation) measured 2 and 6 months later, were compared with pre-intervention concentrations. Although no effects of writing condition were found, expressive-writing participants who included increasing insight/causation and social words in their writing had higher beta2-microglobulin concentrations and reported more positive changes at follow-up. Care must be taken, however, not to overinterpret such findings, because salivary beta2-microglobulin may not necessarily indicate improved systemic immune control of HIV infection.

Several studies have assessed the immune effects of emotional disclosure using Epstein-Barr virus (EBV) activation as a marker for effective immunity. EBV is a latent herpes virus that infects a high proportion of the population and spends much of the time hidden unexpressed in certain nerve cells. Under conditions of physical or psychological stress, EBV activates, and this process is accompanied by an increase in circulating antibodies specific for the virus. Because effective control of EBV is T lymphocyte-mediated rather than antibody-mediated, the appearance of high titers of EBV-specific antibodies is generally taken as an indication of ineffective immune control of the virus. Esterling and colleagues (Esterling, Antoni, Kumar, Scheiderman, 1990) investigated whether emotional disclosure would have any impact on EBV-positive volunteers by testing whether not disclosing emotional material would correlate with poor control of the virus. The degree of emotional disclosure in essays written about stressful life events was inversely correlated with EBV antibody titers indicating better immune control of the virus was associated with emotional disclosure. Further, those participants who had repressive interpersonal styles had high antibody titers irrespective of the level of disclosure, whereas those not characterized as repressors only had high titers if they did not disclose emotions in their essays. Subsequently, these researchers compared written and spoken emotional expression with writing about superficial topics (Esterling, Antoni, Fletcher, Margulies, & Schneiderman, 1994) and found that both oral and written trauma expression resulted in lower EBV antibody titers after the intervention. The oral group achieved the greatest improvements in cognitive change, self-esteem, and adaptive coping strategies. Further, the ability of participants to involve themselves in the disclosure process and abandon their avoidance of the stressful topic during the course of the study predicted lower anti-EBV antibody titers, and these associations were more pronounced for individuals who disclosed older and more troublesome events (Lutgendorf, Antoni, Kumar, & Schneiderman, 1994).

The effects of emotional disclosure interventions on immune responses to vaccines have also been investigated. A study of healthy medical students inoculated with hepatitis B vaccine following four daily sessions of writing emotionally about traumatic events or descriptively about mundane topics revealed small but significant differences in antibody response between the two groups at 4 and 6 months after writing (Petrie et al., 1995). The emotional disclosure group displayed higher antiviral antibody titers than the descriptive writing group, suggesting that the disclosure process was influencing the ability of B lymphocytes to generate a primary antibody response over a prolonged period. In another laboratory-based disclosure intervention, Stetler and colleagues (Stetler, Chen, & Miller, 2006) assessed whether African Americans who wrote about their experiences of racial discrimination would show greater levels of antibody production in response to an influenza vaccine compared with those who wrote about a neutral topic. Interestingly, participants in the racism-disclosure group produced significantly lower antibody levels to 2 of 3 viral strains, and post hoc analysis indicated that participants who were unsure about whether their events were due to racism or due to other factors had reduced levels of antibody to 1 viral strain. The researchers concluded that attributional ambiguity sometimes associated with racism may inhibit the benefits of disclosure interventions for these types of stressors.

Cancer

Cancer is a term for a heterogeneous cluster of diseases in which there is a defect in normal cell growth regulation. The immune system certainly plays a part in controlling aberrant neoplastic (cancer) cells and although natural killer (NK) cells appear to be one crucial immune element for cancer control and recovery, the involvement and importance of other immune factors is less clear and may vary among different cancers.

A diagnosis of cancer is usually a source of considerable stress, and cancer patients are often reticent about disclosing their experience of the condition. In a study of 300 women with breast cancer, Henderson and colleagues (Henderson, Davison, Pennebaker, Gatchel, & Baum, 2002) assessed how much and with whom the women discussed their cancer in the month following diagnosis. Seven percent reported little or no disclosure to anyone besides their spouse or doctor, and between 20 and 30% reported little or no disclosure to entire subgroups of their social network (family, friends, and health professionals). Interestingly, greater disclosure about their disease was associated with younger participants, greater disease severity, optimism, and attitudes oriented toward disclosure. Can interventions designed to promote emotional disclosure, therefore, benefit cancer patients? Several studies have addressed this question. Using a group of 42 terminally ill patients with metastatic renal cell carcinoma randomly assigned to an expressive-writing or neutral-writing group, de Moor and colleagues (2002) found that, although there were no group differences in symptoms of distress, perceived stress, or mood disturbance, patients in the expressive-writing group reported significantly less sleep disturbance, better sleep quality and sleep duration, and less day-time dysfunction compared with those in the neutral writing group. In a small group of men with diagnosed prostate cancer, patients in an expressive disclosure group showed improvements in physical symptoms and health care utilization, but not in psychological variables nor in disease-relevant aspects of immunocompetence compared with a control group (Rosenberg et al., 2002). In a cohort of breast cancer patients, women who coped through expressing emotions about cancer and their experience of it, had enhanced physical health and vigor, decreased distress, and fewer medical appointments for cancer-related morbidities during the 3 months after medical treatment compared with those women who were low in emotional expression (Stanton et al., 2000). Expressive coping was also related to improved quality of life for those who perceived their social contexts as highly receptive. Subsequently, the same researchers extended this work by assessing the effects of emotional disclosure interventions on breast cancer patients (Stanton et al., 2002). Early-stage breast cancer patients were randomly assigned to write over four sessions about their deepest thoughts and feelings regarding breast cancer, positive thoughts and feelings regarding their experience with breast cancer, or facts of their breast cancer experience, Assessments 1 and 3 months later revealed that emotionally expressive writing was relatively effective for women low in avoidance, whereas writing about positive thoughts and feelings was more useful for women high in avoidance. Also, compared with control writing participants, the emotional group reported fewer physical symptoms, and both the emotional and positive writing participants had fewer medical appointments for cancer-related morbidities.

Written emotional disclosure has also been found to buffer the effects of social constraints on distress among cancer patients, and avoidance partly mediated these effects (Zakowski, Ramati, Morton, Johnson, & Flanigan, 2004). Further, learning to regulate emotions through emotionally expressive interventions can have a beneficial influence on the emotional experiences and on health in cancer patients, as shown by the work of Cameron and colleagues (Cameron, Booth, Schlatter, Ziginskas, & Harman, 2007). They investigated psychological adjustment in three groups of women recently diagnosed with breast cancer. They compared

54 women involved in a 12-week group intervention with a group of 56 women who refused the intervention, and with a standard-care group of 44 women who were not offered the intervention. The 12-week group intervention included training in relaxation, guided imagery, meditation, emotional expression, and exercises promoting control beliefs and benefit finding. Compared with baseline assessments immediately after diagnosis, the intervention participants reported greater increases in perceived control, emotional well-being, and coping efficacy, and greater decreases in perceived risk of recurrence, cancer worry, anxiety, and emotional suppression over the subsequent 12 months compared with the other two groups. There were also small but significant changes in circulating NK cell numbers in women in the emotional intervention group (Schlatter, 2005).

As was discussed earlier in the HIV studies, it is not emotional expression per se that is salutary; rather, it appears to be the ability of people to reinterpret or reframe their experience as a consequence of emotional expression. This is illustrated by the studies of Bower and colleagues (2003) who assessed cognitive processing using written emotional disclosure in 43 women who had lost a close relative to breast cancer and who wrote about the death weekly for 4 weeks. Although written disclosure did not induce changes in meaning-related goals, women who reported positive changes in them during the study also showed increases in NK cell activity. Bower and colleagues suggested that prioritizing goals, emphasizing relationships, personal growth, and striving for meaning in life may have positive biological correlates but that a single written disclosure may not be sufficient to induce changes. In a more recent study into the effects of expressive writing conducted over 4 consecutive days in women with metastatic breast cancer, a positive relationship between affective language in disclosure and quality of life was evident 3 months after the writing exercise, indicating a cognitive process occurring in expressive writing (Laccetti, 2007). Finally, having a partner assist in the emotional- disclosure process has been reported to benefit patients with gastrointestinal cancer. In a randomized controlled trial, 130 patients and their partners were randomly assigned to receive 4 sessions of either partner-assisted emotional disclosure or a couples cancer education/support intervention (Porter et al., 2009). Although no physiological measures were assessed, compared with education/support, partner-assisted emotional disclosure led to improvements in relationship quality

and intimacy for couples in which the patient initially reported higher levels of holding back from discussing cancer-related concerns.

Wound Healing

Perceived stress and hostility have been found to extend wound healing times in several laboratory-based and clinical studies, and the effects have been attributed to changes in production of pro-inflammatory cytokines associated with the healing process (Broadbent, Petrie, Alley, & Booth, 2003; Glaser et al., 1999; Kiecolt-Glaser et al., 2005; Marucha, Kiecolt-Glaser, & Favagehi, 1998). Patterns of anger expression, such as outward and inward anger expression and lack of anger control, have also been associated with maladaptive alterations in cortisol secretion, immune functioning, and surgical recovery. Two studies have explored the effects of emotional disclosure or emotion-related processes on wound healing. In a sample of 98 volunteers who received standardized blister wounds on their nondominant forearms, those exhibiting lower levels of anger control were more likely to be in the slow healer category (Gouin, Kiecolt-Glaser, Malarkey, & Glaser, 2008). Further, anger control predicted wound repair beyond differences in hostility, negative affectivity, social support, and health behaviors, and participants with lower levels of anger control exhibited higher cortisol reactivity during the blistering procedure. Weinman and colleagues (Weinman, Ebrecht, Scott, & Dyson, 2008) investigated wound healing in a healthy population by recruiting 36 volunteers to be randomly assigned to control (writing about time management) or experimental groups (writing about a traumatic event) following receipt of a small punch-biopsy superficial wound. Using ultrasound to measure wound healing, they found that participants who wrote about traumatic events had significantly smaller wounds 14 and 21 days after the biopsy compared with those who wrote about time management.

Psoriasis

Psoriasis is an immune-mediated inflammation of the skin in which TH1-derived cytokines trigger skin cells to proliferate, resulting in the development of chronic inflamed scaly rashes. Although there is a strong genetic component to psoriasis, the condition is often triggered by infection or stressful events. Two studies have reported some benefits of emotional disclosure for patients with psoriasis. In one, 59 patients were randomly assigned to receive an emotional-disclosure intervention or standard control writing intervention, and disease severity, quality of life, and mood were assessed at baseline and at intervals up to 12 weeks later (Vedhara et al., 2007). Although changes in mood following emotional disclosure predicted improvements in disease severity in patients with psoriasis, the overall degree of improvement did not differ between intervention and control patients. A second study investigated the effect of written-emotional-disclosure interventions in people with psoriasis undergoing narrow band ultraviolet B phototherapy (Paradisi et al., 2010). In a cohort of 40 patients randomly assigned to write about stressful events, to write about major life goals, or to a control group, those allocated to the stressful event-writing group had a longer period of remission after phototherapy.

Emotional Disclosure: What, How, and Why

Since the initial studies of Pennebaker and Beall (Pennebaker & Beall, 1986), much research has employed emotional-disclosure interventions in a wide variety of settings and conditions, using participants drawn from healthy populations and comparing them to those with acute or chronic psychologically based or physiologically based illnesses. A multitude of outcomes have been measured, from behavioral changes through psychological characteristics to physiological and disease effects. Many, but not all, have reported significant benefits of such interventions, and several questions arise. First, can we summarize what works best and under what conditions? Second, how and why does it work? Third, can we make sense of why it works it in terms of psychoneuroimmunology?

Meta-Analyses

Over the last few years, 4 meta-analyses have been published about emotional disclosure. The first, in 1998 (Smyth, 1998), analyzed 13 experimental studies, and the second, in 2004 (Frisina, Borod, & Lepore, 2004), analyzed 9 studies. Both concluded that emotional disclosure does not appear to influence health behaviors but leads to improved physical health, psychological well-being, physiological functioning, and general functioning with significant and positive average effect sizes of 0.230 (Smyth, 1998) and 0.101 (Frisina et al., 2004). A third meta-analysis (Meads & Nouwen, 2005) selected 61 trials for inclusion and examined a wide variety of physical, physiological, immunological, performance, and psychological outcomes, concluding that there was no clear evidence of improvement for emotional disclosure compared

with controls in objectively measured physical health and most other outcomes assessed. The most recent and most extensive meta-analysis, published by Frattaroli (Frattaroli, 2006), included results from 146 published and unpublished studies and used a random-effects analysis rather than a fixed-effects approach as had been used in the first two meta-analyses. Frattaroli's analysis indicated that experimental disclosure is effective, with a positive and significant average effect size of 0.075—much smaller than previously reported effect sizes but comparable to several pharmacological interventions considered medically important (for example, daily aspirin after a heart attack to prevent death from a second heart attack). Further, her analysis also tested an array of moderators and concluded that, "effect sizes tended to be larger when studies included only participants with physical health problems, included only participants with a history of trauma or stressors, did not draw from a college student sample, had participants disclose at home, had participants disclose in a private setting, had more male participants, had fewer participants, paid the participants, had follow-up periods of less than 1 month, had at least three disclosure sessions, had disclosure sessions that lasted at least 15 minutes, had participants who wrote about more recent events, instructed participants to discuss previously undisclosed topics, gave participants directed questions or specific examples of what to disclose, gave participants instructions regarding whether they should switch topics, and did not collect the products of disclosure" (Frattaroli, 2006). Conversely, outcomes of emotional disclosure were not significantly affected by psychological health-selection criteria, participant age, participant ethnicity, participant education level, warning participants in advance that they might disclose traumatic events, spacing of disclosure sessions, valence of the topic, focus of disclosure instructions, time reference of disclosure instructions, and mode of disclosure (handwriting, typing, or talking).

The reason that one of the four meta-analyses (Meads & Nouwen, 2005) did not find any statistically significant effects of emotional disclosure, whereas the other three did, is not obvious from comparing the four analyses, and it may simply reflect the choice of studies included. Alternatively, it might highlight an inherent problem with using meta-analysis to compare studies across such a diverse range of participant groups and incorporating such an extensive variety of outcome measures with the only commonality being the basis of the intervention—emotional disclosure. Meta-analysis is usually conducted on groups of studies with much more similarity than those used here, and computing an overall average-effect size for experimental disclosure might be inappropriate, given the substantial degree of methodological variation across studies (Sloan & Marx, 2004). Further, as Pennebaker pointed out, the assumption that emotional disclosure works the same way in all cases may also be unwarranted (Pennebaker, 2004).

Psychological Theories to Account for Effects

Five psychological processes or theories have been proposed to explain the salutary effects of emotional disclosure. They are disinhibition, cognitive processing, self-regulation, social integration, and exposure. The evidence supporting or opposing each of them has been well reviewed (Frattaroli, 2006) and so will only be summarized briefly here. As discussed earlier, there are immediate postdisclosure changes that are not necessarily linked to more long-term effects, and it is the long-term effects that are of most interest and addressed by these theories. Also, as noted earlier, there is unlikely to be one "perfect" theory to account for all the data, and it is more plausible that more than one theoretical framework will be required to explain all the findings.

Following the early emotional-disclosure publications, explanations of the benefits of experimental disclosure drew from psychoanalytical explanations of the benefits of catharsis, and suggested that inhibiting thoughts and feelings regarding an upsetting event required psychological "work" and was harmful, but conversely, expressing them could reduce stress and improve health outcomes. Indeed, reactivating past trauma-related memory during the disclosure task may evoke various past experiences, memories, and physical sensations, and the consequent short-term distress maybe indicate assimilation of the emotional processes. However, this became a less tenable explanation when Francis and Pennebaker (Francis & Pennebaker, 1992) found that participants who were low in dispositional constraint benefited most from an experimental disclosure intervention, whereas those who were high in this trait benefited less. Further, studies by Greenberg and colleagues (Greenberg, & Stone, 1992) showed that although participants who disclosed more severe traumas subsequently reported fewer physical symptoms than did those disclosing low-severity trauma, health benefits occurred when severe traumas were disclosed, regardless of whether previous disclosure had occurred. Moreover, when

college women, preselected for trauma presence, were randomly assigned to write about real or imaginary traumas, compared with a control group, both trauma groups made significantly fewer health-center visits over the subsequent month (Greenberg, Wortman, & Stone, 1996). Finally, if disinhibition is a mechanism by which experimental disclosure is helpful, traumas inhibited for longer (older and/or undisclosed traumas) would be the best candidates for disclosure, and people who have a tendency to inhibit their thoughts and feelings (men, Asians, people with inhibiting personalities) should benefit most from a disclosure intervention. Meta-analysis results did not show this to be the case (Frattaroli, 2006).

Support for the notion that emotional disclosure promotes cognitive processing has been mentioned in several places earlier in this chapter, and it centers on linguistic analysis identifying changes in causation and insight-related word use (Pennebaker, 1993) or meaning making (Bower et al., 1998; Bower et al., 2003) across disclosure sessions. Some have argued that if cognitive processing is a mechanism for emotional disclosure, allowing more time between sessions should give participants time to process the event and, therefore, result in better outcomes. The fact that the Frattaroli meta-analysis did not find session spacing to be a moderator could be taken as evidence against the cognitive-processing theory. However, this is not convincing, especially given the number of studies that have found an association between linguistic evidence of cognitive processing and positive outcomes. On the other hand, the fact that most positive effects do not occur immediately after disclosure but accrue some time later, perhaps once reinterpretation, reframing, and reconstruction of a coherent narrative of the disclosed experiences has been completed, further reinforces the cognitive-processing explanation.

Improved psychological self-regulation and a stronger sense of self-efficacy resulting from emotional regulation has some persuasive support from several published studies. For example, Cameron and Nicholls (Cameron & Nicholls, 1998) investigated the effectiveness of an expressive writing task designed to foster self-regulatory coping with stressful experiences. They asked student volunteers to express thoughts and feelings about a stressful experience and then to formulate coping plans (self-regulation task), and they compared this group with others instructed to express their thoughts and feelings only (disclosure task) or to write about trivial topics (control task). They found that relative to the control task, those participants who were high scorers on optimism scales in both the self-regulation task and the disclosure task groups reduced illness-related health-center visits during the subsequent month. Among pessimists, however, only the self-regulation task reduced visits. Another study also found support for a self-regulatory component in expressive writing (King, 2001). Here, emotional writing about a traumatic event was compared with writing about life goals in terms of the participant's best possible future self. As well as being less upsetting than writing about trauma, this was associated with an increase in subjective well-being and a comparable decrease in illness compared with a control group, suggesting that some form of cognitive restructuring may be an important facet of effective expressive writing. Further, instructing participants initially to write using first-person pronoun, and then to narrate the same event from a different perspective using second-person pronoun, and finally, to write it again with third-person pronoun from yet another perspective has been reported to have a long-term therapeutic effect in highly anxious people (Seih, Lin, Huang, Peng, & Huang, 2008). Incorporating emotional expression and benefit-finding into theories of cognitive and emotional processing, Cameron and Jago (Cameron & Jago, 2008) suggested an expanded commonsense model of self-regulation that delineates emotion-regulation strategies for coping with illness-related distress. Their model indicates that therapeutic interventions must give appropriate attention to both problem-focused regulation and emotion-regulation processes in order to confer optimal benefits for individuals with physical health conditions.

Social-integration theory argues that experimental disclosure affects the way people interact with their social world, which, in turn, improves their health and well-being. There is some support for social integration being a means by which emotional disclosure works. For example, one study reported that, following emotional disclosure, participants made small changes in their friendship networks and even laughed more than did control participants in the days and weeks following disclosure (Pennebaker & Graybeal, 2001). Finally, the exposure theory of experimental disclosure argues that the expression of thoughts and feelings regarding an upsetting event is similar to exposure therapy used to treat phobias and PTSD. By repeatedly confronting, describing, and reliving the thoughts and feelings about negative experiences within the disclosure process, participants become desensitized by repetition leading to extinction of those thoughts and feelings. Support for this theory has been mixed, with some studies finding that disclosure reduced intrusive and avoidant thoughts about the event (Klein & Boals, 2001), and with others failing to find such a reduction (de Moor et al., 2002; Lepore, 1997).

Interpreting the Effects in a PNI Context

In contrast with possible explanations of the psychological outcomes of emotional disclosure summarized earlier, relatively little has been written to explain the biological outcomes, and there are currently many more questions than answers. For example, if health improvements following disclosure cannot be explained in terms of measurable behavior changes, then what mechanisms might account for them? What happens in the neuroimmune system (or more generally in a person's physiology) as a consequence of writing or talking about emotionally charged events in a particular way? If cognitive processing or self-regulation explain psychological changes, are those explanations germane to biological changes or do we need to invoke completely different explanatory pathways for these? More specifically, why should emotional disclosure result in such diverse immune effects as increased antibody production following vaccination, decreased wound healing rates, improvement in lung function, decreased allergic responsiveness, or decreased autoimmune pathology? Given that there is a range of neuroimmunological mechanisms associated with these effects or conditions, is there likely to be a single molecular biological or cellular physiological pathway underpinning all of them and, if not, how do we explain the full psychoneuroimmune process underlying emotional disclosure?

In terms of psychological effects on immune function in other domains, there is much research (explored in other chapters) showing relationships among such psychological factors as perceived stress, anxiety, and depression, and three important neuroimmune pathways. They are: (1) the autonomic-sympathetic nervous system (SNS) pathway through the adrenal medulla to epinephrine and norepinephrine effects on lymphocyte function, (2) sympathetic innervation of paracortical areas of secondary lymphoid organs and direct neurotransmitter-mediated modulation of helper T lymphocyte cytokine production through these nerves, and (3) endocrine hormonal influences on immune function particularly through hypothalamus-pituitary-adrenal (HPA) cortex activation of corticosteroid production and its regulation of immune inflammatory pathways (and their feedback control mechanisms). Can the biological effects of emotional disclosure, therefore, be entirely explained by perturbations of one or more of these "stress"—or "threat"—response systems?

Some studies certainly indicate that these mechanisms are involved. For example, research by Lutgendorf and colleagues (2008), comparing immune variables in peripheral blood, tumor, and ascites (fluid around the tumor), obtained on the day of surgery from patients with ovarian cancer indicate that depressed and anxious mood are associated with greater impairment of adaptive immunity (as indicated by changes in the balance of TH1 and TH2 cytokines) in peripheral blood and in the tumor microenvironment in these patients. Also, an intriguing body of research by Cole and colleagues (Cole, Kemeny, Weitzman, Schoen, & Anton, 1999) implicates both the autonomic nervous system and HPA axis in the physical health risks associated with social isolation. Using data from a study of psychological factors in functional bowel disease and fibromyalgia, they found that under conditions of high social engagement, socially inhibited individuals showed significantly increased Delayed-Type Hypersensitivity (DTH) responses to intradermal tetanus toxoid. In contrast, under low-engagement conditions, these individuals showed less pronounced DTH responses similar to those of uninhibited individuals. Genomic analyses suggested that physiologic regulation of pro-inflammatory gene expression by endogenous glucocorticoids may be compromised in individuals who experience chronic social isolation and the sensitivity of circulating leukocytes to cortisol regulation might also be diminished in these individuals (Cole, 2008). Further, socially inhibited individuals show increased vulnerability to viral infections and poorer response to antiviral therapy (Cole, Kemeny, Fahey, Zack, & Naliboff, 2003) and this has been linked to increased activity of the SNS. Finally, autonomic innervation of lymphoid organs is also affected by sociability, as demonstrated in experiments with macaques by Sloan and colleagues (Sloan, Capitanio, Tarara, & Cole, 2008). Tissues from low sociable animals showed a two- to threefold greater density of catecholaminergic innervation relative to tissues from high sociable animals, and this was associated with a greater expression of nerve growth factor mRNA, suggesting a molecular mechanism for the observed differences. Moreover, low sociable animals also showed alterations in lymph node expression of the immunoregulatory cytokine genes IFN-gamma and IL4, and lower secondary IgG responses to tetanus vaccination.

Given such results and mindful of the social-integration theory of emotional-disclosure effects discussed earlier, it is conceivable that at least some of the immune-function effects following emotional disclosure might be explained in terms of generalized changes in HPA axis sensitivity, SNS innervation, or both. If so, then we might not expect to observe in the neuroimmune network any sort of correspondence or specificity with the psychological processes underlying emotional disclosure. Rather, we might consider that the physical health changes are, in essence, downstream consequences of changes in sensitivity or activation of the neuroimmune networks controlling responses to "stress," "alarm," or "danger." Elsewhere, I have discussed the notion that our immune systems act to maintain the integrity of our bodies by sensing molecular shapes, determining whether particular shapes are appropriate within the context of our bodies, and coordinating with our nervous systems to maintain the physical process of "self-nonself discrimination" in relation to an ever-changing environment (Booth, 2004, 2005, 2007). Allied to this physiological self-generative process is a psychosocial self that distinguishes us from other humans and arises out of the language that we use to describe and make sense of our relationships. Our psychosocial selves could be considered, therefore, as descriptive narratives of the life stories of our bodies and the events that happen to them (Booth, 2002). Moreover, although we have two levels of self-construction—a psychosocial level and a physiological level—each of us experiences "self" as a coherent whole, and so our psychosocial and physiological selves must operate in a coordinated and coherent manner. Coordination, however, does not mean direct correspondence, and so what happens psychologically is not explicable in physiological terms (or vice versa), even though the two are mutually influential. Instead, to make sense of emotional disclosure and health requires our recognizing an encompassing mind-body dimension in which, for example, we might understand the relationships between sociability and lymphoid innervation discussed earlier as a consequence of a person's psychobiological need to maintain alert vigilance systems in a world perceived as containing high levels of potential threat to self-integrity.

Conclusion

Taken as a whole, research into the benefits of emotionally expressive disclosure indicate that it is not the specificity of the disclosed events that is important, but rather it is the manner in which the disclosure process is carried out and the narrative changes that result. Explaining our experiences in language and constructing narratives and images are a means by which we humans coordinate our living together. They are learned and shared by us as we live and operate within the human sociocultural domain. One of the constructions that each person learns is the notion of "myself"—a particular viewpoint associated with the experience of living in and through one's own particular physical body, and its relation to an environment that includes other humans. The very concept of "myself" is dependent upon dividing the individual from the environment, and is a continual process of "minding"—that is, paying attention to, explaining, and making sense of the experiences of "myself" in relation to the world and to others (Booth, 2004; Maturana, Mpodozis, & Carlos Letelier, 1995; Maturana & Varela, 1987). Because that which we each call "myself" develops out of our immersion in linguistic relationships with others, our humanness or individual human experience is irrevocably woven into the fabric of our social relationships and society. Therefore, activities that diminish our sense or perception of threat and vulnerability sustain our human (and thus our biological) viability. This means that, in terms of emotional disclosure and how it works, effective activities might involve cognitive restructuring, emotional self-regulation, social integration, disinhibition, or extinction through exposure. In essence, it may not matter whether the process is achieved by writing or talking, or whether it involves real or imagined trauma or positive experiences or considerations of goals for a best possible self. Whatever the psychosocial mechanics of the process, the key may be simply whether it diminishes any perceived threat to our self-integrity and reduces our vulnerability. In doing so, the resulting psychosocial self-renovations and reconstructions will be reflected in more controlled activation of neuroimmune alarm responses and more salutary physiological self/nonself discriminating processes.

Future Directions

Several questions remain unanswered in this fascinating field. One concerns the type of people who might benefit from an emotional disclosure process. Are there personality types or groups of people

with particular experiences or illnesses for whom disclosing emotions about past traumatic events is unhelpful? If, as suggested earlier, the process of disclosure is more important than the events disclosed, then it may be that, for such people, an intervention that teaches reflection and narrative reconstruction rather than one the encourages recall of specific past events would be most effective. Indeed, it may be that all the salutary effects of emotional disclosure work through this process and the focus on particular types of events simply serves to engage emotionality to facilitate it. This possibility requires further exploration.

A second question concerns the physiological changes that result from the disclosure process. Given the range of illness conditions found to be affected and the diversity of neuroimmune changes observed, the challenge is to determine whether there are central underlying neuroimmune mechanisms at play here and, if so, what they are. Much of the research points to the sympathetic-autonomic, HPA, and pro-inflammatory/anti-inflammatory neuroimmune circuits being central to the physiological changes that follow effective emotional-disclosure interventions, but it may well be the reactivity or periodicity of these circuits rather than the absolute levels of any component that is relevant.

A final question also relates to the link between pathways (psychological or neuroimmune) and the illnesses or disease processes affected by emotional disclosure. Considering the diversity of conditions that have been investigated to date, one might be forgiven for thinking that emotional disclosure is a panacea for all ills. Although it may be useful in many instances, is it more effective in chronic rather than acute conditions, illnesses with significant involvement of the nervous and/or immune systems, or cyclical rather than stable or degenerative illnesses? Such questions should inform future studies.

Related Chapters

For more information on concepts introduced in this chapter, see also Cohen; and Robles, this volume.

References

Austenfeld, J. L., Paolo, A. M., & Stanton, A. L. (2006). Effects of writing about emotions versus goals on psychological and physical health among third-year medical students. *Journal of Personality, 74*(1), 267–286.

Austenfeld, J. L., & Stanton, A. L. (2008). Writing about emotions versus goals: Effects on hostility and medical care utilization moderated by emotional approach coping processes. *British Journal of Health Psychology, 13*(1), 35–38.

Batten, S. V., Follette, V. M., Rasmussen Hall, M. L., & Palm, K. M. (2002). Physical and psychological effects of written disclosure among sexual abuse survivors. *Behavior Therapy, 33*(1), 107–122.

Bernard, M., Jackson, C., & Jones, C. (2006). Written emotional disclosure following first-episode psychosis: Effects on symptoms of post-traumatic stress disorder. *British Journal of Clinical Psychology, 45*(3), 403–415.

Booth, R. J. (2002). Psychospiritual healing and the immune system in cancer. In C. E. Lewis, R. O'Brien, & J. Barraclough (Eds.), *The psychoimmunology of cancer* (2nd ed., pp. 164–181). Oxford, England: Oxford University Press.

Booth, R. J. (2004). Self, immunity and meaning. *Cybernetics and Human Knowing, 11*(4), 47–61.

Booth, R. J. (2005). Emotional disclosure and psychoneuroimmunology. In K. Vedhara & M. Irwin (Eds.), *Human psychoneuroimmunology* (pp. 319–341). Oxford, England: Oxford University Press.

Booth, R. J. (2007). Are there meaningful relationships between psychosocial self and physiological self? *Attachment: New directions in Psychotherapy and Relational Psychoanalysis, 1*(2), 165–178.

Booth, R. J., & Petrie, K. J. (2002). Emotional expression and health changes: Can we identify biological pathways? In S. Lepore & J. Smythe (Eds.), *The writing cure: How expressive writing promotes health and emotional well-being* (pp. 157–175). Washington, DC: American Psychological Association.

Booth, R. J., Petrie, K. J., & Pennebaker, J. W. (1997). Changes in circulating lymphocyte numbers following emotional disclosure: Evidence of buffering? *Stress Medicine, 13*(1), 23–29.

Bower, J. E., Kemeny, M. E., Taylor, S. E., & Fahey, J. L. (1998). Cognitive processing, discovery of meaning, CD4 decline, and AIDS-related mortality among bereaved HIV-seropositive men. *Journal of Consulting and Clinical Psychology, 66*(6), 979–986.

Bower, J. E., Kemeny, M. E., Taylor, S. E., & Fahey, J. L. (2003). Finding positive meaning and its association with natural killer cell cytotoxicity among participants in a bereavement-related disclosure intervention. *Annals of Behavioral Medicine, 25*(2), 146–155.

Broadbent, E. A., Petrie, K. J., Alley, P. G., & Booth, R. J. (2003). Psychological stress impairs early wound repair following surgery. *Psychosomatic Medicine, 65*(5), 865–889.

Broderick, J. E., Stone, A. A., Smyth, J. M., & Kaell, A. T. (2004). The feasibility and effectiveness of an expressive writing intervention for rheumatoid arthritis via home-based videotaped instructions. *Annals of Behavioral Medicine, 27*(1), 50–59.

Brown, E. J., & Heimberg, R. G. (2001). Effects of writing about rape: Evaluating Pennebaker's paradigm with a severe trauma. *Journal of Trauma & Stress, 14*(4), 781–790.

Burke, P. A., & Bradley, R. G. (2006). Language use in imagined dialogue and narrative disclosures of trauma. *Journal of Traumatic Stress, 19*(1), 141–146.

Cameron, L. D., Booth, R. J., Schlatter, M., Ziginskas, D., & Harman, J. E. (2007). Changes in emotion regulation and psychological adjustment following use of a group psychosocial support program for women recently diagnosed with breast cancer. *Psycho-Oncology, 16*(3), 171–180.

Cameron, L. D., & Jago, L. (2008). Emotion regulation interventions: A common-sense model approach. *British Journal of Health Psychology, 13*(2), 215–221.

Cameron, L. D., & Nicholls, G. (1998). Expression of stressful experiences through writing: Effects of a self-regulation manipulation for pessimists and optimists. *Health Psychology, 17*(1), 84–92.

Campbell, R. S., & Pennebaker, J. W. (2003). The secret life of pronouns: Flexibility in writing style and physical health. *Psychological Science, 14*(1), 60–65.

Cepeda, M. S., Chapman, C. R., Miranda, N., Sanchez, R., Rodriguez, C. H., Restrepo, A. E.,...Carr, D. B. (2008). Emotional disclosure through patient narrative may improve pain and well-being: Results of a randomized controlled trial in patients with cancer pain. *Journal of Pain and Symptom Management, 35*(6), 623–631.

Christensen, A. J., Edwards, D. L., Wiebe, J. S., Benotsch, E. G., McKelvey, L., Andrews, M., & Lubaroff, D. M. (1996). Effect of verbal self-disclosure on natural killer cell activity: Moderating influence of cynical hostility. *Psychosomatic Medicine, 58*(2), 150–155.

Cole, S. W. (2008). Social regulation of leukocyte homeostasis: The role of glucocorticoid sensitivity. *Brain, Behavior, and Immunity, 22*(7), 1049–1055.

Cole, S. W., Kemeny, M. E., Fahey, J. L., Zack, J. A., & Naliboff, B. D. (2003). Psychological risk factors for HIV pathogenesis: Mediation by the autonomic nervous system. *Biological Psychiatry, 54*(12), 1444–1456.

Cole, S. W., Kemeny, M. E., Taylor, S. E., Visscher, B. R., & Fahey, J. L. (1996). Accelerated course of human immunodeficiency virus infection in gay men who conceal their homosexual identity. *Psychosomatic Medicine, 58*(3), 219–231.

Cole, S. W., Kemeny, M. E., Weitzman, O. B., Schoen, M., & Anton, P. A. (1999). Socially inhibited individuals show heightened DTH response during intense social engagement. *Brain, Behavior, and Immunity, 13*(2), 187–200.

Conraads, V. M., Denollet, J., De Clerck, L. S., Stevens, W. J., Bridts, C., & Vrints, C. J. (2006). Type D personality is associated with increased levels of tumour necrosis factor (TNF)-alpha and TNF-alpha receptors in chronic heart failure. *International Journal of Cardiology, 113*(1), 34–38.

Corcos, M., Guilbaud, O., Paterniti, S., Curt, F., Hjalmarsson, L., Moussa, M.,...Jeammet, P. (2004). Correlation between serum levels of interleukin-4 and alexithymia scores in healthy female subjects: Preliminary findings. *Psychoneuroendocrinology, 29*(5), 686–691.

D'Souza, P. J., Lumley, M. A., Kraft, C. A., & Dooley, J. A. (2008). Relaxation training and written emotional disclosure for tension or migraine headaches: A randomized, controlled trial. *Annals of Behavioral Medicine, 36*(1), 21–32.

Dalton, J. J., & Glenwick, D. S. (2009). Effects of expressive writing on standardized graduate entrance exam performance and physical health functioning. *Journal of Psychology, 143*(3), 279–292.

de Moor, C., Sterner, J., Hall, M., Warneke, C., Gilani, Z., Amato, R., & Cohen, L. (2002). A pilot study of the effects of expressive writing on psychological and behavioral adjustment in patients enrolled in a Phase II trial of vaccine therapy for metastatic renal cell carcinoma. *Health Psychology, 21*(6), 615–619.

Dickerson, S. S., Gruenewald, T. L., & Kemeny, M. E. (2004). When the social self is threatened: Shame, physiology, and health. *Journal of Personality, 72*(6), 1191–1216.

Dickerson, S. S., Kemeny, M. E., Aziz, N., Kim, K. H., & Fahey, J. L. (2004). Immunological effects of induced shame and guilt. *Psychosomatic Medicine, 66*(1), 124–131.

Dopp, J. M., Miller, G. E., Myers, H. F., & Fahey, J. L. (2000). Increased natural killer-cell mobilization and cytotoxicity during marital conflict. *Brain, Behavior, and Immunity, 14*(1), 10–26.

Eisenberger, N. I., Kemeny, M. E., & Wyatt, G. E. (2003). Psychological inhibition and CD4 T-cell levels in HIV-seropositive women. *Journal of Psychosomatic Research, 54*(3), 213–224.

Esterling, B. A., Antoni, M. H., Fletcher, M. A., Margulies, S., & Schneiderman, N. (1994). Emotional disclosure through writing or speaking modulates latent Epstein-Barr virus antibody titers. *Journal of Consulting and Clinical Psychology, 62*(1), 130–140.

Esterling, B. A., Antoni, M. H., Kumar, M., & Schneiderman, N. (1990). Emotional repression, stress disclosure responses, and Epstein-Barr viral capsid antigen titers. *Psychosomatic Medicine, 52*(4), 397–410.

Everson-Rose, S. A., & Lewis, T. T. (2005). Psychosocial factors and cardiovascular diseases. *Annual Review of Public Health, 26*, 469–500.

Fowles, D. C. (1980). The three arousal model: Implications of gray's two-factor learning theory for heart rate, electrodermal activity, and psychopathy. *Psychophysiology, 17*(2), 87–104.

Francis, M. E., & Pennebaker, J. W. (1992). Putting stress into words: The impact of writing on physiological, absentee, and self-reported emotional well-being measures. *American Journal of Health Promotion, 6*(4), 280–287.

Frattaroli, J. (2006). Experimental disclosure and its moderators: A meta-analysis. *Psychological Bulletin, 132*(6), 823–865.

Frisina, P. G., Borod, J. C., & Lepore, S. J. (2004). A meta-analysis of the effects of written emotional disclosure on the health outcomes of clinical populations. *Journal of Nervous and Mental Disease, 192*(9), 629–634.

Futterman, A. D., Kemeny, M. E., Shapiro, D., & Fahey, J. L. (1994). Immunological and physiological changes associated with induced positive and negative mood. *Psychosomatic Medicine, 56*(6), 499–511.

Futterman, A. D., Kemeny, M. E., Shapiro, D., Polonsky, W., & Fahey, J. L. (1992). Immunological variability associated with experimentally-induced positive and negative affective states. *Psychological Medicine, 22*(1), 231–238.

Glaser, R., Kiecolt-Glaser, J. K., Marucha, P. T., MacCallum, R. C., Laskowski, B. F., & Malarkey, W. B. (1999). Stress-related changes in proinflammatory cytokine production in wounds. *Archives of General Psychiatry, 56*(5), 450–456.

Gouin, J. P., Kiecolt-Glaser, J. K., Malarkey, W. B., & Glaser, R. (2008). The influence of anger expression on wound healing. *Brain, Behavior, and Immunity, 22*(5), 699–708.

Graham, J. E., Glaser, R., Loving, T. J., Malarkey, W. B., Stowell, J. R., & Kiecolt-Glaser, J. K. (2009). Cognitive word use during marital conflict and increases in proinflammatory cytokines. *Health Psychology, 28*(5), 621–630.

Graham, J. E., Lobel, M., Glass, P., & Lokshina, I. (2008). Effects of written anger expression in chronic pain patients: Making meaning from pain. *Journal of Behavioral Medicine, 31*(3), 201–212.

Greenberg, M. A., & Stone, A. A. (1992). Emotional disclosure about traumas and its relation to health: Effects of previous disclosure and trauma severity. *Journal of Personality and Social Psychology, 63*(1), 75–84.

Greenberg, M. A., Wortman, C. B., & Stone, A. A. (1996). Emotional expression and physical health: Revising traumatic memories or fostering self-regulation? *Journal of Personality and Social Psychology, 71*(3), 588–602.

Henderson, B. N., Davison, K. P., Pennebaker, J. W., Gatchel, R. J., & Baum, A. (2002). Disease disclosure patterns among breast cancer patients. *Psychology & Health, 17*(1), 51–62.

Ishihara, S., Makita, S., Imai, M., Hashimoto, T., & Nohara, R. (2003). Relationship between natural killer activity and anger expression in patients with coronary heart disease. *Heart and Vessels, 18*(2), 85–92.

Ishii, H., Nagashima, M., Tanno, M., Nakajima, A., & Yoshino, S. (2003). Does being easily moved to tears as a response to psychological stress reflect response to treatment and the general prognosis in patients with rheumatoid arthritis? *Clinical and Experimental Rheumatology, 21*(5), 611–616.

Kearns, M. C., Edwards, K. M., Calhoun, K. S., & Gidycz, C. A. (2010). Disclosure of sexual victimization: The effects of Pennebaker's emotional disclosure paradigm on physical and psychological distress. *Journal of Trauma and Dissociation, 11*(2), 193–209.

Keefe, F. J., Anderson, T., Lumley, M., Caldwell, D., Stainbrook, D., McKee, D., ... Uhlin, B. D. (2008). A randomized, controlled trial of emotional disclosure in rheumatoid arthritis: can clinician assistance enhance the effects? *Pain, 137*(1), 164–172.

Kelley, J. E., Lumley, M. A., & Leisen, J. C. (1997). Health effects of emotional disclosure in rheumatoid arthritis patients. *Health Psychology, 16*(4), 331–340.

Kiecolt-Glaser, J. K., Glaser, R., Cacioppo, J. T., MacCallum, R. C., Snydersmith, M., Kim, C., & Malarkey, W. B. (1997). Marital conflict in older adults: Endocrinological and immunological correlates. *Psychosomatic Medicine, 59*(4), 339–349.

Kiecolt-Glaser, J. K., Loving, T. J., Stowell, J. R., Malarkey, W. B., Lemeshow, S., Dickinson, S. L., & Glaser, R. (2005). Hostile marital interactions, proinflammatory cytokine production, and wound healing. *Archives of General Psychiatry, 62*(12), 1377–1384.

Kiecolt-Glaser, J. K., Malarkey, W. B., Chee, M., Newton, T., Cacioppo, J. T., Mao, H. Y., & Glaser, R. (1993). Negative behavior during marital conflict is associated with immunological down-regulation. *Psychosomatic Medicine, 55*(5), 395–409.

King, L. A. (2001). The health benefits of writing about life goals. *Personality & Social Psychology Bulletin, 27*(7), 798–807.

Klein, K., & Boals, A. (2001). Expressive writing can increase working memory capacity. *Journal of Experimental Psychology, 130*, 520–533.

Knapp, P. H., Levy, E. M., Giorgi, R. G., Black, P. H., Fox, B. H., & Heeren, T. C. (1992). Short-term immunological effects of induced emotion. *Psychosomatic Medicine, 54*(2), 133–148.

Kraft, C. A., Lumley, M. A., D'Souza, P. J., & Dooley, J. A. (2008). Emotional approach coping and self-efficacy moderate the effects of written emotional disclosure and relaxation training for people with migraine headaches. *British Journal of Health Psychology, 13*(1), 67–71.

Labott, S. M., Ahleman, S., Wolever, M. E., & Martin, R. B. (1990). The physiological and psychological effects of the expression and inhibition of emotion. *Behavioral Medicine, 16*(4), 182–189.

Laccetti, M. (2007). Expressive writing in women with advanced breast cancer. *Oncology Nursing Forum, 34*(5), 1019–1024.

Lepore, S. J. (1997). Expressive writing moderates the relation between intrusive thoughts and depressive symptoms. *Journal of Personality and Social Psychology, 73*(5), 1030–1037.

Lepore, S. J., & Greenberg, M. A. (2002). Mending broken hearts: Effects of expressive writing on mood, cognitive processing, social adjustment and health following a relationship breakup. *Psychology & Health, 17*(5), 547–560.

Lepore, S. J., & Smyth, J. M. (2002). The writing cure: How expressive writing promotes health and emotional well-being. Washington, DC: American Psychological Association.

Lumley, M. A. (2004). Alexithymia, emotional disclosure, and health: A program of research. *Journal of Personality, 72*(6), 1271–1300.

Lumley, M. A., & Provenzano, K. M. (2003). Stress management through written emotional disclosure improves academic performance among college students. *Journal of Educational Psychology, 95*, 641–649.

Lutgendorf, S. K., Antoni, M. H., Ironson, G., Klimas, N., Fletcher, M. A., & Schneiderman, N. (1997). Cognitive processing style, mood, and immune function following HIV seropositivity notification. *Cognitive Therapy & Research, 21*(2), 157–184.

Lutgendorf, S. K., Antoni, M. H., Kumar, M., & Schneiderman, N. (1994). Changes in cognitive coping strategies predict EBV-antibody titre change following a stressor disclosure induction. *Journal of Psychosomatic Research, 38*(1), 63–78.

Lutgendorf, S. K., Lamkin, D. M., DeGeest, K., Anderson, B., Dao, M., McGinn, S., . . . Lubaroff, D. M. (2008). Depressed and anxious mood and T-cell cytokine expressing populations in ovarian cancer patients. *Brain, Behavior, and Immunity, 22*(6), 890–900.

Malarkey, W. B., Kiecolt-Glaser, J. K., Pearl, D., & Glaser, R. (1994). Hostile behavior during marital conflict alters pituitary and adrenal hormones. *Psychosomatic Medicine, 56*(1), 41–51.

Martin, R. B., Guthrie, C. A., & Pitts, C. G. (1993). Emotional crying, depressed mood, and secretory immunoglobulin A. *Behavioral Medicine, 19*(3), 111–114.

Marucha, P. T., Kiecolt-Glaser, J. K., & Favagehi, M. (1998). Mucosal wound healing is impaired by examination stress. *Psychosomatic Medicine, 60*(3), 362–365.

Maturana, H., Mpodozis, J., & Carlos Letelier, J. (1995). Brain, language and the origin of human mental functions. *Biological Research, 28*(1), 15–26.

Maturana, H. R., & Varela, F. J. (1987). *The tree of knowledge: The biological roots of understanding.* Boston: Shambhala.

Meads, C., & Nouwen, A. (2005). Does emotional disclosure have any effects? A systematic review of the literature with meta-analyses. *International Journal of Technology Assessment in Health Care, 21*(2), 153–164.

Mendes, W. B., Reis, H. T., Seery, M. D., & Blascovich, J. (2003). Cardiovascular correlates of emotional expression and suppression: Do content and gender context matter? *Journal of Personality and Social Psychology, 84*(4), 771–792.

Miller, G. E., Dopp, J. M., Myers, H. F., Stevens, S. Y., & Fahey, J. L. (1999). Psychosocial predictors of natural killer cell mobilization during marital conflict. *Health Psychology, 18*(3), 262–271.

Miller, G. E., Freedland, K. E., Carney, R. M., Stetler, C. A., & Banks, W. A. (2003). Cynical hostility, depressive symptoms, and the expression of inflammatory risk markers for coronary heart disease. *Journal of Behavioral Medicine, 26*(6), 501–515.

Mittwoch-Jaffe, T., Shalit, F., Srendi, B., & Yehuda, S. (1995). Modification of cytokine secretion following mild emotional stimuli. *Neuroreport, 6*(5), 789–792.

Murray, E. J., & Segal, D. L. (1994). Emotional processing in vocal and written expression of feelings about traumatic experiences. *Journal of Trauma & Stress, 7*(3), 391–405.

Norman, S. A., Lumley, M. A., Dooley, J. A., & Diamond, M. P. (2004). For whom does it work? Moderators of the effects of written emotional disclosure in a randomized trial among women with chronic pelvic pain. *Psychosomatic Medicine, 66*(2), 174–183.

O'Cleirigh, C., Ironson, G., Antoni, M., Fletcher, M. A., McGuffey, L., Balbin, E., . . . Solomon, G. (2003). Emotional expression and depth processing of trauma and their relation to long-term survival in patients with HIV/AIDS. *Journal of Psychosomatic Research, 54*(3), 225–235.

O'Cleirigh, C., Ironson, G., Fletcher, M. A., & Schneiderman, N. (2008). Written emotional disclosure and processing of trauma are associated with protected health status and immunity in people living with HIV/AIDS. *British Journal of Health Psychology, 13*(1), 81–84.

Paez, D., Velasco, C., & Gonzalez, J. L. (1999). Expressive writing and the role of alexythimia as a dispositional deficit in self-disclosure and psychological health. *Journal of Personality and Social Psychology, 77*(3), 630–641.

Paradisi, A., Abeni, D., Finore, E., Di Pietro, C., Sampogna, F., Mazzanti, C., . . . Tabolli, S. (2010). Effect of written emotional disclosure interventions in persons with psoriasis undergoing narrow band ultraviolet B phototherapy. *European Journal of Dermatology, 20*(5), 599–605.

Pennebaker, J. W. (1993). Putting stress into words: Health, linguistic, and therapeutic implications. *Behaviour Research and Therapy, 31*(6), 539–548.

Pennebaker, J. W. (2004). Theories, therapies, and taxpayers: On the complexities of the expressive writing paradigm. *Clinical Psychology: Science and Practice, 11*(2), 138–142.

Pennebaker, J. W., Barger, S. D., & Tiebout, J. (1989). Disclosure of traumas and health among Holocaust survivors. *Psychosomatic Medicine, 51*(5), 577–589.

Pennebaker, J. W., & Beall, S. K. (1986). Confronting a traumatic event: Toward an understanding of inhibition and disease. *Journal of Abnormal Psychology, 95*(3), 274–281.

Pennebaker, J. W., Colder, M., & Sharp, L. K. (1990). Accelerating the coping process. *Journal of Personality and Social Psychology, 58*(3), 528–537.

Pennebaker, J. W., Emmanuelle, Z., & Bernard, R. (2001). Disclosing and sharing emotion: Psychological, social and health consequences. In M. S. Stroebe, R. O. Hanson, W. Stroebe, & H. Schut (Eds.), *Handbook of bereavement research: Consequences, coping and care* (pp. 517–543). Washington, DC: American Psychological Association.

Pennebaker, J. W., & Graybeal, A. (2001). Patterns of natural language use: Disclosure, personality and social integration. *Current Directions in Psychological Science, 10*, 90–93.

Pennebaker, J. W., Hughes, C. F., & O'Heeron, R. C. (1987). The psychophysiology of confession: Linking inhibitory and psychosomatic processes. *Journal of Personality and Social Psychology, 52*(4), 781–793.

Pennebaker, J. W., Kiecolt-Glaser, J. K., & Glaser, R. (1988). Disclosure of traumas and immune function: Health implications for psychotherapy. *Journal of Consulting and Clinical Psychology, 56*(2), 239–245.

Pennebaker, J. W., Mayne, T. J., & Francis, M. E. (1997). Linguistic predictors of adaptive bereavement. *Journal of Personality and Social Psychology, 72*(4), 863–871.

Pennebaker, J. W., Mehl, M. R., & Niederhoffer, K. G. (2003). Psychological aspects of natural language use: Our words, our selves. *Annual Review of Psychology, 54,* 547–577.

Petrie, K. J., Booth, R. J., & Pennebaker, J. W. (1998). The immunological effects of thought suppression. *Journal of Personality and Social Psychology, 75*(5), 1264–1272.

Petrie, K. J., Booth, R. J., Pennebaker, J. W., Davison, K. P., & Thomas, M. G. (1995). Disclosure of trauma and immune response to a hepatitis B vaccination program. *Journal of Consulting and Clinical Psychology, 63*(5), 787–792.

Petrie, K. J., Fontanilla, I., Thomas, M. G., Booth, R. J., & Pennebaker, J. W. (2004). Effect of written emotional expression on immune function in patients with human immunodeficiency virus infection: a randomized trial. *Psychosomatic Medicine, 66*(2), 272–275.

Porter, L. S., Keefe, F. J., Baucom, D. H., Hurwitz, H., Moser, B., Patterson, E., & Kim, H. J. (2009). Partner-assisted emotional disclosure for patients with gastrointestinal cancer: Results from a randomized controlled trial. *Cancer, 115*(18), 4326–4338.

Ramírez-Esparza, N., & Pennebaker, J. W. (2006). Do good stories produce good health? Exploring words, language, and culture. *Narrative Inquiry, 16*(1), 211–219.

Richards, J. M., Beal, W. E., Seagal, J. D., & Pennebaker, J. W. (2000). Effects of disclosure of traumatic events on illness behavior among psychiatric prison inmates. *Journal of Abnormal Psychology, 109*(1), 156–160.

Rimé, B., Philippot, P., Boca, S., & Mesquita, B. (1992). Long-lasting cognitive and social consequences of emotion: Social sharing and rumination. In W. Stroebe & M. Hewstone (Eds.), *European review of social psychology* (Vol. 3, pp. 225–258). Chichester, England: Wiley.

Rivkin, I. D., Gustafson, J., Weingarten, I., & Chin, D. (2006). The effects of expressive writing on adjustment to HIV. *AIDS and Behavior, 10*(1), 13–26.

Rosenberg, H. J., Rosenberg, S. D., Ernstoff, M. S., Wolford, G. L., Amdur, R. J., Elshamy, M. R.,...Pennebaker, J. W. (2002). Expressive disclosure and health outcomes in a prostate cancer population. *International Journal of Psychiatry in Medicine, 32*(1), 37–53.

Schlatter, M. C. (2005). Emotional control and breast cancer: Implications for coping, immunocompetence, and the experience of chemotherapy side effects. Auckland, New Zealand: University of Auckland.

Schoutrop, M. J., Lange, A., Hanewald, G., Davidovich, U., & Salomon, H. (2002). Structured writing and processing major stressful events: A controlled trial. *Psychotherapeutics & Psychosomatics, 71*(3), 151–157.

Seih, Y. T., Lin, Y. C., Huang, C. L., Peng, C. W., & Huang, S. P. (2008). The benefits of psychological displacement in diary writing when using different pronouns. *British Journal of Health Psychology, 13*(1), 39–41.

Sheese, B. E., Brown, E. L., & Graziano, W. G. (2004). Emotional expression in cyberspace: Searching for moderators of the Pennebaker disclosure effect via e-mail. *Health Psychology, 23*(5), 457–464.

Sloan, E. K., Capitanio, J. P., Tarara, R. P., & Cole, S. W. (2008). Social temperament and lymph node innervation. *Brain, Behavior, and Immunity, 22*(5), 717–726.

Sloan, D. M., & Marx, B. P. (2004). A closer examination of the structured written disclosure procedure. *Journal of Consulting and Clinical Psychology, 72*(2), 165–175.

Sloan, D. M., & Marx, B. P. (2004). Taking pen to hand: Evaluating theories underlying the written disclosure paradigm. *Clinical Psychology: Science and Practice, 11*(2), 121–137.

Sloan, D. M., Marx, B. P., & Epstein, E. M. (2005). Further examination of the exposure model underlying the efficacy of written emotional disclosure. *Journal of Consulting and Clinical Psychology, 73*(3), 549–554.

Sloan, D. M., Marx, B. P., Epstein, E. M., & Lexington, J. M. (2007). Does altering the writing instructions influence outcome associated with written disclosure? *Behavior Therapy, 38*(2), 155–168.

Smyth, J. M. (1998). Written emotional expression: Effect sizes, outcome types, and moderating variables. *Journal of Consulting and Clinical Psychology, 66*(1), 174–184.

Smyth, J. M., Stone, A. A., Hurewitz, A., & Kaell, A. (1999). Effects of writing about stressful experiences on symptom reduction in patients with asthma or rheumatoid arthritis: A randomized trial. *Journal of the American Medical Association, 281*(14), 1304–1309.

Solano, L., Montella, F., Salvati, S., Di Sora, F., Murgia, F., Figa-Talamanca, L.,...Nicotra, M. (2002). Expression and processing of emotions: Relationships with CD4+ levels in 42 HIV-positive asymptomatic individuals. *Psychology & Health, 16*(6), 689–698.

Spera, S. P., Buhrfeind, E. D., & Pennebaker, J. W. (1994). Expressive writing and coping with job loss. *Academy of Management Journal, 37*(3), 722–733.

Stanton, A. L., Danoff-Burg, S., Cameron, C. L., Bishop, M., Collins, C. A., Kirk, S. B., et al. (2000). Emotionally expressive coping predicts psychological and physical adjustment to breast cancer. *Journal of Consulting and Clinical Psychology, 68*(5), 875–882.

Stanton, A. L., Danoff-Burg, S., Sworowski, L. A., Collins, C. A., Branstetter, A. D., Rodriguez-Hanley, A.,...Twillman, R. (2002). Randomized, controlled trial of written emotional expression and benefit finding in breast cancer patients. *Journal of Clinical Oncology, 20*(20), 4160–4168.

Stetler, C., Chen, E., & Miller, G. E. (2006). Written disclosure of experiences with racial discrimination and antibody response to an influenza vaccine. *International Journal of Behavioral Medicine, 13*(1), 60–68.

Stroebe, M., Schut, H., & Stroebe, W. (2006). Who benefits from disclosure? Exploration of attachment style differences in the effects of expressing emotions. *Clinical Psychology Review, 26*(1), 66–85.

Stroebe, M., Stroebe, W., Schut, H., Zech, E., & van den Bout, J. (2002). Does disclosure of emotions facilitate recovery from bereavement? Evidence from two prospective studies. *Journal of Consulting and Clinical Psychology, 70*(1), 169–178.

Ullrich, P. M., & Lutgendorf, S. K. (2002). Journaling about stressful events: Effects of cognitive processing and emotional expression. *Annals of Behavioral Medicine, 24*(3), 244–250.

van Middendorp, H., & Geenen, R. (2008). Poor cognitive-emotional processing may impede the outcome of emotional disclosure interventions. *British Journal of Health Psychology, 13*(1), 49–52.

van Middendorp, H., Geenen, R., Sorbi, M. J., van Doornen, L. J., & Bijlsma, J. W. (2009). Health and physiological effects of an emotional disclosure intervention adapted for application at home: A randomized clinical trial in rheumatoid arthritis. *Psychotherapy and Psychosomatics, 78*(3), 145–151.

Vedhara, K., Brant, H., Adamopoulos, E., Byrne-Davis, L., Mackintosh, B., Hoppitt, L.,...Pennebaker, J. W. (2010). A preliminary investigation into whether attentional bias influences mood outcomes following emotional disclosure. *International Journal of Behavioral Medicine, 17*(3), 195–206.

Vedhara, K., Morris, R. M., Booth, R., Horgan, M., Lawrence, M., & Birchall, N. (2007). Changes in mood predict disease activity and quality of life in patients with psoriasis following emotional disclosure. *Journal of Psychosomatic Research, 62*(6), 611–619.

Walker, B. L., Nail, L. M., & Croyle, R. T. (1999). Does emotional expression make a difference in reactions to breast cancer? *Oncology Nursing Forum, 26*(6), 1025–1032.

Wegner, D. M., Shortt, J. W., Blake, A. W., & Page, M. S. (1990). The suppression of exciting thoughts. *Journal of Personality and Social Psychology, 58*(3), 409–418.

Weinman, J., Ebrecht, M., Scott, S., Walburn, J., & Dyson, M. (2008). Enhanced wound healing after emotional disclosure intervention. *British Journal of Health Psychology, 13*(1), 95–102.

Wetherell, M. A., Byrne-Davis, L., Dieppe, P., Donovan, J., Brookes, S., Byron, M.,...Miles, J. (2005). Effects of emotional disclosure on psychological and physiological outcomes in patients with rheumatoid arthritis: An exploratory home-based study. *Journal of Health Psychology, 10*(2), 277–285.

Zakowski, S. G., Ramati, A., Morton, C., Johnson, P., & Flanigan, R. (2004). Written emotional disclosure buffers the effects of social constraints on distress among cancer patients. *Health Psychology, 23*(6), 555–563.

Zech, E. (1981). *The impact of the communication of emotional experiences.* Unpublished Doctoral Thesis, University of Louvain, Louvian-la-Neuve, Belgium.

PART 3

Personality and Individual Differences

Temperament/Animal Personality

Kerry C. Michael *and* Sonia A. Cavigelli

Abstract

In humans, the relationship between personality and immunity is an important area of inquiry to better understand mechanisms underlying the diversity of human health and illness trajectories (Segerstrom, 2000; Cohen, this volume). A recent complement to our understanding of human behavior/personality and immune function has been the study of animal immune function as it relates to individual behavioral traits (temperament, personality; Koolhaas et al., 1999; Cavigelli, 2005; Korte, Koolhaas, Wingfield, & McEwen, 2005; Capitanio, 2008). With ample evidence that reliable and stable individual behavioral differences exist in animals and that these differences seem to mimic certain human behavioral traits, we are suddenly afforded a variety of organisms in which to study universal relationships between personality and immune function. The use of animal models additionally allows for a range and depth of evolutionary, developmental, functional and mechanistic investigations that are not possible with humans. We review the utility of animal models in understanding the relationship between personality and immune function.

Key Words: animal, personality, temperament, immune function, disease, health

Introduction

Personalities—that is, stable behavioral response biases in an individual across conditions and time—are an intriguing area of psychological research. Folk medicine has long held that different types of people have differing health outcomes related to personality; modern research is beginning to arrive at a similar conclusion. An early example in modern medicine was the work of Friedman and Rosenman in the 1950s, who postulated that Type A personality was associated with coronary heart disease; later this was clarified to be associated specifically with hostility (Williams, 2001). Since then, the relationship between personality and disease etiology has been more fully investigated and researchers have shown, for example, that individuals with "Type C" personality (characterized by low sociability and denial) have more rapid HIV progression than more sociable individuals (Temoshok et al., 2008), and that

"Type D" individuals (those with a combination of low sociability and high neuroticism) have increased rates of cardiac morbidity and decreased overall health status (Steptoe & Molloy, 2007; Moussavi et al. 2007). On the more optimistic side, positive affect is associated with faster immune recovery from stress (Pressman, this volume). Complementary studies looking at the relationship between specific behavioral traits (e.g. aggression, sociability) and immune function/disease progression have been conducted with animals, and these studies provide further insight into mechanisms underlying the relationship between human personality and disease resistance/susceptibility. These insights lead to the anticipation of a new field of individualized medicine—treatment tailored to the personality and coping styles of the individual patient.

The study of personality as it relates to immune function/disease progression has been exceedingly beneficial in our understanding of individual differences in human health and disease. Many parameters, however, are impossible to study in humans, due to methodological, ethical, and time constraints. For example, understanding the causal relationship between personality and immune function in humans is difficult given the limited kind of experimental manipulations that are possible with humans. However, within the last decade, there has been an explosion of research on animal personality, with studies to understand the evolution, development, function, and mechanisms of consistent individual behavioral differences (e.g. Wilson, Clark, Coleman, & Dearstyne, 1994; Koolhaas et al., 1999; Dingemanse, Both, Drent, & Tinbergen, 2004; Sih, Bell, & Johnson, 2004; Sgoifo, Coe, Parmigiani, & Koolhaas, 2005; Réale, Reader, Sol, McDougall, & Dingemanse, 2007). Animal models provide a tool to study behavior-physiology interactions that are impossible in human work. The typical human lifespan of 70–80 years, for example, means that longitudinal human studies would take several careers to complete; in addition, there is no control over most variables, making such studies intractable (Friedman, 2008). Laboratory rodents, however, have a lifespan of 2–3 years and are completely controlled in living conditions, diet, lifetime experiences, and often even in their genetics. They can be exposed to experiences or substances that are not practical or possible with humans, like early life stress or caloric restriction. Laboratory animals can also be bred for behavioral traits and then examined for the accompanying physiological differences, or vice versa.

Fortunately, many temperamental traits seen in humans have analogues, and probably homologues, in animal models. Limited studies have examined the stability of behavioral traits within an individual over time and across conditions, although this practice is increasing (e.g. Capitanio, 1999; Cavigelli & McClintock, 2003; Leppänen, Ewalds-Kvist, & Selander, 2005; Cavigelli et al., 2007; Cavigelli, Ragan, Michael, Kovacsics, & Bruscke, 2009; Krajl-Fiser, Scheiber, Blejec, Moestl, & Kotrschal, 2007); thus, in this review, we rely heavily on data from inbred strains that have been shown to have relatively consistent behavioral biases. As background, Mehta and Gosling (2008) have provided a comprehensive review of personality in animals, and they have presented a strong and compelling case for the utility of animal models in health and immunology research.

Previous convention has been to avoid use of the term *personality* in animals for fear of anthropomorphizing. More recent research, however, has posited that personality may indeed be objectively assessed in a variety of species. These differing approaches have given rise to various terms used to describe individual differences in animal behavior, such as *behavioral traits, temperament, personality, coping style,* or *behavioral syndromes.* For the sake of continuity, in this chapter we will use the terms *temperament* and *personality* interchangeably and as umbrella terms to refer to behavioral traits that are thought to be stable within an individual over time and across conditions.

Defining Personality

Defining human personality dimensions has been a controversial area of research, and the number of dimensions required to define human personalities is not well-agreed upon (Pervin, 2002). Behavioral theories of personality posit that personality is learned through experience—we act in ways that cause desirable consequences (e.g. Skinner, 1990), and that personality dimensions should relate to behavioral traits. Social cognitive theories, which include constructs like locus of control, self-efficacy, and attributional style, emphasize cognition and expectation factors to define personality dimensions (Bandura, 1977). A relatively recent behavioral model of personality that incorporates some aspects of motivation or cognition is the five-factor model (FFM; Goldberg, 1990; McCrae & Costa, 1999). Behavior theories have always applied equally to humans and nonhuman animals, but new research indicates that the FFM and even such constructs as locus of control are applicable to animals.

Researchers have identified a number of concordances between human personality traits and animal behavior. For example, Gosling and John (1999) conducted a meta-analysis of 19 animal-personality studies on 12 nonhuman species, looking for evidence of personality traits described in the five-factor model (McCrae & John, 1992). They found that extraversion and neuroticism appeared in species from chimpanzees to octopuses, and agreeableness in almost as many. Conscientiousness, however, was found only in chimpanzees, leading to the conclusion that this personality trait evolved much more recently and requires a highly developed cerebral cortex. Budaev (1998) found two overarching traits to be conserved from fish to mammals: activity-exploration, made up of extraversion, novelty-seeking, and proactive coping; and fear-avoidance, consisting of anxiety, behavioral inhibition, and reactive coping. Several other studies of animal personality traits have supported the use of the five-factor model (hyenas—Gosling, 1998; dogs—Ledger & Baxter, 1997; rhesus macaques—Chamove, Eysenck, & Harlow, 1972; Stevenson-Hinde, Stillwell-Barns, & Zunz, 1980; Capitanio, 1999; Figueredo, Cox, & Rhine, 1995; vervet monkeys—McGuire, Raleigh, & Pollack, 1994; chimpanzees—Gold & Maple, 1994; gorillas—Watson & Ward, 1996). Thus, there is ample evidence that certain dimensions or factors used to define human personality types may also apply to animals, supporting the notion that we can gain insight about the relationship between behavioral traits and immune function by expanding our research into the realm of animal models.

Animal personality has been an area of renewed interest to animal behaviorists studying the evolution and ecological relevance of traits in a population. In this research arena, the term *behavioral syndrome* is often used in place of animal personality to refer to a suite of correlated behaviors expressed either within a given behavioral context or across different contexts. These behaviors are thought to evolve as a package, providing a spectrum of individual differences across a population (Price & Langen, 1992). Syndromes produce trade-offs; what is adaptive in an animal's primary context might be maladaptive in a different context (e.g. high aggression in a competitive context versus a noncompetitive context). These syndromes can explain individual differences within a population—as environmental circumstances change, some individuals will be better suited than others, so a variety of behavioral syndromes can be maintained within a population (Dingemanse et al. 2004; Sih, Bell, & Johnson, 2004; Sih, Bell, Johnson, & Ziemba, 2004). Furthermore, social roles or conflict within groups have been argued as other mechanisms that maintains consistent individual behavioral differences within populations (Bergmüller & Taborsky, 2010). Because of these strong arguments that animal personalities exist in wild animal populations, and that there are distinct selection pressures that give rise to distinct behavioral traits among individuals in a population, we look forward to extending the study of animal personality and immune function into natural animal populations to verify that relationships identified in a laboratory context apply to the natural environment, providing further validity to this area of research.

Finally, an overarching concept often used to group different temperament or personality types (e.g. aggression and boldness) into broader cognitive categorical levels is the concept of "coping styles." Coping style is a trait that determines how a creature interprets, reacts to, and controls its environment. Many of the traits seen in both humans and animals can be characterized as belonging to differing coping styles. For example, in the animal literature, two coping styles are frequently used to describe animals with different suites of traits that suggest different interpretations of environmental cues: proactive versus reactive coping. Aggressiveness and novelty seeking are considered to fall into the proactive coping style category while anxiety and fear are considered to indicate a reactive coping style (Koolhaas et al., 1999). These coping styles are referred to as approach or problem-focused and avoidant or emotion-focused coping in the human literature (Lazarus & Folkman, 1984). In addition, certain personality dimensions are associated with coping; for example, emotion-focused coping is correlated with neuroticism in the five-factor theory, whereas problem-focused coping is associated with openness to experience (Penley & Tomaka, 2002; Watson & Hubbard, 1996). These overlaps, different perspectives, and different dimensions used to define personality illustrate the complexity of personality that must be taken into consideration when studying the links between personality and immunology.

The Relationship between Personality and Immune Function

When relating behavioral traits to immunology, it is important to note the significance of bidirectionality. Although much correlational research has been done on the immune differences among individual animals and people of differing temperaments, recent research has investigated the direction of causality, with intriguing evidence that specific immune challenges during infancy in rats can have a significant impact on adult behavior (Bilbo & Schwarz, 2009). On a shorter time scale, further evidence indicates that experimentally induced allergic responses increase anxiety-related behavior in adult rodents (Tonelli et al., 2009). In human research, personality can change when exposed to a disease prime. In one study, participants were shown a slide show of pictures and information about diseases or about architecture. Participants who were exposed to the disease cues rated themselves as less extraverted (Mortensen, Becker, Ackerman, Neuberg, & Kenrick, 2010)—sociability increases disease transmission, so social withdrawal from ill individuals is an adaptive response in a social species (Schaller, 2006). These studies and others demonstrate the influence that the immune system has on the behavioral biases displayed by an organism, and how personality influences the interpretation of cues that alter immune functioning.

In this chapter, we will focus on correlational studies that have shown relationships between animal personality/behavioral biases and immune function, as opposed to more causal studies, because this is where the bulk of information resides. Furthermore, the current review relies heavily on studies conducted with laboratory animals (rodents and primates), because this is where the majority of studies on the relationship between animal behavior and immune function has been conducted. Because of their application to human personality research, we will specifically focus on the personality traits previously mentioned: aggression, fear/anxiety, exploration/novelty-seeking, sociability, coping styles, and depression. With a recent push to understand the existence and maintenance of personality (i.e., complex behavioral syndromes; individual differences) in the natural environment, we expect that there will be an increasing number of studies on animal temperament and immune function in the natural setting in coming years because of renewed interest in stable individual differences in animals within populations and the role of distinct behavioral syndromes in evolutionary processes.

Animal Personality and Immune Function

In the following sections, we review some of the most common behavioral traits that have been identified in animals (aggression, affiliation/sociability, fear/anxiety, and exploration) and review studies that have compared these traits to immune function. Coping styles are presented as one of the more recent, and perhaps comprehensive, methods of categorizing animal personalities. Depression is covered last. Although not a personality trait in itself, it is a reflection of the intersection of environment and coping styles, and it has significant immune implications.

Aggression

Aggressiveness in response to an intruder is a stable trait seen in many vertebrate species (Koolhaas, 2008). In this section, we investigate the immune profiles associated with adaptive aggression versus pathological aggression in laboratory rodents and primates. These two kinds of aggression (defined later) are associated with different hypothalamic-pituitary-adrenal (HPA) axis and sympathetic nervous system activation, and with unique immune profiles.

Although there are many metrics for aggression, the most commonly used test with laboratory rodents is the resident-intruder test in which a novel conspecific is placed into the home cage or territory of a test animal. The common measure in this test is the latency for the test animal to attack the intruder; however, other measures include number and location of bites, the number of attacks, the intensity of attacks, and the duration of attacks (e.g. Jones & Brain, 1987). This test has been used to identify high- and low-aggressive animals to develop inbred strains with distinct stable differences in aggressive behavior, to quantify one aspect of coping styles, and to investigate neurological differences between high- and low-aggressive animals.

Aggression can be both an adaptive and maladaptive response. When threatened by a predator and/or in competition for mates, aggression can be a highly adaptive response, but there is also documentation that excess or ill-placed aggression can be maladaptive. For example, short-attack-latency inbred mice that have been specifically bred for rapid and extreme aggressive behavior toward non-threatening stimuli have been used as a model for human antisocial behavior in males (Sluyter et al., 2003). Excess aggression has also been documented in other species, including water striders, fishing spiders, and bluebirds, and results in increased territory but fewer opportunities to mate, and, thus, excess aggression appears relatively maladaptive and potentially a by-product of selective pressure (summarized in Pennisi, 2005). Here, we differentiate between adaptive aggression, in which an animal defends itself or its territory from attack, and pathological aggression, in which the animal shows excessive aggression out of context. Adaptive aggression is often used as one index of an active coping style—the animal takes the initiative to alter its environment (Benus, Bohus, Koolhaas, & van Oortmerssen., 1991). Pathological aggression, however, seems to confer diminishing advantage. The immune sequelae of these two types of aggression are markedly different; adaptive aggression is associated with greater T-cell and NK cell reactivity, slower tumor growth, and a possible propensity for autoimmune responses, whereas pathological aggression is associated with dampened antibody responses. As postulated by Zuk and Stoehr (2002), it is possible that there is a physiological trade-off between excessively high aggression and strong immune function, likely mediated by testosterone. This seems to be a case of a competition between "eat or be eaten" and "live to fight another day": aggressive animals would have greater access to resources and mates, but may also be more prone to injury and disease (see Wolf, van Doorn, Leimar, & Weissing, 2007).

The difference between health profiles for adaptive and pathologically aggressive animals may be explained by differential HPA activity and the complex interactions between glucocorticoids and the immune system. Although glucocorticoids are often considered globally anti-inflammatory, they can cause several pro-inflammatory effects, such as increased immune cell infiltration at the site of injury and increasing production and release of pro-inflammatory cytokines (de Pablos et al., 2006; Sorrells & Sapolsky, 2010). These seemingly contrary functions are paired with differential sensitivity at various levels of the HPA response (Ebner, Wotjak, Landgraf, & Engelmann, 2005).

Violence, or unnecessary aggression (i.e., pathological aggression), is associated with low basal heart rate and increased sympathetic nervous system (SNS) reactivity in both humans and animals (Böhnke, Bertsch, Kruk, & Naumann, 2010; Natarajan & Caramaschi, 2010; Patrick, 2008; Poutska et al., 2010; Sgoifo et al., 1996) and sometimes with low basal corticosterone (Patrick, 2008). The low basal corticosterone sometimes seen in pathologically aggressive animals may be a result of chronic stress, and, therefore, HPA downregulation (Sheridan, Stark, Avitsur, & Padgett, 2000). If this is the case, the expected immune differences also exist—pathologically aggressive animals generally show lower adaptive immune responses. Adaptive aggression, however, is associated with normal basal corticosterone, HPA reactivity, and heart rate (Caramaschi, de Boer, & Koolhaas, 2008).

Specific selection and breeding of mice into high- and low-aggressive lines has provided additional powerful information, with the best-studied examples coming from NC100 vs. NC900 mouse lines. NC100 mice are low aggressive, and tend to freeze when faced with an unfamiliar conspecific, whereas NC900 mice are quick to attack, even without provocation. Aggressive NC900 mice also show an anxiety-like phenotype (Nehrenberg et al., 2009), indicating that this aggression may be maladaptive in that its primary motivation is as an anxiety-coping mechanism rather than the assumed typical motivation of resource acquisition. Many immune differences exist between these two lines. Male and female NC900 mice have greater mitogen-induced T cell proliferation and IL-2 and IFNγ production in response to concanavalin A (Petitto, Lysle, Gariepy, & Lewis, 1994). When exposed to

the carcinogen 3-methylcholanthrene, the high-aggressive NC900 mice had greater NK cell activity and fewer occurrences of tumor development than the low-aggressive NC100 mice (Petitto et al., 1993). Similar resistance to tumor development has been documented in high-aggressive Balb/c female mice (Amkraut & Solomon, 1972), and male and female OF-1 mice (Vegas, Fano, Brain, Alonso, & Azpiroz, 2006; Azpiroz, De Miguel, Fano, & Vegas, 2008).

An example of pathological aggression is the short attack latency (SAL) versus long attack latency (LAL) mice—inbred strains that were bred from wild mice on the basis of their latency to attack a novel conspecific mouse (van Oortmerssen & Bakker, 1981). The SAL mice have been proposed as a model of personality disorders in men, with the argument that SAL display behavioral characteristics comparable to human antisocial behavior, including rapid, sustained, and unprovoked attacks (e.g., Sluyter et al., 2003). One study compared SAL and LAL behavioral and physiological responses to sensory contact and defeat stress for 25 days, then measured their thymus and spleen weights (Veenema, Meijer, de Kloet, & Koolhaas, 2003). The results were interesting, but confusing. In the sensory-contact task, SAL spleen weight decreased but LAL did not, whereas LAL thymus weights decreased but SAL did not. The LAL also lost weight in both stress conditions, whereas the SAL mice initially lost weight but regained it within 5 days, indicating faster recovery from stress. Compared to the LAL mice, SAL mice had lower corticosterone responses to social stressors, but three times more ACTH production in the control conditions, again indicating that pathological aggression is associated with altered HPA function (Ebner et al., 2005).

Pathological aggression is also seen in primates. In lab-housed adult male rhesus monkeys infected with simian immunodeficiency disorder (SIV; closely related to HIV), those that showed sustained aggression and/or submission during daily encounters with novel social partners (more than 100 seconds of aggressive/submissive behavior during a 5-minute period) had lower basal cortisol, lower anti-SIV IgG, higher viral loads, and shorter life spans than monkeys that did not show sustained levels of these behaviors (Capitanio et al., 2008). In this context, sustained aggression or submission may reflect either poor social skills or, in the case of sustained aggression, a propensity toward pathological aggression. The associated change in immune function may be a result of altered HPA function that results from the chronic stress associated with poor understanding of social interactions (Capitano et al., 2002).

Finally, there is evidence that the actual display of aggressive behavior is not necessary to induce immunological outcomes, suggesting genetic linkages between aggressive propensity and immune function. In one study (Petitto et al., 1999), 45-day-old isolate-housed mice were subjected to the resident-intruder task. Normally, social housing attenuates aggression differences between the NC100 and NC900 line, whereas isolation increases aggression in the NC900 line. NC100 mice of both sexes showed lower NK cell lysis, and group housing did not affect this immune difference between lines, suggesting that expression of aggression or nonaggression may not be necessary for immune-function differences between lines. It is possible that the genes that code for aggression are simply close in proximity to genes that code for these immune parameters, and are, therefore, transmitted together through generations (Petitto et al., 1999).

It is important to keep in mind that the majority of animal-immune research has been conducted in laboratories. Free-range animals often have different physiology than laboratory-housed animals. Laudenslager et al. (1999) captured free-range rhesus macaques to measure endocrine and various parameters of immune function. They found only one relationship between behavior and immune function: Macaques classified as highly irritable (high and fast movement, negative behavioral response to low provocation, low understanding, high aggression, excitable) had higher cytomegalovirus (CMV) antibody titers than low irritable macaques. It should be noted that, in the wild, social interactions are less forced and more voluntary than in laboratory housing conditions because of the increased space and environmental complexity in the natural setting. Increased environmental space and complexity allows individuals to remove themselves from the social group and to actively choose to engage in social interactions. In this context of increased control over the initiation and termination of social interactions, it is possible that underlying physiological processes associated with certain behaviors or behavioral traits are very different than those seen in smaller and more simple laboratory conditions.

In conclusion, normal adaptive aggression and pathological aggression have two unique immune profiles: Adaptive aggression (often further classified as an active coping style) is associated with elevated T-cell and NK cell activation and may predispose animals to autoimmune issues, whereas pathological aggression is associated with low adaptive immunity.

Affiliation/Sociability

Like humans, there are several species that display complex social behavior, and there is evidence that prosocial behavior conveys immune advantages in both animals and humans. Low-sociable people are at greater risk for and have more negative immune trajectories including and autoimmune disease (Kagan, 1994). Research shows that introverted people have greater viral shedding and more severe symptoms after rhinovirus exposure (Broadbent, Broadbent, Philpotts, & Wallace, 1984; Totman, Kiff, Reed, & Craig, 1980, Cohen, Doyle, Turner, Alper, & Skoner, 2003). Introverted or shy individuals are also more likely to suffer from allergies and atopic diseases (Bell, Jasnoski, Kagan, & King, 1990; Gauci, King, Saxarra, Tulloch, & Husband, 1993; Kagan, Snidman, Julia-Sellers, & Johnson, 1991; Muluk, Oğuztürk, Koc, & Ekici, 2003). Low-sociable gay men infected with human immunodeficiency virus (HIV) had faster CD4 T cell decline, higher viral load, and lower response to highly active antiretroviral therapy compared to more social men (Miller, Kemeny, Taylor, Cole, & Visscher, 1997; Cole, Kemeny, Fahey, Zack, & Naliboff, 2003). These human studies have been paralleled in animal research.

In animals, affiliation, sociability, or social affability, is also a powerful predictor of adaptive immune function. Maninger et al. (Maninger, Capitanio, Mendoza, & Mason, 2003) investigated antibody responses to tetanus immunization in high and low sociable adult male rhesus macaques. At baseline, the two behavioral types had similar antibody levels, but after a booster tetanus vaccination and placement into unfamiliar colonies, the highly sociable animals had significantly higher tetanus-specific IgG antibody levels than low-sociable animals. The results suggest that the social stress of relocation into a new group without the ability to quickly carve out a niche in the social hierarchy confers an immunosuppressive level of stress on low-sociable animals. In support of this idea, male cynomolgus monkeys with lower social status were found to be at higher risk for adenovirus infection that higher-status animals (Cohen et al., 1997).

Research done in free-ranging macaques found results in opposition to previously described reports of impaired NK cell and T cell responses in low-sociable macaques; these animals showed no relationship between sociability and immune function (Laudenslager et al., 1999). Social interactions in the wild are much different than those in the laboratory, and these differences must be taken into consideration when analyzing social behavior. Care must also be taken to specifically define personality traits under investigation to be able to compare results across studies.

Evidence suggests that the autonomic nervous system is the link between sociability and immune function. Sloan and colleagues (Sloan, Capitanio, Tarara, & Cole, 2008), for example, assayed 13 lymph nodes pulled from 7 rhesus monkeys. They found that low-social animals had almost three times as much catecholaminergic innervation to the lymph nodes, probably because they had more than twice the expression of nerve-growth factor. These low-social animals were also different in response to tetanus vaccination; after receiving a second "booster" vaccination, they had lower IgG responses than the high-social monkeys. Sloan and colleagues (2008) provided three possible explanations for the immune differences in low-social and high-social animals: (1) Certain animals are more sensitive to threat; exposure to threat alters both physiology and behavior. These animals would then both be low-social and have increased lymph node innervation (Sloan et al., 2008; Sloan et al., 2007). (2) Existing differences in lymph node innervation may cause cytokine release, which then affects the brain in such a way to cause low sociability (Dantzer & Kelley, 2007). (3) High-sociable animals are more exposed to socially transmitted pathogens, which may then influence the development of the immune system (Boyce et al., 1995; Cole, 2006). All these explanations center on the idea that differential immune responses in high-social and low-social animals are driven by differential stress responses by the central nervous system (CNS) (i.e., Kagan, 1994). They also demonstrate the difficulty of determining causality in PNI research; not only can causality not be definitively identified, but it is possible that all these hypotheses are correct to some degree.

Taken together, the research on immune function and sociability indicates that high-social animals are healthier (Sapolsky, 2005). They are less reactive to stress, either because their social position or bonds buffer them from stressors (Ray & Sapolsky, 1992; Virgin & Sapolsky, 1997), or because low-social animals are low-social because they are more reactive to stressors (Abbott et al., 2003). Both of these hypotheses have been supported in human research; we know that high social position protects against stress, and that having close social bonds is related to a lower physiological response to stress (Lepore, Allen, & Evans, 1993; Gerin, Pieper, Levy, & Pickering, 1992; Kamarck, Manuck, & Jennings, 1990). However, it is difficult to directly compare human and animal social behavior because human social behavior tends to be more complex. Even in nonhuman primates, animals are part of a distinct and rigid social hierarchy, whereas a person may be a part of many social hierarchies—at work, at home, at school, among friends—which are constantly shifting.

Sociability shares some overlapping features with other personality traits. High sociability may be an example of a proactive coping style not dissimilar to adaptive aggression—both are active behavioral styles that entail taking control of a social situation. Control, or perception of control, has a major influence over HPA and SNS stress responses (Pruessner et al., 2005). Sociability also serves to allay anxiety and the behavioral and physiological stress responses associated with anxiety.

Fear/Anxiety

Trait anxiety in rodent models is clearly associated with impaired innate and adaptive immune function. Although acute stress or fear is associated with increased innate immune function, particularly in preparation for injury, it seems that chronic anxiety short-circuits this adaptation, most likely through chronically elevated corticosterone or decreased sensitivity to ACTH.

Fear/anxiety in animals is tested in rodents with different protocols in which rodents are exposed to benign but unprotected test arenas. Three of the most common protocols used for laboratory rodents are the elevated plus maze (EPM), the light-dark box (LD), and the open field (OF). All three arenas draw on rodents' preferences for protected areas; the EPM also draws on rodents' avoidance of heights. The open spaces of the test arenas are unprotected, which, in the natural environment would leave a rodent open to overhead predator attacks. On the other hand, for opportunistic foraging species, the space may also hold undiscovered resources. These tests allow researchers to compare the drive to explore with the drive to remain safe. Relative frequency and duration of visits to the closed versus open areas in the EPM, LD, and OF, are used to index anxiety-related behavior—with more time spent in the closed areas indicative of a greater fear/anxiety-related response (Pellow, Chopin, File, &

Briley, 1985, Lister, 1987, Costall, Jones, Kelly, Naylor, & Tomkins, 1989, Carobrez & Bertoglio 2005). These tests have been validated with the use of known anxiolytic compounds.

One rat strain has been bred solely on the basis of anxiety behavior. High anxiety behavior (HAB) and low anxiety behavior (LAB) rats were bred from Wistar stock, based on their anxiety responses in the EPM. Salomé et al. (1999) tested HAB and LAB rats on their corticosterone and IL-6 responses to LPS injection. HABs had greater CORT response, lower basal circulating IL-6, and slightly heavier body weight compared to LABs. However, no differences were found in baseline or 4-hours post-LPS corticosterone, in ACTH at any time point, or in IL-6 responses to LPS. This indicates that HAB rats have greater sensitivity to ACTH and a more sensitive HPA negative feedback loop.

Using male Swiss albino mice, Rammal et al. (Rammal, Bouayed, Falla, Boujenaini, & Soulimani, 2010) tested the association between anxiety and cellular and humoral immunity. Mice were tested in the light-dark box at 10 weeks of age; 10% were classified as anxious and 10% as nonanxious. Immediately following the LD test, anxious mice had decreased number of total lymphocytes, CD4+, and CD8+ cells, and decreased IgA and IgE levels in circulation. If mice were subjected to restraint stress for 2 hours, the anxious ones had a greater decrease in total lymphocyte count. After 15 days of daily 2-hour restraint stress, anxious mice had larger decreases in total lymphocytes, CD8+, and NK cells, and they had larger increases in granulocytes and monocytes. No difference was found in IgG, a marker for adaptive immunity.

In a different Swiss-mouse model, Pérez-Álvarez et al. (2005) characterized mice according to their behavioral response in a T-maze and found that differential behavioral responses predicted differential life spans. Specifically, mice that spent less time in the open arms (indicating greater anxiety-like behavior) had a shorter life span than mice that spent more time in these arms (termed Prematurely Aging Mice—PAM vs. Non-Prematurely Aging Mice—NPAM). In this model, the PAM had increased basal corticosterone, and decreased HPA reactivity to stress compared to the NPAM, and the high-anxious PAM mice also have decreased macrophage and lymphocyte mobility, decreased macrophage phagocytic capacity, decreased lymphocyte proliferation in response to mitogens, and decreased NK cell activity and IL-2 release in response to concanavalin A (Viveros, Arranz, Hernanz, Miquel, &

de la Fuente, 2007). The preceding studies link trait anxiety to immunosenescence.

Anxiety in general is linked to a decrease in immune functioning across the board. This may be due to a sensitized HPA axis. Under normal circumstances, this would be an advantage in stress response and recovery, but when stimulated by repeated acute stressors, it results in generalized immunosuppression.

Exploration

Exploration is another behavioral trait that shares some overlap with other behavioral characteristics. In humans, the parallel trait is referred to as sensation-seeking. This has been characterized and psychometrically tested by Zuckerman with the Sensation-Seeking Scale V (SSS-V; Zuckerman, 1979) and Cloninger with the Tridimensional Personality Questionnaire (TPQ; Cloninger, 1987). Human sensation seekers are prone to injury and are particularly susceptible to drug abuse (Zuckerman, 1994). Similarly, uninhibited/exploratory animals are more likely to choose exploration of novel areas and animals over the safety of the known (Dellu, Mayo, Piazza, Le Moal, & Simon, 1993; Dellu, Piazza, Mayo, Le Moal, & Simon, 1996).

Cavigelli and colleagues have characterized exploratory behavior in Sprague-Dawley rats in two contexts: a novel social arena, and the novel object arena. Both resemble the open field test, except the novel physical arena contains four rat-sized objects to explore, and the novel physical arena contains two cages—one empty and one containing a same-age, same-sex conspecific novel social partner. In these rats, level of exploration tends to be stable traits over time (Cavigelli & McClintock, 2003; Cavigelli et al., 2007, 2009; Cavigelli, Yee, & McClintock, 2006) and is related to immune function. High-locomotion female rats had higher corticosterone, larger adrenal glands, smaller thymuses, and lower circulating TNFα levels during young adulthood, and a shorter lifespan (Cavigelli, Bennett, Michael, & Klein, 2008). In these high-locomotion females, movement was concentrated in the periphery, near arena walls (i.e., thigmotaxis), which was different from male rats that spent more time in the center of the arena (Cavigelli, Michael, West, & Klein, 2011). These locomotion patterns indicate that, for females, locomotion (primarily thigmotactic) may reflect an active coping mechanism for high anxiety. This research provides an interesting counterpoint to research done in male rats, where high locomotion seems to be health-protective (Cavigelli & McClintock, 2003; Cavigelli et al. 2009). Noting the immune differences in shy versus nonshy humans (Bell et al., 1990; Kagan et al., 1994), we have conducted further studies to compare basic immune function between high- and low-exploration male Sprague-Dawley rats, and we have found that low-exploration rats had greater IL-6 response to endotoxin and dampened delayed-type hypersensitivity swelling responses to keyhole limpet hemocyanin reexposure in the hind footpad (Michael, Cavigelli, & Bonneau, in preparation).

These findings indicate a difference in immune function between high- and low-exploration rats that may be because exploratory animals may be more prone to leave the natal group and be exposed to novel antigens and injury it would be adaptive to have an immune system well-suited to respond to novel infectious agents.

Coping Styles

Coping styles are comprised of a conglomeration of traits, and describe a typical pattern of response to a stressor. Generally, there are considered to be two types of coping styles—active and passive. Active (or proactive, or problem-focused) coping involves an active attempt to change environments to minimize adversity. Passive (or reactive, or emotion-focused) coping involves hiding or fleeing from aversive stimuli, or focusing on self-soothing. Active coping animals tend to be less susceptible to tumors and autoimmune diseases, whereas passive-coping animals seem to be better able to mount an immune response to severe injury and to pathogen exposure under stressful conditions.

Many animals, including rats, mice, pigs, lizards, rainbow trout, and even octopuses have been found to have differences in their coping styles (Koolhaas et al., 1999). Koolhaas and colleagues have postulated that having both active and passive animals in a population is evolutionarily advantageous (Koolhaas, 2008). Proactive behavioral control works best under highly predictable conditions, whereas reactive coping style is more appropriate under variable and unpredictable environmental conditions. With this spectrum of possible behaviors, the population as a whole is more likely to survive (Sih, Bell, & Johnson, 2004).

Aggression and sociability both can be described as coping styles. For example, aggressive attacks in the resident-intruder test are often interpreted as a measure of willingness to "make the first move" in a threatening situation—proactively changing a challenging situation rather than simply reacting

to it. Contributing to the idea of aggression as an active coping style, aggressive male rodents are also proactive in other behaviors, like active avoidance, nest building, and defensive burying, whereas low-aggressive males tend toward self-calming behaviors like grooming (Sih, Bell, & Johnson, 2004).

One interesting model for coping style in animals is the Roman High Avoidance (RHA)/Roman Low Avoidance (RLA) rat line (Broadhurst & Bignami, 1965). These Wistar-derived rats, selected for their behavior in the active avoidance shuttle box task, also differ on in anxiety-related behavior, with the RLA rats showing more anxiety-like behavior in the open-field test and the circular corridor. Because RLA rats have increased and lengthened behavioral and HPA responses to stress, and because they focus on "displacement" behaviors like self-grooming or redirected aggression instead of investigating the source of stress, it has been proposed that they use a passive coping style compared to the more problem-focused active coping style of the RHAs (Steimer, la Fleur, & Schulz, 1997, Steimer & Driscoll, 2005). These selected strains were accompanied by some interesting immune differences. Sandi and colleagues (Sandi, Castanon, Vitiello, Neveu, & Morméde, 1991) found higher T cell activity in male and female RLA rats, though no differences in their ability to mount an antibody response to a novel antigen, namely, sheep red blood cells. The RLA rats also had higher NK cell activity, but no differences in B cell responses. Looking for an explanation for these immune differences, Castanon and colleagues (Castanon, Dulluc, le Maol, & Morméde, 1992) investigated prolactin as a link between behavior and immune function. They found that, although there were no differences in basal or stimulated HPA function between the two lines, prolactin was significantly lower in the RLA line. Many immune cells express prolactin receptors, and some secrete prolactin. Prolactin knockout mice do not seem to suffer immune dysfunction (Goffin et al., 1998), indicating a regulatory role for prolactin only under adverse immune conditions (Matera, 1996). In one study, however, prolactin administered in pharmacologic doses to septic mice drastically increased mortality, decreased splenocyte proliferation, and increased splenocyte apoptosis. In addition, prolactin altered the normal immune response to sepsis by inhibiting IL-2 secretion and increasing IFN-γ (Oberbeck et al., 2003). This indicates that the RLA rats may have an immune advantage over the RHA rats in the case of severe injury, whereas RHA rats might be more likely to adapt to severe stressors, lending more support to the theory that a spectrum of behaviors and their attendant physiological differences is adaptive in a population.

Lewis rats are an inbred Wistar-derived line with relatively low baseline corticosterone levels and low corticosterone responses to stress. Because of their low corticosterone secretion, Lewis rats are susceptible to many autoimmune diseases and certain types of tumors. Sajti and colleagues investigated two health outcomes in male and female Lewis rats: tumor angiogenesis (Satji, Kavelaars, et al, 2004) and adjuvant-induced arthritis (Satji, van Meeteren, et al., 2004). They first tested animals in an open field and classified them as high active (HA) or low active (LA); high activity is indicative of active coping style. They found that LA Lewis rats had greater angiogenesis, more lung metastases, and more large (>2mm) tumors compared to the HA Lewis rats (Sajti, Kavelaars, et al., 2004). LA animals were also more susceptible to adjuvant-induced arthritis; severity of inflammation was similar in LA and HA rats, but LA rats had more osteoporosis, periostal new-bone formation, and bone destruction than HA rats. The authors postulated that lower production of IL-10 and IFNγ, both bone-protective cytokines, may be responsible for greater joint destruction in LA rats (Sajti, van Meeteren, et al., 2004). Other strains of rodents show similar results; Vegas and colleagues (2006) found that passive/submissive male OF-1 mice developed more lung metastases than more proactive mice.

In pigs, the test used to determine coping style is called the Backtest, in which pigs are held on their back for one minute. High-resistive (active coping) pigs are defined as those that make more attempts to escape the Backtest, whereas low-resistive (passive coping) pigs make few attempts to escape. In response to keyhole limpet hemocyanin (KLH), a novel antigen, high-resistance pigs had higher KLH-specific lymphocyte proliferation responses than low-resistance pigs (Bolhuis, Parmentier, Schouten, Schrama, & Wiegant, 2003). Similar studies found that low-resistance pigs had a lower cellular immunity but an enhanced or accelerated humoral immunity response in comparison to high-resistance pigs (Hessing, Coenen, Vaiman, & Renard, 1995; Schrama et al., 1997).

As previously mentioned, varied coping styles are not limited to mammals. Øverli and colleagues (2007) reviewed a number of studies on rainbow trout and their cortisol responses to stress.

Low-responsive trout had longer retention of conditioned responses, and were more aggressive/dominant than high-responsive trout. They also were quicker to resume feeding after a stressor. Similar results were found in a lizard, *Anolis carolinensis*. Hanlon and Messenger (1999) have described varying coping methods in octopuses. These results indicate that coping styles are not reserved only for mammals, though little is known about immune responses and coping in these other species.

Coping styles are a description of an animal's response to stressors. Although two animals' behavior might be very similar under normal conditions, behavioral and physiological differences might emerge during periods of stress. Inadequate or misdirected coping can in itself become a stressor (Zozulya, Gabaeva, Sokolov, Surkina, & Kost, 2008). When investigating the interactions between personality traits and immunity, coping styles provide a more comprehensive framework for understanding behavioral traits that often occur together in individuals.

Depression

Unlike the previously described personality styles, depression is not a personality in itself. Depression is an illness, comprised of both innate and learned factors. Depression in humans encompasses a broad range of symptoms, and also has a significant inflammatory component. Common symptoms of major depression include fatigue/hypersomnia, insomnia, weight gain, weight loss, loss of enjoyment or interest, irritability, sadness, anhedonia, and lack of energy. This leads us to one of the limitations of animal personality research, which can also be turned into a lesson. Few of these symptoms are directly measurable in animals, as we cannot ask them how they are feeling today or administer a convenient questionnaire. However, their behavioral changes, similar to those seen in humans, can be indicators of depressive illness.

The studies of Seligman and Maier demonstrated the concept of "learned helplessness" (Seligman & Maier, 1967). In their landmark 1967 study, Seligman and Maier tested the effects of inescapable shock on behavior in dogs. Later, the dogs were exposed to escapable shocks. Control dogs would quickly move to escape the shocks when given means to do so, but two-thirds of the dogs exposed to inescapable shock would not. They would simply sit still and continue to receive the shocks. This learned helplessness has been compared to the anhedonia and hopelessness described by patients with major depression—there is no point in fighting anymore, so they give up.

Two protocols have been widely accepted for testing depressive-like symptoms in laboratory rodents: the forced-swim test (FST) and the sucrose-preference test (SPT). The FST is designed to elicit learned helpless behavior. The rodent is placed in a container of water from which it cannot escape or touch the bottom. The measure taken is the amount of time between the beginning of the test and the cessation of struggling to swim. Shorter latency to cessation of struggle is considered depressive-like behavior. In the SPT, animals are given two water bottles—one with plain water and the other with a sucrose solution. Most animals will show a preference for the sucrose solution. In anhedonia, however, the drive for pleasant stimuli is reduced, so animals that do not show preference for the sucrose solution are considered anhedonic. Other behavioral markers of depression in animals include anorexia, changes in sleep patterns, and social withdrawal in social species.

Interest in the psychoneuroimmunology of depression was sparked by the observation that cancer patients receiving interferon-alpha reported developing depression (Renault et al., 1987). Several studies since then have shown that depression in humans is associated with inflammation (e.g., Dantzer, O'Connor, Freund, Johnson, & Kelley, 2008). However, other biological and experiential factors also contribute in large part to the development of depression, such as serotonin transporter genes and childhood abuse. Because of this complex etiology, determining causality is difficult in humans. Animal models allow behavioral and physiological experimental manipulations and control over an animal's entire lifespan and, thus, provide one method to study immune mechanisms associated with depression.

One very interesting study investigated the effects of live *Escherichia coli* infection in neonatal male Sprague-Dawley rats (Bilbo et al., 2008). The pups were infected subcutaneously with live *E. coli* at 4 days of age, which roughly corresponds with the third trimester of human pregnancy. Because merely the injury associated with injection may cause an immune response, control rats were injected with phosphate-buffered saline. As adults, the *E. coli*-exposed rats had attenuated depressive-like behavioral changes following stress—less anorexia, greater sucrose intake, and less social withdrawal—compared to control rats. This was not related to any changes in serotonin, but it may have been related to corticosterone; the *E. coli*-exposed rats had attenuated corticosterone responses to stress. The results of this study were in opposition to what previous similar studies had found using lipopolysaccharide (LPS), a common nonpathogenic antigen found in *E. coli* cell walls (e.g. Musson, Morrison, & Ulevitch, 1978). This indicates that, although LPS is the epitope that is detected by Toll-like receptors, some process unique to live infection stimulates a different behavioral and possibly a different immune response.

The Flinders line of rats provides an interesting model for the study of depression and immunity. These strains were derived from Sprague-Dawley rats, and inbred based on their airway sensitivity to methacholine, a muscarinic receptor-agonist that, when inhaled, causes bronchial constriction similar to that seen in asthma (Russell, Overstreet, Messenger, & Helps, 1982). These two lines are referred to as the Flinders sensitive line (FSL) and the Flinders resistant line (FRL). The FSL rats have many symptoms consistent with depression, such as reduced appetite and body weight, reduced activity in novel environments, increased withdrawal and inhibitory behaviors when exposed to stressors, anhedonia (demonstrated by low frequency bar pressing for water or food reward), and slow completion of a food-motivated nonmatching-to-sample learning procedure compared to control rats (Overstreet & Russell 1982, Overstreet, Janowsky, Gillin, Shiromani, & Sutin, 1986; Overstreet, 1993, Overstreet, Pucilowski, Rezvani, & Janowsky, 1995; Bushnell et al. 1995). In addition, FSL sleep patterns are somewhat similar to those seen in depressed humans—REM sleep is increased in FSL rats, and latency to REM is decreased (Benca et al. 1996, Shiromani et al. 1988). The Flinders lines are not a perfect model of human depression, but in addition to these behavioral analogies, FSL rat immune function is comparable to that seen in human depression (e.g. reduced Th1 immune function with normal Th2 function). For example, FSL rats had reduced basal NK cell activity, reduced primary antibody response, and splenocyte production of IFN-gamma and IL-6 in response to keyhole limpet hemocyanin, indicating an increased susceptibility to infection (Friedman, Irwin, & Overstreet, 1996; Friedman, Becker, Overstreet, & Lawrence, 2002). As expected, FSL rats had more hyperresponsive airways (a typical allergy symptom) than FRL or control rats (Djurić et al. 1998). FSL rats, however, have similar IgE levels to FRL rats—a surprising finding, as allergies in humans are mediated by IgE. Despite similar IgE activity, exposure to a choline agonist or a generic antigen (ovalbumin) did cause greater inflammation and immune cell proliferation in FSL compared to FRL rats (Djurić, Overstreet, Bienenstock, & Perdue, 1995).

Depression is not a personality trait itself, but a reaction to external events seen through the lens of personality and coping styles. In evolutionary terms, it may even be a vestige of an adaptive trait (Raison, Capuron, & Miller,., 2006). With more insight into the etiology of inflammation and depression through the use of animal models, further strides can be made in the prevention and treatment of this disorder.

Conclusion

Personality research in animals has proceeded in leaps and bounds in recent years. Traits previously thought to belong only to humans have been identified in species from primates to invertebrates. These personality traits are linked to systematic differences in immune function among individuals, much as they are in humans. Although animal psychoneuroimmunology research is a fascinating field in its own right, these animal models are also compelling for their potential to be applied to human research. Together with human research, animal models provide an exciting and promising avenue to further examine the mechanistic links between personality and health outcomes. To strengthen the contribution of this research area, we suggest the following key research topics to focus on in future studies.

Future Directions

1. Are there sex differences in the relationship between behavior and immune function? The majority of studies that have investigated the relationship between animal temperament and immune function have been conducted with male animals. Although this research bias has been decreasing in the past decades, there is still a strong bias toward more research with male subjects. Given differential social roles for male and female animals and a host of different physiological processes between the sexes, the relationship between personality and immune function may be quite different between males and females.

2. Given a renewed interest in the evolution and ecological significance of animal personalities in the natural habitat, it will be important to determine if there are different immunological biases associated with different behavioral biases in the natural environment. For example, bolder or more aggressive animals that are more prone to emigrate from the natal group and therefore more susceptible to wounding, may benefit more from certain kinds of immunological bias like increased wound-healing abilities or increased ability to fight off parasites, whereas less exploratory or aggressive animals may benefit more from immunological biases that protect them from socially transmitted pathogens.

3. What are the mechanisms that lead animals with one behavioral bias to have a specific immunological bias that is different from animals with a different behavioral bias? For example, are behavioral and immunological biases linked at the genetic level? Or, do behavioral traits lead to biases in physiological processes (e.g., increased HPA function, increased sympathetic activity, etc.) that then influence immune-system function? The study of animal behavior and immune function provides an interesting complement to research on human personality and immune function; longitudinal and experimental studies can be conducted with animals to answer mechanistic questions about how personality and immune function are related.

4. Further work is required to determine which behavioral traits are universally displayed across a variety of species and to determine the evolutionary pressures that lead to selection of certain behavioral traits. Furthermore, if personality traits are defined as stable/consistent individual differences in behavior, and it is this consistency over time and across conditions that is an important aspect of why personality is related to physiological processes like immune function, then it is important to verify the degree of behavioral stability in a study population.

5. Finally, this area of research requires further studies on how activation of specific immune responses during sensitive development periods can have long-term influences on behavioral traits. This kind of work is best conducted with animal models, but the implications for our understanding of how human personality develops would be great.

Related Chapters:

For more information on concepts introduced in this chapter, see also Cavigelli; Cohen; Pressman; and Cole, this volume.

References

Abbott, D. H., Keverne, E. B., Bercovitch, F. B., Shively, C. A., Mendoza, S. P., & Saltzman, W. et al. (2003). Are subordinates always stressed? A comparative analysis of rank differences in cortisol levels among primates. *Hormones and Behavior, 43,* 67–82.

Amkraut, A., & Solomon, G. F. (1972). Stress and murine sarcoma virus (Moloney)-induced tumors. *Cancer Research, 32,* 1428–1433.

Azpiroz, A., De Miguel, Z., Fano, E., & Vegas, O. (2008). Relations between different coping strategies for social stress, tumor development and neuroendocrine and immune activity in male mice. *Brain Behavior and Immunity, 22,* 690–698.

Bandura, A. (1977). Self-efficacy: Toward a unifying theory of behavioral change. *Psychological Review, 84,* 191–215.

Bell, I. R., Jasnoski, M. L., Kagan, J., & King, D. S. (1990). Is allergic rhinitis more frequent in young adults with extreme shyness? A preliminary survey. *Psychosomatic Medicine, 52,* 517–525.

Benca, R. M., Overstreet, D. E., Gilliland, M. A., Russell, D., Bergmann, B. M., & Obermeyer, W. H. (1996). Increased basal REM sleep but no difference in dark induction or light suppression of REM sleep in flinders rats with cholinergic supersensitivity. *Neuropsychopharmacology, 15,* 45–51.

Benus, R. F., Bohus, B., Koolhaas, J. M., & van Oortmerssen, G. A. (1991). Heritable variation for aggression as a reflection of individual coping strategies. *Cellular and Molecular Life Sciences, 47,* 1008–1019.

Bergmüller, R., & Taborsky, M. (2010). Animal personality due to social niche specialization. *Trends in Ecology and Evolution, 25,* 504–511.

Bilbo, S. D., & Schwarz, J. M. (2009). Early-life programming of later-life brain and behavior: A critical role for the immune system. *Frontiers in Behavioral Neuroscience, 3,* 14.

Bilbo, S. D., Yirmiya, R., Amat, J., Paul, E. D., Watkins, L. R., & Maier, S. F. (2008). Bacterial infection early in life protects against stressor-induced depressive-like symptoms in adult rats. *Psychoneuroendocrinology, 33,* 261–269.

Böhnke, R., Bertsch, K., Kruk, M. R., & Naumann, E. (2010). The relationship between basal and acute HPA axis activity and aggressive behavior in adults. *Journal of Neural Transmission, 117,* 629–637.

Bolhuis, J. E., Parmentier, H. K., Schouten, W. G., Schrama, J. W., & Wiegant, V. M. (2003). Effects of housing and individual coping characteristics on immune responses of pigs. *Physiology and Behavior, 79,* 289–296.

Boyce, W. T., Chesney, M., Alkon, A., Tschann, J. M., Adams, S., Chesterman, B., et al. (1995). Psychobiologic reactivity to stress and childhood respiratory illnesses: Results of two prospective studies. *Psychosomatic Medicine, 57,* 411–422.

Broadbent, D. E., Broadbent, M. H., Phillpotts, R. J., & Wallace, J. (1984). Some further studies on the prediction of experimental colds in volunteers by psychological factors. *Journal of Psychosomatic Research, 28,* 511–523.

Broadhurst, P. L., & Bignami, G. (1965). Correlative effects of psychogenetic selection: A study of the Roman high and low avoidance strains of rats. *Behavioral Research and Therapy, 2,* 273–280.

Budaev, S. V. (1998). How many dimensions are needed to describe temperament in animals? A factor reanalysis of two data sets. *International Journal of Comparative Psychology, 11,* 17–29.

Bushnell, P. J., Levin, E. D., & Overstreet, D. H. (1995). Spatial working and reference memory in rats bred for autonomic sensitivity to cholinergic stimulation: Acquisition, accuracy, speed, and effects of cholinergic drugs. *Neurobiology of Learning and Memory, 63,* 116–132.

Capitanio, J. P. (1999). Personality dimensions in adult male rhesus macaques: Prediction of behaviors across time and situation. *American Journal of Primatology, 47,* 299–320.

Capitanio, J. P. (2008). Personality and disease. *Brain Behavior and Immunity, 22,* 647–650.

Capitanio, J. P, Abel, K., Mendoza, S. P., Blozis, S. A., McChesney, M. B., Cole, S. W., & Mason, W. A. (2008). Personality and serotonin transporter genotype interact with social context to affect immunity and viral set-point in simian immunodeficiency virus disease. *Brain Behavior and Immunity, 22,* 676–689.

Caramaschi, D., de Boer, S. F., & Koolhaas, J. M. (2008). Is hyper-aggressiveness associated with physiological hypoarousal? A comparative study on mouse lines selected for high and low aggressiveness. *Physiology and Behavior, 95,* 591–598.

Carobrez, A. P., & Bertoglio, L. J. (2005). Ethological and temporal analyses of anxiety-like behavior: The elevated plus-maze model 20 years on. *Neuroscience and Biobehavioral Reviews, 29,* 1193–1205.

Castanon, N., Dulluc, J., le Moal, M., & Mormède, P. (1992). Prolactin as a link between behavioral and immune differences between the Roman rat lines. *Physiology and Behavior, 51,* 1235–1241.

Cavigelli, S. A. (2005). Animal personality and health. *Behaviour, 142,* 1223–1244.

Cavigelli, S. A., Bennett, J. M., Michael, K. C., & Klein, L. C. (2008). Female temperament, tumor development and life span: Relation to glucocorticoid and tumor necrosis factor alpha levels in rats. *Brain Behavior and Immunity, 22,* 727–35.

Cavigelli, S. A., & McClintock, M. K. (2003). Fear of novelty in infant rats predicts adult corticosterone dynamics and an early death. *Proceedings of the National Academy of Sciences, 100,* 16131–16136.

Cavigelli, S. A., Michael, K. C., West, S. G., Klein, L. C. (2011). Behavioral responses to physical vs. social novelty in male and female laboratory rats. *Behavioural Processes, 88,* 56–59.

Cavigelli, S. A., Ragan, C. M., Michael, K. C., Kovacsics, C. E., & Bruscke, A. P. (2009). Stable behavioral inhibition and glucocorticoid production as predictors of longevity. *Physiology and Behavior, 98,* 205–214.

Cavigelli, S. A., Stine, M. M., Kovacsics, C. E., Jefferson, A., Diep, M. N., & Barrett, C. E. (2007). Behavioral inhibition and glucocorticoid dynamics in a rodent model. *Physiology and Behavior, 92,* 897–905.

Cavigelli, S. A., Yee, J. R., & McClintock, M. K. (2006). Infant temperament predicts life span in female rats that develop spontaneous tumors. *Hormones and Behavior, 50,* 454–462.

Chamove, A. S., Eysenck, H., & Harlow, H. F. (1972). Personality in monkeys: Factor analysis of rhesus social behaviour. *Quarterly Journal of Experimental Psychology, 24,* 496–504.

Cloninger, C. R. A. (1987) A systematic method for clinical description and classification of personality variants: A proposal. *Archives of General Psychiatry, 44,* 573–588.

Cohen, S., Doyle, W. J., Turner, R., Alper, C. M., & Skoner, D. P. (2003). Sociability and susceptibility to the common cold. *Psychological Science, 14,* 389–395.

Cohen, S., Line, S., Manuck, S. B., Rabin, B. S., Heise, E. R., & Kaplan, J. R. (1997). Chronic social stress, social status, and susceptibility to upper respiratory infections in nonhuman primates. *Psychosomatic Medicine, 59,* 213–221.

Cole, S. W. (2006). The complexity of dynamic host networks. In T. S. Deisboeck & K. Y. Kresh(Eds.), *Complex systems science in biomedicine.* New York: Springer.

Cole, S. W., Kemeny, M. E., Fahey, J. L., Zack, J. A., & Naliboff, B. D. (2003). Psychological risk factors for HIV pathogenesis: Mediation by the autonomic nervous system. *Biological Psychiatry, 54,* 1444–1456.

Costall, B., Jones, B. J., Kelly, M. E., Naylor, R. J., & Tomkins, D. M. (1989). Exploration of mice in a black and white test box: Validation as a model of anxiety. *Pharmacology, Biochemistry and Behavior, 32,* 777–785.

Dantzer, R., & Kelley, K. W. (2007). Twenty years of research on cytokine-induced sickness behavior. *Brain Behavior and Immunity, 21,* 153–160.

Dantzer, R., O'Connor, J. C., Freund, G. G., Johnson, R. W., & Kelley, K. W. (2008). From inflammation to sickness and depression: When the immune system subjugates the brain. *Nature Reviews Neuroscience, 9,* 46–56.

Dellu, F., Mayo, W., Piazza, P. V., Le Moal, M., & Simon, H. (1993). Individual differences in behavioral responses to novelty in rats: Possible relationship with the sensation seeking trait in man. *Personality and Individual Differences, 15,* 411–418.

Dellu, F., Piazza, P. V., Mayo, W., Le Moal, M., & Simon, H. (1996). Novelty-seeking in rats: Biobehavioral characteristics and possible relationship with the sensation seeking trait in man. *Neuropsychobiology, 34,* 136–145.

de Pablos, R. M., Villarán, R. F., Argüelles, S., Herrera, A. J., Venero, J. L., Ayala, A., et al. (2006). Stress increases vulnerability to inflammation in the rat prefrontal cortex. *Journal of Neuroscience, 24,* 5709–5719.

Dingemanse, N. J., Both, C., Drent, P. J., & Tinbergen, J. M. (2004). Fitness consequences of avian personalities in a fluctuating environment. *Proceedings of the Royal Society of London B, 271,* 847–852.

Djurić, V. J., Cox, G., Overstreet, D. H., Smith, L., Dragomir, A., & Steiner, M. (1998). Genetically transmitted cholinergic hyperresponsiveness predisposes to experimental asthma. *Brain, Behavior, and Immunity, 12,* 272–284.

Djurić, V. J., Overstreet, D. H., Bienenstock, J., & Perdue, M. H. (1995). Immediate hypersensitivity in the Flinders rat: Further evidence for a possible link between susceptibility to allergies and depression. *Brain, Behavior, and Immunity, 9,* 196–206.

Ebner, K., Wotjak, C. T., Landgraf, R., & Engelmann, M. (2005). Neuroendocrine and behavioral response to social confrontation: Residents versus intruders, active versus passive coping styles. *Hormones and Behavior, 47,* 14–21.

Figueredo, A. J., Cox, R. L., & Rhine, R. J. (1995). A generalizability analysis of subjective personality assessments in the stumptail macaque and the zebra finch. *Multivariate Behavioral Research, 30,* 167–197.

Friedman, E. M., Becker, K. A., Overstreet, D. H., & Lawrence, D. A. 2002. Reduced primary antibody responses in a genetic animal model of depression. *Psychosomatic Medicine, 64,* 267–273.

Friedman, E. M., Irwin, M. R., & Overstreet, D. H. 1996. Natural and cellular immune responses in Flinders sensitive and resistant line rats. *Neuropsychopharmacology, 15,* 314–322.

Friedman, H. S. (2008). The multiple linkages of personality and disease. *Brain Behavior and Immunity, 22,* 668–675.

Gauci, M., King, M. G., Saxarra, H., Tulloch, B. J., & Husband, A. J. (1993). A Minnesota Multiphasic Personality Inventory profile of women with allergic rhinitis. *Psychosomatic Medicine, 55,* 533–540.

Gerin, W., Pieper, C., Levy, R., & Pickering, T. G. (1992). Social support in social interaction: A moderator of cardiovascular reactivity. *Psychosomatic Medicine, 54,* 324–336.

Goffin, V., Bouchard, B., Ormandy, C. J., Weimann, E., Ferrag, F., Touraine, P., et al. (1998). Prolactin: A hormone at the crossroads of neuroimmunoendocrinology. *Neuroimmunomodulation, 840,* 498–509.

Gold, K. C., & Maple, T. J. (1994). Personality assessment in the gorilla and its utility as a management tool. *Zoo Biology, 13,* 509–522.

Goldberg, L. R. (1990). An alternative description of personality: The Big-Five factor structure. *Journal of Personality and Social Psychology, 59,* 1216–1229.

Gosling, S. D. (1998). Personality dimensions in spotted hyenas (Crocuta crocuta). *Journal of Comparative Psychology, 112,* 107–118.

Gosling, S. D., & John, O. P. (1999). Personality dimensions in non-human animals: A review. *Current Directions in Psychological Science, 8,* 69–75.

Hanlon, R. T., & Messenger J. B. (1999). Cephalopod behaviour. Cambridge, UK: Cambridge University Press.

Hessing, M. J., Coenen, G. J., Vaiman, M., & Renard, C. (1995). Individual differences in cell-mediated and humoral immunity in pigs. *Veterinary Immunology and Immunopathology, 45,* 97–113.

Jones, S. E., & Brain, P. F. (1987). Performances of inbred and outbred laboratory mice in putative tests of aggression. *Behavior Genetics, 17,* 87–96.

Kagan, J. (1994). Galen's prophecy: Temperament in human nature. New York: Basic Books.

Kagan, J., Snidman, N., Julia-Sellers, M., & Johnson, M. O. (1991). Temperament and allergic symptoms. *Psychosomatic Medicine, 53,* 332–340.

Kamarck, T. W., Manuck, S. B., & Jennings, J. R. (1990). Social support reduces cardiovascular reactivity to psychological challenge: A laboratory model. *Psychosomatic Medicine, 52,* 42–58.

Koolhaas, J. M. (2008). Coping style and immunity in animals: Making sense of individual variation. *Brain Behavior and Immunity, 22,* 662–667.

Koolhaas, J. M., Korte, S. M., De Boer, S. F., Van Der Vegt, B. J., Van Reened, C. G., Hopster, H., et al. (1999). Coping styles in animals: Current status in behavior and stress-physiology. *Neuroscience & Biobehavioral Reviews, 23,* 925–935.

Korte, S. M., Koolhaas, J. M., Wingfield, J. C., & McEwen, B. S. (2005). The Darwinian concept of stress: Benefits of allostasis and costs of allostatic load and the trade-offs in health and disease. *Neuroscience and Biobehavioral Reviews, 29,* 3–38.

Kralj-Fiser, S., Scheiber, I. B. R., Blejec, A., Moestl, E., & Kotrschal, K. (2007). Individualities in a flock of free-roaming greylag geese: Behavioral and physiological consistency over time and across situations. *Hormones and Behavior, 51,* 239–248.

Laudenslager, M. L., Rasmussen, K. L., Berman, C. M., Lilly, A. A., Shelton, S. E., Kalin, N. H., & Suomi, S. J. (1999). A preliminary description of responses of free-ranging rhesus monkeys to brief capture experiences: Behavior, endocrine, immune, and health relationships. *Brain Behavior and Immunity, 13,* 124–137.

Lazarus, R., & Folkman, S. (1984). *Stress, appraisal and coping.* New York: Springer.

Ledger, R. A., & Baxter, M. R. (1997). The development of a validated test to assess the temperament of dogs in a rescue shelter. In D. S. Mills & S. E. Heath (Eds.), *Proceedings of the first international conference on veterinary behavioural medicine.* (pp. 87–92). Birmingham: UFAW.

Lepore, S. J., Allen, K. A., & Evans, G. W. (1993). Social support lowers cardiovascular reactivity to an acute stressor. *Psychosomatic Medicine, 55,* 518–524.

Leppänen, P. K., Ewalds-Kvist, S. B., & Selander, R. K. (2005). Mice selectively bred for open-field thigmotaxis: Life span and stability of the selection trait. *Journal of General Psychology, 132,* 187–204.

Lister, R. G. (1987). The use of a plus-maze to measure anxiety in the mouse. *Psychopharmacology (Berlin), 92,* 180–185.

Maninger, N., Capitanio, J. P., Mendoza, S. P., & Mason, W. A. (2003). Personality influences tetanus-specific antibody response in adult male rhesus macaques after removal from natal group and housing relocation. *American Journal of Primatology, 61,* 73–83.

Matera, L. (1996). Endocrine, paracrine and autocrine actions of prolactin on immune cells. *Life Sciences, 59,* 599–614.

McCrae, R. R., & Costa, P. T. (1999). A five-factor theory of personality. In L. A. Pervin & O. P. John (Eds.), *Handbook of personality: Theory and research.* New York: Guilford.

McCrae, R. R., & John, O. P. (1992). An introduction to the five-factor model and its applications. *Journal of Personality, 60,* 175–215.

McGuire, M. T., Raleigh, M. J., & Pollack, D. B. (1994). Personality features in vervet monkeys: The effect of sex, age, social status, and group composition. *American Journal of Primatology, 33,* 1–13.

Mehta, P. H., & Gosling, S. D. (2008). Bridging human and animal research: A comparative approach to studies of personality and health. *Brain, Behavior, and Immunity, 22,* 651–661.

Michael, K. C., Cavigelli, S. A., & Bonneau, R. H. (in preparation). Temperament-associated immune differences in neophobic versus neophilic rats. Unpublished data.

Miller, G. E., Kemeny, M. E., Taylor, S. E., Cole, S. W., & Visscher, B. R. (1997). Social relationships and immune processes in HIV seropositive gay and bisexual men. *Annals of Behavioral Medicine, 19,* 139–151.

Mortensen, C. R., Becker, D. V., Ackerman, J. M., Neuberg, S. L., & Kenrick, D. T. (2010). Infection breeds reticence: The effects of disease salience on self-perceptions of personality and behavioral avoidance tendencies. *Psychological Science, 21,* 440–447.

Moussavi, S, Chatterji, S., Verdes, E., Tandon, A., Patel, V., & Ustun, B. (2007). Depression, chronic diseases, and decrements in health: Results from the World Health Surveys. *Lancet, 370,* 851–858.

Muluk, N. B., Oğuztürk, O., Koç, C., & Ekici, A. (2003). Minnesota multiphasic personality inventory profile of patients with allergic rhinitis. *Journal of Otolaryngology, 32,* 198–202.

Musson, R. A., Morrison, D. C., & Ulevitch, R. J. (1978). Distribution of endotoxin (lipopolysaccharide) in the tissues of lipopolysaccharide-responsive and –unresponsive mice. *Infection and Immunity, 21,* 448–457.

Natarajan, D., & Caramaschi, D. (2010). Animal violence demystified. *Frontiers in Behavioral Neuroscience, 5,* 9.

Nehrenberg, D. L., Rodriguiz, R. M., Cyr, M., Zhang, X., Lauder, J. M., Gariépy, J. L., & Westel, W. C. (2009). An anxiety-like phenotype in mice selectively bred for aggression. *Behavioral Brain Research, 201,* 179–191.

Oberbeck, O., Schmitz, D., Wilsenack, K., Schüler, M., Biskup, C., Schedlowski, M., … et al. (2003). Prolactin modulates survival and cellular immune functions in septic mice. *Journal of Surgical Research, 113,* 248–256.

Øverli, Ø., Sørensen, C., Pulman, K. G., Pottinger, T. G., Korzan, W., Summers, C. H., & Nilsson, G. E. (2007). Evolutionary background for stress-coping styles: Relationships between physiological, behavioral, and cognitive traits in non-mammalian vertebrates. *Neuroscience & Biobehavioral Reviews, 31,* 396–412.

Overstreet, D.H. (1993). The Flinders sensitive line rats: A genetic animal model of depression. *Neuroscience and Biobehavioral Reviews, 17,* 51–68.

Overstreet, D. H., Janowsky, D. S., Gillin, J. C., Shiromani, P. J., & Sutin, E. L. (1986). Stress-induced immobility in rats with cholinergic supersensitivity. *Biological Psychiatry, 21,* 657–664.

Overstreet, D. H., & Russell, R. W. (1982). Selective breeding for diisopropyl fluorophosphate-sensitivity: Behavioural effects of cholinergic agonists and antagonists. *Psychopharmacology (Berl), 78,* 150–155.

Overstreet, D. H., Pucilowski, O., Rezvani, A. H., & Janowsky, D. S. (1995). Administration of antidepressants, diazepam and psychomotor stimulants further confirms the utility of Flinders Sensitive Line rats as an animal model of depression. *Psychopharmacology (Berl), 121,* 27–37.

Patrick, C. J. (2008). Psychophysiological correlates of aggression and violence: An integrative review. *Philosophical Transactions—Royal Society: Biological Sciences, 363,* 2543–2555.

Pellow, S., Chopin, P., File, S. E., & Briley, M. (1985). Validation of open: Closed arm entries in an elevated plus-maze as a measure of anxiety in the rat. *Journal of Neuroscience Methods, 14,* 149–167.

Penley, T. A., Tomaka, J. (2002). Associations among the Big Five, emotional responses, and coping with acute stress. *Personality and Individual Differences, 32,* 1215–1228.

Pennisi, E. (2005). Strong personalities can pose problems in the mating game. *Science, 309,* 694–695.

Pérez-Álvarez, L., Baeza, I., Arranz, L., Marco, E. M., Borcel, E., Guaza, C., et al. (2005). Behavioral, endocrine and immunological characteristics of a murine model of premature aging. *Developmental & Comparative Immunology, 29,* 965–976.

Pervin, L. A. (2002). *Current controversies and issues in personality* (3rd ed.). New York: Wiley.

Petitto, J. M., Gariepy, J. L., Gendreau, P. L., Rodriguiz, R., Lewis, M. H., & Lysle, D. T. (1999). Differences in NK cell function in mice bred for high and low aggression: Genetic linkage between complex behavioral and immunological traits? *Brain Behavior and Immunity, 13,* 175–186.

Petitto, J. M., Lysle, D. T., Gariepy, J. L., Clubb, P. H., Cairns, R. B., Lewis, & M. H. (1993). Genetic differences in social behavior: Relation to natural killer cell function and susceptibility to tumor development. *Neuropsychopharmacology, 8,* 35–43.

Petitto, J. M., Lysle, D. T., Garièpy, J. L., & Lewis, M. H. (1994). Association of genetic differences in social behavior and cellular immune responsiveness: Effects of social experience. *Brain Behavior and Immunity, 8,* 111–122.

Poustka, L., Maras, A., Hohm, E., Fellinger, J., Holtmann, M., Banaschewski, T., et al. (2010). Negative association between plasma cortisol levels and aggression in a high-risk community sample of adolescents. *Journal of Neural Transmission, 117*, 621–627.

Price, T., & Landgren, T. (1992). Evolution of correlated characters. *Trends in Ecology & Evolution, 7*, 307–310.

Pruessner, J. C., Baldwin, M.W., Dedovic, K., Renwick, R., Mahani, N. K., Lord, C., et al. (2005). Self-esteem, locus of control, hippocampal volume, and cortisol regulation in young and old adulthood. *Neuroimage, 28*, 815–826.

Raison, C. L., Capuron, L., & Miller, A. H. (2006). Cytokines sing the blues: Inflammation and the pathogenesis of depression. *Trends in Immunology, 27*, 24–31.

Rammal, H., Bouayed, J., Falla, J., Boujenaini, N., & Soulimani, R. (2010). The impact of high anxiety level on cellular and humoral immunity in mice. *NeuroImmunoModulation, 17*, 1–8.

Ray, J., & Sapolsky, R. (1992). Styles of male social behavior and their endocrine correlates among high-raking wild baboons. *American Journal of Primatology, 28*, 231–250.

Réale, D., Reader, S. M., Sol, D., McDougall, P. T., & Dingemanse, N. J. (2007). Integrating animal temperament within ecology and evolution. *Biological Reviews, 82*, 291–318.

Renault, P. F., Hoofnagle, J. H., Park, Y., Mullen, K. D., Peters, M., Jones, D. B., Rustgi, V., & Jones, E. A. (1987). Psychiatric complications of long-term interferon alpha therapy. *Archives of Internal Medicine, 147*, 1557–1580.

Russell, R. W., Overstreet, D. H., Messenger, M., & Helps, S. C. (1982). Selective breeding for sensitivity to DFP: Generalization of effects beyond criterion variables. *Pharmacology, Biochemistry and Behavior, 17*, 885–891.

Sajti, E., Kavelaars, A., van Meeteren, N., Teunis, M., Gispen, W. H., & Heijnen, C. (2004). Tumor angiogenesis and metastasis formation are associated with individual differences in behavior of inbred Lewis rats. *Brain Behavior and Immunity, 18*, 497–504.

Sajti, E., van Meeteren, N., Kavelaars, A., van der Net, J., Gispen, W. H., & Heijnen, C. (2004). Individual differences in behavior of inbred Lewis rats are associated with severity of joint destruction in adjuvant-induced arthritis. *Brain Behavior and Immunity, 18*, 505–514.

Salome, N., Tasiemski, A., Dutriez, I., Wigger, A., Landgraf, R., & Viltart, O. (1999). Immune challenge induces differential corticosterone and IL-6 responsiveness in rats bred for extremes in anxiety-related behavior. *Neuroscience, 151*, 1112–1118.

Sandi, C., Castanon, N., Vitiello, S., Neveu, P. J., & Mormède, P. (1991). Different responsiveness of spleen lymphocytes from two lines of psychogenetically selected rats (Roman high and low avoidance). *Journal of Neuroimmunology, 31*, 27–33.

Sapolsky, R. M. (2005). The influence of social hierarchy on primate health. *Science, 308*, 648–652.

Schaller, M. (2006). Parasites, behavioral defenses, and the socialpsychological mechanisms through which cultures are evoked. *Psychological Inquiry, 17*, 96–101.

Schrama, J. W., Schouten, J. M., Swinkels, J. W., Gentry, J. L., de Vries Reilingh, G., & Parmentier, H. K. (1997). Effect of hemoglobin status on humoral immune response of weanling pigs differing in coping styles. *Journal of Animal Science, 75*, 2588–2596.

Segerstrom, S. (2000). Personality and the immune system: Models, methods, and mechanisms. *Annals of Behavioral Medicine, 22*, 180–190.

Seligman, M. E. P., & Maier, S. F. (1967). Failure to escape traumatic shock. *Journal of Experimental Psychology, 74*, 1–9.

Sgoifo, A., Coe, C., Parmigiani, S., & Koolhaas, J. (2005). Individual differences in behavior and physiology: Causes and consequences. *Neuroscience and Biobehavioral Reviews, 29*, 1–2.

Sgoifo, A., de Boer, S. F., Haller, J., & Koolhaas, J. M. (1996). Individual differences in plasma catecholamine and corticosterone stress responses of wild-type rats: Relationship with aggression. *Physiology and Behavior, 60*, 1403–1407.

Sheridan, J. F., Stark, J. L., Avitsur, R., & Padgett, D. A. (2000). Social disruption, immunity, and susceptibility to viral infection. Role of glucocorticoid insensitivity and NGF. *Annals of the New York Academy of Sciences, 917*, 894–905.

Shiromani, P. J., Overstreet, D., Levy, D., Goodrich, C. A., Campbell, S. S., & Gillin, J. C. (1988). Increased REM sleep in rats selectively bred for cholinergic hyperactivity. *Neuropsychopharmacology, 1*, 127–133.

Sih, A., Bell, A., & Johnson, J. C. (2004). Behavioral syndromes: An ecological and evolutionary overview. *Trends in Ecology and Evolution, 19*, 372–378.

Sih, A., Bell, A. M., Johnson, J. C., & Ziemba, R. E. (2004). Behavioral syndromes: An integrative overiew. *Quarterly Review of Biology, 79*, 241–277.

Skinner, B. F. (1990). Can psychology be a science of mind? *American Psychologist, 45*, 1206–1210.

Sloan, E. K., Capitanio, J. P., Cole, S. W. (2007). Stress-induced remodeling of lymphoid innervation. *Brain Behavior and Immunity, 22*, 15–21.

Sloan, E. K., Capitanio, J. P., Tarara, R. P., & Cole, S. W. (2008). Social temperament and lymph node innervation. *Brain Behavior and Immunity, 22*, 717–726.

Sloan, E. K., Capitanio, J. P., Tarara, R. P., Mendoza, S. P., Mason, W. A., & Cole, S. W. (2007). Social stress enhances sympathetic innervation of primate lymph nodes: Mechanisms and implications for viral pathogenesis. *Journal of Neuroscience, 27*, 8857–8865.

Sluyter, F., Arseneault, L., Moffitt, T. E., Veenema, A. H., de Boer, S., & Koolhaas, J. M. (2003). Toward an animal model for antisocial behavior: Parallels between mice and humans. *Behavior Genetics, 33*, 563–574.

Sorrells, S. F., & Sapolsky, R. M. (2010). Glucocorticoids can arm macrophages for innate immune battle. *Brain Behavior and Immunity, 24*, 17–18.

Steimer, T., & Driscoll, P. (2005). Inter-individual vs line/strain differences in psychogenetically selected Roman High-(RHA) and Low-(RLA) Avoidance rats: Neuroendocrine and behavioural aspects. *Neuroscience and Biobehavioral Review, 29*, 99–112.

Steimer, T., la Fleur, S., & Schulz, P. E. (1997). Neuroendocrine correlates of emotional reactivity and coping in male rats from the Roman high (RHA/Verh)- and low (RLA/Verh)-avoidance lines. *Behavior Genetics, 27*, 503–512.

Steptoe, A., & Molloy, G. J. (2007). Personality and heart disease. *British Heart Journal, 93*, 783–784.

Stevenson-Hinde, J., Stillwell-Barns, R., & Zunz, M. (1980). Subjective assessment of rhesus monkeys over four successive years. *Primates, 21*, 66–82.

Temoshok, L. R., Waldstein, S. R., Wald, R. L., Garzino-Demo, A., Synowski, S. J., Sun, L., & Wiley, J. A. (2008). Type C coping, alexithymia, and heart rate reactivity are associated independently and differentially with specific immune mechanisms linked to HIV progression. *Brain Behavior and Immunity, 22*, 781–792.

Tonelli, L. H., Katz, M., Kovacsics, C. E., Gould, T. D., Joppy, B., Hoshino, A., et al. (2009). Allergic rhinitis induces anxiety-like behavior and altered social interaction in rodents. *Brain Behavior and Immunity, 23,* 784–793.

Totman, R., Kiff, J., Reed, S. E., & Craig, J. W. (1980). Predicting experimental colds in volunteers from different measures of recent life stress. *Journal of Psychosomatic Research, 24,* 155–163.

Van Oortmerssen, G. A., Bakker, T. C. M. (1981). Artificial selection for short and long attack latencies in wild *Mus musculus domesticus. Behavioral Genetics, 11,* 115–126.

Veenema, A. H., Meijer, O. C., de Kloet, E. R., Koolhaas, J. M. (2003). Genetic selection for coping style predicts stressor susceptibility. *Journal of Neuroendocrinology, 15,* 256–267.

Vegas, O., Fano, E., Brain, P. F., Alonso, A., & Azpiroz, A. (2006). Social stress, coping strategies and tumor development in male mice: Behavioral, neuroendocrine and immunological implications. *Psychoneuroendocrinology, 31,* 69–79.

Virgin, C. E. Jr., Sapolsky, R. M. (1997). Styles of male social behavior and their endocrine correlates among low-ranking baboons. *American Journal of Primatology, 42,* 25–39.

Viveros, M. P., Arranz, L., Hernanz, A., Miquel, J., & de la Fuente, M. (2007). A model of premature aging in mice based on altered stress-related behavioral response and immunosenescence. *NeuroImmunoModulation, 14,* 157–162.

Watson, D., & Hubbard, B. (1996). Adaptational style and dispositional structure: Coping in the context of the Five-Factor Model. *Journal of Personality, 64,* 737–774.

Watson, S. L., & Ward, J. P. (1996). Temperament and problem solving in the small-eared bushbaby (Otolemur garnetii). *Journal of Comparative Psychology, 110,* 377–385.

Williams, R. B. (2001). Hostility: Effects on health and the potential for successful behavioral approaches to prevention and treatment. In A. Baum, T. A. Revenson, & J. E. Singer (Eds.), *Handbook of health psychology.* Mahwah, NJ: Erlbaum.

Wilson, D. S., Clark, A. B., Coleman, K., Dearstyne, T. (1994). Shyness and boldness in humans and other animals. *Trends in Ecology and Evolution, 9,* 442–446.

Wolf, M., van Doorn, G. S., Leimar, O., & Weissing, F. J. (2007). Life-history trade-offs favour the evolution of animal personalities. *Nature, 31,* 581–584.

Zozulya, A. A., Gabaeva, M. V., Sokolov, O. Y., Surkina, I. D., & Kost, N. V. (2008). Personality, coping style, and constitutional neuroimmunology. *Journal of Immunotoxicology, 5,* 221–225.

Zuckerman, M. (1979) *Sensation seeking: Beyond the optimal level of arousal.* Hillsdale, NJ: Erlbaum.

Zuckerman, M. (1994). *Behavioral expression and biological bases of sensation seeking.* Cambridge, England: Cambridge University Press.

Zuk, M., Stoehr, A. M. (2002). Immune defense and host life history. *The American Naturalist, 160,* 9–22.

Personality and Human Immunity

Sheldon Cohen, Denise Janicki-Deverts, Crista N. Crittenden, *and* Rodlescia S. Sneed

Abstract

We review evidence on the role of personality traits in immune function including studies of enumerative and functional immune markers and of host resistance to infectious illness. We begin by discussing a series of pathways through which traits may influence immunity: immune-altering behaviors; concomitant activation of physiological systems; aggravation or attenuation of the activating effects of environmental demands or stressors; or selection into environments that alter immunity. We focus on the "Big Five" personality factors—extraversion, agreeableness, neuroticism, conscientiousness, and openness to experience but also address other trait characteristics that do not cleanly fit into the Big Five typology including dispositional optimism, trait positive affect, hostility, and social inhibition. We conclude that the literature on personality and immunity is in its infancy and not developed enough to make any definitive conclusions. We can say that there is evidence of possible associations with immunity across all the traits, with existing data suggesting some reliable associations. We suggest the importance of future works being based in trait-specific theory and outline a number of important methodological concerns.

Key Words: personality, Big Five, extraversion, agreeableness, neuroticism, conscientiousness, openness to experience, optimism, positive affect, hostility, social inhibition, immunity, immune function, host resistance, infectious disease

Introduction

The terms "personality" and "personality trait" generally refer to stable individual differences in a person's characteristic patterns of behavior, thoughts, and feelings. A prototypic text on personality discusses dozens if not hundreds of possible personality traits. However, the literature addressing the role of personality in immunity is much more constrained, focusing on less than a dozen personality factors. One of the major theories of personality posits five superordinate independent traits (McCrae & Costa, 1987; Goldberg, 1992). The so called "Big Five" are extraversion, agreeableness, neuroticism, conscientiousness, and openness to experience. Here we review the existing literature examining the association of each of the Big Five factors with human

immunity, as well as literature on four other trait characteristics that have been studied in relation to immunity: trait positive affect, optimism, hostility, and social inhibition.

How Could Personality Traits Influence Immunity?

A trait may influence the likelihood of an *immune altering behavior*. For example, persons high in conscientiousness are more likely to take care of themselves (refrain from smoking, drink alcohol moderately, exercise, get sufficient sleep) hence increasing the possibility of a better functioning immune system. Some traits covary with levels of nervous or endocrine system *activation* through which they may modulate immunity. For example, neuroticism is thought to be a manifestation of high levels of cortical activation. Relatedly, a trait could operate by either *aggravating or attenuating the activating effects of environmental demands or stressors.* Neuroticism is thought to aggravate stress responses and optimism to reduce them. Personality traits may also result in a tendency to *select environments that alter immunity.* For example, those high in hostility tend to seek out and create social conflicts and, in turn, experience their activating properties. In contrast, agreeable persons are most likely to seek out positive interactions with others. Of course, there is also the possibility that associations between traits and immunity occur because either stable differences in our immune function influence our behavior or third factors, such as sex, age, genetics, or differences in the function of other physiological systems influence both our personalities and our immune responses.

Most of the literature we review is focused on the main effects of personality characteristics on measures of basal immunity. However, because personality may influence immunity by exacerbating or attenuating the activating effects of stress, we also discuss evidence on stress-by-personality interactions.

How is Personality Measured in this Literature?

There are two standard strategies for assessing personality. The most common is to ask people about the extent to which various statements or adjectives describe "how they usually are." These assessments are most often collected at a single point in time. Although rare, a better strategy would be to collect these data at two or more points, the further apart the better, and average the scores. This approach maximizes the stable aspects of responses to the items and minimizes responses that might reflect experiences/feelings surrounding the time of questionnaire administration. Overall, this retrospective methodology is often criticized as heavily reflecting a person's reconstruction of their memory for their own behavior based on their beliefs and recent experiences rather than accurately reflecting how they usually behave. An alternative approach uses the same items but asks people to rate the extent to which the items reflect how they are right now (or over a short period like a day). With this procedure the instrument is administered on multiple days, optimally covering a relatively long interval, and the personality score is based on average response over the repeated

administrations of the scale. This strategy both avoids the retrospective reconstruction and the potential threats to reliability inherent in basing a personality score on an assessment administered at only one point in time. Although the single assessment retrospective technique is the one used most often in the personality and immunity literature, averaging over multiple state reports is also used in a handful of studies.

Which Immune Outcomes are Addressed in this Literature?

As difficult, if not more difficult, than defining and measuring personality in an integrated and comprehensive manner, is addressing how one should define and assess immune competence. We will not directly address the definition of immunocompetence and its appropriate measurement here for two reasons. First, we expect these issues to appear in multiple chapters in this volume, but more importantly, there are relatively few immune outcomes used in this literature, and, hence, what is important in this context is the nature of these specific outcomes.

The most common measures of immunity used in this literature include enumerations of leukocytes, antibody response to immunization, natural killer (NK) cell cytotoxicity, mitogen-stimulated lymphocyte proliferation, delayed-type hypersensitivity (DTH), antibody level to herpes viruses, stimulated production of pro-inflammatory cytokines, and circulating markers of inflammation. Although some of these measures are (at least in theory) interpretable in terms of their implications for host resistance (e.g., greater NK cytotoxicity, greater lymphocyte proliferation), others (e.g., numbers of leukocytes when counts fall within normal ranges, stimulated production of pro-inflammatory cyto-kines) are not.

Our review goes beyond the standard immune measures in that we also address literatures on the role of personality in the onset or exacerbation of infectious disease. The major function of the immune system is identifying and destroying infectious agents. As we have noted, individual measures of either enumerative or functional immunity seldom have straightforward implications for overall immunocompetence. Consequently, we view host resistance to infection as the ultimate downstream marker of immunocompetence. Infectious diseases that have been studied in relation to personality traits include the common cold, HIV/AIDS, and genital herpes.

Can We Make Causal Inferences?

Work on the role of personality and immunity is challenging to interpret in regard to the direction of causal inference. Personality is not generally thought to be manipulable, and, hence, experiments are not possible. Because traits are stable over long periods, it is assumed that related immunity would also be stable and hence prospective studies would be no more useful (no change to predict) than cross-sectional studies. The exception is studies that examine a critical point in the development of the immune system (when immunity would change). Exclusion of alternative causal explanations is, however, possible by controlling for third factors (e.g., sex, age, genetics, various physiological states) that may contribute both to personality and immunity, and we place special emphasis on appropriate use of this technique.

The Big Five Personality Factors

The Big Five traits are most often assessed by the Neuroticism Extraversion Openness Personality Inventory (NEO PI; Costa & McCrae, 1985), or one of its revisions: the NEO PI-R and the 60-item NEO Five-Factor Inventory (NEO-FFI) (Costa & McCrae, 1992), or a version of the Goldberg trait adjective scales (Goldberg, 1992). Extraversion and neuroticism are also often assessed using the Eysenck Personality Inventory (EPI; Eysenck & Eysenck, 1968) or the Eysenck Personality Questionnaire (EPQ; Eysenck & Eysenck, 1975).

Each of the Big Five is thought to be composed of six constituent facets or subtraits (Costa & McCrae, 1995). The NEO scale (but not others) allows the assessment of subtraits as well as factors. Although most of the studies we report in this section are focused on the associations of the factors with immune markers, some investigations assess subtrait scores. Which level of analysis (factor or subtrait) is best is debatable. Many believe that a focus that is limited to the five factors results in the loss of explanatory power (Paunonen & Ashton, 2001). Others, however, argue that the use of only the five factors allows for a more intuitive and easier interpretation of results (Carver & Scheier, 2008). Within the literature reviewed here, most studies are limited to the factor level. However, we will briefly define the subtraits for each factor and will review any results reported at the subtrait level.

Extraversion

Extraversion/introversion is the extent to which individuals are sociable and outgoing. Subtraits of extraversion include friendliness, gregariousness, assertiveness, activity level, excitement seeking, and cheerfulness. Eysenck (1967) hypothesized that extraverts are motivated to seek out social activity and other forms of external stimulation in order to compensate for low levels of basal cortical arousal, whereas introverts avoid social interaction and other forms of external excitation in order not to further heighten an already hyperaroused basal state.

SUSCEPTIBILITY TO INFECTIOUS DISEASE

Some of the earliest work to explore the immunological correlates of extraversion examined the importance of this personality characteristic in predicting susceptibility to infectious disease. Totman, Kiff, Reed, and Craig, (1980) employed a viral challenge design to address the question of whether extraversion is associated with the likelihood of developing signs and symptoms of upper respiratory infection (URI). Following completion of the EPI, 52 healthy volunteers (mean age 30.9 years, range 18 to 49; 67% female) were exposed to one of two rhinoviruses that cause the common cold (Rhinovirus [RV] 2 or RV31). During the 5 days after exposure, the investigators collected nasal secretions on a daily basis to assess the amount of virus shedding (replication), an indication of having been infected with challenge virus. They also collected daily self-reported symptoms, and they monitored for the presence of fever and the number of tissues used. Analyses controlling for viral antibody level to the challenge virus before exposure showed that those with *lower* scores on the extraversion scale (i.e., those who were more introverted) shed more virus, and reported more cold symptoms than those with higher scores (i.e., those who were more extraverted). Extraversion was not, however, related to fever or tissue usage.

Similar findings were reported by Broadbent, Broadbent, Phillpotts, and Wallace (1984). These authors examined 173 men and women (over several different studies) who had completed the EPQ and were then exposed to either RV9, a combination of RV9 and RV14, or either of two strains of influenza virus (A/Munich [H1N1] or A/California [H1N1]). Nasal virus shedding, number of tissues used, and the weight of nasal secretions in the 5 days following virus exposure were employed as markers of illness susceptibility. The analysis aggregated data across the rhinovirus studies, and controlled for virus strain and viral-specific prechallenge antibody. Introverts (scoring < 13) shed more virus than extraverts (>13), but no associations were found with tissue use or nasal secretion. Among the influenza studies, extraversion was not correlated with any of the markers of illness susceptibility.

In another viral challenge study that focused on the effects of social ties on susceptibility to the common cold, extraversion was examined as a control variable (Cohen, Doyle, Skoner, Rabin, & Gwaltney, 1997). After completing a modified version of Goldberg's trait adjective scales, 276 healthy adults between the ages of 18 and 55 (mean age 29.1 ± 9.1 years; 55% female) were experimentally exposed to one of two rhinoviruses (RV39 or Hanks), and then sequestered in a hotel for 5 days. Infection was defined as viral shedding or a fourfold or greater increase (from previral exposure to 4 weeks postexposure) in virus-specific antibody titer. Disease expression was defined objectively as increased mucus production or decreased nasal mucociliary clearance function (a marker of congestion). Colds were defined as the combination of infection and expressing signs of illness. Those scoring below the median on the extraversion scale were more likely to develop a cold even after controlling for prechallenge antibody, body mass index (BMI), season of the year, age, race, sex, virus type, and education.

Cohen, Doyle, Turner, Alper, and Skoner (2003a) again made use of the viral-challenge paradigm to examine the association of extraversion and cold risk in a different sample of 334 healthy adults (mean age 28.8 ± 10.4 years; 52% female). Participants completed the Goldberg scales and were then exposed to one of two rhinoviruses (RV39 or RV23) and sequestered for 5 days. Colds were defined using the objective criteria described earlier, and the same 8 control variables were included in the analysis. Consistent with the findings from Cohen et al. (1997), higher extraversion scores were associated with fewer colds for both viruses.

ANTIBODY RESPONSE TO VACCINATION

Pressman, Cohen, Miller, Barkin, Rabin, and Treanor (2005) recruited 37 male and 46 female college freshmen for a study examining the role of psychosocial factors in antibody response to a trivalent influenza vaccine. Participants were 18 to 25 years of age (96.4% were 18–19 years old). Extraversion was assessed 5 to 6 days prior to immunization using the Goldberg trait adjective scales. Participants were immunized in conjunction with university-wide flu vaccine clinics. Vaccine antibody levels were assessed at baseline (day of immunization) and again one and four months postimmunization. Extraversion was not related to vaccine antibody response at either the 1-month or 4-month follow-up.

ENUMERATIVE MEASURES OF IMMUNITY

Two published studies have addressed the question of whether extraversion is associated with circulating numbers of total lymphocytes and lymphocyte subsets. In the first of these, Miller, Cohen, Rabin, Skoner, and Doyle (1999) observed no association between scores on Goldberg's extraversion scale and numbers of circulating total T lymphocytes (CD3+), helper T lymphocytes (CD4+), cytotoxic/suppressor T lymphocytes (CD8+), B cells (CD19+), or NK cells (CD3-CD16+ CD56+) in the 276 healthy men and women (ages 18 to 55 years) who participated in the Cohen et al. (1997) study.

The second study, by comparison, did find an association between extraversion and enumerative immune measures. Using an elderly adult sample comprised of 11 medicated depressives (mean age 71 ± 8 years; 73% female), 10 unmedicated depressives (mean age 76 ± 7 years; 70% female), and 23 nondepressed controls (mean age 70 ± 7 years; 30% female), Bouhuys, Flentge, Oldehinkel, and van den Berg (2004) examined the association of extraversion, as assessed by the EPQ, with counts of CD3+, CD8+, and CD3-CD16+CD56+ cells, and the CD4+/CD8+ ratio. The authors found that greater extraversion was related to greater CD3-CD16+CD56+ counts and *lower* CD4+/CD8+ ratios, independent of depression group and age. However, extraversion was not related to either total CD3+ or CD8+ counts.

IMMUNE FUNCTION MEASURED IN VITRO

Gonzales-Quijano, Martin, Millan, and Lopez-Calderon (1998) examined the role of extraversion in lymphocyte proliferative response to phytohaemagglutinin (PHA) in a sample of 28 male undergraduate students in Madrid, Spain (mean age 19 ± 0.2 years). Extraversion was assessed with a Spanish version of the Sixteen Personality Factors (16PF) Questionnaire (Cattell, 2005). The authors found that proliferative responses decreased with decreasing levels of extraversion. In studies described in the previous section, Miller, Cohen, et al. (1999) found lower extraversion to be associated with reduced NK cell cytotoxicity in a relatively large sample of healthy young to middle aged adults, whereas Bouhuys et al. (2004) found no association of extraversion with lipopolysaccharide (LPS)-stimulated production of the pro-inflammatory cytokine interleukin (IL)-6 in a small sample that consisted primarily of depressed elderly.

HIV

Ironson, O'Cleirigh, Weiss, Schneiderman, and Costa (2008) examined whether extraversion was related to the average rate of change in CD4+ counts and viral load over a 4-year period in a sample of 104 HIV patients (mean age 38 ± 8.5 years; 32% female). All participants were free of AIDS-defining illnesses and had midrange CD4+ counts (150 to 500) at baseline. Data on all variables including extraversion, as measured by the NEO PI-R and blood samples for measurement of CD4+ cells and viral load were collected every 6 months over 4 years. Covariates included antiretroviral use, medication adherence, baseline CD4+ or viral load, race, sex, age, education, and time since baseline. Greater extraversion was associated with both a lower average rate of increase in viral load and a slower average rate of decline in CD4+ cell count over the 4-year period.

HERPES RECURRENCES

In a sample of 116 men and women with previously diagnosed culture-positive HSV2 (genital herpes) (mean age 35.3 years, range 21–69; 59% female), Cassidy, Meadows, Catalon, and Barton (1997) examined whether extraversion was related prospectively to number of genital herpes recurrences over a 6-month period. Extraversion was measured using the EPQ, and recurrence was determined by patient report. Results indicated no association between extraversion and symptom recurrence.

MODERATING THE EFFECTS OF STRESS ON IMMUNITY

In their sample of 28 male undergraduates, Gonzalez-Quijano and colleagues (1998) also explored the possibility that extraversion might buffer the expected attenuation of lymphocyte proliferative response following exposure to psychological stress. Stress was assessed with a questionnaire that asked participants to list the number of major life changes that occurred over the previous year. There was no interaction between stressful life events and extraversion and, hence, no evidence for extraversion buffering the effects of stress.

CONCLUSIONS

Studies of extraversion suggest that it may play a role in host resistance. Data from prospective

(viral-challenge) cold studies are quite consistent in indicating that introverted persons are more susceptible to developing colds following experimental exposure to rhinovirus than their more extraverted counterparts. The single influenza study, however, failed to observe an association between extraversion and URI risk. In a single study of persons with HIV, greater extraversion was associated with a slower rate of decline in CD4+ cells in addition to a smaller increase in viral load.

The evidence in relation to immune markers is limited, but when associations were found, they were in the expected direction. Greater extraversion was associated with increased lymphocyte proliferative response and greater NK cell cytotoxicity. However, extraversion was unrelated to stimulated IL-6 production or to antibody response to a trivalent influenza vaccine. Moreover, among persons infected with HSV2, extraversion did not predict symptom recurrence. In general, extraversion appears not to be related to enumerative measures in healthy populations, although Bouhuys et al. (2004) found greater extraversion to be associated with greater numbers of NK cells, and lower CD4+/CD8+ ratios in their older adult sample.

Why is there more consistency in extraversion's association with host resistance than with its associations with specific markers of immunity? Host resistance is a downstream response that integrates the dynamic and interactive roles of various aspects of functional immunity. A change in any *relevant* component of the immune response might (under the right conditions) result in a change in host resistance. However, many of the immune measures studied in this literature may have little or no implications for host resistance and hence we may not even expect them to be correlated with host resistance or for that matter with extraversion just because it predicts host resistance.

Neuroticism

Neuroticism reflects the extent to which individuals tend to experience negative emotional states, including anxiety, depression, and anger (Costa & McCrae, 1992). Accordingly, this construct also has been referred to as trait negative affectivity (NA), negative emotional style (NES), and negative emotionality. Individuals who score high on measures of neuroticism view the world as threatening, are easily distressed, and have difficulty coping with stressful situations, whereas those who score low on neuroticism are calm, emotionally stable, and cope well in the face of stress. Accordingly, the neuroticism subtraits include anxiety, depression, anger, self-consciousness, immoderation, and vulnerability to stress.

Eysenck (1967) theorized that neurotic tendencies derive from an innate predisposition toward low-threshold, high-intensity, and long-lasting autonomic activation in response to sensory stimuli. Accordingly, some interpret high levels of neuroticism as being analogous to a high-stress condition with accompanying sympathetic and hypothalamic-pituitary-adrenal (HPA) activation (Miller, Cohen, et al., 1999). Moreover, because higher levels of neuroticism are thought to be associated with increased stress-related activation, neuroticism is also thought to exacerbate stress effects on immune function.

As discussed earlier, neuroticism frequently is assessed by questionnaire. Another approach is the assessment of individuals' levels of negative mood daily for a week or more, and then creating a summary measure (average across days) of *typical* NA or NES.

SUSCEPTIBILITY TO INFECTIOUS DISEASE

In their sample of 334 healthy men and women, Cohen, Doyle, Turner, Alper, and Skoner (2003b) used an interview measure to examine the association of NES with susceptibility to the common cold. During the month prior to being exposed to either of two rhinoviruses (RV39 or RV23), participants were interviewed nightly over a period of seven days. Interviewers asked participants to rate nine negative adjectives in regard to how accurately each of the adjectives described how they were feeling that day. Adjectives represented three subcategories of negative emotion: depression (sad, depressed, unhappy), anxiety (on edge, nervous, tense), and hostility (hostile, resentful, angry). NES scores were computed by averaging participants' daily negative mood scores across the seven days. Following exposure to the challenge virus, participants were sequestered in a hotel for five days, and monitored for the development of infection and signs of illness. NES was unrelated to the risk of developing a cold.

Cohen, Alper, Doyle, Treanor, and Turner (2006) replicated these findings in a different sample of 193 healthy adults (mean age 37.3 ± 8.8 years, 51% female), using a modified version of the procedures employed in their previous study (Cohen et al., 2003b). NES again was measured by nightly telephone interview, but over the course of *two* weeks, and asking participants to rate their mood based on six, rather than nine adjectives (sad, unhappy, on edge, tense, hostile, angry). Participants subsequently were exposed to either RV39 or to A Texas/36/91 (H1N1) influenza virus, sequestered in a hotel for five (RV39) or six (influenza) days and monitored for signs and symptoms of URI. Colds were defined using the criteria described earlier. Consistent with their earlier findings, NES was unrelated to colds, regardless of the criteria used to define them.

ANTIBODY RESPONSE TO VACCINATION

Marsland, Cohen, Rabin, and Manuck (2001) examined whether neuroticism was associated with antibody response to Hepatitis B (HBV) vaccine in 84 healthy, HBV seronegative graduate students (mean age 24 years, range 21–33; 39% female). Participants received three doses of HBV vaccine: baseline, six weeks postenrollment, and six months postenrollment. Five weeks after the initial HBV vaccination, participants completed a battery of psychological questionnaires. Neuroticism was measured using subscales from four instruments: anxiety and depression from the POMS Affect Scale; emotional stability from the Goldberg trait adjective scales; unpleasant affect and activated unpleasant affect from the Larsen and Diener Circumplex (Larsen & Diener, 1992); and positive loading for stress from the Mackay Circumplex (Mackay, Cox, Burrows, & Lazzerini, 1978). Antibody response to HBV vaccine was measured following the second vaccination, and participants were identified as being low ($n = 40$) or high ($n = 41$) antibody responders. Results of logistic regression analysis controlling for age, sex, and BMI showed that neuroticism independently predicted antibody response to HBV vaccine such that greater neuroticism was associated with a greater likelihood of being in the low response group.

Phillips, Carroll, Burns, and Drayson (2005) examined whether neuroticism, as assessed by the EPQ, was associated with antibody response to a trivalent influenza vaccine in a sample of 57 healthy university students (mean age 19.8 ± 2.3 years; 46% female). After completing demographic and psychological questionnaires, participants received an influenza vaccination containing three viral strains: A/Panama (H3N2); A/New Caledonia (H1N1); and B/Shangdong. Baseline antibody titers were assessed prior to vaccination, and antibody response to vaccination was measured 5 weeks and 5 months later. Although neuroticism was unrelated to baseline antibody titers, persons scoring higher on neuroticism had lower antibody titers to A/Panama at both 5 weeks and 5 months. Neuroticism was unrelated to antibody response to the A/New Caledonia and B/Shangdong viral strains.

In a study of the role of neuroticism in the vaccine response of children, Morag, Morag, Reichenberg, Lerer, and Yirmiya (1999) studied 240 female students (mean age 12.4 ± 0.2 years) recruited from 8 public schools in Israel. Two weeks prior to vaccination, neuroticism was assessed using the Junior EPI (Eysenck, 1965). Baseline rubella antibody titers were determined 2 weeks later, immediately prior to vaccination with a live-attenuated rubella virus. Participants were divided into a seronegative group (no immunity prior to vaccination; $n = 60$) and a seropositive group (immunity prior to vaccination; $n = 180$). Infection with rubella, as determined by a fourfold increase in antibody titers to the virus, was assessed 10.5 weeks later. Only infected participants were included in analyses. Among those in the seronegative group, higher neuroticism was associated with reduced antibody production following viral infection. By comparison, neuroticism was unrelated to antibody titers in the seropositive group in which, as expected, there was considerably less change in antibody in response to the vaccine.

As described in the extraversion section, Pressman and colleagues (2005) examined the role of personality in immune response to influenza vaccination in 83 college freshman. The authors found that neuroticism, as measured by the Goldberg emotional stability scale, was not related to vaccine antibody response at either the 1- or 4-month follow-ups.

ENUMERATIVE MEASURES OF IMMUNITY

Two of the studies described in the extraversion section also examined the association of neuroticism with circulating lymphocyte counts (Bouhuys et al., 2004; Miller, Cohen et al., 1999), and in neither study was neuroticism related to total lymphocytes or lymphocyte subsets. Shea, Burton, and Girgis (1993) also examined the association of neuroticism with lymphocyte counts (total lymphocytes, CD3+, CD4+, CD8+, and CD4+/CD8+ ratio) in a sample of 39 female undergraduates (from a sample of 220) who scored extremely high and extremely low on both the Willoughby Neuroticism scale (Willoughby, 1932) and an absorption questionnaire. Again, neuroticism was unrelated to cell numbers.

IMMUNE FUNCTION MEASURED IN VITRO

Two studies described earlier also addressed the role of neuroticism in functional immunity. Miller, Cohen et al. (1999) found no association between neuroticism and NK cell cytotoxicity in a sample of healthy adults. In contrast, Bouhuys et al. (2004)

found higher neuroticism scores to be associated with greater stimulated IL-6 production in a sample including mostly depressed elderly.

Three additional studies examined the role of trait anxiety, a well-studied subtrait of neuroticism, in cellular immune function. In their previously described cross-sectional study of 28 male undergraduates, Gonzalez-Quijano and colleagues (1998) did not find an association between anxiety and lymphocyte proliferative response to PHA. By comparison, Arranz, Guayerbas, and De la Fuente (2007) found anxiety to be associated with several in vitro measures of immune function, including proliferative response, in a sample of 66 healthy Spanish women (mean age 43.3 ± 2.1 years). Anxiety was assessed with the Beck Anxiety Inventory (Beck, Epstein, Brown, & Steer, 1988), and participants were divided into high (score of >30) and low (score of <9) anxiety groups. Functional immune measures included PHA-stimulated lymphocyte proliferation; PHA-stimulated lymphocyte productions of tumor necrosis factor (TNF)-α, and IL-2; chemotaxis; lymphocyte adherence capacity (ability of lymphocytes to adhere to endothelial cells); phagocytosis; and NK cell cytotoxicity. When compared to those with low anxiety, highly anxious women showed *decreases* in PHA-stimulated lymphoproliferation, stimulated IL-2, lymphocyte chemotaxis, phagocytosis, and NK cell activity, and *increases* in stimulated TNF-α. The groups did not differ in adherence capacity.

Esterling, Antoni, Kumar, & Schneiderman (1993) used circulating levels of antibody to Epstein-Barr virus (EBV) to examine whether trait anxiety was associated with cellular immune function in a sample of 54 EBV seropositive undergraduate students (age range 17–25 years). EBV is a latent virus that is held in check by the cellular immune system. Poorer cellular immunity is thought to result in activation of the virus, and in turn an increase in the production of viral specific antibody. Thus, in contrast to vaccination studies wherein higher viral antibody concentrations are indicative of well-functioning humoral immunity, here, higher concentrations of circulating antibody are suggestive of *impaired* cellular immunity. They reported that greater anxiety, as measured by the Taylor Manifest Anxiety Scale (Taylor, 1953), was associated with greater EBV antibody levels and, thus, poorer cellular immunity.

Finally, in their sample of 39 female undergraduates, Shea and colleagues (Shea et al., 1993) examined the association of neuroticism with DTH skin responses to seven antigens: tetanus, diphtheria, streptococcus, tuberculin, candida, trichophyton, and proteous, as well as to a glycerin control. Those high in neuroticism showed greater induration (i.e., *better* cellular immunity) in response to streptococcus, candida, and tuberculin than those low in neuroticism.

CIRCULATING MARKERS OF INFLAMMATION

In a sample of 855 relatively healthy middle-aged adults (mean age 45 ± 7 years; 50% female), Marsland, Prather, Peterson, Cohen, and Manuck (2008) examined whether trait NA, as assessed with the Multidimensional Personality Questionnaire—Short Form (MPQ-SF; Tellegen, 1982) was associated with circulating concentrations of IL-6 and C-reactive protein (CRP). Greater NA was associated with greater circulating concentrations of both IL-6 and CRP, independent of age, sex, race, years of education, and medical conditions or medications known to influence inflammation.

Similar results were reported by Sutin, Terracciano, Deiana, Naitza, Ferrucci, Uda et al. (2009) in a sample of 5,119 residents of the Italian island of Sardinia (mean age 39.3 ± 14.7 years; 55% female). Higher levels of neuroticism as assessed by the Italian version of the NEO PI-R (Terracciano, 2003) were associated with higher concentrations of both IL-6 and CRP independent of age, sex, BMI, aspirin use, and disease burden (sum of current diseases).

HIV

Tomakowsky, Lumley, Markowitz, and Frank (2001) examined the cross-sectional association of trait NA, as assessed by the Positive and Negative Affect Schedule (PANAS), with HIV disease status, as indicated by CD4+ cell count, in a sample of 78 HIV-infected men (mean age 39 ± 7.8 years) who were free of AIDS-defining illnesses. Negative affectivity was not associated with CD4+ count. Similarly, in their 4-year prospective study of personality and disease progression in persons with HIV, Ironson and colleagues (2008) found no association between neuroticism, as assessed by the NEO PI-R, and change in either CD4+ cell count or viral load.

HERPES RECURRENCES

In their prospective study of personality and genital herpes symptom recurrence described earlier, Cassidy and colleagues (1997) found that neuroticism was unrelated to number of recurrences over a 6-month period.

MODERATING THE EFFECTS OF STRESS ON IMMUNITY

Borella, Bargellini, Rovesti, Pinelli, Vivoli, Solfrini, et al. (1999) examined whether neuroticism moderates the effects of a brief naturalistic stressor (first semester at an Italian military academy) on NK cell function. Stressors of this sort tend to be associated with decreases in NK cell cytoxicity (Segerstrom & Miller, 2004). Neuroticism was assessed in 39 male cadets using a composite measure combining the Goldberg emotional stability scale, the Trait Anxiety Scale from the State-Trait Anxiety Inventory, and the neuroticism items from the EPI. Results supported an exacerbating effect of neuroticism on the stress-related changes in NK cell cytotoxicity, such that those with high neuroticism scores experienced a decline in NK cell activity from the beginning of the semester to final examinations, whereas those with midrange scores showed no change in cytotoxicity. Interestingly, low neuroticism scores were associated with an *increase* in NK cell cytotoxicity from the beginning to the end of the semester. All findings were independent of coffee consumption and smoking status.

CONCLUSIONS

The most consistent evidence to support an association between neuroticism and immunity derives from the vaccination studies, wherein three of four studies found greater neuroticism to be associated with attenuated antibody response (Marsland et al., 2001; Morag et al., 1999; Phillips et al., 2005). By comparison, neuroticism was unrelated to developing a common cold following experimental exposure to any of several cold viruses (Cohen et al., 2006; Cohen et al., 2003b). The research has also consistently failed to show any association between neuroticism and enumerative measures. Whether neuroticism is associated with *functional measures* of immunity, however, is less clear. Arranz et al. (2007) found higher levels of neuroticism to be associated with poorer lymphocyte proliferation, NK cell cytotoxicity, phagocytosis, chemotaxis, and stimulated IL-2 production. Both Arranz et al. (2007) and Bouhuys et al. (2004) found higher levels of neuroticism to be associated with *greater* stimulated production of two pro-inflammatory cytokines, TNF-α and IL-6, respectively, and Shea et al. (1993) observed *greater* DTH responses among young women who scored high relative to low in neuroticism. By comparison,

Gonzales-Quijano et al. (1998) observed no association between neuroticism and lymphocyte proliferation, and Miller, Cohen et al. (1999) observed no association with NK cell cytotoxicity. Neuroticism also was unrelated to HIV progression, as indicated by either CD4+ counts or viral load, or to genital herpes recurrence. Sex differences in the association of neuroticism with immune activity might account for these inconsistent findings. For example, Arranz et al. (2007) and Shea et al. (1993) employed entirely female samples, whereas Gonzalez-Quijano et al. (1998) and Tomakowsky et al. (2001) studied only men. In regard to integrating stress in the relationship between neuroticism and immunity, the single published study (Borella et al., 1999) suggests that stress and neuroticism may have a synergistic, dysregulating effect on immune functioning.

With only three studies, it is hard to interpret the impact of the neuroticism subtrait, anxiety, on immunity. Overall, the results were mixed, with anxiety predicting poorer cellular immunity in some cases but not in others. Moreover, since the associations of anxiety and immunity were not compared to other subtraits or even to neuroticism, little can be said about whether it is *the* or merely *a* central component of neuroticism in terms of its potential to influence immunity.

Conscientiousness

Conscientiousness is a personality trait that includes as its subtraits self-efficacy, orderliness, dutifulness, achievement-striving, self-discipline, and cautiousness. Individuals with high levels of conscientiousness demonstrate greater self-discipline, greater adherence to ethical/moral standards, and a strong sense of order (e.g., neatness, organization). Further, they strive for achievement and are cautious in their actions. Conscientiousness is most likely to influence immunity through its relationship with better health practices and adherence to medication regimens. The association between conscientiousness and immunity has been addressed in only four studies, two of which have their methods described in detail in previous sections (Cohen et al., 1997; Pressman et al., 2005).

SUSCEPTIBILITY TO INFECTIOUS DISEASE

In Cohen and colleagues' (1997) prospective study of psychosocial factors and susceptibility to the common cold in healthy adults, conscientiousness, as measured with Goldberg's trait adjectives, was unrelated to the likelihood of developing a cold following experimental exposure to one of two viruses.

ANTIBODY RESPONSE TO VACCINATION

In their prospective study of healthy young adults that also assessed personality with the Goldberg scales, Pressman and colleagues (2005) found no association between conscientiousness and antibody response to influenza vaccine either 1 or 4 months after immunization.

CIRCULATING MARKERS OF INFLAMMATION

In contrast, findings from Sutin and colleagues' (2009) study of 5,119 Italian men and women suggest that conscientiousness might be associated with reduced inflammation in healthy adults. In this large sample, lower conscientiousness scores on the NEO PI-R were associated with higher concentrations of both IL-6 and CRP, independent of age, sex, BMI, aspirin use in the last two weeks, and disease burden. Less smoking among those scoring higher in conscientiousness partially mediated the relationship between IL-6 levels and five conscientiousness subcomponents: competence, dutifulness, achievement striving, self-discipline, and deliberation. The mediation tests for the association of total conscientiousness with IL-6, and analyses with CRP as the outcome, were not reported.

HIV

O'Cleirigh, Ironson, Weiss, and Costa (2007) used a prospective design to examine the association of conscientiousness with HIV disease progression among 119 HIV-positive adults (mean age 37 years; 34% female). Conscientiousness, assessed with the NEO PI-R, CD4+ cell counts, and viral load were measured at baseline and one year later. Covariates included age, race, sex, antiretroviral medication use, and baseline CD4+ or viral load levels. Higher conscientiousness at baseline was related to a slower decline in CD4+ levels and an attenuated increase in viral load from baseline to 1-year follow-up. None of the potential mediators tested (depression, perceived stress, coping style, and medication adherence) explained the association of conscientiousness with either outcome. In their longitudinal analysis of 104 surviving participants from this sample, Ironson and colleagues (2008) found that greater conscientiousness was associated with a slower average rate of increase in viral load over the course of 4 years. In this case, however, conscientiousness was not related to changes in CD4+ count.

CONCLUSIONS

To date, available information on the relation of conscientiousness to immunity is insufficient to draw any meaningful conclusions. Conscientiousness appears not to be related to the likelihood of developing a cold following experimental exposure to viruses that cause URI, nor to antibody response to influenza vaccination. However, lower levels of conscientiousness may be associated with elevated circulating markers of inflammation. Among HIV patients, conscientiousness has been associated with slower increases in viral load, and inconsistently with a slower decline in CD4+ cells. It is not clear, however, whether these associations are mediated by better health behaviors (e.g., diet, physical activity, smoking) and medication adherence among more conscientious persons or is via some other pathway.

Agreeableness

Agreeableness refers to being concerned with and contributing to the maintenance of relationships with other persons. Persons who score high on agreeableness tend to be pleasant and accommodating, and place considerable importance on maintaining harmony in their interpersonal relationships. Agreeable persons also tend to hold optimistic views of human nature. Subtraits of agreeableness include trust, morality, altruism, cooperation, modesty, and sympathy. Agreeableness has rarely been examined in relation to immunity. The findings summarized next derive from four studies (all described earlier) that were conducted with healthy adults, and one HIV study. In most cases, agreeableness was one of several personality characteristics that were examined or was included as a control variable. Two healthy population studies examined whether Goldberg's agreeableness subscale was related to susceptibility to the common cold (Cohen et al., 1997; Cohen et al., 2003a). Whereas the earlier study conducted in a sample of 193 found no relation between agreeableness and cold susceptibility, the later study, conducted in a larger sample of 334, found greater agreeableness to be associated with greater resistance (Cohen et al., 2003a). Other outcomes examined in healthy adults included antibody response to vaccination (Pressman et al., 2005), enumerative measures of immunity (i.e., total lymphocytes and lymphocyte subsets; Miller, Cohen et al., 1999) and NK cell cytotoxicity (Miller, Cohen et al., 1999). Agreeableness was unrelated to any of these outcomes. The HIV study similarly found no associations between agreeableness and changes in CD4+ counts or viral load across 4 years (Ironson et al., 2008).

Openness

Openness to experience, or simply openness, refers to the extent to which individuals are appreciative of new or different ideas and experiences. Persons scoring high on measures of openness tend to be curious, imaginative, and reflective, whereas those scoring low on openness tend to be more conventional and less given to abstract thought. Subtraits of openness include imagination, artistic interests, emotionality, adventurousness, intellect, and liberalism. To date, only three studies have examined whether openness is associated with measures of immunity in samples of healthy adults, and only one study in persons with HIV. All of these studies were described previously, and all examined openness as a secondary variable. Among the studies conducted in healthy populations, the assessed immune outcomes were susceptibility to the common cold (Cohen et al., 1997), antibody response to vaccination (Pressman et al., 2005), and circulating markers of inflammation (Sutin et al., 2009). In none of these studies was openness associated with immune outcomes. In the HIV study, neither changes in CD4+ counts nor viral load were associated with openness across the 4-year follow-up (Ironson et al., 2008).

Other Personality Characteristics

In addition to the Big Five personality characteristics, four other personality traits have been examined in regard to associations with immune function: dispositional optimism, trait positive affect, hostility, and social inhibition. We discuss these traits separately from the Big Five because none is encompassed by a single Big Five category. For example, hostility is thought to include dimensions of both agreeableness and neuroticism; trait positive affect, agreeableness and extraversion; social inhibition, agreeableness, extraversion, and neuroticism; and optimism, possibly all five factors.

Dispositional Optimism

Dispositional optimism reflects the extent to which individuals hold generalized favorable expectancies for their future, and pessimism reflects the extent to which they hold unfavorable expectancies (Carver, Scheier, & Segerstrom, 2010). Optimism is most often assessed by the Life Orientation Test (LOT; Scheier & Carver, 1985; revised version

LOT-R; Scheier, Carver, & Bridges, 1994). Higher scores on this questionnaire suggest strong agreement with the expectation of favorable experiences and strong disagreement with the expectation of unfavorable experiences. The LOT also contains subscales that can be used to assess optimism and pessimism separately. Another approach to optimism focuses on attributional styles—how people explain events. In this approach, optimistic justifications of *negative experiences* are attributed to factors outside the self (external), that are not likely to occur consistently (unstable), and are limited to specific life domains (specific). In contrast, optimistic interpretations of *positive experiences* would be labeled as the opposite: internal, stable, and global. Pessimistic attributional styles are defined as the opposite of the optimistic styles. Attributional styles are assessed by the Attributional Style Questionnaire (ASQ; Peterson et al., 1982) or the Content Analysis of Verbatim Explanations (CAVE; Peterson, Luborsky, & Seligman, 1983) technique, in which interview answers or archival data are content analyzed for attributional styles. The attributional style measures are only modestly associated with measures of generalized expectancies (Ahrens & Haaga, 1993; Peterson & Vaidya, 2001). Thus, expectancy and attribution measures cannot be considered interchangeable.

ENUMERATIVE MEASURES OF IMMUNITY

Kamen-Siegel, Rodin, Seligman, and Dwyer (1991) examined whether pessimistic attributional style, as measured by the CAVE, was associated with percentages of CD3+, CD4+, and CD8+ cells in 26 men and women between the ages of 62 and 83 years (mean age 70.4 years). Analyses that controlled for lag in days between CAVE interview and blood tests, general health, and depressive symptoms revealed that pessimistic explanatory style was correlated with low CD4+/CD8+ ratios, and was accounted for largely by the association between more pessimistic style and a higher percentage of CD8+ cells. No results were reported for analyses predicting CD3+ cells.

Brennan & Charnetski (2000) investigated whether attributional style, as assessed by the ASQ, was associated with total salivary secretory immunoglobulin A (sIgA) concentrations. In a sample of 112 undergraduates (mean age 18.8 years, range 16 to 23; 63% female). Neither total ASQ scores nor scores on the optimistic style subscale were related to sIgA. However, higher scores on the pessimistic style subscale were associated with lower sIgA levels.

IMMUNE FUNCTION MEASURED IN VITRO

Kamen-Siegel and colleagues (1991) also examined whether pessimistic attributional style was associated with PHA-stimulated lymphocyte proliferation. A more pessimistic style was associated with a lower proliferative response, but only when stimulated with a 0.5μg/mL dose of PHA and not 10.0μg/mL or 1.0μg/mL. In a study of the potential role of optimism in response to an immunization, Kohut, Cooper, Nickolaus, Russell, and Cunnick (2002) administered the LOT to 56 healthy men and women aged 62 years and older (63% female) who were vaccinated with a trivalent influenza vaccine. Blood for immune assessments was drawn 14 weeks postvaccination. Outcomes included influenza-specific lymphocyte proliferation and influenza vaccine-stimulated productions of IL-2, IL-10, and IFN-γ. Optimism was unrelated to any of these measures.

ANTIBODY RESPONSE TO VACCINATION

Kohut et al. (2002) also examined whether optimism was related to IgG and IgM antibody response to the trivalent influenza vaccine. The LOT was not related to response of either antibody.

CIRCULATING MARKERS OF INFLAMMATION

Two recent studies examined whether optimism is associated with circulating markers of inflammation. In a sample of 36 healthy nonsmoking postmenopausal women (mean age 60.7 ± 6.7 years), O'Donovan, Lin, Dhabhar, Wolkowitz, Tillie, Blackburn, and Epel (2009) found that higher scores on the pessimism subscale of the LOT-R were associated with higher IL-6 concentrations, independent of age, caregiver status, and optimism subscale scores. Optimism, by comparison, was unrelated to IL-6 even when adjusting only for age. In another multivariate model that included a group of hypothesized mediators (neuroticism, perceived stress, physical activity, and sleep quality) in addition to age, caregiver status, and optimism, the association of pessimism with IL-6 was slightly reduced; evidence consistent with the hypothesis that one or more of these variables (or their combination) may act as pathways linking optimism to IL-6 concentrations.

Roy, Diez-Roux, Seeman, Ranjit, Shea, and Cushman (2010) also tested the hypothesis that lower optimism and higher pessimism each would be related to greater circulating markers of inflammation. However, in addition to IL-6, Roy and colleagues measured CRP, fibrinogen, and homocysteine. Participants were drawn from the 6,195 men and women (mean age 62.2 years, range 45 to 84; 53% female) who took part in the first MultiEthnic Study of Atherosclerosis (MESA) follow-up examination ($n = 5,220$ to 5,358, depending on outcome). Bivariate analysis showed that higher scores on the pessimism subscale of the LOT-R were associated with higher concentrations of all four inflammatory markers, independent of age, race, and sex. By comparison, lower scores on the optimism subscale showed only a marginal association with higher homocysteine, and were unrelated to IL-6, CRP, and fibrinogen. The authors further explored the associations of pessimism with inflammatory markers by conducting three additional sets of multivariate analyses. In the first, which controlled for age, sex, fasting, recent infections, and medication use, greater scores on the pessimism subscale remained an independent predictor of greater IL-6, CRP, and fibrinogen, respectively, but not of homocysteine. In the second model, including additional controls for race, education, income, depression, cynical distrust, smoking status, exercise, and diet, the associations of pessimism with CRP and fibrinogen remained, but the association with IL-6 lost significance. A final model entered three potential mediators, BMI, diabetes, and hypertension as additional controls. The results were consistent with the hypothesis that one or more (or a combination) of these variables act as pathways linking optimism to inflammatory response. In contrast, the association between pessimism and fibrinogen was reduced only minimally, a finding inconsistent with mediation in this case.

TELOMERE LENGTH IN LEUKOCYTES

In addition to examining an association between optimism and pessimism with IL-6, O'Donovan et al. (2009) also explored the association of these traits with telomere length in leukocytes. Telomeres are regions of repetitive DNA that form at the ends of chromosomes and function to protect the chromosome terminus from deterioration subsequent to repeated replication. Leukocyte telomere length may serve as an indicator of immunosenescence, with shorter telomeres indicating more DNA replications, and thus more aged or compromised immunity. Age-adjusted analyses showed higher pessimism subscale scores to be associated with shorter telomeres. Optimism scores, by comparison, were unrelated to telomere length. When entered into a model that controlled for age, caregiver status, optimism, perceived stress, neuroticism, BMI, exercise,

and sleep, pessimism remained an independent correlate of telomere length.

HIV

Several studies have explored the relation of optimism to disease progression in HIV-infected individuals. Ironson and colleagues (2005) examined the prospective association of optimism with change in CD4+ counts and viral load among 177 HIV-infected adults (mean age 37.5 years; 30% female) with midrange CD4+ counts and no AIDS defining illnesses at baseline. Dispositional optimism was measured at baseline using a composite of the LOT and the LOT-R. CD4+ counts, viral load, and potential psychosocial (depression, perceived stress, coping) and behavioral mediators (medication adherence, substance use, sleep, exercise, condom use, proactive disease behaviors) were measured every 6 months over a 2-year period. Covariates included time since study entry, viral load or CD4+ count at study entry, use of antiviral medications, race, sex, age, education, route of infection, and sexual orientation. Greater optimism at baseline was associated with both a slower average decline in CD4+ counts and a slower average increase in viral load across the two years of follow-up. Further, analyses were consistent with less depression, more proactive disease behavior (e.g., information seeking, health behavior change), and less avoidant coping among those with greater optimism partially mediating the association of optimism with CD4+ count, and less depression alone playing a mediating role in the association of optimism with viral load.

Milam, Richardson, Marks, Kemper, and McCutchan (2004) explored similar research questions in a prospective study conducted among 412 HIV-infected men and women attending 6 public HIV clinics in California (mean age 39.0 ± 7.9 years; 12% female). All participants were on antiretroviral therapy at study entry. Optimism and pessimism were measured at baseline using separate subscales of the LOT-R. Other baseline measurements included age, race, sex, diagnosis date, exercise, diet, tobacco use, depression, illicit drug use, viral load, and CD4+ count. Viral load and CD4+ count were measured again 18 months later, as was antiretroviral adherence. Greater pessimism at baseline was associated with a greater increase in viral load over 18 months. This association was not explained by any of the behavioral variables. By comparison, although greater optimism was related cross-sectionally to lower viral load at baseline, optimism did not predict viral load at follow-up. Neither pessimism nor optimism was linearly related to follow-up CD4+ counts. However, optimism showed a curvilinear association with CD4+ counts such that individuals with moderate optimism scores displayed higher counts than those with either low or high scores. This association was not explained by health behaviors or depression.

In the sample of HIV-positive men described in the section on neuroticism, Tomakowsky and colleagues (2001) examined both cross-sectional and prospective associations of optimism with disease progression using two models of optimism: dispositional optimism, as measured by the LOT, and optimistic attributional style, as measured by the Expanded Attributional Style Questionnaire (EASQ; Peterson & Villanova, 1988). All 78 men were included in the cross-sectional analyses, and a subset of these men ($n = 47$) who had survived and remained in treatment at the clinic 2 years after the initial enrollment were included in the 2-year prospective follow-up analyses. Health status at baseline and follow-up was assessed with CD4+ cell counts. Fully adjusted models controlled for demographics, length of diagnosis, antiretroviral drug use, and negative affectivity. Prospective models included additional control for baseline CD4+ counts. Surprisingly, results indicated that those scoring higher on optimistic explanatory style displayed *more advanced* disease at baseline and experienced a greater *decline* in health status over the subsequent two years. Optimism as measured by the LOT was neither cross-sectionally nor prospectively associated with HIV disease progression.

MODERATING THE EFFECTS OF STRESS ON IMMUNITY

In a three-month prospective study conducted among 39 healthy white women (mean age 32.0 ± 6.6 years), Cohen, Kearney, Zegans, Kemeny, Neuhaus, and Stites (1999) evaluated whether dispositional optimism buffers the effects of stress on lymphocyte percentages and NK cell cytotoxicity. Dispositional optimism was evaluated using total LOT scores. Participants' experiences of acute stress (less than one week) and persistent stress (more than one week) were assessed with weekly stress logs. Enumerative measures included percentages of CD4+ and CD8+ cells. In light of evidence suggesting that phenotypically different CD8+ cells may have different functions, the authors also measured two subsets of CD8+ cells, CD8+CD11b+ and CD8+CD11b-, to explore whether these subsets show differential responses to stress. The authors

observed interactions of optimism with acute stress in the prediction of CD8+CD11b+ cell percentages, and with persistent stress in the predictions of CD8+CD11b- percentages and NK cell cytotoxicity. Only in the case of acute stress, however, was the moderating effect consistent with a buffering role for optimism—that is, acute stress-related increases in CD8+CD11b+ cells were less pronounced at higher relative to lower levels of optimism. Unexpectedly, the persistent stress-associated decreases in CD8+CD11b- percentages and NK cell cytotoxicity were *more* pronounced at higher levels of optimism.

Using data from 59 male university students (age range 18 to 30), Brydon, Walker, Wawrzyniak, Chart, and Steptoe (2009) examined whether optimism would moderate the combined effects of psychological and immune (i.e., vaccination for typhoid) challenge on immunity. After the assessment of optimism using the LOT-R, participants were randomized into one of four conditions: vaccine/stress; placebo/stress; vaccine/rest; and placebo/rest. Vaccination (or placebo) was administered 30 minutes prior to laboratory stress (or rest). The stress condition involved both a Stroop task and a public-speaking task. Circulating serum IL-6 and typhoid antibody were both measured before vaccination. IL-6 was measured again 3 hours after vaccination, and antibody to the vaccine 3 weeks later. The results were consistent with a stress-buffering hypothesis. Among persons in the combined vaccine/stress and placebo/stress conditions, IL-6 increased from baseline to posttask at low levels of optimism, and the magnitude of this increase became less apparent as LOT-R total scores increased. Among persons in the vaccine-stress group only, the expected acute stress-associated increase in antibody production was evident at high but not low levels of optimism.

In three studies, Segerstrom and colleagues (Segerstrom 2006; Segerstrom, 2001; Segerstrom, Taylor, Kemeny, & Fahey, 1998) evaluated the potential moderating role of optimism in immune response to the stress of attending law school. In none of these studies, however, did optimism show the expected moderating effect.

The first study evaluated 50 first-year law students at the University of California at Los Angeles (Segerstrom et al., 1998). Data were collected during low (two weeks prior to law school orientation and the first day of classes) and high (during midsemester) stress periods. Dispositional optimism was measured using the LOT. Additional measures included coping skills, mood, and health behaviors. Immune measures included the numbers of CD4+, CD8+, CD19+, and CD3-CD16+CD56+ cells and NK cell cytotoxicity. Dispositional optimism did not moderate any changes in immune parameters during this stressful academic period.

In the second study, Segerstrom (2001) used two separate samples of law students to investigate whether optimism interacts with relocation status in predicting changes in immune parameters during the first semester of law school. She posited that students who do not relocate to attend school experience greater social-academic conflict than those who do relocate because they are trying to balance their current social situations with academic demands. Thus, being a "nonrelocator" might be considered a high-stress condition. The first of the two samples was comprised of 48 of the UCLA students examined in Segerstrom et al. (1998), and the immune outcomes were the same as those described earlier. The second sample was comprised of 22 first-year University of Kentucky law-school students (median age 24.5; 45.5% female), and the immune outcome was delayed-type hypersensitivity (DTH), as indicated by induration response to intradermally injected antigen. In both samples, LOT total scores were used to assess dispositional optimism. Although significant interactions between optimism and relocation status emerged in both samples, in neither case did the nature of the interactions support a buffering effect of optimism. Contrariwise, those higher in optimism showed poorer immune responses in the face of the presumed stress of not relocating.

The third study (Segerstrom, 2006) also evaluated the extent to which optimism interacted with relocation status to predict DTH response. The sample was comprised of 46 first-year law-school students (mean age 23, SD 1.9; 61% female). The Life Orientation Test-Revised (LOT-R) was used to assess dispositional optimism. Significant interactions between optimism and relocation status also emerged here. Among students who did not relocate, dispositional optimism was associated with smaller DTH responses. Among students who did relocate, dispositional optimism was associated with larger DTH response. Again, although optimism interacted with relocation status, optimism did not appear to have a buffering effect. Further, like the two samples reported on in Segerstrom (2001), higher optimism was associated with poorer immune responses among those who did not relocate.

CONCLUSIONS

When examined collectively, research on dispositional optimism and immunity suggests that greater pessimism rather than less optimism may be the more important dimension of personality in regard to predicting individuals' predispositions toward immune dysregulation. The link between pessimism and immunity has been demonstrated across several immune outcomes, with greater pessimism being associated with increased likelihood of exhibiting a pro-inflammatory phenotype, poorer cell-mediated immunity, reduced humoral immunity, and accelerated immunosenescence. There is evidence that at least some of the tie between pessimism and inflammatory markers may be mediated by lifestyle and risk behaviors and possibly perceived stress.

Evidence for links between optimism and immunity is weaker. None of the studies reviewed here observed a main effect association between optimism and immune outcomes in healthy adult samples, regardless of whether optimism was measured using total LOT scores, the optimism subscale of the LOT, or the optimistic-style subscale of the ASQ. By comparison, the HIV studies found associations between both optimism and pessimism with HIV disease status and progression, but the directions of these associations were inconsistent and often counterintuitive. For example, greater optimism has been associated cross-sectionally with lower viral load and lower CD4+ counts, and with less CD4+ decline over time, whereas optimistic attributional style has been associated cross-sectionally with *higher* CD4+ counts, and with *greater* CD4+ decline over time.

In contrast to the studies examining main effect associations of optimism with immune-related outcomes, there is evidence to suggest that optimism moderates the effects of stress on immunity. The findings of these studies, however, are difficult to interpret. Two studies provided support for the buffering hypothesis by showing that real life acute stress-related elevations in CD8+CD11b+ percentages and laboratory stress-related increases in IL-6, respectively, are reduced among persons with higher levels of optimism. These findings, however, appear to be the exception rather than the rule, because most of the studies we discuss here either reported no moderating effect of optimism or even an *accentuating* effect of optimism on stress-related changes in immunity. It is noteworthy that these studies all had relatively small samples ($Ns = 22–59$) and may have been underpowered to detect stress-buffering effects (Cohen & Edwards, 1989).

Trait Positive Affect/Positive Emotional Style

Positive affect (PA) is the experience of feelings that indicate a positive engagement or interaction with one's environment (Clark, Watson, & Leeka, 1989). Trait PA (also called *positive emotional style* [PES]) is a dispositional characteristic that reflects one's tendency to experience PA (Cohen et al., 2003b). An important aspect of the research on trait PA/PES and immunity is its emphasis on establishing whether associations of PES with immunity are independent of those of trait NA or neuroticism.

ANTIBODY RESPONSE TO VACCINATION

In a study described earlier in the section on neuroticism, Marsland, Cohen, Rabin, and Manuck (2006) also examined whether trait PA was associated with antibody response to Hepatitis B (HBV) vaccine in 84 healthy, HBV seronegative graduate students (mean age 24 years, range 21–33; 39% female). PA was measured using subscales from the POMS Affect Scale, the Goldberg Big Five Factor Scales (Goldberg, 1992), the Larsen and Diener Circumplex (Larsen & Diener, 1992) and from the Mackay Circumplex (Mackay, Cox, Burrows, & Lazzerini, 1978). Results of logistic regression analysis controlling for age, sex, BMI and depression showed that trait PA independently predicted antibody response to HBV vaccine such that greater PA was associated with less likelihood of being in the low-response group. This effect was also independent of neuroticism (trait NA) and of other dimensions of personality that are closely related to PA such as optimism and extraversion.

SUSCEPTIBILITY TO INFECTIOUS DISEASE

The majority of this work has focused on the role of this personality characteristic in resistance to URI. In the initial study, Cohen and colleagues (2003b) used two methods to assess PES in the sample of 334 healthy men and women described in the extraversion and neuroticism sections. The first was a brief retrospective questionnaire that was administered six weeks prior to viral exposure and on which participants rated how accurately each of nine adjectives reflecting positive mood states (e.g., happy, enthusiastic, calm) described how they "usually" feel. The second was a multiple interview-based summary measure of daily mood. During the month prior to viral exposure, participants were interviewed by telephone on seven nights and asked to rate the same nine adjectives that were included in the questionnaire in regard to how accurately

each of the adjectives described how they were feeling that day. Positive emotional style scores were computed by averaging participants' daily positive mood scores across the seven days.

Higher scores on the interview-based PES measure were related in a dose-response manner to a lower risk of developing a cold. This association was independent of preexposure viral-specific-antibody level, age, race, sex, education, BMI, season of the year, and virus type. Results were also independent of trait NA. Inclusion of potential health-behavior mediators (smoking status, alcohol intake, exercise, and sleep quality) into the model did not diminish the association. Higher scores on the questionnaire measure of PES showed a similar association with reduced cold risk.

In a later paper based on data from the same sample, Doyle, Gentile, and Cohen (2006) examined the possibility that the aforementioned reported association of PES with signs of clinical illness may have been mediated by *local* (in nasal secretions) release of pro-inflammatory cytokines (IL-1β, IL-6, and IL-8). Results showed that higher scores on the interview measure of PES were associated with lower production of IL-6 in response to infection. Moreover, IL-6 accounted for 25–44% of the association of PES with signs of clinical illness, thus suggesting a mediational role for IL-6 in the association of PES with the expression of clinical colds. PES was not related to either IL-1β or IL-8.

In the sample of 193 healthy men and women described in the section on neuroticism, Cohen and colleagues replicated the association between higher PES and fewer colds using a modified version of the interview-based PES measure (Cohen et al., 2006). Prior to exposure to either RV39 or the A/Texas/36/91 (H1N1) influenza virus, participants were interviewed nightly over a period of *two* weeks and asked to report on their mood using the nine-adjective PA scale employed in Cohen et al. (2003b). Positive emotional style scores were computed by averaging daily mood scores across the two weeks. The remainder of the protocol was identical to the previous study, and the primary outcome was the development of a cold. Similar to the previous findings, increases in PES were associated with decreases in objectively diagnosed illness independent of age, sex, race, education, BMI, virus type, antibody levels, and NA.

IMMUNE FUNCTION MEASURED IN VITRO

Prather, Marsland, Muldoon, and Manuck (2007) explored whether trait PA is associated with stimulated production of pro- and anti-inflammatory cytokines in vitro in a sample of 146 community volunteers (mean age 45.2 ± 6.2 years; 42.5% female). PA was assessed with the trait version of the PANAS. Productions of three pro-inflammatory cytokines (IL-1β, IL-6, TNF-α) and one anti-inflammatory cytokine (IL-10) were measured following stimulation in whole blood with LPS in vitro. Higher trait PA was associated with lower productions of IL-6 and IL-10, but was not related to production of either IL-1β or TNF-α. A significant PA-by-sex interaction in the prediction of IL-10 revealed that the decrease in IL-10 production with increasing PA was apparent only in men. No PA-by-sex interactions were found for IL-6.

CONCLUSIONS

The data support a reliable association of greater trait PA (PES) with less expression of signs of illness in persons experimentally exposed to rhinoviruses. In addition, a single study suggests that PA is associated with a better secondary response to HBV vaccine. Another indicates the possibility of trait PA modulating lymphocyte production of pro-inflammatory cytokines. However, as there are no norms for appropriate levels of cytokine production in vitro, the implication of this association for immunocompetence is unclear.

Hostility

Hostility is often defined in terms of its cognitive, affective, and behavioral components. The cognitive component encompasses cynicism as well as hostile attributions, the affective component includes negatively charged emotions such as anger and annoyance, and the behavioral component includes verbal and physical aggression (Barefoot et al., 1991; Smith, 1992). Two of the more frequently used instruments to measure hostility are the Cook-Medley Hostility Scale (Ho; Cook & Medley, 1954; Barefoot, Dodge, Peterson, Dahlstrom, & Williams, 1989) and the Buss-Perry Aggression Questionnaire (BPAQ; Buss & Perry, 1992). Both scales are comprised of subsets of items reflecting the cognitive, affective, and behavioral dimensions of hostility. However, whereas the constructs measured by the Cook-Medley Ho are referred to as cynicism, hostile affect, and aggression, analogous constructs measured by the BPAQ are referred to as hostility, anger, physical aggression, and verbal aggression.

Much of the interest in exploring whether hostility is related to immune function stems from the well-established association of hostility with risk for cardiovascular disease (CVD) (e.g., Everson-Rose et al., 2006; Smith, 1992; Suls & Wan, 1993). Activities of the immune system, in particular inflammation, have come to be recognized as important contributors to the pathogenesis of atherosclerotic CVD (Ross, 1999). In light of evidence implicating inflammation in CVD pathogenesis, and evidence showing associations between the components of hostility and atherosclerotic CVD (Everson-Rose et al., 2006; Miller, Freedland, Carney, Stetler, & Banks, 2003), there has been considerable interest in the association between hostility and markers of inflammation.

STIMULATED PRO-INFLAMMATORY CYTOKINE PRODUCTION

In a sample of 62 healthy, nonsmoking men (mean age 25.4 ± 5.9 years), Suarez, Lewis, and Kuhn (2002) tested the hypothesis that greater levels of hostility, assessed with the BPAQ, would be associated with greater LPS-stimulated production of TNF-α. In analyses that controlled for age, race, education, and alcohol use, BPAQ total scores, as well as scores on the hostility and physical aggression subscales, were each associated with greater stimulated TNF-α production. The anger and verbal aggression subscales were not related to stimulated TNF-α.

In a later study of 44 healthy, nonsmoking premenopausal women (mean age 33.5 ± 8.2 years), Suarez, Lewis, Krishnan, and Young (2004) examined the association of cynical hostility, as assessed by the Cook-Medley Ho, with stimulated productions of three pro-inflammatory cytokines (IL-1α, IL-1β, TNF-α) and three chemokines involved in the recruitment of leukocytes to locations of injury (IL-8, monocyte chemotactic protein [MCP]-1, macrophage inflammatory protein [MIP]-1α). Analyses controlling for race, BMI, total cholesterol, and alcohol consumption indicated that greater hostility was associated with greater stimulated productions of IL-1α and IL-1β, but in contrast to the authors' previous finding in men (Suarez et al., 2002), not with production of TNF-α. Greater hostility also was associated with greater stimulated IL-8, but was unrelated to productions of either of the other two chemokines.

More recently, Janicki-Deverts, Cohen, & Doyle (2010) examined the association of hostility, as assessed by the Cook-Medley Ho, with stimulated productions of three pro-inflammatory (IL-2, TNF-α, INF-γ) and three anti-inflammatory (IL-4, IL-5, IL-10) cytokines in a sample of 153 healthy men and women (mean age 37.3 ± 8.8 years; 51% female). The authors found that greater hostility was related to greater stimulated production of the pro-inflammatory cytokines TNF-α and IFN-γ, but was unrelated to production of IL-2 or to any of the anti-inflammatory cytokines. Further analysis of the subcomponents of hostility—cynicism, hostile affect, and aggression—showed that greater cynicism was related to greater productions of all three of the pro-inflammatory cytokines independent of age, sex, race, socioeconomic status, BMI, and health behaviors. Neither hostile affect nor aggression was related to any of the stimulated cytokine measures. These findings suggest that cynicism may be the key aspect of hostility associated with increases in stimulated pro-inflammatory cytokine production.

CIRCULATING MARKERS OF INFLAMMATION

Five published studies have examined the association of hostility with circulating markers of inflammation. Four of these used the Cook-Medley Ho to assess hostility, examined pro-inflammatory cytokines and/or CRP as outcomes, and included several control variables in their analyses. Suarez (2003) examined the association of hostility with IL-6 in 90 healthy, nonsmoking men (mean age 26.1 ± 6.8 years), and controlled for age, BMI, fasting total cholesterol, HDL cholesterol, resting diastolic blood pressure, and depressive symptoms. Miller, Freedland, Carney, Stetler, and Banks (2003) studied the relation of hostility to IL-1β, IL-6, and TNF-α in 100 healthy men and women (mean age 30.2 ± 10.0 years; 68% female), and controlled for demographic variables, smoker status, BMI, waist-hip ratio, cholesterol, mean arterial pressure, oral contraceptive use, and depressive symptoms. Stewart, Janicki-Deverts, Muldoon, and Kamarck (2008) examined the association of hostility with IL-6 and CRP in 316 healthy, older adults (mean age 60.6 ± 4.8 years; 49.1% female), and controlled for age, sex, race, education, BMI, blood pressure, cholesterol, triglycerides, glucose, insulin, health behaviors, and depressive symptoms. Most recently, Brummett, Boyle, Ortel, Becker, Siegler and Williams (2010) examined circulating IL-6 and CRP concentrations in 525 younger adults (mean age 30.3 ± 9.0 years; 58% female) who were selected based on being either low (score of 9 or less) or high (score of 14 or more) in hostility, and controlled for age, race, sex, BMI, and sibship (some of the participants were related). Although Stewart and colleagues (2008) found greater hostility to be

associated with greater IL-6 (but not greater CRP), none of the remaining studies observed an association between hostility and any of the measured circulating inflammatory markers.

In contrast to most of the aforementioned findings, Marsland and colleagues (2008) found hostility to be related to circulating markers of inflammation in their sample of 855 middle-aged adults (see study description in the neuroticism section). The authors used both the Cook-Medley Ho and the BPAQ to measure hostility, and created composite measures of the cognitive, affective, and behavioral dimensions by averaging standardized scores of the analogous subscales of the two hostility inventories. Circulating IL-6 and CRP concentrations were examined as outcomes. Results of analyses that controlled for age, sex, race, years of education, medical conditions, or medications known to influence inflammation, and trait NA revealed that higher scores on each of the three hostility subscales were associated with higher circulating concentrations of both inflammatory markers. The inclusion of health practices (BMI, smoking, exercise) as covariates reduced the association of *hostile cognitions* and *hostile affect* with IL-6 and CRP, consistent with the hypothesis that higher levels of BMI and smoking and lower levels of exercise may mediate these associations. By comparison, similar analyses did not support the hypothesis that health practices mediated the associations of *hostile behavioral tendencies* with IL-6 and CRP.

MODERATING THE EFFECTS OF STRESS ON IMMUNITY

As suggested earlier, it is possible that hostility moderates the immune system's response when individuals are subjected to stress. Findings from laboratory research suggest that exposure to acute psychological stressors—of either an interpersonal or noninterpersonal nature—gives rise to detectible changes in immunity (Segerstrom & Miller, 2004). Assuming that hostility may be associated with greater sensitivity to social stressors, one hypothesis that has been explored is that hostility should be associated with increased immune reactivity in response to interpersonal stress.

Mills, Dimsdale, Nelesen, and Dillon (1996) investigated whether changes in white blood cell (WBC) counts after participating in a public-speaking task (defending oneself against a false shoplifting accusation) differed depending on relative levels of hostility. A sample of 104 healthy adults (mean age 39.7 ± 10 years; 31% female) completed the

Buss-Durkee Hostility Inventory (BDHI; Buss & Durkee, 1957) and the Cook-Medley Ho within 48 hours of completing the stress task. Two factors related to the affective component of hostility were derived from BDHI scores, experience of anger (BD-experience), and expression of anger (BD-expression), and Cook-Medley Ho scores were used to measure total hostility (CM-hostility). Both before and after the task, participants completed the Spielberger State Anger Questionnaire, and blood was drawn for assessment of immune parameters (counts of CD3+, CD4+, CD8+, and CD19+ cells, two subsets of NK cells [CD56+ and CD57+], and total WBCs). The stress task was associated with increases over baseline in total WBCs, CD8+, CD57+, and CD56+ cells, and decreases in CD4+ and CD19+ cells. Cook-Medley total hostility moderated the effect of the stress task on CD57+ cell counts, and BD-expression scores moderated the effect of stress on CD19+ and CD56+ counts, but the nature of these effects were contradictory. Whereas the stressor-associated increase in CD57+ cells was *amplified* among those with higher CM-hostility scores, the stress-related changes in CD19+ and CD56+ counts were *reversed* among those with higher BD-expression scores—that is, CD19+ cells increased and CD56+ cells decreased subsequent to stress among those with higher scores. Neither anger responses to the task nor BD-experience were associated with changes in any of the immune measures.

Christensen, Edwards, Wiebe, Benotsch, McKelvey, Andrews, and Lubaroff (1996) addressed whether hostility might influence changes in immune cell *function* in response to an interpersonal stress task. Forty-three male undergraduates completed a battery of psychological questionnaires that included the Cook-Medley Ho. Participants were then randomly assigned to one of two public-speaking conditions: a self-disclosure condition that required participants to describe an intimate and troubling personal experience; or a non-self-disclosure (low-stress control) condition wherein participants read from a passage describing a hypothetical student's stressful experience. NK cytotoxicity was measured before and after the task. The results were consistent with the hypothesis that hostility moderates response to interpersonal stressors. Those with low levels of hostility responded to the interpersonal stressor with a small increase in NK cytotoxicity (relative to the low stress control), whereas those with high levels of hostility responded with a substantial increase in NK cytotoxicity.

Miller, Dopp, Myers, Stevens, and Fahey (1999) explored the possibility that hostility might moderate the association of negative emotional response to interpersonal stress with immunologic reactivity. To address this question, 41 couples (wives mean age 31.0 ± 7.5 years; husbands mean age 31.9 ± 7.7 years) took part in a marital conflict discussion. Hostility was measured before the discussion using the Cook-Medley Ho and counts of CD4+, CD8+, and CD3⁻CD16+CD56+ cells, and NK cell cytotoxicity were measured both before and after the discussion. Emotional response during the discussion was coded by trained observers. The results were consistent with hostility moderating stress response to interpersonal stressors, but only for men. In low-hostility husbands, *decreased* anger was associated with a small increase in NK cell cytotoxicity at mid-discussion, with no difference at the end of recovery. In contrast, for high-hostility husbands, anger expression was associated with a substantial *increase* in NK cell cytotoxicity during the discussion and a decline after the discussion. In high hostile men, higher levels of anger also covaried with greater increases in CD3⁻CD16+CD56+ counts. Anger was unrelated to immune parameters among wives, irrespective of their levels of hostility.

Although the laboratory studies suggest a possible moderating role for hostility in the immune system's response to acute stress, data from a single field study failed to observe a moderating effect of hostility on functional immune response (lymphocyte proliferation) to a relatively short-lived real-life stressor. Lee, Meehan, Robinson, Smith, and Mabry (1995) used the five-item hostility subscale of the Brief Symptoms Inventory to measure hostility in 89 male first-year United States Air Force Academy cadets. Hostility was assessed on three occasions, 2 weeks prior to arrival at the Academy (pre-orientation), orientation, and 4 weeks postorientation (i.e., during a stressful training period). Proliferative response was measured on two occasions—orientation and 4 weeks later—by stimulating mononuclear leukocytes with PHA, phorbyl 12-myristate 13-acetate (PMA), or anti-CD3 antibody. There were no cross-sectional associations between hostility and proliferative response during either orientation or training nor were there any lagged correlations between hostility at either pre-orientation or orientation and proliferative response during training.

CONCLUSIONS

There is reasonably reliable evidence that greater hostility (particularly cynicism) is associated with greater stimulated production of pro-inflammatory cytokines. Less clear is its relation to circulating inflammatory markers. In this case, three small studies of primarily young samples found no relation between hostility and several markers of inflammation. However, two studies showed strong associations of hostility with IL-6 (Marsland et al., 2008; Stewart et al., 2008) and CRP (Marsland et al., 2008). The use of what may be a more reliable assessment of hostility and a larger and older adult sample may account for the discrepancy in findings between Marsland et al. (2008) and most of the other studies. Age is an especially important issue—and one that may explain Stewart et al.'s (2008) significant finding, because inflammation and, in turn, the variability of inflammatory markers within a sample increase with age. The average ages of participants in the three studies that found no association between hostility and inflammatory markers were all less than 31 years, whereas the average ages of the Stewart et al. (2008) and Marsland et al. (2008) samples were 61 and 45 years, respectively.

The evidence suggests the possibility that hostility moderates the effects of experimental stress—in particular interpersonal stress, on NK cell cytotoxicity. Both studies of NK cell cytotoxicity showed stress-induced increases in immune function to be most apparent among the most hostile. Findings for changes in CD56+ counts are more difficult to interpret. For example, while Mills and colleagues (1996) found those who scored higher on *trait anger expression* decreased in CD56+ cells during acute stress, Miller and colleagues (1999) found highly hostile men who *expressed anger during laboratory stress* increased in CD56+ cells.

Social Inhibition

Social inhibition* is a tendency to suppress the expression of emotions in social interactions, to demonstrate extreme sensitivity to social criticism, and to withdraw in uncertain or challenging situations (Asendorpf, 1993). Although social inhibition has been recognized as an enduring trait, no published and validated measures of this personality characteristic are presently available. Accordingly, the studies we describe below either employed study-specific measures or measures of closely related personality constructs.

DELAYED-TYPE HYPERSENSITIVITY RESPONSE

Cole, Kemeny, Weitzman, Schoen, and Anton (1999) evaluated the role of social inhibition in DTH responses to tetanus toxoid during social engagement. Participants were 36 men and women (86% female) with either functional bowel disease (FBD; 55%), fibromyalgia (15%), or both disorders (30%), who were enrolled in a study assessing the effectiveness of hypnosis and education interventions in immune function among persons with FBD. Social inhibition was measured using the UCLA Rejection Sensitivity Scale (UCLARS; Cole, 1996), and by combining items from the Restricted Expression, Social Apprehensiveness, and Intimacy Problems scales of the Dimensional Assessment of Personality and Psychopathology (DAPP; Livesley, Jackson, & Schroeder, 1992). The first DTH inoculation was administered during the low-social-engagement baseline period, and induration responses were read 48 hours later. Inoculations were then repeated 4 weeks later, during the high-social-engagement intervention period, and 6 weeks later, following completion of the intervention. Induration responses were read 48 hours after each inoculation with the larger of the two values taken as a measure of the maximal response during the intervention period. Socially inhibited participants (upper 15% of scores) displayed *greater* induration responses than their less-inhibited counterparts during the high-engagement intervention period but not during the low-engagement baseline, when the groups did not differ. The authors attributed the *improved* cellular immune response to inhibition-related "hyperresponsivity."

HIV

Eisenberger, Kemeny, and Wyatt (2003) used a cross-sectional design to examine whether emotional expression was associated with CD4+ cell levels in a sample of 61 HIV-positive low-income minority women (mean age 37.2 ± 8.4 years). All participants took part in a 3- to 5-hour face-to-face interview that included open and closed-ended questions. *Emotional expression* was based on the percentage of negative (e.g., sad, hurt, hate, guilty) and positive (e.g., happy, joy, peaceful) emotion terms used during the coping with HIV component of the interview and *emotional inhibition* on the percentage of inhibition words used (e.g., inhibit, restrain, withhold, suppress, avoid). A blood draw at the time of the interview was used to evaluate CD4+ levels. Control variables included age, socioeconomic status, race, level of depression, recreational drug use, exercise, nutrition, sleep patterns, smoking, disease duration, HIV-related symptoms, HIV-related medication use, and sexually transmitted diseases. Emotional expression—either positive or negative, was unrelated to CD4+ levels. However, greater emotional inhibition was associated with lower CD4+ levels.

Fincham, Smit, Carey, Stein, and Seedat (2008) used a cross-sectional design to evaluate the relationship between behavioral inhibition and CD4+ counts among 454 HIV-positive South Africans (mean age 33.7 ± 7.6 years; 75% female). Behavioral inhibition was assessed using the 30-item Retrospective Self-Report of Childhood Inhibition scale (RSRCI; Reznick, Hegeman, Kaufman, Woods, & Jacobs, 1992), which is comprised of two subscales: a social fears subscale and a general fearfulness subscale. CD4+ counts were obtained from participant medical records within four weeks of the interview assessment. Covariates included age, sexual orientation, antiretroviral drug use, race, and disease duration. CD4+ counts were not associated with the RSRCI total scale or either of its subscales.

In a sample of 54 asymptomatic HIV-infected gay men (median age 41 years, range 26–55), Cole, Kemeny, Fahey, Zack, and Naliboff (2003) examined whether social inhibition influences changes in viral load and CD4+ cell counts over the course of 11 to 18 months, and if so, whether sympathetic nervous system (SNS) activity constitutes a possible explanatory mechanism. Social inhibition was measured using a composite of scales assessing introversion (extraversion subscale of the NEO-FFI; Costa & McCrae, 1992), social avoidance (DAPP social apprehensiveness and intimacy problems subscales; Cole et al., 1999; Livesley et al., 1992), emotional inexpression (Emotional Expressiveness Questionnaire; King & Emmons, 1990; DAPP restricted expression subscale), hostility (Cook-Medley Ho), and agreeableness (NEO-FFI). SNS activation was approximated using a composite score measuring skin conductance, brachial artery systolic blood pressure, and electrocardiogram data collected before, during, and after a serial subtraction stress task. HIV progression was assessed in terms of response to antiretroviral treatment (change in viral load and CD4+ count between baseline and follow-up). Control variables included age, race, income, education, substance use, sexual activity, infection duration, antiretroviral treatment, and baseline viral load or CD4+ count. Individuals scoring in the upper half of the social inhibition distribution had greater viral loads at baseline than those scoring below the median. Further, social inhibition was associated with poorer responses to antiretroviral treatment such that, relative to those who were less inhibited, inhibited persons demonstrated smaller CD4+ increases and smaller viral load declines following treatment with the antiretroviral medication. Socially inhibited persons also showed greater SNS activity in response to the stress task. Mediation analyses indicated that SNS activity accounted for 72% of the relationship between social inhibition and virologic response and 92% of CD4+ recovery following antiretroviral treatment.

CONCLUSIONS

The substantial differences in how social inhibition is measured across studies make it difficult to integrate the results. Even so, there is suggestive evidence that social inhibition is associated with poorer progression of disease among HIV-positive men. Evidence that this association may be mediated by SNS activation is also provocative.

Chapter Summary

The literature on personality and immunity is in its infancy. The lack of consistency of results across and within traits, and in what outcomes have been studied, makes it difficult to determine how reliable or meaningful associations are and whether different traits are important for different outcomes. Another limitation is the relative lack of evidence on the mediating pathways linking personality to various immune outcomes. It is only by understanding how specific traits may influence immunity that we could generalize existing findings to outcomes that have not yet received attention.

Overall, it is impossible to summarize this literature in any meaningful way. We can say that there is promising evidence across all the traits, with existing evidence at least suggesting some reliable associations and directions that future work might take to fill in voids in the literature.

Suggestions for Future Work

There is a clear need for adopting a *strong theoretical stance* in studying the association between personality traits and immunity. We have presented a general discussion of pathways that might link traits to immune function, but each trait has its own specific characteristics and each requires its own model. Such models should identify pathways and, in turn, outcomes that are most likely to be effected. For example, conscientiousness may be most closely tied to outcomes that respond to engagement in health-promoting behaviors and adherence to medical regimens, whereas extraversion might be more closely tied to outcomes influenced by physiological activation. Moreover, studies need to be designed in response to these models. This includes not only appropriate choice of outcomes, but also assessment and testing of proposed mediating pathways.

As discussed earlier, each of the Big Five personality characteristics is comprised of several subtraits. For example, extraversion includes friendliness, gregariousness, assertiveness, activity level, excitement seeking, and cheerfulness. For the most part, personality subtraits are not individually studied in the literature. Future research might investigate the relative importance of factor subtraits in regard to immune function, and whether all subtraits of a given personality factor influence immunity via similar and/or complementary mechanisms. Distinguishing subtraits that are responsible for associations with immune outcomes can help in understanding the basis for personality driven immunity, and it can help identify responsible mechanisms. Although not a Big Five factor, the work focusing on distinguishing the role of different aspects of hostility in immunity provides a good model. Here it seems that cynicism may be the driving force, suggesting that a particular component of hostility—general feelings of belief and trust in others—may be the important characteristic to focus on.

Stronger methodological approaches are also required. Especially in studies of markers of immunity, there is a tendency to use available samples, often students. However, in many cases *young healthy adults are inappropriate* because there is relatively little variance in their immune function and especially in markers of underlying disease such as chronic underlying inflammation (circulating CRP and IL-6). Moreover, the older one gets, the longer he or she has been exposed to the pathways linking personality to immunity, such as smoking or SNS activation. Similarly, and often because of the high cost of conducting studies, the sample sizes are small when considering the probable effect sizes and the noise often inherent in assessing functional immunity. Underpowered studies can mislead the field about the importance of addressing specific questions. Finally, there is a need to carefully consider controls for third factor variables in correlational studies. Personality traits and immunity both vary with demographics, with health, and with physical status (e.g., body mass); reasonable attempts to assess and control for these variables are imperative.

Finally, an important hypothesis concerns the potential role of personality in moderating the effects of stress on immunity. Here again, the development of appropriate theoretical approaches to each trait is essential. Why would we expect a trait to buffer or exacerbate the effects of stress? Should moderating effects look the same in healthy versus unhealthy (e.g., HIV) —or younger versus older, or male versus female—populations? Should there be some kind of match between the type of stressor and type of trait? For example, hostility (a characteristic of social behavior) may exacerbate effects of social but not nonsocial stressors. Moreover, tests of interactions generally require large samples for adequate power. Finally, it is noteworthy that chronic and life-threatening diseases themselves often are major stressors, and associations between a personality trait and disease status or its progression may actually be driven by its moderating effects of the stress experience as opposed to a direct (main) effect on disease.

Related Chapters

For more information on concepts introduced in this chapter, see also Suarez; Pressman; and Booth, this volume.

Author Note

Preparation of this chapter was supported by AI066367, HL092858 and a minority supplement from the National Institute of Allergy and Infectious Diseases.

References

Ahrens, A. H., & Haaga, D. A. F. (1993). The specificity of attributional style and expectations to positive and negative affectivity, depression, and anxiety. *Cognitive Therapy and Research, 17,* 83–98.

Arranz, L., Guayerbas, N., & De la Fuente, M. (2007). Impairment of several immune functions in anxious women. *Journal of Psychosomatic Research, 62,* 1–8.

Asendorpf, J. B. (1993). Social inhibition: A general–developmental perspective. In H. C. Traue & J. W. Pennebaker (Eds.), *Emotion, inhibition, and health* (pp. 80–99). Seattle, WA: Hogrefe & Huber.

Barefoot, J. C., Dodge, K. A., Peterson, B. L., Dahlstrom, W. G., & Williams, R. B. (1989). The Cook-Medley Hostility Scale: Item content and ability to predict survival. *Psychosomatic Medicine, 51,* 46–57.

Barefoot, J. C., Peterson, B. L., Dahlstrom, W. G., Siegler, I. C., Anderson, N. B., & Williams, R. B. J. (1991). Hostility patterns and health implications: Correlates of Cook-Medley Hostility Scale scores in a national survey. *Health Psychology, 10*(1), 18–24.

Beck, A. T., Epstein, N., Brown, G., & Steer, R. A. (1988). An inventory for measuring clinical anxiety: Psychometric properties. *Journal of Consulting and Clinical Psychology, 56,* 893–897.

Borella, P., Bargellini, A., Rovesti, S., Pinelli, M., Vivoli, R., Solfrini, V., et al. (1999). Emotional stability, anxiety, and natural killer activity under examination stress. *Psychoneuroendocrinology, 24,* 613–627.

Bouhuys, A. L., Flentge, F., Oldehinkel, A. J., & van den Berg, M. D. (2004). Potential psychosocial mechanisms linking depression to immune function in elderly subjects. *Psychiatry Research, 127*(3), 237–245.

Brennan, F. X., & Charnetski, C. J. (2000). Explanatory style and immunoglobulin A (IgA). *Integrative Psychological and Behavioral Science, 35*(4), 251–255.

Broadbent, D. E., Broadbent, R., Phillpotts, J., & Wallace, J. (1984). Some further studies on the prediction of experimental colds in volunteers by psychological factors. *Journal of Psychosomatic Research, 28,* 511–523.

Brummett, B. H., Boyle, S. H., Ortel, T. L., Becker, R. C., Siegler, I. C., & Williams, R. B. (2010). Associations of depressive symptoms, trait hostility, and gender with C-reactive protein and interleukin-6 response after emotion recall. *Psychosomatic Medicine, 72*(4), 333–339.

Brydon, L., Walker, C., Wawrzyniak, A. J., Chart, H., & Steptoe, A. (2009). Dispositional optimism and stress-induced changes in immunity and negative mood. *Brain, Behavior, and Immunity, 23*(6), 810–816.

Buss, A., & Durkee, A. (1957). An inventory for assessing different kinds of hostility. *Journal of Consulting Psychology, 21,* 343–349.

Buss, A. H., & Perry, M. P. (1992). The aggression questionnaire. *Journal of Personality & Social Psychology, 63,* 452–459.

Carver, C. S., & Scheier, M. (2008). *Perspectives on personality* (6th ed.). Boston, MA: Allyn & Bacon.

Carver, C. S., Scheier, M. F., & Segerstrom, S. C. (2010). Optimism. *Clinical Psychology Review, 30,* 879–889.

Cassidy, L., Meadows, J., Catalon, J., & Barton, S. (1997). Are reported stress and coping style associated with frequent recurrence of genital herpes? *Genitourinary Medicine, 73,* 263–266.

Cattell, H. E. P. (2005). *Spanish-American 16PF questionnaire technical manual: A pan-Spanish psychological assessment.* Champaign, IL: Institute for Personality and Ability Testing.

Christensen, A. J., Edwards, D. L., Wiebe, J. S., Benotsch, E. G., McKelvey, L., Andrews, M., et al. (1996). Effect of verbal self-disclosure on natural killer cell activity: Moderating influence of cynical hostility. *Psychosomatic Medicine, 58*(2), 150–155.

Clark, L. A., Watson, D., & Leeka, J. (1989). Diurnal variation in the positive affects. *Motivation and Emotion, 13,* 205–234.

Cohen, S., Alper, C. M., Doyle, W. J., Treanor, J. J., & Turner, R. B. (2006). Positive emotional style predicts resistance to illness after experimental exposure to rhinovirus or influenza A virus. *Psychosomatic Medicine, 68,* 809–815.

Cohen, S., Doyle, W. J., Skoner, D. P., Rabin, B. S., & Gwaltney, J. M., Jr. (1997). Social ties and susceptibility to the common cold. *Journal of the American Medical Association, 277,* 1940–1944.

Cohen, S., Doyle, W. J., Turner, R. B., Alper, C. M., & Skoner, D. P. (2003a). Sociability and susceptibility to the common cold. *Psychological Science, 14,* 389–395.

Cohen, S., Doyle, W. J., Turner, R. B., Alper, C. M., & Skoner, D. P. (2003b). Emotional style and susceptibility to the common cold. *Psychosomatic Medicine, 65,* 652–657.

Cohen, S., & Edwards, J. R. (1989). Personality characteristics as moderators of the relationship between stress and disorder. In R. W. J. Neufeld (Ed.), *Advances in the investigation of psychological stress.* New York: Wiley.

Cohen, F., Kearney, K. A., Zegans, L. S., Kemeny, M. E., Neuhaus, J. M., & Stites, D. P. (1999). Differential immune system changes with acute and persistent stress for optimists vs pessimists. *Brain, Behavior, and Immunity, 13*(2), 155–174.

Cole, S. W. (1996). *UCLA Rejection Sensitivity Scale*: Unpublished psychometric instrument.

Cole, S. W., Kemeny, M. E., Fahey, J. L., Zack, J. A., & Naliboff, B. D. (2003). Psychological risk factors for HIV pathogenesis: Mediation by the autonomic nervous system. *Biological Psychiatry, 54,* 1444–1456.

Cole, S. W., Kemeny, M. E., Weitzman, O. B., Schoen, M., & Anton, P. A. (1999). Socially inhibited individuals show heightened DTH response during intense social engagement. *Brain, Behavior, and Immunity, 13*(2), 187–200.

Cook, W., & Medley, D. (1954). Proposed hostility and pharasaic-virtue scales for the MMPI. *Journal of Applied Psychology, 38,* 414–418.

Costa, P. T., & McCrae, R. R. (1985). *The NEO personality inventory manual.* Odessa, FL: Psychological Assessment Resources.

Costa, P. T., & McCrae, R. R. (1995). Domains and facets: Hierarchical personality assessment using the Revised NEO Personality Inventory. *Journal of Personality Assessment, 64,* 21–50.

Costa, P. T. J., & McCrae, R. R. (1992). *Revised NEO personality inventory (NEO-PI-R) and the NEO five-factor inventory (NEO-FFI) professional manual.* Odessa, FL: Psychological Assessment Resources.

Doyle, W. J., Gentile, D. A., & Cohen, S. (2006). Emotional style, nasal cytokines, and illness expression after experimental rhinovirus exposure. *Brain, Behavior, and Immunity, 20,* 175–181.

Eisenberger, N. I., Kemeny, M. E., & Wyatt, G. E. (2003). Psychological inhibition and CD4 t-cell levels in HIV-seropositive women. *Journal of Psychosomatic Research, 54,* 213–224.

Esterling, B. A., Antoni, M. H., Kumar, M., & Schneiderman, N. (1993). Defensiveness, trait anxiety, and Epstein-Barr viral capsid antigen antibody titers in healthy college students. *Health Psychology, 12*(2), 132–139.

Everson-Rose, S. A., Lewis, T. T., Karavolos, K., Matthews, K. A., Sutton-Tyrrell, K., & Powell, L. H. (2006). Cynical hostility and carotid atherosclerosis in African American and white women: The Study of Women's Health Across the Nation (SWAN) heart study. *American Heart Journal, 152*(5), 952. e957–952.e913.

Eysenck, H. J. (1967). *The biological basis of personality.* Springfield, IL: Thomas.

Eysenck, H. J., & Eysenck, S. B. G. (1968). *Manual of the Eysenck personality inventory.* San Diego, CA: Educational and Industrial Testing Service.

Eysenck, H. J., & Eysenck, S. B. G. (1975). *Manual of the Eysenck personality questionnaire.* San Diego, CA: Educational and Industrial Testing Service.

Eysenck, S. B. G. (1965). *Manual of the junior Eysenck personality inventory.* London: University of London Press.

Fincham, D., Smit, J., Carey, P., Stein, D. J., & Seedat, S. (2008). The relationship between behavioural inhibition, anxiety disorders, depression and CD4 counts in HIV-positive adults: A cross-sectional controlled study. *AIDS Care, 20*(10), 1279–1283.

Goldberg, L. R. (1981). Language and individual differences: The search for universals in personality lexicons. In L. Wheeler (Ed.), *Review of personality and social psychology* (Vol. 2). Beverly Hills, CA: Sage.

Goldberg, L. R. (1992). The development of markers for the Big Five Factor structure. *Psychological Assessment, 4,* 26–42.

Gonzales-Quijano, M. I., Martin, M., Millan, S., & Lopez-Calderon, A. (1998). Lymphocyte response to mitogens: Influence of life events and personality. *Neuropsychobiology, 38,* 90–96.

Ironson, G., Balbin, E., Stuetzle, R., Fletcher, M. A., O'Cleirigh, C., Laurenceau, J. P., et al. (2005). Dispositional optimism and the mechanisms by which it predicts slower disease progression in HIV: Proactive behavior, avoidant coping, and depression. *International Journal of Behavioral Medicine, 12*(2), 86–97.

Ironson, G. H., O'Cleirigh, C., Weiss, A., Schneiderman, N., & Costa, P. T. (2008). Personality and HIV disease progression: Role of NEO-PI-R openness, extraversion, and profiles of engagement. *Psychosomatic Medicine, 70*(2), 245–253.

Janicki-Deverts, D., Cohen, S., & Doyle, W. J. (2010). Cynical hostility and stimulated Th1 and Th2 cytokine production. *Brain, Behavior, and Immunity, 24*(1), 58–63.

Kamen-Siegel, L., Rodin, J., Seligman, M. E. P., & Dwyer, J. (1991). Explanatory style and cell-mediated immunity in elderly men and women. *Health Psychology, 10,* 229–235.

King, L. A., & Emmons, R. A. (1990). Conflict over emotional expression: Psychological and physical correlates. *Journal of Personality & Social Psychology, 58*(5), 864–877.

Kohut, M. L., Cooper, M. M., Nickolaus, M. S., Russell, D. R., & Cunnick, J. E. (2002). Exercise and psychosocial factors modulate immunity to influenza vaccine in elderly individuals. *Journals of Gerontology: Series A. Biological Sciences and Medical Sciences, 57,* 557–562.

Larsen, R. J., & Diener, E. (1992). Promises and problems with the circumplex model of emotions. In M. S. Clark (Ed.), *Emotion* (pp. 25–59). Newburg Park, CA: Sage.

Lee, D. J., Meehan, R. T., Robinson, C., Smith, M. L., & Mabry, T. R. (1995). Psychosocial correlates of immune responsiveness and illness episodes in US Air Force Academy cadets undergoing basic cadet training. *Journal of Psychosomatic Research, 39*(4), 445–457.

Livesley, W. J., Jackson, D. N., & Schroeder, M. L. (1992). Factorial structure of traits delineating personality disorders in clinical and general population samples. *Journal of Abnormal Psychology, 3,* 432–440.

Mackay, C., Cox, T., Burrows, G., & Lazzerini, T. (1978). An inventory for the measurement of self-reported stress and arousal. *Journal of Social and Clinical Psychology, 17,* 283–284.

Marsland, A. L., Cohen, S., Rabin, B. S., & Manuck, S. B. (2001). Associations between stress, trait negative affect, acute immune reactivity, and antibody response to hepatitis B injection in healthy young adults. *Health Psychology, 20*(1), 4–11.

Marsland, A. L., Prather, A. A., Peterson, K. L., Cohen, S., & Manuck, S. B. (2008). Antagonistic characteristics are positively associated with inflammatory markers independently of trait negative emotionality. *Brain, Behavior, and Immunity, 22,* 753–761.

Marsland, A. L., Cohen, S., Rabin, B. S., & Manuck, S. B. (2006). Trait positive affect and antibody response to hepatitis B vaccination. *Brain, Behavior, and Immunity, 20,* 261–269.

McCrae, R. R., & Costa, P. T., Jr. (1987). Validation of the five-factor model of personality across instruments and observers. *Journal of Personality and Social Psychology, 52,* 81–90.

Milam, J. E., Richardson, J. L., Marks, G., Kemper, C. A., & McCutchan, A. J. (2004). The roles of dispositional optimism and pessimism in HIV disease progression. *Psychology & Health, 19*(2), 167–181.

Miller, G. E., Cohen, S., Rabin, B. S., Skoner, D. P., & Doyle, W. J. (1999). Personality and tonic cardiovascular, neuro-endocrine and immune parameters. *Brain, Behavior, and Immunity, 13,* 109–123.

Miller, G. E., Dopp, J. M., Myers, H. F., Stevens, S. Y., & Fahey, J. L. (1999). Psychosocial predictors of natural killer cell mobilization during marital conflict. *Health Psychology, 18*(3), 262–271.

Miller, G. E., Freedland, K. E., Carney, R. M., Stetler, C. A., & Banks, W. A. (2003). Cynical hostility, depressive symptoms, and the expression of inflammatory risk markers for coronary heart disease. *Journal of Behavioral Medicine, 26*(6), 501–515.

Mills, P. J., Dimsdale, J. E., Nelesen, R. A., & Dillon, E. (1996). Psychologic characteristics associated with acute stressor-induced leukocyte subset redistribution. *Journal of Psychosomatic Research, 40*(4), 417–423.

Morag, M., Morag, A., Reichenberg, A., Lerer, B., & Yirmiya, R. (1999). Psychological variables as predictors of rubella antibody titers and fatigue: A prospective, double blind study. *Journal of Psychiatric Research, 33*(5), 389–395.

O'Cleirigh, C., Ironson, G., Weiss, A., & Costa, P. T. (2007). Conscientiousness predicts disease progression (CD4 number and viral load) in people living with HIV. *Health Psychology, 26*(4), 473–480.

O'Donovan, A., Lin, J., Dhabhar, F. S., Wolkowitz, O., Tillie, J. M., Blackburn, E., et al. (2009). Pessimism correlates with leukocyte telomere shortness and elevated interleukin-6 in post-menopausal women. *Brain, Behavior, and Immunity, 23,* 446–449.

Paunonen, S. V., & Ashton, M. C. (2001). Big Five factors and facets and the prediction of behavior. *Journal of Personality and Social Psychology, 81,* 524–539.

Peterson, C., Luborsky, L., & Seligman, M. E. P. (1983). Attributions and depressive mood shifts: A case study using the symptom-context method. *Journal of Abnormal Psychology, 92,* 96–103.

Peterson, C., Semmel, A., von Baeyer, C., Abramson, L. Y., Metalsky, G. I., & Seligman, M. E. P. (1982). The Attributional Style Questionnaire. *Cognitive Therapy and Research, 6*(3), 287–299.

Peterson, C., & Vaidya, R. S. (2001). Explanatory style, expectations, and depressive symptoms. *Personality and Individual Differences, 31,* 1217–1223.

Peterson, C., & Villanova, P. (1988). An expanded Attributional Style Questionnaire. *Journal of Abnormal Psychology, 97*(1), 87–89.

Phillips, A. C., Carroll, D., Burns, V. E., & Drayson, M. (2005). Neuroticism, cortisol reactivity, and antibody response to vaccination. *Psychophysiology, 42*(2), 232–238.

Prather, A. A., Marsland, A. L., Muldoon, M. F., & Manuck, S. B. (2007). Positive affective style covaries with stimulated IL-6 and IL-10 production in a middle-aged community sample. *Brain, Behavior, and Immunity, 21*(8), 1033–1037.

Pressman, S., Cohen, S., Miller, G. E., Barkin, A., Rabin, B. S., & Treanor, J. J. (2005). Loneliness, social network size, and immune response to influenza vaccination in college freshmen. *Health Psychology, 24,* 297–306.

Reznick, J. S., Hegeman, I. M., Kaufman, E. R., Woods, S. W., & Jacobs, M. (1992). Retrospective and concurrent self-report of behavioural inhibition and their relation to adult mental health. *Development and Psychopathology, 4,* 301–321.

Ross, R. (1999). Mechanisms of disease: Atherosclerosis—An inflammatory disease. *The New England Journal of Medicine, 340,* 115–126.

Roy, B., Diez-Roux, A. V., Seeman, N., Ranjit, N., Shea, S., & Cushman, M. (2010). Association of optimism and pessimism with inflammation and hemostasis in the Multi-Ethnic Study of Atherosclerosis (MESA). *Psychosomatic Medicine, 72*(2), 134–140.

Scheier, M. F., & Carver, C. S. (1985). Optimism, coping, and health: Assessment and implications of generalized outcome expectancies. *Health Psychology, 4*(3), 219–247.

Scheier, M. F., Carver, C. S., & Bridges, M. W. (1994). Distinguishing optimism from neuroticism (and trait anxiety, self-mastery, and self-esteem): A reevaluation of the Life Orientation Test. *Journal of Personality & Social Psychology, 67*(6), 1063–1078.

Segerstrom, S. C. (2001). Optimism, goal conflict, and stressor-related immune change. *Journal of Behavioral Medicine, 24*(5), 441–467.

Segerstrom, S. C. (2006). How does optimism suppress immunity? Evaluation of three affective pathways. *Health Psychology, 25,* 653–657.

Segerstrom, S. C., & Miller, G. E. (2004). Psychological stress and the human immune system: A meta-analytic study of 30 years of inquiry. *Psychological Bulletin, 104,* 601–630.

Segerstrom, S. C., Taylor, S. E., Kemeny, M. E., & Fahey, J. L. (1998). Optimism is associated with mood, coping, and immune change in response to stress. *Journal of Personality & Social Psychology, 74*(6), 1646–1655.

Shea, J. D. C., Burton, R., & Girgis, A. (1993). Negative affect, absorption, and immunity. *Physiology & Behavior, 53*(3), 449–457.

Smith, T. W. (1992). Hostility and health: Current status of a psychosomatic hypothesis. *Health Psychology, 11,* 139–150.

Stewart, J. C., Janicki-Deverts, D., Muldoon, M. F., & Kamarck, T. W. (2008). Depressive symptoms moderate the influence of hostility on serum interleukin-6 and C-reactive protein. *Psychosomatic Medicine, 70,* 197–204.

Suarez, E. C. (2003). Joint effect of hostility and severity of depression symptoms on plasma interleukin-6 concentration. *Psychosomatic Medicine, 65,* 523–527.

Suarez, E. C., Lewis, J. G., Krishnan, R. R., & Young, K. H. (2004). Enhanced expression of cytokines and chemokines by blood monocytes to in vitro lipopolysaccharide stimulation are associated with hostility and severity of depressive symptoms in healthy women. *Psychoneuroendocrinology, 29,* 1119–1128.

Suarez, E. C., Lewis, J. G., & Kuhn, C. (2002). The relation of aggression, hostility, and anger to lipopolysaccharide-stimulated tumor necrosis factor (TNF)-alpha blood monocytes from normal men. *Brain, Behavior, and Immunity, 16,* 675–684.

Suls, J., & Wan, C. K. (1993). The relationship between trait hostility and cardiovascular reactivity: A quantitative review and analysis. *Psychophysiology, 30*(6), 615–626.

Sutin, A. R., Terracciano, A., Deiana, B., Naitza, S., Ferrucci, L., Uda, M., et al. (2010). High neuroticism and low conscientiousness are associated with interleukin-6. *Psychological Medicine, 40,* 1485–1493.

Taylor, J. A. (1953). A personality scale of manifest anxiety. *Journal of Abnormal and Social Psychology, 48*(2), 285–290.

Tellegen, A. (1982). *Brief manual for the Differential Personality Questionnaire.* Unpublished manuscript. Minneapolis, MN: University of Minnesota.

Terracciano, A. (2003). The Italian version of the NEO PI-R: Conceptual and empirical support for the use of targeted rotation. *Personality and Individual Differences, 35,* 1859–1872.

Tomakowsky, J., Lumley, M. A., Markowitz, N., & Frank, C. (2001). Optimistic explanatory style and dispositional optimism in HIV-infected men. *Journal of Psychosomatic Research, 51*(4), 577–587.

Totman, R., Kiff, J., Reed, S. E., & Craig, J. W. (1980). Predicting experimental colds in volunteers from different measures of recent life stress. *Journal of Psychosomatic Research, 24,* 155–163.

Willoughby, R. R. (1932). Some properties of the Thurstone Personality Schedule and a suggested revision. *Journal of Social Psychology, 3,* 401–424.

The Association Between Measures of Inflammation and Psychological Factors Associated with an Increased Risk of Atherosclerotic Cardiovascular Disease: Hostility, Anger and Depressed Mood and Symptoms

Edward C. Suarez

Abstract

Inflammation is acknowledged as a risk factor for the onset and development of cardiovascular disease (CVD). This has led some to hypothesize that inflammation is a possible mechanism that may mediate, in part, the relation of CVD to factors associated with increased CVD risk—hostility, anger, and depression. This chapter reviews the empirical evidence of the associations between biomarkers of inflammation and hostility, anger and depression, alone and in combination. Before doing so, I present a brief description and review of the role of inflammation in disease development and the methods used to measure inflammation at point-of-care and in research laboratories. Lastly, I review preliminary data suggesting that gender and adiposity may potentially mediate and moderate the relationship between depression and inflammation.

Key Words: Inflammation, cytokines, hostility, anger, depression, depressive symptoms, cardiovascular. disease, gender

Notae vero inflammationis sunt quattuor: rubor et tumour
cum calore et dolore [There are four signs of inflammation—
redness, swelling, heat and pain]
—Aulus Cornelius (Celsus), *De Medicina*

Introduction

It was not long ago that atherosclerotic cardiovascular disease (ACVD) was primarily thought to be a lipid-storage disease. The build-up of atherosclerotic plaque as a result of the deposit of lipids within the artery wall was considered a key mechanism leading to atherosclerosis. As the plaque grew in size, blood supply was diminished resulting in cardiovascular events such as myocardial infarction (MI). In the last three decades, however, accumulating evidence suggests that atherosclerosis is more complex than lipid accumulation. In fact, atherosclerosis is now understood to be the result of complex interactions among lipid constituents and specific cellular and molecular responses associated with inflammation (Ross, 1986; Libby et al., 2009). These interactions result in a chronic and evolving inflammatory fibro-proliferative response against harmful factors acting on the vascular wall (Ross, 1999). That inflammation plays a significant role at all stages of ACVD has led researchers to examine the degree to which traditional and emerging risk factors of ACVD are associated with markers of inflammation and how such empirical evidence can help guide medical treatment (Libby et al., 2006).

That inflammation contributes significantly to the onset and development of ACVD has led some to speculate whether inflammation is associated with key psychological factors associated with disease, such as hostility, depression, and anger. In this chapter, I review initial evidence supporting the relation of hostility, anger, and depression to various biomarkers of inflammation, including circulating markers associated with disease risk (Rozanski, Blumenthal, & Kaplan, 1999) and in vitro measures of cellular mediated immunity. I review published studies linking inflammatory markers to hostility, depression, and anger, alone and in combination. In so doing, I also discuss preliminary evidence suggesting that the relation of psychological factors to inflammatory biomarkers may be moderated by gender and adiposity (Shelton & Miller, 2011). To better understand the relation of psychological factors to ACVD, it is important to understand the role of inflammation in disease onset and progression.

Risk Factors of Heart Disease

Reflecting the multicausal nature of ACVD, there is an abundance of evidence identifying various factors associated with a heightened risk of heart disease. This constellation of risk factors includes both nonmodifiable factors, such as increasing age, being male, and a family history of heart disease, and modifiable factors, such as smoking, elevated cholesterol, high blood pressure, physical inactivity, obesity, and diabetes mellitus. The extent to which exposure to modifiable risk factors incurs disease risk in asymptomatic patients is significant (Greenland et al., 2003). However, there are studies that have shown that coronary heart disease (CHD) can develop in individuals who do not have elevated cholesterol, a key modifiable risk factor (e.g.,Ridker, Rifai, Rose, Buring, & Cook, 2002). These latter observations have led some to suggest that traditional risk factors account for "only 50%" of the CHD. This frequently cited percentage has been shown to be inaccurate and that a more reasonable estimate of the contributions of traditional risk factors to CHD ranges from 75% to 98% (Magnus & Beaglehole, 2001; Kannel & Vasan, 2009). Given this, the question about the significance of the contribution of psychological and behavioral stress factors to CHD risk requires careful consideration within the context of the contribution of traditional risk factors (Rozanski et al., 1999). Although appearing relatively straightforward, such an evaluation is complex, given that exposure to many of the modifiable traditional risk factors, such as smoking, sedentary lifestyle, obesity, and poor dietary habits in adulthood are predicted by the level of hostility, anger, and depression in adolescence and early adulthood (Miller, Markides, Chiriboga, & Ray, 1995; Kahler, Strong, Niaura, & Brown, 2004; Weiss, Mouttapa, Cen, Johnson, & Unger, 2011; Camacho, Roberts, Lazarus, Kaplan, & Cohen, 1991). Such findings

have led some to postulate that the influence of psychological stress on disease may be via unhealthy behaviors such as smoking (Mainous et al., 2010).

It has also been proposed that sympathetic arousal may be a biologically plausible patho-physiological mechanism underlying the association between psychological factors and ACVD. Although most of this evidence stems from animal studies (Kaplan et al., 1983; Kaplan, Pettersson, Manuck, & Olsson, 1991), human studies have also shown that the magnitude of physiological responses to psychological stressors and the degree of physiological recovery are associated with markers of early ACVD. In light of this evidence, it has been suggested that psychological factors contribute to the onset and progression of cardiovascular disease via excessive and repeated episodes of sympathetic mediated hyperresponsivity to interpersonal stressors (Treiber et al., 2003; Brotman, Golden, & Wittstein, 2007). That inflammation is recognized to be a critical factor in ACVD has led to the hypothesis that psychological factors are associated with inflammation as a result of sympathoadrenalmedullary mediated responses to psychological stressors. Specifically, it is thought that excessive sympathetic arousal triggers an inflammatory response characterized by cellular and molecular phenotypic changes on peripheral leukocytes and release of pro-inflammatory cytokines that promote tethering of cellular leukocytes and subsequent leukocyte migration into the intima (Ross, 1999). This cascade of events from stress to inflammation may be particularly salient in hostile individuals where frequent bouts of anger have been shown to evoke excessive sympathetic arousal that could potentially trigger an inflammatory response (Suarez, Sasaki, Lewis, Williams, & Adams, 1996; Greeson et al., 2009).

The notion that psychological factors are associated with an immune response is not particularly novel. A number of studies have linked psychological distress to immunosuppression (Dantzer & Kelley, 1989). What is emerging, however, is that psychological distress may also evoke immune activation and specifically activation of the inflammatory response system. A number of animal studies have shown that stressful manipulations, such as immobilization, isolation, and open field, have been shown to increase circulating markers of inflammation. However, it was not until the 1990s that researchers began to examine the relation of psychosocial stress factors to biomarkers of inflammation. Initial studies showed that, among healthy adults, acute laboratory stressors alone increased cellular-adhesion molecules (Mills & Dimsdale, 1996). During the same time period, my laboratory showed that anger arousal during the Anger Recall Interview was associated with an increase in the expression of cytokines by peripheral blood monocytes from high-hostility, but not low-hostility, women (Suarez et al., 1996). Combined, these studies provided initial evidence that stress responses, and specifically emotional responses characterized by arousal of negative affect such as anger, could induce cellular and molecular changes consistent with an inflammatory phenotype. As reviewed in this chapter, these preliminary findings have been subsequently replicated and expanded to include other biomarkers of inflammation.

Conceptualizations of Depression, Hostility, and Anger in Cardiovascular Research

In addressing the hypothesis that psychological stress evokes an inflammatory responses it is important to define what constitutes stress. Unlike traditional risk factors such as cholesterol, blood pressure, and weight that are intrinsically well delineated and characterized, defining the concept of stress presents a greater challenge. This is due to the fact that the concept of stress encompasses diverse conceptualizations that reflect different dimensions. For researchers, stress is conceptualized as the organism's response to challenge. For the man or woman on the street, however, the term "stress" is frequently used to describe heightened emotional and mental responses to everyday events. In today's society, the phrase "I am stressed out" is the catch-all phrase to communicate to others that one is experiencing negative emotions, such as anger, tension, and anxiety, and/or changes in behaviors such as sleep, eating, and physical activities. Needless to say, the degree to which individuals report "being stressed" reflects their subjective evaluations of their emotional and physical state.

The same can be said of researchers when using the terms depression, hostility and anger. In the case of hostility and anger, researchers often used these two concepts interchangeably, but while they are related, they are distinct constructs (Smith, 1994). Similar conceptual ambiguity occurs when researchers refer to depression, especially in the cardiovascular disease literature. Review of published studies reveals that the term *depression* is used to refer to both a clinical diagnosis of depression and elevated levels of depressive symptoms. Differences in measurement instruments may also contribute to conceptual ambiguity. Hostility, for example has

at least 26 measures used in cardiovascular studies (Matthews, Jamison, & Cottington, 1985). Like hostility, there are at least 24 measures of anger (Martin, Watson, & Wan, 2000). These self-report measures of anger purport to assess dimensions of anger that reflect affective, cognitive, and behavioral components. The confusion between the constructs of anger and hostility goes beyond mere operationalization and extends to what is being assessed even when studies used the same instrument. Specifically, in studies that have used the same questionnaire, some researchers have described the measure as tapping aggression while others have identified it as a measure of anger and hostility (Martin et al., 2000).

To circumvent the conundrum regarding the conceptualization and operationalization of the hostility and anger constructs, some researchers have used statistical modeling to examine dimensions of hostility and anger (e.g., Martin et al., 2000; Suarez & Williams, 1990). Researchers using this approach have reported two- and three-factor models. Although the three-factor model attempts to discriminate the specific dimensions of hostility and anger, the two-factor model attempts to conceptualize hostility and anger within the context of the five-factor model of personality. The two-factor model is particularly relevant because it conceptualizes and discriminates the neurotic and antagonistic dimensions of hostility while including measures of anger (Suarez & Williams, 1990), dimensions that are consistent with the five-factor model of personality (Digman, 1990). In our study, indicators of neurotic hostility included the experience of anger subscales from the Buss-Perry Hostility Inventory (BPHI) (Bernstein & Gesn, 1997), neuroticism (one of the five factors) from the NEO-Personality Inventory (PI) (Costa & McCrae, 1985), and the propensity to suppress the outward expression of anger from Spielberger's Anger Expression Scale (Spielberger et al., 1985). Indicators of antagonistic hostility, on the other hand, were BPHI physical and verbal anger expression subscales and NEO-PI agreeableness (negatively weighted) or antagonism. As described in the following sections, neurotic and antagonistic hostility appear to be differentially correlated with measures of inflammation (Suarez, Lewis, & Kuhn, 2002).

For the most part, the conceptualization of depression in most cardiovascular studies reflects categorization of level of severity based on clinical diagnosis and depressive subtypes. As described in the Diagnostic and Statistical Manual of Mental

Disorder (DSM)—IV, clinical criteria for major depressive disorders (MDD) emphasize duration, depressed mood and anhedonia in conjunction with other symptoms (Beck, Steer, & Garbin, 1988; Brown, Shulberg, & Madonia, 1995). Specifically, MDD is defined as depressed mood and anhedonia in addition to 5 to 9 specific depressive symptoms lasting for a period of at least 2 weeks. Individuals who do not meet the full criteria for MDD often receive a diagnosis of minor depression (MinD) or subsyndromal or subthreshold depression (SSD). A diagnosis of MinD is indicated when an individual presents 2 to 4 depressive symptoms during a 2-week period and requires one of these symptoms to be either depressed mood or loss of interest or pleasure. A history of MDD excludes the possibility of MinD. Subthreshold depression, on the other hand, is defined as a depressive state having two or more symptoms of depression of the same quality as in MDD, excluding depressed mood and anhedonia (Judd, Rapaport, Paulus, & Brown, 1994). For SSD, the symptoms must be present for more than 2 weeks and be associated with social dysfunction. Lastly, another category often noted in the cardiovascular literature is dysthymic disorder. A diagnosis of dysthymia indicates a depressed mood existing for a period of at least 2 years. Although categorical diagnoses have relevance to psychiatric treatment, the use of diagnoses in CVD research may lead researchers to underestimate the effects of depression and depressive symptomatology on health (Musselman, Evans, & Nemeroff, 1998). That the relation of depression to cardiovascular disease is linear argues for examining the risk of disease along a continuum (Rozanski, Blumenthal, Davidson, Saab, & Kubzansky, 2005). Such differences limit the generalizability of findings from studies that only examine the relation of cardiovascular risk and inflammation to diagnostic categories to a larger percentage of the population that exhibits symptoms of depression not meeting clinical criteria but that is at an elevated risk for disease. Although the issues raised in the preceding section are beyond the scope of this chapter, it is important that the reader be cognizant of the complexities of the constructs being reviewed in this chapter and how these terms may serve as a proxy for various dimensions of the psychological construct and its severity. In this chapter, I emphasize three psychological factors that have received considerable attention in the CVD literature (Rozanski et al., 1999). These factors are depression, anger, and hostility. Although other stress measures have been linked to CVD (e.g., social isolation, anxiety), the emphasis on these three factors is based on the evidence from case-control, cross-sectional and prospective cohort studies of initially healthy individuals linking hostility, anger, and depression to various cardiovascular endpoints (Smith, 1992; Everson-Rose & Lewis, 2005; Ford et al., 1998; Chang, Ford, Meoni, Wang, & Klag, 2002; Chida & Steptoe, 2009). As described in the following sections, the majority of cardiovascular studies have examined the effects of these factors to CVD in isolation. As with the clustering of traditional and emerging risk factors (Dandona, Aljada, Chaudhuri, Mohanty, & Garg, 2005), it also widely acknowledged that these psychological factors tend to cluster within individuals (Suls & Bunde, 2005). There is also evidence to suggest that trait measures of hostility and anger predict future increases in depressive symptoms (Stewart et al., 2010; Busch, 2009). These latter observations are in line with the notion that daily life stressors can precipitate increases in anger, depressive mood, and depressive symptoms, aspects that are associated with hostility as a trait. Further strengthening the likelihood of these factors clustering, emerging evidence suggests that hostility, anger, and depression may share a common underlying biological pathway—dysregulation of the serotonin system (5-HT) (Kamarck et al., 2009). Given the evidence, it is puzzling why the majority of studies have focused on a single factor in isolation (Suls & Bunde, 2005). To address this issue, I will present preliminary data to suggest that the combination of these three factors may not only be the best predictor of disease incidence and risk (Rozanski et al., 1999; Boyle, Michlek, & Suarez, 2007), but also changes in markers of inflammation (Boyle, Jackson, & Suarez, 2007).

Hostility

Hostility is frequently used interchangeably with anger, and although these two concepts are distinct, the use of these terms often is confusing. For the purpose of this chapter, I will consider anger a negative emotion, whereas hostility will be conceptualized as a personality trait characterized by negative beliefs and attitudes about others, such as cynicism, mistrust, and the attribution of hostile intent (Barefoot & Lipkus, 1994). What is evident from the definition is that the construct of hostility is multidimensional, one that reflects cognitive, affective, and behavioral components (Barefoot & Lipkus, 1994). The multidimensional aspects of this construct are also reflected in frequently used measures—from self-report paper-and-pencil measures, such as the Cook and Medley Hostility Scale (Cook & Medley, 1954) and the Buss-Perry Hostility Inventory (BPHI) (Bernstein & Gesn, 1997), to the Structured Interview Potential for Hostility (Dembroski, MacDougall, Costa, & Grandits, 1989). Although they vary to some degree, for the most part these instruments appear to tap cognitive and behavioral dimensions of hostility. What is most important to know is that the previously mentioned questionnaires have been linked to CVD in some but not all studies (Miller, Smith, Turner, Guijarro, & Hallet, 1996).

Anger

In the literature, anger, can refer to either an emotional state or a psychological trait. When used as a trait, anger i refers to a person's predisposition to experience frequent and pronounced episodes of the emotional state of anger. As an emotional state, anger reflects a transitory subjective experience of angry affect. As with hostility, anger is often associated with aggression, but there is a distinction between these two concepts. In this chapter, aggression is defined as the physical and verbal actions resulting from anger. Not surprisingly, measures of hostility and trait anger are associated with both aspects of aggression, yet these correlations range from 0.30–0.50, suggesting that the shared variance between personality traits and aggression is moderate at best. Similarly, the shared variance among measures of verbal and physical aggression and anger expression is comparable to that between traits and aggression, suggesting that these terms encompass different aspects of anger. This is particularly the case for anger suppression, as measures of aggression do not correlate with measures of anger suppression.

Depression

In the cardiovascular literature, depression has been used to refer to an assortment of phenomena ranging from a categorical diagnosis to severity of depressive symptoms (Davidson, Rieckmann, & Rapp, 2005). As with hostility and anger, assessment of depression includes both clinical interviews and self-report scales with varying groupings of symptoms that reflect the broad use of the term *depression*. To guide the reader, the following sections will differentiate studies that used clinical diagnosis from those using continuous measures of symptom severity.

The Joint Effects of Psychological Factors and Cardiovascular Risk

A number of prospective studies have shown that depression, hostility, and anger independently predict the risk of coronary heart disease (CHD) (for review, see Rozanski et al., 2005; Smith & Ruiz, 2002; Yusuf et al., 2004). Moreover, the risk of CHD associated with the factors appears to be proportional to the degree of severity (e.g., Smith & Ruiz, 2002; Lesperance, Frasure-Smith, Talajic, & Bourassa, 2002). For the most part, methodological and statistical approaches employed by these studies have emphasized each factor in isolation (Suls & Bunde, 2005). As with the clustering of traditional risk factors that define the metabolic syndrome, psychological factors of hostility, anger, depression, and anxiety show high covariation, and there is the tendency for these factors to cluster within at-risk populations (e.g., Kareinen, Viitanen, Halonen, Lehto, & Laakso, 2001). Suls and Bunde (2005) have suggested that the conceptual and measurement overlap of these factors demands the development of more complex affect-disease models, models that will have direct implications for interpretation of prior studies, statistical analyses, prevention, and intervention in health psychology and behavioral medicine. In my laboratory, we have made a concerted effort to examine the joint effect of these factors not only on measures of disease (Boyle et al., 2007; Lemogne et al., 2010) but also on putative risk factors including inflammation (Suarez et al., 2002; Suarez, 2003). A similar approach was adopted by the researchers of the INTERHEART study who examined the effects of feeling irritable, perceived stress, depressive symptoms, recent stressful life events and locus of control (Rosengren et al., 2004). The case-control study was conducted in over 24,000 adults from 52 countries. Results indicated that people with myocardial infarction (MI cases) reported the experience of all stress factors and this association was independent of smoking, age, sex, ethnic group, and geographic region (Rosengren et al., 2004). Given these findings, it is reasonable to examine not only the effect of a single factor but their combined effects on health outcomes.

The notion that the presence of a mosaic of interrelated factors defines a subgroup of individuals and patients at heightened risk for new and recurring cardiac events has been reported in a number of studies. This is evident by reports from the THROMBO study of nondiabetic patients who had a documented myocardial infarction (Moss et al., 1999) suggesting that combinations of inflammatory and thrombotic factors identifies a subgroup of patients who are at elevated risk for recurrent events (Corsetti, Zareba, Moss, Rainwater, & Sparks, 2006). It has even been suggested that understanding the interaction between metabolic and inflammatory pathways may lead to improved therapeutic strategies (Fernandez-Real & Ricart, 2003). It is my opinion that this is also the case for psychological risk factors and potential pathophysiological and behavioral pathways contributing to ACVD. Although this chapter includes studies that report "main" effects, I will stress the importance of the interaction or joint effect among these three factors and how their interaction may be the best correlate and predictor of inflammation and CVD risk.

Inflammation and Disease

The body's primary response to infections, irritation, or injury is inflammation, a nonspecific immune response characterized by the release of an arsenal of mediators that include bioactive amines, eicosanoids, cytokines, chemokines, and growth factors (Silva, 1994). In response to this arsenal of mediators, the classic clinical symptoms of acute inflammation emerge: pain (*dolore*), heat (*calore*), redness (*rubor*), swelling (*tumour*) and loss of function (*function leasa*). The protective actions of inflammation are usually localized to the area of trauma or to the invading microbe and these actions aim to destroy, dilute, or wall off the injurious agent and the injured tissue. The inflammatory response guides immune system components to the site of the injury or infection by manifesting an increase in blood supply and increasing vascular permeability. These actions are also accompanied by the exudation of fluids including plasma protein, chemotatic peptides, and leukocyte migration in the inflammatory site. In tissue damage, the acute inflammatory response is a critical mechanism in isolating the damaged area, and mobilizing effector cells and molecules to the site while promoting healing. In infection, inflammatory responses protect the body by creating a barrier that prevents the pathogen from damaging the host. In these scenarios, inflammation occurs as a defensive response to trauma or invasion of the host by foreign material.

Advances in the understanding of inflammation and disease pathogenesis has led many to conclude that inflammation may contribute to many chronic diseases as diverse as diabetes, Alzheimer's disease, cataracts, cancer, and atherosclerosis. It is from this conclusion and a wealth of clinical and experimental evidence that today's view of atherosclerosis has emerged. The predominant thought is that the atherosclerotic process is fundamentally an inflammatory-fibroproliferative process (Ross, 1999), one that many now believe to be an inflammatory disease (Pearson et al., 2003). Toward understanding how inflammation contributes and characterizes atherosclerotic disease, I will briefly describe the processes contributing to atherosclerosis and subsequent clinical disease and the role of inflammation.

Inflammation, Atherosclerosis, and Atherosclerotic Lesions

The pathogenesis of atherosclerosis is believed to initiate as a result of injury to the artery wall and, specifically, to the lining of the artery or endothelium (Ross, Glomset, & Harker, 1977). It is speculated that injury can be caused by exposure to a number of different risk factors of atherosclerosis such as smoking, hypercholesterolemia, hypertension, elevations of homocysteine and other toxic factors as well as mechanical factors that occur at bifurcation sites. Although more controversial, it has been suggested that injury to the endothelium may also be infection-initiated (Saikku et al., 1992). Depending on the causative factor(s), the injury leads to inflammation (Libby & Theroux, 2005), endothelial dysfunction (Bonetti, Lerman, & Lerman, 2003), abnormal cellular interactions (Ross et al., 1977) and increases in oxidative stress and the production of reactive oxygen species (ROS) (Griendling & FitzGerald, 2003). Although the inflammatory response may be initially appropriate, if it becomes excessive and chronic it contributes to further injury and damage to the tissue. Prolonged inflammation is thought to promote further changes in the artery that advance the development of the atherosclerotic lesion that are differentiated by characteristic morphology (Stary et al., 1995). These morphological differences, however, are all characterized by inflammation.

Models of atherosclerosis in animals and humans have focused on the effects of hypercholesterolemia and the retention of atherogenic lipoprotein particles in the subendothelium (Skalen et al., 2002). It has been suggested that infiltration of these particles evokes an inflammatory response in the artery wall. Once in the endothelium, modification of the cholesterol particles leads to the release of phospholipids that can activate endothelial cells, a process that more likely occurs in lesion-prone areas of the arterial tree. As a result, monocytes and lymphocytes are recruited and accumulated due to the expression of specific leukocyte adhesion molecules by the vascular endothelium (Nakashima, Raines, Plump, Breslow, & Ross, 1998). The role of inflammation is not solely noted in the early stages of atherosclerosis but it also plays a role in more advanced lesions (Rosenfeld et al., 2000). In humans, inflammation is noticed in both activated plaques in patients with acute coronary syndrome but also in silent plaques.

It has been suggested that lesions of atherosclerosis (atheromata) may be arbitrarily divided into three categories: the early lesion or fatty streak, the intermediate or fibrofatty lesion, and the advanced or complicated lesion or fibrous plaque (Stary et al., 1994; Ross, 1999; Virmani, Kolodgie, Burke, Farb, & Schwartz, 2000). Models of atherosclerosis in hypercholesterolemic nonhuman primates have shown that one of the earliest events in atherosclerosis is the entrance of lipids into the intima (Faggiotto, Ross, & Harker, 1984). Soon thereafter, there is an increased adherence of monocytes and lymphocytes to the intimal surface, evidence for the initial involvement of the immune system and specifically cellular components of the inflammatory responses (Faggiotto et al., 1984; Faggiotto & Ross, 1984). The early lesion or fatty streak is characterized by a yellow discoloration on the surface of the artery that is caused by lipid accumulation in foam cells, most of which are lipid-filled macrophages making up the bulk of the lesion (Hansson, 2001; Daugherty, Rateri, & Lu, 2008). Studies of these early lesions have shown that earliest fatty streaks consist entirely of lipid-laden, monocyte-derived macrophages together with T-lymphocytes (Emeson & Robertson, 1988; Jonasson, Holm, Skalli, Bondjers, & Hansson, 1986). With progression, smooth muscle cells appear and the accumulation of macrophages and T lymphocytes are superimposed or are intermixed with the accumulations of smooth muscle and connective tissue. Extension of the proatherogenic processes contributing to early lesions leads to further thickening of the intima and subsequent intrusion of the intima into the lumen of the artery (Jonasson et al, 1986).

Assessment of Inflammation in Clinical and Research Settings

The knowledge that inflammation played an important role in atherosclerotic cardiovascular disease (ACVD) stimulated the development of more sophisticated and sensitive laboratory tests to measure inflammation. In vivo measures of immunity such as white blood cell count and fibrinogen were used in early studies of the association of inflammation to CVD (Meade et al., 1986; Kannel, Wolf, Castelli, & D'Agostino, 1987; Yarnell et al., 1991). Although useful in initially demonstrating the relationship between inflammation and CVD, these initial findings stimulated the development of other platforms to assess inflammation. The challenge was that the degree of inflammation suspected of contributing to heart disease was not associated with acute trauma or clinical diseases, but with low levels of inflammation that required highly sensitive assays. Out of this need came the development of the highly sensitive C-reactive protein (CRP) assay. Although CRP was discovered in 1930, it was not until the 1940s that CRP was described as an acute-phase reactant that was elevated among patients with conditions that were characterized by inflammation (McCarty, 1947). In the 1980s and 1990s, prospective and cross-sectional studies linked CRP to atherosclerosis (Kuller, Tracy, Shaten, & Meilahn, 1996). The challenge, however, was that the CRP levels associated with cardiovascular risk were often below the detectable levels of the available assay. This led to the development and validation of a high-sensitivity (hs) assay to measure CRP. The commercial availability of hsCRP assay allowed physicians and researchers to evaluate in vivo inflammation with greater sensitivity.

The hsCRP assay joined other in vivo tests used to examine immune-system status and responses in situ. Other assays include humoral measure of complement, alpha1-acid glycoprotein, alpha1-antitrypsin haptoglobin, and immunoglobulin plasma measures of circulating cytokines and their soluble receptors. Acute phase proteins include not only CRP and fibrinogen but also serum ferritin, serum albumins, serums amyloid A, and transferrin protein that are continually produced in the liver.

The selection of assay in the clinical setting is frequently guided by the relevance to diagnosis and the availability of the assay. In contrast, the selection of assay in research settings rests on various factors that include the specific aims of the study, characteristics of the study population (e.g., age, gender, health status, medication use), sampling rates (e.g., hours or days versus years or decades), and storage (e.g., fresh samples versus frozen). In addition to procedures used to measure humoral factors, research procedures to assess inflammations include enumerative and functional measures. Enumerative procedures are those techniques such as flow cytometry that measure the number and percentages of various immune cells by gating on specific cellular surface markers (e.g., CD14, CD56, CD11/CD18) or by measuring intracellular cytokine expression by specific circulating cells such as CD14+ monocytes (Suarez, Krishnan, & Lewis, 2003).

There has been a concerted effort by industry to develop commercially available assays that are appropriately standardized so as to allow comparisons of results across studies ("C-reactive protein testing," 2009). A cursory review of articles published in recent years show that the most frequently used commercial assays to assess circulating levels of inflammatory biomarkers as they relate to CVD were: (a) soluble adhesion molecules such as E-selectin, P-selectin, intracellular adhesion molecules-1, and vascular cell adhesion molecules-1; (b) cytokines such as interleukin (IL)-1beta, IL-6, IL-8 and IL-10, and tumor necrosis factor-alpha; (c) acute-phase reactants such as fibrinogen, high sensitivity C-reactive protein, serum amyloid A; (d) white blood cell counts (e.g., total white blood cells, number of mononuclear blood cells). Although all the individual biomarkers have been associated with CVD in prospective studies (e.g., Woodward, Rumley, Tunstall-Pedoe, & Lowe, 1999; Ridker, Hennekens, Roitman-Johnson, Stampfer, & Allen, 1998; Hwang et al., 1997; Ridker & Haughie, 1998; Luc et al., 2003), the most often used has been high sensitivity C-reactive protein (hsCRP) (Ridker, 2007).

Although not exhaustive, the assays just listed allow for clinicians and researchers to assess circulating blood levels of biomarkers associated with inflammation with relative ease. Markers of inflammation such as white blood cells are simple to perform. In the case of hsCRP, commercially available assay kits also have allowed for ease of comparisons of results among research studies. What is important to understand is that, for the most part, the preceding listed measures of circulating biomarkers are nonspecific measures of inflammation. In other words, elevated levels of these inflammatory biomarkers do not reflect any specific factor that contributes to inflammation. Thus, elevated IL-6 and hsCRP may reflect the impact of factors ranging from adiposity, smoking, and exercise, to underlying inflammatory disease, to an acute infection or injury. Thus, it is important to interpret the results of any tests within the context of the individual's overall health status and vitals such as weight, age, and medications. This is particularly important in studies of patient populations in which elevations in acute phase proteins are likely to be noted.

Additional Measures of Inflammation in Research Settings

As previously described, measures of inflammation as it relates to CVD can be done using various methods that have quickly become commonly used in both clinical and research laboratories. Other measures of inflammation, however, are more complex and involve time-consuming procedures, some of which require that the test be conducted on fresh blood samples and not frozen. For the most part, the purpose of conducting these laboratory tests is to assess the complexity of the inflammatory system by quantifying cellular and molecular characteristics of the various components of the inflammatory response. The use of fluorescence flow cytometry and enzyme-linked immunosorbent assay (ELISA), alone or in conjunction with in vitro stimulation procedures, are often used to examine changes in cell populations, complexity, phenotype, and health, as well as production and expression of various cellular markers that allow for more detailed characterization of the inflammatory response.

Evidence for the Relation of Hostility, Anger, and Depression to Biomarkers of Inflammation

The preceding sections have provided a brief introduction to the concept of inflammation and a review of the most frequently examined psychological factors associated with CVD. In this section, I will review the evidence for the associations among measures of inflammation and depression, hostility and anger, alone and in combination. Although negative findings have been reported, the weight of the evidence from both cross-sectional and longitudinal studies in patient populations and healthy subjects suggests a relationship between markers of inflammation and psychological factors. What is clearly apparent is that the majority of studies have focused on depression. This may reflect the fact that researchers have long been interested in the effects of depression and immune function, and specifically the influence of depression on immune responses to infections and injury. Consistent with this notion, meta-analysis by Herbert and Cohen found that depression was significantly associated with decreases in immune parameters (Herbert & Cohen, 1993). In that same year, Smith proposed the macrophage-T-lymphocyte hypothesis of major depression (Smith, 1991). Smith posited that depression evoked immune activation and specifically inflammation, but that inflammation was a putative factor for depression (Smith, 1991). This novel hypothesis not only stimulated researchers to review the data already at hand (Maes, Smith, & Simon, 1995), but also to propose new studies to examine the relation of depression to biomarkers of inflammation.

In contrast to the large number of studies examining depression, far fewer studies have examined anger and hostility as they relate to inflammation. Of those studies that have assessed anger and hostility, the rationale for such assessment reflects evidence linking hostility and anger to CVD. However, as widely acknowledged, the influence of the immune system on the central nervous system (CNS) is reciprocal, in other words, bidirectional. It is not surprising that cytokines may facilitate the expression of aggressive behavior. Such a possibility reflects the fact that cytokines are present in the brain regions that are known to be associated with aggression and rage behaviors (Zalcman & Siegel, 2006). Although few in number, the results are remarkably consistent in documenting an association between inflammatory biomarkers and measures of anger and hostility, alone or in combination with depression (e.g., Suarez, 2004).

It is important to note that the majority of studies linking psychological factors to measures of inflammation have been cross-sectional in design. Few studies have examined the temporal relationship between depression and inflammation, and only one study has examined the sequential relation of anger and hostility preceding inflammation.

Depression

The notion that inflammation is associated with depression has been a topic of interest for many reasons, one of which is the biologically plausible hypothesis that inflammation may explain, in part, the depression-CVD association (Shimbo, Chaplin, Crossmna, Haas, & Davidson, 2005). This hypothesis rests on the notion that depression, via various mechanisms of action that include both biological and behavioral pathways, leads to a pro-inflammatory state characterized by enhanced cellular-mediated immunity (i.e., increases in monocytes and natural killer cells, increases in macrophage/monocyte derived cytokines, and increases in circulation complement and other acute phase proteins) (Maes, 2011), mechanisms contributing to the etiology of CVD (Shimbo et al., 2005). Although many have focused on the notion that depression precedes inflammation, others have speculated that depression is an inflammatory disease and that inflammation is a putative risk factor for the onset of depression and depressive symptoms (Maes, Smith, & Scharpe, 1995; Smith, 1991). Such a possibility leads to the notion that inflammation precedes depression and CVD, suggesting that the covariation often observed between depression and CVD is more likely an epiphenomenon (Shimbo et al., 2005). These two alternative hypotheses have been the target of considerable research efforts in determining the strength and directionality of the association between inflammation and depression.

A number of studies have examined the bidirectional nature of this association (Glover, Shaw, Williams, & Fildes, 2010; Adler, Marques, & Calil, 2008). In direct evidence for the potential impact of inflammation on depression stems from studies documenting elevated rates of depression in patients with inflammatory diseases including cardiovascular disease (Irwin, 2002). More direct evidence for a causal relation comes from studies where interferon-alpha and/or interleukin-2 were administered as part of treatment. For the most part, the evidence from those studies suggests that administration of INF-alpha or interleukin-2 evokes changes in mood and behaviors associated with depression (Capuron & Miller, 2004; Capuron, Ravaud, & Dantzer, 2000). Similar causal pathways have been demonstrated in studies of healthy adults with no history of depression or current symptoms of depression. In those studies, administration of low amounts of endotoxin and interleukin-2 reliably produced "sickness-like" behaviors that are consistent with depression (DellaGioia & Hannestad, 2010).

The temporal and relative strength of the association between inflammation and depression also underlies a third model suggesting that depression and inflammation are independent risk factors of CVD (Shimbo et al., 2005). In this case, the shared variance between depression and inflammation, even if significant, would not diminish the unique contributions of each factor to disease onset and progression. Two studies have explored the unique contributions of inflammation and depression or depressed mood in predicting future CHD (Empana et al., 2005) and CVD mortality risk (Kop et al., 2010). In both studies, measures of depression were significantly correlated with circulating inflammatory biomarkers such as CRP and IL-6. However, depression and inflammation were both significant predictors in multivariate analysis that included traditional risk factors. These results suggest that inflammation, although associated with depression, does not explain the significant relationship between depression and CVD and that depression does not increase the risk of CVD via inflammation alone. These preliminary findings need to be interpreted cautiously given the acknowledged limitations of the studies including the temporal relation of inflammation to episodic depression events. In both studies, depression was measured only at one time point. Interpretation of the results must also take into account that the study populations were relatively homogenous with respect to gender, race (Empana et al., 2005), and age (Kop et al., 2010), factors that are known to influence inflammation (O'Connor et al., 2009) and thus potentially moderate the relationship between depression and CHD.

OVERALL FINDINGS

A meta-analysis that included over 80 studies examined the relation of a diagnosis of depression (e.g., MDD) to approximately 40 measures of inflammation (Zorrilla et al., 2001). Using fixed-effect and random-effect modeling, these authors concluded that major depression "*may* be associated with immune activation reminiscent of an acute phase" (italic as used by study authors, p. 210). An acute phase response is a nonspecific and systemic immune reaction that is initiated by inflammatory processes and specifically cytokines from macrophages and circulating monocytes (Baumann & Gauldie, 1994).

As I noted in the preceding sections, studies that examine the effects of MDD cannot address whether markers of inflammation are associated with symptom severity of depression along a continuum. It is well recognized that an elevated risk of coronary disease is not restricted to a diagnosis of depression but extends to include severity of depressive symptoms that do not meet criteria for a clinical diagnosis (Wulsin & Singal, 2003). This dose-response association is similar to the associations of traditional risk factors to coronary risk and in particular, the case of low-density lipoprotein where a 1 mmol drop leads to a 25% reduction in the relative risk of vascular events (Yusuf, 2002). A similar dose-response has been shown for blood pressure, where reduction in blood pressure shows benefit across a wide range of hypertensive and nonhypertensive patients (Blood Pressure Lowering Treatment Trialist's Collaboration, 2003). Such observations lend support to the "lower is better" hypothesis (Heart Protection Study Collaborative Group, 2002). If incremental increases in depressive symptom severity are associated with increases in CVD risk, then it important to examine the relation of symptom severity to inflammation along a continuum.

CROSS-SECTIONAL STUDIES

There are a number of studies that have examined the cross-sectional relationship between markers of inflammation and severity of depressive symptoms along a continuum. Although various measures of severity of depressive symptoms have been used, the most often used instruments have been the Beck Depression Inventory (BDI) (Beck et al., 1988) and the Center for Epidemiologic Studies Depression (CESD) scale, both well-validated self-report scales. Other measures include the Hamilton Depression Rating Scale (HAM-D). For the most part, these studies have suggested that severity of depressive symptoms is associated with circulating levels of inflammatory biomarkers (Suarez, 2004; Hamer & Chida, 2009; Kobrosly & van Wijngaarden, 2010; Panagiotakos et al., 2004; Kop et al., 2002; Marsland, Sathanoori, Muldoon, & Manuck, 2007; Elovainio et al., 2009) in most but not all studies (Pan et al., 2008; Steptoe, Kunz-Ebrecht, & Owen, 2003). Reflecting the dose-dependent association between severity of depressive symptom and CVD (Rugulies, 2002), a recent meta-analysis suggested that inflammation increases incrementally, tracking increases in severity of depressive symptoms (Kobrosly & Wijngaarden, 2010). Studies included in the meta-analysis by Howren et al. (Howren, Lamkin, & Suls, 2009) primarily assessed CRP and IL-6, with considerably fewer studies measuring IL-1 and IL-1 receptor antagonist (ra). Using these inflammatory markers, the authors reported that depression and severity of depression were associated with inflammatory markers in both clinic- and community-based samples with the association showing a dose-related association (Howren et al., 2009). It was noted, however, that the effect size was larger for MDD than for severity of depressive symptoms.

Most published studies have used CRP and IL-6 as measures of inflammation (Howren et al., 2009). What is also important to note is that the most often used biomarkers of inflammation, CRP and IL-6, are nonspecific indicators of inflammation. Although circulating concentrations of these two biomarkers are known to predict CVD endpoints (Ridker, 2009; Ridker, Rifai, Stampfer, & Hennekens, 2000), the role of inflammation in atherosclerosis and its sequelae is thought to involve cellular and molecular responses associated with peripheral blood monocytes, monocyte-derived macrophages, and T lymphocytes. In atherosclerosis, it is hypothesized that the development and progression of atherosclerotic lesions involves monocyte-derived macrophages and T lymphocytes (Ross, 1999). Similarly, the basic premise of the monocyte-T-lymphocyte hypothesis of depression as proposed by Smith (1991) and expanded by Maes et al. (1995) emphasizes activation of peripheral blood monocytes and T lymphocytes as key cellular components in the development of depression. That role of peripheral monocytes and T lymphocytes in both depression and cardiovascular disease has prompted researchers to determine if depression is associated with monocyte and T lymphocyte function. In my laboratory, we have shown that severity of depressive symptoms is positively associated with stimulated expression of IL-1alpha, IL-1beta, IL-8, monocyte chemotactic protein (MCP)-1 and TNF-a (Suarez et al., 2003; Suarez, Lewis, Krishnan & Young, 2004) on peripheral monocytes from healthy controls. These initial observations have been partially replicated by Marsland et al. who showed that stimulated production of IL-8 by peripheral monocytes was positively associated with severity of depressive symptoms in a large community sample of healthy adults (Marsland et al., 2007). Together, these findings are consistent with one animal study that showed that exposure to chronic mild stress leading to mild anhedonia (operationalized as a reduction in sucrose intake with concomitant reduction in water intake) evoked increases in plasma levels of TNF-alpha and IL-1b (Grippo, Francis, Beltz, Felder, & Johnson, 2005). I note that the relationship between severity of depressive symptoms and IL-8 may be particularly important given that macrophages from atherosclerotic plaque show an enhanced capacity to produce IL-8 (Astolopoulos, Davenport, & Tipping, 1996).

The observations of an association between severity of depression and monocytic cytokines in community samples extends earlier reports of differences in monocyte function between healthy controls and patients with major depression (Schlatter, Ortuño, & Cervera-Enguix, 2004). In that study, Schlatter et al. showed that relative to healthy nondepressed controls, subjects with MDD and dysthymia showed greater stimulated production of IL-1beta and IL-6 by peripheral monocytes as well as elevated burst activity and phagocytosis (Schlatter et al., 2004). Overall, the evidence suggests that increased monocytic production of IL-1b, IL-6, and TNF-alpha reflect key and early markers of immune activation

and subsequent systemic inflammation associated with MDD and severity of depressive symptom (Maes, 1995).

PROSPECTIVE STUDIES

The evidence described in the preceding section emerges from cross-sectional studies of the relationship between inflammation and various aspects of depression. Although these studies provide positive support for this association, they do not address the issue of directionality. To best address this issue, it is necessary to examine this association in prospective studies (Howren et al., 2009). As of 2011, only a few studies have directly evaluated the temporal relationship between inflammatory biomarkers and depression (Boyle et al., 2007; Matthews et al., 2007; Stewart, Rand, Muldoon, & Kamarck, 2009; Von Känel, Bellingrath, & Kudielka, 2009; van den Biggelaar et al., 2007; Gimano et al., 2009; Kiecolt-Glaser et al., 2003; Hamer, Molloy, de Oliveira, & Demakakos, 2009) in healthy subjects and in patient populations (Shaffer et al., 2011; Wirtz, 2010).

Most of these prospective studies have examined whether depression precedes or predicts inflammation. For example, Kiecolt-Glaser (Kiecolt-Glaser et al., 2003) examined changes in IL-6 over a 6-year period in a group comparison study of older adults who were current or previous caregivers and noncaregivers. Relative to noncaregivers, caregivers showed increases in IL-6 during the 6-year follow-up period. These increases, however, were not associated with depressive symptoms as measured by the BDI (Kiecolt-Glaser et al., 2003). In contrast, Matthews et al. (2007) showed that in women going through the menopausal transition, depression predicted 5-year increases in fibrinogen even after adjusting for potential confounders including body mass index (BMI). The relation of depression at baseline to longitudinal changes in fibrinogen and CRP were also examined in adult men and women enrolled in the English Longitudinal Study of Aging (Hamer et al., 2009). Hamer et al. showed that depression, measured using the CESD, predicted 2-year changes in both CRP and fibrinogen. Using mediational analysis, Hamer et al. were able to demonstrate that the effects of depression on changes in CRP over time were both direct and indirect through behavioral risk factors. For fibrinogen, the association was completely accounted for by health behaviors. Lastly, in a large sample of healthy Vietnam veterans, Boyle et al. (2007) used the Minnesota Multiphasic Personality Inventory (MMPI) depression scale (Nelson & Cicchetti,

1991) to examine whether depression, alone and in combination with anger and hostility, predicted changes in C3 and C4 complement over a 10-year period. Results indicated that depression, both alone and in combination with anger and hostility, predicted increases in C3 complement but not C4 complement in a model adjusted for health, behavioral, and sociodemographic variables (including BMI).

Only one study has examined whether inflammation precedes changes in depression. Van den Biggelaar et al. (2007) examined the relation of depression, assessed by the 15-item Geriatric Depression Scale, and cognitive functioning, assessed by the Mini-Mental State Examination, to baseline inflammation in 85-year-old participants enrolled in a prospective population-based study of inhabitants in Leiden, the Netherlands (Leiden-85-plus study). Measures of inflammation include both in vivo CRP and albumin, and in vitro stimulated production of IL-1beta, IL-1ra, IL-6, and IL-10. Results indicated that higher baseline CRP preceded accelerated increases in depressive symptoms. Similarly, elevated production of IL-1beta predicted increases in depressive symptoms, and IL-1ra, the natural antagonist to IL-1beta, preceded smaller increases in depressive symptoms. None of the inflammatory markers predicted changes in cognitive decline.

Lastly, the remaining studies have examined the bidirectional nature of the relationship between depression and inflammation. These studies directly tested whether depression precedes inflammation and whether inflammation precedes depression. In a study of healthy adult men and women, Stewart et al. (2009) showed that severity of depressive symptoms, assessed at entry using the BDI-II, predicted changes in IL-6, but not in CRP, over a 6-year follow-up period. In contrast, baseline IL-6 and CRP failed to predict 6-year changes in BDI-II score. Such a pattern of results suggest that depression may influence downstream inflammation, but that inflammation may not evoke increases in severity of depressive symptoms in apparently older healthy adults.

IN PATIENT POPULATIONS

Two studies have examined the temporal relationship between depression and markers of inflammation in patient populations (Shaffler et al., 2011; Wirtz et al., 2010). In a sample of heart failure (HF) patients, Wirtz et al (2010) examined the relation of severity of depressive symptoms using the BDI to peripheral markers of inflammation, CRP, IL-6, and the soluble intracellular adhesion molecule-1 (sICAM-1). After controlling for baseline BDI, cardiovascular risk factors, HF severity and medications, baseline sICAM-1 predicted 12-month increases in BDI scores. C-reactive protein and IL-6 did not predict changes in BDI scores at 12-month follow-up.

Using path analysis, Shaffer et al. examined the relation of CRP to BDI score in a sample of adults with acute coronary syndrome (ACS) (Shaffer et al., 2011). Baseline measures were taken at the time of an acute cardiac event and at 1- and 3-months post cardiac event. Results indicated that baseline BDI score and the score for the cognitive-affective subscale predicted a smaller decrease in CRP from baseline to 1-month. Similar analysis failed to show that the somatic affective symptoms subscale predicts changes in CRP. Baseline CRP did not predict changes in BDI score at 1- and 3-months.

LIMITATIONS

For the most part, studies examining the association between depression and inflammation are cross-sectional studies. As widely acknowledged, a cross-sectional design cannot be used to examine directionality. Only seven longitudinal-prospective studies have examined the relation of depression predicting measures of inflammation at follow-up (Boyle et al., 2007; Stewart et al., 2009; Gimeno et al., 2009; Hamer et al., 2009). In addition to study design, significant variability is noted in other methodological design features across studies. These include differences in study populations (healthy controls versus patients), measures of depression (self report and clinical ratings), and measures of inflammation (acute phase proteins, humoral inflammatory measures, cellular function). Study populations appear to fall in one of three categories: community samples of apparently healthy subjects; psychiatric populations of subjects with major depressive disorder and other depression-related diagnosis; and subject with inflammatory diseases such as CVD, chronic obstructive pulmonary disease (COPD), and arthritis. Depression measures also vary, ranging from studies using well-validated clinical and self-report measures of depression and depressive symptomatology to those that use unvalidated measures. Lastly, measures of inflammation include: (a) in vivo measures such as CRP, interleukin (IL)-6, fibrinogen, and, to a lesser extent, measures of circulating cytokines such as IL-1beta, soluble IL-2 receptor, and tumor necrosis factor (TNF)-alpha;

and (b) in vitro techniques used to evaluate cellular and functional responses to mitogen stimulation. Regardless of these differences in methodology, the majority of studies have emphasized the directional hypothesis that depression precedes inflammation, whereas fewer studies have examined the possibility that inflammation precedes depression (Miller, Maletic, & Raison, 2009).

HOSTILITY AND ANGER

Relative to studies of depression and inflammation, fewer studies have examined the relation of hostility and anger to inflammation. With the exception of two studies (Boyle et al., 2007; Elovainio et al., 2011), the studies have been cross-sectional in design and, for the most part, study populations have been healthy subjects recruited from the community. Other methodological characteristics common across studies include the use of the Cook-Medley Hostility Scale and CRP and IL-6 as inflammatory markers. Although all studies have examined hostility or anger, some have examined the joint effect of hostility with depression and in combination with anger (Suarez, 2003; Suarez, 2004; Suarez et al., 2004; Graham et al., 2006; Miller, Freedland, Carney, Stetler, & Banks, 2003; Stewart, Janicki-Deverts, Muldoon, & Kamarck, 2008). In light of these findings, the next sections will review the cross-sectional and longitudinal studies.

CROSS-SECTIONAL STUDIES

The initial study reporting a relationship between hostility, anger, and inflammation was conducted in my laboratory (Suarez, Lewis, & Kuhn, 2002). In that study of healthy men, we assessed hostility and anger using the Buss-Perry Aggression Questionnaire (BPAQ) (Bernstein & Gesn, 1997). The BPAQ yields a total score as well as scores on subscales of hostility, anger, verbal, and physical aggression. Inflammation was assessed using lipopolysaccharide (LPS)-stimulated expression of TNF-alpha on peripheral monocytes. Results indicated that greater stimulated production of TNF-alpha was associated with BPAQ total score as well as scores on the hostility, physical, and verbal aggression subscales (Suarez et al., 2002). These associations were observed in an analysis that controlled for demographic and biological factors known to increase inflammation. Thus, hostile men, and especially those who reported high levels of verbal aggression and physical aggression, exhibited greater in vitro production of TNF-alpha.

The 2002 Suarez study was soon followed by a study published in 2003 that showed that hostility, alone and in combination with BDI-measured severity of depressive symptom, predicted elevated concentration of IL-6 in healthy men (Suarez, 2003). In analysis that included demographic, behavioral, and biological factors, higher hostility scores were associated with higher IL-6, but only in those subjects with high BDI scores. Conversely, depressive-symptom severity was associated with higher IL-6, but only among hostile men. The observation that hostility interacts with severity of depressive symptoms to predict IL-6 was subsequently replicated by Stewart et al. (2008). Stewart et al. measured hostility using the CMHO and severity of depressive symptoms using the BDI-II. As observed in the Suarez study, hostility was associated with higher levels of CRP and IL-6, but only among those subjects who report high levels of depressive symptoms.

Longitudinal Studies

Although a test of the depression by hostility interaction was not conducted, Graham et al. (2006) examined the relation of hostility to changes in CRP and IL-6 over a 6-year follow-up period of older caregivers and noncaregivers. Administration of CMHO and BDI scales was conducted at yearly intervals during the 6-year follow-up period. Using structural equation modeling, Graham et al. developed and used a latent hostility factor with yearly CMHO scores as measured indicators. Graham et al. observed that hostility latent factor predicted CRP, but not IL-6 level, independent of demographic, behavioral, and biomedical factors as well as caregiver status. It was noted that inclusion of BDI score in the structural equation model attenuated the relation between hostility and CRP, even though depressed mood was associated with hostility but not with either CRP or IL-6. This pattern of observations led the authors to postulate that depressed mood may have an indirect effect on CRP via hostility, a pathway that is consistent with previous observations that hostility moderates the relationship between severity of depressive symptoms and markers of inflammation.

Not all studies have reported significant main effects for hostility or anger, and one study testing the interaction between hostility and depression resulted in a different form of the interaction. In a study of 100 healthy adults where half of the sample had a diagnosis of MDD, Miller et al. (2003) reported a significant hostility by severity of depressive-symptoms interaction predicting circulating levels of IL-6 and TNF-alpha. The form of the interaction, however, was dramatically different from what had been previously reported (Suarez, 2003). Using the Cook-Medley Hostility BDI, Miller et al. showed that increases in hostility were associated with higher circulating TNF-alpha and IL-6, but only among those subjects with reporting *low* levels of depressive symptoms. Hostility was not significantly associated with either marker in subjects reporting *moderate* to *high* levels of depressive symptoms. Differences in the form of the interaction as reported by Suarez (2003) and Miller et al. (2003) may reflect subject characteristics. In the Miller et al. study, half the subjects had previously been diagnosed with MDD, whereas none of the subjects in the Suarez study had a diagnosis of MDD. Such differences may account in part for the variation in the form of the interaction.

The previously described studies assessed not only hostility but also depression. This allowed for some, but not all, to examine the hostility-depressed mood interaction. Other studies, however, have only examined the main effect of hostility. In 2005, Coccaro (2006) examined the relation of hostility and aggression to CRP in healthy young adults meeting clinical criteria for personality disorder. Using the Buss-Durkee Hostility Inventory (BDHI), Coccaro showed that subjects with elevated CRP scored higher on the hostility and aggression subscales of the BDHI. Controlling for possible confounding variables did not eliminate the significance of the relationships. The results reported by Coccaro replicated and extended earlier work by Suarez (Suarez et al., 2002) showing that subscales of the BPHI, and specifically those measuring the dimensions of hostility and physical and verbal aggression, predicted biomarkers of inflammation.

Similarly, Shivpuri et al. (2011) examined the main effect of dimensions of anger and hostility on soluble intracellular adhesion molecule (sICAM). Subjects were apparently healthy middle-aged Mexican-American women. Anger was assessed using the Speilberger Trait Anger Scale, which yields a total anger score and scores on two subscales: anger temperament and anger reaction. Anger temperament is conceptualized as the predisposition toward quick, unprovoked or minimally provoked anger. Anger reaction, on the other hand, refers to anger aroused in response to frustration, criticism, or unfair treatment. Hostility was measured using the 6-item cynicism scale from the Cook-Medley. Results indicated no association between trait anger total score or score on the anger temperament and sICAM-1. Anger reaction was marginally associated with sICAM-1. Cynical hostility was significantly associated with sICAM-1, even after controlling for demographic, biological, and behavioral covariates. The reported analysis did not test the interaction between hostility and dimensions of anger. However, based on a request by this author to the investigators, Shivpuri et al. examined the interaction between hostility and anger. Results showed that although the hostility by total anger and the hostility by anger-reaction interactions were not significant, the hostility by anger temperament was significant in predicting sICAM. Decomposition of the significant two-way interaction revealed that hostility was not associated with sICAM for those subjects reporting low ($p = .98$) and moderate ($p = .06$) levels of angry temperament. Only among those subjects who reported that they are quick to anger, even when unprovoked or minimally provoked, was hostility significantly associated with sICAM ($p = .005$) (personal communication, June 30, 2011). These novel findings add to the proposed hypothesis that hostility, in conjunction with anger, predicts levels of inflammation.

In most psychoimmunological studies, the primary measures of inflammation have been CRP and IL-6. A number of studies, however, have employed more comprehensive approaches to the measurement of inflammation. For example, both Janicki-Deverts et al. (Janicki-Deverts, Cohen, & Doyle, 2010) and Mommersteeg et al. (Mommersteeg, Vermetten, Kavelaars, Geuze, & Heijnen, 2008) assessed degree of inflammation using in vitro stimulated production of pro-inflammatory and anti-inflammatory cytokines. Janicki-Deverts et al. (2010) examined the relation of hostility to stimulated production of Th1 cytokines IL-2, TNF-alpha, INF-gamma, and Th2 cytokines IL-4, IL-5, and IL-10 in a sample of healthy men and women. Hostility was assessed using the 20-item CMHO scale and severity of depressive symptoms was measured using the CESD. The primary analysis used the total CMHO score, whereas exploratory analysis examined the relation of the cynicism, hostile affect, and aggression subscales of the CMHO to inflammatory biomarkers. When controlling for confounding variables including depression, results revealed that the total CMHO score predicted both stimulated production of TNF-alpha and INF-gamma, replicating and extending the initial findings reported by Suarez et al. (Suarez, Krishnan, & Lewis, 2003). In contrast, CMHO failed to predict Th2 cytokines. Results of the exploratory analysis suggested that all three Th1 cytokines were associated with scores on the cynicism subscale but not on the subscales of hostile affect and aggressive responding. The authors concluded that hostility, and particularly the cognitive component of hostility, was significantly associated with greater stimulated production of inflammatory cytokines and not with a production of anti-inflammatory cytokines. Although the authors noted that the inclusion of CESD score in the model did not attenuate the strength of the associations between hostility, cynicism, and Th1 cytokines, they did not test whether the interaction of CMHO by CESD predicted inflammation.

Mommersteg et al. (2008) also examined the relation of CMHO hostility to an array of stimulated production of pro-inflammatory and anti-inflammatory cytokines. Using a multiplex platform, Mommersteg et al. measured stimulated levels of IL-2, TNF-alpha, INF-gamma, IL-4, IL-5 IL-10, IL-6, chemokines, MCP-1, RANTES, IP-10, and MIF in healthy male military personnel prior to combat deployment. To reduce the number of statistical tests, Mommersteg et al. conducted a factor analysis with an oblique rotation on the array of immune markers. Results indicated a four-factor structure: a pro-inflammatory factor with IL-2, TNF-alpha, and INF-gamma as positive indicators, an anti-inflammatory factor with IL-4, IL-5, and IL-10 as negative indicators, an IL-6/chemokine factor with IL-6MCP-1, and IR10 as indicators, and a one-item factor migration inhibitory factors (MIF). Using factor scores derived from linear combinations, Mommersteg et al. showed that hostility was positively associated with both the "pro-inflammatory" and "anti-inflammatory" factor scores and negatively associated with the IL-6/chemokine factor score. As noted by the authors, that both anti-inflammatory and pro-inflammatory factors were positively associated with hostility was "remarkable." Such surprising findings may reflect the difficulty in interpretation of negative loadings (Lawley & Maxwell, 1963), and in this case, the interpretation of the negative factor loadings defining the anti-inflammatory factor. As published, the anti-inflammatory factor was defined by large negative loadings for IL-4, IL-5, and IL-10. Using these loadings, larger negative factors scores reflect higher stimulated production of these cytokines. In contrast, smaller negative scores would reflect lower stimulated production. Given this interpretation of the factor score, a positive association between the anti-inflammatory factor score and CMHO

scores suggests that hostile men (those with higher CMHO scores) showed lower production of anti-inflammatory cytokines (smaller negative factor scores) indicative of a blunted anti-inflammatory response to LPS. Men with low-hostility scores, on the other hand, would exhibit greater stimulated production of anti-inflammatory cytokines corresponding to a larger negative factor score. There is no doubt that negative loadings are difficult to interpret, and this is an excellent example of the conceptualization of the factors. However, this should not get in the way of what are important findings as they relate to hostility and inflammation.

The proposed alternative interpretation of the factors loadings deviates from that proposed by the study authors, suggesting that hostility was associated with "greater" production of anti-inflammatory cytokines. Given the negative loadings and the positive beta-value for the anti-inflammatory factor score predicting hostility suggests that hostile men showed "smaller" stimulated production of anti-inflammatory cytokines and low-hostility men showed larger stimulated production. This interpretation, in combination with the observation that high CMHO scores were associated with greater stimulated production of pro-inflammatory cytokines, suggests that hostile men show an imbalance in the pattern of pro-inflammatory to anti-inflammatory cytokines. Such an imbalance has been noted in cardiology studies that have used factor analysis to derive linear combinations of inflammatory and anti-inflammatory factors. As an example, an anti-inflammatory factor, defined by positive loadings on IL-10 and high-density-lipoprotein (HDL) cholesterol, was the best prospective predictor of adverse cardiac events in a one-year follow-up of patients with acute coronary syndrome (ACS) (Tziakas et al., 2007). In contrast to the Mommersteg et al. study, Tziakas et al. defined the anti-inflammatory factor by *positive* loadings on IL-10 and HDL, allowing for a more straightforward interpretation of the factor.

The proposed interpretation of the factor analysis and its impact on the interpretation of the results provides new evidence that hostile persons show an imbalance between levels of anti-inflammatory cytokines and levels of pro-inflammatory cytokines. Not surprisingly, this is not the only biological imbalance noted in hostile persons. Studies have shown differences in sympathovagal balance in hostile persons that is characterized by a shift toward sympathetic dominance (Demaree & Everhart, 2004; Sloan et al., 1994). In one study, sympathovagal balance was negatively associated with stimulated expression of IL-6 by peripheral mono-cytes in women but not men (O'Connor, Motivala, Valladares, Olmstead, & Irwin, 2007). Together, these data support the general hypothesis that the increased risk of CVD associated with hostility may be due to biological imbalances across various physiological systems that include immune and nervous systems. Such an interpretation is parsimonious with previous findings suggesting that inflammatory and anti-inflammatory balance predicts the progression of the atherosclerotic lesion.

Although only measuring one cytokine, Sjogren et al. (Sjogren, Leanderson, Kristenson, & Ernerudh, 2006) examined the relation of IL-6 levels in saliva, serum, and supernatants of peripheral blood mononuclear cells (PBMC) before and after stimulation with LPS to psychosocial measures of hostility (CMHO), severity of depressive state (Major Depressive Scale), vital exhaustion (Maastricht Vital Exhaustion Scale), hopelessness (2-items from the Kuopio study), and self-esteem/coping (Pearlin's scale). Correlational analysis controlling for demographic, health, and behavioral factors revealed that *serum* IL-6 was *positively* correlated with cynicism, hostile affect, hopelessness, severity of depressed mood, and vital exhaustion. In contrast, *stimulated* production of IL-6 was *negatively* correlated with cynicism, severity of depressed mood, and vital exhaustion. The results using serum IL-6 replicate and extend previous observations of the relation of hostility and depressed mood to IL-6. However, that cynicism and depressed mood are negatively associated with stimulated production of IL-6 is in contrast to reports of positive associations among these measures. At this time, it is not clear why the pattern of correlations differs so dramatically between psychological factors and in vivo and in vitro measures of IL-6. It is possible that salivary, serum, and stimulated production reflect different regulatory mechanisms. What is apparent is that in vivo and in vitro IL-6 are not correlated and reflect different aspects of the immune system.

PROSPECTIVE STUDIES

To date, there are two prospective studies that examined whether hostility and anger precede inflammation (Boyle et al., 2007; Elovainio et al., 2011). In a study of Vietnam male veterans, Boyle et al. (2007) showed that MMPI-derived measures of hostility and anger independently predicted 10-year increases in C3, but not C4, complement. These associations were significant even when demographic, health, and behavioral factors were

included in the statistical analysis. What was also noted was that, compared to the unique association between C3 and each psychological factor, the shared variance among hostility, anger, and depression was the best predictor of C3 changes over time. These latter findings underscore the need to focus on the interaction among psychological factors that are known to cluster in individuals in light of the potential importance of the nature of these interactions regarding development of CVD (Boyle, Michalek, & Suarez, 2007).

Elovainio et al. (2011) examined the relation of cynical hostility, assessed using seven items of the cynicism scale from the CMHO, to CRP measured 9 years later. Subjects were Finnish children and adolescents participating in the Young Finns Study. Hostility was measured at baseline when subjects were 3 to 18 years and CRP was measured 9 years later when subjects were 24 to 39 years of age. After controlling for demographic, metabolic, and behavioral factors, and baseline level of CRP, cynical hostility was associated with CRP in women but not in men. In this same study, hostility only predicted aspects of the metabolic syndrome in women but not in men. Given that CRP is associated with the metabolic syndrome, the gender-disparity observed in the relationship between hostility and both factors is not surprising. Findings from Elavainio et al. extend observations from a cross-sectional study of healthy men and women who showed that hostility and anger were associated with insulin resistance, fasting glucose, and fasting insulin in women but not in men (Suarez, 2006).

OVERALL FINDINGS

Cross-sectional and prospective studies suggest that depressive mood, hostility, and anger are positively associated with both in vivo and in vitro *measures of* inflammation in both healthy adults and minors and in patient populations. For the most part, these associations appear to be independent of sociodemographic, behavioral, and biological factors known or suspected of being associated with CVD and inflammation. The most consistent finding among studies is that the relation of anger, hostility, and depression to measures of inflammation are complex. Moreover, the presence of more than one psychological factor is potentially synergistic. Thus, a number of studies have shown that depression and hostility interacted to predict inflammation in many cross-sectional studies. Similarly, one study showed that hostility and angry temperament predicted inflammation. Lastly, there is emerging evidence that hostility, anger, and depression identify a group at particularly high risk for CHD, a group that showed consistent elevations in C3 over at 10-year period.

Such complex interactions are not unexpected as related to the development and progression of ACVD. It is acknowledged that ACVD is a multicausal disease that reflects the influences of many factors, both unmodifiable factors, such as gender, age, family history, and modifiable factors, such as lipids, weight, and physical activity. For example, it is well-established that inflammation and lipoprotein constituents are independently associated with CVD risk (Ridker & Morrow, 2003). Recent studies have focused their efforts on examining the interactions among these factors with the assumption being that the presence of these two factors would identify a high-risk subgroup (Corsetti et al., 2006). The results of that study showed that high CRP and cholesterol identified a subgroup at particularly high risk (hazard ratio = 2.24, 95% CI 1.12, 4.49, p = .03) for a recurrent evident. What was surprising was that HDL, usually associated with a protective effect, was associated with increased risk in this particular subgroup. Similarly, Ridker et al. (Ridker, Hennekens, Buring, & Rifai, 2000) showed that the combination of total cholesterol and IL-6 predicted CV risk in women, with higher IL-6 having a marginal effect in women with low total cholesterol. In contrast, in women with median cholesterol, high IL-6 was associated with greater risk, and in women with high cholesterol, high IL-6 has significant effects.

The same can be said for hostility, anger, and depression. One study has shown that the shared variance of these three factors is the best predictors of incident CHD over a 20+ year follow-up period. Similarly, in the presence of depression, lack of social integration has an additive effect on cardiac events (Naqvi, Naqvi, & Merz, 2005). Thus, it may be the case that the interaction of hostility, anger, and depression is not the only one that may identify a subgroup at heightened risk, but other interactions, such as depression by social isolation, may show similar predictive power.

RECOMMENDATION

Future studies examining the relation of psychological factors to inflammation should adopt an approach that emphasizes tests of higher-order interactions. In the case of anger, hostility, and depression, such an approach is reasonable, given

the likelihood that dysregulation of the serotonergic system may underlie anger, hostility, and depression. Aside from the possibility of a shared biological mechanism, it is well established that these factors tend to cluster in individuals. Similar to current approaches in cardiovascular research in which subgroups at heightened risk for disease are characterized by the presence of more than one risk factors, the presence of two or more psychological factors may identify a subgroup of individuals who are particularly at high risk for disease.

POTENTIAL MODERATORS AND MEDIATORS

Whatever approach is examined, whether researchers emphasize main effects or interaction, some have speculated that the relation of psychological factors to inflammation is moderated or mediated by traditional risk factors, such as gender, adiposity, and insulin resistance. Few studies, however, have examined these moderating effects.

GENDER

Danner et al. (Danner, Kasl, Abramson, & Vaccarino, 2003) examined the relation of a lifetime history of major depressive episode to CRP in over 6,000 participants from the Third National Health and Nutrition Examination Survey. Among men, a history of depression was associated with elevated CRP, but this was not observed in women.

In another study, the Zung Self-Rating Depression Scale was used to examine the relation of depression to CRP in a sample of adult men and women free of cardiovascular disease (Panagiotakos et al., 2004). Although women scored significantly higher on the Zung Depression Scale than men, depression was similarly correlated to CRP, white blood cell count, and fibrinogen in both men and women. Differences in life styles and demographic characteristics appeared to partially be responsible for this association, however, control of these factors did significantly attenuate the relationship.

In two studies conducted in my laboratory, we have shown that BDI scores were similarly associated with stimulated levels of cytokines production by peripheral monocytes in men and women (Suarez et al., 2003; Suarez et al., 2004). The fact that these were independent studies did not allow for the BDI by gender interaction to be evaluated. Comparison of results, however, showed that BDI score predicted TNF-alpha and IL-8 in both men and women. Beck Depression Inventory predicted IL-1alpha and IL-1beta in men but not in women, suggesting that BDI may be a more robust predictor of inflammation in men.

Gender may also moderate the relation of anger and hostility to CVD and measures of inflammation. A recent meta-analysis (Chida & Steptoe, 2009) indicated that although there was an overall effect of hostility and anger on measures of CVD in healthy populations, this association was stronger in healthy men. Those findings contrast the results from the study by Elovainio et al., who showed that cynical hostility predicted increases in CRP over a 9-year follow-up period but only in women and not in men.

Given that women report greater severity of depressive symptoms and men report greater levels of hostility and anger, it is recommended that future studies examine gender-related interactions to confirm or exclude the possibility that the relationship between psychological factors and measures of inflammation is different or similar in men and women.

ADIPOSITY

Adiposity is related to increased risk of abdominal adiposity and obesity in later life. Since adiposity is positively associated with inflammation, some have suggested that adiposity may mediate the relation of depression to future inflammation. Some, but not all, studies have reported that controlling for adiposity attenuates the relationship between depression and IL-6 and CRP. For example, Miller et al. used structural equation modeling and cross-sectional data to show that, in a sample of healthy men and women, depression was associated with increases in weight that mediated the relation of depression to CRP and IL-6 (Miller, Freedland, Carney, Stetler, & Banks, 2003). Similar observations were reported by Ladwig et al., (Ladwig, Marten-Mittag, Lowel, Doring, & Koenig, 2003) who showed that in a large sample of healthy middle-aged men, hostility was positively associated with CRP, but only in those men who were obese, defined by body mass index (BMI) equal or greater than 30 kg/m². A similar relationship was observed in obese female patients scheduled for obesity surgery. Dixon et al. (2008) showed that the strongest predictor of elevated CRP was BMI, followed by female gender, estrogen therapy, higher BDI score, and insulin resistance. Given that all subjects were obese, no interaction was tested.

Not all studies have shown that obesity or adiposity mediates the depression-inflammation pathway. A small study of 63 obese women with and without depression showed no difference in BMI, TNF-alpha, and leptin among nondepressed,

mild depression, and severe depression groups (Olszanecka-Glinianowicz et al., 2009).

It is important to note that the evidence for the mediating role of adiposity in the depression-inflammation pathway has been shown solely in studies using circulating inflammatory biomarkers and specifically CRP and IL-6. In studies that have used in vitro measures, the influence of measures of adiposity has been negligible, and the inclusion of these indicators in statistical models does not attenuate the relation of depressed mood to cytokine production (Suarez et al., 2003; Marsland et al., 2007; Suarez, Lewis, Krishnan, & Young, 2004). This is not unexpected given that levels of circulating inflammatory proteins are more strongly influenced by adiposity and factors beyond monocyte/macrophages and T lymphocytes (Shelton & Miller, 2011). Whatever the case may be, it is recommended that future studies examine the moderating and mediating effects of adiposity in the relation of depression to inflammation.

The role of adiposity has not been examined in the relation of hostility and anger to inflammation. Like depression, hostility has been related to increased weight over time (Siegler, Peterson, Barefoot, & Williams, 1992). It is possible that the relationship between hostility and inflammation is similarly mediated by adiposity. To date, no study has examined this hypothesis. Future studies should examine whether adiposity mediates the relation of hostility to inflammation.

Additional Recommendations for Future Studies

It is likely that the association between measures of inflammation and psychological factors is complex and that simple main-effect and additive models do not capture potential interactions among psychological factors as well as the potential moderating and mediating effects of biological, social, and demographic factors. With few exceptions, most studies have examined one psychological construct in isolation with post-hoc or exploratory analysis deconstructing the factor into its various components. Although such an approach is statistically sound, it fails to reflect the dynamic interplay among interrelated factors. As underscored by Suls and Bunde, there is significant construct and measurement overlap between these three factors (Suls et al., 2005). In echoing their recommendations, it is advised that future studies develop more complex models to be used in examining the relation of psychological factors to disease outcomes and putative mechanisms. Toward attaining this goal, the assessment of multiple psychological dimensions can provide more precise conceptualization and yield better empirical descriptions than those afforded by any single measure no matter how reliable.

One emerging hypothesis that has garnished some attention is that certain genetic polymorphisms may explain the link between psychological factors and inflammation (Almeida et al., 2009; Lotrich, Ferrell, Rabinovitz, & Pollock, 2010). For example, in hepatitis patients without MDD, the A allele in the promoter region of the TNF-alpha gene (A-308G), associated with higher plasma levels, was associated with increases in labile anger following treatment with interferon-alpha (Lotrich et al., 2010). The A allele was not associated with worsening depression. Interestingly, the serotonin transporter polymorphism did not predict labile anger.

Another study examined the polymorphisms of the CRP gene in a large sample of men and women (Almeida et al., 2009). Results from this study had already indicated that higher concentrations of CRP (>= 3 mg/l) were associated with a twofold increase in the odds of depression. Investigators then examined whether polymorphisms of the CRP gene associated with higher basal and simulated increases in CRP (rs1130864 C > T variant) and those associated with lower basal and stimulated production (rs1205 G > A variant) would be associated with the severity of depressive symptoms assessed using the 15-item Geriatric Depression Scale (GDS-15). In contrast to the expected association, the odds of having higher GDS-15 scores was associated with the rs1205 G > A genetic polymorphism associated with lower CRP. Although surprising given that greater severity of depressive symptoms was associated with higher CRP concentration, the result of the genetic analysis may reflect potential confounding with other factors such as age and medical co-morbidities. It may be the case that shared genetic influences between CRP and depression may be observed only in samples of medically healthier individuals.

Conclusion

The prevailing understanding of atherosclerosis is that it is an inflammatory disease. In light of this, studies have identified various biomarkers of inflammation that are associated with CVD risk in healthy men and women and recurrent events in CHD patients. These associations have led many to examine the relation of inflammatory biomarkers to psychological factors associated with CVD. Most studies have focused on measures of depression with the results suggesting that depression, whether operationalized as a clinical diagnosis or as a continuum of severity of depressed symptoms, is associated with biomarkers on inflammation in both cross-sectional and longitudinal studies. Although the data are equivocal, there is evidence to suggest that this association is bidirectional in that depression precedes inflammation and inflammation precedes depression.

Although fewer studies have examined the role of hostility and anger, the available evidence suggests that hostility and anger are independently associated with inflammation. What is emerging is that the interaction of depression, hostility, and anger identifies a subgroup that shows levels of inflammation higher than those with only one or two of these factors. It is recommended that future studies examine the joint effects among these factors and with others.

Related Chapters

For more information on concepts introduced in this chapter, see also Cohen, this volume.

References

Adler, U. C., Marques, A. H., & Calil, H. M. (2008). Inflammatory aspects of depression. *Inflammation & Allergy Drug Targets, 7,* 19–23.

Almeida OP, Norman PE, Allcock R, et al.: Polymorphisms of the CRP gene inhibit inflammatory response and increase susceptibility to depression: The Health in Men Study. *International Journal of Epidemiology.* 2009, *38*:1049–1059.

Anonymous (2009). C-reactive protein testing comes of age. Measuring low-grade inflammation can help refine cardiovascular risk. *Harvard Heart Letter,19,* 2.

Apostolopoulos, J., Davenport, P., & Tipping, P. G. (1996). Interleukin-8 production by macrophages from atheromatous plaques. *Arteriosclerosis, Thrombosis, and Vascular Biology, 16,* 1007–1012.

Barefoot, J. C., & Lipkus, I. M. (1994). The assessment of anger and hostility. In A. W. Sigman & T. W. Smith (Eds.), *Anger, hostility and the heart* (pp. 43–66). Hillsdale, NJ: Erlbaum.

Baumann, H., & Gauldie, J. (1994). The acute phase response. *Immunology Today, 15,* 74–80.

Beck, A. T., Steer, R. A., & Garbin, M. G. (1988). Psychometric properties of the Beck Depression Inventory: Twenty-five years of evaluation. *Clinical Psychology Review, 8,* 77–100.

Bernstein, I. H., & Gesn, P. (1997). On the dimensionality of the Buss/Perry Aggression Questionnaire. *Behaviour Research & Therapy, 35,* 563–568.

Blood Pressure Lowering Treatment Trialists' Collaboration. (2003). Effects of different blood-pressure-lowering regimens on major cardiovascular events: Results of prospectively-designed overviews of randomised trials. *The Lancet,362,* 1527–1535.

Bonetti, P. O., Lerman, L. O., & Lerman, A. (2003). Endothelial dysfunction: A marker for atherosclerotic risk (review). *Arteriosclerosis, Thrombosis, and Vascular Biology, 23,*168–175.

Boyle, S. H., Jackson, W. G., & Suarez, E. C. (2007). Hostility, anger, and depression predict increases in C3 over a 10-year period. *Brain, Behavior, and Immunity, 21,* 816–823.

Boyle, S. H., Michalek, J. E., & Suarez, E. C. (2007). Covariation of psychological attributes and incident coronary heart disease in US Air Force veterans of the Vietnam War. *Psychosomatic Medicine, 68,* 844–850.

Brotman, D. J., Golden, S. H., & Wittstein, I. S. (2007). The cardiovascular toll of stress. *The Lancet, 370,* 1089–1100.

Brown, C., Shulberg, H. C., & Madonia, M. J. (1995). Assessing depression in primary care practice with the Beck Depression Inventory and the Hamilton Rating Scale for Depression. *Psychological Assessment, 7,* 59–65.

Busch, F. N. (2009). Anger and depression. *Advanced Psychiatric Treatment, 15,* 271–278.

Camacho, T. C., Roberts, R. E., Lazarus, N. B., Kaplan, G. A., & Cohen, R. D. (1991). Physical activity and depression: Evidence form the Alameda County Study. *Journal of Epidemiology, 134,* 220–231.

Capuron, L., & Miller, A. H. (2004). Cytokines and psychopathology: Lessons from interferon-alpha. *Biological Psychiatry, 56,* 819–824.

Capuron, L., Ravaud, A., & Dantzer, R. (2000). Early depressive symptoms in cancer patients receiving interleukin 2 and/or interferon alfa-2b therapy. *Journal of Clinical Oncology, 18,* 2143–2151.

Chang, P. P., Ford, D. E., Meoni, L. A., Wang, N. Y., & Klag, M. J. (2002). Anger in young men and subsequent premature cardiovascular disease: The precursors study. *Archives of Internal Medicine, 162,* 901–906.

Chen, C. C., Lu, F. H., Wu, J. S., & Chang, C. J. Correlation between serum lipid concentrations and psychological distress. *Psychiatry Research, 102,* 153–162.

Chida, Y., & Steptoe, A. (2009). The association of anger and hostility with future coronary heart disease: A meta-analytic review of prospective evidence. *Journal of the American College of Cardiology, 53,* 936–946.

Coccaro, E. F. (2006). Association of C-reactive protein elevation with trait aggression and hostility in personality disordered subjects: A pilot study. *Journal of Psychiatric Research, 40,* 460–465.

Cook, W. W., & Medley, D. M. (1954). Proposed hostility and pharisaic-virtue scales for the MMPI. *Journal of Applied Psychology, 38,* 414–418.

Corsetti, J. P., Zareba, W., Moss, A. J., Rainwater, D. L., & Sparks, C. E. (2006). Elevated HDL is a risk factor for recurrent coronary events in a subgroup of nondiabetic postinfarction patients with hypercholesterolemia and inflammation. *Atherosclerosis, 187,* 191–197.

Costa, P. T., Jr., & McCrae, R. R. (1985). *The NEO personality inventory manual.* Odessa, FL: Psychological Assessment Resources.

Dandona, P., Aljada, A., Chaudhuri, A., Mohanty, P., & Garg, R. (2005). Metabolic syndrome: A comprehensive perspective based on interactions between obesity, diabetes, and inflammation. *Circulation, 111,* 1448–1454.

Danner, M., Kasl, S. V., Abramson, J. L., & Vaccarino, V. (2003). Association between depression and elevated C-reactive protein. *Psychosomatic Medicine, 65,* 347–356.

Dantzer, R., & Kelley, K. W. (1989). Stress and immunity: An integrated view of relationships between the brain and the immune system. *Life Sciences, 44,* 1995–2008.

Daugherty, A., Rateri, D. L., & Lu, H. (2008). As macrophages indulge, atherosclerotic lesions bulge. *Circulation Research, 102,* 1445–1447.

Davidson, K. W., Rieckmann, N., & Rapp, M. A. (2005). Definitions and distinctions among depressive syndromes and symptoms: Implications for a better understanding of the depression–cardiovascular disease association. *Psychosomatic Medicine, 67,* S6–S9.

DellaGioia, N., & Hannestad, J. (2010). A critical review of human endotoxin administration as an experimental paradigm of depression. *Neuroscience & Biobehavioral Reviews, 34,* 130–143.

Dembroski, T., MacDougall, J., Costa, P., & Grandits, G. (1989). Components of hostility as predictors of sudden death and myocardial infarction in the Multiple Risk Factor Intervention Trial. *Psychosomatic Medicine, 51,* 514–522.

Demaree, H. A., & Everhart, D. E. (2004). Healthy high-hostiles: Reduced parasympathetic activity and decreased sympathovagal flexibility during negative emotional processing. *Personality and Individual Differences, 36,* 457–469.

Digman, J. M. (1990). Personality structure: Emergence of the five-factor model. *Annual Review of Psychology, 41,* 417–440.

Dixon, J. B., Hayden, M. J., Lambert, G. W., Dawood, T., Anderson, M. L., Dixon, M. E., & O'Brien, P. E. (2008). Raised CRP levels in obese patients: Symptoms of depression have an independent positive association. *Obesity, 16,* 2010–2015.

Elovainio, M., Aalto, A.-M., Kivimaki, M., Pirkol, S., Sundvall, J., Lonnqvist, J., & Reunanen A. (2009). Depression and C-reactive protein: Population-based health 2000 study. *Psychosomatic Medicine, 71,* 423–430.

Elovainio, M., Merjonen, P., Pulkki-Råback, L., Kivimaki, M., Jokela, M., Mattson, N., et al. (2011). Hostility, metabolic syndrome, inflammation and cardiac control in young adults: The Young Finns Study. *Biological Psychology, 87,* 234–240.

Emeson, E. E., & Robertson, A. L. (1988). T lymphocytes in aortic and coronary intimas: Their potential role in atherogenesis. *American Journal of Pathology, 130,* 369–376.

Empana, J. P., Sykes, D. H., Luc, G., Juhan-Vague, I., Arveiler, D., & Ferrieres, J. (2005). Contributions of depressive mood and circulating inflammatory markers to coronary heart disease in healthy European men: The prospective epidemiological study of myocardial infarction (PRIME). *Circulation, 111,* 2299–2305.

Everson-Rose, S. A., & Lewis, T. T. (2005). Psychosocial factors and cardiovascular diseases. *Annual Review of Public Health, 26,* 469–500.

Faggiotto, A., & Ross, R. (1984). Studies of hypercholesterolemia in the nonhuman primate, II: Fatty streak conversion to fibrous plaque. *Arteriosclerosis, Thrombosis, and Vascular Biology, 4,* 341–356.

Faggiotto, A., Ross, R., & Harker, L. (1984). Studies of hypercholesterolemia in the nonhuman primate, I: Changes that lead to fatty streak formation. *Arteriosclerosis, Thrombosis, and Vascular Biology, 4,* 323–340.

Fernandez-Real, J. M., & Ricart, W. (2003). Insulin resistance and chronic cardiovascular inflammatory syndrome. *Endocrine Reviews, 24,* 278–301.

Ford, D. E., Mead, L. A., Chang, P. P., Cooper-Patrick, L., Wang, N. Y., & Klag, M. J. (1998). Depression is a risk factor for coronary artery disease in men: The precursors study. *Archives of Internal Medicine, 158,* 1422–1426.

Gimeno, D., Kivimäki, M., Brunner, E. J., Elovainio, M., De Vogli, R., Steptoe, A., et al. (2009). Associations of C-reactive protein and interleukin-6 with cognitive symptoms of depression: 12-year follow-up of the Whitehall II study. *Psychological Medicine, 39,* 413–423.

Glover, A. T., Shaw, S. M., Williams, S. G., & Fildes, J. E. (2010). Can inflammation be an independent predictor of depression? *Brain, Behavior, & Immunity, 24,* 173; author reply 174–175.

Graham, J. E., Robles, T. F., Kiecolt-Glaser, J. K., et al. (2006). Hostility and pain are related to inflammation in older adults. *Brain, Behavior, and Immunity Stress, Genetics, and Immunity, 20,* 389–400.

Greenland, P., Knoll, M. D., Stamler, J., Neaton, J. D., Dyer, A. R., Garside, D. B., & Wilson, P. W. (2003). Major risk factors as antecedents of fatal and nonfatal coronary heart disease events. *JAMA: The Journal of the American Medical Association, 290,* 891–897.

Greeson, J. M., Lewis, J. G., Achanzar, K., Zimmerman, E., Young, K. H., & Suarez, E. C. (2009). Stress-induced changes in the expression of monocytic beta2-integrins: The impact of arousal of negative affect and adrenergic responses to the Anger Recall Interview. *Brain, Behavior, and Immunity, 23,* 251–256.

Griendling, K. K., & FitzGerald, G. A. (2003). Oxidative stress and cardiovascular injury, part II: Animal and human studies. *Circulation, 108,* 2034–2040.

Grippo, A. J., Francis, J., Beltz, T. G., Felder, R. B., & Johnson, A. K. (2005). Neuroendocrine and cytokine profile of chronic mild stress-induced anhedonia. *Physiology & Behavior, 84,* 697–706.

Hamer, M., & Chida, Y. (2009). Associations of very high C-reactive protein concentration with psychosocial and cardiovascular risk factors in an ageing population. *Atherosclerosis, 206,* 599–603.

Hamer, M., Molloy, G. J., de Oliveira, C., & Demakakos, P. (2009). Persistent depressive symptomatology and inflammation: To what extent do health behaviours and weight control mediate this relationship? *Brain, Behavior, and Immunity, 23,* 413–418.

Hansson, G. K. (2001). Immune mechanisms in atherosclerosis. *Arteriosclerosis, Thrombosis, and Vascular Biology, 21,* 1876–1890.

Heart Protection Study Collaborative Group. (2002). MRC/BHF heart protection study of cholesterol lowering with simvastatin in 20[punctuation space]536 high-risk individuals: A randomised placebocontrolled trial. *The Lancet, 360,* 7–22.

Herbert, T. B., & Cohen, S. (1993). Depression and immunity: A meta-analytic review. *Psychological Bulletin, 113,* 472–486.

Howren, M. B., Lamkin, D. M., & Suls, J. (2009). Associations of depression with C-reactive protein, IL-1, and IL-6: A meta-analysis. *Psychosomatic Medicine, 71,* 171–186.

Hwang, S.-J., Ballantyne, C. M., Sharrett, A. R., Smith, L. C., Davis, C. E., Gotto, A. M. Jr., & Boerwinkle, E. (1997). Circulating adhesion molecules VCAM-1, ICAM-1, and E-selectin in carotid atherosclerosis and incident coronary heart disease cases: The atherosclerosis risk In communities (ARIC) study. *Circulation, 96,* 4219–4225.

Irwin, M. (2002). Psychoneuroimmunology of depression: Clinical implications. *Brain, Behavior, and Immunity, 16,* 1–16.

Janicki-Deverts, D., Cohen, S., & Doyle, W. J. (2010). Cynical hostility and stimulated Th1 and Th2 cytokine production. *Brain, Behavior, and Immunity, 24,* 58–63.

Jonasson, L., Holm, J., Skalli, O., Bondjers, G., & Hansson, G. K. (1986). Regional accumulations of T cells, macrophages, and smooth muscle cells in the human atherosclerotic plaque. *Arteriosclerosis, Thrombosis, and Vascular Biology, 6,* 131–138.

Judd, L. L., Rapaport, M. H., Paulus, M. P., & Brown, J. L. (1994). Subsyndromal symptomatic depression: A new mood disorder. *Journal of Clinical Psychiatry, 55,* 18–28.

Kahler, C. W., Strong, D. R., Niaura, R., & Brown, R. A. (2004). Hostility in smokers with past major depressive disorder: Relation to smoking patterns, reasons for quitting, and cessation outcomes. *Nicotine and Tobacco Research, 6,* 809–818.

Kamarck, T. W., Haskett, R. F., Muldoon, M., Flory, J. D., Anderson, B., Bies, R., et al. (2009). Citalopram intervention for hostility: Results of a randomized clinical trial. *Journal of Consulting & Clinical Psychology, 77,* 174–188.

Kannel, W. B., Wolf, P. A., Castelli, W. P., & D'Agostino, R. B. (1987). Fibrinogen and risk of cardiovascular disease: The Framingham Study. *JAMA, 258,* 1183–1186.

Kannel, W. B., & Vasan, R. S. (2009). Adverse consequences of the 50% misconception. *American Journal of Cardiology, 103,* 426–427.

Kaplan, J. R., Manuck, S. B., Clarkson, T. B., Lusso, F. M., Taub, D. M., & Miller, E. W. (1983). Social stress and atherosclerosis in normocholesterolemic monkeys. *Science, 220,* 733–735.

Kaplan, J. R., Pettersson, K., Manuck, S. B., & Olsson, G. (1991). Role of sympathoadrenal medullary activation in the initiation and progression of atherosclerosis. *Circulation, 84,* VI23–32.

Kareinen, A., Viitanen, L., Halonen, P., Lehto, S., & Laakso, M. (2001). Cardiovascular risk factors associated with insulin resistance cluster in families with early-onset coronary heart disease. *Arteriosclerosis, Thrombosis, and Vascular Biology, 21,* 1346–1352.

Kiecolt-Glaser J. K., Preacher K. J., MacCallum R. C., Atkinson, C., Malarkey, W. B., and Glaser, R. (2003). Chronic stress and age-related increases in the pro-inflammatory cytokine IL-6. *Proceedings of the National Academy of Sciences, 100,* 9090–9095.

Kobrosly, R., & van Wijngaarden, E. (2010). Associations between immunologic, inflammatory, and oxidative stress markers with severity of depressive symptoms: An analysis of the 2005–2006 National Health and Nutrition Examination Survey. *Neurotoxicology, 31,* 126–133.

Kop, W. J., Gottdiener, J. S., Tangen, C. M., Fried, L. P., McBurnie, M. A., Walston, J., et al. (2002). Inflammation and coagulation factors in persons > 65 years of age with symptoms of depression but without evidence of myocardial ischemia. *American Journal of Cardiology, 89,* 419–424.

Kop, W. J., Stein, P. K., Tracy, R. P., Barzilay, J. I., Schulz, R., & Gottdiener, J. S. (2010). Autonomic nervous system dysfunction and inflammation contribute to the increased cardiovascular mortality risk associated with depression. *Psychosomatic Medicine, 72,* 626–635.

Kuller, L., Tracy, R. P., Shaten, J., & Meilahn, E. N. (1996). Relationship of C-reactive protein and coronary heart disease in the MRFIT nested case-control study multiple risk factor intervention trial. *American Journal of Epidemiology, 144,* 537–547.

Ladwig, K. H., Marten-Mittag, B., Lowel, H., Doring, A., & Koenig, W. (2003). Influence of depressive mood on the association of CRP and obesity in 3205 middle aged healthy men. *Brain, Behavior, and Immunity, 17,* 268–275.

Lawley, D. N., & Maxwell, A. E. (1963). *Factor analysis as a statistical method*. London: Butterworths.

Lemogne, C., Nabi, H., Zins, M., Cordier, S., Ducimetier, P., Goldberg, M., and Consoli, S. M. (2010). Hostility may explain the association between depressive mood and mortality: Evidence from the French GAZEL cohort study. *Psychother Psychosom, 79*, 164–171.

Lesperance, F., Frasure-Smith, N., Talajic, M., & Bourassa, M. G. (2002). Five-year risk of cardiac mortality in relation to initial severity and one-year changes in depression symptoms after myocardial infarction. *Circulation, 105*, 1049–1053.

Libby, P., Okamoto, Y., Rocha, V. Z., & Folco, E. (2006). Inflammation in atherosclerosis: Transition from theory to practice. *Circulation Journal, 74*, 213–220.

Libby, P., Ridker, P. M., & Hansson, G. K. (2009). Inflammation in atherosclerosis: From pathophysiology to practice. *Journal of the American College of Cardiology, 54*, 2129–2138.

Libby, P., & Theroux, P. (2005). Pathophysiology of coronary artery disease. *Circulation, 111*, 3481–3488.

Lotrich, F. E., Ferrell, R. E., Rabinovitz, M., & Pollock, B. G. (2010). Labile anger during interferon alfa treatment is associated with a polymorphism in tumor necrosis factor-alpha. *Clinical Neuropharmacology, 33*, 191–197 110.1097/WNF.1090b1013e3181de8966

Luc, G., Bard, J. M., Juhan-Vague, I., Ferrieres, J., Evans, A., Amouyel, P., et al. (2003). C-reactive protein, interleukin-6, and fibrinogen as predictors of coronary heart disease: The PRIME Study. *Arteriosclerosis, Thrombosis and Vascular Biology, 23*, 1255–1261.

Maes, M. (1995). Evidence for an immune response in major depression: A review and hypothesis. *Progress in Neuro-Psychopharmacology and Biological Psychiatry, 19*, 11–38.

Maes, M. (2011). Depression is an inflammatory disease, but cell-mediated immune activation is the key component of depression. *Progress in Neuro-Psychopharmacology and Biological Psychiatry, 35*, 664–675.

Maes, M., Smith, R., & Scharpe, S. (1995). The monocyte-t-lymphocyte hypothesis of major depression. *Psychoneuroendocrinology, 20*, 111–116.

Maes, M., Smith, R., & Simon, S. (1995). The monocyte-T-lymphocyte hypothesis of major depression. *Psychoneuroendocrinology, 20*, 111–116.

Magnus, P., & Beaglehole, R. (2001). The real contribution of the major risk factors to the coronary epidemics: Time to end the "only-50%" myth. *Archives of Internal Medicine, 161*, 2657–2660.

Mainous, A. G., Everett, C. J., Diaz, V. A.,Player, M. S., Gebregziabher, M., & Smith, D. W. (2010). Life stress and atherosclerosis: A pathway through unhealthy lifestyle. *International Journal of Psychiatry in Medicine, 40*, 147–161.

Marsland, A. L., Sathanoori, R., Muldoon, M. F., & Manuck, S. B. (2007). Stimulated production of interleukin-8 covaries with psychosocial risk factors for inflammatory disease among middle-aged community volunteers. *Brain, Behavior, and Immunity, 21*, 218–228.

Martin, R., Watson, D., & Wan, C. K. (2000). A three-factor model of trait anger: Dimensions of affect, behavior, and cognition. *Journal of Personality, 68*, 869–897.

Matthews, K. A., Jamison, W., & Cottington, E. M. (1985). Assessment of type A, anger, and hostility: A review of measures through 1982. In A. Ostfeld, & E. Eaker (Eds.), *Proceedings of the NHLBI workshop on measuring psychosocial variables in epidemiologic studies of cardiovascular disease*. NIH Publication No. 85–2270. Bethesda: NIH.

Matthews, K. A., Schott, L. L., Bromberger, J., Cyranowski, J., Everson-Rose, S. A., & Sowers, M. F. (2007). Associations between depressive symptoms and inflammatory/hemostatic markers in women during the menopausal transition. *Psychosomatic Medicine, 69*, 124–130.

McCarty, M. (1947). The occurence during acute infections of a protein not normally present in blood. *The Journal of Experimental Medicine, 85*, 491–498.

Meade, T. W., Mellows, S., Brozovic, M., Miller, G. J., Chakrabarti, R. R., North, W. R., et al. (1986). Haemostatic function and ischaemic heart disease: Principal results of the Northwick Park Heart Study. *Lancet, 2*, 533–537.

Miller, A. H., Maletic, V., & Raison, C. L. (2009). Inflammation and its discontents: The role of cytokines in the pathophysiology of major depression. *Biological Psychiatry, 65*, 732–741.

Miller, G. E., Freedland, K. E., Carney, R. M., Stetler, C. A., & Banks, W. A. (2003a). Pathways linking depression, adiposity, and inflammatory markers in healthy young adults. *Brain, Behavior, and Immunity, 17*, 276–285.

Miller, G. E., Freedland, K. E., Carney, R. M., Stetler, C. A., & Banks, W. A. (2003b). Cynical hostility, depressive symptoms, and the expression of inflammatory risk markers for coronary heart disease. *Journal of Behavioral Medicine, 26*, 501–515.

Miller, T., Markides, K., Chiriboga, D., & Ray, L. (1995). A test of the psychosocial vulnerability and health behavior models of hostility: Results from an 11-year follow-up study of Mexican Americans. *Psychosomatic Medicine, 57*, 572–581.

Miller, T. Q., Smith, T. W., Turner, C. W., Guijarro, M. L., & Hallet, A. J. (1996). A meta-analytic review of hostility and physical health. *Psychological Bulletin, 119*, 322–348.

Mills, P. J., & Dimsdale, J. E. (1996). The effects of acute psychologic stress on cellular adhesion molecules. *Journal of Psychosomatic Research, 41*, 49–53.

Mommersteeg, P. M. C. Vermetten, E., Kavelaars, A., Geuze, E., & Heijnen, C. J. (2008). Hostility is related to clusters of T-cell cytokines and chemokines in healthy men. *Psychoneuroendocrinology, 33*, 1041–1050.

Moss, A. J., Goldstein, R. .E., Marder, V. J., Sparks, C. E., Oakes, D., Greenberg, H., et al. (1999). Thrombogenic factors and recurrent coronary events. *Circulation, 99*, 2517–2522.

Musselman, D. L., Evans, D. L., & Nemeroff, C. B. (1998). The relationship of depression to cardiovascular disease. *Archives of General Psychiatry, 55*, 580–592.

Nakashima, Y., Raines, E. W., Plump, A. S., Breslow, J. L., & Ross, R. (1998). Upregulation of VCAM-1 and ICAM-1 at atherosclerosis-prone sites on the endothelium in the apoE-deficient mouse. *Arteriosclerosis, Thrombosis, and Vascular Biology, 18*, 842–851.

Naqvi, T. Z., Naqvi, S. S. A., & Merz, C. N. B. (2005). Gender differences in the link between depression and cardiovascular disease. *Psychosomatic Medicine, 67*, S15–S18.

Nelson, L. D., & Cicchetti, D. (1991). Validity of the MMPI depression scale for outpatients. *Psychological Assessment: A Journal of Consulting and Clinical Psychology, 3*, 55–59.

O'Connor, M.-F., Bower, J. E., Cho, H. J., Creswell, J. D., Dimitrov, S., Hamby, M. E., et al. (2009). To assess, to control, to exclude: Effects of biobehavioral factors on circulating inflammatory markers. *Brain, Behavior, and Immunity, 23*, 887–897.

O'Connor, M.-F., Motivala, S. J., Valladares, E. M., Olmstead, R., & Irwin, M. R. (2007). Sex differences in monocyte expression of IL-6: Role of autonomic mechanisms. *American Journal of Physiology: Regulatory, Integrative and Comparative Physiology, 293,* R145–R151.

Olszanecka-Glinianowicz, M., Zahorska-Markiewicz, B., Kocelak, P., Janowska, J., Semik-Grabarczyk, E., Wikarek, T., et al. (2009). Is chronic inflammation a possible cause of obesity-related depression? *Mediators of Inflammation, 2009,* 439107.

Pan, A., Ye, X., Franco, O. H., Yu, Z., Wang, J., Qi, Q., et al. (2008). The association of depressive symptoms with inflammatory factors and adipokines in middle-aged and older Chinese. *PLoS ONE [Electronic Resource], 3,* e1392.

Panagiotakos, D. B., Pitsavos, C., Chrysohoou, C., Tsetsekou, E., Papageorgiou, C., Christodoulou, G., et al. (2004). Inflammation, coagulation, and depressive symptomatology in cardiovascular disease-free people: The ATTICA study 10.1016/j.ehj.2004.01.018. *European Heart Journal,25,* 492–499.

Pearson, T. A., Mensah, G. A., Alexander, R. W., Anderson, J. L., Cannon, R. O., 3rd, Criqui, M., et al. (2003). Markers of inflammation and cardiovascular disease: Application to clinical and public health practices. A statement for the healthcare professionals from the Center from Disease Control and Prevention and the American Heart Association. *Circulation, 107,* 499–511.

Ridker, P. M. (2007). C-reactive protein and the prediction of cardiovascular events among those at intermediate risk: Moving an inflammatory hypothesis toward consensus. *Journal of the American College of Cardiology.* Doi: j.jacc.2007.2002.2052

Ridker, P. M. (2009). C-reactive protein: Eighty years from discovery to emergence as a major risk marker for cardiovascular disease. *Clinical Chemistry, 55,* 209–215.

Ridker, P. M., & Haughie, P. (1998). Prospective studies of C-reactive protein as a risk factor for cardiovascular disease. [Review] [26 refs]. *Journal of Investigative Medicine, 46,* 391–395.

Ridker, P. M., Hennekens, C. H., Buring, J., & Rifai, N. (2000). C-reactive protein and other markers of inflammation in the prediction of cardiovascular disease in women. *New England Journal of Medicine, 342,* 836–843.

Ridker, P. M., Hennekens, C. H., Roitman-Johnson, B., Stampfer, M. J., & Allen, J. (1998). Plasma concentration of soluble intercellular adhesion molecule 1 and risks of future myocardial infarction in apparently healthy men. *The Lancet, 351,* 88–92.

Ridker, P. M., & Morrow, D. A. (2003). C-reactive protein, inflammation, and coronary risk. *Cardiology Clinics, 21,* 315–325.

Ridker, P. M., Rifai, N., Rose, L., Buring, J., & Cook, N. R. (2002). Comparison of C-reactive protein and low-density lipoprotein cholesterol levels in the prediction of first cardiovascular events. *New England Journal of Medicine, 347,* 1557–1565.

Ridker, P. M., Rifai, N., Stampfer, M. J., & Hennekens, C. H. (2000). Plasma concentration of interleukin-6 and the risk of future myocardial infarction among apparently healthy men. *Circulation,101,* 1767–1772.

Rosenfeld, M. E., Polinsky, P., Virmani, R., Kauser, K., Rubanyi, G., & Schwartz, S. M. (2000). Advanced atherosclerotic lesions in the innominate artery of the apoE knockout mouse. *Arteriosclerosis, Thrombosis, and Vascular Biology, 20,* 2587–2592.

Rosengren, A., Hawken, S., Ounpuu, S., Sliwa, K., Zubaid, M., Almahmeed, W. A., et al. (2004). Association of psychosocial risk factors with risk of acute myocardial infarction in 11119 cases and 13648 controls from 52 countries (the INTERHEART study): Case-control study.[see comment]. *Lancet, 364,* 953–962.

Ross, R. (1986). The pathogenesis of atherosclerosis: An update. *New England Journal of Medicine, 314,* 488–500.

Ross, R. (1999a). Atherosclerosis: An inflammatory disease. *New England Journal of Medicine, 340,* 115–126.

Ross, R. (1999b). Atherogenesis. In J. I. Gallin & R. Snyderman (Eds.), *Inflammation: Basic principles and clinical correlates* (pp. 1083–1096). Philadelphia: Lippincott Williams & Wilkin.

Ross, R., Glomset, J., & Harker, L. (1977). Response to injury and atherogenesis. *American Journal of Pathology, 86,* 675–684.

Rozanski, A., Blumenthal, J. A., Davidson, K. W., Saab, P. G., & Kubzansky, L. (2005). The epidemiology, pathophysiology, and management of psychosocial risk factors in cardiac practice: The emerging field of behavioral cardiology. *Journal of the American College of Cardiology, 45,* 637–651.

Rozanski, A., Blumenthal, J. A., & Kaplan, J. R. Impact of psychological factors on the pathogenesis of cardiovascular disease and implication for therapy. *Circulation, 99,* 2129–2217.

Rugulies, R. (2002). Depression as a predictor of coronary heart disease. *American Journal of Preventive Medicine, 23,* 51–61.

Saikku, P., Leinonen, M., Tenkanen, L., Linnanmaki, E., Ekman, M. R., Manninen, V., et al. (1992). Chronic chlamydia pneumoniae infection as a risk factor for coronary heart disease in the Helsinki Heart Study. *Annals of Internal Medicine, 116,* 273–278.

Schlatter, J., Ortuño, F., & Cervera-Enguix, S. (2004). Monocytic parameters in patients with dysthymia versus major depression. *Journal of Affective Disorders,78,* 243–247.

Shaffer, J. A., Edmondson, D., Chaplin, W. F., Schwartz, J. E., Shimbo, D., Burg, M. M., et al. (2011). Directionality of the relationship between depressive symptom dimensions and C-reactive protein in patients with acute coronary syndromes. *Psychosomatic Medicine, 73,* 370–377.

Shelton, R. C., & Miller, A. H. (2011). Inflammation in depression: Is adiposity a cause? *Dialogues in Clinical Neuroscience, 13,* 41–53.

Shimbo, D., Chaplin, W., Crossman, D., Haas, D., & Davidson, K. W. (2005). Role of depression and inflammation in incident coronary heart disease events. *The American Journal of Cardiology, 96,* 1016–1021.

Shivpuri, S., Gallo, L. C., Mills, P. J., et al. (2011). Trait anger, cynical hostility and inflammation in latinas: Variations by anger type? *Brain, Behavior, and Immunity, 25,* 1256–1263.

Siegler, I. C., Peterson, B. L., Barefoot, J. C., & Williams, R. B. (1992). Hostility during late adolescence predicts coronary risk factors at mid-life. *American Journal of Epidemiology, 136,* 146–154.

Silva, M. R. (1994). A brief survey of the history of inflammation: 1978. *Agents and Actions, 43,* 86–90.

Sjögren, E., Leanderson, P., Kristenson, M., & Ernerudh, J. (2006). Interleukin-6 levels in relation to psychosocial factors: Studies on serum, saliva, and in vitro production by blood mononuclear cells. *Brain, Behavior, and Immunity, 20,* 270–278.

Skalen, K., Gustafsson, M., Rydberg, E. K., Hulten, L. M., Wiklund, O., Innerarity, T. L., & Boren, J. (2002).

Subendothelial retention of atherogenic lipoproteins in early atherosclerosis. *Nature, 417,* 750–754.

Sloan, R. P., Shapiro, P. A., Bigger, J. T., Bagiella, E., Steinman, R. C., & Gorman, J. M. (1994). Cardiac autonomic control and hostility in healthy subjects. *The American Journal of Cardiology, 74,* 298–300.

Smith, R. S. (1991). The macrophage theory of depression. *Medical Hypotheses, 35,* 298–306.

Smith, T. W. (1992). Hostility and health: Current status of a psychosomatic hypothesis. *Health Psychology, 11,* 139–150.

Smith, T. W. (1994). Concepts and methods in the study of anger, hostility, and health. In A. W. Siegman & T. W. Smith (Eds.), *Anger, hostility and the heart* (pp. 23–42). Hillsdale, NJ: Erlbaum.

Smith, T. W., & Ruiz, J. M. (2002). Psychosocial influences on the development and course of coronary heart disease: Current status and implications for research and practice. *Journal of Consulting & Clinical Psychology, 70,* 548–568.

Spielberger, C. D., Johnson, E. H., Russell, S. F., et al.(1985). The experience and experience of anger: Construction and validation of anger of an anger expression scale. In M. A. Chesney & R. H. Rosenman (Eds.), *Anger and hostility in cardiovascular and behavioral disorders* (pp. 5–30). Washington, DC: Hemisphere Publishing.

Stary, H. C., Chandler, A. B., Dinsmore, R. E., Fuster, V., Glagov, S., Insull, W. Jr., et al. (1995). A definition of advanced types of atherosclerotic lesions and a histological classification of atherosclerosis: A report from the Committee on Vascular Lesions of the Council on Arteriosclerosis, American Heart Association. *Arteriosclerosis, Thrombosis, and Vascular Biology, 15,* 1512–1531.

Stary, H. C., Chandler, A. B., Glagov, S., Guyton, J. R., Insull, W. Jr., Rosenfeld, M. E., et al. (1994). A definition of initial, fatty streak, and intermediate lesions of atherosclerosis: A report from the Committee on Vascular Lesions of the Council of Arteriosclerosis, American Heart Association. *Arteriosclerosis and Thrombosis, 14,* 840–856.

Steptoe, A., Kunz-Ebrecht, S. R., & Owen, N. (2003). Lack of association between depressive symptoms and markers of immune and vascular inflammation in middle-aged men and women. *Psychological Medicine, 33,* 667–674.

Stewart, J. C., Fitzgerald, G. J., & Kamarck, T. W. (2010). Hostility now, depression later? Longitudinal associations among emotional risk factors for coronary artery disease. *Annals of Behavioral Medicine, 39,* 258–266.

Stewart, J. C., Janicki-Deverts, D., Muldoon, M. F., & Kamarck, T. W. (2008). Depressive symptoms moderate the influence of hostility on serum interleukin-6 and C-reactive protein. *Psychosomatic Medicine, 70,* 197–204.

Stewart, J. C., Rand, K. L., Muldoon, M. F., & Kamarck, T. W. (2009). A prospective evaluation of the directionality of the depression-inflammation relationship. *Brain, Behavior, and Immunity, 23,* 936–944.

Suarez, E. C., Lewis, J. G., & Kuhn, C. (2002). The relation of aggression, hostility, and anger to lipopolysaccharide-stimulated tumor necrosis factor (TNF)-alpha by blood monocytes from normal men. *Brain, Behavior, and Immunity, 16,* 675–684.

Suarez, E. C. (2003). The joint effect of hostility and depressive symptoms on plasma interleukin-6 in apparently healthy men. *Psychosomatic Medicine, 65,* 523–527.

Suarez, E. C. (2004). C-reactive protein is associated with psychological risk factors of cardiovascular disease in apparently healthy adults. *Psychosomatic Medicine, 66,* 684–691.

Suarez, E. C. (2006). Sex differences in the relation of depressive symptoms, hostility, and anger expression to indices of glucose metabolism in nondiabetic adults. *Health Psychology, 25,* 484–492.

Suarez, E. C., Krishnan, R. R., & Lewis, J. G. (2003). The relation of severity of depressive symptoms to monocyte-associated pro-inflammatory cytokines and chemokines in apparently healthy men. *Psychosomatic Medicine, 65,* 362–368.

Suarez, E. C., Lewis, J. G., Krishnan, R. R., & Young, K. H. (2004). Enhanced expression of cytokines and chemokines by blood monocytes to in vitro lipopolysaccharide stimulation are associated with hostility and severity of depressive symptoms in healthy women. *Psychoneuroendocrinology, 29,* 1119–1128.

Suarez, E. C., Lewis, J. G., & Kuhn, C. (2002). The relation of aggression, hostility, and anger to lipopolysaccharide-stimulated tumor necrosis factor (TNF)-[alpha] by blood monocytes from normal men. *Brain, Behavior, and Immunity, 16,* 675–684.

Suarez, E. C., Sasaki, M., Lewis, J. G., Williams, R. B., & Adams, D. O. (1996). Anger- increases expression of interleukin-1 on monocytes in high hostile women. *Psychosomatic Medicine, 58,* 87.

Suarez, E. C., & Williams, R. B. (1990). The relationships between dimensions of hostility and cardiovascular reactivity as a function of task characteristics. *Psychosomatic Medicine, 52,* 558–570.

Suls, J., & Bunde, J. (2005). Anger, anxiety, and depression as risk factors for cardiovascular disease: The problems and implication of overlapping affective dispositions. *Psychological Bulletin, 131,* 260–300.

Treiber, F. A., Kamarck, T., Schneiderman, N., Sheffield, D., Kapuku, G., & Taylor, T. (2003). Cardiovascular reactivity and development of preclinical and clinical disease states. *Psychosomatic Medicine, 65,* 46–62.

Tziakas, D. N., Chalikias, G. K., Kaski, J. C., Kekes, A., Hatzinikolaou, E. I., Stakos, D. A., et al. (2007). Inflammatory and anti-inflammatory variable clusters and risk prediction in acute coronary syndrome patients: A factor analysis approach. *Atherosclerosis, 193,* 196–203.

van den Biggelaar, A. H. J., Gussekloo, J., de Craen, A. J. M., Frolich, M., Stek, M. L., van der Mast, R. C., & Westendorp, R. G. (2007). Inflammation and interleukin-1 signaling network contribute to depressive symptoms but not cognitive decline in old age. *Experimental Gerontology, 42,* 693–701.

Virmani, R., Kolodgie, F. D., Burke, A. P., Farb, A., & Schwartz, S. M. (2000). Lessons from sudden coronary death: A comprehensive morphological classification scheme for atherosclerotic lesions. *Arteriosclerosis, Thrombosis, and Vascular Biology, 20,* 1262–1275.

Von Känel, R., Bellingrath, S., & Kudielka, B. M. (2009). Association between longitudinal changes in depressive symptoms and plasma fibrinogen levels in school teachers. *Psychophysiology, 46,* 473–480.

Weiss, J. W., Mouttapa, M., Cen, S., Johnson, C. A., & Unger, J.: Longitudinal effects of hostility, depression, and bullying on adolescent smoking initiation. *Journal of Adolescent Health, 48,* 591–596.

Wirtz, P. H., Redwine, L. S., Linke, S., Hong, S., Rutledge, T., Greenberg, B. H., & Mills, P. J. (2010). Circulating levels of soluble intercellular adhesion molecule-1 (sICAM-1) independently predict depressive symptom severity after

12 months in heart failure patients. *Brain, Behavior, and Immunity, 24,* 366–369.

Woodward, M., Rumley, A., Tunstall-Pedoe, H., & Lowe, G. D. (1999). Associations of blood rheology and interleukin-6 with cardiovascular risk factors and prevalent cardiovascular disease. *British Journal of Haematology, 104,* 246–257.

Wulsin, L. R., & Singal, B. M. (2003). Do depressive symptoms increase the risk for the onset of coronary disease? A systematic quantitative review. *Psychosomatic Medicine, 65,* 201–210.

Yarnell, J. W., Baker, I. A., Sweetnam, P. M., Bainton, D., O'Brien, J. R., Whitehead, P. J., & Elwood, P. C. (1991). Fibrinogen, viscosity, and white blood cell count are major risk factors for ischemic heart disease: The Caerphilly and Speedwell collaborative heart disease studies. *Circulation, 83,* 836–844.

Yusuf, S. (2002). Two decades of progress in preventing vascular disease. *The Lancet, 360,* 2–3.

Yusuf, S., Hawken, S., Ounpuu, S., et al. (2004). Effect of potentially modifiable risk factors associated with myocardial infarction in 52 countries (the INTERHEART study): Case-control study.[see comment]. *Lancet, 364,* 937–952.

Zalcman, S. S., & Siegel, A. (2006). The neurobiology of aggression and rage: Role of cytokines. *Brain, Behavior, and Immunity, 20,* 507–514.

Zorrilla, E. P., Luborsky, L., McKay, J. R., et al. (2001). The relationship of depression and stressors to immunological assays: A meta-analytic review. *Brain, Behavior, & Immunity, 15,* 199–226.

PART 4

Social Relationships

CHAPTER 1

Marriage

Theodore F. Robles *and* Heidi S. Kane

Abstract

For most adults, marriage is a key social relationship that provides economic, social, psychological, and health benefits. At the same time, low marital quality and high conflict have detrimental effects on health. This chapter reviews evidence for immune mechanisms that may explain how marital functioning influences health. Poor marital functioning is related to enhanced innate immunity and diminished adaptive immunity, in a similar direction as the effects of chronic stress. Biobehavioral mechanisms that explain how marital functioning influences immunity include health behaviors; psychological mechanisms including depression, social rejection, and social support; and neuroendocrine mechanisms. Female gender and older age may magnify the effects of marital functioning on immunity, although more research is needed. Key directions for future research on marriage and immunity include further explicating biopsychosocial mechanisms, expanding the sociodemographic range of couples in marriage and immunity research, studying couples outside the laboratory, and incorporating couples intervention research.

Key Words: marriage, immunity, neuroendocrine, marital quality, marital satisfaction, interpersonal relationships, couples, gender, social rejection, social support

Introduction

Each year, the periodical *U.S. News and World Report* publishes a list of "50 ways to improve your life." The suggestions typically range from financial advice ("Put your Cash in Safe Accounts," 2009) to health behaviors ("Walk the Cravings Away," 2009). In 2004, number 34 was "Get Married," which highlights how important marriage is for health and well-being, including increased earning potential, resources for raising a family, and fulfilling needs for security and belonging (Kulman, 2004). Indeed, across a number of surveys, married individuals report greater happiness and life satisfaction (Mastekaasa, 1994), and they have a lower risk of clinical depression than their unmarried counterparts (Robins & Regier, 1991). In addition to these benefits, marriage confers benefits for physical health. For example, nonmarried individuals have higher rates of mortality compared to their married counterparts (Johnson, Backlund, Sorlie, & Loveless, 2000), and morbidity among married persons is lower compared to unmarried persons across a variety of health conditions, including cancer, heart attacks, and surgery (Chandra, Szklo, Goldberg, & Tonascia, 1983; Goodwin, Hunt, Key, & Samet, 1987; Gordon & Rosenthal, 1995). All told, these benefits have led many to extol the virtues of marriage, ranging from the *U.S. News and World Report* list, to the Healthy Marriage Initiative promoted by the U.S. Department of Health and Human Services Administration for Children and Families (www.acf.hhs.gov/healthymarriage).

At the same time, marriages characterized by low marital satisfaction and high conflict have damaging effects on physical health. People in troubled marriages have worse mental and physical well-being compared to people in satisfactory and happy marriages. The most dramatic examples of the relationship between marital *quality* and health come from studies of patients with existing chronic medical conditions. Low marital quality, typically measured through self-report, predicted earlier mortality over long-term (between 4 and 8 years) follow-up in end-stage renal disease and congestive heart failure patients (Coyne et al., 2001; Kimmel et al., 2000; Rohrbaugh, Shoham, & Coyne, 2006). Beyond mortality, low marital quality is also related to increased risk of coronary events (including cardiac death, acute myocardial infarction, and revascularization procedures) in patients with cardiovascular disease (Orth-Gomer et al., 2000) and in a large 9,000-person cohort of British civil servants (De Vogli, Chandola, & Marmot, 2007), increased illness symptoms over longitudinal follow-up (4 years) in healthy married couples (Wickrama, Lorenz, & Conger, 1997), and increased pain flares in patients with rheumatoid arthritis (Zautra et al., 1998).

Our goal in this chapter is to describe the immune mechanisms that explain how marital functioning influences health. The focus of this chapter will be studies that specifically examine the role of marital functioning (as opposed to aspects of the broader social network, such as social support or conflict across the social network) on immunity. Moreover, our focus is on psychoneuroimmunology (PNI) research in married individuals, rather than research on marital status and immunity (e.g., Sbarra, 2009). We initially outline the theoretical frameworks that describe marital influences on health, followed by reviewing the literature on marital factors and immune function, organizing the findings by the useful distinction between innate and adaptive immunity used in previous reviews of stress and immune function (Segerstrom & Miller, 2004). We then describe the biobehavioral mechanisms that explain how marital functioning can modulate immune function, and moderating variables that can influence the link between marital quality and immunity. Importantly, we describe how the extant PNI research has potential or actual implications for clinical health outcomes. We conclude by discussing future directions for research on marriage and immunity.

Marriage, Health, and Immunity: Theoretical Frameworks

Several explanatory frameworks emerged over the last 30 years to explain how marital functioning impacts health, most of which derive from the *stress/social support hypothesis* (Burman & Margolin,

1992). The stress/social support hypothesis suggested that stress and support in marriages influences health through the individual's cognitions, emotions, health behaviors, coping behaviors, and most relevant for this chapter, biological systems. Kiecolt-Glaser and Newton updated this framework, adding several important moderating and mediating pathways, including mental health and psychopathology, and individual differences in personality such as hostility (Kiecolt-Glaser & Newton, 2001). In addition, they proposed that the effect of marital quality on biological systems and health is moderated by gender-related traits, cognitive schemas, and social roles, which explains why marital quality has stronger effects on health for women compared to men (discussed in the *Moderators* section). In a similar vein, Slatcher proposed that positive aspects of marital functioning can buffer against the negative impacts of stress on health, whereas negative aspects of marital functioning can exacerbate the effects of stress on health (Slatcher, 2010). We summarize these conceptual frameworks in Figure 11.1.

Focusing more specifically on how marital functioning can impact biological systems, we proposed viewing marital functioning, particularly negative aspects of marital functioning, as stressors that can lead to detrimental effects on the biological systems through the same pathways as chronic stressors in the allostatic load framework (McEwen, 1998; Robles & Kiecolt-Glaser, 2003). For instance, marital conflict is a common occurrence, with an average frequency of 1–2 times per month (McGonagle, Kessler, & Schilling, 1992), and the topics of conflict can range widely (work-home balance, home maintenance, parenting, etc.). Thus, marital conflicts can serve as "repeated hits" described in the allostatic model. Moreover, couples often have the same arguments over the same problems over time; some couples may show physiological adaptation over time, so that increases in neuroendocrine and autonomic mediators during those arguments gradually decrease with each subsequent discussion, whereas other couples may not show the same physiological adaptation. For example, after the fifth argument about the broken dishwasher, increases in norepinephrine are the same as the very first time the couple talked about the problem. Another pathway leading to cumulative damage to physiological systems is a failure to shut off physiological responses once the stressor has terminated, also described as recovery. As we discuss below, in more hostile couples, autonomic nervous system responses to marital conflict remain elevated well after the discussion

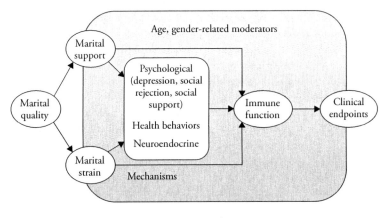

Summary of:
Burman & Margolin, 1992
Kiecolt-Glaser & Newton, 2001
Slatcher, 2010

Figure 11.1 Summary of prevailing models of marital functioning, immunity, and healthy

ends (Malarkey, Kiecolt-Glaser, Pearl, & Glaser, 1994). A final pathway is the inability to mount adequate biological responses to a stressor, which may result from disruption in the normal functioning of stress-responsive systems. Thus, a variety of plausible psychological and biological pathways can explain how poor marital functioning can negatively impact immune function and health, which we describe after reviewing the literature on marital functioning and immunity.

Marriage and Immune Function

The dual challenge of recruiting married couples, particularly unhappy couples, and conducting PNI studies in humans has contributed to the relatively small literature on marriage and immunity compared to other areas of PNI research. At the same time, the literature that does exist represents significant innovations in both methodology and data on interpersonal functioning and immune function. Borrowing from previous reviews (Segerstrom & Miller, 2004), the studies reviewed next are organized in terms of the two primary divisions of the immune system, innate and adaptive immunity.

Innate Immunity

The first published marital interaction and PNI study examined several immune parameters in newlywed couples, including one of the mainstays of early PNI research, natural killer (NK) cell function (Kiecolt-Glaser et al., 1993). Marital interaction studies involve having couples talk to each other in a semistructured way (usually regarding problems

in their relationship, also known as marital conflict) for 20–30 minutes while being audio- and videorecorded (Heyman, 2001). In the Kiecolt-Glaser study, videorecordings were subsequently coded for the presence of hostile/negative behaviors, which included criticism, making negative attributions for the spouse's behavior, and interrupting. Blood samples for immune measures were obtained on arrival to the research unit, approximately 2 hours before the actual marital interaction, and when the couples left the research unit the next morning. The behavioral coding allowed for classifying couples as either high or low in negative behaviors. High negative couples had higher NK cytotoxicity when arriving at the research unit, and a larger decrease in NK cytotoxicity 24 hours later (Kiecolt-Glaser et al., 1993). In a later marital interaction study, self-reported hostile traits emerged as a potential moderator; among men high in cynical hostility, greater anger (assessed using behavioral coding) displayed during conflict was related to increased NK cytotoxicity and greater NK numbers during and 25 minutes after the discussion (Miller, Dopp, Myers, Stevens, & Fahey, 1999). In addition, increased NK cytotoxicity during the discussion was due to greater numbers of circulating NK cells, rather than increased per-cell cytotoxicity (Dopp, Miller, Myers, & Fahey, 2000), and NK cells that lacked the cell adhesion molecule L-selectin (CD62L- cells) were selectively mobilized into the bloodstream rather than L-selectin positive cells. Taken together, these data suggest that negative aspects of marital functioning, including couples who tend to exhibit hostile behavior during marital conflict, and higher hostility in men, are related to greater short-term increases in NK cytotoxicity, which may be due to increased circulation of NK cells in the bloodstream. This response is consistent with NK cell responses observed in response to acute physical and psychological stressors (Segerstrom & Miller, 2004), although the increases in NK cytotoxicity may not last over a 24-hour period (Kiecolt-Glaser et al., 1993).

More recent attention to the role of inflammation in PNI research (Kiecolt-Glaser, McGuire, Robles, & Glaser, 2002) led to examining marital functioning and systemic and localized inflammation (Kiecolt-Glaser et al., 2005). In a study of marital interaction and wound healing, 42 married couples participated in two separate visits to a hospital research unit, during which couples provided repeated blood samples over a 24-hour period to monitor systemic inflammation, and blister wounds were administered to examine wound healing and localized inflammation. Marital interactions occurred during each visit, with one involving a standard problem-solving/conflict discussion, and the other involving a discussion in which one spouse described an aspect of themselves that they wanted to change while the other spouse was asked to respond as he/she normally would. This latter discussion is considered a support discussion, as the normative response by one partner is providing social support to the partner describing aspects of themselves they want to change. Couples were videorecorded, and, as before, the recordings were coded for the presence of negative and hostile behaviors. Couples who showed greater negative behaviors across both discussions had a larger increase in circulating interleukin (IL)-6 and tumor necrosis factor (TNF)-α during the conflict visit compared to the support visit. Couples with low levels of negative behaviors showed no differences in circulating pro-inflammatory cytokines between visits.

Additional studies from the same sample yielded several notable findings, including greater circulating IL-6 during the conflict compared to the support visit for individuals who reported high levels of attachment avoidance (Gouin et al., 2009). Individuals with high attachment avoidance are uncomfortable with interpersonal intimacy and prefer not to rely or depend on other people. In another report, audiorecordings of the discussions were transcribed and analyzed for the use of words indicating causal reasoning (words like *because* or *why*), insight (*think, realize, know*), and other thinking-related words (*should, ought*). During the conflict visit, greater use of these "cognitive words" were related to lower circulating IL-6 and TNF-α levels, and an interesting effect emerged such that husbands had lower IL-6 levels when their wives used greater cognitive words during conflict (Graham et al., 2009). These data suggest that the language couples use while talking to each other about relationship problems can influence their own levels of inflammation, and the way in which partners (in this study wives) talk to their spouses can influence their spouses' inflammation.

At the same time, systemic inflammation may not reflect inflammation at local sites of injury or infection (Kuhns, DeCarlo, Hawk, & Gallin, 1992), which was also demonstrated in the blister-wound-healing study. Although the conflict discussion was characterized by larger increases in systemic pro-inflammatory cytokine levels (in high hostile couples), pro-inflammatory cytokines at the wound site showed larger increases after the support discussion compared to the conflict discussion (Kiecolt-Glaser et al., 2005). Moreover, high-hostility couples showed lower production of TNF-α in blister fluid compared to low-hostility couples.

Taken together, these findings suggest that negative marital functioning is related to elevated circulating pro-inflammatory cytokine levels over a 24-hour period, and to the importance of both individual differences in attachment orientations and the actual spoken content during marital interactions for short-term inflammation levels. However, negative marital functioning is actually related to lower inflammation at local sites, where inflammation contributes to the wound-healing process. Finally, although the findings for systemic inflammation suggest elevations in circulating pro-inflammatory cytokines related to negative marital functioning, increases in cytokines occurred in the context of an administered blister wound; whether such changes would occur if a wound was not administered is unknown.

Adaptive Immunity

The first marital functioning and PNI study recruited married individuals and examined links between self-reported marital quality and several adaptive immune measures. Lower marital quality was related to a lower CD4/CD8 cell ratio in men (Kiecolt-Glaser et al., 1988), and poorer adaptive immunity on several functional measures, including poorer lymphocyte proliferation, in women (Kiecolt-Glaser et al., 1987), and for both men and women, greater Epstein Barr Virus (EBV) antibody titers, which indicate poorer cellular immune control of the latent virus (Kiecolt-Glaser et al., 1987; Kiecolt-Glaser, et al., 1988). In the newlywed-marital-interaction study, high-negative-behavior subjects during conflict showed larger declines in blastogenic response to PHA and Con A and lymphocyte proliferation to mitogen (CD3 receptor) over a 24-hour period compared to low-negative-behavior subjects (Kiecolt-Glaser et al., 1993). Moreover, high-negative-behavior subjects had higher EBV antibody titers compared to low-negative-behavior subjects. Beyond functional measures, high-negative subjects showed changes in enumerative measures, including larger increases in circulating T-cells and a larger increase in the CD4/CD8 ratio. A later study in a small sample of distressed couples showed that, in wives, participating in a conflict discussion decreased lymphocyte proliferation to PHA after the task (Mayne, O' Leary, McCrady, Contrada, & Labouvie, 1997). Moreover, larger increases in hostile mood during the task were related to larger decreases in lymphocyte proliferation.

Similar patterns emerged in a sample of older couples who were married an average of 42 years. In this study, individuals were grouped into a high- or low-immune-response categories based on several measures (EBV antibody titers, lymphocyte proliferation to PHA, and ConA). Individuals with lower responses displayed greater negative behavior during conflict in the laboratory, and they reported greater negative behavior during conflicts outside the lab (Kiecolt-Glaser et al., 1997).

These initial studies, like most PNI research in the early 1990s focused on measures of immunity outside the context of illness or disease. Several later studies showed that marital quality was related to immune measures with relevance to clinical outcomes. In a sample of women with rheumatoid arthritis, women who reported spousal criticism showed increased soluble IL-2R levels during a stressful week compared to a baseline week, whereas women who reported more positive spousal interaction and less spousal criticism or negativity on daily diary measures showed no increase in adaptive immune responses during the stressful week compared to a baseline week (including no increase in cell numbers or soluble IL-2R levels, which were positively correlated with pain symptoms) (Zautra et al., 1998). Finally, several studies have established relationships between chronic stress and immune responses to influenza virus vaccination (Kiecolt-

Glaser, Glaser, Gravenstein, Malarkey, & Sheridan, 1996; Vedhara et al., 1999), and in that vein, a recent study found that antibody titers against the A/Panama influenza vaccine component one month after influenza virus vaccination were lower for individuals reporting low marital satisfaction (Phillips et al., 2006).

Summary

Overall, poorer marital functioning, assessed through self-reports and behavioral data, shows relationships with innate and adaptive immunity that are similar to the effects of chronic stress. For innate immunity, marital conflict is related to short-term increases in NK cytotoxicity for men high in hostility, primarily due to increased cellularity; over longer periods (more than several hours), greater negative behaviors are related to lower NK cytotoxicity. In addition, poorer marital functioning is related to larger increases in circulating inflammatory markers in response to interpersonal discussions, which may be amplified by conflict interactions. Both individual differences in attachment avoidance and language use during discussions appear to moderate these relationships. In contrast, local production of pro-inflammatory cytokines at wound sites is greater during less conflictual discussions, and it is generally lower for less hostile couples. For specific immunity, lower marital quality is related to diminished adaptive immunity, including lower lymphocyte proliferation, higher EBV antibody titers, and poorer antibody response to one component of an influenza virus vaccine. One exception is context of the autoimmune disease rheumatoid arthritis, in which lower marital functioning is related to increased activity of specific immunity in autoimmune disease.

Mechanisms

In this section, we review potential mechanisms that explain how marital functioning can influence immune function. We note that these mechanisms are not mutually exclusive and all likely operate additively and potentially interactively to impact immunity.

Behavioral Mechanisms

One limitation to the overall literature on marital functioning and immunity is that in order to reduce potential confounds for immune measures (Kiecolt-Glaser & Glaser, 1988; O'Connor et al., 2009), these studies have typically recruited healthy individuals who practice very few health-compromising behaviors such as smoking and excessive alcohol use. That said, health behaviors are a very likely mechanism, particularly in couples who are not represented by the samples studied thus far. Indeed, married partners influence each other's behavior across many contexts, including health-promoting behaviors (physical activity, diet, adherence with physician recommendations) and health-compromising behaviors (alcohol use, tobacco use, problematic eating). In general, couples tend to be similar or concordant on health behaviors including diet, smoking, and illegal drug use (Meyler, Stimpson, & Peek, 2007). Individuals whose spouses had a greater frequency of health-promoting behaviors prior to marriage (including regular exercise, routine physical examinations, and healthy eating) were more likely to perform those behaviors themselves during the first four years of marriage, even after adjusting for sociodemographic factors (Homish & Leonard, 2008). At the same time, the way in which partners attempt to influence each others' health behaviors may play a role in the success of those methods, and marital functioning likely contributes to whether a partner coerces or motivates their spouse to change his or her behavior. For instance, positive control behaviors such as modeling a behavior were related to greater intent to change health behaviors (in the direction of more healthy behaviors), whereas negative control behaviors, such as inducing fear, had no effect (Lewis & Butterfield, 2007). Beyond health behaviors associated with "lifestyle," marital functioning also influences adherence to physician recommendations, which can also influence immune function depending on the intervention in question. For example, in a prospective study, lower marital quality predicted worse self-reported adherence with diabetes-self-care recommendations by a physician (Trief, Ploutz-Snyder, Britton, & Weinstock, 2004). Greater marital conflict predicted worse adherence with continuous positive airway- pressure treatment in patients with obstructive sleep apnea (Baron, Smith, Czajkowski, Gunn, & Jones, 2009). Unfortunately, at this point, no studies have explicitly examined how marital functioning influences health behaviors and how those health behaviors subsequently impact immunity.

In addition to adherence, two promising areas for examining how marital functioning influences immune function through health behaviors are diet and sleep—two behaviors that married couples most likely participate in together compared to other behaviors. Given that psychological stress can influence food choices, the metabolic response to

high-fat, high-sugar foods, and that both psychological stress and nutrient consumption (including omega 3 & 6 fatty acids and antioxidants) can influence inflammation, marriage is a natural context to study how both psychological stress and diet work additively and interactively to promote inflammation (Kiecolt-Glaser, 2010). Besides eating together, most couples sleep together (61% in a 2005 National Sleep Foundation poll; National Sleep Foundation, 2005), and beyond the aforementioned social control on health behaviors, another way marital functioning may influence sleep is through shared life events and transitions that affect marriages and sleep, particularly transitions to parenthood and chronic illness in the family. A recent review of extant data (Troxel, Robles, Hall, & Buysse, 2007) suggests that poor marital quality is correlated with poor sleep, including reduced subjective sleep quality and increased self-reported sleep problems, and sleep problems themselves, such as sleep disordered breathing and obstructive sleep apnea, are related to poorer marital quality. Most importantly, although no studies have directly established sleep as a mediator of the impact of marital quality on immunity, sleep problems (including partial sleep deprivation and insomnia) are clearly related to immune dysregulation (Irwin, 2008).

Psychological Mechanisms

Depression has historically received significant attention in the PNI literature as one possible psychological pathway through which psychological factors influence immune function (Irwin, 2008; Miller, 1998). Interestingly, martial dysfunction has consistent associations with depressive symptoms and syndromal depression (Beach, Fincham, & Katz, 1998). Furthermore, depression is reliably associated with immune function dysregulation, including amplifying inflammatory responses (Glaser, Robles, Sheridan, Malarkey, & Kiecolt-Glaser, 2003) and increasing systemic inflammation (Howren, Lamkin, & Suls, 2009), and diminished adaptive immunity (Zorrilla et al., 2001). At the same time, the association between marital quality, depression, and immunity is complex. For example, the association between marital quality and depression is bidirectional; low martial quality predicts the onset of depression and conversely depression predicts decreases in martial quality over time (Davila, Bradbury, Cohan, & Tochluk, 1997; Davila, Karney, Hall, & Bradbury, 2003). Beyond marital conflict leading to increased depression (Beach et al., 1998), depressed individuals tend to increase marital discord by behaving in ways that elicit negative interactions (Davila et. al., 1997; Davila et. al., 2003) and by perceiving more interactions as rejecting (see later). Indeed, in a longitudinal study of newlyweds (Davila et. al., 1997), dysphoric wives reported increases in marital discord a year later (controlling for initial marital discord), and this association was mediated by negative elicitation, receipt, and provision of support during a support discussion. Further complicating these relationships is that the association between depression and immunity is also bidirectional (Miller, 1998). Thus, even in longitudinal studies, disentangling whether depressive symptoms explain the link between marital functioning and immunity or whether marital functioning explains the link between depressive symptoms and immunity can be difficult. Moreover, marital functioning and depressive symptoms may work additively or interactively to influence immunity. Unfortunately, because prior studies recruited relatively healthy samples of married couples, none of the literature to date has directly addressed depressive symptoms as a mediator.

One specific psychological mechanism related to depressive symptoms that may explain the effects of marital dysfunction on immunity is social rejection. Social rejection, social evaluative threat (indicating the possibility of rejection), and rejection-related emotions such as shame are associated with increased systemic inflammation (Dickerson, Gable, Irwin, Aziz, & Kemeny, 2009; Dickerson, Kemeny, Aziz, Kim, & Fahey, 2004; Kemeny, 2009; Slavich, O'Donovan, Epel, & Kemeny, 2010). Furthermore, social-rejection-related experiences are thought to be particularly central to the elicitation of increased inflammatory activity (Dickerson, this volume; Dickerson et al., 2009; Kemeny, 2009; Slavich et al., 2010).

Within the context of martial interactions, hostile and critical behaviors (especially during conflict) may elicit feelings of rejection and perceptions of negative evaluation that are reliably associated with increased inflammatory activity. Marriage (i.e., adult romantic relationships) serves as the primary social or attachment bond in adulthood (e.g., Hazan & Shaver, 1994) making the disruption of these bonds especially distressing. Therefore, the perception of rejection or negative evaluation from a marital partner would also be especially threatening. Furthermore, because couple members are quite familiar with what kinds of comments would be the most derogating or devaluing, rejection from a partner may be especially hurtful. Perceptions of

rejection or negative evaluation during martial interactions might serve as viable pathway for understanding how marital quality and, in particular, conflict interactions affect immunity, particularly inflammation. Future research should examine this possibility within the context of marriage through studies that explicitly assess the degree to which partners feel rejected or evaluated during martial interactions or experimentally manipulate partner rejection and assess changes in inflammation.

The stress/social support hypothesis proposed that although marriages are a source of strain, depression, and social rejection, they are also a source of social support, which is another psychological pathway through which marital functioning may influence immunity. Social support from marital partners can reduce (or buffer) stress appraisals and physiological responses to stress when that support is provided in a responsive way (Coan, Schaefer, & Davidson, 2006; Kirschbaum, Klauer, Filipp, & Hellhammer, 1995). Even in the absence of a current stressor, merely interacting with spouses who are supportive and comforting may serve as a psychosocial resource that attenuates stress appraisals of later stressors. For example, interacting with others perceived as comforting, supportive, and close on a daily basis is associated with attenuated neural activity in brain regions that are associated with social threat during a laboratory rejection task (Eisenberger, Taylor, Gable, Hilmert, & Lieberman, 2007). Furthermore, activation in the same regions is associated with increased inflammation (Slavich et. al., 2010). Interestingly, social-support discussions in martial-interaction studies are not associated with immune activity and are often used as a control or comparison group (e.g., Kiecolt-Glaser et al., 2005). However, consistent with the stress-buffering hypothesis, social- support processes may elicit effects on the immune system within the context of stressful situations, although this concept needs further exploration.

In addition, social support can increase intimacy and associated positive emotions, which may also serve as another potential psychological mediator between marital quality and immunity. One potential pathway through which intimacy and closeness affects immunity is through effects of neuroendocrine hormones associated with affiliation (described in further detail later). Also, feelings of closeness and intimacy may also play a stress-buffering role, by reducing physiological stress reactivity. Preliminary evidence suggests that daily variations in intimacy (as measured by instances of physical affection) are associated with reduced cortisol reactivity to work-related problems, and this association was mediated by positive affect (Ditzen, Hoppmann, & Klumb, 2008). In addition, recent work has demonstrated that trait positive affect is associated with increases with improved adaptive immunity to infectious challenge (Marsland, Cohen, Rabin, & Manuck, 2006), faster skin-barrier recovery (Robles, Brooks, & Pressman, 2009), and increased inflammation fostering tissue repair after radiation in cancer patients (Sepah & Bower, 2009). Therefore, an indirect pathway through which social support can influence immunity is by maintaining healthy, happy relationships (Kane et al., 2007; Pasch & Bradbury, 1998); by enhancing intimacy and positive affect; by promoting positive interactions (Collins & Feeney, 2000); and by decreasing vulnerability to depression (Monroe, Bromet, Connell, & Steiner, 1986), all of which, in turn, influence immunity. For example, in the study previously described, positive interactions with partners and lower reported criticism attenuated rheumatoid arthritis disease activity during a stressful week (Zautra et al., 1998). In general, research on marital functioning and health, including immunity, has primarily focused on the "stress" side of the stress/social-support hypothesis. Only recently has attention begun to swing on how the "social-support" side of the stress/social-support hypothesis influences physiology and immune function, and this will be an important avenue for future research.

Neuroendocrine Mechanisms

As with most, if not all, of the PNI literature, the neuroendocrine mechanisms that explain how marital functioning influences health primarily involve the hypothalamic-pituitary-adrenal (HPA) axis and the autonomic nervous system (Robles & Kiecolt-Glaser, 2003). Following a compelling finding showing that a particularly destructive pattern of marital-interaction behavior—wife making a demand followed by husband's withdrawing from the discussion—was related to elevated cortisol levels in wives over a 24-hour period (Kiecolt-Glaser et al., 1996), several independent studies showed that lower marital quality is related to flatter diurnal cortisol slopes (Adam & Gunnar, 2001; Robles, Shaffer, Malarkey, & Kiecolt-Glaser, 2006; Saxbe, Repetti, & Nishina, 2008), which likely contribute to immune dysregulation. Regarding the autonomic nervous system, greater negative behavior during marital interaction was related to higher circulating catecholamines during and after discussions in both

newlywed (Malarkey et al., 1994) and older adult couples (Kiecolt-Glaser, et al. 1997). Interestingly, in newlywed couples, elevated levels of catecholamines and adrenocorticotropic hormone during the first year of marriage were related to higher rates of marital dissolution (divorce/separation) and lower marital satisfaction in intact couples 10 years later (Kiecolt-Glaser, Bane, Glaser, & Malarkey, 2003). Poor marital functioning is also related to another set of measures related to the autonomic nervous system: cardiovascular function at rest and in response to stress (reviewed in Robles & Kiecolt-Glaser, 2003). For example, greater relationship quality is related to lower ambulatory blood pressure in naturalistic settings (Holt-Lunstad, Birmingham, & Jones, 2008).

Although research on marital functioning has not explicitly examined interactions between neuroendocrine changes and immune function, other work suggests those connections are likely. Regarding innate immunity, similar to work by Miller and Dopp and colleagues, acute laboratory stress was related to large increases in circulating L-selectin negative NK cells (Bosch, Berntson, Cacioppo, & Marucha, 2005); evidence for the role of catecholamines comes from pharmacological studies where a β-adrenergic agonist (isopreteronol) increased circulating L-selectin negative NK cells, an effect that was blocked by propranolol (Mills, Goebel, Rehman, Irwin, & Maisel, 2000). In terms of inflammation, exposure to acute stressors increases inflammatory-marker levels across a number of studies, but the exact mechanisms (beyond the intracellular mechanisms that beget inflammation) through which this occurs have not been fully outlined (Steptoe, Hamer, & Chida, 2007).

Regarding adaptive immunity, in older women, greater sympathetic cardiovascular responses to acute stress were related to higher EBV antibody titers compared to women who showed lower sympathetic cardiovascular responses (Cacioppo et al., 2002). In another study, cells infected with EBV had greater reactivation of the latent virus when exposed to repeated "pulses" of dexamethasone rather than a constant high level of the glucocorticoid agonist (Cacioppo et al., 2002). This *in vitro* finding suggests that repeated exposures to surges of glucocorticoids, such as those encountered during repeated marital conflicts over time, may be related to poorer cellular immune control of latent EBV infection.

Beyond the prototypical neuroendocrine pathways that have been featured throughout PNI research, more recent work suggests an additional set of neuroendocrine pathways that are related to both social affiliation and immune regulation: oxytocin- and vasopressin-mediated pathways. Elevated levels of circulating oxytocin are related to better relationship quality (broadly defined to include ratings of support and actual provision of support) across several studies (Grewen, Girdler, Amico, & Light, 2005; Light, Grewen, & Amico, 2005). Although not directly linked to interpersonal romantic relationship functioning, lower circulating vasopressin is related to early neglect in children, suggesting that poor interpersonal functioning may be related to lower vasopressin levels (Fries, Ziegler, Kurian, Jacoris, & Pollak, 2005). Following up on literature showing that oxytocin and vasopressin can modulate proinflammatory cytokine levels and also wound healing in animal models, Gouin and colleagues examined relationships between marital functioning, oxytocin and vasopressin, and immunity. Extending previous work on interpersonal relationships and oxytocin, greater positive behaviors during a social support discussion were related to greater peripheral oxytocin levels (Gouin et al., 2010). Moreover, lower negative behaviors were related to greater peripheral vasopressin levels. In terms of interactions with inflammation, higher vasopressin levels were related to higher circulating TNF-α. Although this particular finding was opposite to what one might expect given the previous literature, the authors noted that prior work on oxytocin and vasopressin effects on inflammation used exogenous administration at often pharmacological levels of the hormones, whereas this study examined endogenous levels. As research on the role of oxytocin and vasopressin systems continues to progress, continued integration with understanding marital and immune functioning will be a fruitful area for future work.

Moderators

Research to date suggests that, in general, poor marital quality is related to enhanced innate immunity and diminished adaptive immunity. However, this relationship likely varies across different groups of individuals; that is, several factors may moderate the relationship between marital functioning and immunity, particularly gender and age.

Although men derive greater health benefits by being married compared to women, marital quality appears to have larger effects for women compared to men (Kiecolt-Glaser & Newton, 2001). For innate immunity, several studies have reported no moderating effects for gender (Gouin et al.,

2009; Kiecolt-Glaser et al., 2005; Kiecolt-Glaser et al., 1993), whereas others have shown larger (or at least significant) effects for men and not women (Graham et al., 2009; Miller et al., 1999). For adaptive immunity, some studies have reported no moderating effects for gender (Kiecolt-Glaser et al. 1997), larger effects for women (Kiecolt-Glaser et al., 1993), or larger effects for men and not women (Mayne et al., 1997). Although these patterns are not as consistent with the larger pattern observed in marriage and health research, we note that small sample sizes limit the ability to test moderating effects. Moreover, marriage and immunity research involves relatively short-term effects on biological processes and outcomes (minutes to months), whereas research on marital quality and health typically examines biological processes that reflect long-term influences (e.g., ambulatory blood pressure, atherosclerotic processes) and outcomes (morbidity and mortality).

The effects of gender on the link between marital functioning and health involve a variety of potential cultural, psychosocial, and biological mechanisms; the latter include gender differences in health behaviors, the relative contribution of sex hormones, and gender differences in regulation of stress-response systems. Cultural and psychosocial processes are particularly notable, as they bear directly on the types of stressors that are traditionally experienced by wives in contemporary society. Drawing on prior research, Kiecolt-Glaser and Newton (2001) identified the gender-related personality trait of communion (characterized by a motivation to focus on and attend to others instead of oneself), degree of relational interdependence in self-representations, and exposure to stress through normative gender-based marital and parental roles as possible explanations for why women are more vulnerable to the influence of martial quality on their health. For example, communion is more characteristic of women than men, and it is positively associated with increased vulnerability to interpersonal stressors (Helgeson, 1994). Additionally, they proposed that because women tend to have relationally interdependent self-representations (i.e., their sense of self, construal of social information and self-regulation are tied to close relationships) (e.g., Cross & Madson, 1997a; Cross & Madson, 1997b), they are more aware of and influenced by the emotional quality of marital interactions. In contrast, men are insulated from these vulnerabilities to marital quality because their self-representations are less associated with the marital relationship making them less attuned to and influenced by the emotional quality of the relationship. Finally, social norms regarding wives' roles in the home typically lead to greater wives' contributions to household and parenting duties, despite increasingly equal contributions to household income between husbands and wives in many families. Thus, although discussions of gender differences in marital quality and immune function, and marital quality and health, more broadly, may often involve discussing biological mechanisms, cultural and psychosocial aspects of gender must also be taken into account because they are difficult to separate from biological sex in most studies.

In addition to gender, age likely plays an important role in the relationship between marital functioning and immunity, although this has not been formally tested in research to date. That said, the effects of marital functioning on immune function do persist in older couples (Kiecolt-Glaser et al., 1997). Age is a likely moderating factor for several reasons. The immune system changes with age, including increased systemic inflammation and diminished adaptive immunity (Graham, Christian, & Kiecolt-Glaser, 2006). For couples who remain together over long periods of time, negative marital functioning likely evolves into a chronic stressor of very long duration (Robles & Kiecolt-Glaser, 2003). Moreover, with age comes the potential for other burdens on married couples, particularly if one spouse becomes chronically ill. Indeed, caring for a spouse with progressive dementia is related to poorer immune function of the caregiver. with major negative consequences for health (Kiecolt-Glaser, Dura, Speicher, Trask, & Glaser, 1991; Kiecolt-Glaser, Marucha, Malarkey, Mercado, & Glaser, 1995). In the United States, the baby-boomer generation has the highest proportion of married adults; thus, continuing to explore how age influences links between marital functioning, immune function, and health will have important public-health consequences for a large segment of the population.

Consequences for Acute and Chronic Conditions

With a few important exceptions, most work on marital functioning and immunity has been limited to "X → Y" relationships between marital functioning and immunity without examining the full X → Y → Z model (Kemeny, 2003) in which psychosocial factors are related to immunity and subsequent health outcomes. Indeed, as PNI research has established over the last three decades, any number of psychological stimuli can cause changes in immune function, but many of those changes may not have measurable impact on health or disease (Kiecolt-Glaser, Cacioppo, Malarkey, & Glaser, 1992). In this section, we highlight potential and, in some cases, actual evidence suggesting that immune dysregulation related to marital functioning may have clinically relevant health consequences. We review several short-term health outcomes, including wound healing and upper respiratory infections, and one chronic disease—atherosclerosis.

Wound Healing

Both acute and chronic psychological stress can delay wound healing (Walburn, Vedhara, Hankins, Rixon, & Weinman, 2009), and interpersonal stressors can be a particularly potent type of stressor. Couples receiving blister wounds on two separate days showed 72% slower healing during a day involving a marital-conflict discussion compared to a day involving a nonconflict discussion. Moreover, individuals in high-hostile behavior couples based on behavioral ratings on both days showed 60% slower healing compared to low-hostile behavior couples. In terms of potential mechanisms, individuals in high-hostile couples showed fewer cells in blister chamber fluid, which provides a window into immune cell migration into the blister wound site, compared to individuals in low-hostile couples (Kiecolt-Glaser et al., 2005). Another potential mechanism is oxytocin levels, as previous animal work showed that treatment with oxytocin in social isolated rodents sped wound healing (Detillion, Craft, Glasper, Prendergast, & DeVries, 2004). However, in the blister-wound study, oxytocin levels (treated as a continuous predictor) were not related to wound healing, although individuals in the upper quartile for oxytocin healed blister wounds faster compared to individuals in the lower quartile (Gouin et al., 2010). Moreover, women in the upper quartile for vasopressin healed faster compared to women in the lower quartile. These data provide compelling evidence that marital quality can impact a clinical outcome, and may suggest one mechanism through which marital functioning can delay related outcomes such as surgical recovery (Kiecolt-Glaser, Page, Marucha, MacCallum, & Glaser, 1998; Kulik & Mahler, 2006).

Upper respiratory infections

Chronic interpersonal stressors are related to greater susceptibility to the common cold (Cohen et al., 1998); thus, marital quality may be related to the likelihood of developing upper respiratory infections like the cold or flu. Although no studies have directly examined marital quality in viral challenge studies, one recent study suggests that marital quality may reduce the ability to fight off viral infection. In an influenza virus vaccination study, antibody titers against the A/Panama component one month after vaccination were lower for individuals reporting low marital satisfaction (Phillips et al., 2006). Coupled with other findings on marital functioning and adaptive immunity, these studies suggest that low marital quality may impair the ability to eradicate upper respiratory infections. Moreover, the data on marital functioning and innate immunity potentially suggest that if poor marital quality is associated with enhanced innate immune responses, such persons may have exaggerated symptoms when they are infected. Indeed, levels of pro-inflammatory cytokines in the respiratory compartment are linked to psychosocial factors, including low positive affect and perceived stress (Cohen, Doyle & Skoner, 1999; Doyle, Gentile, & Cohen, 2006), and they account for a significant proportion of the variance in upper respiratory infection symptoms (Doyle, et al., 2006). Thus, we would expect individuals in low-quality marriages to experience more respiratory infections of longer duration and greater severity, and we are currently exploring this in our current work.

Atherosclerosis

The strongest evidence for links between marital functioning, biological processes, and health comes from cardiovascular disease research. Low marital quality is related to elevated cardiovascular risk factors (e.g., "good" and "bad" cholesterol, triglycerides; Gallo, Troxel, Matthews, & Kuller, 2003), predicts elevated ambulatory blood pressure (Holt-Lunstad et al., 2008), and predicts faster progression of atherosclerosis across several studies (Gallo et al., 2003). Moreover, among patients with existing cardiovascular disease, poor marital functioning predicts longer hospital stays following coronary artery bypass graft surgery (Kulik & Mahler, 2006), risk of recurrent cardiac events (e.g., a second myocardial infarction after a first myocardial infarction) (Orth-Gomer et al., 2000), and mortality in prospective longitudinal studies (Rohrbaugh et al., 2006). Although immune mechanisms have not been directly implicated in the observed health outcomes in these studies, several immune markers, including plasma levels of C-reactive protein and interleukin-6, have emerged as potential surrogate markers for cardiovascular disease risk, particularly

risk of initial clinical events (Ridker, Brown, Vaughan, Harrison, & Mehta, 2004). Importantly, inflammatory mediators may play important mechanistic roles in the progression of atherosclerosis and the instability of plaques in existing disease (Libby & Theroux, 2005). Given the preliminary data on short-term elevations in pro-inflammatory cytokines during marital conflict days compared to non-conflict days in high-hostile couples (Kiecolt-Glaser et al., 2005), and the wealth of data on marital functioning in cardiovascular disease reviewed earlier, understanding the role of immune mechanisms in cardiovascular disease will be a fruitful avenue in future marriage-and-health research.

Conclusion

Despite a relatively small number of studies, research on marital functioning and immunity provides some of the most compelling PNI data to date on social influences on the immune system in humans, particularly in the context of a *specific* social relationship. Marriages are both a source of support and stress, and although most data clearly suggests that negative aspects of marital functioning are related to immunity, this is, in part, due to the historical focus on marital strain rather than marital support in the broader marriage literature. As a stressor, negative aspects of marital functioning should influence physiology in much the same way as other stressors in broader conceptualizations of stress and health (McEwen, 1998). Indeed, the literature on marriage and immunity shows a pattern similar to the broader literature on stress and immunity: short-term elevations in innate immunity, including NK cytotoxicity and systemic inflammation; and diminished adaptive immunity, particularly functional measures of cell-mediated and humoral immunity.

The biobehavioral mechanisms through which marital functioning can influence immunity are similar to other processes described in PNI research. One unique aspect of these mechanisms is that they operate in a dyadic manner—that is, spouses influence each others' health behaviors, and, more recently, there is evidence suggesting that spouses have significant covariation in basal HPA function (Saxbe & Repetti, 2010). In addition, the support component of marriages suggests that additional neuroendocrine pathways involved in affiliation and attachment may play a role in modulating immunity. Beyond influencing mediators, gender may play a key role in moderating the relationship between marital functioning and immunity for a variety of reasons beyond biological sex, notably cultural and psychosocial factors linked to gender. Age is also a key moderator, given how relationships and immune function change over the life course and the cumulative impact of the marital strain over time.

Although fully explicating mediators and moderators remains an important empirical question for future research, recent work clearly establishes the clinical implications of marital functioning and health. Increased marital strain can delay wound healing and diminish protections afforded by influenza virus vaccination. Extant data suggest that marital function may contribute to susceptibility and responses to upper respiratory infections, a fairly common but also costly health concern. In terms of chronic illness, research amassed over the past decade clearly showing prospective relationships between marital functioning and cardiovascular disease risk, morbidity, and mortality. Thus far, the specific immune mechanisms have not been definitively outlined for these outcomes; that is, no study has definitively shown an $X \rightarrow Y \rightarrow Z$ relationship, but the existing data suggests that such relationships are quite plausible. Although we focused on a few health conditions, other chronic health conditions that have immune system involvement are also excellent candidates for exploring relationships between marriage and immunity, including autoimmune disease (Zautra et al., 1998), breast cancer (Yang & Schuler, 2009), and chronic pain (Leonard, Cano, & Johansen, 2006).

Future Directions

Although research on marital functioning and immunity emerged during the first decade of modern PNI research, studies have been relatively few compared to other areas in the field. The many prevailing questions in understanding how marital quality affects immune function makes the field a fertile one. Here we identify some future directions for moving forward.

Further Explicating Mechanisms

Much like our understanding of how psychological stress influences innate and adaptive immunity, future work in marriage and immunity should continue to identify specific biobehavioral mechanisms. We suggest turning attention to behavioral mechanisms that were described previously, notably sleep and nutrition, as well as adherence in chronically ill populations. Moreover, although negative aspects of marital functioning have detrimental effects on immunity, how behaviors like hostility

and criticism specifically impact spouses to influence immunity is not clear. For example, does criticism increase feelings of rejection, which uniquely increases systemic inflammation? Or does criticism increase stress appraisals from stressors occurring outside the marriage? Finally, at a biological level, evidence suggests that our typical models of P to N to I operate in the context of marriages, we do not have definitive evidence that, for example, increases in norepinephrine during marital conflict explain changes in immunity that result from conflict. Moreover, the field still needs clear evidence for intracellular changes that occur during negative marital interactions. Although most of these suggestions are in the "N to I" category, also worth noticing is a growing literature on neural circuitry activated during interpersonal interactions between couples. Although we previously described research on social rejection, thus far, that work has not focused on rejection that occurs specifically within couples. On the other hand, research on social support has involved intimate couples, and several studies now suggest that support provided by one intimate partner to another can activate neural regions that are responsive to threat and that regulate peripheral physiology (Coan et al., 2006). Integrating this "P to N" work with immune outcomes would provide a fuller picture of how intimate relationships influence physiology.

Expanding the Range of Couples

Research on marriage involving samples that are not obtained through population-based strategies designed to provide maximum generalizablity (e.g., random-digit dialing, large samples over 1,000), or samples that are seeking marital therapy, faces a persistent obstacle: recruiting unhappy couples (Karney et al., 1995). As we discussed earlier, this issue is further compounded when rigorous exclusion and inclusion criteria necessary to minimize confounds in PNI research are added. Thus, the marriage and immunity research reviewed in this paper comes from mostly healthy, highly satisfied couples with restricted ranges in socioeconomic status and ethnicity. On one hand, this likely means that most research on marital functioning and immunity understates the effect of marital functioning (Kiecolt-Glaser & Newton, 2001). At the same time, the degree to which the findings reviewed in this paper generalize to populations that were not sampled is an empirical question.

Generalizability is important not only from a scientific perspective, but also from a public-health perspective. Federal efforts to promote marriage are primarily targeted toward low-income individuals and minorities, in part to reduce health disparities. Thus, the question of how marital functioning impacts health is probably most crucial for disadvantaged populations. Low education, poor mental health, and domestic violence are all associated with poor marital functioning (Rauer, Karney, Garvan, & Hou, 2008), as well as low socioeconomic status. The extent to which marital support can promote health and marital strain can erode health remains unknown. Thus, we suggest future work on marital functioning and immunity should begin to recruit samples in ways that can address the generalizability concerns. One way to do so is increasing efforts to recruit a broad range of participants across socio-economic strata, perhaps with oversampling lower strata, and ethnicity. Although such recruitment presents challenges, they are not insurmountable (Rogge et al., 2006). Another way to increase generalizability is conducting marriage and immunity research that focuses on specific chronic disease populations. The burden of chronic illness often falls to more disadvantaged individuals, and couples who may not sign up for a study of "marriage" may sign up for a study of "how diabetes affects your life."

Studying Couples in Their Natural Contexts

The most influential studies of marital functioning and immunity have taken place inside the laboratory; their influence is due in large part to the ability to observe behavior as it happens. At the same time, studying couples in their actual settings can provide valuable insights in understanding how marital functioning influences physiology. Thus far, naturalistic studies of marital functioning and physiology have focused on neuroendocrine mediators, primarily due to the ease of obtaining biological samples through saliva (Saxbe, 2008). Combining these designs, in which couples complete daily diary or ecological momentary-assessment measures, with immunological measures can provide a larger snapshot of couples' functioning over longer periods of time than a 30-minute discussion. Moreover, although methodologically and logistically challenging, observing couples in their home environment is increasingly possible through technological advances, including videorecording families at home (Campos, Graesch, Repetti, Bradbury, & Ochs, 2009) and minimally obtrusive electronically activated recordings (Mehl, 2007).

Thus far, we have discussed studying couples in their everyday contexts. Another important context

in which to study couples is in the external stressors that impinge upon couples (Story & Bradbury, 2004). Thus far, research on marriage and immunity has considered marital functioning as the stressor. External stressors, ranging from financial problems to difficulties with children, can place strain on marriages (Karney & Bradbury, 1995; Story & Bradbury, 2004), and the impact of these stressors on the link between marital functioning and immunity has not yet been fully explored. Doing so requires assessing the presence of episodic and chronic stressors in couples, which can be easily done using methods previously used in PNI research such as life-stress interviews (Cohen et al., 1998; Miller & Chen, 2006). Moreover, married couples face normative challenges, like transitions to parenthood, school transitions, employment or location changes, and transitions that accompany older age like empty nesting and retirement. Studying samples facing a common challenge provides an opportunity to examine how normative events impact marital functioning and immunity, and how marital functioning might influence how stressful events impact immunity. Beyond adding the aforementioned features to research designs, we also repeat a prior suggestion for more longitudinal studies (Robles & Kiecolt-Glaser, 2003), which provide the best opportunity to study couples in their naturalistic contexts.

Incorporating Intervention Studies

We close by cautioning that a major limitation of research on marital functioning and health is that the primary research designs involve observational studies. Thus, the question of whether happier couples are healthier, or whether healthier couples are happier cannot be easily disentangled. Experimentally manipulating marital functioning can only be accomplished in the long run through interventions. Fortunately, empirically supported marital-therapy interventions are available with well-documented effects on marital quality (Baucom, Shoham, Mueser, Daiuto, & Stickle, 1998). Randomized controlled trials of marital therapy interventions thus provide an excellent context for examining how experimentally manipulated changes in marital functioning might impact immune function and other health outcomes. Ultimately, although PNI research on marriage and immunity provides us with valuable insights into how interpersonal relationships influence biology, the public health relevance for this work will be decided by whether interventions to prevent marital distress or change marital functioning have significant impacts on immune function and health.

Author Note

This research was supported by a William T. Grant Foundation Research Grant and National Institutes of Health grant AG032494 to the first author, and training grant MH015750 to the second author.

Related Chapters

For more information on concepts introduced in this chapter, see also Dickerson; and Pressman, this volume.

References

Adam, E. K., & Gunnar, M. R. (2001). Relationship functioning and home and work demands predict individual differences in diurnal cortisol patterns in women. *Psychoneuroendocrinology, 26,* 189–208.

Baron, K. G., Smith, T. W., Czajkowski, L. A., Gunn, H. E., & Jones, C. R. (2009). Relationship quality and CPAP adherence in patients with obstructive sleep apnea. *Behavioral Sleep Medicine, 7,* 22–36.

Baucom, D. H., Shoham, V., Mueser, K. T., Daiuto, A. D., & Stickle, T. R. (1998). Empirically supported couple and family interventions for marital distress and adult mental health problems. *Journal of Consulting and Clinical Psychology, 66,* 53–88.

Beach, S. R. H., Fincham, F. D., & Katz, J. (1998). Marital therapy in the treatment of depression: Toward a third generation of therapy and research. *Clinical Psychology Review, 18,* 635–661.

Bosch, J. A., Berntson, G. G., Cacioppo, J. T., & Marucha, P. T. (2005). Differential mobilization of functionally distinct natural killer subsets during acute psychologic stress. *Psychosomatic Medicine, 67,* 366–375.

Burman, B., & Margolin, G. (1992). Analysis of the association between marital relationships and health problems: An interactional perspective. *Psychological Bulletin, 112,* 39–63.

Cacioppo, J. T., Kiecolt-Glaser, J. K., Malarkey, W. B., Laskowski, B. F., Rozlog, L. A., & Poehlmann, K. M. (2002). Autonomic and glucocorticoid associations with the steady-state expression of latent Epstein-Barr virus. *Hormones and Behavior, 42,* 32–41.

Campos, B., Graesch, A. P., Repetti, R. L., Bradbury, T. N., & Ochs, E. (2009). Opportunity for interaction? A naturalistic observation study of dual-earner families after work and school. *Journal of Family Psychology, 23,* 798–807.

Chandra, V., Szklo, M., Goldberg, R., & Tonascia, J. (1983). The impact of marital status on survival after an acute myocardial infarction: A population-based study. *American Journal of Epidemiology, 117,* 320–325.

Coan, J. A., Schaefer, H. S., & Davidson, R. J. (2006). Lending a hand: Social regulation of the neural response to threat. *Psychological Science, 17,* 1032–1039.

Cohen, S., Doyle, W. J., & Skoner, D. P. (1999). Psychological stress, cytokine production, and severity of upper respiratory illness. *Psychosomatic Medicine, 61,* 175–180.

Cohen, S., Frank, E., Doyle, W. J., Skoner, D. P., Rabin, B. S., & Gwaltney, J. M. (1998). Types of stressors that increase susceptibility to the common cold in healthy adults. *Health Psychology, 17,* 214–223.

Collins, N. L., & Feeney, B. C. (2000). A safe haven: An attachment theory perspective on support seeking and caregiving in intimate relationships. *Journal of Personality and Social Psychology, 78,* 1053–1073.

Coyne, J. C., Rohrbaugh, M. J., Shoham, V., Sonnega, J. S., Nicklas, J. M., & Cranford, J. A. (2001). Prognostic importance of marital quality for survival of congestive heart failure. *American Journal of Cardiology, 88,* 526–529.

Cross, S. E., & Madson, L. (1997a). Elaboration of models of the self: Reply to Baumeister and Sommer (1997) and Martin and Ruble (1997). *Psychological Bulletin, 122,* 51–55.

Cross, S. E., & Madson, L. (1997b). Models of the self: Self-construals and gender. *Psychological Bulletin, 122,* 5–37.

Davila, J., Bradbury, T. N., Cohan, C. L., & Tochluk, S. (1997). Marital functioning and depressive symptoms: Evidence for a stress generation model. *Journal of Personality and Social Psychology, 73,* 849–861.

Davila, J., Karney, B. R., Hall, T. W., & Bradbury, T. N. (2003). Depressive symptoms and marital satisfaction: Within-subject associations and the moderating effects of gender and neuroticism. *Journal of Family Psychology, 17,* 557–570.

De Vogli, R., Chandola, T., & Marmot, M. G. (2007). Negative aspects of close relationships and heart disease. *Archives of Internal Medicine, 167,* 1951–1957.

Detillion, C. E., Craft, T. K., Glasper, E. R., Prendergast, B. J., & DeVries, A. C. (2004). Social facilitation of wound healing. *Psychoneuroendocrinology, 29,* 1004–1011.

Dickerson, S. S., Gable, S. L., Irwin, M. R., Aziz, N., & Kemeny, M. E. (2009). Social-evaluative threat and proinflammatory cytokine regulation: An experimental laboratory investigation. *Psychological Science, 20,* 1237–1244.

Dickerson, S. S., Kemeny, M. E., Aziz, N., Kim, K. H., & Fahey, J. L. (2004). Immunological effects of induced shame and guilt. *Psychosomatic Medicine, 66,* 124–131.

Ditzen, B., Hoppmann, C., & Klumb, P. (2008). Positive couple interactions and daily cortisol: On the stress-protecting role of intimacy. *Psychosomatic Medicine, 70,* 883–889.

Dopp, J. M., Miller, G. E., Myers, H. F., & Fahey, J. L. (2000). Increased natural killer-cell mobilization and cytotoxicity during marital conflict. *Brain, Behavior, and Immunity, 14,* 10–26.

Doyle, W. J., Gentile, D. A., & Cohen, S. (2006). Emotional style, nasal cytokines, and illness expression after experimental rhinovirus exposure. *Brain, Behavior, and Immunity, 20,* 175–181.

Eisenberger, N. I., Gable, S. L., & Lieberman, M. D. (2007). Functional magnetic resonance imaging responses relate to differences in real-world social experience. *Emotion, 7,* 745–754.

Fries, A. B. W., Ziegler, T. E., Kurian, J. R., Jacoris, S., & Pollak, S. D. (2005). Early experience in humans is associated with changes in neuropeptides critical for regulating social behavior. *Proceedings of the National Academy of Sciences of the United States of America, 102,* 17237–17240.

Gallo, L. C., Troxel, W. M., Kuller, L. H., Sutton-Tyrrell, K., Edmundowicz, D., & Matthews, K. A. (2003). Marital status, marital quality, and atherosclerotic burden in postmenopausal women. *Psychosomatic Medicine, 65,* 952–962.

Gallo, L. C., Troxel, W. M., Matthews, K. A., & Kuller, L. H. (2003). Marital status and quality in middle-aged women:

Associations with levels and trajectories of cardiovascular risk factors. *Health Psychology, 22,* 453–463.

Glaser, R., Robles, T. F., Sheridan, J., Malarkey, W. B., & Kiecolt-Glaser, J. K. (2003). Mild depressive symptoms are associated with amplified and prolonged inflammatory responses following influenza vaccination in older adults. *Archives of General Psychiatry, 60,* 1009–1014.

Goodwin, J. S., Hunt, W. C., Key, C. R., & Samet, J. M. (1987). The effect of marital status on stage, treatment, and survival of cancer patients. *Journal of the American Medical Association, 34,* 20–26.

Gordon, H. S., & Rosenthal, G. E. (1995). Impact of marital status on outcomes in hospitalized patients. *Archives of Internal Medicine, 155,* 2465–2471.

Gouin, J., Carter, C. S., Pournajafi-Nazarloo, H., Glaser, R., Malarkey, W. B., & Loving, T. J. (2010). Marital behavior, oxytocin, vasopressin, and wound healing. *Psychoneuroendocrinology, 35,* 1082–1090.

Gouin, J., Glaser, R., Loving, T. J., Malarkey, W. B., Stowell, J. R., & Houts, C. (2009). Attachment avoidance predicts inflammatory responses to marital conflict. *Brain, Behavior, and Immunity, 23,* 898–904.

Graham, J. E., Christian, L. M., & Kiecolt-Glaser, J. K. (2006). Stress, age, and immune function: Toward a lifespan approach. *Journal of Behavioral Medicine, 29*(4), 389–400.

Graham, J. E., Glaser, R., Loving, T. J., Malarkey, W. B., Stowell, J. R., & Kiecolt-Glaser, J. K. (2009). Cognitive word use during marital conflict and increases in proinflammatory cytokines. *Health Psychology, 28,* 621–630.

Grewen, K. M., Girdler, S. S., Amico, J., & Light, K. C. (2005). Effects of partner support on resting oxytocin, cortisol, norepinephrine, and blood pressure before and after warm partner contact. *Psychosomatic Medicine, 67,* 531–538.

Hazan, C., & Shaver, P. R. (1994). Attachment as an organization framework for research on close relationships. *Psychological Inquiry, 5,* 1–22.

Heyman, R. E. (2001). Observation of couple conflicts: Clinical assessment applications, stubborn truths, and shaky foundations. *Psychological Assessment, 13,* 5–35.

Holt-Lunstad, J., Birmingham, W., & Jones, B. Q. (2008). Is there something unique about marriage? The relative impact of marital status, relationship quality, and network support on ambulatory blood pressure and mental health. *Annals of Behavioral Medicine, 35,* 239–244.

Homish, G. G., & Leonard, K. E. (2008). Spousal influence on general health behaviors in a community sample. *American Journal of Health Behavior, 32,* 754–763.

Howren, M. B., Lamkin, D. M., & Suls, J. (2009). Associations of depression with C-reactive protein, IL-1, and IL-6: A meta-analysis. *Psychosomatic Medicine, 71,* 171–186.

Irwin, M. R. (2008). Human psychoneuroimmunology: 20 years of discovery. *Brain, Behavior, and Immunity, 22,* 129–139.

Johnson, N. J., Backlund, E., Sorlie, P. D., & Loveless, C. A. (2000). Marital status and mortality: The National Longitudinal Mortality Study. *Annals of Epidemiology, 10,* 224–238.

Kane, H. S., Jaremka, L. M., Guichard, A. C., Ford, M. B., Collins, N. L., & Feeney, B. C. (2007). Feeling supported and feeling satisfied: How one partner's attachment style predicts the other partner's relationship experiences. *Journal of Social and Personal Relationships, 24,* 535–555.

Karney, B. R., & Bradbury, T. N. (1995). The longitudinal course of marital quality and stability: A review of theory, method, and research. *Psychological Bulletin, 118,* 3–34.

Karney, B. R., Davila, J., Cohan, C. L., Sullivan, K. T., Johnson, M. D., & Bradbury, T. N. (1995). An empirical investigation of sampling strategies in marital research. *Journal of Marriage and the Family, 57,* 909–920.

Kemeny, M. E. (2003). An interdisciplinary research model to investigate psychosocial cofactors in disease: Application to HIV-1 pathogenesis. *Brain, Behavior, and Immunity, 17,* S62–72.

Kemeny, M. E. (2009). Psychobiological responses to social threat: Evolution of a psychological model in psychoneuroimmunology. *Brain, Behavior, and Immunity, 23,* 1–9.

Kiecolt-Glaser, J. K. (2010). Stress, food, and inflammation: Psychoneuroimmunology and nutrition at the cutting edge. *Psychosomatic Medicine, 72,* 365–369.

Kiecolt-Glaser, J. K., Bane, C., Glaser, R., & Malarkey, W. B. (2003). Love, marriage, and divorce: Newlyweds' stress hormones foreshadow relationship changes. *Journal of Consulting and Clinical Psychology, 71,* 176–188.

Kiecolt-Glaser, J. K., Cacioppo, J. T., Malarkey, W. B., & Glaser, R. (1992). Acute psychological stressors and short-term immune changes: What, why, for whom, and to what extent? *Psychosomatic Medicine, 54,* 680–685.

Kiecolt-Glaser, J. K., Dura, J. R., Speicher, C. E., Trask, O. J., & Glaser, R. (1991). Spousal caregivers of dementia victims: Longitudinal changes in immunity and health. *Psychosomatic Medicine, 53,* 345–362.

Kiecolt-Glaser, J. K., Fisher, L., Ogrocki, P., Stout, J. C., Speicher, C. E., & Glaser, R. (1987). Marital quality, marital disruption, and immune function. *Psychosomatic Medicine, 49,* 31–34.

Kiecolt-Glaser, J. K., & Glaser, R. (1988). Methodological issues in behavioral immunology research with humans. *Brain, Behavior, and Immunity, 2,* 67–78.

Kiecolt-Glaser, J. K., Glaser, R., Cacioppo, J. T., MacCallum, R. C., Snydersmith, M., & Kim, C. (1997). Marital conflict in older adults: Endocrinological and immunological correlates. *Psychosomatic Medicine, 59,* 339–349.

Kiecolt-Glaser, J. K., Glaser, R., Gravenstein, S., Malarkey, W. B., & Sheridan, J. (1996). Chronic stress alters the immune response to influenza virus vaccine in older adults. *Proceedings of the National Academy of Sciences of the United States of America, 93,* 3403–3047.

Kiecolt-Glaser, J. K., Kennedy, S., Malkoff, S., Fisher, L., Speicher, C. E., & Glaser, R. (1988). Marital discord and immunity in males. *Psychosomatic Medicine, 50,* 213–229.

Kiecolt-Glaser, J. K., Loving, T. J., Stowell, J. R., Malarkey, W. B., Lemeshow, S., & Dickinson, S. L. (2005). Hostile marital interactions, proinflammatory cytokine production, and wound healing. *Archives of General Psychiatry, 62,* 1377–1384.

Kiecolt-Glaser, J. K., Malarkey, W. B., Chee, M., Newton, T., Cacioppo, J. T., & Mao, H. (1993). Negative behavior during marital conflict is associated with immunological downregulation. *Psychosomatic Medicine, 55,* 395–409.

Kiecolt-Glaser, J. K., Marucha, P. T., Malarkey, W. B., Mercado, A. M., & Glaser, R. (1995). Slowing of wound healing by psychological stress. *Lancet, 346,* 1194–1196.

Kiecolt-Glaser, J. K., McGuire, L., Robles, T. F., & Glaser, R. (2002). Emotions, morbidity, and mortality: New perspectives from psychoneuroimmunology. *Annual Review of Psychology, 53,* 83–107.

Kiecolt-Glaser, J. K., & Newton, T. (2001). Marriage and health: His and hers. *Psychological Bulletin, 127,* 472–503.

Kiecolt-Glaser, J. K., Newton, T., Cacioppo, J. T., MacCallum, R. C., Glaser, R., & Malarkey, W. B. (1996). Marital conflict and endocrine function: Are men really more physiologically affected than women? *Journal of Consulting and Clinical Psychology, 64,* 324–332.

Kiecolt-Glaser, J. K., Page, G. G., Marucha, P. T., MacCallum, R. C., & Glaser, R. (1998). Psychological influences on surgical recovery: Perspectives from psychoneuroimmunology. *American Psychologist, 53,* 1209–1218.

Kimmel, P. L., Peterson, R. A., Weihs, K. L., Shidler, N., Simmens, S. J., & Alleyne, S. (2000). Dyadic relationship conflict, gender, and mortality in urban hemodialysis patients. *Journal of the American Society of Nephrology, 11,* 1518–1525.

Kirschbaum, C., Klauer, T., Filipp, S. H., & Hellhammer, D. H. (1995). Sex-specific effects of social support on cortisol and subjective responses to acute psychological stress. *Psychosomatic Medicine, 21,* 525–531.

Kuhns, D. B., DeCarlo, E., Hawk, D. M., & Gallin, J. I. (1992). Dynamics of the cellular and humoral components of the inflammatory response elicited in skin blisters in humans. *Journal of Clinical Investigation, 89,* 1734–1740.

Kulik, J. A., & Mahler, H. I. M. (2006). Marital quality predicts hospital stay following coronary artery bypass surgery for women but not men. *Social Science & Medicine, 63,* 2031–2040.

Kulman, L. (2004, December 19). 34. Get married. *U.S. News and World Report* Retrieved from http://health.usnews.com/usnews/health/articles/041227/27getwell_3.htm

Leonard, M. T., Cano, A., & Johansen, A. B. (2006). Chronic pain in a couples context: A review and integration of theoretical models and empirical evidence. *Journal of Pain, 7,* 377–390.

Lewis, M. A., & Butterfield, R. M. (2007). Social control in marital relationships: Effect of one's partner on health behaviors. *Journal of Applied Social Psychology, 37,* 298–319.

Libby, P., & Theroux, P. (2005). Pathophysiology of coronary artery disease. *Circulation, 111,* 3481–3488.

Light, K. C., Grewen, K. M., & Amico, J. A. (2005). More frequent partner hugs and higher oxytocin levels are linked to lower blood pressure and heart rate in premenopausal women. *Biological Psychology, 69,* 5–21.

Malarkey, W. B., Kiecolt-Glaser, J. K., Pearl, D., & Glaser, R. (1994). Hostile behavior during marital conflict alters pituitary and adrenal hormones. *Psychosomatic Medicine, 56,* 41–51.

Marsland, A. L., Cohen, S., Rabin, B. S., & Manuck, S. B. (2006). Trait positive affect and antibody response to hepatitis B vaccination. *Brain, Behavior, and Immunity, 20,* 261–269.

Mastekaasa, A. (1994). Marital status, distress, and well-being: An international comparison. *Journal of Comparative Family Studies, 25,* 183–206.

Mayne, T. J., O' Leary, A., McCrady, B., Contrada, R., & Labouvie, E. (1997). The differential effects of acute marital distress on emotional, physiological and immune functions in maritally distressed men and women. *Psychology and Health, 12,* 277–288.

McEwen, B. S. (1998). Protective and damaging effects of stress mediators. *New England Journal of Medicine, 388,* 171–179.

McGonagle, K. A., Kessler, R. C., & Schilling, E. A. (1992). The frequency and determinants of marital disagreements in a community sample. *Journal of Social and Personal Relationships, 9,* 507–524.

Mehl, M. R. (2007). Eavesdropping on health: A naturalistic observation approach for social health research. *Social and Personality Psychology Compass, 1,* 359–380.

Meyler, D., Stimpson, J. P., & Peek, M. K. (2007). Health concordance within couples: A systematic review. *Social Science and Medicine, 64,* 2297–2310.

Miller, A. H. (1998). Neuroendocrine and immune system interactions in stress and depression. *Psychiatric Clinics of North America, 21,* 443–463.

Miller, G. E., & Chen, E. (2006). Life stress and diminished expression of genes encoding glucocorticoid receptor and b2-adrenergic receptor in children with asthma. *Proceedings of the National Academy of Sciences of the United States of America, 103,* 5496–5501.

Miller, G. E., Dopp, J. M., Myers, H. F., Stevens, S. Y., & Fahey, J. L. (1999). Psychosocial predictors of natural killer cell mobilization during marital conflict. *Health Psychology, 18,* 262–271.

Mills, P. J., Goebel, M. U., Rehman, J., Irwin, M. R., & Maisel, A. S. (2000). Leukocyte adhesion molecule expression and T cell naive/memory status following isoproterenol infusion. *Journal of Neuroimmunology, 102,* 137–144.

Monroe, S. M., Bromet, E. J., Connell, M., & Steiner, S. C. (1986). Social support, life events, and depressive symptoms: A 1-year prospective study. *Journal of Consulting and Clinical Psychology, 54,* 424–431.

National Sleep Foundation. (2005, March). 2005 Sleep in America poll. Retrieved from http://www.sleepfoundation.org/sites/default/files/2005_summary_of_findings.pdf

O'Connor, M. F., Bower, J. E., Cho, H. J., Creswell, J. D., Dimitrov, S., & Hamby, M. E. ... Irwin, M. R. (2009). To assess, to control, to exclude: Effects of biobehavioral factors on circulating inflammatory markers. *Brain, Behavior, and Immunity, 23,* 887–897.

Orth-Gomer, K., Wamala, S. P., Horsten, M., Schenck-Gustafsson, K., Schneiderman, N., & Mittleman, M. A. (2000). Marital stress worsens prognosis in women with coronary heart disease: The Stockholm Female Coronary Risk Study. *JAMA, 284,* 3008–3014.

Pasch, L. A., & Bradbury, T. N. (1998). Social support, conflict, and the development of marital dysfunction. *Journal of Consulting and Clinical Psychology, 66,* 219–230.

Phillips, A. C., Carroll, D., Burns, V. E., Ring, C., Macleod, J., & Drayson, M. (2006). Bereavement and marriage are associated with antibody response to influenza vaccination in the elderly. *Brain, Behavior, and Immunity, 20,* 279–289.

Rauer, A. J., Karney, B. R., Garvan, C. W., & Hou, W. (2008). Relationship risks in context: A cumulative risk approach to understanding relationship satisfaction. *Journal of Marriage and the Family, 70,* 1122–1135.

Ridker, P. M., Brown, N. J., Vaughan, D. E., Harrison, D. G., & Mehta, J. L. (2004). Established and emerging plasma biomarkers in the prediction of first atherothrombotic events. *Circulation, 109,* IV6–19.

Robins, L., & Regier, D. (1991). *Psychiatric disorders in America.* New York: Free Press.

Robles, T. F., Brooks, K. P., & Pressman, S. D. (2009). Trait positive affect buffers the effects of acute stress on skin barrier recovery. *Health Psychology, 28,* 373–378.

Robles, T. F., & Kiecolt-Glaser, J. K. (2003). The physiology of marriage: Pathways to health. *Physiology and Behavior, 79,* 409–416.

Robles, T. F., Shaffer, V. A., Malarkey, W. B., & Kiecolt-Glaser, J. K. (2006). Positive behaviors during marital conflict:

Influences on stress hormones. *Journal of Social and Personal Relationships, 23,* 305–325.

Rogge, R. D., Cobb, R. J., Story, L. B., Johnson, M. D., Lawrence, E. E., & Rothman, A. D. (2006). Recruitment and selection of couples for intervention research: Achieving developmental homogeneity at the cost of demographic diversity. *Journal of Consulting and Clinical Psychology, 74,* 777–784.

Rohrbaugh, M. J., Shoham, V., & Coyne, J. C. (2006). Effect of marital quality on eight-year survival of patients with heart failure. *The American Journal of Cardiology, 98,* 1069–1072.

Saxbe, D. E. (2008). A field (researcher's) guide to cortisol: Tracking HPA axis functioning in everyday life. *Health Psychology Review, 2,* 163–190.

Saxbe, D. E., & Repetti, R. L. (2010). For better or worse? Coregulation of couples' cortisol levels and mood states. *Journal of Personality and Social Psychology, 98,* 92–103.

Saxbe, D. E., Repetti, R. L., & Nishina, A. (2008). Marital satisfaction, recovery from work, and diurnal cortisol among men and women. *Health Psychology, 27,* 15–25.

Sbarra, D. A. (2009). Marriage protects men from clinically meaningful elevations in C-reactive protein: Results from the National Social Life, Health, and Aging Project (NSHAP). *Psychosomatic Medicine, 71,* 828–835.

Segerstrom, S. C., & Miller, G. E. (2004). Psychological stress and the human immune system: A meta-analytic study of 30 years of inquiry. *Psychological Bulletin, 130,* 601–630.

Sepah, S. C., & Bower, J. E. (2009). Positive affect and inflammation during radiation treatment for breast and prostate cancer. *Brain, Behavior, and Immunity, 23,* 1068–1072.

Slatcher, R. B. (2010). Marital functioning and physical health: Implications for social and personality psychology. *Social and Personality Psychology Compass, 4,* 455–469.

Slavich, G. M., O'Donovan, A., Epel, E. S., & Kemeny, M. E. (2010). Black sheep get the blues: A psychobiological model of social rejection and depression. *Neuroscience and Biobehavioral Review, 35,* 39–45.

Steptoe, A., Hamer, M., & Chida, Y. (2007). The effects of acute psychological stress on circulating inflammatory factors in humans: A review and meta-analysis. *Brain, Behavior, and Immunity, 21,* 901–912.

Story, L. B., & Bradbury, T. N. (2004). Understanding marriage and stress: Essential questions and challenges. *Clinical Psychology Review, 23,* 1139–1162.

Trief, P. M., Ploutz-Snyder, R., Britton, K. D., & Weinstock, R. S. (2004). The relationship between marital quality and adherence to the diabetes care regimen. *Annals of Behavioral Medicine, 27,* 148–154.

Troxel, W. M., Robles, T. F., Hall, M., & Buysse, D. J. (2007). Marital quality and the marital bed: Examining the covariation between relationship quality and sleep. *Sleep Medicine Reviews, 11,* 389–404.

Vedhara, K., Cox, W. M., Wilcock, G. K., Perks, P., Hunt, M., & Anderson, S. (1999). Chronic stress in elderly careers of dementia patients and antibody response to influenza vaccination. *Lancet, 353,* 627–631.

Walburn, J., Vedhara, K., Hankins, M., Rixon, L., & Weinman, J. (2009). Psychological stress and wound healing in humans: a systematic review and meta-analysis. *Journal of Psychosomatic Research, 67,* 253–271.

Wickrama, K. A. S., Lorenz, F. O., & Conger, R. D. (1997). Marital quality and physical illness: A latent growth curve analysis. *Journal of Marriage and the Family, 59,* 143–155.

Yang, H. C., & Schuler, T. A. (2009). Marital quality and survivorship: Slowed recovery for breast cancer patients in distressed relationships. *Cancer, 115,* 217–228.

Zautra, A. J., Hoffman, J. M., Matt, K. S., Yocum, D., Potter, P. T., & Castro, W. L. (1998). An examination of individual differences in the relationship between interpersonal stress and disease activity among women with rheumatoid arthritis. *Arthritis Care and Research, 11,* 271–279.

Zorrilla, E. P., Luborsky, L., McKay, J. R., Rosenthal, R., Houldin, A., & Tax, A. (2001). The relationship of depression and stressors to immunological assays: A meta-analytic review. *Brain, Behavior, and Immunity, 15,* 199–226.

Social Support and Immunity

Bert N. Uchino, Allison A. Vaughn, McKenzie Carlisle, *and* Wendy Birmingham

Abstract

Social support has been reliably related to lower rates of morbidity and mortality across a number of diseases. However, little is known about the more specific pathways and mechanisms responsible for such links. In this chapter, we argue that part of the link between social support and health is explained by immune-system alternations that, in turn, influence broad-based disease outcomes. Recent studies suggest that social support is related to lower IL-6 and better immune function in biologically relevant contexts (e.g., vaccinations, cancer patients). The implications of these findings are discussed in light of a broad model hypothesizing that social support may influence health outcomes via behavioral (e.g., health behaviors), psychological (e.g., stress appraisals), and neuroendocrine-immune mechanisms. Important future research areas are also emphasized, especially the need to uncover the psychological pathways by which social support may be health-promoting.

Key Words: social support, social networks, functional support, immune function, inflammation, mechanisms, health

Introduction

> The prospective mortality data are made more compelling by their congruence with growing evidence from experimental and clinical research on animals and humans that variations in exposure to social contacts produce psychological or physiological effects that could, if prolonged, produce serious morbidity and even mortality. (House, Landis, & Umberson, 1988, p. 542)

It has been well-established that social relationships influence health and disease (Barth, Schneider, & von Kanel, 2010; Berkman, Glass, Brissette, & Seeman, 2000; Cohen, 1988; House et al., 1988; Holt-Lunstad, Smith, & Layton, 2010; Uchino, 2004) and that social support can protect health from the detrimental effects of stress (Berkman et al., 2000; Cohen & Wills, 1985). In fact, House and colleagues (1988) argued that the protective influence of social support was evident across

different diseases and recent reviews are consistent with this early conclusion (Berkman et al., 2000; Holt-Lunstad et al., 2010; Uchino, 2004). In this chapter, we argue that the links between social support and broad-based mortality is consistent with the possibility that these associations are mediated, in part, via immune system alterations. The immune system is the major bodily defense against infectious and malignant disease (Abbas & Lichtman, 2003). Research has also clearly documented the influence of immune processes (e.g., inflammation) on cardiovascular disease (Ross, 1999; Libby, 2002). Thus, a focus on the immune system provides an integrative biological approach to modeling the mechanisms linking social support to major chronic and acute disease outcomes.

In this chapter, we review evidence linking social support to immune-system alternations and its implications for understanding the mechanisms linking relationships to disease. We first provide a brief review of links between social support and physical health outcomes. Next, different operationalizations of support are examined along with its theoretical implications. In the main part of this chapter, we provide an updated review of research linking social support to immune function. We discuss these findings in light of an integrative mechanistic model of immune system involvement linking social support to physical health. Finally, key future research directions are discussed based on the available literature.

Social Support and Physical Health

One of the most important studies linking relationships to health was published by Berkman and Syme (1979). These researchers linked questions about the extent of peoples' social connections to overall mortality and found that people who were less socially integrated had higher mortality rates. This paper was influential because it was able to rule out possible alternative explanations (e.g., results due to poorer initial health status) and hence provided the most compelling empirical links at the time between social relationships and mortality. A second important study by Blazer (1982) extended this work showing that one' perceptions of support was also related to lower mortality; and that these associations were apparent even when considering the extent of individuals' social connections. These early epidemiological studies provided part of the basis for the influential conclusion of House and colleagues (1988) that social relationships were not only related to disease, but perhaps played a causal role in the development of health problems.

Recent research on social support and health is consistent with the conclusions of House and colleagues (1988). In perhaps the most compelling evidence to date on the health effects of social support, Holt-Lunstad and colleagues (2010) conducted a meta-analysis of 148 studies comprised of over 308,000 participants. They found evidence that social support was related to about a 50% lower risk for future all-cause mortality (Holt-Lunstad et al., 2010). These links were not moderated by age, gender, initial health status, cause of death, and length of follow-up period. Consistent with House and colleagues (1988), the links between social relationships and mortality appeared comparable to standard risk factors including smoking, exercise, and even obesity (Holt-Lunstad et al., 2010).

Research examining links between social support and specific causes of mortality is also consistent with a beneficial influence of social ties across different diseases. A recent meta-analysis found that individuals low in functional support had a greater risk of mortality from cardiovascular disease (Barth et al., 2010). Although more research is needed, social support from network members also appears to predict lower cancer mortality (Ell, Nishimoto, Medianski, Mantell, & Hamovitch, 1992; Weihs et al., 2005), with these associations most evident for breast cancer outcomes (Nausheen, Gidron, Peveler, & Moss-Morris, 2009). Finally, social support is also linked to mortality from infectious diseases (Lee & Rotheram-Borus, 2001; Patterson et al., 1996). However, there is less research linking social support to such outcomes, and there are some notable counter findings to be discussed later in this review (Blomkvist et al., 1994). Overall, however, social support appears to influence the course of HIV infection, especially later in the course of disease (Ironson & Hayward, 2008).

Definitions of Social Support and Its Implications for Health

The epidemiological studies described earlier have operationalized social support in a number of ways (Cohen, 2004; Uchino, 2009). A broad but generally accepted definition of social support includes both the *structure* of a person's network and the *functions* that these network members serve (Thoits, 2011). Structural social support is usually defined as the degree to which one is integrated into social networks (e.g., spouse, parents, siblings, children, friends, or group memberships). Such social integration measures can include the *number* of network members, the *type* of relationship (spouse versus acquaintance) and/or the *amount of contact* the individual has with the network members.

Much of the conceptual work on social integration and health has its roots in the ideas of symbolic interactionism (Mead, 1934). Symbolic interactionism highlights the importance of society for normal personal and social development. According to this perspective, we form our sense of self or identity in the context of meaningful social ties and roles (Stryker & Burke, 2000). Researchers have applied these ideas to the health domain by arguing that social integration provides the basis for a strong sense of self-identity, appropriate norms for behavior, and greater meaning or worth to life (Thoits, 1983, Umberson, 1987). Such social integration sets the stage for social control as it increases the possibility that others will exert direct (e.g., verbal) or indirect (e.g., life meaning) control over one's health (Lewis & Rook, 1999; Umberson, 1987).

The specific measures of social integration that are most health relevant are still being debated, but it appears that composite measures that examine integration across a number of roles are more strongly related to mortality (Holt-Lunstad et al., 2010).

Functional support, in comparison, is usually examined along two dimensions: what support an individual *perceives* may be available to him/her, and the support an individual actually *receives*, which, in turn, is predicted to be most health relevant when individuals are under stress (Cohen & Wills, 1985). The perception or receipt of support includes specific components such as emotional support (e.g., listening to your problems, offering a shoulder to cry on), informational support (e.g., giving you advice), tangible support (e.g., loaning you money or giving you a ride when your car breaks down), and belonging support (e.g., having people to do things with). It is important to note that the perceived availability and receipt of support are not always related in a clear-cut manner and have often been associated with different effects on well-being (Antonucci & Israel, 1986; Cutrona, 1986; Dunkel-Schetter & Bennett, 1990) and, perhaps, on physical health (Uchino, 2004). For instance, perceived support appears to have stronger links to mortality than receiving support (e.g., Holt-Lunstad et al., 2010, Uchino, 2004). We will return to a discussion of measurement issues and its conceptual implications based on the results of our recent review detailed next.

Evidence Linking Social Support to Immune Function

Most of the epidemiological literature linking social support to health outcomes has focused on structural measures of support (Holt-Lunstad et al., 2010). In comparison, most of the research examining links between social support and immunity has examined functional measures of perceived support. In an earlier review, we examined 16 studies that directly tested such associations (Uchino, Cacioppo, & Kiecolt-Glaser, 1996). Since that time, this literature has more than doubled. Most of this recent literature continues to examine functional measures of perceived support, however, the types of immune measures utilized has changed since our initial review. Most of the prior research had examined more general assessments including quantitative measures of cell counts or percentages (e.g., helper T-cells) and/or functional measures such as the ability of natural killer cells to lyse a susceptible tumor cell line (i.e., natural killer cell activity,

NKCA). Many of the recent studies have focused on links between social support and inflammation. In addition, there is a greater focus on examining social support in more biologically relevant contexts (e.g., vaccination, cancer patients). As reviewed later, these studies continue to suggest that social support predicts immune function, but they highlight a different set of immune mechanisms compared to prior work.

As a brief review, in our earlier paper the results of the 16 existing studies were consistent with links between social support and better immune system function (Uchino et al., 1996). Of these studies, 8 used only functional assays (e.g., NKCA, proliferative response to mitogens), 3 used only quantitative assays (most commonly cell counts), and 5 used both quantitative and functional immunological measures. Importantly, the data linking social support to functional immune measures at the time was one of the largest effect sizes in our meta-analysis, and this effect was particularly strong in older-adult populations. The later finding is significant because alterations in immune function may have direct health consequences in this population since aging is associated with a downregulation of immune function and infectious illnesses are a leading cause of death in the elderly (Effros & Walford, 1987; Haynes & Maue, 2009).

Recent research on social support and immunity appears to have taken a significant turn; one that is partially based on two trends in psychoneuroimmunology (PNI) research. First, the involvement of immune-mediated inflammation on diverse disease processes (e.g., cardiovascular, Libby, 2002) has led to increased emphasis on processes related to natural immunity. Such an emphasis is consistent with broad links between social support and all-cause mortality (Uchino, 2004). Second, there has been greater attention to modeling biologically significant outcomes in PNI work and the tendency to see more vaccination studies or chronic disease patients in social support work is a step in this direction. A smaller set of studies continues to test the possibility that social support may buffer stress-related immune changes and that social networks may have negative influences on immune outcomes in some contexts.

Social Support and Inflammation

One of the most active recent areas has been studies linking social support to inflammation (Costanzo et al., 2005; Coussons-Read, Okun, & Nettles, 2007; Friedman et al., 2005; Loucks et al.,

2006; Lutgendorf, Anderson, Sorosky, Buller, & Lubaroff, 2000; Marsland, Sathanoori, Muldoon, & Manuck, 2007; Marucha, Crespin, Shelby, & Andersen, 2005; McDade, Hawkley, & Cacioppo, 2006; Miyazaki et al., 2005; Von Ah, Kang, & Carpenter, 2007). Of these studies, most have examined IL-6, which has both pro- and anti-inflammatory influences (Papanicolaou, Wilder, Manolagas, & Chrousos, 1998; Hawkley, Bosch, Engeland, Marucha, & Cacioppo, 2007). IL-6 is a potent stimulator of CRP release as well as the HPA axis and elevated levels of IL-6 appear to be related to a number of disease processes such as diabetes, cardiovascular disease, osteoporosis, and some cancers (Barton, 2005; Danesh et al., 2008; Kristiansen & Mandrup-Poulsen, 2005; Papanicoloau et al., 1998; Ridker, Rifai, Stampfer, & Hennekens, 2000).

The existing data are consistent with a link between social support and lower levels of IL-6, implicating this as one potential inflammatory pathway involved in the health benefits of support (Costanzo et al, 2005; Friedman et al., 2005; Loucks et al., 2006; Lutgendorf et al., 2000). For instance, Loucks and colleagues (2006) examining data from the Framingham Heart Study found that social integration as indexed by the social network index was related to lower IL-6 levels after adjustments for age and health behaviors in men. These data are also apparent in cancer patients as functional support has been associated with lower levels of IL-6 in plasma (Lutgendorf et al., 2000) and ascitic fluid surrounding tumors (Costanzo et al., 2005).

The links between social support and other inflammatory cytokines have not been investigated in sufficient numbers of studies to draw firm conclusions. For instance, the link between social support and CRP levels has only been examined in a few studies and shows weak or no association with support (Coussons-Read et al., 2007; Loucks et al., 2006; McDade et al., 2006). Although the studies are few, these data are surprising in light of links between support and IL-6, which is a potent stimulator of CRP release. However, it is possible that IL-6 may have independent links to disease processes beyond that of CRP (Ridker et al., 2000). It is also important to note that these studies are heterogeneous in terms of populations (e.g., healthy, pregnant) and sample sizes utilized. The use of stringent statistical control in these studies may have also limited power to detect smaller effect sizes because health behaviors may be pathways by which social support influences inflammation (e.g., Segerstrom, 2009). Future research will have to test more specific

models (or test these controls in stages) so that the influence of social support on health-relevant inflammatory processes can be determined in light of current perspectives (Uchino, 2004).

There have been a few studies that examined links between social support and other cytokines. For instance, Miyazaki and colleagues (2005) found that perceived support from home or work was associated with greater Th1 dominance as indexed by inteferon-gamma/IL-4. Perceived support was also linked in a community sample to lower stimulated levels of IL-8, which is an important chemokine for inflammatory cells (Marsland et al., 2007). However, no link was found between perceived support and stimulated levels of TNF-alpha in this study (Marsland et al., 2007). In another study, changes in social activities were associated with greater stimulated levels of TNF-alpha in cancer patients (Marucha et al., 2005). The differences in these findings for TNF-alpha may reflect the sample because localized infusions of TNF-alpha confer therapeutic benefits in cancer patients (Dranoff, 2004). Clearly, more work is needed in this area, especially with regard to the more classic pro-inflammatory cytokines such as TNF-alpha and IL-1. However, the available evidence suggests that low social support is related to higher levels of IL-6, which is a global predictor of future health problems (Hong, Angelo, & Kurzrock, 2007; Kiecolt-Glaser, McGuire, Robles, & Glaser, 2002; Papanicoloau et al., 1998).

Social Support and Biologically Significant Contexts

There has also been a systematic effort to link social support to more biologically relevant outcomes. One particularly active area examined whether social support predicts better antibody (Ab) responses to vaccination (Gallagher, Phillips, Ferraro, Drayson, & Carroll, 2008a; Gallagher, Phillips, Ferraro, Drayson, & Carroll, 2008b; Moynihan et al., 2004; Phillips, Burns, Carroll, Ring, & Drayson, 2005; Phillips, Carroll, Burns, Ring, Macleod, & Drayson, 2006; Pressman et al., 2005). This would be an important association because higher Ab responses to vaccination reflect the outcome of an integrative immune response and predicts lower rates of infection (Beyers, Palache, Baljet, & Masurel, 1989; Haynes & Maue, 2009). In one of the first studies in this area, Glaser, Kiecolt-Glaser, Bonneau, Malarkey, & Hughes (1992) examined links between perceived support and a Hepatitis B vaccine given to medical students.

Results revealed that support was associated with higher Ab titers and T-lymphocyte responses to the vaccine. Subsequent work has shown that social support is related to greater Ab responses to influenza (Moynihan et al., 2004; Phillips et al., 2005; Pressman et al., 2005) and pneumococcal (Gallagher et al., 2008a; Gallagher et al., 2008b) vaccines. However, no association has been found between social support and meningococcal or Hepatitis A vaccines (Gallagher et al., 2008b; Phillips et al., 2005).

These studies provide some preliminary data linking social support to a biologically significant outcome. However, there are several issues that are relevant to discuss. Perhaps the most promising data come from studies examining social support and influenza vaccination. However, these data suggest that the links are only apparent on certain strains as perceived support and network size appear to largely predict better immune responses to the Type A strain of the flu vaccine (Moynihan et al., 2004; Phillips et al., 2005; Pressman et al., 2005). The reasons behind this specificity are not clear and may be related to variations in prior exposure or antigenic drift (Moynihan et al., 2004; Pressman et al., 2005). Nevertheless, the links to Type A (especially New Caledonia) appear reliable, and future work will need to model the factors that may be responsible for such links.

One other issue to discuss is that these studies are thought to provide links between social support and a biologically significant endpoint. However, many of these studies do not use established clinical cutoffs for examining links to support. For instance, a clinically protected response (seroconversion) is generally defined as a fourfold increase in Ab titers. This is important because it is less clear if small relative differences in Ab titers confer protection. Of the existing studies, only Glaser et al. (1992) and Phillips et al. (2005) appear to have examined seroconversion rates and both reported that social support was related to being a vaccine "responder." One difficulty in showing clinically relevant differences, however, is that, due to prior exposure or the use of relatively healthy participants, many individuals may seroconvert and hence little variability may be found. Future work should include older adults who show significantly more variability in their seroconversion rates (Haynes & Maue, 2009) or utilize more novel antigens in younger adults. The 2009–2010 vaccination program to the novel H1N1 flu virus would be a good candidate, and it is possible that such data are forthcoming.

In order to examine a more biologically significant disease context there has also been much recent interest in examining links between social support and immune function in cancer patients. This is important because the immune system plays an important role in the control and course of cancer outcomes (Dunn, Bruce, Ikeda, Old, & Schreiber, 2002). In an influential early study in this area, Levy and colleagues (1990) examined links between perceived support and NKCA in 61 stage I and II breast-cancer patients. These researchers found that higher levels of perceived emotional support from the spouse/intimate other or physician predicted greater NKCA in these cancer patients.

Subsequent work has demonstrated a link between social support and aspects of immune function in cancer patients (Lutgendorf et al., 2002, 2005; 2008; Marucha et al., 2005; Turner-Cobb et al., 2004). For instance, social network size appeared to buffer the effects of stressful life events on delayed type hypersensitivity (DTH) responses in breast-cancer patients (Turner-Cobb et al., 2004). A systematic and innovative program of research by Lutgendorf and colleagues has also started to delineate more precise immunologic pathways that might link social support to cancer progression. These researchers have found that perceived support was related to higher NKCA in both blood and the tumor microenvironment (Lutgendorf et al., 2005). In addition, perceived support has been related to lower levels of growth factors (e.g., vascular endothelial growth factor, matrix metalloproteinase) in the blood and tumors of ovarian cancer patients (Lutgendorf et al., 2002, 2008). These findings are important because such growth factors play a role in tumor angiogenesis (Kerbel, 2000). Of course, the direct biological relevance of these findings to cancer progression will need to be examined by modeling these pathways and their ability to predict the course of disease (Levy et al., 1990).

The recent studies on social support and immune function in cancer patients highlight an important gap in this line of work. Most chronic disease processes can be separated in terms of factors that lead to its development (i.e., incidence) in comparison to factors that influence its clinical course. The studies examining social support and immune function in healthy populations suggest that there may be a theoretical link to lower cancer incidence via processes such as better immunosurveillance (Burnett, 1970). However, stronger inferences might be possible if one focuses on populations that might be of greater risk using relevant biomarkers. In one of the only studies we are aware of in the social support literature, Stone and colleagues (Stone, Mezzacappa, Donatone, & Gonder, 1999) found that perceived social support was related to lower prostate-specific antigen levels in men during a community screening. More studies are needed to examine links between social support and different stages of cancer risk that might be mediated by immune processes.

A second population in which immune alterations may be more health relevant are older adults. As noted earlier, aging is associated with decrements in immune function, and infectious diseases are a leading cause of death in older adults (Haynes & Maue, 2009; Yoshikawa, 2000). This is important because in the United States alone, the proportion of individuals over age 65 will increase from 12.4% in 2000 to 19.6% in 2030. These statistics reflect worldwide changes where there will be an almost doubling of older adults over age 65 by 2030 (CDC, 2003). To this point, there is recent evidence linking social support to immunosenescence (Bosch, Fischer, & Fischer, 2009). As individuals age, the thymus shrinks, with a resulting decline in naive T-cells (Haynes & Maue, 2009). As a result, individuals are more reliant on the existing pool of T-cells to generate an immune response. Over time, this leads to an accumulation of T-lymphocytes that are at a late stage of differentiation (e.g., CD27-, CD28-) and this is one important marker of immunosenescence (Bosch et al., 2009). In an intriguing study of 537 workers, Bosch and colleagues (2009) examined links between perceived support at work and T-lymphocytes with a late-stage marker. Importantly, these authors found that perceived support at work was associated with lower levels of late stage CD8+ cells. It is worth repeating that the influence of social support on immune function appears particularly evident in older adults (Uchino et al., 1996) and might be a population of particular interest for interventions.

Stress-Buffering Model

There have been a number of recent studies that have continued to test the influential stress-buffering model of support on immunity (Bosch et al., 2009; Kang, Coe, Karaszewski, & McCarthy, 1998; Marsland et al., 2007; Turner-Cobb et al., 2004; Von Ah et al., 2007). Cohen and Wills (1985) argue that one methodological requirement for an adequate test of the buffering model is to show a main effect of stress on the outcome, and all these studies reported such an effect. Importantly, a majority of these studies reported some evidence for a buffering

effect of support for individuals high in life stress on measures of DTH (Turner-Cobb et al., 2004), NKCA (Kang et al., 1998); and immunosenescence (Bosch et al., 2009). However, there is also some heterogeneity in these studies (Marsland et al., 2007), so more data will be needed to draw stronger conclusions. Nevertheless, the existing research is consistent with this important model on immune outcomes (also see Kiecolt-Glaser, Dura, Speicher, Trask, & Glaser, 1991).

Potential Negative Influences of Larger Social Networks

Most research suggests that social support has beneficial links to immune function. However, in some contexts, larger social networks may be detrimental (Hamrick, Cohen, & Rodriquez, 2002; Segerstrom, 2008). These findings are consistent with an early review suggesting that larger networks were associated with faster disease progression in HIV+ individuals (to be discussed later; Miller & Cole, 1998). Potential mechanisms linking larger social networks to increased risk for infection include greater exposure to viruses or interpersonal stress due to social responsibilities (Hamrick et al., 2002). A more recent explanation for some of these findings has been made by Segerstrom (2008) who argues for an ecological explanation in which immune function may be compromised for the sake of gaining or maintaining important social resources. Consistent with this reasoning, she found that individuals with larger social networks who stayed at home for law school (and hence had more pressure to maintain their relationships in the face of great academic responsibilities) showed lower DTH responses compared to those who went away to law school (Segerstrom, 2008). More data are needed on this issue, however, and disentangling potential explanations will require prospective studies that measure the precise mediators that might be operating, such as network exposure, interpersonal conflict, social emotions (e.g., guilt), and/or energetic resources.

As noted earlier, there is also some evidence linking larger social networks to faster disease progression in HIV+ individuals (Miller & Cole, 1998). It is important to note, however, that some studies have not replicated this finding (Uchino, 2004). Moreover, it has also been found that patients with advanced-stage HIV infections survived longer if they have larger social networks (Patterson et al., 1996). These data suggest that stage of disease may be particularly important, as Patterson and colleagues (1996) found evidence for social support's beneficial influence later in the course of disease but that larger social networks predicted a faster progression to AIDS-defining symptoms in early-stage HIV patients (also see Ironson & Hayward, 2008). The mechanisms responsible for such stage-specific findings remain to be elucidated, but they include riskier behaviors and greater exposure to HIV-related caregiving and bereavement (Kemeny et al., 1995; Miller & Cole, 1998). The later possibilities may be consistent with the ecological explanation of Segerstrom (2008).

It is also important to note that studies examining links between functional support and immune function in HIV+ individuals have also shown mixed findings (Uchino, 2004). Several have failed to find a significant association between social support and aspects of immune function in HIV+ men (Goodkin et al., 1992; Perry, Fishman, Jacobsberg, & Frances, 1992). However, several other studies have reported an association between social support and helper T-cell counts (a marker of disease progression) in HIV+ men (Fekete et al., 2009; Persson, Gullberg, Hanson, Moestrup, & Ostergren, 1994; Theorell et al., 1995). One of the more long-term studies on this issue examined the association between social support and changes in helper T-cells across a five year period (Theorell et al., 1995). Results of this study showed perceived social support became a more powerful predictor of helper T-cells as time progressed. Thus, there is also more consistent evidence linking functional support to beneficial influences on immunity in HIV+ populations later in the stage of disease (Ironson & Hayward, 2008).

A Broad Model Linking Social Support to Immune-Mediated Diseases

We must further understand the psychological and biological processes or mechanisms linking social relationships to health, either as extensions of the social processes just discussed... or as independent mechanisms. In the latter regard, psychological and sociobiological theories suggest that the mere presence of, or sense of relatedness with, another organism may have relatively direct motivational, emotional, or neuroendocrine effects that promote health either directly or in the face of stress or other health hazards but that operate independently of cognitive appraisal or behavioral coping and adaptation. (House, Landis, & Umberson, 1988, pp. 543–544)

Consistent with our prior review (Uchino et al., 1996), the recent literature continues to suggest the plausibility of links between social support and immune function. Furthermore, these links appear across both structural and functional measures of support, although most of the research has focused on functional measures of perceived support. This recent literature is also important because many of these studies contain data on potential theoretical mechanisms at different levels of analysis. However, it is fair to say that most of the studies reviewed earlier were focused on simply documenting a link between social support and immunity. We believe that we are now at the stage at which theory testing of important pathways should be a primary research objective for social support investigators. In fact, the quote by House and colleagues (1988) over 22 years ago argued for the importance of such an approach, while anticipating some of the problems faced in examining psychological mediation to be discussed later. In this section, we first outline a broad model linking social support to health. We then discuss the evidence for major pathways linking social support to health outcomes with particular attention paid to mechanisms examined in the existing social-support and immunity literature.

Depicted in Figure 12.1 is a broad model linking social support to immunity and health, based on different theoretical perspectives (Berkman et al., 2000; Cohen, 1988; Gore, 1981; Lin, 1986; Thoits, 1995; Umberson, 1987) and the available literature linking social support to physical health (also see Uchino, 2004). Accordingly, structural and functional measures of support may ultimately influence morbidity and mortality through two distinct but not necessarily independent pathways. One pathway involves behavioral processes including health behaviors and adherence to medical regimens as outlined by social control and social identity theorists (Lewis & Rook, 1999; Umberson, 1987). The other major pathway involves psychological processes that are linked to appraisals, emotions or moods (e.g., depression), and feelings of control (Cohen, 1988; Gore, 1981; Lin, 1986). Note that the behavioral and psychological levels are linked because each has been shown to exert an influence over the other. For instance, feelings of stress can adversely impact the practice of health behaviors (e.g., Ng & Jeffery, 2003), whereas health behaviors, such as exercise, can have beneficial effects on feelings of stress (e.g., Rejeski, Thompson, Brubaker, & Miller, 1992). Finally, these psychological and behavioral pathways may have reciprocal influence on social-support

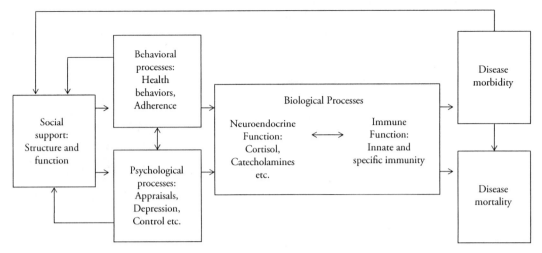

Figure 12.1 A broad model highlighting the major pathways by which social support may influence physical-health outcomes.

processes. For instance, psychological distress may influence perceptions of support and contribute to negative social interactions (Alferi, Carver, Antoni, Weiss, & Duran, 2001; Coyne, 1976).

Of central importance to this review is that the links between social support and disease are hypothesized to be mediated through relevant immunologic processes. These changes are thought to have important reciprocal links with neuroendocrine processes (Berkman et al., 2000; Uchino et al., 1996). Although not a focus of this review, it is important to note that the feedback loop between morbidity and social support highlights the unique challenges faced by individuals diagnosed with disease that can impact their social network (see Bolger, Foster, Vinokur, & Ng, 1996; Holahan & Moos, 1990). For instance, family members may be threatened by the potential loss of the close relationship or having to bear witness to their loved ones' distress. This may result in network members withdrawing in an attempt to cope with an overwhelming situation (Bolger et al., 1996).

Behavioral Pathways

As shown in Figure 12.1, a major pathway potentially linking social support to immune function and subsequent health involves health behaviors and cooperation with medical regimens (DiMatteo, 2004; Umberson, 1987). According to social control and social identity theorists, social support is health promoting because it facilitates healthier behaviors such as exercise, eating right, and not smoking; as well as greater adherence to medical regimens. This can happen in a direct (e.g., health-

related informational support) or indirect (e.g., life-meaning) manner (DiMatteo, 2004; Lewis & Rook, 1999; Umberson, 1987).

The broader literature on social support and health has mostly focused on establishing that any links were not due to health behaviors such as smoking and exercise because these factors have been shown to predict mortality in their own right (Holt-Lunstad et al., 2010). Many of these studies suggest that social support effects are still significant when considering these health behaviors (Ceria et al., 2001; Kaplan et al., 1994; Penninx et al., 1997). Of course, social control theorists do not conceptualize health behaviors as alternative explanations, and research does suggest that at least some of the association between social support and mortality may be due to such health practices (Uchino, 2004). Although social support proved to predict mortality above and beyond what was predicted by these health behaviors, some of these studies did find that the association between social support and all-cause mortality was weaker when these health behaviors were considered. For instance, the Alameda County Study found that the risk associated with a lack of social integration, although significant, was reduced when considering a set of behavioral risk factors including smoking, exercise, and eating breakfast (Seeman, Kaplan, Knudsen, Cohen, & Guralnik, 1987). These findings suggest that at least a part of the complex association between social support and disease may be due to health behaviors.

Many of the recent existing research linking social support to immune function has typically included at least some health behavior assessments (e.g., Friedman et al., 2005; Loucks et al., 2006; Lutgendorf et al., 2000; Marsland et al., 2007; Phillips et al., 2005; Pressman et al., 2005). Consistent with the mortality work described earlier, most of these studies suggest that links between social support and immune outcomes are still significant while considering health behaviors including sleep, smoking, and alcohol consumption (e.g., Friedman et al., 2005; Lutgendorf et al., 2000; Phillips et al. 2005; Pressman et al., 2005). It is important to note, however, that there is some evidence for partial mediation in some of these studies (Loucks et al., 2006; Marsland et al., 2007). For instance, Marsland and colleagues (2007) found that perceived support predicted lower IL-6 and IL-8 levels in univariate analyses. However, statistically controlling for a block of variables that included health behaviors rendered nonsignificant the links between support and IL-6. It is also possible that some of the studies described earlier may have found evidence for partial mediation although none directly tested for it using more recent (and powerful) tests for mediation (see MacKinnon, 2008). Thus, a health-behavior pathway remains viable based on existing models and data.

According to social control and identity theorists, social support may also promote greater cooperation with medical regimens through direct or indirect social control of a persons' behavior with subsequent effects on health. Functional support theorists also highlight how emotional support may help initiate and maintain healthy behavioral change. There is relatively strong evidence based on a recent meta-analysis that social support predicts cooperation with medical regimens in chronic disease patients (DiMatteo, 2004). In one study, researchers in the Multiple Risk Factor Intervention Trial (MRFIT) included a comprehensive assessment of both structural and functional measures of social support (O'Reilly & Thomas, 1989). Results of this study showed that informational, emotional, and available support for risk reduction predicted a more healthy profile. It is also interesting that individuals who reduced their risk reported higher levels of conflict within their network. This may be seen as consistent with the social control hypothesis that predicts beneficial effects of social control on physical health, but increased psychological distress due to social control efforts (Lewis & Rook, 1999).

A behavioral pathway involving cooperation with medical regimens is particularly salient for chronic disease populations and several of the recent support-immunity studies examined cancer patients

(Costanzo et al., 2005; Lutgendorf et al., 2000, 2005; Marucha et al., 2005; Turner-Cobb et al., 2004). However, none of these studies appeared to examine cooperation with regimens as a mediator of links between social support and immunologic outcomes. This is an important gap because of reliable links between social support and cooperation with medical regimens in chronic disease patients (DiMatteo, 2004). For instance, one study found that nonadherent HIV+ participants showed clinically higher viral loads compared to adherent participants (Gonzalez, Penedo, Antoni, Duran, Fernandez, et al., 2004). Importantly, social support was predictive of greater adherence, and positive states of mind partially mediated this relationship (Gonzalez et al., 2004). The general lack of attention to this behavioral mechanism highlights an important pathway in need of future evaluation in studies of social support, immunity, and health.

Psychological Pathways

It is commonly hypothesized that social support may influence health outcomes via relevant psychological processes such as stress appraisals, depression, and feelings of control (Cohen, 1988; Uchino, 2004). In fact, there is a robust literature linking perceived support to psychological outcomes including lower stress, depression, loneliness, and higher life satisfaction (Barrera, 2000; Wills & Shinar, 2000). Such psychological factors also appear to have reliable effects on immune function (Herbert & Cohen, 1993; Lyubomirsky, King, & Diener, 2005; Segerstrom & Miller, 2004). Hence, it seems plausible that these psychological processes might mediate links between social support and health. Epidemiological studies, however, have provided little direct evidence on the psychological pathways linking social support to health outcomes (House, 2001). Laboratory studies examining the influence of received support on cardiovascular reactivity would be an ideal paradigm to examine these processes due to the well-controlled context. However, to date most of these studies, although showing reductions in cardiovascular reactivity, have not been able to show that appraisals or emotions mediated such links (e.g., Gerin et al., 1992).

A number of studies examining links between social support and immunity included measures of these psychological processes (Baron et al., 1990; Kiecolt-Glaser, Dura, Speicher, Trask, & Glaser, 1991; Loucks et al., 2006; Lutgendorf et al., 2000, 2005; Marsland et al., 2007; Segerstrom, 2008; Stone et al., 1999; Thomas, Goodwin, & Goodwin,

1985). In general, there is very little evidence in these studies that the influence of social support on immunity is statistically mediated by life stress, subjective distress, or depression. As noted earlier, the quote by House and colleagues over 22 years ago foreshadowed this possibility. Is it the case that the links between social support and health are independent of cognitive appraisals and other psychological processes?

There are several explanations for the existing state of the literature that warrant serious consideration, especially in light of long-standing suggestions that elucidating such psychological pathways be a primary research agenda (Davidson & Shumaker, 1987; Cohen, 1988). One possibility is that heightened measurement error may limit our tests of mediation. However, many of these studies used well-validated measures of psychological processes (e.g., profile of mood states, Lutgendorf et al., 2000). In addition, this explanation would seem inconsistent with the null findings for laboratory studies that usually result in larger effect sizes and less measurement error (Thorsteinsson & James, 1999). A second possibility is that none of these studies used more recently recommended tests for mediation (e.g., bootstrapping, MacKinnon, 2008). As noted by MacKinnon (2008), testing for mediation using the criteria of Baron and Kenny (1986) or the Sobel test is quite conservative and more likely to result in such null findings.

Although we certainly believe that researchers need to test mediation by minimizing measurement error and using more sensitive statistical techniques, it is time to also expand the way we currently think about testing mediation of social support effects in the health domain. As a result, we would like to discuss several ideas on a more exploratory basis that will need future inquiry. First, it is possible that greater attention to the context of support processes may provide a more sensitive test of mediation. Thoits (2011) has argued for a distinction between primary and secondary groups in understanding links between social support and health. Primary group members are typically long-lasting, informal, and consist of close or "significant others." Secondary group members can be short- or long-lasting, but are characterized by more formal roles, are less personal, and members can exit or enter such groups on their own discretion (also see Granovetter, 1973). Thoits (2011) predicts that emotional support is more effective coming from primary group members given the closeness characterizing these relationships, whereas informational support is less likely to be effective,

given that such group members lives are also disrupted by the stressor (which may create impatience, anger, resentment, etc.). In addition, such primary social ties are less likely to have direct experience with the stressor (i.e., experiential dissimilarity) and, hence, their attempts at providing informational support may be off track, ingenuous, or ineffective. Secondary group members, in comparison, may be better sources of informational support, given their past experience (typically in context, e.g., asking a co-worker about a job problem). This perspective suggests that a more sensitive test of psychological mechanisms would need to take into account the support context (e.g., the type of group member, experiential similarity).

A second contextual issue that may shed greater light on mechanisms is reflected by work on relational regulation theory (Lakey & Orehek, 2010). These authors have argued that support perceptions develop primarily in the context of daily, mundane interactions (e.g., talking about sports, music, gossip). These interactions help to regulate individuals on a daily basis and serve as the initial basis for expectations about support from particular relationships. This perspective suggests that greater attention to such daily life interactions (as opposed to stressful contexts) may provide a better understanding of the interpersonal and psychological processes associated with support, which may then have implications for health.

Recent work on the neural basis of social psychological processes (e.g., Cacioppo et al., 2007; Lieberman, 2007) may also have implications for psychological mediation of social support and health links. It is clear that self-report measures of psychological processes reflect complex information processing pathways that may rely on separable neural substrates (Eisenberger, Gable, & Lieberman, 2007a). Some of these neural substrates are more closely linked to health-relevant physiological alterations than others (e.g., amygdala, anterior cingulate cortex; Gianaros et al., 2005; Wang et al., 2005). Future work informed by this expanding literature identifying brain processes linked to health-related psychological pathways may provide a more direct test of social support influences involved in appraisals, emotions, and peripheral physiology (Eisenberger, Taylor, Gable, Hilmert, & Lieberman, 2007b).

It is also possible that one is unlikely to find evidence for a single dominant psychological pathway given the complexity of links between social support and physical health that unfold over time (Uchino,

2004). Most prior work has typically examined one potential pathway at a time based on the Baron and Kenny (1986) procedures. However, there are other techniques that will allow for an examination of multiple pathways that may be a more accurate way of modeling support influences as depicted in Figure 12.1. The multiple-mediators approach, based on additive models, have had some success in documenting pathways between SES and health outcomes (Evans & Kim, 2010). In addition, structural equation modeling (SEM) allows for a test of multiple pathways via overall model fit as well as individual pathways (Bollen, 1989). Although SEM models are more reliably estimated based on larger sample sizes, recent developments may allow for such modeling using considerable smaller samples (i.e., Bayesian approach, Lee & Shi, 2000; Lee & Song, 2004). Of course, these models need to take into account the sequence of events that lead to physical health changes so longitudinal designs would be important to incorporate into future studies.

Finally, most of the existing studies on social support and health have examined conscious reports of support. It is possible that at least some of the psychological pathways may be less conscious (more automatic), and related cognitive paradigms may provide an alternative test of mechanisms. This possibility is consistent with the general view that people construct working models of their relationships with others as an automatic organizational guide in navigating complex and important social worlds (Baldwin, 1992; Ogilvie & Ashmore, 1991), and simply calling to mind feelings of connectedness and support can attenuate physiological reactivity to a stressor task (Ratnasingam & Bishop, 2007; Smith, Ruiz, & Uchino, 2004). For instance, Smith and colleagues (2004) used a *supraliminal* prime by having participants write about a supportive tie or casual acquaintance (e.g., what you appreciate about this person) and then having them perform psychological stressors. Results revealed that writing about a supportive tie was associated with lower cardiovascular reactivity to a subsequent speech stressor compared to writing about an casual acquaintance (also see Ratnasingam & Bishop, 2007). In addition, the links between supportive ties and lower cardiovascular reactivity were mediated by decreases in state anxiety levels using this paradigm.

Despite the difficulties in examining the psychological processes mediating support influences, there are preliminary studies indicating that social support may mediate effects of other psychosocial variables (Dixon et al., 2001; Marsland et al.,

2007). For instance, stress can lead to disruptions in perceived support which might then negatively influence immune function. Such a mediational pathway was examined by Marsland and colleagues (2007) who showed that the links between perceived stress and depression on stimulated IL-8 levels were mediated by perceived support. In addition, Dixon and colleagues (2001) found that perceived support predicted lower herpesvirus Ab titers. However, stronger evidence was found that perceived support mediated the links between loneliness and higher herpesvirus Ab titers than vice versa. These findings suggest that the testing of alternative models is warranted. Importantly, such models do not diminish the importance of social support as an explanatory variable but provide data on its antecedent process, which, in turn, places it in a larger psychosocial context. Nevertheless, prior work has not had much success modeling the psychological processes responsible for links between support and health. We believe it is time for researchers to start thinking more broadly on how to model these links. Such research may ultimately pay dividends as insight into these pathways can suggest novel intervention approaches. For instance, simply activating support schemas on a regular basis may be sufficient to influence physiological function and perhaps long-term health (Smith et al., 2004).

Biological Pathways

A final common pathway by which social support may influence health is based on reciprocal neuroendocrine-immune interactions. Cells of the immune system (e.g., lymphocytes) have functional receptors for endocrine hormones, which provide a mechanism by which social support may influence immunity (Sanders, Kasprowicz, Kohm, & Swanson, 2001). It is evident that immune cells have receptors for a variety of hormones including EPI, norepinephrine (NE), ACTH, cortisol, opioids, growth hormone, prolactin, and estrogen that provide a pharmacological basis for neuromodulation (Sanders et al., 2001).

A major neuroendocrine pathway possibly linking support to immune processes include activation of the hypothalamic pituitary adrenal (HPA) axis. The major influence of HPA hormones on immune processes appears inhibitory (Munck, Guyre, & Holbrook, 1984). For instance, glucocorticoids typically inhibit the activity of immune cells, including the synthesis and release of many cytokines (Kaltsas & Chrousos, 2007; Sapolsky, Romero, & Munck, 2000). Although inconsistencies arose in earlier studies, more recent work is consistent with a link between social support and lower cortisol levels (Grant, Hamer, & Steptoe, 2009; Floyd et al., 2007). More specifically, these recent studies have improved upon prior work by measuring salivary cortisol over several points in time instead of just a single point in time (Grant et al., 2009; Heinrichs, Baumgartner, Kirschbaum, & Ehlert, 2003; Turner-Cobb et al., 2000).

The strongest evidence, however, would be studies that directly examine if cortisol mediates links between social support and aspects of immune function. Direct evidence to this point, however, is rare and existing studies testing this proposition have not provided evidence for mediation (Bosch et al., 2009; Cohen et al., 1997; Lutgendorf et al., 2000; Pressman et al., 2005). The reasons behind these inconsistencies are unclear but may reflect the general issues in examining mediational pathways in social support and health work (see earlier). However, there is some evidence that a more sensitive test of cortisol as a mediational pathway may be obtained when examining individuals exposed to chronic stress or with compromised immune systems (Cacioppo et al., 1998; Glaser, Kutz, MacCallum, & Malarkey, 1995; Vedhara et al., 1999).

Activation of the sympathetic nervous system (SNS) is another potential neuroendocrine mechanism linking social support to immunity. Sympathetic nerve fibers innervate both primary and secondary lymphoid organs (Felton, Ackerman, Wiegand, & Felton, 1987), providing a direct mechanism by which the SNS may influence aspects of immunity. Sympathetic nervous system agonists also increase the production of IL-6 and β_2-adrenegic blockade eliminates these effects (Soszynski, Lozak, Conn, Rudolph, & Kluger, 1996). Importantly, there is some evidence that social support is associated with lower catecholamine levels (Seeman, Berkman, Blazer, & Rowe, 1994; Grewen, Girdler, Amico, & Light, 2005). As was the case for cortisol, however, there is presently little direct evidence that social support is linked to immunity via SNS hormones (Bosch et al., 2009; Cohen et al., 1997). However, in one study, it was found that individuals high in biobehavioral risk (i.e., low social support and high depression) had increased activity of beta-adrenergic transcription factors (Lutgendorf et al., 2009). Moreover, intratumor (but not plasma) NE concentrations were higher for such individuals. These data suggest that plasma levels of SNS hormones may provide a less sensitive test of neuroendocrine mediation of social support influences on immunity although more data are needed testing these neuroendocrine mechanisms more generally.

There are a number of other neuroendocrince pathways of relevance to links between social support and immunity. There are documented links between opioid processes and immunity (Bayer et al. 1990; Shavit, Ben-Eliyahu, Zeidel, & Beilin, 2004). In addition, although most research has focused on the SNS, there is evidence to indicate that parasympathetic nervous system (PNS) influences on immune function may also be important (Haas & Schauenstein, 1997; Tracey, 2002). In response to inflammation, activation of the PNS serves to blunt the inflammatory response in "real time." This reflex serves to limit pro-inflammatory processes that if left unchecked can in some cases be more dangerous than the initial pathogen (e.g., septic shock). Finally, researchers have argued that some of the benefits of social support may be mediated by its influence on the hormone oxytocin (Grewen et al., 2005; Knox & Uvnas-Moberg, 1998), possibly due to its links to the aforementioned cholinergic anti-inflammatory pathway (Clodi et al., 2008). However, the viability of these neuroendocrine pathways as direct mechanisms linking social support to immunity remain largely untested.

Conclusions

There is consistent evidence linking social support to immune processes that might explain links to physical health outcomes. However, these data still represent just the first wave of work examining such links. In the next section, we argue that there are five general future directions that will be critical for the evolution of social support as a risk factor that might gain acceptance in both the social and biomedical sciences. These directions represent what we believe to be important "second generation" questions. The most important of these would be elucidating, by relevant theory, the mechanisms by which social support influences immunity and health. We have proposed a broad model to facilitate such work, and it is our hope that the next generation of studies will bring us closer to the ultimate goal of being able to more fully utilize this work to inform relevant intervention approaches.

Future Directions

Question 1: What are the mechanisms linking social support to immunity and health? There appear to be reliable links between social support and immunity. At least part of this link may be due to behavioral mechanisms. The most examined behavioral pathway includes health behaviors as many studies have assessed it to rule out this potential factor. However, according to existing models, health behaviors may be part of the phenomena in which support encourages (directly or indirectly) individuals to engage in healthier practices. In fact, at least part of the link between social support and immunity may be driven by health behaviors (Loucks et al., 2006; Marsland et al., 2007), although more explicit tests of such pathways remain to be conducted. This literature is also particularly silent about the possibility that social support links to immunity in chronic disease populations might be mediated by cooperation with medical regimens.

The literature has been particularly weak in terms of demonstrating psychological mediation of links between social support and immunity. There is a large basic literature linking social support to mental health that should be health-relevant (e.g., depression, stress, Berkman et al., 2000; Wills & Shinar, 2000). As noted earlier, future research may have to expand on the types of assessments and methods used to determine such psychological pathways. For instance, greater consideration of the support context and/or the use of statistical techniques that can simultaneously consider multiple pathways (e.g., SEM). In the absence of such mechanistic information, theoretical progress will be hindered and interventions may not be optimized.

Question 2: What is the role of model testing in social support research? Most of the prior research has been mainly focused on documenting links between social support and immunity. However, the next generation of studies needs to capitalize on the existing theoretical models linking social support to health outcomes. The most tested model is the buffering model of support on immunity (e.g., Bosch et al., 2009; Kiecolt-Glaser et al., 1991). However, other complementary models have been available for some time (Gore, 1981; Lin, 1986; Umberson, 1987). For instance, the matching hypothesis is an important variant of the stress-buffering model and suggests that buffering effects are more likely when the type of support matches the type of stress (e.g., emotional support for relatively uncontrollable stressors; Cutrona & Russell, 1990). A strong test of the matching hypothesis requires a more extensive examination of stressor characteristics, and such assessments are available (Almeida & Horn, 2004). In addition, an important relatively unexplored model is the stress-prevention model (Gore, 1981; Lin, 1986). This model suggests that social support is important because it decreases one's actual

exposure to stress over time (Lin, 1986; Russell & Cutrona, 1991). There are also promising recent perspectives that need further tests (e.g., ecological model, Segerstrom, 2008). Importantly, providing explicit tests of these models will also aide in answering Question 1, because these models highlight particular mechanisms. Model testing is also likely to positively influence an important goal of utilizing support interventions to facilitate healthy outcomes in different populations given the reciprocal links between theory and application (Lewin, 1951).

Question 3: What measures of social support are most health-relevant and why? One basic issue that is a source of discussion in the support literature is the breadth of the construct. Social support is usually defined as including both the structure of an individual's social life (e.g., group memberships, existence of familial ties) and the more explicit functions they may serve (e.g., provision of useful advice, emotional support). However, many researchers have called for greater specificity in how support is measured and defined (House et al., 1988; Vaux, 1988). In our view, this diversity of approaches is both a strength and a weakness of social support research. It is a strength in that it illustrates the generality of links between social ties and health and because particular measures of support may have different implications for the mechanisms linking it to physical-health outcomes (House et al., 1988). An important weakness of this approach, however, is that there is no generally accepted model of how these measures are related in ways that are health relevant, which hinders integrating the results of different studies (Cohen, 2004; Thoits, 2011).

The research reviewed earlier suggests that both structural and functional measures of support predict better immune function. It is important to note, however, that most of this literature has examined functional measures of perceived support that are more strongly linked to beneficial mental and physical health outcomes than received support (e.g., Uchino, 2009; Wills & Shinar, 2000). In addition, there is evidence linking structural measures of support to worse immune function in some contexts (Hamrick et al., 2002; Segerstrom, 2008). Recent theoretical work is aimed at explaining such measurement-based findings (Cohen, 2004; Segerstrom, 2008; Thoits, 2011; Uchino, 2009). For instance, we have recently argued that measures of perceived and received support are separable constructs, and one important reason they might be linked to different outcomes is that they have different origins (or antecedent processes). As argued by Sarason, Sarason, and Shearin (1986), measures of perceived support may have their origins in early familial transactions (e.g., caring, positive involvement) that set the basis for supportive relational schemas that co-develop with other positive psychosocial processes (e.g., self-esteem, less hostility; also see Flaherty & Richman, 1986). However, received support is more likely to represent a situational factor that is sought or provided in response to stress (Barrera, 2000). Thus, the context plays an important role about whether received support is beneficial or detrimental (e.g., receiving the "right" type of support, partner responsiveness, visibility of support, Bolger & Amarel, 2007; Maisel & Gable, 2009). Due to these emerging issues, future research should include different measures of support that are most conceptually linked to the population and processes of interest (see Cohen, 2004; Cohen, Gordon, & Gottlieb, 2000; Segerstrom, 2008; Thoits, 2011; Uchino, 2009).

Question 4: How are these diverse physiological processes coordinated? It is clear that social support is related to multiple physiological changes across systems (Uchino, 2006). Such data are consistent with a general health-promoting role of social support. In the search for more integrative processes, an important future question will pertain to how these systems are coordinated. One promising integrative mechanism relates to the central brain processes that might be responsible for such links (Coan, Schaefer, & Davidson, 2006; Eisenberger et al., 2007b). In one study, Eisenberger and colleagues (2007b) examined the associations between perceptions of social support using daily experience sampling, and its links to brain activity as indexed by functional magnetic resonance imaging (fMRI) during a social exclusion task (i.e., cyberball) and cortisol reactivity during social stress (tier social-stress task). Results replicated prior work showing that social support was associated with lower cortisol reactivity to stress. In addition, this association was statistically mediated by lower neural activity in the dorsal anterior cingulate cortex (dACC) and Broadmanns area 8 (part of frontal cortex) as evidenced during the cyberball task. There was also some evidence of further mediation via the hypothalamus.

The data linking social support to these brain processes as indexed by fMRI are also important because of potential links to existing models such as the stress-buffering model of support. For instance, stress reliably activates the dACC as well as the amygdala (Critchley et al., 2003; Wang et al., 2005). These structures are particularly important for the processing and subsequent biological responses associated with negative emotional states (Gianaros et al., 2005; Mohanty et al., 2007). Thus, insight into brain mechanisms may provide a theoretical bridge to understanding how links between social support and peripheral physiological responses are coordinated. It is also possible that such data may provide more guidance to Question 1 given the emerging perspective on brain mechanisms responsible for important psychological processes (e.g., self-regulation; Cacioppo et al., 2007).

Question 5: Should there be consideration of both positive and negative relationship processes? Finally, as we begin to explore greater links between social support and immunity, the importance of a more comprehensive view of relationships in a health context takes on added importance. As noted earlier, depending on the context, receiving support may have detrimental influences on health (Bolger & Amarel, 2007). Although relationships can be a source of life-affirming love and support, there is a potential "dark side" to relationships in terms of conflict, control, abuse, and jealousy (Rook, 1998). There is a smaller but robust literature on the health risks associated with negativity in relationships (De Vogli, Chandola, & Marmot, 2007; Matthews & Gump, 2002), including its association to immune processes (Kiecolt-Glaser et al., 2005). The simple existence of social ties and links to various groups and organizations does not guarantee that they are health-promoting. It is clear that social ties may also serve as significant sources of stress or become models for deviant or unhealthy behaviors (Burg & Seeman, 1994).

Even close relationships are not uniformly positive (Braiker & Kelley, 1979; Major, Zubek, Cooper, & Richards, 1997; Rook, 1984) and negativity in relationships predicts poorer health outcomes (De Vogli et al., 2007). The joint contribution of positivity *and* negativity to the study of social relationships and health has not been adequately examined, because most studies examine relationship positivity or negativity in isolation (Uchino, Holt-Lunstad, Uno, & Flinders, 2001). However, positive and negative aspects of social relationships tend to be distinct, separable factors (Finch et al., 1989; Newsom, Nishishiba, Morgan, & Rook, 2003; Pierce, Sarason, & Sarason, 1991). We have shown that positive and negative aspects of relationships can co-occur within relationships (i.e., ambivalence; Uchino et al., 2001). In addition, such ambivalent ties are not an isolated feature of individuals' social networks and appear associated with detrimental influences on health-relevant physiological processes (Uchino et al., 2007). The full conceptual implications of such findings remain to be explored, but they suggest the importance of a more comprehensive view of relationships that considers both positive and negative aspects.

Related Chapters

For more information on concepts introduced in this chapter, see also Effros, this volume.

References

Abbas, A. K., & Lichtman, A. H. (2003). *Cellular and molecular immunology* (5th ed.). Philadelphia: Harcourt Brace.

Alferi, S. M., Carver, C. S., Antoni, M. H., Weiss, S., & Duran, R. E. (2001). An exploratory study of social support, distress, and life disruption among low-income Hispanic women under treatment for early stage breast cancer. *Health Psychology, 20,* 41–46.

Almeida, D. M., & Horn, M. C. (2004). Is daily life more stressful during middle adulthood? In O. G. Brim, C. D. Ryff, & R. C. Kessler (Eds.), *How healthy are we? A national study of well-being at midlife* (pp. 425–451). Chicago: University of Chicago Press.

Antonucci, T. C., & Israel, B. A. (1986). Veridicality of social support: A comparison of principal and network members' responses. *Journal of Consulting and Clinical Psychology, 54,* 432–437.

Baldwin, M. W. (1992). Relational schemas and the processing of social information. *Psychological Bulletin, 112*(3), 461–484.

Baron, R. M., & Kenny, D. A. (1986). The moderator-mediator distinction in social psychological research: Conceptual, strategic, and statistical considerations. *Journal of Personality and Social Psychology, 51,* 1173–1182.

Baron, R. S., Cutrona, C. E., Hicklin, D., Russell, D. W., & Lubaroff, D. M. (1990). Social support and immune function among spouses of cancer patients. *Journal of Personality and Social Psychology, 59,* 344–352.

Barrera, M., Jr. (2000). Social support research in community psychology. In J. Rappaport & E. Seidman (Eds.), *Handbook of community psychology* (pp. 215–245). New York: Kluwer Academic/Plenum.

Barth, J., Schneider, S., & von Kanel, R. (2010). Lack of social support in the etiology and prognosis of coronary heart disease: A systematic review and meta-analysis. *Psychosomatic Medicine, 72,* 229–238.

Barton, B. E. (2005). Interleukin-6 and new strategies for the treatment of cancer, hyperproliferative diseases and paraneoplastic syndromes. *Expert Opinion on Therapeutic Targets, 9,* 737–752.

Bayer, B. M., Daussin, S., Hernandez, M., & Irvin, L. 1990. Morphine inhibition of lymphocyte activity is mediated by an opioid dependent mechanism. *Neuropharmacology, 29,* 369–374.

Berkman, L. F., Glass, T., Brissette, I., & Seeman, T. E. (2000). From social integration to health: Durkheim in the new millennium. *Social Science and Medicine, 51,* 843–857.

Berkman, L. F., & Syme, S. L. (1979). Social networks, host resistance, and mortality: A nine-year follow-up study of Alameda county residents. *American Journal of Epidemiology, 109,* 186–204.

Beyers, W. E. P., Palache, A. M., Baljet, M., & Masurel, N. (1989). Antibody induction by influenza vaccines in the elderly: A review of the literature. *Vaccine, 7,* 385–394.

Blazer, D. G. (1982). Social support and mortality in an elderly community population. *American Journal of Epidemiology, 115,* 684–694.

Blomkvist, V., Theorell, T., Jonsson, H., Schulman, S., Berntorp, E., & Stigendal, L. (1994). Psychosocial self-prognosis in relation to mortality and morbidity in hemophiliacs with HIV infection. *Psychotherapy and Psychosomatics, 62,* 185–192.

Bollen, K. A. (1989). *Structural equations with latent variables.* New York: Wiley.

Bolger, N., & Amarel, D. (2007). Effects of social support visibility on adjustment to stress: Experimental evidence. *Journal of Personality and Social Psychology, 92*(3), 458–475.

Bolger, N., Foster, M., Vinokur, A. D., & Ng, R. (1996). Close relationships and adjustment to a life crisis: The case of breast cancer. *Journal of Personality and Social Psychology, 70,* 283–294.

Bollen, K. A. (1989). *Structural equations with latent variables.* Mahwah, NJ: Wiley.

Bosch, J. A., Fischer, J. E., & Fischer, J.C. (2009). Psychologically adverse work conditions are associated with CD8+ T cell differentiation indicative of immunesenescence. *Brain, Behavior, and Immunity, 23,* 527–534.

Braiker, H. B., & Kelley, H. H. (1979). Conflict in the development of close relationships. In R. L. Burgess & T. L. Huston (Ed.), *Social exchange in developing relationships* (pp. 135–168). New York: Academic Press.

Burg, M. M., & Seeman, T. E. (1994). Families and health: The negative side of social ties. *Annals of Behavioral Medicine, 16,* 109–115.

Burnett, F. M., (1970). The concept of immunological surveillance. *Progress in Experimental Tumor Research, 13,* 1–27.

Cacioppo, J. T., Amaral, D. G., Blanchard, J. J., Cameron, J. L., Carter, C. S., Crews, D., et al. (2007). Social neuroscience: Progress and implications for mental health. *Perspectives on Psychological Science, 2,* 99–123.

Cacioppo, J. T., Berntson, G. G., Malarkey, W. B., Kielcolt-Glaser, J. K., Sheridan, J. F., Poehlmann, K. M., et al. (1998). Autonomic, neuroendocrine, and immune responses to psychological stress: The reactivity hypothesis. *Annals of the New York Academy of Sciences, 840,* 664–673.

Center for Disease Control (2003). Public health and aging: Trends in aging—United States and worldwide. *MMWR, 52,* 101–106.

Ceria, C. D., Masaki, K. H., Rodriguez, B. L., Chen, R., Yano, K., & Curb, J. D. (2001). The relationship of psychosocial factors to total mortality among older Japanese-American men: The Honolulu heart program. *Journal of the American Geriatric Society, 49,* 725–731.

Clodi, M., Vila, G., Geveregger, R., Riedl, M., Stulnig, T.M., Struck, J., et al. (2008). Oxytocin alleviates the neuroendocrine and cytokine response to baterial endotoxin in healthy men. *American Journal of Physiology: Endocrinology and Metabolism, 295,* E686–691.

Coan, J. A., Schaefer, H. S., & Davidson, R. J. (2006). Lending a hand: Social regulation of the neural response to threat. *Psychological Science, 17,* 1032–1039.

Cohen, S. (1988). Psychosocial models of the role of social support in the etiology of physical disease. *Health Psychology, 7,* 269–297.

Cohen, S. (2004). Social relationships and health. *American Psychologist, 59,* 676–684.

Cohen, S., Doyle, W. J., Skoner, D. P., Rabin, B. S., & Gwaltney, J. M., Jr. (1997). Social ties and susceptibility to the common cold. *Journal of the American Medical Association, 277,* 1940–1944.

Cohen, S., Gordon, L., & Gottlieb, B. (2000). *Social support measurement and intervention: A guide for health and social scientists.* New York: Oxford University Press.

Cohen, S., & Wills, T. A. (1985). Stress, social support, and the buffering hypothesis. *Psychological Bulletin, 98,* 310–357.

Costanzo, E. S., Lutgendorf, S. K., Sood, A. K., Anderson, B., Sorosky, J., & Lubaroff, D. M. (2005). Psychosocial factors and interleukin-6 among women with advanced ovarian cancer. *Cancer, 104,* 305–313.

Coussons-Read, M. E., Okun, M. L., & Nettles, C. D. (2007). Psychosocial stress increases inflammatory markers and alters cytokine production across pregnancy. *Brain, Behavior and Immunity, 21,* 343–350.

Coyne, J. C. (1976). Depression and the response of others. *Journal of Abnormal Psychology, 85,* 186–193.

Critchley, H. D., Mathias, C. J., Josephs, O., O'Doherty, J., Zanini, S., Dewar, B.-K., et al. (2003). Human cingulated cortex and autonomic control: Converging neuroimaging and clinical evidence. *Brain, 126,* 2139–2152.

Cutrona, C. E. (1986). Behavioral manifestations of social support: A microanalytic investigation. *Journal of Personality and Social Psychology, 51,* 201–208.

Cutrona, C. E., & Russell, D. W. (1990). Type of social support and specific stress: Towards a theory of optimal matching. In B. R. Sarason, I. G. Sarason, & G. R. Pierce (Eds.), *Social support: An interactional view* (pp. 319–366). New York: Wiley.

Danesh, J., Kaptoge, S., Mann, A. G., Sarwar, N., Wood, A., Angleman, S. B., et al. (2008). Long-term interleukin-6 levels and subsequent risk of coronary heart disease: Two new prospective studies and a systematic review. *PLoS Medicine, 5,* 600–610.

Davidson, D. M., & Shumaker, S. A. (1987). Social support and cardiovascular disease. *Arteriosclerosis, 7,* 101–104.

De Vogli, R., Chandola, T., & Marmot, M. G. (2007). Negative aspects of close relationships and heart disease. *Archives of Internal Medicine, 167,* 1951–1957.

DiMatteo, M. R. (2004). Social support and patient adherence to medical treatment: A meta-analysis. *Health Psychology, 23,* 207–218.

Dixon, D., Cruess, S., Kilbourn, K., Klimas, N., Fletcher, M. A., Ironson, G., et al. (2001). Social support mediates loneliness and human herpesvirus type 6 (HHV-6) antibody titers. *Journal of Applied Social Psychology, 31,* 1111–1132.

Dranoff, G. (2004). Cytokines in cancer pathogenesis and cancer therapy. *Nature Reviews Cancer, 4,* 11–22.

Dunkel-Schetter, C., & Bennett, T. L. (1990). Differentiating the cognitive and behavioral aspects of social support. In B. R. Sarason, I. G. Sarason, & G. R. Pierce (Eds.), *Social support: An interactional view* (pp. 267–296). New York: Wiley.

Dunn, G. P., Bruce, A. T., Ikeda, H., Old, L. J., & Schreiber, R. D. (2002). Cancer immunoediting: From immunosurveillance to tumor escape. *Nature Immunology, 3,* 991–998.

Effros, R. B., & Walford, R. L. (1987). Infection and immunity in relation to aging. In E. A. Goidl (Ed.), *Aging and the immune response* (pp. 45–65). New York: Marcel Dekker.

Eisenberger, N. I., Gable, S. L., & Lieberman, M. D. (2007). Functional magnetic resonance imaging responses relate to differences in real-world social experience. *Emotion, 7,* 745–754.

Eisenberger, N. I., Taylor, S. E., Gable, S. L., Hilmert, C. J., & Lieberman, M. D. (2007). Neural pathways link social support to attenuated neuroendocrine stress responses. *NeuroImage, 35,* 1601–1612.

Ell, K., Nishimoto, R., Medianski, L., Mantell, J., & Hamovitch, M. (1992). Social relations, social support and survival among patients with cancer. *Journal of Psychosomatic Research, 36,* 531–541.

Evans, G. W., & Kim, P. (2010). Multiple risk exposure as a potential explanatory mechanism for the socioeconomic status-health gradient. *Annals of the New York Academy of Sciences, 1186,* 174–189.

Fekete, E. M., Antoni, M. H., Lopez, C. R., Durán, R. E., Penedo, F. J., Bandiera, F. C., et al. (2009). Men's serostatus disclosure to parents: Associations among social support, ethnicity, and disease status in men living with HIV. *Brain, Behavior, and Immunity, 23,* 693–699.

Felton, D. L., Ackerman, K. D., Wiegand, S. J., & Felton, S. Y. (1987). Noradrenergic sympathetic innervation of the spleen: I. Nerve fibers associate with lymphocytes and macrophages in specific compartments of the splenic white pulp. *Journal of Neuroscience Research, 18,* 28–36.

Finch, J. F., Okun, M. A., Barrera, M., Zautra, A. J., & Reich, J. W. (1989). Positive and negative social ties among older adults: Measurement models and the prediction of psychological distress and well-being. *American Journal of Community Psychology, 17,* 585–605.

Flaherty, J. A., & Richman, J. A. (1986). Effects of childhood relationships on the adult's capacity to form social supports. *American Journal of Psychiatry, 143,* 851–855.

Floyd, K., Mikkelson, A. C., Tafoya, M. A., Farinelli, L., La Valley, A. G., Judd, J., et al. (2007). Human affection exchange XIV: Relational affection predicts resting heart rate and free cortisol secretion during acute stress. *Behavioral Medicine, 32,* 151–156.

Friedman, E. M., Hayney, M. S., Love, G. D., Urry, H. L., Rosenkranz, M. A., Davidson, et al. (2005). Social relationships, sleep quality, and interleukin-6 in aging women. *PNAS, 102,* 18757–18762.

Gallagher, S., Phillips, A. C., Ferraro, A. J., Drayson, M. T., & Carroll, D. (2008a). Social support is positively associated with the immunoglobulin M response to pneumococcal vaccination. *Biological Psychology, 78,* 211–215.

Gallagher, S., Phillips, A. C., Ferraro, A. J., Drayson, M. T., & Carroll, D. (2008b). Psychosocial factors are associated with the antibody response to both thymus-dependent and thymus-independent vaccines. *Brain, Behavior, and Immunity, 22,* 456–460.

Gerin, W., Pieper, C., Levy, R., & Pickering, T. G. (1992). Social support in social interaction: A moderator of cardiovascular reactivity. *Psychosomatic Medicine, 54,* 324–336.

Gianaros, P. J., Derbyshire, S. W. G., May, J. C., Siegle, G. J., Gamalo, M. A., & Jennings, J. R. (2005). Anterior cingulated activity correlates with blood pressure during stress. *Psychophysiology, 42,* 627–635.

Glaser, R., Kiecolt-Glaser, J. K., Bonneau, R., Malarkey, W., Hughes, J. (1992). Stress-induced modulation of the immune response to recombinant hepatitis B vaccine. *Psychosomatic Medicine, 54,* 22–29.

Glaser, R., Kutz, L. A., MacCallum, R. C., & Malarkey, W. B. (1995). Hormonal modulation of Epstein-Barr virus replication. *Neuroendocrinology, 62,* 356–361.

Gonzalez, J. S., Penedo, F. J., Antoni, M. H., Duran, R. E., Fernandez, M. I., McPherson-Baker, S., et al. (2004). Social support, positive states of mind, and HIV treatment adherence in men and women living with HIV/AIDS. *Health Psychology, 23,* 413–418.

Goodkin, K., Blaney, N. T., Feaster, D., Fletcher, M., Baum, M. K., Mantero-Atienza, E., et al. (1992). Active coping style is associated with natural killer cell cytotoxicity in asymptomatic HIV-1 seropositive homosexual men. *Journal of Psychosomatic Research, 36,* 635–650.

Gore, S. (1981). Stress-buffering functions of social supports: An appraisal and clarification of research models. In B. Dohrenwend & B. Dohrenwend (Eds.), *Stressful life events and their context* (pp. 202–222). New York: Prodist.

Granovetter, M. S. (1973). The strength of weak ties. *American Journal of Sociology, 78,* 1360–1380.

Grant, N., Hamer, M., & Steptoe, A. (2009). Social isolation and stress-related cardiovascular, lipid, and cortisol responses. *Annals of Behavioral Medicine, 27,* 29–37.

Grewen, K. M., Girdler, S. S., Amico, J., & Light, K. C. (2005). Effects of partner support on resting oxytocin, cortisol, norepinephrine, and blood pressure before and after warm partner contact. *Psychosomatic Medicine, 67,* 531–538.

Haas, H. S., & Schauenstein, K. (1997). Neuroimmunomodulation via limbic structures: The neuroanatomy of psychoimmunology. *Progress in Neurobiology, 51,* 195–222.

Hamrick, N., Cohen, S., & Rodriguez, M. S. (2002). Being popular can be healthy or unhealthy: Stress, social network diversity and incidence of upper respiratory infection. *Health Psychology, 21,* 294–298.

Hawkley, L. C., Bosch, J. A., Engeland, C. G., Marucha, P. T., & Cacioppo, J. T. (2007). Loneliness, dysphoria, stress and immunity: A role for cytokines. In N. P. Plotnikoff, R. E. Faith, & A. J. Murgo (Eds.), *Cytokines: Stress and immunity* (pp. 67–86). Bocan Raton, LA: CRC Press.

Haynes, L., & Maue, A. C. (2009). Effects of aging on T cell function. *Current Opinions in Immunology, 21,* 414–417.

Heinrichs, M., Baumgartner, T., Kirschbaum, C., & Ehlert, U. (2003). Social support and oxytocin interact to suppress cortisol and subjective responses to psychosocial stress. *Biological Psychiatry, 54,* 1389–1398.

Herbert, T. B., & Cohen, S. (1993). Depression and immunity: A meta-analytic review. *Psychological Bulletin, 113,* 472–486.

Holahan, C. J., & Moos, R. H. (1990). Life stressors, resistance factors, and improved psychological functioning: An extension of the stress resistance paradigm. *Journal of Personality and Social Psychology, 58,* 909–917.

Holt-Lunstad, J., Smith, T. B., Layton, B. (2010). Social relationships and mortality: A meta-analysis. *PLoS Medicine, 7,* e1000316.

Hong, D. S., Angelo, L. S., & Kurzrock, R. (2007). Interleukin-6 and its receptor in cancer: Implications for translational therapeutics. *Cancer, 110,* 1911–1928.

House, J. S. (2001). Social isolation kills, but how and why? *Psychosomatic Medicine, 63,* 273–274.

House, J. S., Landis, K. R., & Umberson, D. (1988). Social relationships and health. *Science, 241,* 540–545.

Ironson, G., & Hayward, H. (2008). Do positive psychosocial factors predict disease progression in HIV-1? A review of the evidence. *Psychosomatic Medicine, 70,* 546–554.

Kaltsas, G. A., & Chrousos, G. P. (2007). The neuroendocrinology of stress. In J. T. Cacioppo, L. G. Tassinary, & G. G. Berntson (Eds.), *Handbook of Psychophysiology* (pp. 303–318). New York: Cambridge University Press.

Kang, D. H., Coe, C. L., Karaszewski, J., & McCarthy, D. O. (1998). Relationship of social support to stress responses and immune function in healthy and asthmatic adolescents. *Research in Nursing and Health, 21,* 117–128.

Kaplan, G. A., Wilson, T. W., Cohen, R. D., Kauhanen, J., Wu, M., & Salonen, J. T. (1994). Social functioning and overall mortality: Prospective evidence from the Kuopio ischemic heart disease risk factor study. *Epidemiology, 5,* 495–500.

Kemeny, M. E., Weiner, H., Duran, R., Taylor, S. E., Visscher, B., & Fahey, J. L. (1995). Immune system changes after the death of a partner in HIV-positive gay men. *Psychosomatic Medicine, 57,* 547–54.

Kerbel, R. (2000). Tumor angiogenesis: Past, present, and the near future. *Carcinogenesis, 21,* 505–515.

Kiecolt-Glaser, J. K., Dura, J. R., Speicher, C. E., Trask, O. J., & Glaser, R. G. (1991). Spousal caregivers of dementia victims: Longitudinal changes in immunity and health. *Psychosomatic Medicine, 53,* 345–362.

Kiecolt-Glaser, J. K., Loving, T. J., Stowell, J. R., Malarkey, W. B., Lemeshow, S., Dickinson, S. L., & Glaser, R. (2005). Hostile marital interactions, proinflammatory cytokine production, and wound healing. *Archives in General Psychiatry, 62,* 1377–1384.

Kiecolt-Glaser, J. K., McGuire, L., Robles, T. F., & Glaser, R. (2002). Emotions, morbidity, and mortality: New perspectives from psychoneuroimmunology. *Annual Review of Psychology, 53,* 83–107.

Knox, S. S., & Uvnas-Moberg, K. (1998). Social isolation and cardiovascular disease: An atherosclerotic pathway? *Psychoneuroendocrinology, 23,* 877–890.

Kristiansen, O. P., & Mandrup-Poulsen, T. (2005). Interleukin-6 and diabetes: The good, the bad, or the indifferent? *Diabetes, 54,* S114–124.

Lakey, B., & Orehek, E. (2011). Relational regulation theory: A new approach to explain the link between perceived social support and mental health. *Psychological Bulletin, 118,* 482–495. Lee, M., & Rotheram-Borus, M. J. (2001). Challenges associated with increased survival among parents living with HIV. *American Journal of Public Health, 91,* 1303–1309.

Lee, S. Y., & Shi, J. Q. (2000). Bayesian analysis of structural equation model with fixed covariates. *Structural Equation Modeling, 7,* 411–430.

Lee, S. Y., & Song, X. Y. (2004). Evaluation of the bayesian and maximum likelihood approaches in analyzing structural equation models with small sample sizes. *Multivariate Behavioral Research, 39,* 653–686.

Levy, S. M., Herberman, R. B., Whiteside, T., Sanzo, K., Lee, J., & Kirkwood, J. (1990). Perceived social support and tumor estrogen/progesterone receptor status as predictors of natural killer cell activity in breast cancer patients. *Psychosomatic Medicine, 52,* 73–85.

Lewin, K. (1951). *Field theory in social science.* New York: Harper and Bros.

Lewis, M. A., & Rook, K. S. (1999). Social control in personal relationships: Impact on health behaviors and psychological distress. *Health Psychology, 18,* 63–71.

Libby, P. (2002). Inflammation in atherosclerosis. *Nature, 420,* 868–874.

Lieberman, M. D. (2007). Social cognitive neuroscience: A review of core processes. *Annual Review Psychology, 58,* 259–289.

Lin, N. (1986). Modeling the effects of social support. In N. Lin, A. Dean, & W. Ensel (Eds.), *Social support, life events, and depression* (pp. 173–209). Orlando, FL: Academic Press.

Loucks, E. B., Sullivan, L. M., D'Agostino, R. B., Larson, M. G., Berkman, L. F., & Benjamin, E. J. (2006). Social networks and inflammatory markers in the Framingham Heart Study. *Journal Of Biosocial Science, 38,* 835–842.

Lutgendorf, S. K., Anderson, B., Sorosky, J., Buller, R., & Lubaroff, D. (2000). Interleukin-6 and use of social support in gynecologic cancer patients. *International Journal of Behavioral Medicine, 7,* 127–142.

Lutgendorf, S. K., DeGeest, K., Sung, C. Y., Arevalo, J. M. G., Penedo, F., Lucci, J. A. III, et al. (2009). Depression, social support, and beta-adrenergic transcription control in human ovarian cancer. *Brain, Behavior, and Immunity, 23,* 176–183.

Lutgendorf, S. K., Johnsen, E., Cooper, B., Anderson, B., Buller, R., & Sood, A. K. (2002). Vascular endothelial growth factor and social support in patients with ovarian cancer. *Cancer, 95,* 808–815.

Lutgendorf, S. K., Lamkin, D. M., Jennings, N. B., Arevalo, J. M. G., Penedo, F., DeGeest, K., et al. (2008). Biobehavioral influences on matrix metalloproteinase expression in ovarian carcinoma. *Clinical Cancer Research, 14,* 6839–6846.

Lutgendorf, S. K., Sood, A. K., Anderson, B., McGinn, S., Maiseri, H., Dao, M., et al. (2005). Social support, psychological distress, and natural killer cell activity in ovarian cancer. *Journal of Clinical Oncology, 23,* 7105–7113.

Lyubomirsky, S., King, L., & Diener, E. (2005). The benefits of positive affect: Does happiness lead to success? *Psychological Bulletin, 131,* 803–855.

MacKinnon, D. P. (2008). *Introduction to statistical mediational analyses.* New York: Erlbaum.

Maisel N., & Gable, S. L. (2009). The paradox of received social support: The importance of responsiveness. *Psychological Science, 20,* 928–932.

Major, B., Zubek, J. M., Cooper, M. L., & Richards, C. (1997). Mixed messages: Implications of social conflict and social support within close relationships for adjustment to a stressful life event. *Journal of Personality and Social Psychology, 72,* 1349–1363.

Marsland, A. L., Sathanoori, R., Muldoon, M. F., & Manuck, S. B. (2007). Stimulated production of interleukin-8 covaries with psychosocial risk factors for inflammatory disease among middle-aged community volunteers. *Brain, Behavior and Immunity, 21,* 218–228.

Marucha, P. T., Crespin, T. R., Shelby, R. A., & Andersen, B. L. (2005). TNF-alpha levels in cancer patients relate to social variables. *Brain, Behavior, and Immunity, 19,* 521–525.

Matthews, K. A., & Gump, B. B. (2002). Chronic work stress and marital dissolution increase risk of post-trial mortality in men from the multiple risk factor intervention trial. *Archives of Internal Medicine, 162,* 309–315.

McDade, T. W., Hawkley, L. C., & Cacioppo, J. T. (2006) Psychosocial and behavioral predictors of inflammation in middle-aged and older adults: The Chicago health, aging, and social relations study. *Psychosomatic Medicine, 68,* 376–381.

Mead, G. H. (1934). *Mind, self, and society.* Chicago: University of Chicago Press.

Miller, G. E., & Cole, S. W. (1998). Social relationships and the progression of human immunodeficiency virus infection: A review of evidence and possible underlying mechanisms. *Annuals of Behavioral Medicine, 20,* 181–189.

Miyazaki, T., Ishikawa, T., Nakata, A., Sakurai, T., Miki, A., Kawakami, N., et al. (2005). Association between perceived social support and Th1 dominance. *Biological Psychology, 70,* 30–37.

Mohanty, A., Engels, A. S., Herrington, J. D., Heller, W., Ho, M. R., Banich, M. T., et al. (2007). Differential engagement of anterior cingulate cortex subdivisions for cognitive and emotional function. *Psychophysiology, 44,* 343–351.

Moynihan, J. A., Larson, M. R., Treanor, J., Duberstein, P. R., Power, A., Shore, B., & Ader, R. (2004). Psychosocial factors and the response to influenza vaccination in older adults. *Psychosomatic Medicine, 66,* 950–953.

Munck, A., Guyre, P. M., & Holbrook, N. J. (1984). Physiological functions of glucocorticoids in stress and their relation to pharmacological actions. *Endocrine Reviews, 5,* 25–44.

Nausheen, B., Gidron, Y., Peveler, R., & Moss-Morris, R. (2009). Social support and cancer progression: A systematic review. *Journal of Psychosomatic Research, 67,* 403–415.

Newsom, J. T., Nishishiba, M., Morgan, D. L., & Rook, K. S. (2003). The relative importance of three domains of positive and negative social exchanges: A longitudinal model with comparable measures. *Psychology and Aging, 18,* 746–754.

Ng, D. M., & Jeffery, R. W. (2003). Relationships between perceived stress and health behaviors in a sample of working adults. *Health Psychology, 22,* 638–642.

Ogilvie, D. M., & Ashmore, R. D. (1991). Self-with-other representation as a unit of analysis in self-concept research. In R. C. Curtis (Ed.), *The relational self: Theoretical convergences in psychoanalysis and social psychology* (pp. 282–314). New York: Guilford Press.

O'Reilly, P., & Thomas, H. E. (1989). Role of support networks in maintenance of improved cardiovascular health status. *Social Science and Medicine, 28,* 249–260.

Papanicolaou, D. A., Wilder, R. L., Manolagas, S. C., & Chrousos, G. P. (1998). The pathophysiologic roles of interleukin-6 in human disease. *Annals of Internal Medicine, 128,* 127–137.

Patterson, T. L., Shaw, W. S., Semple, S. J., Cherner, M., McCutchan, J. A., Atkinson, J., et al. (1996). Relationship of psychosocial factors to HIV progression. *Annals of Behavioral Medicine, 18,* 30–39.

Penninx, B. W. J. H., van Tilburg, T., Kriegsman, D. M. W., Deeg, D. J. H., Boeke, A. J. P., & van Eijk, J. T. M. (1997). Effects of social support and personal control resources on mortality in older age: The longitudinal aging study Amsterdam. *American Journal of Epidemiology, 146,* 510–519.

Perry, S., Fishman, B., Jacobsberg, L., & Frances, A. (1992). Relationships over 1 year between lymphocyte subsets and psychosocial variables among adults with infection by human immunodeficiency virus. *Archives of General Psychiatry, 49,* 396–401.

Persson, L., Gullberg, B., Hanson, B. S., Moestrup, T., & Ostergren, P. O. (1994). HIV infection: Social network, social support, and CD4 lymphocyte values in infected homosexual men in Malmo, Sweden. *Journal of Epidemiology and Community Health, 48,* 580–585.

Phillips, A. C., Burns, V. E., Carroll, D., Ring, C., & Drayson, M. (2005). The association between life events, social support and antibody status following thymus-dependent and thymus-independent vaccinations in healthy young adults. *Brain, Behavior and Immunity,19,* 325–333.

Phillips, A. C., Carroll, D., Burns, V. E., Ring, C., Macleod, J., & Drayson, M. (2006). Bereavement and marriage are associated with antibody response to influenza vaccination in the elderly. *Brain, Behavior and Immunity, 20,* 279–289.

Pierce, G. R., Sarason, I. G., & Sarason, B. R. (1991). General and relationships-specific perceptions of social support: Are two constructs better than one? *Journal of Personality and Social Psychology, 61,* 1028–1039.

Pressman, S. D., Cohen, S., Miller, G. E., Barkin, A., Rabin, B. S., & Treanor, J. J. (2005). Loneliness, social network size, and immune response to influenza vaccination in college freshmen. *Health Psychology, 24,* 297–306.

Ratnasingam, P., & Bishop, G. D. (2007). Social support schemas, trait anger, and cardiovascular responses. *International Journal of Psychophysiology, 63,* 308–316.

Rejeski, W. J., Thompson, A., Brubaker, P. H., & Miller, H. S. (1992). Acute exercise: Buffering psychosocial stress responses in women. *Health Psychology, 11,* 355–362.

Ridker, P. M., Rifai, N., Stampfer, M. J., & Hennekens, C. H. (2000). Plasma concentration of interleukin-6 and the risk of future myocardial infarction among apparently healthy men. *Circulation, 101,* 1767–1772.

Rook, K. S. (1984). The negative side of social interaction: Impact on psychological well being. *Journal of Personality and Social Psychology, 46,* 1097–1108.

Rook, K. S. (1998). Investigating the positive and negative sides of personal relationships: Through a lens darkly? In B. H. Spitzberg & W. R. Cupach (Eds.), *The dark side of close relationships* (pp. 369–393). Mahwah, NJ: Erlbaum.

Ross, R. (1999). Mechanisms of disease: Atherosclerosis—An inflammatory disease. *New England Journal of Medicine, 340,* 115–126.

Russell, D. W., & Cutrona, C. E. (1991). Social support, stress, and depressive symptoms among the elderly: Test of a process model. *Psychology and Aging, 6,* 190–201.

Sanders, V. M., Kasprowicz, D. J., Kohm, A. P., & Swanson, M. A. (2001). Neurotransmitter receptors on lymphocytes and other lymphoid cells. In R. Ader, D. L. Felten, & N. Cohen (Eds.), *Psychoneuroimmunology* (Vol. 1, 3rd ed., pp. 161–196). New York: Academic Press.

Sapolsky, R. M., Romero, M., & Munck, A. U. (2000). How do glucocorticoids influences stress responses? Integrating permissive, suppressive, stimulatory, and preparative actions. *Endocrine Reviews, 21,* 55–89.

Sarason, I. G., Sarason, B. R., & Shearin, E. N. (1986). Social support as an individual difference variable: Its stability, origins, and relational aspects. *Journal of Personality and Social Psychology, 50,* 845–855.

Seeman, T. E., Berkman, L. F., Blazer, D., & Rowe, J. W. (1994). Social ties and support and neuroendocrine function: The MacArthur studies of successful aging. *Annals of Behavioral Medicine, 16,* 95–106.

Seeman, T. E., Kaplan, G. A., Knudsen, L., Cohen, R., & Guralnik, J. (1987). Social network ties and mortality among the elderly in the Alameda County Study. *American Journal of Epidemiology, 126,*714–723.

Segerstrom, S. C. (2008). Social networks and immunosuppression during stress: Relationship conflict or energy conservation? *Brain, Behavior, and Immunity, 22,* 279–284.

Segerstrom, S. (2009). Biobehavioral controls: Threats to psychoneuroimmunology research? *Brain, Behavior, and Immunity, 23,* 885–886.

Segerstrom, S. C., & Miller, G. E. (2004). Psychological stress and the human immune system: A meta-analytic study of 30 years of inquiry. *Psychological Bulletin, 130,* 601–630.

Shavit, Y., Ben-Eliyahu, S., Zeidel, A., & Beilin, B. (2004). Effects of fentanyl on natural killer cell activity and on resistance to tumor metastasis in rats: Dose and timing study. *Neuroimmunomodulation, 11,* 255–260.

Smith, T. W., Ruiz, J. M., & Uchino, B. N. (2004). Mental activation of supportive ties, hostility, and cardiovascular reactivity to laboratory stress in young men and women. *Health Psychology, 23,* 476–485.

Soszynski, D., Lozak, W., Conn, C. A., Rudolph, K., & Kluger, M. J. (1996). Beta- adrenoceptor antagonists suppress elevation in body temperature and increase in plasma IL-6 in rats exposed to open field. *Neuroendocrinology, 63,* 459–467.

Stone, A. A., Mezzacappa, E. S., Donatone, B. A., & Gonder, M. (1999). Psychosocial stress and social support are associated with prostate-specific antigen levels in men: Results from a community screening program. *Health Psychology, 18,* 482–486.

Stryker, S., & Burke, P. J. (2000). The past, present, and future of an identity theory. *Social Psychology Quarterly, 63,* 284–297.

Theorell, T., Blomkvist, V., Jonsson, H., Schulman, S., Berntorp, E., & Stigendal, L. (1995). Social support and the development of immune function in human immunodeficiency virus infection. *Psychosomatic Medicine, 57,* 32–36.

Thoits, P. A. (1983). Multiple identities and psychological well-being: A reformulation and test of the social isolation hypothesis. *American Sociological Review, 48,* 174–187.

Thoits, P. A. (1995). Stress, coping, and social support processes: Where are we? What next? *Journal of Health and Social Behavior, 35,* 53–79.

Thoits, P. (2011). Mechanisms linking social ties and support to physical and mental health. *Journal of Health and Social Behavior, 52,* 145–165.

Thomas, P. D., Goodwin, J. M., & Goodwin, J. S. (1985). Effects of social support on stress-related changes in cholesterol level, uric acid level, and immune function in an elderly sample. *American Journal of Psychiatry, 142,* 735–737.

Thorsteinsson, E. B., & James, J. E. (1999). A meta-analysis of the effects of experimental manipulations of social support during laboratory stress. *Psychology and Health, 14,* 869–886.

Tracey, K. J. (2002). The inflammatory reflex. *Nature, 420,* 853–859.

Turner-Cobb, J. M., Koopman, C., Rabinowitz, J. D., Terr, A. I., Sephton, S. E., & Spiegel, D. (2004). The interaction of social network size and stressful life events predict delayed-type hypersensitivity among women with metastatic breast cancer. *International Journal of Psychophysiology, 54,* 241–249.

Turner-Cobb, J. M., Sephton, S. E., Koopman, C., Blake-Mortimer, J., & Spiegel, D. (2000). Social support and salivary cortisol in women with metastatic breast cancer. *Psychosomatic Medicine, 62,* 337–345.

Uchino, B. N. (2004). *Social support and physical health: Understanding the health consequences of relationships.* New Haven, CT: Yale University Press.

Uchino, B. N. (2006). Social support and health: A review of physiological processes potentially underlying links to disease outcomes. *Journal of Behavioral Medicine, 29,* 377–387.

Uchino, B. N. (2009). Understanding the links between social support and physical health: A lifespan perspective with emphasis on the separability of perceived and received support. *Perspectives in Psychological Science, 4,* 236–255.

Uchino, B. N., Cacioppo, J. T., & Kiecolt-Glaser, J. K. (1996). The relationship between social support and physiological processes: A review with emphasis on underlying mechanisms and implications for health. *Psychological Bulletin, 119,* 488–531.

Uchino, B. N., Holt-Lunstad, J., Uno, D., Campo, R., & Reblin, M. (2007). The social neuroscience of relationships: An examination of health relevant pathways. In E. Harmon-Jones & P. Winkielman (Eds.), *Social neuroscience: Integrating biological and psychological explanations of social behavior* (pp. 474–492). New York: Guilford.

Uchino, B. N., Holt-Lunstad, J., Uno, D., & Flinders, J. B. (2001). Heterogeneity in the social networks of young and older adults: Prediction of mental health and cardiovascular reactivity during acute stress. *Journal of Behavioral Medicine, 24,* 361–382.

Umberson, D. (1987). Family status and health behaviors: Social control as a dimension of social integration. *Journal of Health and Social Behavior, 28,* 306–319.

Vaux, A. (1988). *Social support: Theory, research, and intervention.* New York: Praeger.

Vedhara, K., Cox, N. K. M., Wilcock, G. K., Perks, P., Hunt, M., Anderson, S., et al. (1999). Chronic stress in elderly carers of dementia patients and antibody response to influenza vaccination. *Lancet, 353,* 627–631.

Von Ah, D., Kang, D. H., & Carpenter, J. S., (2007). Stress, optimism, and social support: Impact on immune responses in breast cancer. *Research in Nursing and Health, 30,* 72–83.

Wang, J., Rao, H., Wetmore, G. S., Furlan, P. M., Korczykowski, M., Dinges, D. F., & Detre, J. A. (2005). Perfusion functional MRI reveals cerebral blood flow pattern under psychological stress. *PNAS, 102,* 17804–17809.

Weihs, K. L., Simmens, S. J., Mizrahi, J., Enright, T. M., Hunt, M. E., & Siegel, R. S. (2005). Dependable social relationships predict overall survival in Stages II and III breast carcinoma patients. *Journal of Psychosomatic Research, 59,* 299–306.

Wills, T. A., & Shinar, O. (2000). Measuring perceived and received social support. In S. Cohen, L. Gordon, & B. Gottlieb (Eds.), *Social support measurement and intervention: A guide for health and social scientists* (pp. 86–135). New York: Oxford University Press.

Yoshikawa, T. T. (2000). Epidemiology and unique aspects of aging and infectious diseases. *Clinical Infectious Diseases, 30,* 931–933.

Socioeconomic Status, Inflammation, and Immune Function

Andrew Steptoe

Abstract

Socioeconomic status (SES) is a major determinant of health and well-being in childhood, adult life, and old age, with people of lower SES, as defined by education, occupation, income, and neighborhood deprivation being at higher risk for a range of communicable and noncommunicable diseases. Psychoneuroimmunological processes may contribute to links between SES and health outcomes. There is extensive population evidence that SES is inversely associated with chronic inflammation indexed by markers such as C-reactive protein, interleukin-6, and fibrinogen. Both childhood and adult SES contribute to this pattern. Evidence for SES differences in acquired immunity is more sparse, but it also implicates lower SES in the dysregulation of immune responses. There is limited experimental data from humans showing that lower SES is associated with heightened inflammation following acute stress. There is an inverse correlation between SES and seropositivity for common infections acquired early in the life course that may in turn contribute to low-grade inflammation in adult life. SES differences in immunity and inflammation are also mediated in part by variations in health-related behaviors such as smoking and energy balance, and by direct stress-related processes. Research linking SES, psychosocial adversity, immune function, and health outcomes longitudinally is needed, together with intervention studies that explore the impact of modifying links in the causal chain.

Key Words: heightened inflammation, impaired immune function, low socioeconomic status

Introduction

It has been recognized since the earliest times that poverty is associated with ill health and premature death, and influential writers in the nineteenth century of both fiction (such as Charles Dickens) and social philosophy (including Friedrich Engels) inveighed against the hazards of poverty and unemployment (Adler & Stewart, 2010). The quantification of the associations between health and income and education was pioneered in the United States by Kitagawa and Hauser (1973). In Great Britain, the Whitehall studies established that economic and occupational gradients, and not only poverty, are relevant to health and survival, even when universal health care is available (Marmot, Shipley, & Rose, 1984). Jemal et al (2008) showed that death

rates in the United States in 2001 from the leading 15 causes among people aged 25–64 were almost all inversely related to education, irrespective of race. It was estimated that 48% of deaths in white, black, and Hispanic men and 38% of deaths in women would have been avoided if all sectors of society had the same rates as those of college graduates.

Social gradients are apparent not only in mortality, but in the occurrence of a range of other health outcomes including coronary heart disease, diabetes, depression, and asthma (Adler & Rehkopf, 2008; Clark, DesMeules, Luo, Duncan, & Wielgosz, 2009; Lorant et al., 2003; Wright & Subramanian, 2007). There are also socioeconomic gradients in functional disability among people with inflammatory conditions such as polyarthritis (Harrison et al., 2009). The impact of socioeconomic status (SES)[1] is recognized as a worldwide problem. An analysis of 22 (mostly European) countries documented higher rates of death and poorer self-rated health in almost all countries with lower SES, as defined by education, occupational class, or income, albeit with variations in the magnitude of differences (Mackenbach et al., 2008). The World Health Organization Commission on the Social Determinants of Health assembled evidence from around the world documenting the powerful effects of socioeconomic circumstances, and it recommended actions at several levels relating to factors such as living conditions, work practices, access to health case, and health equity (CSDH, 2008).

Gradients in health related to SES are apparent throughout life. A review of 106 studies showed overwhelming evidence of SES gradients in birth outcomes such as low birth weight and preterm birth (Blumenshine, Egerter, Barclay, Cubbin, & Braveman, 2010). Hospitalization for infectious illness in infants aged less than two years is inversely related to parental education and income (Thrane, Sondergaard, Schonheyder, & Sorensen, 2005). In childhood and adolescence, mental illness and biological risk factors are social graded, as is risk of accidents, drug abuse, and sexually transmitted infection (Goodman, 1999; Goodman, McEwen, Huang, Dolan, & Adler, 2005; Newbern, Miller, Schoenbach, & Kaufman, 2004). Childhood SES also appears to have an impact on adult health independently of adult social disadvantage (Cohen, Janicki-Deverts, Chen, & Matthews, 2010). Thus, reviews of prospective and case-control studies indicate that that childhood SES has consistent effects on adult mortality and cardiovascular and respiratory disease incidence, even after adult SES is taken into account, although some associations are quite modest (Galobardes, Lynch, & Smith, 2008; Galobardes, Smith, & Lynch, 2006; Pollitt, Rose, & Kaufman, 2005). This is also true in the dental-health arena; an analysis of the Dunedin birth cohort study showed that low childhood SES defined by parental occupational status was associated with a greater adult incidence of gingivitis and dental caries independently of adult SES (Poulton et al., 2002).

The evidence relating SES with health is observational, and even longitudinal studies over long time periods cannot establish causality. Although much of the evidence is consistent with lower SES influencing future health and premature mortality, the reverse may also be the case. Smith (2009) has demonstrated that poor health in childhood has an adverse effect on adult socioeconomic trajectories in terms of future occupation, wealth, and income, whereas, in adult life, major health events also have a negative impact on wealth, income, and paid employment (Smith, 2004).

Explanations for social inequalities in health can be developed at several levels of analysis, and theories emphasizing cultural, economic, material, and psychosocial factors have all proved illuminating. Nevertheless, influences on physical health risk must ultimately impact on the biology of the individual (Steptoe & Marmot, 2002). This chapter focuses on inflammation and immune function as potential mediating processes linking SES with health outcomes. The emphasis on inflammatory factors reflects modern understanding of their role in major chronic health problems such as coronary heart disease, diabetes, rheumatoid conditions, depression, and some cancers. The evidence relating SES with inflammatory and immune factors derives from observational studies and experimental research on stress-induced responses in humans. Animal research makes only a limited contribution in the light of difficulties in translating work on social hierarchies in animal species to human SES (Kaplan, Chen, & Manuck, 2009; Sapolsky, 2005). In addition to summarizing the evidence relating SES with immune function, this chapter outlines potential mediating mechanisms such as genetic factors, exposure to infection, health behaviors, and differential exposure to chronic life stress. Throughout the chapter, there is a focus on life-course influences, in the light of evidence that early life experience may have enduring effects on adult inflammatory and immune responses relevant to health, together with a recognition that these factors will have their greatest impact at older ages, as susceptibility to chronic disease increases.

Conceptualization of Socioeconomic Status

Some consideration of how SES is conceptualized and measured is important because several different methods are in common use, and they may not have the same association with health outcomes (Adler & Rehkopf, 2008). Many conceptualizations of social status and social class have their origins with Karl Marx and Max Weber in the nineteenth century. Marx argued that class was defined by the relationship between the individual and the means of production in capitalist societies. By contrast,

Weber proposed that societies are structured hierarchically along several dimensions, resulting in people having different life chances, created through ability to trade skills, education, or other attributes for social advantage (Galobardes, Lynch, & Smith, 2007). These different views are embodied in the emphasis placed on structural factors and human agency in societal relations.

Education, income, and occupation are the commonest measures of SES in adult life (Galobardes et al., 2007), whereas studies of children typically use parental education or occupation. Each has advantages and limitations. Occupational class is fairly straightforward to measure, and it can be categorized crudely (with the distinction between white collar and blue collar workers), or by using more elaborate stratified systems based on the nature of work (e.g., professional occupations), managerial capacity, and other factors. In traditional Western cultures, occupation defines the person's "place" in society, reflected in standard of living, housing, interests, and social outlook. However, occupational classifications are better suited to men than women, and many people may be excluded from an occupational classification because they are too young or too old to be working, are unemployed, or chose not to be in paid employment. People also change their occupations in different periods of their lives, and the increase in part-time work complicates the issue still further. There are also important variations in how theorists conceptualize the social status of different occupations, and these lead to different associations with health (Muntaner et al., 2010).

Measures of income provide a good indication of the person's financial resources and relate to material standard of living. Assessment of individual income is often insufficient, and household income is more relevant in many cases (Krieger, Williams, & Moss, 1997). Data tend to be less complete and accurate than for some other measures, either because people are unwilling to disclose all their income, forget to take all sources into account, or are ignorant of all the income streams of their households. As people move beyond working age, wealth rather than income may be more important (Banks, Karlsen, & Oldfield, 2003). Wealth reflects economic resources accumulated over a lifetime, including major items such as property, cars, and investments. Both income and wealth are not fixed, of course, but may fluctuate at different life stages and different phases of the economic cycle.

Education is easier to measure than income or wealth, and being typically assessed in terms of the person's highest attainment or number of years of schooling. Since education is usually completed early in life, it is less influenced by adult health than occupation or income. It may also have specific attributes that set it apart from other SES indicators. Reynolds and Ross (1998) have pointed out that education can be regarded in two ways: the first as a symbolic marker of social class, reflecting the social opportunities and level of job status and income that the adult will enjoy; the second as providing specific skills, training the person in cognitive flexibility and enhancing ability to function effectively in complex environments. According to the latter view, education may have positive effects over and above the access it provides to privileged economic positions in society (Mirowsky & Ross, 2003). However, since most people complete their education in early adult life, its impact may be superseded in later years by current circumstances and access to material resources. Education is a relatively fixed characteristic of the individual, so it cannot easily accommodate changes in SES in adult life. It is linked with intelligence and academic ability, which may themselves impact on health (Batty, Kivimaki, & Deary, 2010; Gottfredson, 2004). There are also important cohort effects, since the meaning of educational qualification changes in different decades. For example, the proportion of people with college degrees has increased severalfold over the past 50 years, meaning that the sector of the population classified as highly educated has become correspondingly broader.

The life-course approach typically involves assessing SES indicators in childhood as well as adult life. Parental educational attainment or occupational status (white or blue collar) are typically used to index childhood SES, whereas the person's own education is often measured as an indication of adolescent or early adult SES. Life-course methods are powerful because measures at different phases of people's lives can be used to disentangle the nature of the influence of prior life experience (Kuh & Ben-Shlomo, 2004). One possibility is that there is an accumulation of risk, so that exposure to low SES in early life contributes to cumulative social disadvantage that could affect risk factors such as inflammation and immune dysfunction in adult life. A second notion is that there are sensitive periods, such that early life low SES or social adversity has a specific impact on later outcomes. In the context of psychoneuroimmunology, an instance of this process may be exposure to early-life infection, discussed later in the chapter. A third way that life-course methods can be used is to examine social mobility, and to assess whether someone who moves from an affluent early life environment to more deprived conditions in adult life (or vice versa) is at particular risk (Loucks et al., 2010).

In addition to these "individual-level" indicators, the last decade has witnessed vigorous growth in the use of area-level indicators based on socioeconomic circumstances measured at the neighborhood, city, state, or even national level. This development has stemmed from the recognition that health and well-being are determined not only by individual and family characteristics, but by social and environmental factors related to the place where the person lives, works or studies. The environment a person lives in might have adverse effects both because of physical characteristics such as patterns of land use, occupational density, access to recreational spaces or shops selling healthy products, and because of social environmental factors such as safety, social capital, traffic density, and aesthetic qualities (Mujahid & Diez Roux, 2010). For example, Diez Roux et al. (2001) used data from the Atherosclerosis Risk in Communities (ARIC) study to show that risk of coronary heart disease (CHD) over a 9-year follow-up period was predicted by living in socioeconomically disadvantaged neighborhoods, even after controlling for standard cardiovascular risk factors and for personal income, education, and occupation. An important issue in this work is whether findings are due to compositional effects (the characteristics of people within the area), or contextual effects (features of the area itself).

Another measure that has grown in popularity over the past decade is self-rated social status (Adler, Epel, Castellazzo, & Ickovics, 2000; Singh-Manoux, Adler, & Marmot, 2003). This is typically measured with a social-status "ladder." For example, the respondent may be shown a ladder with 10 rungs, and be told, "Think of this ladder as representing where people stand in our society. At the top of the ladder are the people who are the best off—those who have the most money, most education, and best jobs. At the bottom are the people who are the worst off—who have the least money, least education, and the worst jobs or no jobs. The higher up you are on this ladder, the closer you are to the people at the very top, and the lower you are, the closer you are to people at the very bottom." Respondents are asked to indicate which rung they occupy. Adler et al. (2000) demonstrated that subjective social status

was more closely related to health-related factors and psychological functioning than objective indicators. It has been argued that such ratings reflect the person's perception of social position, and may provide an integrated estimate of the impact of different components of social status including education, income, and satisfaction with standard of living, depending not only on current circumstances but also on the past and expectations of future prospects (Singh-Manoux et al., 2003).

These general measures may not be appropriate for all sectors of the population. For example, education may not be a good marker in ethnic minority or migrant groups, because some people take more mundane jobs than would be expected from their level of attainment. Income may also be misleading because of the impact of the informal economy. Some authorities have advocated the use of standard of living indicators in minority ethnic groups, arguing that possession of vehicles, electronic equipment, and other consumables may provide a better indication of socioeconomic circumstances than conventional measures (Nazroo, 2003).

It may be that different social-status markers are relevant at different stages of life. Figure 13.1 outlines one such proposal, adapted from Adler and Stewart (2010). Parental education and socioeconomic position are particularly relevant in early life, but, as people grow up, their own educational attainment becomes more prominent. During early and midadult life, it is occupation and income that provide the most direct indicators of socioeconomic circumstances. Later in life, when people retire, their accumulated wealth is more significant, although income remains important. It should be noted that health at each life stage may have an impact on future SES as well as the reverse.

Observational Studies of SES and Immune Processes

Research relating SES with immune and inflammatory processes is still limited, but the largest effort to date has focused on cross-sectional observational studies of plasma or serum concentrations of inflammatory markers. The primary markers include C-reactive protein, fibrinogen, and interleukin (IL) 6, partly because they are easy to measure and partly because they relate to physical health outcomes such as CHD and mental-health conditions such as depression. The research that has been published broadly supports the hypothesis that lower SES is associated with greater chronic inflammation, but studies vary considerably in the strength

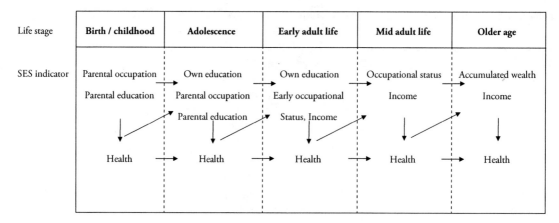

Life stage	Birth / childhood	Adolescence	Early adult life	Mid adult life	Older age
SES indicator	Parental occupation Parental education	Own education Parental occupation Parental education	Own education Early occupational Status, Income	Occupational status Income	Accumulated wealth Income
	Health	Health	Health	Health	Health

Figure 13.1 Outline of a life course perspective on the measurement of individual-level socioeconomic position. Adapted from Adler and Stewart (2010).

of effects. A central element of observational studies is the extent to which potential confounding factors are controlled statistically. In order to establish a robust association between SES and inflammation, it is necessary to demonstrate that effects are not due to extraneous differences between SES groups in the study, such as age, gender, or the presence of illnesses that stimulate inflammatory responses.

Fibrinogen was the first inflammatory marker to be studied extensively. Substantial evidence supports the notion that plasma fibrinogen is an independent risk factor for CHD as well as being implicated in nonvascular mortality (Danesh et al., 2005). In the 1980s, several early reports from cardiovascular epidemiological studies such as the Coronary Artery Risk Development in Young Adults (CARDIA) study and the Whitehall study documented associations between elevated plasma fibrinogen and low SES defined by education, income, and occupation (Folsom et al., 1993; Markowe et al., 1985; Wilson et al., 1993). C-reactive protein is also related to CHD (Kaptoge et al., 2010), although the functional significance of the association continues to be debated (Danesh & Pepys, 2009). A systematic review of articles published up to 2006 identified 26 studies, almost all of which showed inverse associations between C-reactive protein and SES (Nazmi & Victora, 2007). IL-6 is a risk factor for CHD (Danesh et al., 2008), as well as being associated with other health outcomes such as frailty and type 2 diabetes (Kiecolt-Glaser et al., 2003; Tilg & Moschen, 2008).

Table 13.1 summarizes recent findings from 14 recent large-scale (*n* > 500) population studies, including major US studies such as the National Health and Nutrition Examination Survey (NHANES),

CARDIA, and the Multi-Ethnic Study of Atherosclerosis (MESA), together with studies in the United Kingdom, Finland, and Greece. The samples in these studies have ranged from 704 to more than 14,000, with most involving education and income as markers of SES. Results have been somewhat varied across different inflammatory markers, gender, and ethnic groups. In some cases, associations have been observed after controlling for demographic, health, and behavioral factors, whereas, in others, associations have disappeared when preexisting health and behavior have been taken into account. The extent to which factors such as smoking and body mass index (BMI) are confounders or are part of the pathway linking SES with inflammation, continues to be debated. However, it is striking that associations between C-reactive protein and SES have been rather consistent, and in many cases survive adjustment for health and lifestyle factors (Alley et al., 2006; Friedman & Herd, 2010; Loucks et al., 2006; Muennig, Sohler, & Mahato, 2007; Panagiotakos et al., 2005). Associations with fibrinogen have been less consistent, whereas many of the associations with IL-6 are confounded with behavioral risk factors (Koster et al., 2006; Loucks et al., 2006; Ranjit et al., 2007).

In addition to work on C-reactive protein, fibrinogen and IL-6, other inflammatory markers have been investigated to a limited extent. For example, Loucks et al (2006) showed inverse associations between education and soluble intercellular adhesion molecule 1 (ICAM-1) and monocyte chemoattractant protein-1 (MCP-1), whereas social class, education, and occupation have been related to von Willebrand factor (Ramsay et al., 2008; Steptoe, Kunz-Ebrecht, Rumley, & Lowe, 2003;

Table 13.1 SES and inflammatory markers in population studies

Study	Participants	Measures	Key outcomes
Alley et al., 2006 NHANES	7,634 US adults age >20 years. Mean age 45.8, 51% women. 72.3% white, 7.1% Hispanic, 9.8% black, 10.8% other.	SES: Family income above or below the poverty level. Inflammatory marker: CRP.	(1) Poverty associated with 82% elevated odds of very high CRP, adjusting for demographics (age, sex, race/ethnicity). (2) Poverty associated with 33% elevated odds of very high CRP, adjusting for demographics, illness and immune activation (recent illness, leukocyte count, asthma, chronic bronchitis, rheumatoid arthritis). (3) Poverty associated with 27% elevated odds of very high CRP, adjusting for demographics, illness and immune activation, and health behaviors (obesity, smoking, heavy drinking, exercise).
Brunner et al (1996) Whitehall II study	3,297 UK adults, age 45–55 years, 36% women.	SES: Employment grade. Inflammatory marker: fibrinogen.	(1) Lower occupational grade associated with higher fibrinogen in both men and women. (2) Association remains significant in men after adjustment for age, ethnicity, BMI, smoking, alcohol, and physical activity.
Dowd & Goldman, 2006 SEBAS study	972 Taiwanese adults, age 54 and older.	SES: Education and income. Inflammatory marker: IL-6.	(1) Greater education associated with lower IL-6 in men. (2) No association of IL-6 with income in men. (3) No associations with education or income in women.
Friedman & Herd, 2010 MIDAS study	704 US adults. Mean age 57.9. 53.6% women, 25.1% nonwhite.	SES: Education and income. Inflammatory markers: CRP, fibrinogen, and IL-6.	(1) CRP significantly elevated only in the lowest-income quintile, adjusting for age, gender, race, health status (BMI, chronic conditions, medications), and health behaviors (smoking, alcohol, caffeine, physical activity). (2) Fibrinogen not associated with income or education, adjusting for age, gender, race, health status, and health behaviors. (3) IL-6 significantly elevated only in the lowest-income quintile, adjusting for age, gender, race, health status, and health behaviors.
Gimeno et al, 2008 Cardio-vascular Risk in Young Finns study	1,484 Finnish adults age 24–39.	SES: Education and occupation. Inflammatory marker: CRP.	(1) CRP inversely associated with education but not income in age and sex-adjusted analyses.
Gruenwald et al., 2009 CARDIA study	3,266 US adults, 28.9% white women, mean age 45.7. 26.3% black women, mean age 44.7. 26.6% white men, mean age 45.7. 18.2% black men, mean age 44.6.	SES: Education and income. Inflammatory markers: CRP and IL-6.	(1) White women: CRP and IL-6 inversely associated with education and income, but not significant after adjusting for health covariates. (2) Black women: CRP and IL-6 inversely associated with education and income. CRP by education remained significant adjusting for health status, behavioral and psychosocial co-variates. IL-6 by income and education remained significant adjusting for health status only. (3) White men: CRP and IL-6 inversely associated with education and income. Effects significant after adjustment for health status, behavioral and psychosocial covariates. (4) Black men: CRP and IL-6 inversely associated with income. Effects significant after adjustment for health status, behavioral and psychosocial covariates. No associated with education.

(continued)

Table 13.1 (continued)

Study	Participants	Measures	Key outcomes
Koster et al., 2006 Health ABC study	3,044 US adults, mean age 74.2, 51.4% women, 58.5% white.	SES: Education, family income, and financial assets. Inflammatory markers: CRP IL-6 and TNFα.	(1) CRP inversely related to education and income. Not significant after adjusting for prevalent diseases or behavioral factors. (2) IL-6 inversely related to income. Significant after adjusting for prevalent diseases, but not behavioral factors. (3) TNFα highest in middle SES groups.
Loucks et al., 2006 Framingham Offspring Study	2,729 US adults, mean age 62. 53.4% women.	SES: Education and income. Inflammatory markers: CRP and IL-6.	(1) CRP inversely associated with education adjusting for age, gender, income, clinical cardiovascular risk factors and depression. (2) IL-6 inversely associated with education adjusting for age, gender, and income, but not after controlling for clinical risk factors. (3) CRP and IL-6 inversely associated with income, adjusting for age and gender.
Muenning et al., 2007 NHANES	14,015 US adults for CRP. 5,087 for fibrinogen. Ages not specified.	SES: Education and family income. Inflammatory markers: CRP, fibrinogen.	(1) CRP inversely associated with education and income, adjusted for age, race, gender, BMI, smoking, physical activity, family history. (2) Fibrinogen, no association.
O'Reilly et al., (2006) WOSCOPS	5,245 men age 45–64.	SES: Social deprivation score. Inflammatory marker: CRP.	(1) CRP positively related to social deprivation, adjusting for age, smoking, BMI, and medication.
Panagiotakos et al, (2005) ATTICA study	3,042 Greek men and women, age 20–87. 49.8% men.	SES: Education and income combined. Inflammatory markers: CRP, fibrinogen, IL-6, TNF-α.	(1) CRP, fibrinogen and IL-6 all inversely associated with SES after adjustment for age, gender, smoking, medication, BMI, diet and physical activity.
Petersen et al., 2008 AHAB Study	851 US adults. Mean age 44.9, 49.8% men. 77% white, 23% black.	SES: Education and income combined. Neighborhood characteristics. Inflammatory markers: CRP and IL-6.	(1) Higher individual SES associated with lower IL-6, and higher community SES with lower CRP and IL-6, after adjustment for age, gender, and race. (2) Individual SES no longer associated with IL-6 after adjustment for BMI, smoking, sleep, alcohol, and physical activity. (3) Community SES still associated with IL-6 but not CRP after adjustment for lifestyle factors.
Ramsay et al., 2008 British Regional Heart Study	3,682 British men age 60–79.	SES: Registrar General social class classification. Inflammatory markers: CRP. Fibrinogen, IL-6.	(1) CRP, fibrinogen and IL-6 associated with lower SES in age-adjusted analyses, but not after controlling for behavioral risk factors (BMI, smoking, alcohol, and physical activity).
Ranjit et al., 2007 MESA study	6,814 US adults. Mean age 62.1, 47% women, 38.5% white, 11.8% Chinese, 27.8% black, 21.9% Hispanic.	SES: Household income and years of education. Inflammatory markers: CRP and IL-6.	(1) CRP associated with low education only among white and black participants in age- and sex-adjusted analyses. Effect significant in white participants only after full adjustment (age, sex, infection, medications, psychosocial, behavioral, and metabolic co-variates). (2) CRP associated with low income in white participants only.

Table 13.1 (continued)

Study	Participants	Measures	Key outcomes
			In fully adjusted analyses, association significant in white and Chinese participants. (3) IL-6 inversely associated with education among white and black participants in age- and sex-adjusted analyses, but not after full adjustment. (4) IL-6 associated with low income in all ethnic groups in age- and sex-adjusted analyses. However, in fully adjusted analyses association only significant in white and Chinese participants.

AHAB—University of Pittsburgh Adult Health and Behavior study; MESA—Multi-Ethnic Study of Atherosclerosis; MIDUS—Mid-Life Development in the United States study; SEBAS—Taiwanese social environment and biomarkers of aging study; WOSCOPS—West of Scotland Coronary Prevention Study
CRP = C-reactive protein; IL-6 = interleukin 6; TNFα = tumor necrosis factor alpha

Wamala et al., 1999). Large scale observational studies of immune measures apart from inflammatory markers are sparse. Evans et al (2000) studied secretion of salivary immunoglobulin A (sIgA) in just under 2,000 participants in a health survey in Scotland. Higher SES as defined by occupational class was related to greater sIgA secretion independently of age and gender, but the effect were attenuated after controlling for smoking. A study of 127 healthy middle-aged men and women from the Whitehall II cohort, or group, found that low SES (defined by occupational grade) was associated with a raised number of circulating T and B lymphocytes and natural killer (NK) cells (Owen, Poulton, Hay, Mohamed-Ali, & Steptoe, 2003). Another approach is to assess antibody responses to latent viruses as indicators of cell-mediated immune function. Dowd and Aiello (2009) analyzed SES variations in the ability to maintain cytomegalovirus (CMV) in a quiescent state. Using data from the third NHANES, they found that CMV antibody levels among individuals who are seropositive were negatively related to education and income, after control for health status, smoking, and BMI. These findings have been extended to children, with evidence that poverty in childhood is associated with increased CMV antibody titers (Dowd, Palermo, & Aiello, 2012). Lower SES may also act to reduce the benefit of protective factors such as social support; Fagundes et al (2012) reported that greater social support was associated with lower antibody titers to Epstein-Barr virus among women awaiting evaluation following an abnormal mammogram or newly diagnosed with breast cancer, but only in higher SES participants as defined by education. Taken together, these results suggest that lower SES

individuals experience downregulation of cell-mediated immunity.

Life Course and Longitudinal Associations

The studies discussed in the previous section were cross-sectional, making it impossible to determine the temporal relationship between SES, inflammation, and immune function. Although it appears unlikely that inflammation and immune activation could "cause" variations in SES, some of the health consequences of inflammation and immune disturbance might contribute to reductions in SES. Alternatively, common underlying factors might result both in lower SES and inflammation. Two complementary research strategies add to this literature. The first is to conduct longitudinal studies in adult populations, assessing whether SES at one time point is associated with changes in inflammatory markers over time. There has been little research of this type to date, but one example comes from an analysis of neighborhood deprivation in the MESA study (Nazmi, Diez Roux, Ranjit, Seeman, & Jenny, 2010). Cross-sectionally, C-reactive protein, IL-6, and fibrinogen were all greater in people living in more deprived neighborhoods, even after individual SES (income and education) were taken into account. Interestingly, over an average period of just under four years, the increase of IL-6 was greater in participants from more deprived neighborhoods, after adjustment for individual SES, BMI, waist circumference, smoking, physical activity, alcohol, medication, diabetes, and impaired glucose tolerance.

The second strategy has been to carry out life-course studies, investigating the extent to which early-life SES predicts inflammation in adult life.

Evidence relating childhood SES with concurrent inflammation early in life is mixed (Dowd, Zajacova, & Aiello, 2010; Gimeno et al., 2008), but childhood circumstances may nonetheless influence immune function in later life. A number of major population studies of life-course SES and adult inflammation are summarized in Table 13.2. In general, they show that lower SES early in life predicts inflammation in adult life, and in several cases the effects remain significant after the participants' adult SES is taken into account (Brunner et al., 1996; Loucks et al., 2010; Nazmi, Oliveira,

et al., 2010; Phillips et al., 2009; Tabassum et al., 2008). However, in many studies, the effects are markedly attenuated or disappear completely when adult risk factors such as smoking, BMI, and physical inactivity are taken into account. This suggests that adult health behaviors may be on the pathway linking childhood SES with adult inflammation.

An advantage of these studies is that they can be used to investigate socioeconomic trajectories. If lower SES is causally linked with inflammation, then one might expect that people who move from a

Table 13.2 Life course SES and adult inflammation in population studies

Study	Participants	Measures	Key outcomes
Brunner et al., 1996 Whitehall II study	3,297 UK adults, age 45–55 years, 36% women.	SES (childhood): Father's occupational class, adult height, own education. SES (adult): Employment grade. Inflammatory marker: fibrinogen.	(1) Lower father's occupational class associated with higher fibrinogen in both sexes. Effect remains significant in men after adjustment for own employment grade. (2) Lower occupational grade associated with higher fibrinogen in both men and women (see Table 13.1). Effect remains significant in men after adjustment for childhood SES, age, ethnicity, BMI, smoking, alcohol, and physical activity.
Gimeno et al., 2008 Cardiovascular Risk in Young Finns study	1,484 Finnish adults, tested in childhood (age 3–9), adolescence (age 12–18), and adulthood (age 24–39).	SES (childhood): Parental education and occupation. SES (adult): Own education and occupation. Inflammatory marker: CRP	(1) Childhood SES not associated with adult CRP. (2) Adult CRP associated with participants' education but not occupational status (see Table 13.1).
Lawlor et al., 2005 British Women's Health and Heart Study	3,745 UK adult women, age 60–79. 15.2% have coronary heart disease.	SES (childhood): Parental occupation, household amenities. SES (adult): Husband's occupational class or own occupation if single, education, adult housing tenure, car access. Inflammatory markers: CRP and fibrinogen.	(1) Childhood manual social class associated with higher CRP and fibrinogen. (2) Adult SES indicators associated with CRP and fibrinogen. (3) Cumulative effect of adverse SES on CRP and fibrinogen.
Loucks et al., 2010 Framingham Offspring Study	1,413 US adults, mean age 61.2, 54% women.	SES (childhood): Parental education and occupation. SES (adult): Own education and occupation. Inflammatory markers: CRP, IL-6, fibrinogen, ICAM-1, MCP-1, sTNFR2 and others.	(1) Cumulative SES associated with CRP, IL-6, fibrinogen, ICAM-1, MCP-1, sTNFR2 and other markers adjusting for age and gender. (2) Associations are more consistent for adult than parental SES. (3) Few effects remain significant after adjustment for adult risk factors (smoking, BMI, blood pressure, cholesterol, fasting glucose, medication, and depression).

Table 13.2 (continued)

Study	Participants	Measures	Key outcomes
Nazmi et al., 2010 The 1982 Pelotas (Brazil) Birth Cohort Study	4,297 adults, age 22.7 years, 75% white.	SES (childhood): Family income at birth, maternal education. SES (adult): Family income and education. Inflammatory marker: CRP.	(1) Lower early life SES associated with greater CRP levels in men aged 23 independent of adult SES. (2) Associations in men remain significant after adjusting for BMI, waist circumference, smoking, diet, physical activity, alcohol and stress. (3) Lower maternal education but not family income associated with greater CRP in women, but not after adjusting for lifestyle factors. Weaker associations of adult SES with CRP, and not significant after adjustment for lifestyle factors.
Phillips et al., 2009 AHAB study	811 US adults, Mean age 44.8, 51% women, 87% white, 13% black.	SES (childhood): Parental education. SES (adult): Own education. Inflammatory marker: CRP.	(1) Parental and own educational attainment inversely associated with CRP in women, but not men, adjusting for age and race. (2) Associations between CRP and parental education remain significant after adjustment for lifestyle risk factors (smoking, alcohol consumption, sleep, exercise, BMI) and own education. (3) Both mothers' and fathers' education associated with CRP levels in women.
Pollitt et al., 2008 ARIC study	11,842 US adults, age 45–64 years, 76.7% white, 23.3% black.	SES (childhood): Parental education and occupation. SES (adult): Education and occupation. SES (neighborhood): Neighborhood characteristics. Inflammatory markers: CRP, fibrinogen, WBC.	(1) Lower cumulative SES significantly associated with elevated fibrinogen and WBC but not CRP in white participants, after adjustment for BMI, smoking, alcohol, lipids, hypertension, diabetes, and family history. Weaker effects in blacks. (2) Adult education, occupation, and neighborhood SES also associated with fibrinogen and WBC but not CRP after adjustment for covariates.
Tabassum et al., 2008 958 British Birth Cohort	8,795 UK adults, age 42 years, 48% women.	SES (childhood): Social class (occupational classification) at birth. SES (adult): Social class at ages 23 and 42. Inflammatory markers: CRP and fibrinogen.	(1) CRP and fibrinogen both associated with childhood and adult social class. (2) Associations between inflammation and childhood social class remain significant after adjustment for adult class, and vice versa. (3) Cumulative risk scores associated with CRP and fibrinogen after adjustment for smoking, BMI and physical activity.

AHAB—University of Pittsburgh Adult Health and Behavior study; ARIC—Atherosclerosis Risk in Communities study; WBC—White blood cell count

higher SES category in childhood to a lower position in adult life might be at increased risk. Such effects were indeed reported by Loucks et al (2010) in the Framingham Offspring Study, where individuals from affluent backgrounds whose own occupations were lower status showed greater elevations in IL-6, ICAM-1, and soluble TNF receptor levels.

Research on early-life SES and the life course overlaps with work on early-life adversity. A small but important literature is emerging that relates harsh early-life experience with adult inflammation. Taylor et al (2006) analyzed 3,248 adults from the CARDIA study who had completed retrospective questionnaire measures of early family environment. Risky family environments were indicated by reports of not feeling loved, having been verbally or physically abused, or having lived with a substance abuser. Early-life stress was associated with higher C-reactive protein, primarily through its impact on adult psychological factors such as depression and limited social contacts. Interestingly, early-life adversity was more common among individuals who had been of lower SES in childhood, suggesting this might be part of the mechanism linking low SES and inflammation. In the same vein, an analysis from the MIDUS biomarker study found that early-life adversity was associated with elevated IL-6, fibrinogen, and endothelial leukocyte adhesion molecule-1 and ICAM-1, but only in the smaller group of African Americans and not the larger white group (Slopen et al., 2010).

These studies involved retrospective assessments of early childhood adversity. A stronger design was used by Danese and colleagues (Danese et al., 2008; Danese, Pariante, Caspi, Taylor, & Poulton, 2007) in their analyses of the Dunedin birth cohort. This study had measures of childhood maltreatment assessed at the time, and it showed associations with elevated C-reactive protein and fibrinogen at age 32. In contrast to the CARDIA results, these associations were independent of childhood and adult SES.

A somewhat different design was used by Miller and Chen (2010), who administered Taylor's early-life family measure to 135 young women aged 15–19 years. Blood was drawn four times over a 1.5-year period, and trajectories of changes in circulating IL-6 and IL-6 production after stimulation with lipopolysaccharide were assessed. The trajectory of IL-6 stimulated production over time was greater among individuals who had experienced early harsh family environments, but serum IL-6 was unaffected. Socioeconomic status (indexed by parental education) was not related to inflammatory responses.

The data from studies of early-life SES present quite a consistent picture (Table 13.2). Most investigators have found associations between low SES early in life and adult inflammation, although effects are typically less strong than the relationship with adult SES. Perhaps this is not surprising, because adult SES is related to ongoing psychosocial challenges that are likely to have biological consequences (Steptoe & Marmot, 2002). Psychosocial adversity in early life appears to predict elevations in inflammatory markers in adult life. However, even though adversity in early life is more common among lower SES individuals, the evidence that it mediates SES effects is, at present, inconclusive.

Experimental Studies of SES and Immune Processes

The population-based studies described in the previous section provide good evidence for links between SES and inflammation, but have less information about other aspects of immune function. Interpretation of the findings is inevitably limited by the observational nature of the data, the difficulty of measuring all relevant confounders, and by the challenges of maintaining uniform methods of data collection and processing in large-scale studies. For example, bloods should only be analyzed in these studies from participants who are free of any current illness such as upper respiratory tract (URI) infection, so as to avoid the short-term inflammatory effects of acute illness. In some cases, the levels of inflammation are so high in some individuals as to suggest that screening of participants has not been sufficiently stringent.

A complementary strategy is to carry out experimental studies, investigating the impact of SES on acute immune and inflammatory responses to stress. Such studies can be carried out under controlled conditions, so the effects of extraneous factors such as current health, physical activity, and symptoms can be taken into account. Research on acute inflammatory stress responses has blossomed over the past decade following the realization that increases in plasma concentrations of biomarkers such as IL-6 and interleukin 1 receptor antagonist (IL-1Ra) are slower to emerge than is the case for many other biological responses (Steptoe, Hamer, & Chida, 2007). Consequently, it is wise to continue sampling for 1.5 to 2 hours following stress exposure in order to measure changes in these variables.

Our group carried out a series of analyses of the Whitehall Psychobiology Study, in which 235 men and women aged 45–59 years were administered a standardized laboratory stress protocol (Steptoe, Owen, Kunz-Ebrecht, & Mohamed-Ali, 2002). Participants were recruited in a stratified fashion based on grade of employment, a robust marker of SES in this population. We found that the number of cells expressing CD45 (total lymphocytes), CD3 (pan T-lymphocytes), and CD16CD56 (NK cells) was greater in lower SES than in higher SES participants, and it increased following behavioral stress (Owen et al., 2003). These differences were independent of changes in hemoconcentration that also occurred following stress. There were, however, no differences in stress reactivity across SES groups. The analyses of circulating IL-6, IL1-Ra, and tumor necrosis factor (TNF)α showed a similar pattern, with higher concentrations in lower SES participants, increases following stress, but little difference in stress reactivity by SES (Steptoe et al., 2002). A new study has largely replicated these findings with a larger sample of 543 healthy older participants, again recruited from the Whitehall II epidemiological cohort. Results for IL-6 are summarized in Figure 13.2, where it is evident that lower SES participants had higher concentrations of plasma IL-6 than the higher SES group, with participants in the intermediate grades showing values that fell between the other two groups. There were significant increases in IL-6 in all groups, so that, following stress, the absolute levels of IL-6 were greater among lower SES participants (after adjustment for age, gender, BMI, and smoking). However, no differences in stress responsivity were observed.

One explanation for the lack of differences in stress response might be the duration of sampling. As noted earlier, increases in circulating levels of inflammatory markers emerge progressively over time, and in this study the final blood sample was 75 minutes after stress. Another study tested this possibility by extending sampling to 2 hours following stress in a smaller comparison of higher and lower SES groups (Brydon, Edwards, Mohamed-Ali, & Steptoe, 2004). We found that plasma IL-6 continued to increase between 75 and 120 minutes after stress in lower SES participants, so that differences between SES groups were significant by the final sample.

At present, therefore, findings from acute stress studies present a somewhat inconclusive picture. Plasma concentrations of inflammatory markers are inversely related to SES, and increase in response to acute stress. However, differences in stress responsivity have been observed only inconsistently, probably because of the limited duration of sampling times following stress.

Socioeconomic Status, Immune Function, and Health Outcomes

Inflammation and some other aspects of immune function appear to differ across SES groups both at rest and in response to stress, with greater inflammation and immune activation among lower SES individuals. The question can then be asked: Do these differences account for SES variations in health outcomes or physical-illness markers? There has been limited research thus far that has investigated this possibility. A study of 3,921 middle-aged Swedish men and women assessed whether differences in C-reactive protein concentration accounted for SES variations in subclinical atherosclerosis (Rosvall, Engstrom, Janzon, Berglund, & Hedblad, 2007). There were differences in C-reactive protein between

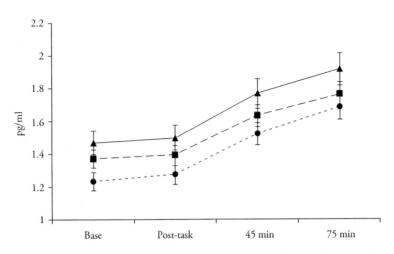

Figure 13.2 Mean plasma interleukin 6 at the end of 30 minutes rest (base), immediately after challenging behavioral tasks (posttask) and 45 minutes and 75 minutes later in healthy older men and women categorized into lower (▲, solid line), intermediate (■, dashed line), and higher (●, dotted line) SES groups. Values adjusted for age, gender, body mass index, and smoking status. Error bars are standard error of the mean.

SES groups, but these made only a minor contribution to variations in atherosclerosis. However, the differences in subclinical atherosclerosis (indicated by carotid intima-medial thickness and the presence of carotid plaque) by SES were modest, limiting the ability of the study to examine mediation by inflammatory markers. An analysis of the Whitehall II epidemiological cohort examined factors accounting for SES differences in CHD incidence over a 13 year period (Marmot, Shipley, Hemingway, Head, & Brunner, 2008). It was found that plasma concentrations of CRP, IL-6, and fibrinogen accounted for 18%, 14%, and 13%, respectively, of the SES gradient in CHD. In combination with the metabolic syndrome, inflammation was responsible for around one-third of the excess CHD in the lower compared with higher SES groups.

Another condition in which SES differences in inflammation appears to be directly relevant to health outcomes is childhood asthma. Chen et al (2006) measured cytokines relevant to asthma (IL-4, IL-5, and IL-13) in a small group of children with asthma and in a group of controls. They found that lower SES was associated with raised IL-5, IL-13, and eosinophil counts in children with asthma but not in controls. Lower SES was also related to heighted chronic self-reported stress, and chronic stress and threat perception statistically mediated the relationship between SES and inflammation. In a subsequent study, 38 children with asthma were assessed during a conflict discussion with a parent (Chen, Strunk, Bacharier, Chan, & Miller, 2010). Airway-inflammation responses to the discussion were greater in lower SES children than higher SES children, suggesting that lower SES children with asthma may be more sensitive to heightened airway inflammation in response to stress.

Psychoneuroimmunological processes may also be involved in SES differences in infectious illness, though in this case the interpretation of literature is complicated. A greater incidence of infectious illness in lower SES populations could be due to differential in exposure to pathogens because of differences in the healthiness of living conditions, atmospheric pollution, water contamination, and access to vaccination. Cohen's studies of experimentally administered infectious agents overcome these problems. In two separate analyses, Cohen's group has investigated whether low SES increases susceptibility to common cold viruses. They found that childhood SES, operationalized as the number of years of participants' childhoods during which their parents owned their own home, was related to susceptibility to infection independent of adult SES, baseline immunity, and other factors (Cohen, Doyle, Turner, Alper, & Skoner, 2004). Interestingly, the increased vulnerability was only present for individuals whose parents had not owned a home during their childhood rather than adolescent years, suggesting that low SES early in life is particularly problematic. In a second study, it was found that low ratings of subjective SES measured with the social-status ladder predicted risk of acquiring a cold following virus administration independent of relevant covariates (Cohen et al., 2008). Neither education nor income was related to risk of the common cold, though this might have been due to the specific characteristics of the volunteers who took part in the study.

It is evident that, although immune processes do appear to relate SES with clinical illness, the evidence base is slender. Further studies are urgently needed to investigate this issue more fully.

Mechanisms Relating Immunity and Inflammation with Social Status

Theoretically, several different mechanisms might be responsible for SES differences in immunity and inflammation. The main possibilities are outlined here.

Genetic Factors

Many of the diseases related to SES have strong hereditary components, and there are genetic influences not only on inflammatory and immune processes but also on some of the psychosocial factors that are related to health risk such as depression, aggressive dispositions, and biological-stress responsivity. Mackenbach (2005) has suggested that there might be genetic factors that influence attributes such as cognitive ability and mental and bodily fitness that, in turn, affect educational and occupational success, while also determining adult health. For example, a population study in Rotterdam showed that shared genetic factors contributed to the co-occurrence of lower SES and depressive symptoms (Lopez-Leon et al., 2009). There is also evidence that polymorphisms in the serotonin transporter gene are related to SES, and may be relevant to neurobehavioral pathways related to health (Manuck, Flory, Ferrell, & Muldoon, 2004).

One specific example of the way these processes might be relevant to SES and immunity is through cognitive ability and intelligence. It has emerged over recent years that low childhood cognitive ability predicts increased risk of a range of adult diseases, including cardiovascular problems and arthritis (Der, Batty, & Deary, 2009; Hart et al., 2003). Phillips et al. (2010) have shown that cognitive ability early in life is associated with a marker of inflammation in adult life (erythrocyte sedimentation rate). Greater cognitive ability is partly genetically determined, and also relates to adult SES. It is conceivable, therefore, that genetically determined cognitive ability could influence both adult SES and inflammatory processes. However, it should be remembered that there have been marked and rapid changes over time in the social distribution of illnesses such as coronary heart disease that are difficult to reconcile with the timescale of genetic influences. There is also uncertainty in this literature about whether childhood cognitive ability is related to adult health outcomes independent of SES or through influencing the individual's socioeconomic circumstances (Batty et al., 2008; Shipley, Der, Taylor, & Deary, 2008).

History of Infection and Exposure to Pathogens

It is probable that exposure to infections early in life can increase risk of noncommunicable disease in adult life through the activation of low-grade inflammatory responses. Experimental studies with animals show that early exposure to endotoxins modifies later inflammatory and HPA axis function (Shanks, Larocque, & Meaney, 1995; Shanks et al., 2000). Lower SES may increase risk of exposure to pathogens, or reduce resistance to infections, making such a history more likely. Thus, lower SES is related to greater crowding, poorer heating, and ventilation in the home, greater exposure to particulate matter from traffic and industrial plants, and greater exposure to parental smoking in the home (Cohen et al., 2010; Evans & Kantrowitz, 2002).

There is accumulating evidence that lower SES is associated with seropositivity in adult life to pathogens that were likely acquired in childhood. In the Whitehall II study, we found that a cumulative index of seropositivity to CMV, *Chlamydia pneumoniae* (*C. pneumoniae*), and herpes simplex virus 1 (HSV-1) was inversely related to SES as defined by grade of employment, with CMV making the greatest contribution (Steptoe, Shamaei-Tousi, et al., 2007). Seropositivity to CMV was associated with lower SES indexed by education or income in NHANES III, with differences being present from age 6 onward (Dowd, Aiello, & Alley, 2009). These effects were extended to show educational gradients for seropositivity to a wider set of pathogens including *Helicobacter pylori* (*H. pylori*), HSV-1

and hepatitis B in NHANES (Zajacova, Dowd, & Aiello, 2009), and an analysis in MESA showed that low education and low income were associated with seropositivity for *H. pylori*, CMV, HSV-1 and *C.pneumoniae* (Aiello et al., 2009). It is important to recognize that these differences do not simply arise from the contrast between people who live in poverty or extreme deprivation and the rest of the population. They are graded effects, with intermediate levels of seropositivity in people who are intermediate in terms of their SES.

These findings raise the possibility that infections acquired early in life might contribute to SES differences in low grade inflammation that contributes to adult health outcomes. Individual pathogens are relevant to specific disorders, but, in addition, the concept of an aggregate pathogen burden is gaining currency, particularly in relation to cardiovascular disease. Positive serostatus for a range of pathogens has been associated with coronary artery disease in case-control and longitudinal cohort studies (Espinola-Klein et al., 2002; Kiechl et al., 2001; Spahr et al., 2006). Pathogen burden has also been related to cardiovascular risk markers such as endothelial dysfunction and insulin resistance in some studies (Fernandez-Real et al., 2006; Prasad et al., 2002). It is notable that cumulative pathogen burden has been associated with a flatter cortisol profile over the day, suggesting active disturbance of neuroendocrine regulation of immune function (Steptoe, Gylfe, Shamaei-Tousi, Bergstrom, & Henderson, 2009). The extent to which these processes contribute to SES differences in cardiovascular disease risk is currently under active investigation (Simanek, Dowd, & Aiello, 2008; Steptoe, Shamaei-Tousi, et al., 2007).

Access to Health Care

There is debate about access to quality health care by different social groups, with evidence for differential rates of access both to primary health care and more elaborate interventions at more advanced stages of disease (e.g. Casale, Auster, Wolf, Pei, & Devereux, 2007; Pappas, Hadden, Kozak, & Fisher, 1997). These patterns are certainly important in SES health disparities, but whether they are relevant to links between immune function and SES is less certain. It could be that SES differences in uptake of immunization programs, or in seeking medical support during episodes of infectious illness, could result in long-term differences in inflammation and immune regulation. At present, however, there is no direct evidence for the operation of such pathways.

Health behaviors

There are pronounced socioeconomic gradients in many countries in behaviors relevant to communicable and noncommunicable diseases, including cigarette smoking, alcohol consumption, physical activity, and nutrition (Steptoe, Gardner, & Wardle, 2010). There is also a relatively consistent social gradient in overweight and obesity among women (Ogden, Lamb, Carroll, & Flegal, 2010). Health behaviors are strongly related to many immune and inflammatory processes. For example, smoking stimulates increased concentrations of C-reactive protein, IL-6, fibrinogen, and white-blood-cell counts (Yanbaeva, Dentener, Creutzberg, Wesseling, & Wouters, 2007); adiposity is strongly related to inflammation and immune regulation (Musaad & Haynes, 2007; Xu et al., 2003); physical inactivity is associated with inflammatory markers and immune function (PAGA Committee, 2008); and alcohol has powerful immunomodulatory effects (Szabo & Mandrekar, 2009). There is widespread evidence that smoking, excessive alcohol consumption, and nutritional deficits increase risk of a variety of infections. It is, therefore, plausible that some of the variation in inflammation and immunity with SES is mediated through differences in health behavior. Direct research on this issue is limited. However, it is notable that many of the studies detailed in Table 13.1 included behaviors such as smoking, sleep disturbance, alcohol consumption, and adiposity as covariates, and still found independent relationships between SES and inflammation. On the other hand, a proportion of the variance in inflammation by SES is typically accounted for by health behaviors, and in some studies the associations were no longer significant after behaviors had been taken into account. Yet it can be argued that differences in health behaviors are part of the pathway through which SES impacts health. Habitual behaviors are definitely relevant to the socioeconomic gradient in inflammation and immunity.

Direct Psychophysiological Processes

Another possibility is that lower SES individuals show greater inflammation and disturbed immune function because of heightened psychophysiological responsivity. As noted earlier, the evidence directly exploring differential psychoneuroimmunological responsivity across the socioeconomic spectrum is limited at present. However, it should be noted that many of the psychosocial factors addressed elsewhere in this *Handbook* that are related to immune function are themselves graded socioeconomically.

For example, exposure to chronic individual and neighborhood adversity is inversely related to SES, with heightened work stress, domestic and neighborhood strain, neighborhood deprivation, and financial strain in less privileged SES groups (Diez Roux & Mair, 2010; Matthews, Gallo, & Taylor, 2010; Steptoe & Marmot, 2003). Lower SES is also associated with fewer social resources, more depressive symptoms, greater hostility, and less adaptive coping responses. If these factors influence immune function, then such effects will be graded socially, providing a mechanism through which SES, immune function, and inflammation are interrelated.

Ultimately, several different interrelated mechanisms linking SES with inflammation and immunity may be operating simultaneously. Take, for example, the report from Poulton et al. (2002) that lower SES in childhood was associated with poorer dental health (plaque, gingival bleeding) in adult life. This could be mediated in part by stress-related differences in immune defenses across SES groups, but variations in oral health behaviors also probably play a substantial role, as might differential exposure to infectious organisms in participants growing up in different socioeconomic circumstances.

Conclusions and Future Directions

The study of socioeconomic gradients in immunity and inflammation is an active field of research involving several types of investigation. Untangling these links will help us better understand how social circumstances and childhood and adult life influence health outcomes, and provide broader options for intervention. Both studies of adults and investigations that take account of the life course are valuable. Consensus is being reached on some research questions, but others remain unresolved. Among the key goals of the next generation of research will be robust studies linking SES with immune disturbance and health outcomes longitudinally, and investigations that tease out the relative importance of direct psychobiological processes, pathogen exposure, and health behaviors as pathways mediating SES differences in inflammation and immunity. We also need intervention studies that can establish causality and identify ways for breaking the links between lower SES and immune dysfunction. The combination of large scale observational studies, more focused experiments, and laboratory investigations is essential to encompass this complex multidisciplinary issue.

Related Chapters

For more information on concepts introduced in this chapter, see also Uchino; and Suarez, this volume.

Note

1. The term socioeconomic status is used throughout this chapter. Many authorities prefer the terms socioeconomic position or socioeconomic disparity, but SES is used here as the commonest descriptor of social economic inequality in studies of health.

References

Adler, N. E., Epel, E. S., Castellazzo, G., & Ickovics, J. R. (2000). Relationship of subjective and objective social status with psychological and physiological functioning: preliminary data in healthy white women. *Health Psychology, 19*, 586–592.

Adler, N. E., & Rehkopf, D. H. (2008). U.S. disparities in health: descriptions, causes, and mechanisms. *Annual Review of Public Health, 29*, 235–252.

Adler, N. E., & Stewart, J. (2010). Health disparities across the lifespan: meaning, methods, and mechanisms. *Annals of the New York Academy of Sciences, 1186*, 5–23.

Aiello, A. E., Diez-Roux, A., Noone, A. M., Ranjit, N., Cushman, M., Tsai, M. Y., et al. (2009). Socioeconomic and psychosocial gradients in cardiovascular pathogen burden and immune response: the multi-ethnic study of atherosclerosis. *Brain Behavior and Immunity, 23*, 663–671.

Alley, D. E., Seeman, T. E., Ki Kim, J., Karlamangla, A., Hu, P., & Crimmins, E. M. (2006). Socioeconomic status and C-reactive protein levels in the US population: NHANES IV. *Brain Behavior and Immunity, 20*, 498–504.

Banks, J., Karlsen, S., & Oldfield, Z. (2003). Socio-economic position. In M. Marmot, J. Banks, R. Blundell, C. Lessof, & J. Nazroo (Eds.), *Health, wealth and lifestyles of the older population in England* (pp. 71–125). London: Institute for Fiscal Studies.

Batty, G. D., Kivimaki, M., & Deary, I. J. (2010). Intelligence, education, and mortality. *British Medical Journal, 340*, c563.

Batty, G. D., Shipley, M. J., Mortensen, L. H., Boyle, S. H., Barefoot, J., Gronbaek, et al. (2008). IQ in late adolescence/ early adulthood, risk factors in middle age and later all-cause mortality in men: The Vietnam Experience Study. *Journal of Epidemiology and Community Health, 62*, 522–531.

Blumenshine, P., Egerter, S., Barclay, C. J., Cubbin, C., & Braveman, P. A. (2010). Socioeconomic disparities in adverse birth outcomes: A systematic review. *American Journal of Preventive Medicine, 39*, 263–272.

Brunner, E., Davey Smith, G., Marmot, M., Canner, R., Beksinska, M., & O'Brien, J. (1996). Childhood social circumstances and psychosocial and behavioural factors as determinants of plasma fibrinogen. *Lancet, 347*, 1008–1013.

Brydon, L., Edwards, S., Mohamed-Ali, V., & Steptoe, A. (2004). Socioeconomic status and stress-induced increases in interleukin-6. *Brain Behavior and Immunity, 18*, 281–290.

Casale, S. N., Auster, C. J., Wolf, F., Pei, Y., & Devereux, R. B. (2007). Ethnicity and socioeconomic status influence use of primary angioplasty in patients presenting with acute myocardial infarction. *American Heart Journal, 154*, 989–993.

Chen, E., Hanson, M. D., Paterson, L. Q., Griffin, M. J., Walker, H. A., & Miller, G. E. (2006). Socioeconomic status and inflammatory processes in childhood asthma: the role of psychological stress. *Journal of Allergy and Clinical Immunology, 117*, 1014–1020.

Chen, E., Strunk, R. C., Bacharier, L. B., Chan, M., & Miller, G. E. (2010). Socioeconomic status associated with exhaled nitric oxide responses to acute stress in children with asthma. *Brain Behavior and Immunity, 24*, 444–450.

Clark, A. M., DesMeules, M., Luo, W., Duncan, A. S., & Wielgosz, A. (2009). Socioeconomic status and cardiovascular disease: Risks and implications for care. *Nature Reviews Cardiology, 6*, 712–722.

Cohen, S., Alper, C. M., Doyle, W. J., Adler, N., Treanor, J. J., & Turner, R. B. (2008). Objective and subjective socioeconomic status and susceptibility to the common cold. *Health Psychology, 27*, 268–274.

Cohen, S., Doyle, W. J., Turner, R. B., Alper, C. M., & Skoner, D. P. (2004). Childhood socioeconomic status and host resistance to infectious illness in adulthood. *Psychosomatic Medicine, 66*, 553–558.

Cohen, S., Janicki-Deverts, D., Chen, E., & Matthews, K. A. (2010). Childhood socioeconomic status and adult health. *Annals of the New York Academy of Sciences, 1186*, 37–55.

CSDH. (2008). *Closing the gap in a generation: Health equity through action on the social determinants of health. Final Report of the Commission on Social Determinants of Health.* Commission on Social Determinants of Health: WHO.: http://whqlibdoc.who.int/hq/2008/WHO_IER_CSDH_08.1_eng.pdf.

Danese, A., Moffitt, T. E., Pariante, C. M., Ambler, A., Poulton, R., & Caspi, A. (2008). Elevated inflammation levels in depressed adults with a history of childhood maltreatment. *Archives of General Psychiatry, 65*, 409–415.

Danese, A., Pariante, C. M., Caspi, A., Taylor, A., and Poulton, R. (2007). Childhood maltreatment predicts adult inflammation in a life-course study. *Proceedings of the National Academy of Sciencies U S A, 104*, 1319–1324.

Danesh, J., Kaptoge, S., Mann, A. G., Sarwar, N., Wood, A., Angleman, S. B., et al. (2008). Long-term interleukin-6 levels and subsequent risk of coronary heart disease: Two new prospective studies and a systematic review. *PLoS Medicine, 5*, e78.

Danesh, J., Lewington, S., Thompson, S. G., Lowe, G. D., Collins, R., Kostis, J. B., et al. (2005). Plasma fibrinogen level and the risk of major cardiovascular diseases and nonvascular mortality: an individual participant meta-analysis. *Journal of the American Medical Associaion, 294*, 1799–1809.

Danesh, J., & Pepys, M. B. (2009). C-reactive protein and coronary disease: Is there a causal link? *Circulation, 120*, 2036–2039.

Der, G., Batty, G. D., & Deary, I. J. (2009). The association between IQ in adolescence and a range of health outcomes at 40 in the 1979 US National Longitudinal Study of Youth. *Intelligence, 37*, 573–580.

Diez Roux, A. V., & Mair, C. (2010). Neighborhoods and health. *Annals of the New York Academy of Sciences, 1186*, 125–145.

Diez Roux, A. V., Merkin, S. S., Arnett, D., Chambless, L., Massing, M., Nieto, F. J., et al. (2001). Neighborhood of residence and incidence of coronary heart disease. *New England Journal of Medicine, 345*, 99–106.

Dowd, J. B., & Goldman, N. (2006). Do biomarkers of stress mediate the relation between socioeconomic status and health? *Journal of Epidemiology and Community Health, 60*, 633–639.

Dowd, J. B., & Aiello, A. E. (2009). Socioeconomic differentials in immune response. *Epidemiology, 20*, 902–908.

Dowd, J. B., Aiello, A. E., & Alley, D. E. (2009). Socioeconomic disparities in the seroprevalence of cytomegalovirus infection in the US population: NHANES III. *Epidemiology and Infection, 137,* 58–65.

Dowd, J. B., Zajacova, A., & Aiello, A. E. (2010). Predictors of inflammation in U.S. children aged 3–16 years. *American Journal of Preventive Medicine, 39,* 314–320.

Dowd, J. B., Palermo, T. M., & Aiello, A. E. (2012). Family poverty is associated with cytomegalovirus antibody titers in U.S. children. *Health Psychology, 31,* 5–10.

Espinola-Klein, C., Rupprecht, H. J., Blankenberg, S., Bickel, C., Kopp, H., Rippin, G., et al. (2002). Impact of infectious burden on extent and long-term prognosis of atherosclerosis. *Circulation, 105,* 15–21.

Evans, G. W., & Kantrowitz, E. (2002). Socioeconomic status and health: The potential role of environmental risk exposure. *Annual Review of Public Health, 23,* 303–331.

Evans, P., Der, G., Ford, G., Hucklebridge, F., Hunt, K., & Lambert, S. (2000). Social class, sex, and age differences in mucosal immunity in a large community sample. *Brain Behavior and Immunity, 14,* 41–48.

Fagundes, C. P., Bennett, J. M., Alfano, C. M., Glaser, R., Povoski, S. P., Lipari, A. M., et al. (2012). Social support and socioeconomic status interact to predict Epstein-Barr virus latency in women awaiting diagnosis or newly diagnosed with breast cancer. *Health Psychology, 31,* 11–19.

Fernandez-Real, J. M., Lopez-Bermejo, A., Vendrell, J., Ferri, M. J., Recasens, M., & Ricart, W. (2006). Burden of infection and insulin resistance in healthy middle-aged men. *Diabetes Care, 29,* 1058–1064.

Folsom, A. R., Qamhieh, H. T., Flack, J. M., Hilner, J. E., Liu, K., Howard, B. V., et al. (1993). Plasma fibrinogen: Levels and correlates in young adults. The Coronary Artery Risk Development in Young Adults (CARDIA) study. *American Journal of Epidemiology, 138,* 1023–1036.

Friedman, E. M., & Herd, P. (2010). Income, education, and inflammation: Differential associations in a national probability sample (The MIDUS study). *Psychosomatic Medicine, 72,* 290–300.

Galobardes, B., Lynch, J., & Smith, G. D. (2007). Measuring socioeconomic position in health research. *British Medical Bulletin, 81–82,* 21–37.

Galobardes, B., Lynch, J. W., & Smith, G. D. (2008). Is the association between childhood socioeconomic circumstances and cause-specific mortality established? Update of a systematic review. *Journal of Epidemiology and Community Health, 62,* 387–390.

Galobardes, B., Smith, G. D., & Lynch, J. W. (2006). Systematic review of the influence of childhood socioeconomic circumstances on risk for cardiovascular disease in adulthood. *Annals of Epidemiology, 16,* 91–104.

Gimeno, D., Ferrie, J. E., Elovainio, M., Pulkki-Raback, L., Keltikangas-Jarvinen, L., Eklund, C., et al. (2008). When do social inequalities in C-reactive protein start? A life course perspective from conception to adulthood in the Cardiovascular Risk in Young Finns Study. *International Journal of Epidemiology, 37,* 290–298.

Goodman, E. (1999). The role of socioeconomic status gradients in explaining differences in US adolescents' health. *American Journal of Public Health, 89,* 1522–1528.

Goodman, E., McEwen, B. S., Huang, B., Dolan, L. M., & Adler, N. E. (2005). Social inequalities in biomarkers of cardiovascular risk in adolescence. *Psychosomatic Medicine, 67,* 9–15.

Gottfredson, L. S. (2004). Intelligence: Is it the epidemiologists' elusive "fundamental cause" of social class inequalities in health? *Journal of Personality and Social Psychology, 86,* 174–199.

Gruenewald, T. L., Cohen, S., Matthews, K. A., Tracy, R., & Seeman, T. E. (2009). Association of socioeconomic status with inflammation markers in black and white men and women in the Coronary Artery Risk Development in Young Adults (CARDIA) study. *Social Science and Medicine, 69,* 451–459.

Harrison, M. J., Farragher, T. M., Clarke, A. M., Manning, S. C., Bunn, D. K., & Symmons, D. P. (2009). Association of functional outcome with both personal- and area-level socioeconomic inequalities in patients with inflammatory polyarthritis. *Arthritis and Rheumatism, 61,* 1297–1304.

Hart, C. L., Taylor, M. D., Davey Smith, G., Whalley, L. J., Starr, J. M., Hole, D. J., et al. (2003). Childhood IQ, social class, deprivation, and their relationships with mortality and morbidity risk in later life: Prospective observational study linking the Scottish Mental Survey 1932 and the Midspan studies. *Psychosomatic Medicine, 65,* 877–883.

Jemal, A., Thun, M. J., Ward, E. E., Henley, S. J., Cokkinides, V. E., & Murray, T. E. (2008). Mortality from leading causes by education and race in the United States, 2001. *American Journal of Preventive Medicine, 34,* 1–8.

Kaplan, J. R., Chen, H., & Manuck, S. B. (2009). The relationship between social status and atherosclerosis in male and female monkeys as revealed by meta-analysis. *American Journal of Primatology, 71,* 732–741.

Kaptoge, S., Di Angelantonio, E., Lowe, G., Pepys, M. B., Thompson, S. G., Collins, R., et al. (2010). C-reactive protein concentration and risk of coronary heart disease, stroke, and mortality: An individual participant meta-analysis. *Lancet, 375,* 132–140.

Kiechl, S., Egger, G., Mayr, M., Wiedermann, C. J., Bonora, E., Oberhollenzer, F., et al.. (2001). Chronic infections and the risk of carotid atherosclerosis: Prospective results from a large population study. *Circulation, 103,* 1064–1070.

Kiecolt-Glaser, J. K., Preacher, K. J., MacCallum, R. C., Atkinson, C., Malarkey, W. B., & Glaser, R. (2003). Chronic stress and age-related increases in the proinflammatory cytokine IL-6. *Procedings of the National Academy of Sciencies U S A, 100,* 9090–9095.

Kitagawa, E. M., & Hauser, P. M. (1973). *Differential mortality in the United States: A study in socioeconomic epidemiology.* Cambridge, MA: Harvard University Press.

Koster, A., Bosma, H., Penninx, B. W., Newman, A. B., Harris, T. B., van Eijk, J. T., et al. (2006). Association of inflammatory markers with socioeconomic status. *Journal of Gerontology A Biological Science and Medical Science, 61,* 284–290.

Krieger, N., Williams, D. R., & Moss, N. E. (1997). Measuring social class in US public health research: Concepts, methodologies, and guidelines. *Annual Review of Public Health, 18,* 341–378.

Kuh, D., and Ben-Shlomo, Y. (Eds.). (2004). *A life course approach to chronic disease epidemiology* (2nd ed.) Oxford, England: Oxford University Press.

Lawlor, D. A., Ebrahim, S., & Davey Smith, G. (2005). Adverse socioeconomic position across the lifecourse increases coronary heart disease risk cumulatively: Findings from the British women's heart and health study. *Journal of Epidemiology and Community Health, 59,* 785–793.

Lopez-Leon, S., Choy, W. C., Aulchenko, Y. S., Claes, S. J., Oostra, B. A., Mackenbach, et al. (2009). Genetic factors influence the clustering of depression among individuals with lower socioeconomic status. *PLoS One, 4,* e5069.

Lorant, V., Deliege, D., Eaton, W., Robert, A., Philippot, P., & Ansseau, M. (2003). Socioeconomic inequalities in depression: a meta-analysis. *American Journal of Epidemiology, 157,* 98–112.

Loucks, E. B., Sullivan, L. M., Hayes, L. J., D'Agostino, R. B., Sr., Larson, M. G., Vasan, R. S., et al. (2006). Association of educational level with inflammatory markers in the Framingham Offspring Study. *American Journal of Epidemiology, 163,* 622–628.

Loucks, E. B., Pilote, L., Lynch, J. W., Richard, H., Almeida, N. D., Benjamin, E. J., et al. (2010). Life course socioeconomic position is associated with inflammatory markers: The Framingham Offspring Study. *Social Science and Medicine, 71,* 187–195.

Mackenbach, J. P. (2005). Genetics and health inequalities: Hypotheses and controversies. *Journal of Epidemiology and Community Health, 59,* 268–273.

Mackenbach, J. P., Stirbu, I., Roskam, A. J., Schaap, M. M., Menvielle, G., Leinsalu, M., et al. (2008). Socioeconomic inequalities in health in 22 European countries. *New England Journal of Medicine, 358,* 2468–2481.

Manuck, S. B., Flory, J. D., Ferrell, R. E., & Muldoon, M. F. (2004). Socio-economic status covaries with central nervous system serotonergic responsivity as a function of allelic variation in the serotonin transporter gene-linked polymorphic region. *Psychoneuroendocrinology, 29,* 651–668.

Markowe, H. L., Marmot, M. G., Shipley, M. J., Bulpitt, C. J., Meade, T. W., Stirling, Y., et al. (1985). Fibrinogen: a possible link between social class and coronary heart disease. *British Medical Journal, 291,* 1312–1314.

Marmot, M. G., Shipley, M. J., Hemingway, H., Head, J., & Brunner, E. J. (2008). Biological and behavioural explanations of social inequalities in coronary heart disease: the Whitehall II study. *Diabetologia, 51,* 1980–1988.

Marmot, M. G., Shipley, M. J., & Rose, G. (1984). Inequalities in health: Specific explanations of a general pattern? *Lancet, i,* 1003–1006.

Matthews, K. A., Gallo, L. C., & Taylor, S. E. (2010). Are psychosocial factors mediators of socioeconomic status and health connections? A progress report and blueprint for the future. *Annals of the New York Academy of Sciences, 1186,* 146–173.

Miller, G. E., & Chen, E. (2010). Harsh family climate in early life presages the emergence of a proinflammatory phenotype in adolescence. *Psychological Science, 21,* 848–856.

Mirowsky, J., & Ross, C. E. (2003). *Education, Social Status and Health.* New York: Aldine De Gruyter.

Muennig, P., Sohler, N., & Mahato, B. (2007). Socioeconomic status as an independent predictor of physiological biomarkers of cardiovascular disease: Evidence from NHANES. *Preventive Medicine, 45,* 35–40.

Mujahid, M. S., & Diez Roux, A. V. (2010). Neighborhood factors and health. In A. Steptoe (Ed.), *Handbook of Behavioral Medicine.* New York: Springer.

Muntaner, C., Borrell, C., Vanroelen, C., Chung, H., Benach, J., Kim, I. H., et al. (2010). Employment relations, social class and health: a review and analysis of conceptual and measurement alternatives. *Social Science and Medicine, 71,* 2130–2140.

Musaad, S., & Haynes, E. N. (2007). Biomarkers of obesity and subsequent cardiovascular events. *Epidemiological Review, 29,* 98–114.

Nazmi, A., Diez Roux, A., Ranjit, N., Seeman, T. E., & Jenny, N. S. (2010). Cross-sectional and longitudinal associations of neighborhood characteristics with inflammatory markers: Findings from the multi-ethnic study of atherosclerosis. *Health and Place, 16,* 1104–1112.

Nazmi, A., & Victora, C. G. (2007). Socioeconomic and racial/ethnic differentials of C-reactive protein levels: a systematic review of population-based studies. *BMC Public Health, 7,* 212.

Nazmi, A., Oliveira, I. O., Horta, B. L., Gigante, D. P., & Victora, C. G. (2010). Lifecourse socioeconomic trajectories and C-reactive protein levels in young adults: Findings from a Brazilian birth cohort. *Social Science and Medicine, 70,* 1229–1236.

Nazroo, J. Y. (2003). The structuring of ethnic inequalities in health: economic position, racial discrimination, and racism. *American Journal Public Health, 93,* 277–284.

Newbern, E. C., Miller, W. C., Schoenbach, V. J., & Kaufman, J. S. (2004). Family socioeconomic status and self-reported sexually transmitted diseases among black and white american adolescents. *Sexually Transmitted Diseases, 31,* 533–541.

Ogden, C. L., Lamb, M. M., Carroll, M. D., & Flegal, K. M. (2010). *Obesity and socioeconomic status in adults: United States 1988–1994 and 2005–2008.* Hyattsville, MD: National Center for Health Statistics.

O'Reilly, D. S., Upton, M. N., Caslake, M. J., Robertson, M., Norrie, J., McConnachie, A., et al. (2006). Plasma C reactive protein concentration indicates a direct relation between systemic inflammation and social deprivation. *Heart, 92,* 533–535.

Owen, N., Poulton, T., Hay, F. C., Mohamed-Ali, V., & Steptoe, A. (2003). Socioeconomic status, C-reactive protein, immune factors, and responses to acute mental stress. *Brain Behavior and Immunity, 17,* 286–295.

P. A. G. A. Committee, (2008). *Physical activity guidelines advisory committee report, 2008.* Washington, DC: Department of Health and Human Services.

Panagiotakos, D. B., Pitsavos, C., Manios, Y., Polychronopoulos, E., Chrysohoou, C. A., & Stefanadis, C. (2005). Socioeconomic status in relation to risk factors associated with cardiovascular disease, in healthy individuals from the ATTICA study. *European Journal of Cardiovascular Prevention and Rehabilitation, 12,* 68–74.

Pappas, G., Hadden, W. C., Kozak, L. J., & Fisher, G. F. (1997). Potentially avoidable hospitalizations: Inequalities in rates between US socioeconomic groups. *American Journal of Public Health, 87,* 811–816.

Petersen, K. L., Marsland, A. L., Flory, J., Votruba-Drzal, E., Muldoon, M. F., & Manuck, S. B. (2008). Community socioeconomic status is associated with circulating interleukin-6 and C-reactive protein. *Psychosomatic Medicine, 70,* 646–652.

Phillips, A. C., Batty, G. D., van Zanten, J. J., Mortensen, L. H., Deary, I. J., Calvin, C. M., et al. (2010). Cognitive ability in early adulthood is associated with systemic inflammation in middle age: The Vietnam experience study. *Brain Behavior and Immunity, 25,* 298–301.

Phillips, J. E., Marsland, A. L., Flory, J. D., Muldoon, M. F., Cohen, S., & Manuck, S. B. (2009). Parental education is related to C-reactive protein among female middle aged community volunteers. *Brain Behavior and Immunity, 23*, 677–683.

Pollitt, R. A., Rose, K. M., & Kaufman, J. S. (2005). Evaluating the evidence for models of life course socioeconomic factors and cardiovascular outcomes: a systematic review. *BMC Public Health, 5*, 7.

Pollitt, R. A., Kaufman, J. S., Rose, K. M., Diez-Roux, A. V., Zeng, D., & Heiss, G. (2008). Cumulative life course and adult socioeconomic status and markers of inflammation in adulthood. *Journal of Epidemiology and Community Health, 62*, 484–491.

Poulton, R., Caspi, A., Milne, B. J., Thomson, W. M., Taylor, A., Sears, M. R., et al. (2002). Association between children's experience of socioeconomic disadvantage and adult health: A life-course study. *Lancet, 360*, 1640–1645.

Prasad, A., Zhu, J., Halcox, J. P., Waclawiw, M. A., Epstein, S. E., & Quyyumi, A. A. (2002). Predisposition to atherosclerosis by infections: Role of endothelial dysfunction. *Circulation, 106*, 184–190.

Ramsay, S., Lowe, G. D., Whincup, P. H., Rumley, A., Morris, R. W., & Wannamethee, S. G. (2008). Relationships of inflammatory and haemostatic markers with social class: Results from a population-based study of older men. *Atherosclerosis, 197*, 654–661.

Ranjit, N., Diez-Roux, A. V., Shea, S., Cushman, M., Ni, H., & Seeman, T. (2007). Socioeconomic position, race/ethnicity, and inflammation in the multi-ethnic study of atherosclerosis. *Circulation, 116*, 2383–2390.

Reynolds, J. R., & Ross, C. E. (1998). Social stratification and health: education's benefit beyond economic status and social origins. *Social Problems, 45*, 221–247.

Rosvall, M., Engstrom, G., Janzon, L., Berglund, G., & Hedblad, B. (2007). The role of low grade inflammation as measured by C-reactive protein levels in the explanation of socioeconomic differences in carotid atherosclerosis. *European Journal of Public Health, 17*, 340–347.

Sapolsky, R. M. (2005). The influence of social hierarchy on primate health. *Science, 308*, 648–652.

Shanks, N., Larocque, S., & Meaney, M. J. (1995). Neonatal endotoxin exposure alters the development of the hypothalamic-pituitary-adrenal axis: Early illness and later responsivity to stress. *Journal of Neuroscience, 15*, 376–384.

Shanks, N., Windle, R. J., Perks, P. A., Harbuz, M. S., Jessop, D. S., Ingram, C. D., et al. (2000). Early-life exposure to endotoxin alters hypothalamic-pituitary-adrenal function and predisposition to inflammation. *Procedings of the National Academy of Sciences U S A, 97*, 5645–5650.

Shipley, B. A., Der, G., Taylor, M. D., & Deary, I. J. (2008). Cognition and mortality from the major causes of death: The Health and Lifestyle Survey. *Journal of Psychosomatic Research, 65*, 143–152.

Simanek, A. M., Dowd, J. B., & Aiello, A. E. (2008). Persistent pathogens linking socioeconomic position and cardiovascular disease in the US. *International Journal of Epidemiology, 38*, 775–787.

Singh-Manoux, A., Adler, N. E., & Marmot, M. G. (2003). Subjective social status: its determinants and its association with measures of ill-health in the Whitehall II study. *Social Science and Medicine, 56*, 1321–1333.

Slopen, N., Lewis, T. T., Gruenewald, T. L., Mujahid, M. S., Ryff, C. D., Albert, M. A., et al. (2010). Early life adversity and inflammation in african americans and whites in the midlife in the United States survey. *Psychosomatic Medicine, 72*, 694–701.

Smith, J. P. (2004). Unraveling the SES-health connection. *Population and Development Review, 30*, 108–132.

Smith, J. P. (2009). The impact of childhood health on adult labor market outcomes. *Review of Economics and Statistics, 91*, 478–489.

Spahr, A., Klein, E., Khuseyinova, N., Boeckh, C., Muche, R., Kunze, M., et al. . (2006). Periodontal infections and coronary heart disease: Role of periodontal bacteria and importance of total pathogen burden in the Coronary Event and Periodontal Disease (CORODONT) study. *Archives of Internal Medicine, 166*, 554–559.

Steptoe, A., Gardner, B., & Wardle, J. (2010). The role of health behaviour. In D. French & K. Vedhara & A. A. Kaptein & J. Weinman (Eds.), *Health Psychology* (2nd ed., pp. 13–32). Chichester: BPS Blackwell.

Steptoe, A., Gylfe, A., Shamaei-Tousi, A., Bergstrom, S., & Henderson, B. (2009). Pathogen burden and cortisol profiles over the day. *Epidemiology and Infection, 137*, 1816–1824.

Steptoe, A., Hamer, M., & Chida, Y. (2007). The effects of acute psychological stress on circulating inflammatory factors in humans: A review and meta-analysis. *Brain Behavior and Immunity, 21*, 901–912.

Steptoe, A., Kunz-Ebrecht, S., Rumley, A., & Lowe, G. D. (2003). Prolonged elevations in haemostatic and rheological responses following psychological stress in low socioeconomic status men and women. *Thrombosis and Haemostasis, 89*, 83–90.

Steptoe, A., & Marmot, M. (2002). The role of psychobiological pathways in socio-economic inequalities in cardiovascular disease risk. *European Heart Journal, 23*, 13–25.

Steptoe, A., & Marmot, M. (2003). Burden of psychosocial adversity and vulnerability in middle age: associations with biobehavioral risk factors and quality of life. *Psychosomatic Medicine, 65*, 1029–1037.

Steptoe, A., Owen, N., Kunz-Ebrecht, S., & Mohamed-Ali, V. (2002). Inflammatory cytokines, socioeconomic status, and acute stress responsivity. *Brain Behavior and Immunity, 16*, 774–784.

Steptoe, A., Shamaei-Tousi, A., Gylfe, A., Henderson, B., Bergstrom, S., & Marmot, M. (2007). Socioeconomic status, pathogen burden and cardiovascular disease risk. *Heart, 93*, 1567–1570.

Szabo, G., & Mandrekar, P. (2009). A recent perspective on alcohol, immunity, and host defense. *Alcohol Clinical and Experimental Research, 33*, 220–232.

Tabassum, F., Kumari, M., Rumley, A., Lowe, G., Power, C., & Strachan, D. P. (2008). Effects of socioeconomic position on inflammatory and hemostatic markers: a life-course analysis in the 1958 British birth cohort. *American Journal of Epidemiology, 167*, 1332–1341.

Taylor, S. E., Lehman, B. J., Kiefe, C. I., & Seeman, T. E. (2006). Relationship of early life stress and psychological functioning to adult C-reactive protein in the coronary artery risk development in young adults study. *Biological Psychiatry, 60*, 819–824.

Thrane, N., Sondergaard, C., Schonheyder, H. C., & Sorensen, H. T. (2005). Socioeconomic factors and risk of hospitalization with infectious diseases in 0- to 2-year-old Danish children. *European Journal of Epidemiology, 20*, 467–474.

Tilg, H., & Moschen, A. R. (2008). Inflammatory mechanisms in the regulation of insulin resistance. *Molecular Medicine, 14*, 222–231.

Wamala, S. P., Murray, M. A., Horsten, M., Eriksson, M., Schenck-Gustafsson, K., Hamsten, A., et al. (1999). Socioeconomic status and determinants of hemostatic function in healthy women. *Arteriosclerosis, Thrombosis and Vascular Biology, 19*, 485–492.

Wilson, T. W., Kaplan, G. A., Kauhanen, J., Cohen, R. D., Wu, M., Salonen, R., et al. (1993). Association between plasma fibrinogen concentration and five socioeconomic indices in the Kuopio Ischemic Heart Disease Risk Factor Study. *American Journal of Epidemiology, 137*, 292–300.

Wright, R. J., & Subramanian, S. V. (2007). Advancing a multilevel framework for epidemiologic research on asthma disparities. *Chest, 132*, 757S–769S.

Xu, H., Barnes, G. T., Yang, Q., Tan, G., Yang, D., Chou, C. J., et al. (2003). Chronic inflammation in fat plays a crucial role in the development of obesity-related insulin resistance. *Journal of Clinical Investigation, 112*, 1821–1830.

Yanbaeva, D. G., Dentener, M. A., Creutzberg, E. C., Wesseling, G., & Wouters, E. F. (2007). Systemic effects of smoking. *Chest, 131*, 1557–1566.

Zajacova, A., Dowd, J. B., & Aiello, A. E. (2009). Socioeconomic and race/ethnic patterns in persistent infection burden among U.S. adults. *Journal of Gerontology A Biological Sciences and Medical Sciences, 64*, 272–279.

Social Regulation of Gene Expression in the Immune System

Steven W. Cole

Abstract

Social factors influence health in part by altering the expression of genes in diseased tissue and immune cells. This chapter surveys the emerging field of social genomics, which has begun to identify the types of genes subject to social regulation, the biological signaling pathways mediating those effects, and the genetic polymorphisms that moderate socioenvironmental influences on human gene expression. After highlighting the implications of these dynamics for immune response and host defense, this chapter considers the evolutionary basis for the deep functional connections between social behavior and immune response.

Key Words: genetics, genomics, social factors, gene-environment interactions

Introduction

Over the past three decades, scientists have increasingly come to understand both the nature of disease and the human immune response in terms of gene expression (Janeway, Travers, Walport, & Shlomchik, 2001). If we want to understand how psychological and social factors influence those dynamics, most biologists would expect an answer expressed in terms of the specific genes that are activated in response to socially induced neural and endocrine dynamics, and the role their protein products play in shaping the molecular architecture of our cells and the functional characteristics of our tissues and organs. This chapter surveys the emerging field of social genomics, which has begun to show how social processes influence genome-wide transcriptional profiles in pathogens and cells of the immune system. After summarizing the broad types of genes subject to social regulation in leukocytes, this review maps the neural and endocrine "social signal transduction" pathways that mediate those effects, and considers the role of genetic polymorphisms in modifying individual biological responses

to socioenvironmental conditions. The chapter concludes by considering the teleologic basis for the evolution of deep functional relationships between social behavior and the immune system as an allostatic adaptation to the distinctive health threats associated with social versus solitary existence.

Social Regulation of Gene Expression

The possibility that social factors might regulate gene expression first emerged in the context of biobehavioral health research. Social stress and isolation have long been known to influence individual vulnerability to disease (Seeman, 1996). That effect is particularly strong for viral infections, where adverse social conditions have been linked to increased replication of cold-causing rhinoviruses (Cohen, Doyle, Skoner, Rabin, & Gwaltney, 1997), the AIDS virus, HIV-1 (Cole, 2008a), and some cancer-related viruses (Antoni et al., 2006; Chang et al., 2005). Viruses are little more than small packages of 10–100 genes that hijack the protein production machinery of their host cells (us) to make more copies of themselves. As obligate parasites of our living cells, viruses evolved in a microenvironment structured by our own genome. If social factors can regulate the expression of viral genes, this suggests that social factors are likely to regulate the expression of our own genes as well.

One of the first studies to comprehensively analyze the effects of social conditions on human gene expression assessed genome-wide transcriptional profiles in white blood cells (leukocytes) from healthy older adults who differed in the extent to which they felt socially connected to others (Cole et al., 2007). Long-term social isolation is both a well-established risk factor for physical illness (Seeman, 1996) and a personally generated sociobehavioral phenotype that stems from individual differences in social cognition (Caioppo & Hawkley, 2009), CNS neurobiological sensitivity to threat (Kagan, 1994; Schwartz, Wright, Shin, Kagan, & Rauch, 2003), and increased activity of threat-related peripheral signaling pathways such as the sympathetic nervous system (SNS) (Cole, Kemeny, Fahey, Zack, & Naliboff, 2003; Kagan, 1994; Kagan, Reznick, & Snidman, 1988). Motivated by the epidemiologic evidence in humans and experimental studies documenting adverse effects of social isolation on disease pathogenesis in animal models (summarized in (Cole, 2008b; Cole et al., 2007)), this study sought to identify alterations in immune-cell gene expression that might mediate effects of social conditions on host resistance to infection and inflammation-related diseases such as cardiovascular disease, neurodegenerative disease, and certain types of cancer. Among the 22,283 human genes assayed, 209 showed systematically different levels of expression in people who consistently experienced themselves as lonely and distant from others over a span of 4 years. These transcriptional alterations did not involve a random smattering of all human genes, but focally impacted three specific groups of genes. Genes supporting the early "accelerator" phase of the immune response—inflammation—showed selective upregulation. However, two groups of genes involved in the subsequent "steering" of immune responses were markedly downregulated: those involved in responses to viral infection (particularly Type I interferons), and those involved in the production of antibodies. This initial portrait of a socially sensitive transcriptome provided a molecular framework for understanding how socially isolated individuals could simultaneously show heightened vulnerability to inflammation-driven cardiovascular diseases (i.e., excessive nonspecific immune activity; Caspi, Harrington, Moffitt, Milne, &

Poulton, 2006) and impaired responses to viral infections and vaccines (i.e., insufficient antigen-specific immune responses; Cohen et al., 1997; Cole et al., 2003; Cole, Kemeny, & Taylor, 1997; G. E. Miller, Cohen, Rabin, Skoner, & Doyle, 1999; Pressman et al., 2005). This study also highlighted the key role that CNS interpretation plays in mediating social influences on gene expression in the immune system; leukocyte transcriptional alterations were most strongly linked to a person's subjective sense of isolation, rather than their objective number of social contacts.

Following that initial analysis of subjective social isolation, additional studies rapidly began to identify transcriptional correlates of other socioenvironmental conditions such as low socioeconomic status (SES) (Chen et al., 2009; G. E. Miller et al., 2009) and the chronic threat of social loss (e.g., having a spouse with cancer;) (G. E. Miller et al., 2008). As in the study of chronic loneliness, these other types of social adversity were also associated with leukocyte upregulation of inflammation-related genes and downregulation of Type I interferons. One study focusing specifically on CD14+ monocytes (~5% of total leukoctyes) found an adversity-related transcriptional profile that matched broadly the dynamics observed in the total circulating leukocyte pool (Miller et al., 2008). Another study analyzing loneliness-related differences in gene expression found that those transcripts originated predominately from monocytes and plasmacytoid dendritic cells (Cole, Hawkley, Arevalo, & Cacioppo, 2011). These results suggest that the most evolutionarily ancient cells of the immune system (Hoffmann, Kafatos, Janeway, & Ezekowitz, 1999; Millar & Ratcliffe, 1989) may be the key drivers of the total leukocyte transcriptional response to socioenvironmental adversity. These studies also found evidence that psychological processes play a key role in mediating those transcriptional dynamics in the immune system. For example, among children with asthma, those from lower SES backgrounds tended more often to interpret ambiguous social stimuli as threatening, and that perception of threat was more strongly linked to differential gene expression than was SES per se (Chen et al., 2009).

Subsequent studies have also begun to suggest that socioenvironmental conditions present early in life may induce a sort of "defensive programming" of the developing body that can persist for years after the environmental risk factor itself has abated. For example, one analysis of leukocyte gene expression profiles in young adults found that those who had lived in low SES conditions during early childhood continued to show increased expression of inflammation-related genes, even if they had come to enjoy favorable socioeconomic conditions in adulthood (G. E. Miller et al., 2009). Additional analyses of the same cohort also suggested that high levels of maternal care during early life could potentially mitigate those effects and buffer the impact of low early life SES on inflammatory gene expression in adulthood (Chen, Miller, Kobor, & Cole, 2010). Those findings are consistent with other functional genomics studies in animal models showing that social conditions in early life can persistently alter CNS gene expression in ways that govern behavioral and neuroendocrine responses to future challenges (Champagne & Mashoodh, 2009; Weaver, Meaney, & Szyf, 2006). Thus, the burgeoning literature on social regulation of gene expression may help illuminate the biological basis for developmentally plastic "critical periods" and their transition into long-term molecular "imprints" on physiologic function and disease resistance.

Although leukocyte gene expression profiles can harbor persisting imprints from early socio-environmental conditions, some genes are also subject to short-term plasticity. Two studies suggest that the leukocyte transcriptome shows selective alterations within 30 minutes after the onset of acute social stress (Morita et al., 2005; Nater et al., 2009) (although those dynamics may reflect changes in cell trafficking into the circulating leukocyte pool in addition to any per-cell changes in gene transcription). Other studies that control for cell trafficking dynamics have shown that transient events, such as one night of sleep loss, can alter gene expression profiles in the immune system (Irwin, Wang, Campomayor, Collado-Hidalgo, & Cole, 2006). Recent studies in rhesus macaques have also shown that changes in global social conditions can alter transcriptional profiles in the immune system within a matter of weeks (e.g., 4 weeks of unstable social hierarchy in adulthood (Sloan et al., 2007) or unstable social conditions during the first 12 weeks of life (Cole, Conti, Arevalo, Ruggiero, Heckman, & Suomi, 2012)). The capacity of relatively brief socioenvironmental shocks to induce persisting changes in gene expression stems from the recursive structure of gene regulatory networks, which involve highly interconnected feedback systems that can produce nonlinear "catastrophic" jumps from one regulatory equilibrium to another (Kauffman, 1993; Kim, Shay, O'Shea, & Regev, 2009).

Beyond their remarkable kinetics, social genomic relationships can also penetrate surprisingly deeply into our bodies. Experimental animal studies have shown that social conditions can alter the expression of key neural genes such as *NGF* encoding Nerve Growth Gactor (Sloan et al., 2007), the glucocorticoid receptor gene (Zhang et al., 2006), and the expression of hundreds of genes in CNS structures such as the hippocampus and prefrontal cortex (Karssen et al., 2007; Weaver et al., 2006). This is, perhaps, not too surprising, given the nervous system's key role in perceiving and responding to social stimuli. More surprising is the discovery that key genes involved in the immune system's response to pathogens are also sensitive to social conditions (Sloan et al., 2007). Immune cells exert selective pressure on the evolution of viral genomes by killing human cells that actively express "foreign" viral genes. As a result of immune-mediated selective pressure against viral genomes, and immune cells' functional sensitivity to social conditions, many viruses also appear to have developed a genomic sensitivity to our social conditions as part of their immune-evasion strategy (i.e., activating viral replication during periods of stress-induced immunodeficiency, as reviewed earlier).

However, even biological processes that are subject to little immune-mediated selective pressure may still modulate gene transcription in response to host stress and social conditions. Most human cancers are invisible to the immune system because they express no "foreign" genes for the immune system to attack. Nevertheless, several types of human cancer cells show significant changes in transcription in response to social stress (Antoni et al., 2006; Thaker et al., 2006). One recent study of women with ovarian cancer found that > 220 genes were selectively upregulated in tumors from women with low levels of social support and high depressive symptoms (Lutgendorf et al., 2008). If our socially sensitive immune system is not conveying those effects via natural selection of tumor gene expression, how do social influences reach into the damaged genome of a cancer cell? New insights into the pathways by which social factors regulate gene expression in normal somatic cells and their mutant derivative cancer cells have come from bioinformatic analyses of "social signal transduction."

Social Signal Transduction

Molecular biologists view signal transduction as a microlevel process by which signaling molecules outside the cell interact with receptors to initiate a cascade of biochemical reactions inside the cell, ultimately inducing a protein transcription factor to activate gene expression (Figure 14.1). Transcription factors flag a particular stretch of DNA (the coding region of a gene) for transcription into RNA. Which genes can be activated by a given transcription factor is determined by the nucleotide sequence of the gene's promoter—the stretch of DNA lying upstream of the coding region. For example, the transcription factor NF-κB binds to the nucleotide motif GGGACTTTCC, whereas the CREB transcription factor targets the motif TGACGTCA. These two transcription factors are activated by different receptor-mediated signal transduction pathways, providing distinct molecular channels by which extracellular events can regulate intracellular genomic response. The distribution of transcription factor-binding motifs across our ~22,000 gene promoters constitutes a type of "wiring diagram" that maps microenvironmental processes onto gene expression patterns. Additional layers of negative regulation can also superimpose on the positive activity of transcription factors to further trim the expressed transcriptome. For example, epigenetic modifications of DNA by methylation or histone-mediated sequestration can block transcription factor binding to promoters and thereby "veto" transcriptional stimulation that would otherwise occur (Champagne & Mashoodh, 2009; Weaver et al., 2006; Zhang et al., 2006). Transcription factors can also inhibit gene expression under certain circumstances, particularly when they bind to promoter sequences in a way that impedes access by other transcription factors that would otherwise act to upregulate gene expression.

Given these cell-level microregulatory pathways, how can we account for the effects of macrolevel influences from the social ecology? The key involves the brain's capacity to convert environmental stimuli into changes in cellular function via the regulation of hormones, neurotransmitters, and other signaling molecules that disseminate throughout the body to activate cellular receptors and transcription factors. For example, the SNS and the hypothalamic-pituitary-adrenal (HPA) axis represent two major pathways by which CNS-mediated perceptions of threatening or adverse social conditions can alter gene transcription in a wide array of somatic cells (Sapolsky, 1994; Weiner, 1992). Positive psychological states may also regulate transcription (Dusek

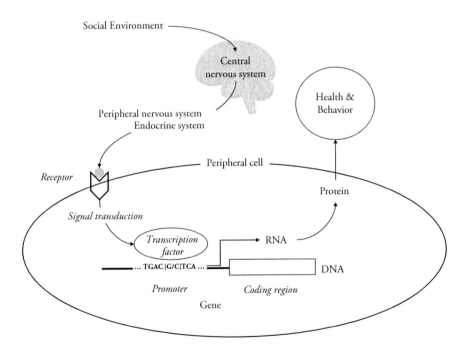

FIGURE 14.1 Social-signal transduction. Socioenvironmental processes regulate human gene expression by activating CNS processes that subsequently influence hormone and neurotransmitter activity in the periphery of the body. Peripheral signaling molecules interact with cellular receptors to activate transcription factors, which bind to characteristic DNA motifs in gene promoters to initiate (or repress) gene expression. Only genes that are transcribed into RNA actually impact health and behavioral phenotypes. Individual differences in promoter DNA sequences (e.g., the [G/C] polymorphism shown here) can affect the binding of transcription factors, and thereby influence genomic sensitivity to socio-environmental conditions. (Adapted from Cole, 2009)

et al., 2008), although their molecular mediators are less well understood.

Links between social experiences and neural/endocrine responses have long been recognized (Sapolsky, 1994; Weiner, 1992), but the breadth of their impact on gene expression has only recently become apparent following the sequencing of the human genome. Early computational analyses of the human genome sequence suggested that promoter DNA sequences might provide for some degree of psychological specificity in transcriptional responses. For example, any gene bearing the motif GGTACAATCTGTTCT in its promoter might potentially be stimulated by stress experiences that induce cortisol release (Henry, 1992; Henry & Stephens, 1977; Sapolsky, 1994; Weiner, 1992), because the cortisol-stimulated glucocorticoid receptor (GR, which also functions as a transcription factor) binds specifically to that DNA motif. In contrast, genes bearing the CREB/ATF promoter motif TGACGTCA would be predicted to activate in response to fight-or-flight stress responses associated with catecholamine release and beta-adrenergic receptor signaling (Dimsdale & Moss, 1980; Frankenhauser, 1975; Weiner, 1992). In the context of Figure 14.2, production of catecholamines by the SNS and the production of cortisol by the HPA axis represent two biologically distinct "social signal transduction pathways," each of which activates a different transcription factor (i.e., CREB and the GR). Because the promoter motifs targeted by those transcription factors are distributed differentially across genes, the two distinct psychological stress experiences that activate those transcription factors may trigger very different transcriptional responses. Genes predicted to be cortisol-responsive disproportionately encode receptors and other molecules involved in cellular "perception" of the physiologic microenvironment. Thus, stress that elevates cortisol may trigger a cellular form of "denial" (altering perception via changes in receptor expression). Putative catecholamine-responsive genes include few receptors, but high concentrations of signal transduction molecules and transcription factors involved in cellular "decision-making" (i.e., converting receptor-mediated perception into changes in gene expression and cellular behavior). Thus, stress that elevates catecholamines induces something more akin to "sublimation" or "reappraisal" (altering cellular responses to perceptions via changes in transcription factor expression).

The sequencing of the human genome has also provided a new analytic infrastructure for mapping the molecular signaling pathways that convert socio-environmental conditions into differential gene expression. One approach to this problem reverses the normal flow of biological information from the environment, through transcription factor activity, and into gene expression (Figure 14.1). This analysis scans the promoters of differentially expressed genes to identify transcription factor-binding motifs that are overrepresented in activated promoters, and thus reflect the specific transcription factors mediating the observed differences in gene expression (Cole, Yan, Galic, Arevalo, & Zack, 2005). Promoter-based bioinformatics have uncovered some surprising differences between the transcriptional signals "sent" by the brain, and the transcriptional signals "heard" by the human genome in peripheral tissues.

In studies of chronic loneliness, threat of social loss, low SES, and the protective effects of early maternal support (Chen et al., 2011; Cole et al., 2007; G. E. Miller et al., 2009; G. E. Miller et al., 2008), promoter analyses indicated that the inflammation-driving NF-κB transcription factor played a central role in orchestrating the observed transcriptional alterations. Results from those studies also suggested that the GR was failing to inhibit the activity of NF-κB as it should (Pace, Hu, & Miller, 2007). Neither study found decreases in circulating cortisol levels that might explain the reduced activity of the GR. If the HPA axis were sending the proper anti-inflammatory cortisol signal, why would the leukocytes of stressed people not downregulate NF-κB transcription of inflammatory genes? The answer appears to involve a reduction in the GR's sensitivity to cortisol—rendering the leukocyte transcriptome deaf to the brain's request to downregulate pro-inflammatory genes.

Although the precise molecular mechanism underlying social stress-induced GR desensitization is not fully defined, it appears that the activity of other physiologic signaling pathways can induce phosphorylation of the GR protein and thereby inhibit its activation by cortisol (Bamberger, Schulte, & Chrousos, 1996; Pace et al., 2007). Animal models of immune regulation show that repeated social threat can induce GR desensitization (Cole, Mendoza, & Capitanio, 2009; Stark, Avitsur, Padgett, & Sheridan, 2001). Recent social genomics studies in humans have shown that chronic loneliness, threat of social loss, and low SES all appear to disconnect this key physiologic negative feedback system that would normally hold harmful inflammation in check (Cole et al., 2007; G. E. Miller et al., 2009; G. E. Miller et al., 2008). One implication of these results is that superficially different types of social adversity might induce a common pattern of regulatory alteration in immune-cell expression of inflammation-related immune-response genes and thereby increase the risk of inflammation-related disease (Seeman, 1996).

Promoter bioinformatics have identified other alterations in transcription factor activity that may connect low SES to inflammatory-gene expression in asthma (Chen et al., 2009), link adverse life circumstances and depressive symptoms to inflammation-related diseases and late-life mortality (Cole, Arevalo, Takahashi, et al., 2010), and connect low social support and depression to altered gene expression in ovarian cancer (Lutgendorf et al., 2008). By relating cell-level changes in gene transcription to neural and endocrine signaling pathways that ultimately convey socioenvironmental influences into the body, studies of social signal transduction are providing a more comprehensive biological portrait of the pathways by which socioenvironmental conditions affect the molecular characteristics of human immune cells.

Socioenvironmental Remodeling of Neuro-immune Interactions

Because RNA transcription shapes the protein complement of our cells, and those proteins mediate cellular function (Figure 14.1), psychological regulation of gene expression implies that the social world can remodel the functional characteristics of the human body. One major goal of social genomics involves determining which specific aspects of human molecular function are most sensitive to socioenvironmental influences. In addition to the marked effects on immune-cell gene expression outlined earlier, neurobiological characteristics appear to be particularly responsive to social regulation, and the nexus of interaction between the nervous and immune systems is especially sensitive as a result. One example involves the regulation of immune cell biology within lymphoid organs by the SNS. All primary and secondary lymphoid tissues contain SNS nerve fibers that regulate immune-cell function via the sympathetic neurotransmitter norepinephrine (NE). This regulatory connection between the nervous and immune systems is sustained by expression of the *NGF* gene encoding Nerve Growth Factor—a key neurotrophic factor supporting the development and maintenance of SNS neural fibers in peripheral tissues (Carlson et al., 1995; Carlson, Johnson, Parrish, & Cass, 1998). In rhesus macaques exposed to low-grade social stress for several months, *NGF* expression increased markedly in secondary lymphoid organs such as lymph nodes (Sloan, Capitanio, & Cole, 2008; Sloan et al., 2007). As a result of that increased *NGF* expression, the number of SNS neural fibers present in the lymph node is also increased substantially, and the CNS thus acquires a greater capacity to regulate the cellular interactions that take place in this critical "convention center" for immune cell coordination and development. That change in neurobiological regulation has the potential to significantly alter the nature of immune response genes expressed in the lymph node.

One consequence of social stress-induced remodeling of lymph node SNS innervation was suppression of leukocyte transcription of the Type I interferon *IFNB*, which plays a critical role in cellular defense against viral infections (Collado-Hidalgo, Sung, & Cole, 2006; Sloan et al., 2007). As a result of those molecular interactions among *NGF*, SNS nerve fibers, and leukocyte suppression of *IFNB*, socially stressed animals showed increased replication of the primate version of HIV-1 (Simian Immunodeficiency Virus) and increased damage to their immune systems as a result (Sloan, Capitanio, & Cole, 2008; Sloan et al., 2007). This series of studies not only provides a comprehensive map of the molecular mechanisms by which socioenvironmental conditions influence the pathogenesis of viral infection (Cole, 2008a; Miller, Chen, & Cole, 2009), but it also exemplifies the self-modifying recursive characteristics of transcription control pathways. To the extent that social signal transduction pathways such as the SNS increase transcription of the very genes that mediate their activity (e.g., upregulating expression of the SNS-sustaining *NGF* gene), the functional alterations that result can become self-staining via positive-feedback loops.

Recursive gene expression dynamics at the micro level (e.g., as in the *NGF*/*IFNB*/SIV example) can significantly influence the long-term temporal dynamics of macrolevel development due to the persistence of their effects on protein expression and cell function. Figure 14.2 illustrates these dynamics in an abstract theoretical form. From a functional genomics perspective, we can think of our physical bodies as machines that convert environmental stimuli into changes in outputs such as behavior and gene expression (RNA). Because the RNA "output" at one time point (e.g., RNA_1) influences the molecular characteristics of the body at future points in time (e.g., $Body_2$)—due to the ~80-day average half-life of transcriptionally induced

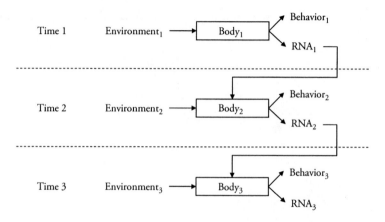

FIGURE 14.2 RNA as a molecular medium of recursive development. Social conditions at one point in time (Environment$_1$) are transduced into changes in behavior (Behavior$_1$) and gene expression (RNA$_1$) via CNS perceptual processes that trigger systemic neural and endocrine responses (mediated by Body$_1$). Those RNA transcriptional dynamics can alter the molecular characteristics of cells involved in environmental perception or response, resulting in a functionally altered Body$_2$. Body$_2$ may respond differently to a given environmental challenge that would the previous Body$_1$, resulting in different behavioral (Behavior$_2$) and transcriptional responses (RNA$_2$). The effect of RNA transcriptional dynamics on persisting cellular protein and functional characteristics provides a molecular framework for understanding how socioenvironmental conditions in the past may continue to affect current behavior and health, and how those historical conditions interact with current environments to shape our future trajectories (e.g., Body$_3$, Behavior$_3$, RNA$_3$). Because gene transcription serves as both a cause of social behavior (by shaping Body) and a consequence of social behavior (a product of Environment x Body), RNA serves as the physical medium for a recursive developmental trajectory that integrates genetic characteristics and historical-environmental regulators to shape individual biological and behavioral responses to current environmental conditions. (Adapted from Cole, 2009)

proteins—that future body may respond to a subsequently encountered Environment$_2$ differently than it would if the body's current molecular characteristics were shaped by a different RNA history. The self-modifying characteristics of social-signal transduction pathways can continue propagating into the future, with Body$_3$ responding to Environment$_3$ differently depending upon the earlier RNA$_2$, and thereby producing a different set of Behavior$_3$ and RNA$_3$ outputs.

In the *NGF/IFNB/*SIV system, for example, the socioenvironmental upregulation of *NGF* at Time$_1$ induces a denser neural network within the lymph node at Time$_2$. That denser neural network provides a stronger signaling pathway by which a stressful event at Time$_2$ can release the SNS neurotransmitter norepinephrine (NE) into the lymph node. As a consequence of increased NE signaling, the immune system mounts a poorer *IFNB* response to a viral infection at Time$_2$ solely because lymph node innervation was remodeled by differing social conditions at Time$_1$. In other words, social stress at Time$_1$ (Environment$_1$) is transmitted through the nervous system (Body$_1$) into behavioral stress responses (Behavior$_1$) and increased *NGF* gene expression (RNA$_1$). Upregulated *NGF* at Time$_1$ increases SNS innervation of the lymph node, and thereby alters the functional relationship between the nervous

and immune systems over the life of the newly expressed proteins/neural fibers (Body$_2$). When that functionally remodeled Body$_2$ encounters a new viral infection in Environment$_2$, the increased SNS neurotransmitter release inhibits transcription of antiviral *IFNB* (RNA$_2$). The antiviral response is impaired, and the resulting increase in viral replication alters both gene expression and health/behavior in the future (RNA$_3$ and Behavior$_3$).

Because gene expression alterations can change the functional characteristics of gene regulation pathways, the experience of Environment$_1$ not only "gets inside the body" but "stays there" in a concrete molecular sense that propagates through multiple gene transcriptional responses, physiologic systems, and time epochs. Recursive social signal transduction dynamics provide one major pathway by which environmental conditions present early in life can exert a persisting impact on biological function over decades (G. E. Miller et al., 2009). Environmental induction of stable epigenetic alterations provides another biological mechanism for long-term change in gene expression (Champagne & Mashoodh, 2009; Zhang et al., 2006). Socioenvironmental conditions can also regulate the molecular composition of CNS cells, and thereby alter psychological, behavioral, and neuroendocrine-mediated transcriptional responses to future environments (Zhang et al., 2006). Each of these biological mechanisms can propagate a transient change in gene expression into a self-perpetuating cycle that persists even after its initial environmental stimulus has abated. As a result, your body may respond very differently to a challenge today than it would have had you experienced a different history of environmental exposures and transcriptional responses.

Because the molecular composition of our cells constitutes the physical machinery by which we perceive and respond to the world around us ("Body" in Figure 14.2), and that molecular composition is itself subject to remodeling by socioenvironmental influences, gene expression constitutes both a cause and a consequence of behavior. RNA can be construed as the physical medium of a recursive developmental system in which social, behavioral, and health *outcomes* at one point in time also constitute *inputs* that shape our future responses to the environment (e.g., as in recursive models of human capability development, wherein functional capacities developed at Time$_1$ impact the ability to capitalize on environmental opportunities at Time$_2$ (Heckman, 2007)). Given the key role of neuroendocrine responses in mediating these effects, the most decisive influences likely involve our psychological reactions to social conditions rather than the properties of the external condition per se. After all, it is the subjective perception of conditions as threatening or uncertain that directly triggers SNS and HPA responses (Henry, 1992; Henry & Stephens, 1977; Sapolsky, 1994; Weiner, 1992). Our genome's social sensitivity ultimately stems from the capacity of social conditions to affect CNS perceptions (e.g., of safety versus threat; Dickerson & Kemeny, 2004), and thereby trigger biological stress responses that alter gene transcription.

The Role of Genetic Polymorphism

With genes and environments now operating in parallel to shape our RNA-driven bodies, the integration of those two streams of influence has become a central challenge in biological analyses of human health and behavior. The regulatory paradigm outlined in Figure 14.1 provides a framework for analyzing the interplay of those factors in the context of Gene x Environment interactions. For example, variations in the DNA sequence of promoters can affect the binding of environmentally activated transcription factors, and thereby buffer the effects of adverse social environments on immunologic responses (e.g., averting SNS induction of the pro-inflammatory cytokine *IL6*)(Cole et al.,

2012). These "regulatory polymorphisms" in DNA sequence essentially add or remove a connection within the complex wiring diagram of a cell.

Figure 14.3 illustrates one example in which the most prevalent version of the human *IL6* gene shows substantial transcriptional activation in response to the SNS neurotransmitter NE. In the wiring diagram of the ancestral human genome, SNS activation is connected to *IL6* transcription because the GATA1 transcription factor stimulated by NE can bind with high affinity to the GATG motif present in the *IL6* promoter. However, people whose *IL6* promoters bear the variant *C*ATG allele are much less susceptible to stress-induced up-regulation of *IL6* because NE-activated GATA1 does not bind efficiently to that alternative DNA motif. The G > C substitution essentially disconnects the regulatory circuit linking stressful experience to *IL6* transcription via SNS activation of GATA1. Presumably as a result of that differential transcriptional response to SNS activation, people bearing G vs. C allele *IL6* promoters show differing social epidemiologic relationships between stressful life circumstances and the incidence of inflammation-related disease and mortality. Stressful conditions sufficient to induce symptoms of depression are associated with a significant increase in inflammation-related mortality risk in people bearing 2 copies of the GATA1-sensitive *IL6* G allele promoter (Cole, Arevalo, Takahashi, et al., 2010). However, heterozygotes and those homozygous for the GATA1-insensitive C allele show no relationship between stress/depression and mortality. The *IL6* regulatory polymorphism blocks the capacity of adverse environmental conditions to activate the expression of this key disease-related gene, and thus renders carriers less vulnerable to socio-environmentally-mediated health risks.

Regulatory polymorphisms may have little effect on behavioral or biological phenotypes if the affected physiologic function continues to be maintained through other redundant regulatory pathways. However, regulatory polymorphisms that affect physiologically influential genes with no functional back-ups can significantly alter relationships between environmental risk factors and survival-related phenotypes such as cardiovascular disease, inflammation-related cancers, or viral infections (Capitanio et al., 2008; S. Cole et al., 2010). Because disease phenotypes influence survival and reproduction (i.e., fitness), individual differences in transcriptional responses to environmental conditions have the potential to shape the evolutionary trajectory of our DNA genome at the population

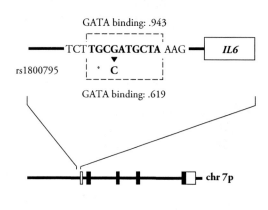

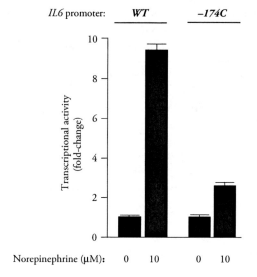

FIGURE 14.3 Effect of the human *IL6* regulatory polymorphism on norepinephrine-induced transcription. The left panel shows bioinformatic analyses comparing the predicted binding of the GATA1 transcription factor (0–1 metric) to either the ancestral G allele of the IL6 promoter or the minor C allele. Affinity values < 0.75 are functionally inactive. The second panel shows the results of in vitro biochemical analyses modeling the effects of stress on IL6 gene expression. IL6 promoter sequences driving the expression of a reporter gene were transfected into human ovarian cancer cells, which were then stimulated with 0 or 10 µM concentrations of the sympathetic nervous system neurotransmitter norepinephrine to activate GATA1. Consistent with the bioinformatic predictions, norepinephrine efficiently activated transcription from the GATA1-sensitive G allele promoter, but had minimal effect on the GATA1-insensitive C allele promoter. The G > C substitution essentially disconnected IL6 transcription from stress-induced regulation by the sympathetic nervous system. (Adapted from Cole et. al, 2010)

level. In integrating the molecular biology of gene structure (DNA), the environmental control of gene expression (RNA), and the social biology of individual behavior and survival, the *IL6* regulatory polymorphism exemplifies the new "environmentally conscious" conception of genetics in which cellular and organismic behaviors constitute the fundamental units of evolutionary selection, and genes and environments depend mutually on one another to shape those behaviors by structuring our brains and bodies.

Evolutionary Basis for Social Regulation of Immune Response Genes

Research in social genomics has now shown that the interpersonal world exerts biologically significant effects on the gene expression profile of immune cells. These effects typically target a nonrandom 1–5% of the genome, though sometimes a different 1–5% depending on the social circumstances and cell type studied. Moreover, the small fraction of genes that are socially sensitive appear to disproportionately influence health and development via the regulation of antiviral responses, inflammation, and cellular reception of hormone and neurotransmitter signals. Ongoing research will more fully map the specific genes that are subject

to social regulation, clarify the types of socioenvironmental conditions that alter their transcription, and further define the psychological and biological pathways mediating those effects. However, even at this early stage of discovery, it is worth asking why we have evolved an immune system that alters its gene expression profiles in response to external social conditions? The answer may very well lie in the implications that external social conditions have for the nature of the pathogens the immune system confronts within the body.

The immune system's evolution has been shaped in large part by its success in defeating infectious pathogens, which have historically dominated our fitness and mortality outcomes (Finch, 2010). Many infectious diseases are intrinsically social in that they are conveyed to us primarily from our conspecifics. This is especially true for viruses and other intracellular pathogens (e.g., intracellular bacteria), which are often highly restricted in the types of host organisms they can infect. Most human viruses cannot efficiently infect even other primates, much less the array of other animals we might confront, and vice versa (Knipe et al., 2007). Because most intracellular human pathogens cannot effectively survive anywhere besides the tissues and fluids of other humans, that implies that one of the greatest epidemiologic threats that a human can confront is another human. The near presence of another person drastically alters the "pathogen landscape" confronting our immune system, and physically intimate social contact (e.g., as occurs in mated social life) provides even greater exposure to host-restricted pathogens. Sexual transmission of infectious agents is orders of magnitude more efficient than other person-to-person routes such as airborne aerosols or skin contact (Knipe et al., 2007).

However, not all human pathogens are so fundamentally dependent on conspecific transmission. Many extracellular pathogens such as bacteria and parasitic organisms can survive for long periods of time in or on the surface of other host animals or inanimate objects. To successfully infect a human, however, those pathogens generally need to access the internal tissues of the body—intact skin provides a formidable barrier to their colonization of human cells. However, ingestion or wounding injury can provide those broad host-range pathogens with efficient access to our tissues.

A correspondence thus emerges between historical patterns of pathogen exposure and human socioenvironmental conditions. To the extent that individuals make their way alone, in the absence of friendly conspecifics, "social infections" with intracellular pathogens will rarely occur. However, those lone individuals lack group-mediated protections against wounding by predators or hostile conspecifics (Hamilton, 1964), raising the likelihood of infection by extracellular pathogens. Individuals enmeshed within a group of friendly conspecifics face much greater exposure to infection by host-restricted intracellular and socially transmitted agents such as viruses (Hamrick, Cohen, & Rodriguez, 2002), but the risk of wounding-related infection with broad-range extracellular pathogens is generally ameliorated. To the extent that the individual has secured the even greater fitness opportunities of a mated relationship, the risk of "intimate social infections" by sexually transmitted viruses and bacteria grows even greater. In other words, there exists over the graded series of human social attachment statuses (alone, grouped, mated) a corresponding gradation in the relative exposure to social versus nonsocial infections that maps roughly onto intracellular versus extracellular pathogens.

Gene expression profiles in the immune system bifurcate markedly in response to intracellular versus extracellular pathogens because different types of effector responses are optimal for defeating each type of infection. Intracellular pathogens are best cleared by cell-mediated immune responses (e.g., by macrophages, NK cells, and cytotoxic T lymphocytes), whereas extracellular pathogens are most efficiently cleared by antibody-dependent humoral immune responses. At the transcriptional level, these differing immune response phenotypes are mediated by differing gene expression profiles—for example the activated helper T lymphocyte's production of a Th1 cytokine response promoting cell-mediated immunity versus a Th2 response supporting B cell antibody production (Janeway et al., 2001). Similar transcriptional polarization occurs during activation of other immune effector cells, such as macrophage M1 gene expression profiles, which facilitate classical cell-mediated antimicrobial inflammatory responses, versus M2 profiles, which promote tissue repair and blood vessel growth (Martinez, Gordon, Locati, & Mantovani, 2006; Martinez, Sica, Mantovani, & Locati, 2008; Mills, Kincaid, Alt, Heilman, & Hill, 2000). Optimal immune responses to different types of infections thus require the generation of qualitatively different transcriptional responses by immune cells.

If, as allostatic theories of physiology suggest (Sterling, 2004), natural selection favors a "prepared" genome that actively anticipates physiologic challenges such as pathogen exposure (rather than simply reacting to them post hoc), then cells of the immune system may have evolved the capacity to monitor social threat-dependent physiologic signals such as catecholamines and glucocorticoids that provide a molecular forecast of changing pathogen exposures. Given the ecological association between social isolation or threat and wound-mediated exposure to extracellular pathogens, a forward looking immune system could get a jump start on its microbial adversaries by upregulating pro-inflammatory cytokines and M2/Th2 mediators of humoral immune responses (proximally signaled by threat-associated catecholamine activity) (Henry, 1992; Henry & Stephens, 1977;. Miller et al., 1999; Sloan et al., 2007). In contrast, under more convivial social conditions such as stable community membership or mated life, a forward looking immune system might hedge its bets on pathogen exposure by reducing its basal inflammatory stance and redeploying transcriptional resources toward intracellular pathogens (e.g., Type I interferon-mediated innate antiviral responses, M1/Th1 cytokine profiles).

In short, the combination of (a) allostatic selective forces that favor a forward looking immune system that anticipates threats, and (b) a general ecological correlation between social conditions and pathogen characteristics provides a natural selective pressure for the immunologically responsive portions of the genome to acquire a sensitivity to the neural and endocrine signals that track the human experience of social threat or isolation versus supportive group membership. In that sense, the same "defensive vigilance" program that is theorized to shape general behavioral and physiologic responses to physical or social threat (SNS-mediated fight-or-flight responses in particular) (Henry, 1992; Henry & Stephens, 1977; Weiner, 1992) may also include an immunobiological component in which immune cells alter their basal transcriptional stance to anticipate changing profiles of microbial risk.

Implications of a Socially Sensitive Immune Transcriptome

If, as theorized earlier, the mammalian immune system has evolved a neurally mediated transcriptional sensitivity to external social conditions, that may have some surprising implications for human physiology and disease resistance. For example, to the extent that immunologic transcriptional plasticity is dependent on CNS-mediated transduction of social information, the subjective experience of external social conditions may exert a more pronounced impact on gene expression than do objective social conditions. Subjective estimates of threat are, after all, the proximal physiologic determinants of SNS and HPA activity (Henry, 1992; Henry & Stephens, 1977; Sapolsky, 1994; Weiner, 1992). Consistent with that hypothesis, several studies reviewed earlier have confirmed that subjective perceptions of external social conditions, such as social security versus threat, are more directly related to leukocyte pro-inflammatory transcriptional dynamics than are objective social conditions such as social network size or SES (Chen et al., 2009; Cole et al., 2007; Cole et al., 2011). Similarly, perceptions of past social support (e.g., maternal warmth; Chen et al., 2011) or future social threat (e.g., of social loss due to spousal bereavement by cancer; G. E. Miller et al., 2008) also appear to influence gene expression profiles despite the absence of any current objective variation in environmental conditions.

A neurobiologically sensitive immune system does not, of course, imply that objective socioenvironmental conditions have no influence on the expression of immune response genes. Broad socioenvironmental "ways of living" such as city versus village versus nomadic lifestyles clearly affect the leukocyte transcriptome (Gibson, 2008; Idaghdour, Storey, Jadallah, & Gibson, 2008). However, the capacity of the nervous and endocrine systems to regulate immune cell gene expression implies that what we make of external conditions may often constitute a more proximal determinant of the basal leukocyte transcriptome than are the objective characteristics of those external conditions. Objective properties of external conditions clearly play a role in regulating immune function (e.g., via differential exposure to pathogens), but even when pathogen conditions are held constant, socioenvironmental conditions continue to modulate the leukocyte transcriptome (Cole et al., 2012; Sloan et al., 2007).

The most decisive indication of the dominant role of subjective experience in social regulation of gene expression involves the transcriptional impact of psychologically targeted interventions. Early case-control studies in humans suggested that meditation or intensive total lifestyle interventions could alter gene expression in leukocytes and prostate cancer tissue (Dusek et al., 2008; Ornish et al., 2008). More recent experimental studies have shown that the suppressed Type I interferon/amplified inflammation dynamic, previously linked to adversity, can be counteracted by nonphysical interventions such as cognitive behavioral stress management (e.g., in women confronting the life-threatening adversity of breast cancer; Antoni et al., 2012) or even the provision of a carpet-clad inanimate "surrogate mother" to infant rhesus macaques (Cole et al., 2012). These results underscore the hypothesis that it may be possible to regulate somatic gene expression by altering the socioenvironmental conditions that prevail in everyday life.

Another implication of the key role of subjective perception in mediating leukocyte transcriptional dynamics is that individual differences in perceptual style or subjective theories about the social world should have correlates in immune cell function and health (Cole et al., 2003; Cole, Kemeny, Weitzman, Schoen, & Anton, 1999; Sloan, Capitanio, Tarara, & Cole, 2008). A long line of studies linking introversion in particular to increased risk of viral infections (Broadbent, Broadbent, Phillpotts, & Wallace, 1984; Capitanio, Mendoza, & Baroncelli, 1999; Cohen et al., 1997; Cole et al., 2003; Cole et al., 1997; Totman, Kiff, Reed, & Craig, 1980) might potentially be explained by their common relationship to neural function and leukocyte gene regulation. Much research suggests that socially inhibited phenotypes such as introversion represent the behavioral manifestation of a more general underlying sensitivity to threat that is mediated by individual differences in limbic-system neural function and associated with increases in peripheral SNS activity (Cole et al., 2003; Kagan, 1994; Kagan et al., 1988). Consistent with known SNS effects on antiviral gene expression in particular (Bonneau, 1996; Cole, Korin, Fahey, & Zack, 1998; Collado-Hidalgo et al., 2006; Grebe et al., 2009; Kalinichenko, Mokyr, Graf, Cohen, & Chambers, 1999), individual differences in socially inhibited behavior have been linked to increased viral gene expression in humans and experimental animal models (Capitanio et al., 1999; Cole et al., 2003; Cole et al., 1997) as well as skewing of lymph-node gene expression profile away from antiviral responses and toward Th2 cytokines supporting humoral immunity (Sloan, Capitanio, Tarara, et al., 2008).

Temperament-related differences in immune-system gene expression are also consistent with the observation that self-generated "social interventions," such as concealment of a stigmatized personal identity, appear to help protect dispositionally threat-sensitive individuals from the adverse transcriptional dynamics and health vulnerabilities that would otherwise follow from long-term social threat exposure (Cole et al., 1997). The ethical implications of such social defense mechanisms are chastening (Cole, 2006; Cole et al., 1997), but their capacity to reduce individual vulnerability to viral gene expression underscores the key role of CNS-mediated social processes in shaping transcriptionally mediated host defense against infection.

Perhaps the most striking implication of a socially sensitive immune transcriptome involves its implications for the co-evolution of our pathogens (Knipe et al., 2007; May & Anderson, 1983). If experienced social threat shifts leukocyte gene expression in ways that undermine host defense against viral infections in particular, that should create a socioenvironmental niche within the host body that favors viral replication and transmission, and thereby provides selective pressure for viruses to also evolve their own transcriptional sensitivity to our social adversity. Figure 14.4 illustrates this argument using computational simulations of viral population growth for two versions of a standard latent/active lifestyle in which viruses cease gene expression for extended periods to evade the cellular immune response (latency) and periodically resume replication to spread and infect new host cells (reactivation).

In the first version (V1), the probability of reactivation follows typical quantitative virological theories in being randomly distributed over time. In the second version (V2), the total cumulative probability of reactivation is the same, but the instantaneous reactivation probability spikes during periods of high SNS activity and is correspondingly lower during other periods. The V2 lifestyle models the effects of a virus evolving a transcriptional sensitivity to host cell beta-adrenergic signals from the SNS (e.g., by molecular evolution of a cAMP response element within the promoter of a key viral replication switch gene such as HHV-8 Rta) (Chang et al., 2005). That has the salutary effect (from the virus's perspective) of synchronizing viral reactivation with beta-adrenergic suppression of innate antiviral responses and immune surveillance by cytotoxic T lymphocytes. As a result, more viral gene expression takes place before antiviral responses intervene, and the V2 population outcompetes V1 for host cell niches during periodic bursts of high-efficiency replication relatively unopposed by host antiviral responses. V1 is exposed to the same oscillations in the efficiency of host antiviral responses, but it does not receive as much selective advantage because it does not concentrate its transcriptional activity during the advantaged temporal/physiologic niches created by host adversity (because that virus has not evolved a promoter cAMP response element to listen in on/forecast host cell immune response conditions).

These analyses illustrate the substantial evolutionary incentive for pathogens to acquire a molecular sensitivity to the same neural and endocrine signaling pathways that modulate the human immune response transcriptome. In light of those dynamics, it comes as no surprise that many successful human viruses have evolved promoter DNA sequences and other molecular properties that are sensitive to host-cell signaling from the SNS-induced beta-adrenergic/cAMP/PKA pathway (e.g., HIV-1, Human Herpesvirus 8, Cytomegalovirus, Herpes Simplex Virus 1 and 2) (Berman & Hill, 1985; Bloom, Stevens, Hill, & Tran, 1997; Chang et al., 2005; Cole, Jamieson, & Zack, 1999; Cole et al., 1998; Cole et al., 2001; Millhouse, Kenny, Quinn, Lee, & Wigdahl, 1998; Rader, Ackland-Berglund, Miller, Pepose, & Leib, 1993; Steiner & Kennedy, 1993; Wang, Krause, & Straus, 1995; Wheatley, Dent, Wood, & Latchman, 1992) or the HPA-induced glucocorticoid receptor pathway (e.g., Epstein-Barr virus, Hepatitis B and C Viruses, Human Papillomaviruses) (Bartholomew et al., 1997; Bromberg-White & Meyers, 2003; Cacioppo et al., 2002; Chou, Wang, Lin, & Chi, 1992; Cid

(a)

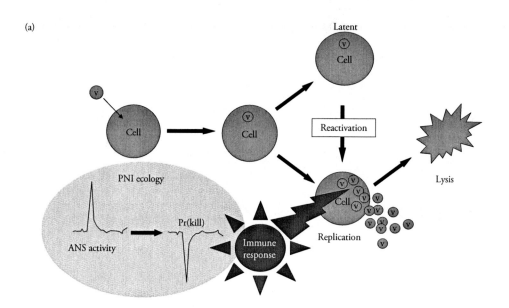

(b)

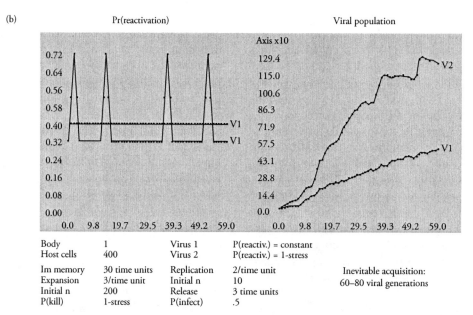

Body	1	Virus 1	P(reactiv.) = constant	
Host cells	400	Virus 2	P(reactiv.) = 1-stress	
Im memory	30 time units	Replication	2/time unit	Inevitable acquisition:
Expansion	3/time unit	Initial n	10	60–80 viral generations
Initial n	200	Release	3 time units	
P(kill)	1-stress	P(infect)	.5	

FIGURE 14.4 Viral evolution into the "host stress niche." (a) Viral evolutionary dynamics are simulated using an agent-based model in which a population of host cells (e.g., 400 here) is subject to infection by a virus (v). Once infected, the virus remains transcriptionally latent in the next time unit, or reactivates viral replication with a specified probability per time unit. Cells that harbor actively replicating viral genomes are subject to detection by an antiviral immune response that results in cell death (lysis) with a fixed probability (0.5 in this case) in each ensuing time epoch, which terminates further viral replication. Prior to immune-mediated lysis, cells that harbor actively replicating virus release new viral particles that can infect neighboring cells at a fixed rate. To model the known sensitivity of the antiviral response to neural and endocrine regulation, the probability of immune-mediated cell lysis periodically decreases (by an empirical average 33% in this case) for a brief period simulating the effects of exogenous adversity. (b) Two competing viral strains are introduced into the model system summarized above. Both have the same total cumulative probability of reactivation per unit time, but V1 reactivates randomly whereas V2 remains latent under basal conditions and shows a transient increased probability of reactivation during periods of physiologic adversity (simulating the effect of a virus evolving a promoter nucleotide motif sensitive to host-cell stress-induced transcription factors such as CREB or the GR). The left panel shows the difference in quantitative reactivation "lifestyles." The right panel shows the relative growth rates for the two viral populations. Note V2's substantial population bursts during periods of stress (corresponding to reduced antiviral immune response), and the resulting "ratcheting up" of the total V2 population. In 10,000 such simulations, the V2 viral population inevitably out-competed the V1 population within 80 viral generations (less than 1 year for a rapidly replicating human virus such as HIV-1, and less than 10 years for a slowly replicating human herpesvirus). These results illustrate the substantial selective pressure for viruses to acquire functional sensitivity to host cell transcription factor signals that are associated with even limited (e.g., 33%) and transient quantitative decrements in the efficiency of host antiviral immune responses.

et al., 1993; Durst, Gallahan, Jay, & Rhim, 1989; Farza et al., 1987; Glaser, Kutz, MacCallum, & Malarkey, 1995; Gloss et al., 1987; Gripon, Diot, Corlu, & Guguen-Guillouzo, 1989; Kamradt, Mohideen, & Vaughan, 2000; Khare, Pater, Tang, & Pater, 1997; Kupfer & Summers, 1990; Lau, Bain, Smith, Alexander, & Williams, 1992; Magy et al., 1999; Mittal, Pater, & Pater, 1993; Mittal, Tsutsumi, Pater, & Pater, 1993; Pater, Hughes, Hyslop, Nakshatri, & Pater, 1988; Pater & Pater, 1991; Piccini, Storey, Romanos, & Banks, 1997; Schuster, Chasserot-Golaz, & Beck, 1991; Schuster, Chasserot-Golaz, Urier, Beck, & Sergeant, 1991; Selvey, Dunn, Tindle, Park, & Frazer, 1994; Tur-Kaspa, Burk, Shaul, & Shafritz, 1986; Tur-Kaspa & Laub, 1990; Tur-Kaspa et al., 1988; Yokosuka, 2000). The magnitude and ubiquity of viral sensitivity to human neural and endocrine signaling likely explains the long-observed effects of socioenvironmental adversity on viral replication and disease pathogenesis (Antoni et al., 2006; Cohen, Janicki-Deverts, & Miller, 2007; Cole, 2008a; Dobbs, Vasquez, Glaser, & Sheridan, 1993; Glaser, Rabin, Chesney, Cohen, & Natelson, 1999).

Viral genomic evolution to capitalize on the human immune system's "stress niche" also provide a pathogen's point of view on the long-standing question regarding whether psychoneuroimmunologic relationships are sufficiently large to be worth worrying about. The simulations in Figure 14.4 were based on quantitative measures of observed transcriptional suppression and cytotoxic T lymphocyte responses from the PNI literature. If the resulting effects on viral evolution are sufficient to matter for viral evolution, they are certainly sufficient to affect human health, both historically, over the course of evolution, and within individual human life spans. These dynamics suggest a sort of evolutionary social arms race in which the evolving vertebrate immune system initially begins to discriminate periods of increased viral risk (i.e., periods of affine social contact) and temporally concentrates its physiologically costly antiviral responses therein; viruses then "discover" that vertebrate transcriptional niche and evolve a complementary transcriptional program to concentrate their reactivation resources outside those periods of relatively high social-signal transduction (i.e., during periods of social isolation/ stress). Ultimately, this suggests a dizzying breadth of connection between the macroenvironmental conditions that shape human social experience and the microbiological and molecular processes that underlie our physical health.

Perhaps the deepest implication of a socially sensitive genome concerns our understanding of individual identity at the molecular biological level. Because socioenvironmental conditions influence gene expression, and those transcriptional dynamics in turn shape the molecular characteristics of our bodies for weeks to months afterward (as noted earlier, the average half-life of a protein in the human body is ~80 days), our bodies are gradually re-programmed over time based on our cumulative life history and environmental exposures. To the extent that the molecular characteristics of our cells define "who we are" molecularly, the social genomic relationships outlined above belie two fundamental tenants of our individualistic conception of the self: continuity and independence. We generally experience ourselves as stable individual beings who live in the world but are fundamentally separate from it. However, the data already reviewed show that the world around us can alter the activity of some of our most fundamentally internal and self-defining features: the activity of our genes. We are who we are transcriptionally *in part* because of who we have spent time with, the trail of physical and social ecologies we have inhabited, and our subjective psychological reactions to our socialenvironmental life histories.

The fundamental permeability of our bodies to our current social conditions and accumulated life histories may seem counterintuitive and perhaps even a bit frightening in the context of the Western individualist conception of identity. After all, this implies that key molecular characteristics of our bodies are shaped by external conditions over which we may have little control. But, from another perspective, social regulation of gene expression also provides a serendipitous opportunity to shape the molecular composition of our bodies, and the specific realization of our DNA-endowed potential, by strategically altering our physical and social environments. These dynamics may be particularly pronounced in the context of the immune system, which is genetically programmed to adapt to the individual's environment and develop different functional potentialities based on the conditions empirically encountered over an individual's life history. What the social-signal transduction pathways outlined earlier imply is that both the molecular characteristics of our pathogenic microenvironment and the macrolevel characteristics of our social and psychological conditions play joint roles in shaping the evolution of our immune-response transcriptomes.

Conclusion

An emerging pattern of results in social genomics research suggests that the mammalian immune system has evolved a set of conserved transcriptional responses to broad dimensions of variation in social conditions, including a propensity to downregulate innate antiviral responses and upregulate inflammatory defenses against wound-related injury during periods of social adversity and a propensity to reverse those dynamics during periods of more affine, supportive, and intimate social contact. Those changes in the basal leukocyte transcriptome correspond to changes in the general probability of exposure to intracellular versus extracellular pathogens (e.g., viruses versus bacteria) as a result of differential social conditions. These dynamics are fundamentally mediated by subjective perceptions of threat versus safety generated by limbic-system neural structures (as opposed to objective characteristics of the external situation) and are molecularly distributed into cellular transcriptional alterations via well known stress-responsive neural and endocrine-response systems such as the SNS and HPA axis.

Socially induced transcriptional dynamics include both acute changes and longer-term remodeling of neurobiological structures that exert a tonic bias on leukocyte gene expression (e.g., increased arborization of SNS nerve fibers in lymphoid organs). The temporal persistence of molecular remodeling and its ability to recursively shape cells' future responses to environmental conditions (including antigenic stimulation) create feedback loops and dynamic regulatory regimes that allow relatively transient exposures early in life to potentially exert an enduring bias over the subsequent evolution of immune responses to infectious diseases and inflammation-related health risks such as cardiovascular disease and cancer later in life.

Social regulation of immune response gene expression appears to have evolved early in mammalian speciation, as indicated by the role of phylogenetically ancient mononuclear phagocytes in mediating such effects, and by the co-evolution of transcriptional counterstrategies against such dynamics by many of our most successful viral parasites. The net result is a human immune system attuned to our social environmental systems in a way that may have optimized historical protection against socially transmitted diseases, but now predisposes us to the development of chronic inflammation and related diseases under contemporary adverse social conditions. By mapping the specific genetic programs activated by distinct modes of social adversity and defining the social signal transduction pathways that mediate such effects, we may potentially be able to rationally target those molecular processes and thereby provide physiologic protection against the detrimental health consequences associated with social deprivation and experienced adversity.

Future Directions

As the field of social genomics continues to develop, some promising new areas of discovery include the following:

1. New social genomic themes in immune response. Suppression of Type I interferons and activation of pro-inflammatory cytokines secondary to glucocorticoid resistance have emerged as consistent gene-regulatory themes in immune cells from people confronting significant life adversity. As the number of leukocyte social genomics studies increase, we have growing statistical power to discover other transcriptional regulatory themes activated by social threat and adversity.

2. New social signal transduction pathways. Early social genomics studies have identified several specific transcription factors that appear to be sensitive to socioenvironmental conditions and mediate their impact on leukocyte transcriptional profiles (e.g., CREB, GR, NF-κB, GATA1). A growing evidence base will likely yield additional regulatory pathways that both shed light on the basic mechanisms of social genomics and can potentially serve as targets for health-protective interventions against the transcriptional effects of adversity.

3. Transcriptional mechanisms of positive psychology and resilience. Which genes and transcription control pathways are sensitive to positive psychological states? Does positive psychology simply buffer the known effects of adversity or does it activate qualitatively distinct transcription factors and genes? What is the evolutionary or teleologic basis for a distinct transcriptional impact of positive psychology?

4. Plasticity of the basal leukocyte transcriptome and immune response. To what extent can psychological or socioenvironmental interventions alter either the basal stance or the intra-organismic evolution of the leukocyte transcriptome? Are such dynamics sufficient to affect the course of emerging or established diseases? Which genes are most sensitive to such interventions, and which interventions are most efficacious in driving persistent changes? Conversely, which aspects of the developing immune-response transcriptome might become persistently biased or locked in by social-signal transduction events early in life?

5. The disease scope of social immunology dynamics. Social regulation of immune system gene expression appears to have evolved as part of an integrated biological and behavioral response to infectious diseases (McDade, 2003; Cole, 2006; Nunn & Altizer, 2006; Finch 2010). However, inflammatory and immune responses contribute (not always helpfully) to a wide variety of other health threats such as cardiovascular disease and cancer. How do social genomics dynamics play out in those contexts?

6. The role of social signal transduction in CNS function. To what extent does social signal transduction remodel gene expression in the CNS? Which genes are targeted and which transcription factors mediate those effects? Although the specific mechanisms and genomic targets are likely to differ from those modulated in immune cells, does the CNS transcriptional response to socioenvironmental conditions serve the same defensive programming ends? Does social isolation or compresence activate neurobiological/behavioral defense programs in the same way that it appears to activate specific immune response modules (e.g., antiviral responses)?

7. Prospects for biological protection from socioenvironmental insults/reprogramming. One of the major motivations for analyzing social regulation of immune function involves the possibility of protecting individual health from the detrimental effects of socioenvironmental adversity (e.g., when it is not feasible or desirable to alter the upstream social conditions). To what extent can pharmacologic strategies mitigate the health risks arising from social genomic dynamics by targeting social-signal transduction pathways (e.g., beta-adrenergic blockade, glucocorticoid antagonism, etc.)?

8. The phylogenetic basis for social-signal transduction. Current evidence in humans, other primates, and model rodent species suggests that there may exist a relatively conserved transcriptionally mediated social sensitivity in vertebrate immune systems. Which leukocyte subtypes predominantly mediate those effects, and how far back in our phylogenetic history do such socially sensitive immune responses extend? Based on the observed transcriptional volatility within mononuclear phagocytes (monocytes, macrophages, and dendritic cells), it is tempting to speculate that these most deeply ancestral immune cells may be particularly sensitive to social, psychological, and neuroendocrine regulation. Are more recently emerging cell types such as T and B lymphocytes, or the ontologically linked NK cells, similarly sensitive? Or do T and B cells receive their predominant socio-neural/endocrine regulation via the mononuclear phagocytes that present antigens to them? In that sense, socioenvironmental information may travel through intercellular networks in parallel with micro-environmental antigen information.

Related Chapters

For more information on concepts introduced in this chapter, see also Cohen, this volume.

References

Antoni, M. H., Lutgendorf, S. K., Blomberg, B., Carvers, C. S., Lechner, S., Diaz, A., et al. (2012). Cognitive-behavioral stress management reverses anxiety-related leukocyte transcriptional dynamics. *Biological Psychiatry, 71*(4), 366–372.

Antoni, M. H., Lutgendorf, S. K., Cole, S. W., Dhabhar, F. S., Sephton, S. E., McDonald, P. G., et al. (2006). The influence of bio-behavioural factors on tumour biology: pathways and mechanisms. *Nature Reviews Cancer., 6*(3), 240–248.

Bamberger, C. M., Schulte, H. M., & Chrousos, G. P. (1996). Molecular determinants of glucocorticoid receptor function and tissue sensitivity to glucocorticoids. *Endocrinology Review., 17*(3), 245–261.

Bartholomew, J. S., Glenville, S., Sarkar, S., Burt, D. J., Stanley, M. A., Ruiz-Cabello, F., et al. (1997). Integration of high-risk human papillomavirus DNA is linked to the down-regulation of class I human leukocyte antigens by steroid hormones in cervical tumor cells. *Cancer Research, 57*(5), 937–942.

Berman, E. J., & Hill, J. M. (1985). Spontaneous ocular shedding of HSV-1 in latently infected rabbits. *Investigative Ophthalmology and Visual Science, 26*(4), 587–590.

Bloom, D. C., Stevens, J. G., Hill, J. M., & Tran, R. K. (1997). Mutagenesis of a cAMP response element within the latency-associated transcript promoter of HSV-1 reduces adrenergic reactivation. *Virology, 236*(1), 202–207.

Bonneau, R. H. (1996). Stress-induced effects on integral immune components involved in herpes simplex virus (HSV)-specific memory cytotoxic T lymphocyte activation. *Brain, Behavior and Immunity, 10*(2), 139–163.

Broadbent, D. E., Broadbent, M. H., Phillpotts, R. J., & Wallace, J. (1984). Some further studies on the prediction of experimental colds in volunteers by psychological factors. *Journal of Psychosomatic Research, 28*, 511–523.

Bromberg-White, J. L., & Meyers, C. (2003). Comparison of the basal and glucocorticoid-inducible activities of the upstream regulatory regions of HPV18 and HPV31 in multiple epithelial cell lines. *Virology, 306*(2), 197–202.

Cacioppo, J. T., & Hawkley, L. C. (2009). Perceived social isolation and cognition. *Trends in Cognitive Sciences, 13*(10), 447–454. Epub 2009 Aug 2031.

Cacioppo, J. T., Kiecolt-Glaser, J. K., Malarkey, W. B., Laskowski, B. F., Rozlog, L. A., Poehlmann, K. M., et al. (2002). Autonomic and glucocorticoid associations with the steady-state expression of latent Epstein-Barr virus. *Hormones and Behavior, 42*(1), 32–41.

Capitanio, J. P., Abel, K., Mendoza, S. P., Blozis, S. A., McChesney, M. B., Cole, S. W., et al. (2008). Personality and serotonin transporter genotype interact with social context to affect immunity and viral set-point in simian immunodeficiency virus disease. *Brain, Behavior and Immunity, 22*(5), 676–689. Epub 2007 Aug 2023.

Capitanio, J. P., Mendoza, S. P., & Baroncelli, S. (1999). The relationship of personality dimensions in adult male rhesus macaques to progression of simian immunodeficiency virus disease. *Brain, Behavior, and Immunity, 13*(2), 138–154.

Carlson, S. L., Albers, K. M., Beiting, D. J., Parish, M., Conner, J. M., & Davis, B. M. (1995). NGF modulates sympathetic innervation of lymphoid tissues. *Journal of Neuroscience, 15*, 5892–5899.

Carlson, S. L., Johnson, S., Parrish, M. E., & Cass, W. A. (1998). Development of immune hyperinnervation in NGF-transgenic mice. *Experimental Neurology, 149*(1), 209–220.

Caspi, A., Harrington, H., Moffitt, T. E., Milne, B. J., & Poulton, R. (2006). Socially isolated children 20 years later: risk of cardiovascular disease. *Archives of Pediatric and Adolescent Medicine, 160*(8), 805–811.

Champagne, F. A., & Mashoodh, R. (2009). Genes in context: gene-environment interplay and the origins of individual differences in behavior. *Current Directions in Psychological Science, 18*(3), 127–131.

Chang, M., Brown, H., Collado-Hidalgo, A., Arevalo, J., Galic, Z., Symensma, T., et al. (2005). Beta-adrenoreceptors reactivate KSHV lytic replication via PKA-dependent control of viral RTA. *Journal of Virology, 79*(21), 13538–13547.

Chen, E., Miller, G. E., Kobor, M. S., & Cole, S. W. (2011). Maternal warmth buffers the effects of low early-life socioeconomic status on pro-inflammatory signaling in adulthood. *Molecular Psychiatry, 16*(7), 729–737.

Chen, E., Miller, G. E., Walker, H. A., Arevalo, J. M., Sung, C. Y., & Cole, S. W. (2009). Genome-wide transcriptional profiling linked to social class in asthma. *Thorax., 64*(1), 38–43. Epub 2008 Nov 2010.

Chou, C. K., Wang, L. H., Lin, H. M., & Chi, C. W. (1992). Glucocorticoid stimulates hepatitis B viral gene expression in cultured human hepatoma cells. *Hepatology, 16*(1), 13–18.

Cid, A., Auewarakul, P., Garcia-Carranca, A., Ovseiovich, R., Gaissert, H., & Gissmann, L. (1993). Cell-type-specific activity of the human papillomavirus type 18 upstream regulatory region in transgenic mice and its modulation by tetradecanoyl phorbol acetate and glucocorticoids. *Journal of Virology, 67*(11), 6742–6752.

Cohen, S., Doyle, W. J., Skoner, D. P., Rabin, B. S., & Gwaltney, J. M. (1997). Social ties and susceptibility to the common cold. *JAMA, 227*, 1940–1944.

Cohen, S., Janicki-Deverts, D., & Miller, G. E. (2007). Psychological stress and disease. *JAMA, 298*(14), 1685–1687.

Cole, S., Arevalo, J., Takahashi, R., Sloan, E. K., Lutgendorf, S., Sood, A. K., et al. (2010). Computational identification of gene-social environment interaction at the human IL6 locus. *Proceedings of the National Academy of Science USA, 107*(12), 5681–5686.

Cole, S. W. (2006). Social threat, personal identity, and physical health in closeted gay men. In A. M. Omoto & H. S. Kurtzman (Eds.), *Sexual orientation and mental health* (pp. 245–268). Washington DC: American Psychological Association.

Cole, S. W. (2008a). Psychosocial influences on HIV-1 disease progression: neural, endocrine, and virologic mechanisms. *Psychosomatic Medicine, 70*(5), 562–568.

Cole, S. W. (2008b). Social regulation of leukocyte homeostasis: The role of glucocorticoid sensitivity. *Brain, Behavior and Immunity, 22*(7), 1049–1055.

Cole, S. W., Conti, G., Arevalo, J. M., Ruggiero, A. M., Heckman, J. J., & Suomi, S. J. (2012). Transcriptional modulation of the developing immune system by early life social adversity. *Under review.*

Cole, S. W., Hawkley, L. C., Arevalo, J. M., & Cacioppo, J. T. (2011) Transcript origin analysis identifies antigen presenting cells as primary targets of socially regulated gene expression in leukocytes. *Proceedings of the National Academy of Sciences USA,* 108, 3080–3085.

Cole, S. W., Hawkley, L. C., Arevalo, J. M., Sung, C. Y., Rose, R. M., & Cacioppo, J. T. (2007). Social regulation of gene expression in human leukocytes. *Genome Biology, 8*(R189), 1–13.

Cole, S. W., Jamieson, B. D., & Zack, J. A. (1999). cAMP externalizes lymphocyte CXCR4: Implications for chemotaxis and HIV infection. *Journal of Immunology, 162*, 1392–1400.

Cole, S. W., Kemeny, M. E., Fahey, J. L., Zack, J. A., & Naliboff, B. D. (2003). Psychological risk factors for HIV pathogenesis: Mediation by the autonomic nervous system. *Biological Psychiatry, 54*, 1444–1456.

Cole, S. W., Kemeny, M. E., & Taylor, S. E. (1997). Social identity and physical health: Accelerated HIV progression in rejection-sensitive gay men. *Journal of Personality and Social Psychology, 72*, 320–336.

Cole, S. W., Kemeny, M. E., Weitzman, O. B., Schoen, M., & Anton, P. A. (1999). Socially inhibited individuals show heightened DTH response during intense social engagement. *Brain, Behavior, and Immunity, 13*, 187–200.

Cole, S. W., Korin, Y. D., Fahey, J. L., & Zack, J. A. (1998). Norepinephrine accelerates HIV replication via protein kinase A-dependent effects on cytokine production. *Journal of Immunology, 161*, 610–616.

Cole, S. W., Mendoza, S. P., & Capitanio, J. P. (2009). Social stress desensitizes lymphocytes to regulation by endogenous glucocorticoids: insights from in vivo cell trafficking dynamics in rhesus macaques. *Psychosomatic Medicine, 71*(6), 591–597. Epub 2009 Jun 2024.

Cole, S. W., Naliboff, B. D., Kemeny, M. E., Griswold, M. P., Fahey, J. L., & Zack, J. A. (2001). Impaired response to HAART in HIV-infected individuals with high autonomic nervous system activity. *Proceedings of the National Academy of Sciences USA., 98*, 12695–12700.

Cole, S. W., Yan, W., Galic, Z., Arevalo, J., & Zack, J. A. (2005). Expression-based monitoring of transcription factor activity: The TELiS database. *Bioinformatics, 21*(6), 803–810.

Collado-Hidalgo, A., Sung, C., & Cole, S. (2006). Adrenergic inhibition of innate anti-viral response: PKA blockade of Type I interferon gene transcription mediates catecholamine support for HIV-1 replication. *Brain, Behavior and Immunity, 20*(6), 552–563. Epub 2006 Feb 2028.

Dickerson, S. S., & Kemeny, M. E. (2004). Acute stressors and cortisol responses: a theoretical integration and synthesis of laboratory research. *Psychology Bulletin, 130*(3), 355–391.

Dimsdale, J. E., & Moss, J. (1980). Plasma catecholamines in stress and exercise. *JAMA, 243*(4), 340–342.

Dobbs, C. M., Vasquez, M., Glaser, R., & Sheridan, J. F. (1993). Mechanisms of stress-induced modulation of viral pathogenesis and immunity. *Journal of Neuroimmunology, 48*(2), 151–160.

Durst, M., Gallahan, D., Jay, G., & Rhim, J. S. (1989). Glucocorticoid-enhanced neoplastic transformation of human keratinocytes by human papillomavirus type 16 and an activated ras oncogene. *Virology, 173*(2), 767–771.

Dusek, J. A., Otu, H. H., Wohlhueter, A. L., Bhasin, M., Zerbini, L. F., Joseph, M. G., et al. (2008). Genomic counter-stress changes induced by the relaxation response. *PLoS ONE., 3*(7), e2576.

Farza, H., Salmon, A. M., Hadchouel, M., Moreau, J. L., Babinet, C., Tiollais, P., et al. (1987). Hepatitis B surface antigen gene expression is regulated by sex steroids and glucocorticoids in transgenic mice. *Proceedings of the National Academy of Science USA, 84*(5), 1187–1191.

Finch, C. E. (2010). Evolution in health and medicine Sackler colloquium: Evolution of the human lifespan and diseases of aging: roles of infection, inflammation, and nutrition. *Proceedings of the National Academy of Science USA, 1,* 1718–1724.

Frankenhauser, M. (1975). Experimental approaches to the study of catecholamines and emotion. In L. Levi (Ed.), *Emotions—Their paramters and measurement.* New York: Raven Press.

Gibson, G. (2008). The environmental contribution to gene expression profiles. *National Review of Genetics, 9*(8), 575–581.

Glaser, R., Kutz, L. A., MacCallum, R. C., & Malarkey, W. B. (1995). Hormonal modulation of Epstein-Barr virus replication. *Neuroendocrinology, 62*(4), 356–361.

Glaser, R., Rabin, B., Chesney, M., Cohen, S., & Natelson, B. (1999). Stress-induced immunomodulation: Implications for infectious diseases. *JAMA, 281*(24), 2268–2270.

Gloss, B., Bernard, H. U., Seedorf, K., Klock, G., von Knebel Doeberitz, M., Bauknecht, T., et al. (1987). The upstream regulatory region of the human papilloma virus-16 contains an E2 protein-independent enhancer which is specific for cervical carcinoma cells and regulated by glucocorticoid hormones. *EMBO Journal, 6*(12), 3735–3743 PMID- 1847520.

Grebe, K. M., Hickman, H. D., Irvine, K. R., Takeda, K., Bennink, J. R., & Yewdell, J. W. (2009). Sympathetic nervous system control of anti-influenza CD8+ T cell responses. *Proceedings of the National Academy of Science USA., 106*(13), 5300–5305. Epub 2009 Mar 5313.

Gripon, P., Diot, C., Corlu, A., & Guguen-Guillouzo, C. (1989). Regulation by dimethylsulfoxide, insulin, and corticosteroids of hepatitis B virus replication in a transfected human hepatoma cell line. *Journal of Medical Virology, 28*(3), 193–199.

Hamilton, W. D. (1964). The genetical evolution of social bahaviour. II. *Journal of Theoretical Biology, 7,* 17–52.

Hamrick, N., Cohen, S., & Rodriguez, M. S. (2002). Being popular can be healthy or unhealthy: stress, social network diversity, and incidence of upper respiratory infection. *Health Psychology, 21*(3), 294–298.

Heckman, J. J. (2007). The economics, technology, and neuroscience of human capability formation. *Proceedings of the National Academy of Science USA., 104*(33), 13250–13255. Epub 12007 Aug 13258.

Henry, J. P. (1992). Biological basis of the stress response. *Integrative Physiological and Behavioral Science, 27*(1), 66–83.

Henry, J. P., & Stephens, P. M. (1977). *Stress, health, and the social environment.* New York: Springer-Verlag.

Hoffmann, J. A., Kafatos, F. C., Janeway, C. A., & Ezekowitz, R. A. (1999). Phylogenetic perspectives in innate immunity. *Science., 284*(5418), 1313–1318.

Idaghdour, Y., Storey, J. D., Jadallah, S. J., & Gibson, G. (2008). A genome-wide gene expression signature of environmental geography in leukocytes of Moroccan Amazighs. *PLoS Genet., 4*(4), e1000052.

Irwin, M. R., Wang, M., Campomayor, C. O., Collado-Hidalgo, A., & Cole, S. (2006). Sleep deprivation and activation of morning levels of cellular and genomic markers of inflammation. *Archives of Internal Medicine, 166*(16), 1756–1762.

Janeway, C. A., Travers, P., Walport, M., & Shlomchik, M. J. (2001). *Immunobiology,* (5th ed.). New York: Garland Science.

Kagan, J. (1994). *Galen's prophecy: Temperament in human nature.* New York: Basic Books.

Kagan, J., Reznick, J. S., & Snidman, N. (1988). Biological bases of childhood shyness. *Science, 240,* 167–171.

Kalinichenko, V. V., Mokyr, M. B., Graf, L. H., Jr., Cohen, R. L., & Chambers, D. A. (1999). Norepinephrine-mediated inhibition of antitumor cytotoxic T lymphocyte generation involves a beta-adrenergic receptor mechanism and decreased TNF-alpha gene expression. *Journal of Immunology, 163*(5), 2492–2499.

Kamradt, M. C., Mohideen, N., & Vaughan, A. T. (2000). RU486 increases radiosensitivity and restores apoptosis through modulation of HPV E6/E7 in dexamethasone-treated cervical carcinoma cells. *Gynecology and Oncology, 77*(1), 177–182.

Karssen, A. M., Her, S., Li, J. Z., Patel, P. D., Meng, F., Bunney, W. E., Jr., et al. (2007). Stress-induced changes in primate prefrontal profiles of gene expression. *Molecular Psychiatry, 12*(12), 1089–1102. Epub 2007 Sep 1025.

Kauffman, S. (1993). *The origins of order: Self-organization and selection in evolution.* Oxford, England: Oxford University Press.

Khare, S., Pater, M. M., Tang, S. C., & Pater, A. (1997). Effect of glucocorticoid hormones on viral gene expression, growth, and dysplastic differentiation in HPV16-immortalized ectocervical cells. *Experimental Cell Research, 232*(2), 353–360.

Kim, H. D., Shay, T., O'Shea, E. K., & Regev, A. (2009). Transcriptional regulatory circuits: predicting numbers from alphabets. *Science., 325*(5939), 429–432.

Knipe, D. M., Howley, P. M., Griffin, D. E., Lamb, R. A., Martin, M. A., Roizman, B., et al. (2007). *Fields virology* (5th ed.). Philadelphia: Lippincott Williams & Wilkins.

Kupfer, S. R., & Summers, W. C. (1990). Identification of a glucocorticoid-responsive element in Epstein-Barr virus. *Journal of Virology, 64*(5), 1984–1990.

Lau, J. Y., Bain, V. G., Smith, H. M., Alexander, G. J., & Williams, R. (1992). Modulation of hepatitis B viral antigen expression by immunosuppressive drugs in primary hepatocyte culture. *Transplantation, 53*(4), 894–898.

Lutgendorf, S. K., Lamkin, D. M., Jennings, N. B., Arevalo, J. M., Penedo, F., DeGeest, K., et al. (2008). Biobehavioral influences on matrix metalloproteinase expression in ovarian carcinoma. *Clinical Cancer Research, 14*(21), 6839–6846.

Magy, N., Cribier, B., Schmitt, C., Ellero, B., Jaeck, D., Boudjema, K., et al. (1999). Effects of corticosteroids on

HCV infection. *International Journal of Immunopharmacology, 21*(4), 253–261.

Martinez, F. O., Gordon, S., Locati, M., & Mantovani, A. (2006). Transcriptional profiling of the human monocyte-to-macrophage differentiation and polarization: new molecules and patterns of gene expression. *Journal of Immunology, 177*(10), 7303–7311.

Martinez, F. O., Sica, A., Mantovani, A., & Locati, M. (2008). Macrophage activation and polarization. *Frontiers in Bioscience, 13*, 453–461.

May, R. M., & Anderson, R. M. (1983). Epidemiology and genetics in the coevolution of parasites and hosts. *Proceedings of the Royal Society, London, B, 219*, 281–313.

McDade, T. W. (2003). Life history theory and the immune system: Steps toward a human ecological immunology. *American Journal of Physical Anthropology, 37*, 100–125.

Millar, D. A., & Ratcliffe, N. A. (1989). The evolution of blood cells: Facts and enigmas. *Endeavour., 13*(2), 72–77.

Miller, G., Chen, E., & Cole, S. W. (2009). Health psychology: Developing biologically plausible models linking the social world and physical health. *Annual Review of Psychology, 60*, 501–524.

Miller, G. E., Chen, E., Fok, A. K., Walker, H., Lim, A., Nicholls, E. F., et al. (2009). Low early-life social class leaves a biological residue manifested by decreased glucocorticoid and increased proinflammatory signaling. *Proceedings of the National Academy of Science USA., 106*(34), 14716–14721. Epub 12009 Jul 14714.

Miller, G. E., Chen, E., Sze, J., Marin, T., Arevalo, J. M., Doll, R., et al. (2008). A functional genomic fingerprint of chronic stress in humans: blunted glucocorticoid and increased NF-kappaB signaling. *Biological Psychiatry., 64*(4), 266–272. Epub 2008 Apr 2028.

Miller, G. E., Cohen, S., Rabin, B. S., Skoner, D. P., & Doyle, W. J. (1999). Personality and tonic cardiovascular, neuroendocrine, and immune parameters. *Brain, Behavior, and Immunity, 13*, 109–123.

Millhouse, S., Kenny, J. J., Quinn, P. G., Lee, V., & Wigdahl, B. (1998). ATF/CREB elements in the herpes simplex virus type 1 latency-associated transcript promoter interact with members of the ATF/CREB and AP-1 transcription factor families. *Journal of Biomedical Science, 5*(6), 451–464.

Mills, C. D., Kincaid, K., Alt, J. M., Heilman, M. J., & Hill, A. M. (2000). M-1/M-2 macrophages and the Th1/Th2 paradigm. *Journal of Immunology, 164*(12), 6166–6173.

Mittal, R., Pater, A., & Pater, M. M. (1993). Multiple human papillomavirus type 16 glucocorticoid response elements functional for transformation, transient expression, and DNA-protein interactions. *Journal of Virology, 67*(9), 5656–5659.

Mittal, R., Tsutsumi, K., Pater, A., & Pater, M. M. (1993). Human papillomavirus type 16 expression in cervical keratinocytes: role of progesterone and glucocorticoid hormones. *Obstetrics and Gynecology, 81*(1), 5–12.

Morita, K., Saito, T., Ohta, M., Ohmori, T., Kawai, K., Teshima-Kondo, S., et al. (2005). Expression analysis of psychological stress-associated genes in peripheral blood leukocytes. *Neuroscience Letters, 381*(1–2), 57–62. Epub 2005 Feb 2016.

Nater, U. M., Whistler, T., Lonergan, W., Mletzko, T., Vernon, S. D., & Heim, C. (2009). Impact of acute psychosocial stress on peripheral blood gene expression pathways in healthy men. *Biological Psychology, 82*(2), 125–132. Epub 2009 Jul 2003.

Nunn, C. L., & Altizer, S. M. (2006). *Infectious diseases in primates: Behavior, ecology and evolution.* Oxford University Press (Series in Ecology and Evolution).

Ornish, D., Magbanua, M. J., Weidner, G., Weinberg, V., Kemp, C., Green, C., et al. (2008). Changes in prostate gene expression in men undergoing an intensive nutrition and lifestyle intervention. *Proceedings of the National Academy of Science USA., 105*(24), 8369–8374. Epub 2008 Jun 8316.

Pace, T. W., Hu, F., & Miller, A. H. (2007). Cytokine-effects on glucocorticoid receptor function: Relevance to glucocorticoid resistance and the pathophysiology and treatment of major depression. *Brain, Behavior and Immunity, 21*(1), 9–19. Epub 2006 Oct 2027.

Pater, M. M., Hughes, G. A., Hyslop, D. E., Nakshatri, H., & Pater, A. (1988). Glucocorticoid-dependent oncogenic transformation by type 16 but not type 11 human papilloma virus DNA. *Nature, 335*(6193), 832–835.

Pater, M. M., & Pater, A. (1991). RU486 inhibits glucocorticoid hormone-dependent oncogenesis by human papillomavirus type 16 DNA. *Virology, 183*(2), 799–802.

Piccini, A., Storey, A., Romanos, M., & Banks, L. (1997). Regulation of human papillomavirus type 16 DNA replication by E2, glucocorticoid hormone and epidermal growth factor. *Journal of General Virology, 78*(Pt 8), 1963–1970.

Pressman, S. D., Cohen, S., Miller, G. E., Barkin, A., Rabin, B. S., & Treanor, J. J. (2005). Loneliness, social network size, and immune response to influenza vaccination in college freshmen. *Health Psychology, 24*(3), 297–306.

Rader, K. A., Ackland-Berglund, C. E., Miller, J. K., Pepose, J. S., & Leib, D. A. (1993). In vivo characterization of site-directed mutations in the promoter of the herpes simplex virus type 1 latency-associated transcripts. *Journal of General Virology, 74*(Pt 9), 1859–1869.

Sapolsky, R. M. (1994). *Why zebras don't get ulcers: A guide to stress, stress-related diseases, and coping.* New York: Freeman.

Schuster, C., Chasserot-Golaz, S., & Beck, G. (1991). Activation of Epstein-Barr virus promoters by a growth-factor and a glucocorticoid. *FEBS Letters, 284*(1), 82–86.

Schuster, C., Chasserot-Golaz, S., Urier, G., Beck, G., & Sergeant, A. (1991). Evidence for a functional glucocorticoid responsive element in the Epstein-Barr virus genome. *Molecular Endocrinology, 5*(2), 267–272.

Schwartz, C. E., Wright, C. I., Shin, L. M., Kagan, J., & Rauch, S. L. (2003). Inhibited and uninhibited infants "grown up": Adult amygdalar response to novelty. *Science., 300*(5627), 1952–1953.

Seeman, T. E. (1996). Social ties and health: the benefits of social integration. *Annals of Epidemiology, 6*(5), 442–451.

Selvey, L. A., Dunn, L. A., Tindle, R. W., Park, D. S., & Frazer, I. H. (1994). Human papillomavirus (HPV) type 18 E7 protein is a short-lived steroid-inducible phosphoprotein in HPV-transformed cell lines. *Journal of General Virology, 75*(Pt 7), 1647–1653.

Sloan, E. K., Capitanio, J. P., & Cole, S. W. (2008). Stress-induced remodeling of lymphoid innervation. *Brain, Behavior and Immunity, 22*(1), 15–21. Epub 2007 Aug 2013.

Sloan, E. K., Capitanio, J. P., Tarara, R. P., & Cole, S. W. (2008). Social temperament and lymph node innervation. *Brain, Behavior and Immunity, 22*(5), 717–726. Epub 2007 Dec 2018.

Sloan, E. K., Capitanio, J. P., Tarara, R. P., Mendoza, S. P., Mason, W. A., & Cole, S. W. (2007). Social stress enhances sympathetic innervation of primate lymph nodes: mechanisms and implications for viral pathogenesis. *Journal of Neuroscience, 27*(33), 8857–8865.

Stark, J., Avitsur, R., Padgett, D. A., & Sheridan, J. F. (2001). Social stress induces glucocorticoid resistance in macrophages. *American Journal of Physiology: Regulatory. Integrative, and Comparitive Physiology, 280*, R1799–R1805.

Steiner, I., & Kennedy, G. E. (1993). Molecular biology of herpes simplex virus type 1 latency in the nervous system. *Molecular Neurobiology, 7*(2), 137–159.

Sterling, P. (2004). Principles of allostasis: Optimal design, predictive regulation, pathophysiology and rational therapeutics. In J. Schulkin (Ed.), *Allostasis, homeostasis, and the costs of physiological adaptation.* Cambridge, England: Cambridge University Press.

Thaker, P. H., Han, L. Y., Kamat, A. A., Arevalo, J. M., Takahashi, R., Lu, C., et al. (2006). Chronic stress promotes tumor growth and angiogenesis in a mouse model of ovarian carcinoma. *Nature Medicine, 12*(8), 939–944. Epub 2006 Jul 2023.

Totman, R., Kiff, J., Reed, S. A., & Craig, J. W. (1980). Predicting experimental colds in volunteers from different measures of recent life stress. *Journal of Psychosomatic Research, 24*, 155–163.

Tur-Kaspa, R., Burk, R. D., Shaul, Y., & Shafritz, D. A. (1986). Hepatitis B virus DNA contains a glucocorticoid-responsive element. *Proceedings of the National Academy of Science USA, 83*(6), 1627–1631.

Tur-Kaspa, R., & Laub, O. (1990). Corticosteroids stimulate hepatitis B virus DNA, mRNA and protein production in a stable expression system. *Journal of Hepatology, 11*(1), 34–36.

Tur-Kaspa, R., Shaul, Y., Moore, D. D., Burk, R. D., Okret, S., Poellinger, L., et al. (1988). The glucocorticoid receptor recognizes a specific nucleotide sequence in hepatitis B virus DNA causing increased activity of the HBV enhancer. *Virology, 167*(2), 630–633.

Wang, K., Krause, P. R., & Straus, S. E. (1995). Analysis of the promoter and cis-acting elements regulating expression of herpes simplex virus type 2 latency-associated transcripts. *Journal of Virology, 69*(5), 2873–2880.

Weaver, I. C., Meaney, M. J., & Szyf, M. (2006). Maternal care effects on the hippocampal transcriptome and anxiety-mediated behaviors in the offspring that are reversible in adulthood. *Proceedings of the National Academy of Science USA., 103*(9), 3480–3485. Epub 2006 Feb 3416.

Weiner, H. (1992). *Perturbing the organism: The biology of stressful experience.* Chicago: University of Chicago Press.

Wheatley, S. C., Dent, C. L., Wood, J. N., & Latchman, D. S. (1992). Elevation of cyclic AMP levels in cell lines derived from latently infectable sensory neurons increases their permissivity for herpes virus infection by activating the viral immediate-early 1 gene promoter. *Brain Research/ Molecular Brain Research, 12*(1–3), 149–154.

Yokosuka, O. (2000). Role of steroid priming in the treatment of chronic hepatitis B. *Journal of Gastroenterology and Hepatology, 15*(Suppl), E41–45.

Zhang, T. Y., Bagot, R., Parent, C., Nesbitt, C., Bredy, T. W., Caldji, C., et al. (2006). Maternal programming of defensive responses through sustained effects on gene expression. *Biological Psychology, 73*(1), 72–89. Epub 2006 Feb 2028.

PART 5

Ecological Approaches

Comparative Psychoneuroimmunology/ Ecoimmunology: Lessons from Simpler Model Systems

Shelley A. Adamo

Abstract

Immune-behavioral interactions are widespread throughout the animal kingdom. For example, decreased feeding after immune activation is common in animals. Work with insects suggests that changes in feeding behavior during an immune response (e.g., illness-induced anorexia) may be a behavioral method of biasing multifunctional physiological pathways toward immune function. Work on insects also suggests that stress hormones help to reconfigure the immune system in order to optimize its performance during the physiological shifts required for "flight-or-fight." The effects of stress hormones on immune function appear maladaptive only when compared to what the animal could do under optimal conditions. Work with insects also cautions against overly simplistic interpretations of immune assay results. A comparative approach to psychoneuroimmunology will increase our understanding of the adaptive function of immune-behavioral interactions. Understanding why these connections exist is of both practical and theoretical importance.

Key Words: insect, invertebrate, stress, octopamine, illness-induced anorexia, sickness behavior, immune assay, immune system, behavior

Introduction. The Benefits of the Comparative Approach for Psychoneuroimmunology

The behavior of people and animals influences their ability to resist disease (Ader, 2007). The effect also runs in the other direction; that is, infection or illness causes predictable changes in behavior (Ader, 2007). Behavior alters immunity and immune activity alters behavior because both the nervous system and immune system have receptors for each other's modulators (e.g., see Sanders and Kavelaars, 2007; Dantzer, 2004). For example, neurons have receptors for immune regulators such as cytokines (Danter, 2007), and immune cells (e.g., macrophages) have receptors for neuromodulators such as norepinephrine (Sanders and Kavelaars, 2007). Moreover, specialized pathways allow signals from immune cells in the periphery to cross the blood-brain barrier to affect central nervous system function (Dantzer, 2004). The existence of these receptors and specialized pathways strongly suggests that bidirectional connections between the immune and nervous system are adaptive; otherwise it is difficult to imagine how these intricate connections evolved. Moreover, connections between the immune system and nervous system exist across phyla (Ottaviani and Franceschi, 1996; Cohen and Kinney, 2007; Adamo 2008a). This ubiquitousness suggests either that these connections have been conserved across hundreds of millions of years or that they have arisen multiple times independently. Either way, their widespread occurrence strongly suggests that these connections serve an important function.

Despite strong circumstantial evidence supporting the functional importance of immune-neural-behavioral interactions, we frequently know more about the mechanisms mediating these interactions than we do about why they exist. This gap in our knowledge prevents a full understanding of psychoneuroimmunological phenomena. More practically, this gap also presents a danger to those designing treatments to remove specific immune-neural interactions (e.g., the effects of glucocorticoids and catecholamines on immune function). Removing a neural-immune connection without knowing its purpose could produce unintended negative consequences.

For example, the adaptive function of appetite loss due to illness (illness-induced anorexia) remains unclear, even though almost all organisms decrease feeding when sick (Adamo, 2006). Superficially, illness-induced anorexia seems maladaptive. An immune response is energetically expensive (Demas, Adamo, & French, 2011); therefore, why curtail energy intake when energy demand is surging? Various hypotheses exist (e.g., Hart, 1988; Aubert, Goodall, & Dantzer, 1995; Exton, 1997; Kyriazakis, Tolkamp, & Hutchings, 1998; Ayres & Schneider, 2009; Adamo, 2010), but a clear understanding of its functional significance remains elusive. In a second example, immune cells have receptors for various hormones (e.g., glucocorticoids; Schoneveld & Cidlowski, 2007). The effects of hormones (e.g., stress hormones) on immune function are typically complex (e.g., norepinephrine, Sanders and Kavelaars, 2007). How do these effects benefit the animal? Researchers have postulated functional explanations for them (e.g., the necessity of preventing immunopathology; Elenkov & Chrousos, 2006); however, the details remain unclear.

Ecological immunologists are also interested in why immune systems and nervous systems influence each other. Combining the approaches of both psychoneuroimmunology and ecological immunology has yielded a number of fruitful insights (e.g., Martin, 2009; Demas et al., 2011). Ecological immunology emphasizes the comparative approach, and ecological immunologists work on a broad variety of vertebrates and invertebrates (Demas et al., 2011). Such a comparative view may help uncover the potential adaptive function of immune-behavioral interactions. For example, examining the adaptive function of the two phenomena discussed earlier in simpler model systems, such as insects, could yield new insights. Immune-behavioral interactions are well-established in insects (Adamo, 2006) and other invertebrates (Ottaviani & Franceschi, 1996), although the mechanisms mediating these interactions (Ottaviani & Franceschi, 1996; Adamo, 2008b; Adamo, 2012) are not

as well understood in invertebrates as they are in vertebrates. Nevertheless, we do know that some of the molecular mechanisms connecting the nervous and immune systems in insects are similar to those used in mammals (Adamo, 2008a). Whether the adaptive functions of these connections are also similar remains to be seen, but knowing their functions in a few species would at least supply testable hypotheses. Insects have an advantage over vertebrates as model systems because their nervous systems, immune systems, and behaviors are simpler than those of vertebrates. For example, insects lack an acquired immune system (although they do have a form of immunological memory) (Pham & Schneider, 2008), making experiments easier to design and interpret. In this chapter, I use a comparative approach, emphasizing work on insects, to review evidence about why immune systems and nervous systems communicate.

Comparative Review of Sickness Behavior from an Ecoimmunological Perspective

Animals across phyla change their behaviors when ill (vertebrates: Aubert, 1999; Dantzer, 2004; Owen-Ashley and Wingfield, 2007; invertebrates: Adamo, 2006). These changes demonstrate a reconfiguration of the animal's motivational state (Aubert, 1999) that is thought to increase the animal's chance of survival (Hart, 1988). Intriguingly, most animals, regardless of taxa, show the same suite of behavioral changes after immune activation. Both vertebrates and invertebrates typically decrease feeding (illness-induced anorexia), locomotion, and reproduction after an immune challenge (Adamo, 2006). However, immune activity does not simply inhibit all behavior. For example, rodents reduce food intake after an immune challenge, but continue to store food (Aubert, Kelley, & Dantzer, 1997; Durazzo, Proud, & Demas, 2008). The ubiquitousness of sickness behavior suggests that it provides some basic advantage to animals.

If these behaviors are adaptive, sickness behavior should be suppressed when the cost of producing it reduces fitness more than the risk of succumbing to an infection. As predicted, sickness behavior is not a mandatory reflex that occurs after every infection, but its presence and severity depends on the ecological context. For example, male song sparrows (*Melospiza molida*) inhibit sickness behaviors (such as a reduction in territorial aggression) when they are immune challenged during the breeding season (Owen-Ashley and Wingfield, 2007). Similarly, illness-induced anorexia is suppressed in food-deprived rats (e.g., Gautron, Mingam, Moranis, Combe, & Laye, 2005). Presumably pro-inflammatory cytokines are still being released by mating birds and hungry rodents. In white-crowned sparrows, testosterone plays a role in the suppression of sickness behaviors during the breeding season (Ashley, Hayes, Bentley, & Wingfield, 2009), although whether it does this by decreasing the release of certain cytokines, preventing transmission of the immune signal to the brain, and/or altering the ability of neuronal cytokine receptors to alter behavior remains unknown. Progress has also been made in determining how fasting reduces illness-induced anorexia. Fasting modulates the effect of immune challenge on neurons in the brain (Gautron et al., 2005).

Although most animals show similar sickness behaviors, there are significant species differences. For example, many animals decrease social behavior when immune challenged (Dantzer, 2004). Rhesus monkeys, however, increase their social behavior after an immune challenge (Willette, Lubach, & Coe, 2007). Studying these "exceptions" could illuminate important information about both the selective pressures shaping sickness behavior as well as the physiology mediating it.

As sickness behavior shows some species specificity, it also shows pathogen specificity in both vertebrates (e.g., fever in humans; Eccles, 2005) and invertebrates (Ayres & Schneider, 2009). For example, crickets exhibit behavioral fever, that is, they migrate to warmer areas when infected with the intracellular parasite *Rickettsiella grylli* (Adamo, 1998). Warmer temperatures lead to increased pathogen mortality and increased host survival. However, the bacterial pathogen *Serratia marcescens* has a much higher heat tolerance than *R. grylli*, and is not negatively affected by the higher temperatures induced by behavioral fever (Adamo, 1998). Interestingly, crickets infected with *S. marcescens* do not exhibit behavioral fever (Adamo, 1998). In mammals as well, fever is not expressed to all pathogens (e.g., cold virus versus influenza virus; Eccles, 2005) even though it is thought to serve an important adaptive function in fighting disease (Kluger, Kozak, Conn, Leon, & Soszynski, 1996). Understanding how the expression of sickness behavior can be suppressed/not initiated by exposure to particular pathogens could have practical importance.

Immune challenge leads to reduced learning in both vertebrates (Dantzer et al., 2008) and insects (Mallon et al., 2003). In rodents, the decline in cognitive ability appears to be induced by immune factors acting on central nervous system sites known to be important for learning and memory (e.g., the hippocampus) (Dantzer, O'Connor, Freund, Johnson, & Kelley, 2008), again suggesting a host response. However, a recent review found that the effects of immune activation (e.g., using lipopolysaccharides) on learning and memory in vertebrates were not straightforward (Cunningham & Sanderson, 2008). Cunningham and Sanderson (2008) suggest that immune-challenged animals are not suffering from a cognitive decline per se, but that the decrease in learning is related more to motivational changes. Moreover, Cunningham and Sanderson (2008) point out that the effect sizes in these studies are often small, raising the question of their biological significance. However, in invertebrates, changes in the floral learning ability of immune-challenged bumblebees suggest that changes in learning during infection could be biologically important (Alghamdi, Dalton, Phillis, Rosato, & Mallon, 2008). One hypothesis is that decreased learning mitigates, or is in response to, an energy drain or other physiological conflict with immune function (e.g., Mallon, Brockman, & Schmid-Hempel, 2003). Therefore, the cognitive decline may enhance immune function, but no mechanisms have been proposed. In bumblebees, immune challenge (i.e., using lipopolysaccharides) decreases learning only when the insects are protein-deficient (Riddell & Mallon, 2006), supporting the notion that the decrease in learning could be an adaptive response to a resource problem. However, in both vertebrates and invertebrates, not all learning is decreased during illness. In fact, some forms of learning are enhanced. For example, the invertebrate *Caenorhabditis elegans* can learn to avoid pathogenic bacteria (Zhang et al. 2005). Exposure to pathogens increases the amount of serotonin in specific chemosensory neurons, leading to enhanced olfactory learning (Zhang et al. 2005). In vertebrates, nausea induces powerful one-trial learning (i.e., conditioned taste aversion; Dantzer, 2004). How, why, and under what conditions learning changes with illness requires more study.

Illness-Induced Anorexia

Illness-induced anorexia, the decline in feeding that occurs during an infection, remains a puzzle. Activating an immune response is energetically demanding in both vertebrates and invertebrates (Demas et al., 2011). Lack of energy (e.g., food deprivation) reduces disease resistance (e.g., Feder, Mello, Garcia, & Azambuja, 1997). Therefore, reducing food intake during an infection seems maladaptive. Yet, it is one of the most widely observed sickness behaviors, found in animals across phyla (Adamo, 2006). In insects, as in vertebrates (Dantzer, 2004), the decrease in feeding can be produced by the injection of an immunogen (e.g., peptidoglycan; Dunn, Bohnert, & Russell, 1994). This observation demonstrates that it is probably a host response.

How the immune system suppresses feeding in invertebrates is not well understood. However, there is some evidence supporting an immune/neural link in insects (Adamo, 2008b). During infection, the biogenic amine octopamine, a compound chemically similar to norepinephrine (Roeder, 2005), is released into the hemolymph (Dunphy and Downer, 1994; Adamo, 2010). The source of this octopamine is unclear. It might be released directly by the immune system via hemocytes (circulating immune cells, Adamo, 2005; Adamo, 2010) and/or indirectly by the central nervous system (Adamo, 2010). Neurons have receptors for octopamine; it is an important neuromodulator in insects (Roeder, 2005). Elevated levels of octopamine in the hemolymph disrupt the neural circuit responsible for swallowing in the caterpillar *Manduca sexta* (Miles and Booker, 2000). The disruption in swallowing reduces feeding, although other effects must also be occurring to produce all the symptoms of illness-induced anorexia in this species (e.g., a decrease in feeding initiation, i.e., feeding motivation; Adamo, 2005). Other biogenic amines (e.g., serotonin) may mediate illness-induced anorexia in other insects (e.g., locusts; Goldsworthy, 2010). Therefore, in vertebrates (Dantzer et al., 2008) and probably in insects, there are mechanisms allowing the immune response to suppress feeding. The evolution of such connections in two widely divergent groups of animals suggests that the ability to depress food intake during infection serves an important function.

Some possible beneficial effects of illness-induced anorexia have been suggested for vertebrates (e.g., Hart, 1988; Exton, 1997; Kyriazakis et al. 1998). However, some of these hypotheses are unlikely to be important in invertebrates. For example Hart (1988) argues that illness-induced anorexia reduces the urge to forage, allowing animals to remain huddled in a shelter, decreasing the cost of fever. Infected insects do not show endogenously generated fever (Moore, 2002), and, therefore, remaining in a shelter would not help them raise their body temperature. Are there hypotheses that could explain the existence of illness-induced anorexia in both groups of animals? The similarity of the behavior across phyla suggests the possibility that it might have a basic, highly conserved, function. However, this does not preclude the possibility that it may also have additional functions that differ between vertebrates and insects.

One of the most common hypotheses for the function of illness-induced anorexia is that it starves pathogens of nutrients, especially micronutrients such as iron (Hart, 1988; Exton, 1997). Both vertebrates and insects upregulate factors such as transferrin that reduce the availability of micronutrients such as iron in the blood (Ong, Ho, Ho, & Ding, 2006). The reduction in iron availability to pathogens is important for immune defense in both groups of animals (Ong et al., 2006). What is less clear is whether illness-induced anorexia plays a critical role in reducing iron availability to pathogens. Supplemental iron in food decreases resistance to pathogens (Smith, Jones, & Smith, 2005), suggesting that reduced iron intake might increase survival. However, infection does not induce a cessation in feeding, it merely reduces it. Brief food deprivation in caterpillars (*Manduca sexta*), similar to that observed during illness-induced anorexia, has no effect on the total iron content of the hemolymph (Adamo, Fidler, & Forestell, 2007). It remains to be shown that illness-induced anorexia has a strong enough effect on iron availability to pathogens that it would be biologically significant.

Enhanced immune function is another common hypothesis for the function of illness-induced anorexia (e.g., Kyriazakis et al., 1998), although how reduced feeding would increase immune function remains unclear. Possibly decreased feeding reduces competition for molecular resources between immune function and digestion. For example, both vertebrates and invertebrates use some of the same molecules for both the immune response and digestion/energy metabolism (e.g., lipid metabolism; vertebrates: Wendel, Paul, & Heller, 2007; invertebrates: Adamo, Roberts, Easy, & Ross, 2008; Adamo, Bartlett, Le, Spencer, & Sullivan, 2010). Decreasing feeding during illness may be a behavioral method of biasing physiological pathways toward immune function and away from digestion (Adamo et al., 2010). These pathways may include highly conserved intracellular signaling pathways involved in stress resistance, metabolism, and immune function. For example, in *Drosophila melanogaster*, during times of energy shortage and stress, antimicrobial peptide production is enhanced via a FOXO-dependent mechanism (Becker et al., 2010). Illness-induced anorexia may be a behavioral way of activating this pathway. This pathway is highly conserved and is also found in humans (Becker et al., 2010).

Diet influences survival after infection in vertebrates (Smith et al., 2005). In insects, force-feeding infected caterpillars (*M. sexta*) decreases survival only if the food has a high lipid content (Adamo et al., 2007). High-fat food also increases mortality in crickets given a bacterial infection (Adamo et al., 2010). Crickets shift their food preference during immune activation and decrease consumption of high-fat foods (Adamo et al., 2010). This shift in food preference should increase their survival after infection. Adamo et al. (2010) suggest that decreased lipid intake is important for optimal immune function in some insects because of a competition between immune function and lipid transport for the same protein, apolipophorin III. By decreasing lipid intake, apolipophorin III can be used for immune defense instead of for lipid transport, resulting in augmented immune function (Adamo et al., 2008). Such physiological conflicts are likely to vary across species, but the basic principle of competition between the immune system and digestion may be the same.

Rodents also show changes in food preference after an immune challenge with lipopolysaccharides. Although rodents eat less overall, they increase the relative amount of carbohydrates consumed after an immune challenge (Aubert et al., 1995), even though increasing carbohydrate consumption should lead to reduced survival, at least to some pathogens (Smith et al., 2005). More studies on vertebrates are needed to resolve whether immune-induced changes in food preferences increase survival after infection. In insects, the effect of immune function on feeding may be dependent on the type of pathogen, the type of immune response activated, and the nutritional ecology of the species.

Work in insects also demonstrates that decreased food intake may increase susceptibility to some pathogens while decreasing susceptibility to others (Ayres and Schneider, 2009). This result is not surprising, given that Ayres and Schneider (2009) found a complex mix of positive and negative effects of food restriction on immune function in *D. melanogaster*. Vertebrates are unlikely to be less complex than insects. Understanding the function of illness-induced anorexia must take into account that it is not always immunoenhancing.

Acute Stress Response and Immune Function in Insects

Stress has complex effects on immunity in animals (Sternberg, 2006). The effects differ depending on factors such as the type of stressor and its duration in both vertebrates and insects (Demas et al., 2011; Adamo, 2012). This section examines the effects of performing flight-or-fight behaviors on immune function in insects. This type of stress is similar to what is commonly called "acute stress" in vertebrates. Acute stress induces changes in immune function in vertebrates, and many of these changes are driven by hormones released during flight-or-fight behavior (Webster, Tonelli, & Sternberg, 2002). Immune cells have receptors for these stress hormones (Webster et al., 2002), suggesting that this connection serves some adaptive function. However, what this adaptive function may be is a matter of debate (Adamo & Parsons, 2006). There are a number of hypotheses (not necessarily mutually exclusive) that attempt to explain why acute stress affects immunity (see Adamo & Parsons, 2006). Part of the difficulty in uncovering clear evidence of an adaptive function for the effects of stress hormones on immune function in the context of acute stress is that: (a) There are a large number of physiological effects (e.g., Webster et al., 2002), and (b) the relevance of many of these effects for disease resistance remains unclear (see Adamo, 2012). A comparative approach may help clarify the problem, especially when this approach encompasses simpler systems (e.g., insects).

Insects show a robust acute stress response (Orchard, Ramirez, & Lange, 1993; Roeder, 1999). Insects such as the flying orthopterans (crickets and locusts) release the neurohormone octopamine during flight-or-fight behavior, followed by the release of the peptide adipokinetic hormone from endocrine glands (corpora cardiaca) (Orchard et al., 1993; Nijhout, 1994). Adipokinetic hormone induces the liberation of energy compounds from the fat body, and this energy release helps to fuel energetically expensive behaviors (Nation, 2008). Octopamine in the hemolymph (blood) has a wide range of effects, such as liberation of energy stores from the fat body (but to a smaller extent than does adipokinetic hormone) that prime the animal for intense physical activity (Roeder, 1999; 2005). The octopaminergic component of the insect stress response may be a stress-response system that has been conserved across phyla. The insect octopaminergic system is similar to the vertebrate sympathetic nervous system (Roeder 2005). Octopamine is the insect equivalent of norepinephrine (Roeder, 2005), and both systems may have evolved from the same ancestral stress system (reviewed in Adamo, 2008a).

Insect hemocytes contain receptors for the stress neurohormone octopamine (Easy & Adamo, unpublished observations), creating a plausible mechanism by which stressful stimuli could influence immune function. Octopamine has a range of effects on hemocytes both in vivo and in vitro (see Adamo, 2008a; Kim, Nalini, Kim, & Lee, 2009; Adamo, 2010). Octopamine tends to upregulate individual immune responses such as phagocytosis (Baines, DeSantis, & Downer, et. al., 1992), although not all its effects enhance immune function (Adamo, 2010). Adipokinetic hormone has also been shown to increase immune function by enhancing phenoloxidase activity after an immune challenge (Goldsworthy, Opoku-ware, & Mullen, 2002).

Despite the fact that the direct effects of octopamine (Adamo, 2008a) and adipokinetic hormone (Goldsworthy et al., 2002) on the immune system are largely immunoenhancing, extended performance of flight-or-fight behaviors results in a decline in disease resistance (Adamo and Parsons, 2006). This result is similar to the window of vulnerability experienced by vertebrates after a period of intense activity (e.g., Nieman, 2007). Injections of either the stress neurohormone octopamine (Adamo and Parsons, 2006) or adipokinetic hormone (Goldsworthy, Opoku-ware, & Mullen, 2005) also induce a decline in disease resistance.

The decline in disease resistance during acute stress in insects appears to be due, at least in part, to a physiological conflict between immune function and lipid transport (Adamo, 2008a). During "flight-or-fight" behaviors, the protein apolipophorin III loses its immune surveillance function (Adamo et. al., 2008a) and is co-opted into lipid transport in order to increase energy supply to the muscles (Figure 15.1, Weers & Ryan, 2006). The result is decreased resistance to bacteria (Adamo et. al., 2008a). In insects, stress hormones may depress immune function indirectly, by redirecting resources (e.g., molecules like apolipophorin III) toward "flight-or-fight" requirements. The direct immune-enhancing effects of octopamine and adipokinetic hormone may act to ameliorate the negative immune effects of this redistribution of resources (Figure 15.2; Adamo, 2009). The effects of octopamine on immune function vary depending on the presence or absence of pathogens suggesting that the effects of stress hormones on immune function also depend on the physiological context in invertebrates (Adamo, 2009), just as they do in vertebrates (Nance and Sanders, 2007). Without the effects of octopamine and adipokinetic hormone on immune function, disease resistance would probably decline even more precipitously during flying or fighting in crickets. This hypothesis explains why octopamine and adipokinetic hormone can have both immuno-suppressive and immunoenhancing effects (Fig. 2, Adamo et al., 2008; Adamo, 2010). Therefore, the data in insects suggests that stress hormones are not globally immunoenhancing or immunosuppressing, but that they help to reconfigure the immune system to optimize its performance given the animal's present physiological state.

In vertebrates there is evidence that at least some of the effects of acute stress on immune function help redistribute immune resources to enhance protection from possible infection through a wound (Dhabhar & Viswanathan, 2005; Dhabhar, 2009). Wounding is a common outcome of flight-or-fight behavior (see Dhabhar, 2002). In insects, acute stress does not reduce the risk of wound infection (Adamo and Parsons, 2006). Moreover, in birds, as opposed to some mammals (Dhabhar & Viswanathan, 2005), acute stress results in a decline in cell-mediated immunity in the skin (Ewenson, Zan, & Flannery, 2003) suggesting a different pattern.

Whether these differences are the result of differences in taxon, methodology, or both remains to be tested. However, a comparison across species can help provide new perspectives on the interactions between acute stress and immunity.

Chronic Stress

In this section I discuss the type of chronic stress that leads to elevated baseline levels of stress hormones. Chronically elevated levels of stress hormones reduce disease resistance in vertebrates (e.g., see Glaser and Kiecolt-Glaser, 2005). The observation that a decline in disease resistance is driven by a receptor-mediated hormonal mechanism suggests that it is an evolved response. Why does long-term exposure to stress hormones reduce immune function? The most common hypothesis is that the effects of chronic stress on immune function represent a maladaptive, pathological version of an adaptive response (i.e., the short-term effect of stress hormones) (Dhabhar & McEwen, 2007). However, this perspective requires the belief that over the course of evolutionary time no vertebrate has managed to desensitize receptors or evolve mechanisms that prevent the negative effects of chronically elevated stress hormone levels on immune function. Yet, there are other examples of adaptive modifications of stress

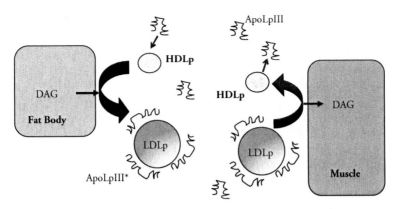

Figure 15.1 Lipid transport in the flying orthoptera (e.g., crickets) (adapted from Weers and Ryan, 2003). During flight-or-fight, lipid transport requirements overwhelm the lipid-carrying capacity of high density lipophorin (HDLp). Under these conditions, apolipophorin III (ApoLpIII) undergoes a conformational change (ApoLpIII*) and joins HDLp to become low density lipophorin (LDLp). The amount of free apolipophorin III (apoLpIII) available to bind to pathogen components declines as it becomes combined with HDLp. Diacylglycerol (DAG)

hormone effects. For example, in semelparous male mammals (those that die after one breeding season), glucocorticoids do not inhibit testosterone production and do not suppress reproduction as they do in other mammals (Boonstra, 2005). However, if chronic stress is an unusual and rare event for most species, then there may be little selection pressure to remove its pathological effects on immune function. In other words, if our ancestors lived in an Eden-like environment, free of all physical stress (e.g., extended periods of cold, hunger, or heat) and lived in perfect harmony with one another (i.e., no bad relationships in the Pleistocene), and if chronic stress is merely a manifestation of modern living,

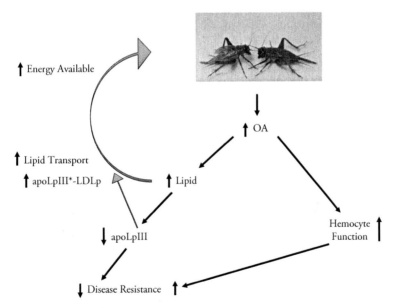

Figure 15.2 Schematic outlining how aggressive behavior could influence disease resistance. Fighting causes the release of octopamine (OA). Octopamine directly and/or indirectly induces the release of lipid from the fat body, stimulating the protein apolipophorin III (apoLpIII) to undergo a conformational change (apoLpIII*). This change is a step in the production of low-density lipophorin (LDLp), resulting in increased lipid transport. However, as apoLpIII transforms into LDLp, the amount of free apoLpIII declines, resulting in reduced immune surveillance and a decline in disease resistance. However, OA also enhances hemocyte function and this may reduce the effect of declining apoLpIII levels. Figure adapted from Adamo (2012).

then evolution may not have had time to select against the negative effects of chronically elevated stress hormones. However, our ancestors did not evolve in Eden, and chronic stress is not the recent product of modern civilization; wild animals also experience chronically elevated stress hormones in response to repeated flight-or-fight situations (e.g., Boonstra, Hik, Singleton, & Tinnikov, 1998). For example, the number of predators preying on snowshoe hares (*Lepus americanus*) varies from year to year (Boonstra et al., 1998). Cortisol levels, an important stress hormone in hares, are chronically elevated during seasons with many predators (Boonstra et al., 1998). The chronically elevated levels of stress hormones have serious negative impacts, including reduced reproduction (Sheriff, Krebs, & Boonstra, 2009). This effect is not limited to vertebrates. Crickets face a wide range of predators (e.g., Sakaluk & Belwood, 1984). As with most animals, predation is a major selective force, and cricket reproductive behavior can be changed by predation risk (Hedrick & Dill, 1993). Repeated simulated predator attacks lead to an increase in the baseline levels of the stress neurohormone octopamine (Adamo & Baker, 2011). These results suggest that upregulation of stress hormone levels may be a widespread response to repeated acute stressors, such as attempted predation. Therefore, people and animals probably have evolved in the presence of chronic stress. This ecoimmunological perspective is changing our views on stress-induced immunosuppression (e.g., Råberg, Grahn, Hasselquist, & Svensson, 1998; Sapolsky, Romero, & Munck, 2000; Dhabhar, 2002; Wingfield, 2003; Segerstrom, 2007; Romero, Dickens, & Cyr, 2009).

ADAPTIVE FUNCTION OF CHRONIC STRESS

How can the effects of chronic stress on immunity have an adaptive function when it reduces disease resistance (e.g., see Glaser and Kiecolt-Glaser, 2005)? For a physiological connection to be adaptive, it must lead to increased successful reproduction relative to other members of the species. In other words, the effects of chronic stress on immune function could be adaptive, even if it leads to increased risk of disease, if it increases the number of offspring the animal has before it dies, relative to its competitors.

Stress hormones appear to do just that in some animals. For example, stress hormones allow males in some species to use all their energy stores (i.e., spend their "somatic capital") on reproduction, even though this leads to an increased risk of death at the end of the breeding season (Boonstra, 2005). Investment in immunity is drastically reduced (Boonstra, 2005). If predation is high, or for some other reason the odds of surviving to the next season are low, it may pay males to put all their energy into one reproductive season (Boonstra, 2005). Chronically elevated stress hormones play an important role in this shift of resources (Boonstra, 2005).

However, in most animals, chronically elevated stress hormones result in both reduced immune function and reduced reproduction (Boonstra, 2005). If the suppression of immune function is not contributing to increased reproduction, how might the effects of chronically elevated stress hormones on immune function be adaptive?

Chronic stress often occurs when the food supply is inadequate. Under these conditions, animals may lack the resources to adequately maintain all systems. Immune function may be downregulated to spare energy for physiological systems more critical for immediate survival and/or reproduction (Sapolsky et al., 2000). For example, in tree lizards, chronic administration of corticosterone for seven days via an implant depresses wound healing in females during reproduction, an energetically expensive task (French McLemore, Vernon, Johnston, & Moore, 2007). In nonreproductive females, corticosterone has no effect on wound healing unless females are food restricted (French et al., 2007). Therefore, corticosterone may suppress immune function only when resources are insufficient to fuel reproduction or other, more immediate, survival needs (French et al., 2007). Suppression may be adaptive under these conditions.

Chronic stress also has negative consequences on immune function in some species, even if food is available and individuals have abundant energy stores. In these species, the depression in immune function may be due to a physiological constraint, not a lack of resources per se. In other words, the web like nature of physiological connections sometimes makes it impossible to maximize two different functions simultaneously. In vertebrates, the effects of stress hormones on immune function are extremely complex (e.g., glucocorticoids; Schoneveld & Cidlowski, 2007), making possible physiological constraints difficult to find. However, in the simpler system of the cricket, constraints may be easier to identify. For example, under chronic stress conditions (e.g., high predator density), crickets may require energy compounds to be more readily available than under good conditions. This switch in energy metabolism may create changes in other physiological pathways, leading to reduced immune function. The reduction could be adaptive because it increases the survival of the individual under these conditions, even though it also depresses disease resistance (also see Wingfield, 2003 for this type of argument). It appears maladaptive only when compared to what the animal could do under perfect conditions (adequate food, proper temperature, no predators or competitors). A similar hypothesis suggests that, after extended periods of chronically high levels of stress hormones, the organism's ability to withstand their effects declines and the result is dysregulation of immune function (e.g., McEwen & Wingfield, 2003; Romero et al., 2009). In other words, the physiological shifts required for survival under suboptimal conditions produces physiological configurations that leave the animal more vulnerable to perturbations such as infection (e.g., Romero et al., 2009). Unfortunately, there are no actual examples of how this occurs (e.g., how and why specific physiological pathways become nonfunctional, or lose their protective function, after continued stimulation by stress hormones). These details may be easier to discover in the insect.

Why the Immune Response Activates the Stress Response

Animals face death at the hands of pathogens, predators, and competitors. Both the stress response and the immune response help the animal survive these extreme challenges. A simplistic view might assume that each response would have its own methods of shifting physiological systems into an optimal state for that response. However, in mammals (Sternberg, 2006), birds (Owen-Ashley & Wingfield, 2007), and insects (Adamo, 2010), the immune response activates components of the stress response, including the release of at least some stress hormones/neurohormones. The use of some of the same mechanism by both responses may be less surprising with the recognition that both require some of the same physiological shifts. To be able to respond to extreme challenges, both responses require the mobilization of energy and the protection of cells against immune-derived insults and stress-induced increases in metabolism (e.g., the release of cytotoxic molecules; Maier, 2003). For example, in crickets and other insects, an immune challenge induces the release of octopamine, a stress neurohormone (Adamo, 2010). Octopamine can activate some intracellular stress responses (Armstrong & Robertson, 2006) as can the immune response (Altincicek, Knorr, & Vilcinskas, 2008),

although whether the immune response relies on octopamine to produce this effect is unknown. The release of octopamine during both the immune and stress responses may help insects survive the damages induced by pathogens, the immune response itself, or the increased metabolic activity that occurs during flight-or-fight. Perhaps it is not surprising that both immune and stress responses use similar hormonal mechanisms to perform the same functions—that is, liberate energy and activate cellular defense mechanisms. The similar requirements of both the immune and stress responses may partially explain their interconnectedness.

In vertebrates, the activation of the stress response during the immune response is thought to dampen an immune response to prevent it from damaging host tissue (Karrow, 2006). This explanation does not fit the data for insects, because octopamine tends to upregulate individual immune responses such as phagocytosis (Baines et al., 1992). Vertebrate immune systems may require more elaborate protection against autoimmunity than do those of invertebrates.

Measurement of Immune Function and Disease Resistance

Immune function is complex and multidimensional. In recognition of this, a large number of different assays have been used to assess it (Luster et al. 1993). Although these assays can provide evidence of a change in immune function, how well they demonstrate an increase or decrease in disease resistance is often unclear (see Keil, Luebke, & Pruett, 2001; Adamo, 2004). A number of ecoimmunological papers have wrestled with the issue of how to interpret immune assays (e.g., Adamo, 2004; Martin, Weil, & Nelson, 2006; Adamo, 2009; Adamo, 2012). There appears to be less published discussion in the psychoneuroimmunological literature on this topic, although there is recognition of the problem (e.g., Robinson, Mathews, & Witek-Janusek, 2002; Wetherell & Vedhara, 2007). Next, I describe how recent work on insects demonstrates some of the difficulties in interpreting immune assay results (Adamo, 2009; Adamo, 2012).

With most immune assays, an increase in function (e.g., increased antibody production to a vaccine) is assumed to correlate with enhanced disease resistance. For some measures, such as antibody production to a vaccine, there is evidence to support this assumption, at least under standard conditions (e.g., Quan et al., 2004). Unfortunately, work on insects has shown that the relationship between a measure of immune function and disease resistance can break down during changes in physiological state. In the cricket, increased octopamine enhances some immune functions, but this enhanced function correlates with reduced resistance to at least some pathogens (Adamo & Parsons, 2006).

These paradoxical effects can occur for a number of reasons. For example, some immune molecules participate in other physiological functions (e.g., apolipophorin III). These multifunctional molecules can lead to physiological trade-offs between the immune system and other physiological systems. These trade-offs can eliminate correlations among immune assays as well as correlations between some immune assays and disease resistance.

Furthermore, because immune systems are composed of multiple physiological pathways, there may be multiple ways for it to be configured. For example, animals have at least two routes for surviving pathogen attack: mechanisms that destroy pathogens (called "resistance"), and mechanisms that allow them to survive the effects of the pathogen ("tolerance"; Schneider & Ayres, 2008). A "tolerant" organism may have relatively high levels of enzymes designed to detoxify bacterial toxins, or upregulated mechanisms designed to protect cells from the consequences of pathogen attack (e.g., heat-shock proteins). An individual emphasizing "resistance" (the ability to destroy pathogens) may show increased production of antimicrobial compounds. Ayres and Schneider (2008) argue that typical measures of immune function assess only half the defensive capacity of the host because mechanisms of "tolerance" are neglected. Some individuals may rely more heavily on one particular pathway (e.g., "tolerance"), whereas another invests more heavily in a different pathway (e.g., "resistance"), but both individuals may still have approximately the same ability to survive most pathogens (e.g., see Schneider & Ayres, 2008). Moreover, the physiological configuration of immune defense may shift among different pathways to provide optimal defense in different situations (Schmid-Hempel & Ebert, 2003). Such shifts will make it difficult to determine the effects of behavior on "immune ability" based on specific immune components. Lower scores on a particular immune assay may signal that immune pathways have been reconfigured, not that there has been a decrease in immune capacity.

Finally, it may be impossible to maximize all physiological pathways involved with immune function simultaneously. Animals must then "choose" a particular immune-systems configuration.

The two pathways may have different costs and benefits, but it may not be obvious which one is the lesser "immune investment" or the least "immunocompetent"—that is, which is the one that results in the least protection from infection and death. For example, the phenoloxidase system is a major immunological pathway in insects and is under heavy inhibition (e.g., serpins; Kanost & Gorman, 2008). Overactivation of this system can kill the host (Kanost & Gorman, 2008), whereas underactivation can also lead to host death by unopposed pathogens (Beck & Strand, 2007). If the relative amount of inhibitors versus activators changes, it could increase or decrease the ease with which the phenoloxidase cascade is activated. Bias toward activation may increase the insect's ability to neutralize pathogens, but it might also lead to greater immunopathology (e.g., a greater risk of its unnecessary deployment). Determining the "optimal" choice (i.e., levels) between two mutually exclusive pathways (e.g., inhibitors versus activators) may be difficult to determine, and is likely to be context- and pathogen-dependent.

Given these complexities, is it possible to make conclusions about disease resistance from measurements of immune function? Immunotoxicologists use host resistance tests to assess the significance of changes in immune function (Descotes, 1999). Typically these tests consist of injecting a known dose of bacteria or other pathogen into an animal. The number of animals that die in control versus those in experimental groups that are given different concentrations of the pathogen is recorded (Robertson, Russell, Preisler, & Savin, 2007). These tests assess the animal's ability to survive a real infection by at least one pathogen. Therefore, it reflects the sum of an even larger range of immune components than typical immune assays by including "tolerance" mechanisms and other assorted physiological systems that contribute to survival after infection. Host-resistance tests have drawbacks as well (Martin, Weil, & Nelson, 2008), but they allow a better estimation of the biological and clinical significance of the change in immune function than individual assays. Obviously host-resistance tests are impossible to conduct in humans. In that case, health outcomes (e.g., wound healing, cancer rates) should be correlated with immune measures (Robinson et al., 2002).

Researchers working with vertebrates that do use live pathogen challenges often use bacterial burden at a particular time point, instead of death, as the end point. Intuitively, it seems reasonable to assume that bacterial clearance would be strongly correlated with survival. However, this is not necessarily the case in insects. In some instances, insects can demonstrate decreased bacterial clearance but increased survival (Schneider and Ayres, 2008). Therefore, especially when changes in physiological state are involved (e.g., a stressed group compared to an unstressed group) conclusions about changes in disease resistance should be made with caution.

Comparative Psychoneuroimmunology: Conclusions and Future Directions

1. A comparative approach can help uncover the adaptive function of immune-behavioral interactions. Unless we know the adaptive function of immune-behavioral interactions, interfering with them could cause unintended negative consequences.

2. Immune-behavioral interactions may vary depending on the ecological context. For example, the effects of cytokines on behavior may differ depending on the animal's life stage (e.g., reproductive status). Therefore, interpretations of psychoneuroimmunological phenomena should take the animal's natural history into consideration.

3. Understanding the function of some psychoneuroimmunological phenomena, such as the effects of stress on health, will require knowing how stress resistance, metabolism, and immune function are interconnected at the molecular level.

4. Without firmly establishing the impact of immune-behavioral interactions on disease resistance, it will be difficult to determine their adaptive function. Unfortunately, the complexity of the immune system makes it difficult to assess to what extent psychoneuroimmunological phenomena alter disease resistance in vertebrates. This limits the conclusions that can be made about the significance of some psychoneuroimmunological phenomena.

References

Adamo, S. A. (1998). The specificity of behavioral fever in the cricket *Acheta domesticus. Journal of Parasitology, 84*(3), 529–533.

Adamo, S. A. (2004). How should behavioural ecologists interpret measurements of immunity? *Animal Behaviour, 68,* 1443–1449.

Adamo, S. A. (2005). Parasitic suppression of feeding in the tobacco hornworm, *Manduca sexta*: Parallels with feeding depression after an immune challenge. *Archives of Insect Biochemistry and Physiology, 60,* 185–197.

Adamo, S. A. (2006). Comparative Psychoneuroimmunology: Evidence from the insects. *Behavioral and Cognitive Neuroscience Reviews, 5*(3), 128–140.

Adamo, S. A. (2008a). Norepinephrine and octopamine: Linking stress and immune function across phyla. *Invertebrate Survival Journal, 5,* 12–19.

Adamo, S. A. (2008b). Bidirectional connections between the immune system and the nervous system in insects. In N. E. Beckage (Ed.), *Insect immunology* (pp. 129–149). San Diego, CA: Academic Press.

Adamo, S. A. (2009). The impact of physiological state on immune function in insects. In J. Rolff & S. E. Reynolds (Eds.), *Insect infection and immunity* (pp. 173–186). Oxford, England: Oxford University Press.

Adamo, S. A. (2010). Why should an immune response activate the stress response? Insights from the insects (the cricket *Gryllus texensis*). *Brain, Behavior and Immunity, 24,* 194–200.

Adamo, S. A. (2012). The importance of physiology for ecoimmunology: lessons from the insects. In *Ecoimmunology* (pp. 413–439), R. J. Nelson and G. E. Demas (Eds.). Oxford, England: Oxford University Press.

Adamo, S. A., Bartlett, A., Le, J., Spencer, N., & Sullivan, K. (2010). Illness-induced anorexia may reduce trade-offs between digestion and immune function. *Animal Behavior, 79,* 3–10.

Adamo, S. A., & Baker, J. L. (2011). Conserved features of chronic stress across phyla: The effects of long-term stress on behaviour and the concentration of the neurohormone octopamine in the cricket, *Gryllus texensis. Hormones and Behavior, 60,* 478–483.

Adamo, S. A., Fidler, T. L., & Forestell, C. A. (2007). Illness-induced anorexia and its possible function in the caterpillar, *Manduca sexta. Brain, Behavior and Immunity, 21,* 293–300.

Adamo, S. A., & Parsons, N. M. (2006). The emergency life-history stage and immunity in the cricket, *Gryllus texensis. Animal Behavior, 72,* 235–244.

Adamo, S. A., Roberts, J. L., Easy, R. H., & Ross, N. W. (2008). Competition between immune function and lipid transport for the protein apolipophorin III leads to stress-induced immunosuppression in crickets. *Journal of Experimental Biology, 211,* 531–538.

Ader, R. (2007). *Psychoneuroimmunology* (4th ed.). New York: Elsevier.

Alghamdi, A., Dalton, L., Phillis, A., Rosato, E., & Mallon, E. B. (2008). Immune response impairs learning in free-flying bumble-bees. *Biology Letters, 4,* 479–481.

Altincicek, B., Knorr, E., & Vilcinskas, A. (2008). Beetle immunity: identification of immune-inducible genes from the model insect *Tribolium castaneum. Developmental and Comparative Immunology, 32*(5), 585–595.

Armstrong, G. A. B., & Robertson, R. M. (2006). A role for octopamine in coordinating thermoprotection of an insect nervous system. *Journal of Thermal Biology, 31,* 149–158.

Ashley, N. T., Hays, Q. R., Bentley, G. R., & Wingfield, J. C. (2009). Testosterone treatment diminishes sickness behavior in male songbirds. *Hormones and Behavior, 56,* 169–176.

Aubert, A. (1999). Sickness and behaviour in animals: a motivational perspective. *Neuroscience and Biobehavioral Reviews, 23,* 1029–1036.

Aubert, A., Goodall, G., & Dantzer, R. (1995). Compared effects of cold ambient temperature and cytokines on macronutrient intake in rats. *Physiology and Behavior, 57*(5), 869–873.

Aubert, A., Kelley, K. W., & Dantzer, R. (1997). Differential effect of lipopolysaccharide on food hoarding behavior and food consumption in rats. *Brain, Behavior and Immunity, 11,* 229–238.

Ayres, J. S., & Schneider, D. S. (2008). A signaling protease required for melanization in *Drosophila* affects resistance and tolerance of infections. *PloS Biology, 6*(12), 2764–2773.

Ayres, J. S., & Schneider, D. S. (2009). The role of anorexia in resistance and tolerance to infections in *Drosophila. PloS Biology, 7*(7), 1–10, e10000150.

Baines, D., DeSantis, T., & Downer, R. G. H. (1992). Octopamine and 5-hydroxytryptamine enhance the phagocytic and nodule formation activities of cockroach (*Periplaneta americana*) haemocytes. *Journal of Insect Physiology, 38,* 905–914.

Beck, M. H., & Strand, M. R. (2007). A novel polydnavirus protein inhibits the insect prophenoloxidase activation pathway. *Proceedings of the National Academy of Sciences of the United States, 104*(49), 19267–19272.

Becker, T., Loch, G., Beyer, M., Zinke, I., Aschenbrenner, A. C., Carrera, P., et al. (2010). FOXO-dependent regulation of innate immune homeostasis. *Nature, 463,* 369–373.

Boonstra, R. (2005). Equipped for life: the adaptive role of the stress axis in male mammals. *Journal of Mammalogy, 86*(2), 236–247.

Boonstra, R., Hik, D., Singleton, G. R., & Tinnikov, A. (1998). The impact of predator-induced stress on the snowshoe hare cycle. *Ecological Monographs, 79*(5), 371–394.

Cohen, N., & Kinney, K. S. (2007). Exploring the phylogenetic history neural-immune system interactions: an update. In R. Aders (Ed.), *Psychoneuroimmunology* (4th ed., Vol. 1, pp. 1–38). New York: Elsevier.

Cunningham, C., & Sanderson, D. J. (2008). Malaise in the water maze: untangling the effects of LPS and IL-1β on learning and memory. *Brain, Behavior and Immunity, 22,* 1117–1127.

Dantzer, R. (2004). Cytokine-induced sickness behavior: A neuroimmune response to activation of the innate immunity. *European Journal of Pharmacology, 500,* 399–411.

Dantzer, R. (2007). Expression and action of cytokines in the brain: Mechanisms and pathophysiological implications. In R. Aders (Ed.), *Psychoneuroimmunology* (4th ed., Vol. 1, pp. 271–280). New York: Elsevier.

Dantzer, R., O'Connor, J. C., Freund, G. G., Johnson, R. W., & Kelley, K. W. (2008). From inflammation to sickness and depression: When the immune system subjugates the brain. *Nature Reviews Neuroscience, 9*(1), 46–57.

Demas, G. E., Adamo, S. A., & French, S. S. (2011). Neuroendocrine-immune crosstalk in vertebrates and invertebrates: implications for host defense. *Functional Ecology, 25,* 29–39.

Descotes, J. (1999). *An introduction to immunotoxicology.* London: Taylor and Francis.

Dhabhar, F. S. (2002). Stress-induced augmentation of immune function—The role of stress hormones, leukocyte trafficking, and cytokines. *Brain, Behavior and Immunity, 16,* 785–798.

Dhabhar, F. S. (2009). Enhancing versus suppressive effects of stress on immune function: Implications for immunoprotection and immunopathology. *Neuroimmunomodulation, 16,* 300–317.

Dhabhar, F. S., & McEwen, B. S. (2007). Bi-directional effects of stress on immune function: possible explanations for salubrious as well as harmful effects. In R. Aders (Ed.),

Psychoneuroimmunology (4th ed., Vol. 2, pp. 723–760). New York: Elsevier.

Dhabhar, F. S., & Viswanathan, K. (2005). Short-term stress experienced at time of immunization induces a long-lasting increase in immunologic memory. *American Journal of Physiology, 289,* R738–R744.

Dunn, P. E., Bohnert, T. J., & Russell, V. (1994). Regulation of antibacterial protein synthesis following infection and during metamorphosis of *Manduca sexta. Annals of the New York Academy of Science, 712,* 117–130.

Dunphy, G. B., & Downer, R. G. H. (1994). Octopamine, a modulator of the haemocytic nodulation response of non-immune *Galleria mellonella. Journal of Insect Physiology, 40,* 267–272.

Durazzo, A., Proud, K., & Demas, G. E. (2008). Experimentally induced sickness decreases food intake, but not hoarding, in Siberian hamsters (*Phodopus sungorus*). *Behavioral Processes, 79,* 195–198.

Eccles, R. (2005). Understanding the symptoms of the common cold and influenza. *Lancet Infectious Diseases, 5*(11), 718–725.

Elenkov, I. J., & Chrousos, G. P. (2006). Stress system—Organization, physiology and immunoregulation. *Neuroimmunodulation, 13*(5–6), 257–267.

Ewenson, E., Zann, R., & Flannery, G. (2003). PHA immune response assay in captive zebra finches is modulated by activity prior to testing. *Animal Behavior, 66,* 797–800.

Exton, M. S. (1997). Infection-induced anorexia: active host defense strategy. *Appetite, 29,* 369–383.

Feder, D., Mello, C. B., Garcia, E. S., & Azambuja, P. (1997). Immune responses in *Rhodnius prolixus*: influence of nutrition and ecdysone. *Journal of Insect Physiology, 43*(6), 513–519.

French, S. S., McLemore, R., Vernon, B., Johnston, G. I. H., & Moore, M. C. (2007). Corticosterone modulation of reproductive and immune systems trade-offs in female tree lizards: Long-term corticosterone manipulations via injectable gelling material. *Journal of Experimental Biology, 210,* 2859–2865.

Gautron, L., Mingam, R., Moranis, A., Combe, C., & Laye, S. (2005). Influence of feeding status on neuronal activity in the hypothalamus during lipopolysaccharide-induced anorexia in rats. *Neuroscience, 134,* 933–934.

Glaser, R., & Kiecolt-Glaser, J. K. (2005). Stress-induced immune dysfunction: implications for health. *Nature Reviews Immunology, 5,* 243–251.

Goldsworthy, G. J. (2010). Locusts as model organisms in which to study immunogen-induced anorectic behavior. *Journal of Insect Physiology 56,* 991–997.

Goldsworthy, G. J., Opoku-ware, K., & Mullen, L. (2002). Adipokinetic hormone enhances laminarin and bacterial lipopolysaccharide-induced activation of the prophenoloxidase cascade in the African migratory locust, *Locusta migratoria. Journal of Insect Physiology, 48,* 601–608.

Goldsworthy, G. J., Opoku-ware, K., & Mullen, L. M. (2005). Adipokinetic hormone and the immune responses of locusts to infection. *Annals of the New York Academy of Science, 1040,* 106–113.

Hart, B. L. (1988). Biological basis of the behavior of sick animals. *Neuroscience and Biobehavioral Reviews, 12,* 123–137.

Hedrick, A. V., & Dill, L. M. (1993). Mate choice by female crickets is influenced by predation risk. *Animal Behavior, 46,* 193–196.

Kanost, M. R., & Gorman, M. J. (2008). Phenoloxidases and insect immunity. In N.E. Beckage (Ed.), *Insect immunology* (pp. 69–96). San Diego, CA: Academic Press.

Karrow, N. A. (2006). Activation of the hypothalamic-pituitary-adrenal axis and autonomic nervous system during inflammation and altered programming of the neuroendocrine-immune axis during fetal and neonatal development: Lessons learned from the model inflammagen, lipopolysaccharide. *Brain, Behavior and Immunity, 20,* 144–158.

Keil, D., Luebke, R. W., & Pruett, S. B. (2001). Quantifying the relationship between multiple immunological parameters and host resistance: probing the limits of reductionism. *Journal of Immunology, 167,* 4543–4552.

Kim, G. S., Nalini, M., KIm, Y., & Lee, D. W. (2009). Octopamine and 5-hydroxytryptamine mediate hemocytic phagocytosis and nodulate formation via eicosanoids in the beet armyworm, *Spodoptera exigua. Archives of Insect Biochemistry and Physiology, 70*(3), 162–176.

Kluger, M. J., Kozak, W., Conn, C. A., Leon, L. R., & Soszynski, D. (1996). The adaptive value of fever. *Infectious Disease Clinics of North America, 10*(1), 1–20.

Kyriazakis, I., Tolkamp, B. J., & Hutchings, M. R. (1998). Towards a functional explanation for the occurrence of anorexia during parasitic infections. *Animal Behaviour, 56,* 265–274.

Luster, M. I., Portier, C., Pait, D. G., Rosenthal, G. J., Germolec, D. R., Corsini, E., et al. (1993). Risk assessment in immunotoxicology: II. Relationships between immune and host resistance tests. *Fundamental and Applied Toxicology, 21,* 71–82.

Maier, S. F. (2003). Bi-directional immune-brain communication: Implications for understanding stress, pain and cognition. *Brain, Behavior and Immunity, 17,* 69–85.

Mallon, E. B., Brockmann, A., & Schmid-Hempel, P. (2003). Immune response inhibits associative learning in insects. *Proceedings of the Royal Society of London B, 270,* 2471–2473.

Martin, L. B. (2009). Stress and immunity in wild vertebrates: Timing is everything. *General and Comparative Endocrinology, 163,* 70–76.

Martin, L. B., Weil, Z. M., & Nelson, R. J. (2006). Refining approaches and diversifying directions in ecoimmunology. *Integrative and Comparative Biology, 46*(6), 1030–1039.

Martin, L. B., Weil, Z. M., & Nelson, R. J. (2008). Seasonal changes in vertebrate immune activity: Mediation by physiological trade-offs. *Philosophical Transactions of the Royal Society B, 363,* 321–339.

McEwen, B. S., & Wingfield, J. C. (2003). The concept of allostasis in biology and biomedicine. *Hormones and Behavior, 43,* 2–15.

Miles, C. I., & Booker, R (2000). Octopamine mimics the effects of parasitism on the foregut of the tobacco hornworm *Manduca sexta. Journal of Experimental Biology, 203,* 1689–1700.

Moore, J. (2002). *Parasites and the behavior of animals.* New York: Oxford University Press.

Nance, D. M., & Sanders, V. M. (2007). Autonomic innervation and regulation of the immune system (1987–2007). *Brain, Behavior and Immunity, 21,* 736–745.

Nation, J. L. (2008). *Insect physiology and biochemistry* (2nd ed.). Boca Raton, FL: CRC Press.

Nieman, D. C. (2007). Exercise and immunity: Clinical studies. In R. Aders (Ed.), *Psychoneuroimmunology* (4th ed., Vol. 1, pp. 661–673). New York: Elsevier.

Nijhout, H. F. (1994). *Insect hormones.* Princeton, NJ: Princeton University Press.

Ong, S. T., Ho, J. Z. S., Ho, B., & Ding, J. L. (2006). Iron-withholding strategy in innate immunity. *Immunobiology, 211,* 295–314.

Orchard, I., Ramirez, J. M., & Lange, A. B. (1993). A multifunctional role for octopamine in locust flight. *Annual Review of Entomology, 38,* 227–249.

Ottaviani, E., & Franceschi, C. (1996). The neuroimmunology of stress from invertebrates to man. *Progress in Neurobiology, 48,* 421–440.

Owen-Ashley, N. T., & Wingfield, J. C. (2007). Acute phase responses of passerine birds: characterization and seasonal variation. *Journal of Ornithology, 148,* S583–S591.

Pham, L. N., & Schneider, D. S. (2008). Evidence for specificity and memory in the insect innate immune response. In N. Beckage (Ed.), *Insect immunology* (pp. 97–127). San Diego, CA: Academic Press.

Quan, F. S., Matsumoto, T., Shin, Y. O., Min, Y. K., Yang, H. M., Othman, T., et al. (2004). Relationships between IgG, IgM, IgE and resistance to reinfection during the early phase of infection with *Clonorchis sinesis* in rats. *Immunological Investigations, 33*(1), 51–60.

Råberg, L., Grahn, M., Hasselquist, D., & Svensson, E. (1998). On the adaptive significance of stress-induced immunosuppression. *Proceedings of the Royal Society of London B, 265,* 1637–1641.

Riddell, C. E., & Mallon, E. B. (2006). Insect psychoneuroimmunology: immune response reduces learning in protein starved bumblebees (*Bombus terrestris*). *Brain, Behavior and Immunity, 20,* 135–138.

Robertson, J. L., Russell, R. M., Preisler, H. K., & Savin, N. E. (2007). *Bioassays with arthropods* (2nd ed.). Boca Raton, FL: CRC Press.

Robinson, F. P., Mathews, H. L., & Witek-Janusek, L. (2002). Issues in the design and implementation of psychoneuroimmunology research. *Biological Research for Nursing, 3,* 165–175.

Roeder, T. (1999). Octopamine in invertebrates. *Progress in Neurobiology, 59,* 1–31.

Roeder, T. (2005). Tyramine and octopamine: ruling behavior and metabolism. *Annual Review of Entomology, 50,* 447–477.

Romero, L. M., Dickens, M. J., & Cyr, N. E. (2009). The reactive scope model—A new model integrating homeostasis, allostasis and stress. *Hormones and Behavior, 55,* 375–389.

Sakaluk, S., & Belwood, J. (1984). Gecko phonotaxis to cricket calling song: a case of satellite predation. *Animal Behaviour, 32,* 659–662.

Sanders, V. M., & Kavelaars, A. (2007). Adrenergic regulation of immunity. In R. Aders (Ed.), *Psychoneuroimmunology* (4th ed., Vol. 1, pp. 63–83). New York: Elsevier.

Sapolsky, R. M., Romero, L. M., & Munck, A. U. (2000). How do glucocorticoids influence stress responses? Integrating permissive, suppressive, stimulatory and preparative actions. *Endocrine Reviews, 21*(1), 55–89.

Schmid-Hempel, P., & Ebert, D. (2003). On the evolutionary ecology of specific immune defense. *Trends in Ecology and Evolution, 18*(1), 27–32.

Schneider, D. S., & Ayres, J. S. (2008). Two ways to survive infection: what resistance and tolerance can teach us about treating infectious diseases. *Nature Reviews Immunology, 8,* 889–895.

Schoneveld, O. J. L. M., & Cidlowski, J. A. (2007). Glucocorticoids and immunity: Mechanisms of regulation. In R. Ader (Ed.), *Psychoneuroimmunology* (4th ed., Vol. 1, pp. 45–61). New York: Elsevier.

Segerstrom, S. C. (2007). Stress, energy and immunity: An ecological view. *Current Directions in Psychological Science, 16*(6), 326–330.

Sheriff, M. J., Krebs, C. J., & Boonstra, R. (2009). The sensitive hare: Sublethal effects of predator stress on reproduction in snowshoe hares. *Journal of Animal Ecology, 78*(6), 1249–1258.

Smith, V. J., Jones, T. P., & Smith, M. S. (2005). Host nutrition and infectious disease: An ecological view. *Frontiers in Ecology and the Environment, 3*(5), 268–274.

Sternberg, E. M. (2006). Neural regulation of innate immunity: A coordinated nonspecific response to pathogens. *Nature Reviews Immunology, 6,* 318–328.

Webster, J. I., Tonelli, L, & Sternberg, E. M. (2002). Neuroendocrine regulation of immunity. *Annual Review of Immunology, 20,* 125–163.

Weers, P. M. M., & Ryan, R. O. (2003). Apolipophorin III: A lipid-triggered molecular switch. *Insect Biochemistry and Molecular Biology, 33*(12), 1249–1260.

Weers, P. M. M., & Ryan, R. O. (2006). Apolipophorin III: Role model apolipoprotein. *Insect Biochemistry and Molecular Biology, 36,* 231–240.

Wendel, M, Paul, R., & Heller, A. R. (2007). Lipoproteins in inflammation and sepsis. II. Clinical aspects. *Intensive Care Medicine, 33,* 25–35.

Wetherell, M. A., & Vedhara, K. (2007). Stress-associated immune dysregulation can affect antibody and T-cell responses to vaccines. In R. Aders (Ed.), *Psychoneuroimmunology* (4th ed., Vol. 2, pp. 897–916). New York: Elsevier.

Willette, A. A., Lubach, G. R., & Coe, C. L. (2007). Environmental context differentially affects behavioral, leukocyte, cortisol, and interleukin-6 responses to low doses of endotoxin in the rhesus monkey. *Brain, Behavior and Immunity, 21,* 807–815.

Wingfield, J. C. (2003). Control of behavioural strategies for capricious environments. *Animal Behaviour, 66,* 807–816.

Zhang, Y., Lu, H., & Bargmann, C. I. (2005). Pathogenic bacteria induce aversive olfactory learning in *Caenorhabditis elegans. Nature, 438*(7065), 179–184.

Seasonal Rhythms in Psychoneuroimmunology

Zachary M. Weil *and* Randy J. Nelson

Abstract

Animals experience substantial and generally predictable, annual changes in environmental conditions. The changing seasons each present different challenges for animals to address. Mechanisms have evolved in many small mammals to confine breeding to the relatively mild conditions of spring and early summer. In addition to adjustments in reproductive function, other physiological systems including many aspects of immune function and stress responses also vary across the year. The goals of this chapter are to review the current state of our knowledge regarding how psychoneuroimmunological processes vary across the year in small mammals. In the second half of the chapter, we will address what is known about seasonal fluctuations in immune function in humans and the consequences of these rhythms for psychiatric, inflammatory, and infectious diseases.

Key Words: seasonality, photoperiodism, immune responses, melatonin, neuroendocrinology

Introduction

Life on earth is characterized by continual and often predictable temporal change. Day is followed by night and winter is followed by spring. Night and spring often require different adaptive responses than day and winter. For virtually all animals, the environment varies markedly as the seasons change. Seasonal changes are dramatic for those of us living in temperate or boreal climates; however, even equatorial regions experience seasons, though they tend to be marked by changes in rainfall rather than ambient temperatures. On most of the planet, food and water availability, predation pressure, thermoregulatory demands, as well as the types and prevalence of parasites and pathogens can all vary markedly across the year. The immunological priorities and energetic budget has to be apportioned differently at different times of the year (Nelson & Demas, 1996; Nelson, Demas, Klein, & Kriegsfeld, 2002). Additionally, dozens of diseases that affect human populations display seasonal rhythms in incidence,

prevalence, or severity (Castrogiovanni, Iapichino, Pacchierotti, & Pieraccini, 1998; Douglas, Russell, & Allan, 1990; Eng & Mercer, 1998; Nelson et al., 2002). Indeed, the seasonality of human illness extends far beyond the well-known fluctuations of infectious diseases (e.g., flu season) into a variety of other diseases (Mikulecky & Cierna, 2005; Torrey, Miller, Rawlings, & Yolken, 2000).

Seasonal changes in immune function and other physiological systems can be broadly categorized into two overlapping and interacting classes. First, there are the direct physiological consequences of environmental conditions. For instance, prolonged exposure to low temperatures and reduced caloric intake can profoundly alter immune cell distribution and function (Cicho, Chadzińska, Ksiek, & Konarzewski, 2002; Konno et al., 1993; Liang, Zhang, & Zhang, 2004; Shephard & Shek, 1998). Additionally, as described later, seasonal variability in exposure to sunlight, allergens, and infections can all profoundly alter immune physiology and behavior. The second class of adaptations is comprised of adjustments that have evolved over multiple generations and serve to adjust physiology and behavior *in advance* of changes in environmental conditions to combat predictable seasonal stressors (Bilbo, Dhabhar, et al., 2002; Prendergast, Bilbo, & Nelson, 2004; Prendergast, Hotchkiss, Bilbo, Kinsey, & Nelson, 2003). Of course, the majority of seasonal phenomena will result from the interactions between endogenous preparatory adaptations and changing environmental conditions.

Many animals use day length (photoperiod) to time seasonal rhythms (Nelson, Denlinger, & Somers, 2009). Photoperiod itself has minimal direct fitness consequences for most animals, but is predictive of changes in environmental conditions (Nelson et al., 2009). Perhaps the best studied of these phenomena is seasonal breeding, wherein small- to medium-sized mammals confine the energetically expensive tasks of pregnancy and lactation to the spring and early summer (Bronson, 1985). Changes in the reproductive neuroendocrine system are tightly coupled to a marked reorganization of the immune system in virtually all seasonal breeders that have been studied (Nelson & Demas, 1996; Nelson et al., 2002). Although individuals of many species, including humans, breed year round (Bronson, 2004), these individuals retain seasonality in the immune system in subtle, but important ways (Killestein et al., 2002; Mann, Akinbami, Gould, & Ansari, 2000; Prendergast et al., 2007). Further, seasonal rhythms in the immune system can have profound consequences for host defense, inflammatory disorders, and psychiatric conditions (Lam & Levitan, 2000; Torrey, Miller, Rawlings, & Yolken, 1997; Torrey, Rawlings, Ennis, Merrill, & Flores, 1996).

In the first half of this chapter, we will review the existing literature on mechanisms of seasonal rhythms in immune responses in experimental animals. We intend to provide an overview of extant knowledge of annual rhythms both in highly seasonal mammals and in those with less overt seasonality. In the second half of this chapter, we will then explore how these types of seasonal rhythms can interact with the human immune system and other core components of psychoneuroimmune phenomena including stress physiology, early-life determinants of adult disease, and the relationship between the immune system and psychiatric disease.

Photoperiodism in the Immune System

As described earlier, animals across taxa have evolved the ability to use day length to time seasonal rhythms of physiology and behavior. Although there are many possible cues that predict changing seasons (e.g., temperature, rainfall, and humidity) they suffer from an inherent noisiness that renders them unreliable in accurately keeping track of the date. Thus, photoperiodism, the ability to measure day length (a virtually noise-free seasonal cue), has become the predominant seasonal timing mechanism among plants and animals (Nelson, Denlinger, & Somers, 2009). In mammals, photic information is transduced from an environmental signal to a physiological one via the nighttime secretion of pineal melatonin. Target tissues, therefore, can attend to the duration (rather than the amplitude) of the nightly elevation in circulating melatonin to monitor changing day length. With only two pieces of information, the day length (or night length) and the direction of change, it is possible to determine the specific date. The immune system may have evolved to "eavesdrop" on the melatonin signal that controls the reproductive system.

In the laboratory, short winter-like photoperiods (e.g., 8 hours of light and 16 hours of dark) or long duration melatonin infusions can induce virtually the full suite of seasonal adaptations including (in rodents) regression of the reproductive tract and modifications in the metabolic, neuroendocrine, and immune systems. Therefore, studying photoperiodic rodents in the laboratory can provide a powerful tool to understand the endogenous adaptations that animals undergo in order to maximize winter survival and reproductive success in the absence (or experimental presence) of the environmental conditions that led to the evolution of these traits originally.

The immune system is a complex and multifaceted collection of cells, tissues, and soluble factors. Overall the immune system tends to defy large generalizations. As a general rule, however, many types of immune responses are enhanced in short winter-like day lengths compared to long summer-like days. There are counterexamples, and the pattern depends in large part on the species, type of immune assay used, and whether the experiments were conducted in the laboratory or in the wild. Nonetheless, immune responses in general and cell-mediated immune responses in particular are enhanced by exposure to short day lengths in cattle (*Bos taurus*), song birds, non-human primates, and dozens of rodent species including Siberian hamsters (*Phodopus sungorus*), Syrian hamsters (*Mesocricetus auratus*), collared lemmings (*Dicrostonyx groenlandicus*), as well as multiple species of wild mice (*Peromyscus spp*) and voles (*Microtus spp*) (Bentley, Demas, Nelson, & Ball, 1998; Bilbo, Dhabhar, et al., 2002; Blom, Gerber, & Nelson, 1994; Dahl, Auchtung, & Kendall, 2002; Demas & Nelson, 1996; Demas & Nelson, 1998c; Drazen, Jasnow, Nelson, & Demas, 2002; Pyter, Weil, & Nelson, 2005; Vaughan et al., 1987; Weil, Martin, & Nelson, 2006). It is important to emphasize that, in these same species, some aspects of the immune system are compromised by short day lengths; thus, it would be inappropriate to state that all immune responses are enhanced by winter-like day lengths (Bilbo, Drazen, Quan, He, & Nelson, 2002; Drazen, Demas, & Nelson, 2001; Yellon, Fagoaga, & Nehlsen-Cannarella, 1999). A more accurate statement is that the immune system priorities are reorganized by day length.

The near ubiquity of these types of data suggests a question: Why should immune responses vary seasonally at all? Logically, it would seem that organisms should maintain the most robust host-defense processes they can without inducing autoimmunity (Nelson & Drazen, 1999). The answer likely has to do with the metabolic costs associated with maintaining self-defense. Because the immune system is energetically costly to maintain and operate, immune defenses must be traded off with other competing physiological priorities (Demas, Chefer, Talan, & Nelson, 1997; Martin, Scheuerlein, & Wikelski, 2003; Prendergast, Hotchkiss, Bilbo, & Nelson, 2004). Specifically, immune responses are often negatively correlated with reproduction (Bentley et al., 1998; Nelson & Demas, 1997; Prendergast, Hotchkiss, et al., 2004; Prendergast, Nelson, & Zucker, 2009). Our lab has been guided by the overarching hypothesis that exposure to short day lengths prophylactically enhances immune responses to maintain immunological homeostasis in the face of seasonal stressors such as low temperatures and reduced food availability. Indeed, in the laboratory, short day lengths buffer animals against the immunosuppressive effects of low temperatures or food restriction (Bilbo & Nelson, 2004; Demas & Nelson, 1998b). An alternative hypothesis has also been considered (for review, see Martin, Weil, & Nelson, 2008) that suggests that short photoperiod-induced elevation in immune responses result from the energy freed up by regression of the reproductive tract (i.e., maintaining peak performance in both the reproductive system and the immune system is physiologically impossible (for a review, see Martin et al., 2008). Most experimental data support the idea of winter immunoenhancement (e.g., Weil, Pyter, Martin, & Nelson, 2006) rather than

a disinhibition mediated by reduction of reproductive function.

Adaptive Immune Defenses

The adaptive immune system, in general, and the cell-mediated components of the adaptive immune system are robustly responsive to changing day length. The adaptive arm of the immune system is responsible for longer-term defenses against microbes and viruses and is characterized by cells that are capable of generating and maintaining immunological memory. In a photoperiodic context, much of the work associated with this branch of the immune system has focused on one of three general approaches: antigen-specific immune responses (1) in vitro and (2) in vivo, and (3) immune-cell counts and dynamics.

Much of the initial immunological investigations into immune defenses in photoperiodic rodents can be traced to observations that short photoperiods increased the size and cellularity of primary immunological tissues such as the spleen and thymus. However, few studies have fully phenotyped the cells in question using modern immunological techniques. When modern phenotyping techniques were employed, short day lengths increased the number of leukocytes in general and lymphocytes in Siberian hamsters (Bilbo, Dhabhar, et al., 2002). Additionally, delayed-type hypersensitivity (DTH) responses, antigen-specific cell-mediated immune response that serves as an index of immune activity in a number of domains including antigen processing and presentation, immunological memory, leukocyte extravasation, and T cell mediated inflammatory responses (Ramshaw, Bretscher, & Parish, 1976; Wachsman, Luo, Aurelian, & Paoletti, 1992) were also significantly enhanced by exposure to short day lengths (Bilbo, Dhabhar, et al., 2002). The same pattern of enhanced DTH responses have been reported in virtually all rodent species studied, including deer mice, voles, lemmings, and hamsters, and it is among the strongest and most consistent example of enhanced winter immune responses (Bilbo, Dhabhar, et al., 2002; Pyter, Neigh, & Nelson, 2005; Pyter, Weil, et al., 2005; Weil, Martin, et al., 2006).

Additional cell-mediated immune responses have been assessed with leukocyte proliferation assays. Leukocyte proliferation assays are conducted in vitro, but presumably map onto the proliferative capacity in vivo. Cells are isolated from immunological tissues or from the general circulation and then stimulated with an antigen that induces division.

These types of proliferative responses are boosted in short day lengths in voles, cotton rats (*Sigmodon hispidus*), and some species of *Peromyscus* (Demas & Nelson, 1998c; Kriegsfeld, Drazen, & Nelson, 2001; Lochmiller, Vesty, & McMurry 1994; Sinclair & Lochmiller, 2000), although leukocyte proliferation is inhibited by short day lengths in Siberian hamsters (Prendergast, Yellon, Tran, & Nelson, 2001). Finally, antibody concentrations both to antigenic stimulation and basal (natural) antibody concentrations are typically higher in short day lengths in several rodent species (Demas & Nelson, 1996; Demas & Nelson, 1998c; Drazen et al., 2002), although other species also exhibit reduced antibody responses to certain antigens (Hadley, Tran, Fagoaga, Nehlsen-Cannarella, & Yellon, 2002; Prendergast, Bilbo, et al., 2004).

Innate Immune Defenses

The innate arm of the immune system is a broadly effective but nonspecific segment of the immune system that serves to provide front-line host defense against invading microbes and parasites. In contrast to many other aspects of the immune system, short day lengths generally suppress various aspects of the innate arm of the immune system. Siberian hamsters exposed to short day lengths display both fewer circulating monocytes and granulocytes and impaired oxidative-burst activity and phagocytosis in those cell types (Yellon, Kim, Hadley, & Tran, 2005).

Do photoperiod-altered innate immune defenses have functional consequences? To address that question Siberian hamsters were treated with lipopolysaccharide (LPS), a component of gram negative bacterial cell-walls that activates the immune system, but it is not a replicating pathogen. Lipopolysaccharide acts almost completely via activation of the toll-like receptor 4 protein (Hoshino et al., 1999). Cytokine production, as well as the induction of sickness behaviors and fever following LPS treatment was then assessed. Siberian hamsters housed in short day lengths attenuated anhedonic, anorexic, and febrile responses to peripheral LPS administration (Bilbo, Drazen, et al., 2002). These behavioral results are mirrored by reduced in vivo and in vitro expression of pro-inflammatory cytokines both at the gene expression and protein levels (Navara, Trainor, & Nelson, 2007; Prendergast et al., 2003). Additionally, in the nervous system, short day lengths abrogate pro-inflammatory cytokine gene expression and cyclooxygenase-2 induction in the hypothalamus (Bilbo, Quan, Prendergast,

Bowers, & Nelson, 2003; Pyter, Samuelsson, Quan, & Nelson, 2005). This short-day reduction in cytokine response is functional because it serves to protect hamsters from lethal LPS-induced endotoxemia (Prendergast et al., 2003).

The specific mediators of photoperiodic adjustments in innate immune responses remain under investigation, though several possibilities have been ruled out. One possibility is that short day lengths reduced the expression or sensitivity of toll-like receptors, the proteins responsible for the detection of LPS and other pathogen associated molecular patterns (Beutler & Poltorak, 2000; Hoshino et al., 1999). However, short photoperiods reduce LPS induced–pro-inflammatory cytokine gene expression in thioglycollate-elicited peritoneal macrophages without altering gene expression of toll-like receptor genes (Navara et al., 2007). Additionally, inflammogens other than LPS, such as muramyl dipeptide and polyinosinepolycytidylic acid, compounds that act via other toll-like receptors (TLRs), also induce more sickness responses in long-day compared to short-day hamsters (Baillie & Prendergast, 2008). Further, administration of pro-inflammatory cytokines, which presumably bypass the TLRs altogether, also induces a more robust sickness response in long compared to short days (Wen & Prendergast, 2007). Thus, short day lengths both decrease the expression of pro-inflammatory cytokines and decrease the sensitivity of target cells to exogenous (and presumably endogenous) cytokines. Future studies should focus on the cellular signaling pathways that link TLRs to cytokine gene expression and cytokine receptor signaling, although the nuclear factor kappa β (NF$\kappa\beta$) pathway seems an attractive target for photoperiodic regulation. An additional possibility, that photoperiod alters immune system to brain communication of inflammatory signals is currently under investigation. Finally, melatonin signaling in the brain is likely to underlie at least part of the altered immune responses because administration of melatonin into the suprachiasmatic nucleus attenuates the behavioral symptoms of LPS, but not the fever or cytokine responses (Freeman, Kampf-Lassin, Galang, Wen, & Prendergast, 2007).

From an adaptive perspective, apparently the high costs of mounting a fever and foregoing food intake outweighed the antimicrobial benefits of the full suite of sickness responses in short day lengths (Bonneaud et al., 2003; Lochmiller & Deerenberg, 2000; Ricklefs & Wikelski, 2002). Reduced food intake is a hallmark of sick animals and facilitates infection recovery at least in part by limiting microbial access to nutrients (Hart, 1990; Horbury, Mercer, & Chappell, 1995; Murray & Murray, 1979). On the other hand, long-term energy restriction can render animals more susceptible to infection and less able to mount effective host defenses. Additionally, mounting a fever is energetically costly meaning that animals must balance the costs of mounting a fever against the reduced food intake that is associated with full expression of sickness behavior. This equation may have led to the evolution of attenuated sickness responses in the short day lengths of winter when food availability is often scarce. One example of this trade-off is that, in cases of negative energy balance, fever is severely inhibited. Twenty-four hour food deprivation is sufficient to nearly totally block the induction of fever in Siberian hamsters (Bilbo & Nelson, 2002). Induction of sickness behaviors with LPS reduces food intake, but it does not alter food hoarding behavior, suggesting that energetic priorities beyond the acute phase of the infection figure into these physiological calculations (Durazzo, Proud, & Demas, 2008).

MECHANISMS

The principal mechanism that underlies the photoperiodic adjustment in immune responses in rodents is the changing duration of elevated pineal melatonin concentrations. Pinealectomy blocks short-day induced bolstering of immune responses (Yellon, Teasley, et al., 1999), and exogenous melatonin (if appropriately timed and of appropriate duration) is sufficient to restore virtually all aspects of the short-day pattern of immune responses (Demas, Klein, & Nelson, 1996; Demas & Nelson, 1998a; Wen, Dhabhar, & Prendergast, 2007). Further, melatonin enhances cell proliferation responses in vitro, apparently by binding directly to melatonin receptors (Drazen, Klein, Yellon, & Nelson, 2000; Drazen & Nelson, 2001). Finally, melatonin actions on the immune system follow a similar time course in common with its actions on the reproductive system. For instance, short-term extension of the melatonin rhythm (i.e., ~1 week) is insufficient to garner major changes in either the reproductive or immune systems although longer exposure induces the short-day phenotype in both systems (Bilbo & Nelson, 2002; Demas & Nelson, 1998a). Further, after prolonged exposure to short day lengths, rodents become refractory to the suppressive effects of short days on their reproductive systems and undergo a "spontaneous" regrowth of their reproductive systems. The enhanced immune responses also recede on the same

time scale (Prendergast & Nelson, 2001). This phenomenon is mediated by the gradual development of insensitivity to melatonin signaling in neuroendocrine tissues. Interestingly, immune cells seem to follow a similar time course because melatonin no longer alters immune responses in vitro in animals that have become reproductively refractory to short day lengths (Prendergast, Wynne-Edwards, Yellon, & Nelson, 2002).

Taken together, it is apparent that melatonin is the primary coordinator of seasonal rhythms, but it remains somewhat equivocal about whether melatonin acts directly on immune cells or exerts its actions via changes in other intervening neuroendocrine systems. One potential neuroendocrine axis that is both altered by photoperiod and produces immunomodulatory hormones is the hypothalamic-pituitary-gonadal (HPG) axis. In general, androgens tend to suppress many types of immune responses, whereas estrogens tend to be immunoenhancing (Folstad & Karter, 1992; Klein, 2008). In short day lengths, circulating sex steroids are nearly undetectable in both sexes. Therefore, it seemed that if sex steroids mediated photoperiod differences in immune responses, then the decrease in circulating androgens in short-day males should be immunoenhancing. The decrease in circulating estrogens in short-day females should have the opposite effect. However, short days enhance immune responses similarly in both sexes (Bilbo & Nelson, 2003; Demas & Nelson, 1998c) and these effects seem to be largely independent of sex steroid hormones (Demas & Nelson, 1998c; Prendergast, Bilbo, & Nelson, 2005), although steroids may have some relatively small modulatory effects (Prendergast, Baillie, & Dhabhar, 2008).

Another neuroendocrine system downstream of the pineal melatonin rhythm is the hypothalamic-pituitary-adrenal (HPA) axis. Glucocorticoid hormone concentrations and HPA reactivity do vary across photoperiod, but the direction of these changes varies across species; there is no consistent relationship between basal corticosterone and immune responses across photoperiodic conditions (Demas & Nelson, 1998c; Pyter, Adelson, & Nelson, 2007; Pyter, Weil, et al., 2005; Ronchi, Spencer, Krey, & McEwen, 1998; Weil, Martin, et al., 2006). Although basal hormone concentrations do not appear to be critical determinants of seasonal variation in immune responses, seasonal variation in immunological responses to stress-induced glucocorticoids are apparent. For instance, acute stressors enhance immune responses and facilitate trafficking of immune cells out of the blood and into tissues responsible for the first line of immunological defense such as the skin and the lymph nodes (Dhabhar & McEwen, 1997; Dhabhar, Satoskar, Bluethmann, David, & McEwen, 2000). This effect is mediated by the stress hormones of the HPA and sympathetic nervous systems (Dhabhar & McEwen, 1997). Short-day hamsters have an increased number of circulating leukocytes, but they also have enhanced stress-induced glucocorticoid responses. When stressed acutely, short-day hamsters display markedly increased trafficking of immune cells out of the blood and boosted inflammatory responses in the skin (Bilbo, Dhabhar, et al., 2002). Similarly, restraint stress enhanced cutaneous wound healing responses in short-, but not long-day Siberian hamsters (Kinsey, Prendergast, & Nelson, 2003). Short day lengths, thus, appear to facilitate stress-induced enhancement of immune responses, but there is also evidence that exposure to short days can buffer animals from the immunosuppressive effects of stressors. For instance, treating female deer mice (*Peromyscus maniculatus*) with 2-deoxy glucose, a glucose analog that inhibits cellular energy utilization, activates the HPA axis and suppresses splenocyte proliferation only in long-day- but not short-day-length deer mice (Demas, DeVries, & Nelson, 1997).

The autonomic nervous system is also a potential intermediate mechanism for photoperiodic modulation of the immune system. The sympathetic nervous system contributes directly to photoperiod changes in immune responses. In Siberian hamster, removal of the adrenal medulla, the principal source of circulating catecholamines, inhibits antibody production but only in long days. On the other hand, denervation of the sympathetic inputs to the spleen significantly attenuates antibody production, but only in short days (Demas, Drazen, Jasnow, Bartness, & Nelson, 2002). Splenic norepinephrine content is increased by short day lengths in Siberian hamsters, and this phenomenon appears to be at least partially responsible for the short-day-induced reduction in lymphocyte proliferation in this species. Adding norepinephrine to lymphocyte cultures attenuates proliferation responses, but only in short day lengths (Demas, Bartness, Nelson, & Drazen, 2003). Taken together, these data indicate that activity of the sympathetic branch is an important component of photoperiodic changes in immune responses. Less is known about the role of the parasympathetic branch in mediating seasonal changes in immune function, although studies in the cardiovascular system indicate that short day lengths

enhance the activity of both parasympathetic and sympathetic branches of the system. Additionally, stress-induced activation of the sympathetic branch and withdrawal of the parasympathetic system are both enhanced in short-day hamsters, suggesting that the parasympathetics may also have immunomodulatory activity (Weil, Norman, DeVries, Berntson, & Nelson, 2009).

Seasonality in Humans and Nonseasonal Animals

Seasonal rhythms in reproduction are very common in animals that have short gestational and lactational periods because these energetically expensive activities can be timed to occur when resources are relatively plentiful. Humans, on the other hand, have extended gestational and lactational periods that may span several years per child. This means that, in humans, it is unlikely that the timing of birth can be optimized to a particular time-of-year. Presumably, this has relaxed the selection pressure for seasonal timing of reproduction such that only minor photoperiodism remains in human reproductive function (Bronson, 2004). The lack of strong reproductive responses to day length among humans does not mean that some seasonality in other systems does not persist (Foster & Roenneberg, 2008). In this section, we will review the current state of our knowledge about seasonality in the immune system and associated neuroendocrine axes and the consequences these phenomena have for human disease dynamics and health.

Seasonality in infectious diseases has been reviewed extensively (Dowell, 2001; Nelson, 2004; Pinner et al., 1996) elsewhere and is beyond the scope of this chapter. However, some of the theoretical considerations are relevant to thinking about seasonality in the immune system. Four general classes of explanations have been proposed to explain the seasonality in infectious disease epidemiology: (1) changes in pathogen/vector prevalence, (2) environmental changes, (3) changes in host/pathogen behavior, or (4) differential strength of host defense (Dowell, 2001). The evidence that immunological parameters vary across the year in humans and other nonphotoperiodic animals is relatively scant but suggestive. The data on numbers of immune cells at different times of the year are highly equivocal with some studies reporting greater T and or B cell numbers in the summer relative to the winter, whereas other studies have reported the opposite results (Abo & Kumagai, 1978; MacMurray, Barker, Armstrong, Bozzetti, & Kuhn, 1983). Still other studies have reported that, although the total numbers of leukocytes are relatively stable across the year, multiple leukocyte subsets including CD3, CD4, CD8, and CD25 positive T cells, as well as CD20 positive B cells all display high amplitude seasonal changes (Maes et al., 1994). Obviously, experimental methodology, composition of the study participants, and latitude of origin are likely to have important input on the direction of these responses. Still, there is little consensus about how immune cell constituents vary in number across the year.

The data on functional immune assays in humans and other primates are less available as compared to laboratory species. Rhesus macaques' mononuclear and T cells show enhanced Th1 cytokines (IL-2 and interferon gamma) when exposed to ionomycin although the Th2 cytokine IL4 did not vary across the year in that same immune cell population. Rhesus peripheral blood mononuclear cells proliferative responses to concanavalin A (ConA), phytohemagglutinin (PHA), and IL-2 were all higher when sampled during the winter than during the summer (Mann et al., 2000). This is of particular interest because exogenous melatonin enhances anti-inflammatory Th1 immune responses (Kuhlwein & Irwin, 2001). In contrast, healthy human lymphocyte responses to ConA, pokeweed mitogen, and PHA responses were elevated during the summer than the winter. However, women only displayed elevated PHA and ConA responses during the summer, but similar winter and summer responses to poke weed mitogen were reported, suggesting that specific immune responses are modulated rather than an overall alteration in blastogenic responses (Boctor, Charmy, & Cooper, 1989). In a study conducted in the former Soviet Union, live attenuated influenza vaccines were administered intranasally. Vaccine-induced fevers were observed in 6.7% (of $n = 360$) volunteers during the winter but only 0.8% (of 197) when participants were inoculated in June.

Although the immunological details are equivocal, the epidemiological data are straightforward. There are strong seasonal components to several diseases that have no direct link to infectious pathogens. In the next section of the chapter we will consider several pathophysiological conditions that have a strong seasonal component and some of the potential mechanisms that may render individuals more susceptible to these diseases,

Cardiovascular Disease

Since the 1930s, it has been known that deaths from cardiovascular disease vary seasonally (Masters,

Dack, & Jaffe, 1937; Rosahn, 1937). Over the subsequent years, several well-controlled studies using modern statistical methods have confirmed that there is a higher incidence of death from cardiovascular disease during winter than summer. Higher winter prevalence of deaths from acute myocardial infarction (AMI) and other types of ischemic heart disease have been reported in Canada (Sheth, Nair, Muller, & Yusuf, 1999), China (Cheng, 1998), Greece (Moschos, Christoforaki, & Antonatos, 2004), the United States (Spencer, Goldberg, Becker, & Gore, 1998), and the United Kingdom (De Lorenzo, Sharma, Scully, & Kakkar, 1999; Pell & Cobbe, 1999). In countries in the southern hemisphere, including New Zealand (Douglas et al., 1990) and Brazil (Sharovsky & Ce sar, 2002), a similar pattern of cardiovascular mortality exists, but it is 180° out of phase with the northern hemisphere (in keeping with a light exposure pattern that is also 180° out of phase with the northern hemisphere). Individuals are 19% less likely to survive out-of-hospital cardiac arrest during winter than summer (Pell, Sirel, Marsden, & Cobbe, 1999). Winter is associated with greater cardiac infarct volume (measured by creatine-kinase concentrations following MI) (Kloner et al., 2001) and a greater risk of hemopericardium following AMI (Biedrzycki & Baithun, 2006), suggesting that pathophysiological differences are affected by seasonal variation and that these factors may contribute to the greater winter mortality.

Several proximate mechanisms have been suggested to underlie the seasonal variation in cardiovascular disease mortality. Seasonal variation is observed in blood lipid content (Gordon et al., 1988; Woodhouse, Khaw, & Plummer, 1993b), coagulation factors (Woodhouse, Khaw, Plummer, Foley, & Meade, 1994), and arterial blood pressure (Brennan, Greenberg, Miall, & Thompson, 1982; Woodhouse, Khaw, & Plummer, 1993a). In elderly patients, there is a pronounced increase in plasma fibrinogen and factor VII clotting activity (FVIIc) during the winter (Crawford, McNerlan, & Stout, 2003; Woodhouse et al., 1993b). Increases in fibrinogen have been linked to vascular disease, as they can promote atherosclerotic plaque formation, and potentially alter the response to endothelial damage, as well as increasing platelet aggregability, and plasma viscosity (Cook & Ubben, 1990). Additionally, respiratory infections, the incidence of which peak in the winter (Nelson et al., 2002), can also exacerbate these biochemical risk factors (e.g., blood hypercoagulability, increased fibrinogen, etc.)

and predispose individuals to inflammatory damage following ischemia.

Seasonal Affective Disorder

Seasonal affective disorder (SAD) or winter depression is a subtype of major depressive disorder that is characterized by recurrent episodes of depression in the autumn and winter. Typical symptoms of SAD include increased sleep, decreased energy, increased appetite, weight gain, and fatigue (Lam & Levitan, 2000). Superficially, this phenomenon seems to incorporate many of the adaptive adjustments to winter that many organisms undergo. There is mounting evidence, however, that dysfunction in the circadian system rather than an adaptive adjustment underlies this disorder (Lam & Levitan, 2000; Rosenthal, 1993). One of the initial theories to explain SAD was that an inappropriate lengthening of the nighttime melatonin rhythm was responsible (Rosenthal, et al., 1984). Indeed, one of the most efficacious treatment regimens for SAD is bright light in the early morning (Rosenthal, et al., 1984). However, the light-treatment effect appears to be mediated via interaction with the circadian system rather than simply lengthening the photoperiod; brief pulses of light are as effective as lengthening the rhythm and the time of day at which they are administered is not the crucial parameter (Rosenthal et al., 1985; Wehr et al., 1986). Further, runaway melatonin production also does not appear to directly mediate SAD as administration of the beta blocker atenolol, a drug that blocks melatonin production, is not an effective SAD therapy (Rosenthal et al., 1988). One possibility that remains understudied is that seasonal alterations in neuroimmune activity are responsible for SAD (Lam, Song, & Yatham, 2004).

The relationship between pro-inflammatory cytokines and affective disorders has been reviewed extensively (e.g., Miller, Maletic, & Raison, 2009; Raison et al., 2010) and elsewhere in this volume. There is a striking resemblance between the behavioral effects of neuroimmune stimulation and depressive disorders; it is known that cytokines can interact with the neurotransmitter systems that modulate mood (Smith, 1991). Many pro-inflammatory cytokines are elevated in the winter relative to the summer in healthy human patients. For instance circulating basal IL-6 concentrations are higher during the winter months, and immune responses tend to be biased toward a higher Th1:Th2 ratio (Kanikowska et al., 2009; Katila, Cantell, Appelberg, & Rimon, 1993). In a study conducted in a population of individuals overwintering in Antarctica, immune responses were biased toward pro-inflammatory Th1 cytokines like interferon-gamma, whereas anti-inflammatory cytokines such as IL-10 were reduced in the winter versus the summer (Shearer et al., 2002). The only study that examined neuroimmune physiology in SAD patients reported greater circulating IL-6 in depressed patients than in healthy controls. However, in this small study, light treatment that is effective at alleviating depression was not sufficient to alter the IL-6 concentration (Leu, Shiah, Yatham, Cheu, & Lam, 2001). An indirect measure of cell-mediated immune responses, the concentration of the pteridine neopterin, was also elevated in SAD patients relative to controls, but it was also not normalized by light therapy (Auerbach & Nar, 1997; Hoekstra, Fekkes, van de Wetering, Pepplinkhuizen, & Verhoeven, 2003).

An additional small subtype of SAD patients that report the opposite pattern of symptom severity wherein depression occurs during the summer months and abates in the fall and winter has been described (Boyce & Parker, 1988; Han et al., 2000). It has been suggested that elevated temperatures during the summer account for this subset of patients. However, there is another compelling and not mutually exclusive possibility that inflammation due to allergens and environmental pollutants drive depressed affect during the summer. Major depressive disorders are strongly co-morbid to asthma and other allergic airway conditions (Fang, Tonelli, Soriano, & Postolache, 2010; Rosenkranz & Davidson, 2009; Wilson et al., 2010). This link is critically important because a preliminary study reported a twofold increase in suicides among young women during the tree pollen season relative to the rest of the year (Postolache et al., 2005). College students in the Washington DC area that reported mood worsening associated with high pollen counts were significantly more likely to meet the diagnosis for summer-type SAD (Guzman et al., 2007).

In the following section, we will discuss the role of season of birth in establishing adult phenotypes in several contexts. It is relevant at this point to describe here the important relationship among season of birth, immune responses, and exposure to allergens. Season of birth is a major risk factor in the development of allergy and asthma. The precise mediators of this phenomenon may be related to the seasonality of infectious diseases and other environmental conditions (Knudsen et al., 2007). However, there is also evidence that the way the immune system responds to allergens, even in neonates, differs at different times of the year. To examine this phenomenon, peripheral blood mononuclear cells (PBMCs) were isolated from neonatal cord blood and then exposed to allergens and other inflammatory stimuli. Exposure to LPS and peptidoglycan produced elevated interferon alpha responses at all times of the year except July-September, whereas CpG produced enhanced responses during this time. Conversely, exposure to allergens, including dust-mite extract and cockroach, produced markedly greater interferon gamma responses during January-March relative to the rest of the year (Gold et al., 2009). Future studies must examine the linkage among neuroimmune dysfunction, season, season of birth, and psychiatric disease.

Season of Birth Effects on the Immune System

Developmental plasticity is a mechanism by which organisms can adapt to meet the demands associated with environmental conditions. One consequence of this set of phenomena is that early life experiences and environmental conditions can have profound, and in some cases permanent, effects on adult phenotype. In humans, early life experiences have been implicated in a range of disorders, from cardiovascular diseases to psychiatric disorders (Gluckman, Hanson, Morton, & Pinal, 2005). For example, the concept of a "thrifty phenotype" has been advanced to link the conditions of fetal malnutrition with metabolic disorders in adulthood. This hypothesis states that early life privation organizes the metabolic machinery in such a way as to maximize survival early in life (Hales & Barker, 1992); this altered phenotype, however, is often associated with disorders such as cardiovascular disease, diabetes, and obesity, particularly when a high fat diet is available later in life (Gluckman et al., 2005).

Season of birth in many cases can be used as a proxy for a set of early-life experiences. Across the globe, resource availability and environmental conditions vary in a predictable fashion over the course of a year. Pathogens, food availability, and ambient temperatures all vary seasonally. Therefore, organisms developing at different times of the year are likely to experience dissimilar environmental conditions. For example, in industrialized countries, the environment during early life has a profound effect on health outcome. Season-of-birth effects have been reported for numerous health conditions including asthma and allergy, inflammatory-bowel disease (Mikulecky & Cierna, 2005), and multiple sclerosis (Sotgiu et al., 2006; Torrey et al., 2000),

among other diseases with an inflammatory component. These seasonal patterns exist despite the fact that most modern societies are buffered from much of the environmental variation that was presumably experienced by our ancestors. In developing countries, the effects of early-life experiences and environmental conditions are readily apparent. For example, in rural villages in the West African country of Gambia, profound seasonality in humans remains extant. Although Gambia lies only 13° north of the equator, seasonal rhythms in rainfall exist that control the timing of the annual harvest. By the time the rains return in July, the previous year's stores of food have been exhausted. Therefore, there is a distinct season of restricted caloric intake that roughly coincides with the annual onset of the rains, termed the "hungry season" (Prentice, Whitehead, Roberts, & Paul, 1981). Pregnant women reduce weight gain during that period (Prentice et al., 1981); in addition, the incidence of maternal and infant disease, mostly malaria and diarrhea, peak during this time (Ceesay et al., 1997). Because there is a pronounced annual rhythm to these conditions, season of birth can be used as a proxy for early-life experience of these factors. There is evidence that this seasonal phenomenon may have effects on immunological development. Children born during the hungry season have attenuated thymic development and are more likely to contract infections later as juveniles (Collinson, Moore Cole, & Prentice, 2003). Perhaps the strongest evidence for a role of seasonality in the regulation of developmental processes and adult phenotype is that individuals born during the hungry season are significantly more likely to die prematurely than are those born when food is more plentiful (Moore et al., 1997). Moreover, a disproportionate number of these early deaths are associated with infections (Moore, et al., 1997). Importantly, it is not apparent whether the effects on phenotype in this population are due to direct actions of malnutrition and early-life infection, or to indirect endogenous changes in developmental trajectory in response to these conditions.

Seasonal Variation in HPA Axis Physiology

Psychoneuroimmunologists have always been interested in the relationship between stress hormones and the immune system. It may be of particular importance to consider the role of seasonal variation in HPA axis physiology as the activity of this key physiological system varies, not just at different times of the day, but also at different times of the year. The precise directionality of seasonal changes in circulating cortisol has varied from study to study with some studies reporting higher 0900 h cortisol concentrations during winter, whereas others reporting no seasonal differences (Labunets, 1996; Malarkey, Pearl, Demers, Kiecolt-Glaser, & Glaser, 1995; Wehr, Giesen, Moul, Turner, & Schwartz, 1995). However, when studies examined cortisol, glucocorticoid sensitivity, and metabolism together, an interesting pattern emerged. Circulating cortisol at 0900 h was higher. Further, dermal glucocorticoid sensitivity, as measured by blanching under fluorescent light, was also significantly higher during the winter (Walker, Best, Noon, Watt, & Webb, 1997). However, cortisol production rate and clearance rate were markedly lower during the winter, suggesting that the winter HPA axis produces a response that is both slow to turn on, slow to turn off, and may have increased effects due to enhanced glucocorticoid sensitivity (Walker et al., 1997). Circulating adrenocorticotrophic hormone (ACTH), the principal cortisol secretagogue, also tends to be enhanced during the winter relative to other times of the year (Kanikowska et al., 2009). HPA axis reactivity also appears to be enhanced during the fall relative to the spring. For example, ACTH levels were increased in medical students prior to autumn, but not prior to spring examinations (Malarkey et al., 1995). Taken together, these data strongly indicate that season of sampling is a critically important variable to consider when designing experiments in stress-PNI research, and that may help explain some of the variability inherent in human clinical research.

Conclusion

This chapter was intended to provide an overview of some of the current state of the knowledge about the interactions among seasonal rhythms in physiological systems and psychoneuroimmunological function. Photoperiodic rodents can provide a tractable animal model system in which to study seasonal phenomena in species that closely time physiological activities to the calendar. These investigations are important because of the relationship between seasonal rhythms and the vulnerability to disease in human populations. Importantly, the science of psychoneuroimmunology is interested in many of the very physiological and immunological processes that we know vary across the year. Therefore, it is important that the field consider how the season during which experiments are conducted bears on the measures under investigation. Further, integrating seasonal information into these experiments may be beneficial in explaining results that appear to be difficult to explain and replicate.

From a theoretical perspective, consideration of seasonal rhythms may enrich our understanding of why the immune system responds to environmental conditions as it does. In all investigations of standard physiology and disease states, it is beneficial for investigators to consider the environmental conditions to which the study species has been exposed over evolutionary time. More specifically there is much to be learned by considering how environmental challenges varied across the year and what physiological steps may have been taken to counteract these challenges. The remnants of those evolutionary "choices" remain relevant to human health today, even though technology has buffered most humans from the most extreme environmental variables.

Future Directions

1. Can we utilize the knowledge we gain from seasonal breeders to better understand both seasonal variation in immune responses in humans and treat diseases related to the immune system at all times of the year?

2. To what extent does seasonal variation in glucocorticoid responses to stress influence the immune system?

3. What is the precise role of annual variation in neuroimmune responses in seasonal affective disorders?

4. Should clinical interventions for diseases related to the immune system and inflammation be different at different times of the year?

5. What does seasonal variation in the immune system teach us about how immunological regulation evolved?

Related Chapters

For more information on concepts introduced in this chapter, see also Suarez; and Bower, this volume.

References

Abo, T., & Kumagai, K. (1978). Studies of surface immunoglobulins on human B lymphocytes. III. Physiological variations of SIg+ cells in peripheral blood. *Clinical and Experimental Immunology, 33*(3), 441–452.

Auerbach, G., & Nar, H. (1997). The pathway from GTP to tetrahydrobiopterin: Three-dimensional structures of GTP cyclohydrolase I and 6-pyruvoyl tetrahydropterin synthase. *Biological Chemistry, 378*(3–4), 185–192.

Baillie, S. R., & Prendergast, B. J. (2008). Photoperiodic regulation of behavioral responses to bacterial and viral mimetics: A test of the winter immunoenhancement hypothesis. *Journal of Biological Rhythms, 23*(1), 81–90.

Bentley, G. E., Demas, G. E., Nelson, R. J., & Ball, G. F. (1998). Melatonin, immunity and cost of reproductive state in male European starlings. *Proceedings of the Royal Society of London. Series B: Biological Sciences, 265*(1402), 1191–1195.

Beutler, B., & Poltorak, A. (2000). Positional cloning of Lps, and the general role of toll-like receptors in the innate immune response. *European Cytokine Network, 11*(2), 143–152.

Biedrzycki, O., & Baithun, S. (2006). Seasonal variation in mortality from myocardial infarction and haemopericardium. A postmortem study. *Journal of Clinical Pathology, 59*(1), 64–66.

Bilbo, S. D., Dhabhar, F. S., Viswanathan, K., Saul, A., Yellon, S. M., & Nelson, R. J. (2002). Short day lengths augment stress-induced leukocyte trafficking and stress-induced enhancement of skin immune function. *Proceedings of the National Academy of Sciences of the United States of America, 99*(6), 4067–4072.

Bilbo, S. D., Drazen, D. L., Quan, N., He, L., & Nelson, R. J. (2002). Short day lengths attenuate the symptoms of infection in Siberian hamsters. *Proceedings of the Royal Society of London. Series B: Biological Sciences, 269*(1490), 447–454.

Bilbo, S. D., & Nelson, R. J. (2002). Melatonin regulates energy balance and attenuates fever in Siberian hamsters. *Endocrinology., 143*(7), 2527.

Bilbo, S. D., & Nelson, R. J. (2003). Sex differences in photoperiodic and stress-induced enhancement of immune function in Siberian hamsters. *Brain, Behavior and Immunity, 17*(6), 462–472.

Bilbo, S. D., & Nelson, R. J. (2004). Photoperiod influences the effects of exercise and food restriction on an antigen-specific immune response in Siberian hamsters. *Endocrinology, 145*(2), 556–564.

Bilbo, S. D., Quan, N., Prendergast, B. J., Bowers, S. L., & Nelson, R. J. (2003). Photoperiod alters the time course of brain cyclooxygenase-2 expression in Siberian hamsters. *Journal of Neuroendocrinology, 15*(10), 958–964.

Blom, J. M., Gerber, J. M., & Nelson, R. J. (1994). Day length affects immune cell numbers in deer mice: Interactions with age, sex, and prenatal photoperiod. *American Journal of Physiology, 267*(2 Pt 2), R596–601.

Boctor, F. N., Charmy, R. A., & Cooper, E. L. (1989). Seasonal differences in the rhythmicity of human male and female lymphocyte blastogenic responses. *Immunological Investigations, 18*(6), 775–784.

Bonneaud, C., Mazuc, J., Gonzalez, G., Haussy, C., Chastel, O., Faivre, B., et al. (2003). Assessing the cost of mounting an immune response. *The American Naturalist, 161*(3), 367–379.

Boyce, P., & Parker, G. (1988). Seasonal affective disorder in the southern hemisphere. *American Journal of Psychiatry, 145*(1), 96–99.

Brennan, P. J., Greenberg, G., Miall, W. E., & Thompson, S. G. (1982). Seasonal variation in arterial blood pressure. *British Medical Journal (Clinical Research Edition), 285*(6346), 919–923.

Bronson, F. H. (2004). Are humans seasonally photoperiodic? *Journal of Biological Rhythms, 19*(3), 180–192.

Bronson, F. H. (1985). Mammalian reproduction: An ecological perspective. *Biology of Reproduction, 32*(1), 1–26.

Castrogiovanni, P., Iapichino, S., Pacchierotti, C., & Pieraccini, F. (1998). Season of birth in psychiatry. A review. *Neuropsychobiology, 37*(4), 175–181.

Ceesay, S. M., Prentice, A. M., Cole, T. J., Foord, F., Weaver, L. T., Poskitt, E. M., et al. (1997). Effects on birth weight and perinatal mortality of maternal dietary supplements in rural Gambia: 5 year randomised controlled trial. *BMJ (Clinical Research Ed.), 315*(7111), 786–790.

Cheng, T. O. (1998). Seasonal incidence of acute myocardial infarction in the Chinese population. *Cardiology, 90*(4), 312.

Cicho, M., Chadzińska, M., Ksiek, A., & Konarzewski, M. (2002). Delayed effects of cold stress on immune response in laboratory mice. *Proceedings of the Royal Society of London. Series B: Biological Sciences, 269*(1499), 1493.

Collinson, A. C., Moore, S. E., Cole, T. J., & Prentice, A. M. (2003). Birth season and environmental influences on patterns of thymic growth in rural Gambian infants. *Acta Paediatrica, 92*(9), 1014–1020.

Cook, N. S., & Ubben, D. (1990). Fibrinogen as a major risk factor in cardiovascular disease. *Trends in Pharmacological Sciences, 11*(11), 444–451.

Crawford, V. L., McNerlan, S. E., & Stout, R. W. (2003). Seasonal changes in platelets, fibrinogen and factor VII in elderly people. *Age and Ageing, 32*(6), 661–665.

Dahl, G. E., Auchtung, T. L., & Kendall, P. E. (2002). Photoperiodic effects on endocrine and immune function in cattle. *Reproduction. Supplement, 59*, 191–201.

De Lorenzo, F., Sharma, V., Scully, M., & Kakkar, V. V. (1999). Cold adaptation and the seasonal distribution of acute myocardial infarction. *QJM, 92*(12), 747–751.

Demas, G. E., Bartness, T. J., Nelson, R. J., & Drazen, D. L. (2003). Photoperiod modulates the effects of norepinephrine on lymphocyte proliferation in Siberian hamsters. *American Journal of Physiology, 285*(4), R873–879.

Demas, G. E., Chefer, V., Talan, M. I., & Nelson, R. J. (1997). Metabolic costs of mounting an antigen-stimulated immune response in adult and aged C57BL/6J mice. *American Journal of Physiology, 273*(5 Pt 2), R1631–1637.

Demas, G. E., DeVries, A. C., & Nelson, R. J. (1997). Effects of photoperiod and 2-deoxy-D-glucose-induced metabolic stress on immune function in female deer mice. *American Journal of Physiology, 272*(6 Pt 2), R1762–1767.

Demas, G. E., Drazen, D. L., Jasnow, A. M., Bartness, T. J., & Nelson, R. J. (2002). Sympathoadrenal system differentially affects photoperiodic changes in humoral immunity of Siberian hamsters (*Phodopus sungorus*). *Journal of Neuroendocrinology, 14*(1), 29–35.

Demas, G. E., Klein, S. L., & Nelson, R. J. (1996). Reproductive and immune responses to photoperiod and melatonin are linked in Peromyscus subspecies. *Journal of Comparative Physiology. A, Sensory, Neural, and Behavioral Physiology, 179*(6), 819–825.

Demas, G. E., & Nelson, R. J. (1996). Photoperiod and temperature interact to affect immune parameters in adult male deer mice (*Peromyscus maniculatus*). *Journal of Biological Rhythms, 11*(2), 94–102.

Demas, G. E., & Nelson, R. J. (1998a). Exogenous melatonin enhances cell-mediated, but not humoral, immune function in adult male deer mice (*Peromyscus maniculatus*). *Journal of Biological Rhythms, 13*(3), 245–252.

Demas, G. E., & Nelson, R. J. (1998b). Photoperiod, ambient temperature, and food availability interact to affect reproductive and immune function in adult male deer mice. *Journal of Biological Rhythms, 13*(3), 253.

Demas, G. E., & Nelson, R. J. (1998c). Short-day enhancement of immune function is independent of steroid hormones in deer mice (*Peromyscus maniculatus*). *Journal of Comparative Physiology. B, Biochemical, Systemic, and Environmental Physiology, 168*(6), 419–426.

Dhabhar, F. S., & McEwen, B. S. (1997). Acute stress enhances while chronic stress suppresses cell-mediated immunity in vivo: A potential role for leukocyte trafficking. *Brain, Behavior and Immunity, 11*(4), 286–306.

Dhabhar, F. S., Satoskar, A. R., Bluethmann, H., David, J. R., & McEwen, B. S. (2000). Stress-induced enhancement of skin immune function: A role for gamma interferon. *Proceedings of the National Academy of Sciences of the United States of America, 97*(6), 2846–2851.

Douglas, A. S., Russell, D., & Allan, T. M. (1990). Seasonal, regional and secular variations of cardiovascular and cerebrovascular mortality in New Zealand. *Australian and New Zealand Journal of Medicine, 20*(5), 669–676.

Dowell, S. F. (2001). Seasonal variation in host susceptibility and cycles of certain infectious diseases. *Emerging Infectious Diseases, 7*(3), 369–374.

Drazen, D. L., Demas, G. E., & Nelson, R. J. (2001). Leptin effects on immune function and energy balance are photoperiod dependent in Siberian hamsters (*Phodopus sungorus*). *Endocrinology, 142*(7), 2768–2775.

Drazen, D. L., Jasnow, A. M., Nelson, R. J., & Demas, G. E. (2002). Exposure to short days, but not short-term melatonin, enhances humoral immunity of male Syrian hamsters (Mesocricetus auratus). *Journal of Pineal Research, 33*(2), 118–124.

Drazen, D. L., Klein, S. L., Yellon, S. M., & Nelson, R. J. (2000). In vitro melatonin treatment enhances splenocyte proliferation in prairie voles. *Journal of Pineal Research, 28*(1), 34–40.

Drazen, D. L., & Nelson, R. J. (2001). Melatonin receptor subtype MT2 (Mel 1b) and not mt1 (Mel 1a) is associated with melatonin-induced enhancement of cell-mediated and humoral immunity. *Neuroendocrinology, 74*(3), 178–184.

Durazzo, A., Proud, K., & Demas, G. E. (2008). Experimentally induced sickness decreases food intake, but not hoarding, in Siberian hamsters (Phodopus sungorus). *Behavioural Processes, 79*(3), 195–198.

Eng, H., & Mercer, J. B. (1998). Seasonal variations in mortality caused by cardiovascular diseases in Norway and Ireland. *Journal of Cardiovascular Risk, 5*(2), 89–95.

Fang, B. J., Tonelli, L. H., Soriano, J.J., & Postolache, T. T. (2010). Disturbed sleep: linking allergic rhinitis, mood and suicidal behavior. *Frontiers in Bioscience, 2*, 30–46.

Folstad, I., & Karter, A. J. (1992). Parasites, bright males and the immunocompetence handicap hypothesis. *American Naturalist, 139*(3), 603–622.

Foster, R., & Roenneberg, T. (2008). Human responses to the geophysical daily, annual and lunar cycles. *Current Biology, 18*(17), R784–R794.

Freeman, D. A., Kampf-Lassin, A., Galang, J., Wen, J. C., & Prendergast, B. J. (2007). Melatonin acts at the suprachiasmatic nucleus to attenuate behavioral symptoms of infection. *Behavioral Neuroscience, 121*(4), 689–697.

Gluckman, P. D., Hanson, M. A., Morton, S. M., & Pinal, C. S. (2005). Life-long echoes—a critical analysis of the developmental origins of adult disease model. *Biology of the Neonate, 87*(2), 127–139.

Gold, D. R., Bloomberg, G. R., Cruikshank, W. W., Visness, C. M., Schwarz, J., Kattan, M., et al. (2009). Parental characteristics, somatic fetal growth, and season of birth influence innate and adaptive cord blood cytokine responses. *Journal of Allergy and Clinical Immunology, 124*(5), 1078–1087.

Gordon, D. J., Hyde, J., Trost, D. C., Whaley, F. S., Hannan, P. J., Jacobs, D. R., et al. (1988). Cyclic seasonal variation in plasma lipid and lipoprotein levels: The Lipid Research Clinics Coronary Primary Prevention Trial Placebo Group. *Journal of Clinical Epidemiology, 41*(7), 679–689.

Guzman, A., Tonelli, L. H., Roberts, D., Stiller, J. W., Jackson, M. A., Soriano, J. J., et al. (2007). Mood-worsening with high-pollen-counts and seasonality: A preliminary report. *Journal of Affective Disorders, 101*(1–3), 269–274.

Hadley, A. R., Tran, L. T., Fagoaga, O. R., Nehlsen-Cannarella, S. L., & Yellon, S. M. (2002). Sex differences in photoperiod control of antigen-specific primary and secondary humoral immunity in Siberian hamsters. *Journal of Neuroimmunology, 128*(1–2), 39–48.

Hales, C. N., & Barker, D. J. (1992). Type 2 (non-insulin-dependent) diabetes mellitus: the thrifty phenotype hypothesis. *Diabetologia, 35*(7), 595–601.

Han, L., Wang, K., Cheng, Y., Du, Z., Rosenthal, N. E., & Primeau, F. (2000). Summer and winter patterns of seasonality in Chinese college students: A replication. *Comprehensive Psychiatry, 41*(1), 57–62.

Hart, B. L. (1990). Behavioral adaptations to pathogens and parasites: five strategies. *Neuroscience and Biobehavioral Reviews, 14*(3), 273–294.

Hoekstra, R., Fekkes, D., van de Wetering, B. J., Pepplinkhuizen, L., & Verhoeven, W. M. (2003). Effect of light therapy on biopterin, neopterin and tryptophan in patients with seasonal affective disorder. *Psychiatry Research, 120*(1), 37–42.

Horbury, S. R., Mercer, J. G., & Chappell, L. H. (1995). Anorexia induced by the parasitic nematode, Nippostrongylus brasiliensis: Effects on NPY and CRF gene expression in the rat hypothalamus. *Journal of Neuroendocrinology, 7*(11), 867–873.

Hoshino, K., Takeuchi, O., Kawai, T., Sanjo, H., Ogawa, T., Takeda, Y., et al. (1999). Cutting edge: Toll-like receptor 4 (TLR4)-deficient mice are hyporesponsive to lipopolysaccharide: evidence for TLR4 as the Lps gene product. *The Journal of Immunology, 162*(7), 3749.

Kanikowska, D., Sugenoya, J., Sato, M., Shimizu, Y., Inukai, Y., Nishimura, N., et al. (2009). Seasonal variation in blood concentrations of interleukin-6, adrenocorticotrophic hormone, metabolites of catecholamine and cortisol in healthy volunteers. *International Journal of Biometeorology, 53*(6), 479–485.

Katila, H., Cantell, K., Appelberg, B., & Rimon, R. (1993). Is there a seasonal variation in the interferon-producing capacity of healthy subjects? *Journal of Interferon Research, 13*(3), 233–234.

Killestein, J., Rep, M. H. G., Meilof, J. F., Ader, H. J., Uitdehaag, B. M. J., Barkhof, F., et al. (2002). Seasonal variation in immune measurements and MRI markers of disease activity in MS. *Neurology, 58*(7), 1077.

Kinsey, S. G., Prendergast, B. J., & Nelson, R. J. (2003). Photoperiod and stress affect wound healing in Siberian hamsters. *Physiology and Behavior, 78*(2), 205–211.

Klein, S. L. (2008). Sex Differences in Infectious and Autoimmune Diseases. In J. B. Becker, J. K. Berkley, N. Geary, E. Hampson, J. P. Herman & E. Young (Eds.), *Sex differences in the brain: From genes to behavior* (pp. 329–353). New York: Oxford University Press.

Kloner, R. A., Das, S., Poole, W. K., Perrit, R., Muller, J., Cannon, C. P., et al. (2001). Seasonal variation of myocardial infarct size. *American Journal of Cardiology, 88*(9), 1021–1024.

Knudsen, T. B., Thomsen, S. F., Ulrik, C. S., Fenger, M., Nepper-Christensen, S., & Backer, V. (2007). Season of birth and risk of atopic disease among children and adolescents. *Journal of Asthma, 44*(4), 257–260.

Konno, A., Utsuyama, M., Kurashima, C., Kasai, M., Kimura, S., & Hirokawa, K. (1993). Effects of a protein-free diet or food restriction on the immune system of Wistar and Buffalo rats at different ages. *Mechanisms of Ageing and Development, 72*(3), 183–197.

Kriegsfeld, L. J., Drazen, D. L., & Nelson, R. J. (2001). In vitro melatonin treatment enhances cell-mediated immune function in male prairie voles (*Microtus ochrogaster*). *Journal of Pineal Research, 30*(4), 193–198.

Kuhlwein, E., & Irwin, M. (2001). Melatonin modulation of lymphocyte proliferation and Th1/Th2 cytokine expression. *Journal of Neuroimmunology, 117*(1–2), 51–57.

Labunets, I. (1996). Age-related biorhythmical dysfunction of the pineal gland, thymus, and hypophysial-adrenal system in healthy subjects. *Aging, 6,* 167–176.

Lam, R. W., & Levitan, R. D. (2000). Pathophysiology of seasonal affective disorder: A review. *Journal of Psychiatry and Neuroscience, 25*(5), 469–480.

Lam, R. W., Song, C., & Yatham, L. N. (2004). Does neuroimmune dysfunction mediate seasonal mood changes in winter depression? *Medical Hypotheses, 63*(4), 567–573.

Leu, S. J., Shiah, I. S., Yatham, L. N., Cheu, Y. M., & Lam, R. W. (2001). Immune-inflammatory markers in patients with seasonal affective disorder: Effects of light therapy. *Journal of Affective Disorders, 63*(1–3), 27–34.

Liang, H., Zhang, J., & Zhang, Z. (2004). Food restriction in pregnant rat-like hamsters (Cricetulus triton) affects endocrine, immune function and odor attractiveness of male offspring. *Physiology and Behavior, 82*(2–3), 453–458.

Lochmiller, R., Vesty, M., & McMurry, S.T. (1994). Temporal variation in humoral and cell-mediated immune response in a *Sigmodon hispidus* population. *Ecology, 75,* 236–245.

Lochmiller, R. L., & Deerenberg, C. (2000). Trade-offs in evolutionary immunology: Just what is the cost of immunity? *Oikos, 88*(1), 87–98.

MacMurray, J. P., Barker, J. P., Armstrong, J. D., Bozzetti, L. P., & Kuhn, I. N. (1983). Circannual changes in immune function. *Life Sciences, 32*(20), 2363–2370.

Maes, M., et al. Seasonal variation in peripheral blood leukocyte subsets and in serum interleukin-6, and soluble interleukin-2 and -6 receptor concentrations in normal volunteers. (1994). *Experientia, 50*(9), 821–829.

Malarkey, W., Pearl, D., Demers, L., Kiecolt-Glaser, J., & Glaser, R. (1995). Influence of academic stress and season on 24-hour mean concentrations of ACTH, cortisol, and [beta]-endorphin. *Psychoneuroendocrinology, 20*(5), 499–508.

Mann, D., Akinbami, M., Gould, K., & Ansari, A. (2000). Seasonal variations in cytokine expression and cell-mediated immunity in male rhesus monkeys. *Cellular Immunology, 200*(2), 105–115.

Martin, L. B., 2nd, Scheuerlein, A., & Wikelski, M. (2003). Immune activity elevates energy expenditure of house sparrows: A link between direct and indirect costs? *Proceedings of the Royal Society of London. Series B, Biological Sciences, 270*(1511), 153–158.

Martin, L. B., Weil, Z. M., & Nelson, R. J. (2008). Seasonal changes in vertebrate immune activity: Mediation by physiological trade-offs. *Philosophical Transactions of the Royal Society of London. Series B, Biological Sciences, 363*(1490), 321–339.

Masters, A. M., Dack, S., & Jaffe, H. L. (1937). Factors and events associated with onset of coronary artery thrombosis. *JAMA, 109,* 546–549.

Mikulecky, M., & Cierna, I. (2005). Seasonality of births and childhood inflammatory bowel disease. *Wiener Klinische Wochenschrift, 117*(15–16), 554–557.

Miller, A. H., Maletic, V., & Raison, C. L. (2009). Inflammation and its discontents: The role of cytokines in the pathophysiology of major depression. *Biological Psychiatry, 65*(9), 732–741.

Moore, S. E., Cole, T. J., Poskitt, E. M., Sonko, B. J., Whitehead, R. G., McGregor, I. A., et al. (1997). Season of birth predicts mortality in rural Gambia. *Nature, 388*(6641), 434.

Moschos, N., Christoforaki, M., & Antonatos, P. (2004). Seasonal distribution of acute myocardial infarction and its relation to acute infections in a mild climate. *International Journal of Cardiology, 93*(1), 39–44.

Murray, M. J., & Murray, A. B. (1979). Anorexia of infection as a mechanism of host defense. *American Journal of Clinical Nutrition, 32*(3), 593–596.

Navara, K. J., Trainor, B. C., & Nelson, R. J. (2007). Photoperiod alters macrophage responsiveness, but not expression of Toll-like receptors in Siberian hamsters. *Comparative Biochemistry and Physiology. A, Comparative Physiology, 148*(2), 354–359.

Nelson, R., & Drazen, D. (1999). Melatonin mediates seasonal adjustments in immune function. *Reproduction Nutrition Development, 39*(3), 383–398.

Nelson, R. J. (2004). Seasonal immune function and sickness responses. *Trends in Immunology, 25*(4), 187–192.

Nelson, R. J., & Demas, G. E. (1996). Seasonal changes in immune function. *Quarterly Review of Biology, 71*(4), 511.

Nelson, R. J., & Demas, G. E. (1997). Role of melatonin in mediating seasonal energetic and immunologic adaptations. *Brain Research Bulletin, 44*(4), 423–430.

Nelson, R. J., Demas, G. E., Klein, S. L., & Kriegsfeld, L. (2002). *Seasonal patterns of stress, immune function and disease.* New York: Cambridge University Press.

Nelson, R. J., Denlinger, D. L., & Somers, D. E. (2009). *Photoperiodism: The biological calendar.* Oxford, UK: Oxford University Press.

Pell, J. P., & Cobbe, S. M. (1999). Seasonal variations in coronary heart disease. *QJM, 92*(12), 689–696.

Pell, J. P., Sirel, J., Marsden, A. K., & Cobbe, S. M. (1999). Seasonal variations in out of hospital cardiopulmonary arrest. *Heart, 82*(6), 680–683.

Pinner, R., Teutsch, S., Simonsen, L., Klug, L., Graber, J., Clarke, M., et al. (1996). Trends in infectious diseases mortality in the United States. *JAMA, 275*(3), 189.

Postolache, T. T., Stiller, J. W., Herrell, R., Goldstein, M. A., Shreeram, S. S., Zebrak, R., et al. (2005). Tree pollen peaks are associated with increased nonviolent suicide in women. *Molecular Psychiatry, 10*(3), 232–235.

Prendergast, B. J., Baillie, S. R., & Dhabhar, F. S. (2008). Gonadal hormone-dependent and -independent regulation of immune function by photoperiod in Siberian hamsters. *American Journal of Physiology, 294*(2), R384–392.

Prendergast, B. J., Bilbo, S. D., & Nelson, R. J. (2004). Photoperiod controls the induction, retention, and retrieval of antigen-specific immunological memory. *American Journal of Physiology, 286*(1), R54–60.

Prendergast, B. J., Bilbo, S. D., & Nelson, R. J. (2005). Short day lengths enhance skin immune responses in gonadectomised Siberian hamsters. *Journal of Neuroendocrinology, 17*(1), 18–21.

Prendergast, B. J., Hotchkiss, A. K., Bilbo, S. D., Kinsey, S. G., & Nelson, R. J. (2003). Photoperiodic adjustments in immune function protect Siberian hamsters from lethal endotoxemia. *Journal of Biological Rhythms, 18*(1), 51.

Prendergast, B. J., Hotchkiss, A. K., Bilbo, S. D., & Nelson, R. J. (2004). Peripubertal immune challenges attenuate reproductive development in male Siberian hamsters (Phodopus sungorus). *Biology of Reproduction, 70*(3), 813–820.

Prendergast, B. J., Kampf-Lassin, A., Yee, J. R., Galang, J., McMaster, N., & Kay, L. M. (2007). Winter day lengths enhance T lymphocyte phenotypes, inhibit cytokine responses, and attenuate behavioral symptoms of infection in laboratory rats. *Brain, Behavior and Immunity, 21*(8), 1096–1108.

Prendergast, B. J., & Nelson, R. J. (2001). Spontaneous "regression" of enhanced immune function in a photoperiodic rodent *Peromyscus maniculatus*. *Proceedings of the Royal Society of London. Series B: Biological Sciences, 268*(1482), 2221–2228.

Prendergast, B. J., Nelson, R. J., & Zucker, I. (2009). Mammalian Seasonal Rhythms: Behavior and Neuroendocrine Substrates. In D. W. Pfaff, A. P. Arnold, S. E. Fahrbach, A. M. Etgen, & R. T. Rubin (Eds.), *Hormones, brain and behavior* (pp. 507–538). San Diego, CA: Academic Press.

Prendergast, B. J., Wynne-Edwards, K. E., Yellon, S. M., & Nelson, R. J. (2002). Photorefractoriness of immune function in male Siberian hamsters (*Phodopus sungorus*). *Journal of Neuroendocrinology, 14*(4), 318–329.

Prendergast, B. J., Yellon, S. M., Tran, L. T., & Nelson, R. J. (2001). Photoperiod modulates the inhibitory effect of in vitro melatonin on lymphocyte proliferation in female Siberian hamsters. *Journal of Biological Rhythms, 16*(3), 224–233.

Prentice, A. M., Whitehead, R. G., Roberts, S. B., & Paul, A. A. (1981). Long-term energy balance in child-bearing Gambian women. *American Journal of Clinical Nutrition, 34*(12), 2790–2799.

Pyter, L. M., Adelson, J. D., & Nelson, R. J. (2007). Short days increase hypothalamic-pituitary-adrenal axis responsiveness. *Endocrinology, 148*(7), 3402–3409.

Pyter, L. M., Neigh, G. N., & Nelson, R. J. (2005). Social environment modulates photoperiodic immune and reproductive responses in adult male white-footed mice (*Peromyscus leucopus*). *American Journal of Physiology, 288*(4), R891–896.

Pyter, L. M., Samuelsson, A. R., Quan, N., & Nelson, R. J. (2005). Photoperiod alters hypothalamic cytokine gene expression and sickness responses following immune challenge in female Siberian hamsters (*Phodopus sungorus*). *Neuroscience, 131*(4), 779–784.

Pyter, L. M., Weil, Z. M., & Nelson, R. J. (2005). Latitude affects photoperiod-induced changes in immune response in meadow voles (*Microtus pennsylvanicus*). *Canadian Journal of Zoology, 83*(10), 1271–1278.

Raison, C. L., Dantzer, R., Kelley, K. W., Lawson, M. A., Woolwine, B. J., Vogt, G., et al. (2010). CSF concentrations of brain tryptophan and kynurenines during immune stimulation with IFN-alpha: Relationship to CNS immune

responses and depression. *Molecular Psychiatry, 15*(4), 393–403.

Ramshaw, I. A., Bretscher, P. A., & Parish, C. R. (1976). Regulation of the immune response. I. Suppression of delayed-type hypersensitivity by T cells from mice expressing humoral immunity. *European Journal of Immunology, 6*(10), 674–679.

Ricklefs, R., & Wikelski, M. (2002). The physiology/life-history nexus. *Trends in Ecology & Evolution, 17*(10), 462–468.

Ronchi, E., Spencer, R. L., Krey, L. C., & McEwen, B. S. (1998). Effects of photoperiod on brain corticosteroid receptors and the stress response in the golden hamster (*Mesocricetus auratus*). *Brain Research, 780*(2), 348–351.

Rosahn, P. D. (1937). Incidence of coronary thrombosis. *JAMA, 109*, 1294–1299.

Rosenkranz, M. A., & Davidson, R. J. (2009). Affective neural circuitry and mind-body influences in asthma. *Neuroimage, 47*(3), 972–980.

Rosenthal, N. (1993). *Winter blues: Seasonal affective disorder: What it is and how to overcome it.* New York: The Guilford Press.

Rosenthal, N. E., Jacobsen, F. M., Sack, D. A., Arendt, J., James, S. P., Parry, B. L., et al. (1988). Atenolol in seasonal affective disorder: A test of the melatonin hypothesis. *American Journal of Psychiatry, 145*(1), 52–56.

Rosenthal, N. E., Sack, D. A., Carpenter, C. J., Parry, B. L., Mendelson, W. B., & Wehr, T. A. (1985). Antidepressant effects of light in seasonal affective disorder. *American Journal of Psychiatry, 142*(2), 163–170.

Rosenthal, N. E., Sack, D. A., Gillin, J. C., Lewy, A. J., Goodwin, F. K., Davenport, Y., et al. (1984). Seasonal affective disorder. A description of the syndrome and preliminary findings with light therapy. *Archives of General Psychiatry, 41*(1), 72–80.

Sharovsky, R., & Cesar, L. A. (2002). Increase in mortality due to myocardial infarction in the Brazilian city of Sao Paulo during winter. *Arquivos Brasileiros de Cardiologia, 78*(1), 106–109.

Shearer, W. T., Lee, B. N., Cron, S. G., Rosenblatt, H. M., Smith, E. O., Lugg, D. J., et al. (2002). Suppression of human anti-inflammatory plasma cytokines IL-10 and IL-1RA with elevation of proinflammatory cytokine IFN-gamma during the isolation of the Antarctic winter. *Journal of Allergy and Clinical Immunology, 109*(5), 854–857.

Shephard, R. J., & Shek, P. N. (1998). Cold exposure and immune function. *Canadian Journal of Physiology and Pharmacology, 76*(9), 828–836.

Sheth, T., Nair, C., Muller, J., & Yusuf, S. (1999). Increased winter mortality from acute myocardial infarction and stroke: The effect of age. *Journal of the American College of Cardiology, 33*(7), 1916–1919.

Sinclair, J. A., & Lochmiller, R. L. (2000). The winter immunoenhancement hypothesis: Associations among immunity, density, and survival in prairie vole (Microtus ochrogaster) populations. *Canadian Journal of Zoology, 78*(2), 254–264.

Smith, R. S. (1991). The macrophage theory of depression. *Medical Hypotheses, 35*(4), 298–306.

Sotgiu, S., Pugliatti, M., Sotgiu, M. A., Fois, M. L., Arru, G., Sanna, A., et al. (2006). Seasonal fluctuation of multiple sclerosis births in Sardinia. *Journal of Neurology, 253*(1), 38–44.

Spencer, F. A., Goldberg, R. J., Becker, R. C., & Gore, J. M. (1998). Seasonal distribution of acute myocardial infarction in the second National Registry of Myocardial Infarction. *Journal of the American College of Cardiology, 31*(6), 1226–1233.

Torrey, E. F., Miller, J., Rawlings, R., & Yolken, R. H. (1997). Seasonality of births in schizophrenia and bipolar disorder: A review of the literature. *Schizophrenia Research, 28*(1), 1–38.

Torrey, E. F., Miller, J., Rawlings, R., & Yolken, R. H. (2000). Seasonal birth patterns of neurological disorders. *Neuroepidemiology, 19*(4), 177–185.

Torrey, E. F., Rawlings, R. R., Ennis, J. M., Merrill, D. D., & Flores, D. S. (1996). Birth seasonality in bipolar disorder, schizophrenia, schizoaffective disorder and stillbirths. *Schizophrenia Research, 21*(3), 141–149.

Vaughan, M. K., Hubbard, G. B., Champney, T. H., Vaughan, G. M., Little, J. C., & Reiter, R. J. (1987). Splenic hypertrophy and extramedullary hematopoiesis induced in male Syrian hamsters by short photoperiod or melatonin injections and reversed by melatonin pellets or pinealectomy. *American Journal of Anatomy, 179*(2), 131–136.

Wachsman, M., Luo, J. H., Aurelian, L., & Paoletti, E. (1992). Protection from herpes simplex virus type 2 is associated with T cells involved in delayed type hypersensitivity that recognize glycosylation-related epitopes on glycoprotein D. *Vaccine, 10*(7), 447–454.

Walker, B., Best, R., Noon, J., Watt, G., & Webb, D. (1997). Seasonal variation in glucocorticoid activity in healthy men. *Journal of Clinical Endocrinology and Metabolism, 82*(12), 4015.

Wehr, T. A., Giesen, H. A., Moul, D. E., Turner, E. H., & Schwartz, P. J. (1995). Suppression of men's responses to seasonal changes in day length by modern artificial lighting. *American Journal of Physiology, 269*(1), 173.

Wehr, T. A., Jacobsen, F. M., Sack, D. A., Arendt, J., Tamarkin, L., & Rosenthal, N. E. (1986). Phototherapy of seasonal affective disorder. Time of day and suppression of melatonin are not critical for antidepressant effects. *Arch Gen Psychiatry, 43*(9), 870–875.

Weil, Z. M., Martin, L. B., 2nd, & Nelson, R. J. (2006). Photoperiod differentially affects immune function and reproduction in collared lemmings (Dicrostonyx groenlandicus). *Journal of Biological Rhythms, 21*(5), 384–393.

Weil, Z. M., Norman, G. J., DeVries, A. C., Berntson, G. G., & Nelson, R. J. (2009). Photoperiod alters autonomic regulation of the heart. *Proceedings of the National Academy of Sciences of the United States of America, 106*(11), 4525–4530.

Weil, Z. M., Pyter, L. M., Martin, L. B., 2nd, & Nelson, R. J. (2006). Perinatal photoperiod organizes adult immune responses in Siberian hamsters (*Phodopus sungorus*). *American Journal of Physiology, 290*(6), R1714–1719.

Wen, J. C., Dhabhar, F. S., & Prendergast, B. J. (2007). Pineal-dependent and -independent effects of photoperiod on immune function in Siberian hamsters (*Phodopus sungorus*). *Hormones and Behavior, 51*(1), 31–39.

Wen, J. C., & Prendergast, B. J. (2007). Photoperiodic regulation of behavioral responsiveness to proinflammatory cytokines. *Physiology and Behavior, 90*(5), 717–725.

Wilson, D. H., Appleton, S. L., Taylor, A. W., Tucker, G., Ruffin, R. E., Wittert, G., et al. (2010). Depression and obesity in adults with asthma: multiple comorbidities and management issues. *Medical Journal of Australia, 192*(7), 381–383.

Woodhouse, P. R., Khaw, K. T., & Plummer, M. (1993a). Seasonal variation of blood pressure and its relationship to ambient temperature in an elderly population. *Journal of Hypertension, 11*(11), 1267–1274.

Woodhouse, P. R., Khaw, K. T., & Plummer, M. (1993b). Seasonal variation of serum lipids in an elderly population. *Age and Ageing, 22*(4), 273–278.

Woodhouse, P. R., Khaw, K. T., Plummer, M., Foley, A., & Meade, T. W. (1994). Seasonal variations of plasma fibrinogen and factor VII activity in the elderly: Winter infections and death from cardiovascular disease. *Lancet, 343*(8895), 435–439.

Yellon, S. M., Fagoaga, O. R., & Nehlsen-Cannarella, S. L. (1999). Influence of photoperiod on immune cell functions in the male Siberian hamster. *American Journal of Physiology, 276*(1 Pt 2), R97–R102.

Yellon, S. M., Kim, K., Hadley, A. R., & Tran, L. T. (2005). Time course and role of the pineal gland in photoperiod control of innate immune cell functions in male Siberian hamsters. *Journal of Neuroimmunology, 161*(1–2), 137–144.

Yellon, S. M., Teasley, L. A., Fagoaga, O. R., Nguyen, H. C., Truong, H. N., & Nehlsen-Cannarella, L. (1999). Role of photoperiod and the pineal gland in T cell-dependent humoral immune reactivity in the Siberian hamster. *Journal of Pineal Research, 27*(4), 243–248.

Motivation

Arnaud Aubert

Abstract

The scientific framework of psychoneuroimmunology was established with the discovery of reciprocal relations between neuroendocrine and immune systems. This bidirectional communication allowed new insights into functions and mechanisms of defensive processes, including the behavioral symptoms of inflammation. The present chapter suggests a motivational analysis of inflammation and related defensive processes. After the description of the fundamental elements concerning the concept of motivation and its relevance for behavioral sciences, the chapter details the characterization of the influence of the immune system on the brain as a motivational system.

Key Words: motivation, inflammation, adaptation, brain, immune system, defensive strategy, ethology

Introduction

Motivation is one of the fundamental concepts of psychoneuroimmunology and health psychology. These disciplines consider health as a physical but also as a social adaptation. This dynamic perspective, as emphasized by the bio-psycho-social model of health, proposes an ideal ground for motivational studies. As a general principle of physiology, neurobiological regulations involve reciprocal influences. Since stress studies showed abundantly how the brain could influence the activity of the immune system (Costa-Pinto & Palermo-Neto, 2010; Ader & Cohen, 1975), the reciprocal impact of the immune system on the brain should not have been a surprise. However, the immune system was considered by biologists as an isolated autonomous entity until the late 1970s. Common physiological and behavioral symptoms on inflammation such as fever, lethargy, hypophagia or curled posture were traditionally considered as the result of the debilitating action of pathogens. However, as the presence of immune mediators—cytokines—and their receptors were revealed in the brain, the general

framework of psychoneuroimmunology was established: the reciprocal and regulated communication of neuroendocrine and immune systems.

In addition to their role in the coordination of the immune response, cytokines are capable of communicating with the brain and modifying brain neurochemistry. For instance, peripheral and central administration of pro-inflammatory cytokines induces norepinephrine release, especially in the hypothalamus, and increases brain concentrations of tryptophan (Dunn, 2006). Moreover, the intracerebroventricular or intrahypothalamic administration of IL-1β (one of the main pro-inflammatory cytokines) induces the onset of a fever and activates the hypothalamo-pituitary-adrenocortical (HPA) axis (Besedovsky & del Rey, 1996). The brain also expresses a large variety of cytokine receptors, either in neurons and glial cells (Conti et al., 2008). Peripherally synthesized cytokines can act on the brain either directly, by entering the brain through circumventricular organs, which offer a passage for these molecules contrary to the cerebral barrier, or indirectly, by active transport through the brain blood barrier (Banks, 2008). Another influence of cytokines on the brain consists in the activation of afferent fibers of the vagus nerve, which project on the nucleus tractus solitarius (Johnston & Webster, 2009). This activation mobilizes, in turn, many brain areas such as the central nucleus of the amygdala, the bed of the nucleus of stria terminalis, and the paraventricular nucleus. Moreover, it has been shown that brain cells (notably astrocytes and microglial cells) can synthesize and release cytokines (Suzumura, 2008).

However, the whole inflammatory condition of a sick individual should not be reduced to the sole action of cytokines. As a global condition, inflammation is more than the sum of the peripheral processes involved in the acute phase response[1] and includes the subjective responses to the inflammatory condition per se and to the appraisal of the effects of this condition on the interactions with physical and social environments. In this present chapter, inflammation is understood as a global—immune, physiological, and subjective—condition.

The following section presents, first, the fundamental elements concerning the concept of motivation and its relevance for behavioral sciences. It then details the characterization of the influence of the immune system on the brain as a motivational system, and finally describes the various aspects of the motivational dynamics of immune-related issues.

The Concept of Motivation

The fundamental agenda of ethology was synthetized by Nikolaas Tinbergen (1963) and consists of four basic perspectives on behavior: causations (i.e., triggering stimuli and events), function (i.e., the adaptive aspects of behavior), ontogenesis (i.e., the setup and maturation of behavior during development), and phylogenesis (i.e., the setup and appearance of behavior in the species). Motivation, a key concept for behavioral sciences, is related to proximate causations (or "immediate" as distinct from "ultimate" evolutionary causes) of behavior. Classically, motivation designates the tendency of an animal to engage in a specific activity at a given time and in certain conditions. Studies from various fields of research such as psychology, ethology, and physiology have established that this tendency is the consequence of internal physiological phenomena (i.e., cues such as hunger, thirst, hormones, endogenous rhythms, state of maturation, past experience of the animal) and external signals (i.e., stimuli, releasing factors). Hence, motivation is characterized as a dynamic state.

Motivation regroups notions as disparate as instinct, force, urge, need, incentive, emotion, or arousal, derived from very different theoretical fields (e.g., psychology, biology, or physics). This heterogeneity is the consequence of the difficulty in establishing a model that would give a general account of the expression of behaviors from their onset to their interruption. However, two main perspectives can be distinguished. The first perspective is centered on the purpose of behaviors and distinguishes "homeostatic" from "nonhomeostatic" motivations. In other words, two forms of motivated behaviors are considered: those related to the control of homeostasis (i.e., physiological balance) and those unrelated to homeostasis. The first category of behaviors includes what are called "primary" motivations (e.g., thirst, hunger). The second category of behaviors includes those that are not directly related to physiological requirements and respond to "secondary" motivation (e.g., play, curiosity).

The second perspective is centered on the nature of triggering stimuli and distinguishes external incentives from internal drives. For example, the threatening presence of a predator is a potent, external incentive cue promoting fear as a motivational state, which in turn supports defensive behaviors such as fleeing. On the opposite, internal incentive cues such as hormonal factors constitute a set of drives. However, it should be noted that almost all behaviors imply the interaction and not only the simple additive effect of both stimulus categories. For example, the quality of food (incentive cues) will interact with one's hunger (internal drive) to shape the final eating behavior.

As an illustration, a classic "psycho-hydraulic" model was proposed by Konrad Lorenz (1963), characterizing motivation as a reservoir in which a liquid, representing inner motivation, accumulates continually. The evacuation end of the reservoir is blocked by a spring-loaded valve connected to a counterweight, representing the stimulus. When the valve is opened by the joint action of the liquid pressure (inner motivation) and action of the counterweight (potency of the external stimulus), the content of the reservoir flows out, representing the animal engaging in the specific motivated behavior with an intensity corresponding to the rate of flow. This model was originally proposed in the context of the instinctive theory of aggression proposed by Lorenz (1963) and was criticized for, among other points, the absence of supporting evidence on the continuous accumulation of inner motivation.

However, this example nonetheless illustrates the dynamic nature of motivation.

The theoretical pitfalls and the complexity of proposing a general model of motivation would suggest abandoning this concept. However, despite these difficulties, motivation remains a necessary concept in the behavioral sciences. The result of avoiding the use of this concept would be a behavioral repertoire of species consisting of a long list of independent stimulus-response couplings. Therefore, motivation appears useful as an intermediate variable (MacCorquodale & Meehl, 1948) allowing adequate decoupling of stimuli from responses. Indeed, a single motivational state can link a set of triggering stimuli to a set of possible responses. That is, according to the context, several stimuli can trigger the same response, whereas a specific stimulus can trigger several responses. Moreover, interactions among different motivational states or dynamics are conceivable and can give accounts of complex situations in which several conflicting stimuli are present at the same time (e.g., food and predatory cues acting simultaneously on a hungry animal). Motivation is finally the process that provides energy for the achievement of behavior (i.e., arousing dimension of behavior), and it orients action on a specific goal (i.e., directional dimension of behavior).

Operationally, several features of behavior will allow the identification of the expression of a motivational system:

1. *Specificity* in the organization of behaviors, because the motivational state is supposed to coordinate a set specific behaviors.
2. *Hierarchy* in the expression of behaviors, because, according to conditions, new adaptive priorities promote a motivational state to the detriment of others.
3. *Flexibility* of the expression of behaviors, because any motivational state is dynamically bound to changes in environmental conditions.

Inflammation as a motivational system

The action of the pro-inflammatory cytokines in the brain induces a variety of behavioral changes. These are commonly experienced during an infectious episode. The most observable nonspecific symptoms include fever, fatigue, drowsiness, and a reduction in appetite, locomotion and libido (Larson & Dunn, 2005).

Adaptive Value of Immune-related Behaviors

Fever appears as one of the main symptoms of infection and inflammation. Up to the 1950s, fever was considered as a deleterious action of pathogens, but since then its adaptive value has been progressively understood. It is now well recognized as a controlled physiological process provoked by the increase of the cerebral thermal set-point regulated by the hypothalamic neurons of the pre-optic area.[2] The adaptive value of fever has been extensively discussed (Kluger, 1991). Its main consequences are an increase of phagocytic cell activity (Atkins, 1960), faster migration of neutrophils to the site of infection (Nahas, Tannieres, & Lennon, 1971), higher rate of replication of T lymphocytes (Duff & Atkins, 1982), and a decrease in the rate of pathogen proliferation.

In vivo experiments confirm the in vitro benefits of fever. The pharmacological deprivation of fever in infected rabbits increased mortality (Vaughn, Veale & Cooper, 1980), whereas a viral overexpression was observable in ferrets treated with antipyretics (Husseini, Sweet, Collie, & Smith, 1982). Finally, infected poikilothermic animals (e.g., desert iguana, *Dipsaurus dorsalis*) which rely exclusively on behavior (i.e., selection of environmental temperature) to regulate body temperature, showed a mortality rate inversely related to the temperature of the room in which they were confined (Vaughn, Bernhaim & Kluger, 1974). The development of a fever is a metabolically costly process (Kluger, 1991). Curled postures, piloerection, and shivering are physical processes supporting fever, either by decreasing thermolysis (i.e., the loss of body heat) or increasing thermogenesis (i.e., the genesis of body heat). The in vitro and in vivo experiments just described, along with the high cost of fever and its generality across species and phyla, emphasize its adaptive value.

The other main clinical sign of infection and inflammation for which adaptive value has been established is the reduction of appetite and food intake. It has been demonstrated that hypophagia facilitates the reduction of plasmatic iron and zinc (Weinberg, 1984) which, in turn, could decrease pathogenic proliferation. The adaptive value of hypophagia has been demonstrated by increased mortality in force-fed mice infected with *Listeria monocytogenes, a Gram-positive bacteria* (Murray & Murray, 1979). Conversely, short food deprivation (2–3 days) before an infectious episode increased survival rate in mice (Wing & Young, 1980).

However, these adaptive features are not sufficient to establish that inflammation corresponds to an organized motivational system, and the three fundamental features evoked earlier have to be established.

Specificity

If inflammation can be described in motivational terms, then behavioral consequences of the action of the immune system on the brain should be more complex than a simple increase or decrease of the different categories of the behavioral repertoire. For example, it has been shown that besides the quantitative decrease of food intake (i.e., hypophagia), stimulation of the immune system induces qualitative changes regarding diet selection (Aubert, Goodall, & Dantzer, 1995). More precisely, Wistar rats were allowed to freely compose their diet from three macronutrient dishes containing carbohydrates, proteins, and lipids. After the administration of interleukin-1β (IL-1β) or lipopolysaccharide (LPS) to activate the immune system, rats ingested relatively more carbohydrates and less protein, whereas the proportion of lipid remained the same. In order to test the specificity of these behavioral changes accompanied by fever, these diets were compared to free-food selection of rats submitted to another thermic challenge, exposure to a cold ambient temperature. Results showed that, unlike immune-stimulated rats, animals exposed to external cold ingested proportionally more lipids. This comparison confirms that food selection in "sick" rats is not the simple consequence of a sensation of cold (due to the difference between external standard temperature and the raised thermal set-point in feverish rats). If the increased proportion of lipid intake in rats exposed to a low ambient temperature corresponds to the increase of long-term potential energy, the increased proportion of carbohydrates intake fits well with the high short-term metabolic demand of fever.

This qualitative approach applies not only to food intake, but also to gustatory emotional reactions that sustain food selection. Such emotional reactions are widely spread across mammalian species and are expressed as specific facial-expression patterns. For example, specific movements of the lower part of the head can be observed in rats in response to pleasant or unpleasant food sources and constitutes measurable hedonic or aversive behavioral sequences (Berridge, 2000). This experimental approach was used to show that bacterial endotoxin (LPS) does not change the reactions provoked by the ingestion of a solution of quinine (aversive) or saccharose (hedonic). However, compared to controls, LPS-treated rats altered reactivity to a complex compound— saccharin—known for its sweet and bitter-like chemical properties (Dess 1993). Indeed, LPS-treated rats expressed more aversive reactions and less hedonic responses to saccharin compared to controls (Aubert & Dantzer, 2005). Moreover, adding an increasing solution of quinine to a palatable solution of saccharose induces an increase in aversive responses and a decrease in hedonic reactions. These changes appeared faster in LPS-treated rats (Aubert & Dantzer, 2005) and were interpreted in terms of negative alliesthesia (Cabanac, 1979), which corresponds to the negative shift in the perceived valence of a stimulus according to physiological condition.

These changes in hedonic dynamics were interpreted as increased finicky-ness in "sick" organisms as a result of the immune system facilitating the rejection of potential toxic food through its influence on the brain. Indeed, bitterness is frequently associated with the presence of potentially toxic chemicals. Whereas these would normally be tolerated by a healthy organism, they could compromise the recovery of an infected organism (Aubert, 1999).

Hierarchy

In order to illustrate the onset of new behavioral priorities as implicated by the motivational perspective of sickness and inflammation, we can consider a series of experiments involving different aspects of maternal behavior in mice. In rodents, newborns are unable to regulate their body temperature and are dependent on maternal influence, not only for maintaining their inner temperature, but also for feeding, as well as urination and defecation (through anogenital lickings by the lactating dam). Maternal behavior is, therefore, critical for the survival of offspring. When pups are dispersed out of the nest, the lactating dam retrieves them. If the expression of this behavior is blocked in any way, the pups' survival is compromised. In parallel, the building of a suitable nest increases the ability of lactating dams to control their pups' body temperature. However, this component of maternal behavior (i.e., nest building) is not always necessary since the contact with the dam's body can be sufficient to regulate a pup's temperature. Under controlled housing conditions (i.e., 24 ± 2°C), lactating mice construct a fully enclosed nest when the necessary material is provided to them, and the dams retrieve their complete litter when it is scattered out of the nest. Under these same conditions, LPS-treated mice, even if they were slightly slower, still retrieve their scattered litter, but cease to engage in nest building, revealing the new priorities defined by inflammation (Aubert, Goodall, Dantzer, & Gheusi, 1997). In other words, immune-stimulated animals still respond to life-threatening situations, but cease to express more "accessory" activities.

Flexibility

To complete the motivational characterization of inflammation, it is necessary to test whether the new behavioral priorities illustrated above remain dynamically linked to the environmental demands. To evaluate the flexibility of immune-related behavioral changes in pup retrieval and nest-building in LPS-treated dams, the ambient temperature was lowered to 6°C (i.e., simulation of winter conditions) in order to increase the adaptive value of nest raw material. When LPS-treated lactating mice were submitted to such conditions, the scattered litter was not only efficiently retrieved as described earlier, but with the same velocity as controls, contrary to retrieving tests in standard thermal conditions. In addition, an enclosed nest was constructed from available raw materials (Aubert et al., 1997).

Besides maternal behavior, another possibility for testing behavioral flexibility in immune-challenged animals is offered by the study of the different components of feeding behavior. As already detailed, the reduction of food consumption (hypophagia) appears adaptive and promotes recovery. Food consumption represents the "consummatory component" of feeding behavior. Another important phase of feeding behavior is the "appetitive component," which precedes the consummatory phase (Bindra, 1948). The appetitive component of feeding behavior organizes activities aiming at locating and acquiring food resources. Hoarding behavior is a fundamental part of this appetitive phase, especially in rodents. This behavior frees the animal from the obligation to eat food where it has been found. Despite the additional energetic expense it represents, the adaptive value of hoarding behavior lies in the fact that it allows not only a safer consummatory phase away from immediate

predatory threat, but it also provides food stocks for delayed consumption and future needs (Whishaw & Kornelson, 1993).

Rats were observed in a seminatural environment that allowed access to distant food through an alley connected to the home cage (Aubert, Kelley, & Dantzer, 1997). Free access to the alley was granted for a limited time (30 minutes daily). This duration was sufficient for rats to hoard their daily ration, but it also sustained appetitive motivation. Observation revealed that, in standard conditions, rats hoarded a comparable amount of food whether they received complementary food at the end of the day or relied only on their hoarding performances to feed. After the administration of LPS, all animals reduced their food intake as expected. However, hoarding decreased according to their food source, and LPS-treated rats relying exclusively on their hoarding hoarded more food than LPS-treated rats receiving a complementary ration (Aubert et al., 1997). These results show that LPS-treated animals keep the ability to anticipate their future needs, and they illustrate how immune activation can differentially modulate primary and secondary feeding motivation.

Altogether, these findings confirm that the behavioral changes of sick and immune-stimulated animals is not the expression of debilitated capabilities (Miller, 1964; Hart, 1988, Dantzer, Bluthé, Kent, & Goodall, 1993), and specify the full characterization of cytokine-induced inflammation as a motivational system (Aubert, 1999). The behavioral expression of immune-stimulated individuals reflects the onset of specific adaptive priorities centered on recuperatory processes and pathogen clearance via facilitation and support of fever development and immune activity. Nevertheless, behavioral flexibility is maintained and allows sick individuals to interrupt these recuperatory processes to respond to immediate threats and challenges.

Motivational Dynamics: A Functional Model

Defining nonspecific symptoms of inflammation (curled posture, social withdrawal, hypophagia, lethargy) as recuperative processes taking place in the context of motivational dynamics parallels a motivational analysis formerly proposed by Richard Bolles and Michael Fanselow, known as the "Perceptive-Defensive-Recuperative" (PDR) model (Bolles & Fanselow, 1980).

These authors proposed a motivational model to account for the dynamic interactions between two motivational systems: pain and fear. The adaptive functions of pain and nociception have been already emphasized as parts of a perceptual system for detecting and focusing attention on breaches in the organism's physical integrity (McMurray, 1955), and endogenous analgesic processes have also been described as part of the system (Cannon, Liebeskind, & Frenk, 1978; Sherman & Liebeskind, 1979). The PDR model was predicated on the observation that if pain is useful in many cases, in other cases, its inhibition is more beneficial. Interestingly, these cases involve immediate threats in which fear appears as the leading motivational system. Fear and pain were, therefore, proposed as two competing motivational systems, each supporting a specific set of adaptive behaviors. Pain focuses attention on nociceptive stimuli and supports recuperative behaviors (e.g., licking and isolating the wound, resting), whereas fear focuses attention on incoming threats and supports defensive behaviors (e.g., fleeing, defensive aggression, hiding). The resulting PDR model describes three stages:

1. *"Perception"*: identification of the trauma and the relevant environmental elements opposing or facilitating recovery. Other information is ignored.

2. *"Defense"*: coping with the opposing forces to recovery and mobilization of resources for immediate preservation.

3. *"Recuperation"*: long-term development of recuperative behaviors and postures in the absence of immediate threat and inhibition of competing activities.

As an experimental illustration of this motivational sequence, rats were injected with a nociceptive formaldehyde solution under the skin of the dorsal part of the rear paw (Fanselow, 1986). Less than 30 minutes after injection, rats expressed typical behavior (rats raised their paw and avoided any contact with the painful area) in response to the aching burning sensation in the treated zone. However, when these rats were injected and then placed in cages previously occupied by highly stressed rats, the typical recuperative postures motivated by pain disappeared, and rats expressed specific defensive behaviors and postures, such as attempts to flee the cage and freezing in a corner of the cage (Blanchard & Blanchard, 1971). Because such defensive behaviors are specific expressions of fear, it appeared that fear and pain were two opposing motivational systems. Moreover, pretreatment with naltrexone (an opiates antagonist) reduced the expression of these defensive behaviors, confirming the analgesic action of fear. (Such a psychogenic analgesia implies endogenous opiates that are well-known antagonists of nociceptive signaling.)

The three-stage PDR model can be applied to the specific changes induced by inflammation. During the first phase, the infected subject is prone to internal changes and physical symptoms, which lead to the expression of specific recuperative postures and behaviors (curled posture, lethargy, social withdrawal, hypophagia). If, during the perception phase, opposing elements are detected (e.g., alarm ultrasonic calls from scattered litter), the sick individual engages first in the defensive phase to cope with the immediate threat (e.g., pup retrieving). In the case of an intensified threat (e.g., colder thermic conditions), these defensive responses are extended (e.g., raw materials are gathered to form an enclosed nest to protect not only the pups but also the sick dam). Once the threats are gone, infected subjects engage in the recuperative phase and deploy specific recovery-promoting postures and behaviors. The fact that most of observations of sick animals have been done under standard housing conditions (and, therefore, during the recuperative stage) is presumably responsible for the attribution of these behaviors to passive debilitative changes.

The PDR motivational model described by Bolles and Fanselow proposes perception and perceptive changes as the keys to behavioral adaptation. Motivation is, therefore, more than an ensemble of physiological conditions and peripheral parameters. Motivation as a global state embraces cognitive aspects of behavior and represents a central state that organizes perception and action (Bolles, 1967).

A Central State Shaping Perception and Action: The Immune System as a Sensory Organ

In 1984, Edwin Blalock proposed that the immune system should be considered a sensory organ (Blalock, 1984). This was surprising in light of classical references to sensory systems as supporting representations of the world through cerebral processing of information. However, according to Blalock, the role of the immune system would be (as in other sensory systems) to link specific phenomena (in this case penetration of nonself elements), with cerebral processing of that information (in this case via action of cytokines in the brain). In other words, the immune system could be a specific sensory organ designed to perceive the presence of threatening microorganisms and inform the brain. The extensive literature describing the links between the immune system and the brain, and more particularly the presence of brain receptors to cytokines, support this germinal perspective.

A main characteristic of perceptual systems is perceptual integration, that is, the interaction between the various perceptual systems in order to support a whole unitary representation of the world at a specific time and under specific conditions. One of the consequences of the sensory perspective of immune system would be to understand to what extent and in which ways the immune system modifies a subject's integration of its world. For example, while facing an infection, the organism can also perceive external threats or events prone to compromise its survival or fitness. What are the proximal mechanisms and the processes underlying the behavioral adjustments suggested by motivational analysis? Based on the established mechanisms linking immunity and brain, the shared mechanisms among stress, emotions, and immunity comprise one of the main avenues to understand these processes and their evolutionary roots.

It has been demonstrated that the activation of the innate immune system induces a nonspecific stimulation of the HPA axis, which is also well known to be involved in stress and emotional arousal. The sensory perspective on the immune system proposed by Blalock and the numerous common mechanisms shared by the innate immune response and stress argue in favor of common evolutionary roots between these two defensive systems. More specifically, it has been proposed that typical *fight-or-flight* stress response would have evolved from the initial immune defensive response (Maier & Watkins, 1998).

Even the most "primitive" organisms can defend against intrusive pathogens. In invertebrates such as sponges (phylum *Porifera*), phagocytic cells (amoebocytes) detect and participate in the elimination of pathogens. Amoebocytes are primitive forms of multipurpose immune cells found in invertebrates, capable of synthesizing and releasing pro-inflammatory cytokines such as IL-1, IL-6 or TNF, and recruiting other amoebocytes (Hughes, Smith, Barnett, Charles, & Stefano, 1991). Moreover, the roots of immune-to-brain communication can also be found in invertebrates, because IL-1 and its receptors are found in neuronal areas. Finally, amoebocytes also release neuroendocrine factors analogous to vertebrates' CRH, ACTH, and corticosteroids (Ottaviani & Franceschi, 1996). Other recent studies of invertebrates confirm the mechanistic and evolutionary relations between stress and immunity and the joint

release of immune and stress mediators either after an external threat or a pathogenic invasion (Adamo, 2008; 2010). For example, in the cricket *Gryllus texensis*, octopamine (a neuroendocrine mediator of stress response in invertebrates) is increased after an immune challenge (Adamo, 2010). Moreover, exposure to a stressful agent increases the number of hemocytes (invertebrates' immune cells; Adamo, 2010). Thus, the stress response represents an evolutionary development of primary defensive responses (i.e., immune defenses) and could have, therefore, evolved by co-opting existing immune mechanisms (Maier & Watkins, 1998).

This evolutionary standpoint of the relations between stress-oriented and immune defenses along with the perceptual perspective on the immune system argue for the investigation of emotional processes as underlying mechanisms to the motivational dynamics described so far.

Motivational Sources in Immune-Challenged Organisms: Emotional and Cognitive Changes

One of the ways to evaluate motivational and emotional resources of immune-challenged subjects is offered by an experimental paradigm involving defensive behavior during an inescapable threat, as in the forced-swim test (Porsolt, Le Pichon, & Jalfre, 1977; Lucki, 1997). The test consists of placing a rodent subject inside an inescapable cylinder, filled with warm water (24–25°C) in a depth sufficient to prevent the subject from supporting itself on its rear paws or even its tail. The standard protocol implies two sessions separated by a 24-hr period. During each session, several parameters can be measured as active defenses (e.g., climbing, swimming, diving) or passive defenses (e.g., tonic floating). In the first test session, subjects develop more or less defensive behaviors (in some cases until exhaustion), which are inevitably inefficient since the water tank is inescapable. The reduction of active defenses in the second test is considered "resignation" of the subject to its forced immersion, and assimilated to a form of depressive-like behavior that is reversible by antidepressant treatments. LPS-injected mice were submitted to forced swim. In the first test, although endotoxin-treated mice expressed all the behavioral symptoms of sickness behavior before testing, they developed a very energetic defensive activity as soon as they were in contact with water. Moreover, contrary to expectations, the defensive sequence developed by LPS-treated mice during the first test was even more active and vigorous than saline controls

(Renault & Aubert, 2006). In the second test, 24 hours later, very different results were obtained, however. Subjects that were previously treated with LPS displayed significantly more passive profiles compared with controls (Renault & Aubert, 2006). It is important to note that mice previously treated with LPS were no longer under the inflammatory effects of endotoxin during the second series of tests, because the inflammatory episode triggered by LPS is time-limited and gone 24 hours after administration.

The subchronic administration of imipramine (a tricyclic antidepressant that inhibits recapture of serotonin and norepinephrine) blocked the increased passivity in the second test, in mice previously treated with LPS. This prevention of the increased loss of active defenses between the two tests (i.e., after having experienced failure of defensive responses under the influence of LPS), argues in favor of an emotional effect rather than a physiological or motor effect. These results emphasize a relation between emotions (at least primary stress-related emotions) and immunity, conditioned by context and situation parameters. The example of the forced swim test reveals that inflammation potentiates the emotional impact faced by subjects (i.e., the perceived intensity of the threat), and not only the threat per se, but also the outcome of the initial coping with the threat (i.e., success or failure).

The processes involved in the emotional consequences of inflammation can be proposed at two levels:

1. At the perceptive and cognitive levels, inflammation as a global individual condition would modify the appraisal of the faced situation and the evaluation of the capacity to cope with it. Borrowing common terminology of health psychology, inflammation would modify—and generally amplify—the intensity and/or valence of perceived stress.

2. At a physiological level, on the basis of the multiple common physiological parameters shared by immune and stress responses (e.g., the HPA axis), inflammation-induced HPA activation would enhance the emotional arousal provoked by a stressful agent (resulting in additive HPA activation). Such a mechanism has already been described as an "excitation transfer," and it has been proposed to account for cross-facilitation between two different behavioral repertoires sharing common supporting processes, such as between exercise-induced sympathetic arousal and

aggression (Zillman, Johnson, & Day, 1974), or sexual and agonistic behaviors in males on the basis of the common involvement of testosterone (Zillman, 1983).

Individual Inflammation in a Social Perspective
The Immune-challenged Organism Facing its Social Environment

Among the numerous possible forms of social interactions, mating is presumably the behavioral category that has been the most extensively studied. One could assume that the strong underlying motivation and important adaptive consequences are the main aspects responsible for the interest in mating. As for feeding, it is possible (and convenient) to dissociate appetitive from consummatory components of sexual behavior. In males of many species (especially mammals), the consummatory phase consists in mounts, intromissions, and ejaculation, whereas the preceding appetitive phase involves distal searches for female partners and proximal mate selection through proceptive behaviors. In females, sexual consummatory phase generally involves postures facilitating intromission, as in the lordosis frequently observed in mammals (Beach, 1976).

The sexual motivation of immune-stimulated mature rats has been studied (Yirmiya, Avitsur, Donchin, & Cohen, 1995), and it has been shown that the effects of either central or peripheral administration of IL-1b depend on gender. An immune challenge in estrous females drastically decreases both appetitive (i.e., partner selection, proceptive behaviors) and consummatory (i.e., lordosis) forms of sexual activities. However, the same modalities of immune activation have only limited effects on males' sexual motivation, although the presence of nonspecific symptoms on inflammation was observed (Yirmiya et al., 1995). The same results were obtained with LPS, confirming that gender-related changes in sexual behaviors are provoked by the global inflammatory state and not due to specific effects of IL-1 on females. The adaptive value of this dramatic decrease in females' sexual motivation during an immune challenge would be the avoidance of highly probable fetal abnormalities or miscarriage occurring along an infectious episode.

Agonistic behaviors represent another fundamental form of intraspecific interactions, and they are involved in many aspects of social life of almost all animal species. Agonistic repertoire consists of offensive and defensive behaviors and postures (Blanchard & Blanchard, 1971). The offensive sequence includes attacks, bites, and chases, whereas the defensive sequence consists mainly of protections and counterattacks. When confronted by an unfamiliar conspecific in a neutral area, male mice receiving an injection of IL-1β drastically decrease their offensive behaviors but not defensive behaviors (Cirulli, De Acetis, & Alleva, 1998). The differences observed here between the two categories of agonistic behaviors can be understood according to their respective survival value. Because offensive behaviors are energetically costly and not related to immediate survival, it is no surprise that the new motivational priorities favor recuperative processes. Conversely, the defensive component of agonistic behaviors is more relevant in terms of immediate survival and protection of physical integrity and takes precedence over recuperative processes. However, because agonistic behaviors are interactively produced, further studies are needed that better consider the social status (or releasing value) of an immune-challenged animal in an agonistic encounter. This contributes directly to the significance of individual sickness for social conspecifics.

The Immune-challenged Organism as Incentive

Sociality implies contacts—limited in some species, very extended in many others. Whereas sociality offers many advantages to individual organisms (e.g., protection, sharing of resources), the relative promiscuity it implies constitutes a potential weakness because it facilitates dissemination of viruses, bacteria, and fungi (Alexander, 1974). In parallel, the immune response to infection and its behavioral extensions aims to protect the organisms from pathogenic damages and facilitates the progressive clearance of invading microorganisms. Even if not sufficient to clear infection, fighting a pathogen prolongs survival, extends the presence of the infected individual in the social group, and increases the pathogenic threat for healthy group mates.

Several strategies are then conceivable to cope with such a risk. The first strategy consists of avoiding potentially infected sexual partners on the basis of "honest" signals (Hamilton & Zuk, 1982). For example, in various bird species, infection or poor health is associated with a loss of carotenoids, which are involved in both immunity and plumage coloration. As vivid coloration plays a significant role in sexual attraction, the double function of carotenoids implies that potentially infected partners (poor health condition) are less attractive

due to their dull coloration of plumage (Hill, 1991; Andersson, 1994).

The sexual attractiveness of immune-activated female rats has been experimentally assessed. Male rats were given the possibility of approaching two females: a control female and an IL-1-treated one. Results showed that male rats spend significantly more time with the control female, avoiding the other (Avistur, Cohen, & Yirmiya, 1997). On the other hand, inflammation does not seem to dramatically reduce attractiveness of males, and only the highest doses of cytokines (e.g., 10µg/kg IL-1b) reduced proceptive behaviors of females toward immune-activated males. Interestingly, the reduced sexual attractiveness of immune-challenged females mirrors the marked decrease in females' sexual motivation. Such gender-dependent differences are easily understood when considering the higher cost of reproduction for females compared to males. Drastic changes in sexual motivation and attractiveness of immune-challenged females echoes the selectivity of females for sexual partners and emphasizes their higher parental investment (Trivers, 1972). On the contrary, the limited effects of immune activation of males' sexual motivation and attractiveness illustrate their higher sexual and lower parental investment and relatively higher priority of mating.

A second social strategy would imply cooperative behaviors toward the infected member of the group in order to facilitate his or her recovery. As an illustration, it has been observed that infected dwarf mongooses *Helogales parvula* have a facilitated access to food resources and receive more allo-grooming from their social-mates (Rasa, 1976). However, it has not been clearly established that these cooperative behaviors aid in the recovery of infected animals.

Finally, a third strategy to limit socially dependent pathogenic risks involves the control of the intensity and frequency of contacts with an infected social mate and, hence, the control of the exposure to the pathogen. Controlled contact involving a limited exposure to pathogen has been discussed as a possibility to promote survival by sensitizing defenses (Hart, 1990). Some evidence of such a strategy has been described in invertebrates. For example, it has been shown that contacts with conspecifics immunized to the pathogenic fungus *Metarhizium anisopliae* increases resistance in naïve *Zootermopsis angusticollis* termites (Traniello, Rosengaus, & Savoie, 2002). These phenomena have been interpreted as a "social transfer" of immunity. However, the molecular basis of such a transfer remains to be elucidated.

In laboratory mice, it has been shown that endotoxin-induced inflammation could modify social behavior of healthy cage mates under specific conditions. First, it has been observed that, in standard conditions, the simple presence of an LPS-treated conspecific did not change the behavior of healthy cage mates. However, if healthy mice were previously exposed to the putrid odor of 1,5-diaminopentane (a toxic bioamine produced by protein hydrolysis during putrefaction of animal tissue, also known as cadaverine), they significantly changed their social repertoire when confronted with an LPS-treated cage mate, whereas control encounters were not significantly influenced by cadaverine (Renault, Gheusi, & Aubert, 2008). These changes consisted in a decrease in the total duration of physical contacts between healthy and LPS-treated mice, as well as modifications in the modalities of social interactions in the form of increased amount of muzzle sniffing and decreased of anogenital sniffing (Renault et al., 2008). These results show, not only that mice are able to perceive inflammation in conspecifics, but also that environmental factors play a key role in the social response to inflammatory cues. The presence of immune-challenged conspecifics motivates, under certain circumstances, not only defensive behaviors (i.e., the decrease in the total duration of contacts), but also a specific pattern of social exploration (i.e., increased muzzle- and decreased anogenital sniffing).

In order to understand the possible function of such a social pattern, the type of information provided by the different areas of the body in rats and mice has to be considered. Exploration of the anogenital area provides information concerning identity (e.g., species, gender, rank, kin). Such information is supported by major urinary proteins (MUP) known for their large genetic variability (Hurst et al., 2001). Major urinary proteins form a chemical signature of individual identity and allow individual recognition and discrimination in social groups. Moreover, the major histocompatibility complex (MHC, notorious in immunology as the molecular system of self-recognition) supports individual olfactive identity, presumably through specific patterns of catabolic products (Singh, Brown, & Roser, 1987; Singh, 2001; Penn & Potts, 1998).

Sniffing of the muzzle area in rodents is known to provide information concerning diet and recent foraging activities through the release of volatile olfactory cues in breath such as carbon sulfurs (Galef & Stein, 1985). This is an important aspect of social life of rats (Galef & Wigmore, 1983) and mice (Valsecchi & Galef, 1989), because muzzle sniffing supports highly adaptive processes such as social transmission of food preferences (STFP). Social transmission of food preferences designates a form of social learning in which a naïve observer will prefer a novel food previously smelled on a "demonstrator" muzzle. Such a social learning has been argued to facilitate the avoidance of potentiate toxic novel food.

In a preliminary study, the influence of the inflammatory condition of the demonstrator mouse on STFP has been tested (Renault & Aubert, 2007). Results revealed that interaction with an LPS-treated "demonstrator" decreases the social transmission of the food preference in healthy "observer" mice relative to that observed in control "demonstrators." Such inhibition could be considered a social form of another kind of food rejection learned from the experience of sickness after ingestion. Such a learning- behavioral process known as "conditioned taste aversion" (CTA), "Garcia effect" or "sauce Béarnaise syndrome," constitutes a valuable defensive strategy to avoid contaminated or toxic food (Garcia & Koelling, 1966; Riley & Freeman, 2004).

If underlying mechanisms of CTA are now relatively well understood, those implicated in the inhibition of STFP remain to be established. Stimulatingly, recent studies report the discovery of a new family of vomero-nasal receptors in rodents (i.e., formyl peptide receptor-like proteins), which respond specifically to immunoactive compounds such as Lipoxin A4 or N-formyl-Met-Leu-Phe peptide (Rivière, Challet, Fluegge, Spehr, & Rodriguez, 2009). Such receptors offer exiting leads to explore the molecular basis of sickness as a social incentive.

Conclusion

Although the neuroendocrine influence on immunity has been acknowledged for a long time, the discovery of the reciprocal influence led to a reconsideration of the organization and the evolution of defensive resources in organisms. Behavioral studies established several psychological and behavioral consequences of inflammation:

• Common behavioral symptoms of inflammation are not the consequence of a debilitation of infected organisms but, rather, correspond to the expression of a motivational system set up by immune mediators—cytokines— in the brain.

- Inflammation as a motivational system supports recuperative processes and pathogen clearance.
- Inflammation-related behaviors respond to fundamental characteristics of motivational systems with specificity, hierarchy, and flexibility.
- Inflammation as a motivational system is more than a peripheral immune condition but also a central state that influences perception and action.
- This central influence is sustained by emotional and cognitive changes.
- Immune-related behaviors share common mechanisms with other (stress-related) defensive behaviors.
- Inflammation acts as an incentive and interacts with various social motivational systems.

Whereas inner drives (involving cytokines) and external incentives (mostly related to immediate threats) have been clearly identified, it should be remembered that understanding the motivational dynamics of immune-related behaviors requires taking into account contextual parameters. The consequences and perspectives of such findings are relevant not only for fundamental fields of research as ethology and behavioral ecology, but also for applied psychological and biomedical research.

Future Directions

- What are the evolutionary roots of immune-related behaviors?
- What are the molecular cues and pathways involved in the identification of infection in a social context?
- What is the nature of emotions released by inflammatory social cues?
- To what extend can inflammation change individual status or identity in social animals?

Notes

1. The acute-phase response corresponds to the onset of the inflammatory response, which is a necessary process for preservation and restoration of damaged tissues. The sequence of events can be described as a cascade. The whole response regroups a local and a systemic component. The local reaction corresponds to an acute inflammation that involves various cell types (e.g., phagocytes, lymphocytes, endothelial cells). The systemic reaction consists in the release of humoral mediators and their action on distant target cells. This reaction includes neurological, endocrine, and metabolic changes. The main changes are the onset of a fever; the alteration of plasmatic levels of several compounds such as iron, copper, and zinc; the activation of acute-phase proteins by the liver; and the increase of circulating leukocytes. The acute-phase response is largely advantageous for the organism because it allows the restoration of homeostasis. The acute-phase response can be experimentally produced by the injection of lipopolysaccharides (LPS): the fragment of membrane of Gram-negative bacteria. Lipopolysaccharides (or bacterial endotoxin) is a potent inducer of cytokines both centrally and peripherally. As such, LPS is a convenient tool to study the behavioral changes that accompany inflammation because they act as a decoy for the immune system that initiates the full defensive sequence, without the presence of any auto-replicative pathogen.

2. The fever is the consequence of the communication between the immune system and the central nervous system. IL-1β is considered as one of the main endogenous pyrogenic agent and acts on the neurons of the hypothalamic pre-optic area to change the thermal set-point through the action of another mediator on inflammation: prostaglandin E2.

References

Adamo, S. A. (2008). Norepinephrine and octopamine: Linking stress and immune function across phyla. *Invertebrate Survival Journal, 5,* 12–19.

Adamo, S. A. (2010). Why should an immune response activate the stress response? Insights from the insects (the cricket Gryllus texensis). *Brain Behavior and Immunity, 24,* 194–200.

Ader, R., & Cohen, N. (1975) Behaviorally conditioned immunosuppression. *Psychosomatic Medicine, 37,* 333–340.

Alexander, M. (1974). *Microbial Ecology.* New York. John Wiley and sons.

Andersson, M. (1994). *Sexual selection.* Princeton, NJ: Princeton University Press.

Atkins, E. (1960). Pathogenesis of fever. *Physiological Reviews, 40,* 580–646.

Aubert, A. (1999). Sickness and behaviour in animals: A motivational perspective *Neuroscience and Biobehavioral Reviews, 23,* 1029–1036.

Aubert, A., & Dantzer, R. (2005). The taste of sickness: Lipopolysaccharide-induced finickiness in rats. *Physiology & Behavior, 84,* 437–444.

Aubert, A., Goodall, G., & Dantzer, R. (1995). Compared effects of cold ambient temperature and cytokines on macronutrient intake in rats. *Physiology & Behavior, 57,* 869–873.

Aubert, A., Goodall, G., Dantzer, R., & Gheusi, G. (1997). Differential effects of lipopolysaccharide on pup retrieving and nest building in lactating mice. *Brain Behavior and Immunity, 11,* 107–118.

Aubert, A., Kelley, K.W., & Dantzer, R. (1997). Differential effect of lipopolysaccharide on food hoarding behaviour and food consumption in rats. *Brain Behavior and Immunity, 11,* 229–238.

Avitsur, R., Cohen, E., & Yirmiya, R. (1997). Effects of Interleukin-1 on sexual attractivity in a model of sickness behavior. *Physiology & Behavior, 63,* 25–30.

Banks, W. A. (2008) Blood-brain barrier transport of cytokines. In C. Phelps & E. Korneva (Eds.), *NeuroImmune biology vol.6: Cytokines and the brain* (pp. 93–110). Amsterdam, The Netherlands: Elsevier Science.

Beach, F. A. (1976). Sexual attractivity, proceptivity and receptivity in female mammals. *Hormones and Behaviour, 7,* 105–138.

Berridge, K. C. (2000). Measuring hedonic impact in animals and infants: Microstructure of affective taste reactivity patterns. *Neuroscience and Biobehavioral Reviews, 24,* 173–198.

Besedovsky, H., & del Rey, A. (1996) Immune- neuro-endocrine interactions: Facts and hypotheses. *Endocrine Review, 17,* 64–102.

Bindra, D. (1948). The nature of motivation for hoarding food. *Journal of Comparative Physiology and Psychology, 41,* 211–218.

Blalock, J. E. (1984). The immune system as a sensory organ. *Journal of Immunology, 132,* 1067–1070.

Blanchard, R. J., & Blanchard, D. C. (1971). Defensive reactions in the rat. *Learning and Motivation, 2,* 351–362.

Bolles, R. C. (1967). *Theory of motivation.* New York: Harper & Row.

Bolles, R. C., & Fanselow M. S. (1980). A perceptual-defensive recuperative model of fear and pain. *Behavioral Brain Sciences, 3,* 291–323.

Cabanac, M. (1979). Sensory pleasure. *Quaterly Review of Biology, 54,* 1–29.

Cannon, J. T., Liebeskind, J. C., & Frenk, H. (1978). Neural and neurochemical mechanisms of pain inhibition. In R. A. Sternbach (Ed.), *The psychology of pain.* New York: Raven Press.

Cirulli, F., De Acetis, L., & Alleva, E. (1998). Behavioral effects of peripheral interleukin-1 administration in adult CD-1 mice: Specific inhibition of the offensive components of intermale agonistic behavior. *Brain Research, 791,* 308–312.

Conti, B., Tabarean, I., Sanchez-Alavez, M., Davis, C., Brownell, S., Behrens, M., & Bartfai, T. (2008). Cytokine receptors in the brain. In C. Phelps & E. Korneva (Eds.), *NeuroImmune biology vol.6: Cytokines and the brain* (pp. 21–38). Amsterdam, The Netherlands: Elsevier Science.

Costa-Pinto, F. A., & Palermo-Neto, J. (2010) Neuroimmune interactions in stress. *Neuroimmunomodulation, 17,* 196–199.

Dantzer, R., Bluthé, R. M., Kent, S., & Goodall, G. (1993). Behavioural effects of cytokines: An insight into mechanisms of sickness behavior. In E. B. deSouza (Ed.), *Neurobiology of cytokines: Methods in neuroscience* (Vol 17, pp. 130–151). New York: Academic Press.

Dess, N. K. (1993). Saccharin's aversive taste in rats: Evidence and implications. *Neuroscience and Biobehavioral Reviews, 17,* 359–372.

Duff, G. W., & Atkins, E. (1982). The detection of endotoxin by in vitro production of endogenous pyrogen: Comparison with limulus amebocyte lysate gelation. *Journal of Immunological Methods, 52,* 323–331.

Dunn, A. J. (2006) Effects of cytokines and infections on brain neurochemistry. *Clinical Neuroscience Research, 6,* 52–68.

Fanselow, M. S. (1986). Conditioned fear-induced opiate analgesia: A competing motivational state theory of stress analgesia. *Annals of the New York Academy of Sciences, 14,* 40–54.

Galef, B. G., & Stein, M. (1985). Demonstrator influence on observer diet preference: Analyses of critical social interactions and olfactory signals. *Animal Learning and Behavior, 13,* 31–38.

Galef, J. B. G., & Wigmore, S. W. (1983). Transfer of information concerning distant foods: A laboratory investigation of the 'information-centre' hypothesis. *Animal Behaviour, 31,* 748–758.

Garcia, J., & Koelling, R. A. (1966). Relation of cue to consequence in avoidance learning. *Psychomic Science, 4,* 123–124.

Hamilton, W. D., & Zuk, M. (1982). Heritable true fitness and bright birds: A role for parasites? *Science, 218,* 384–387.

Hart, B. L. (1988). Biological basis of the behaviour of sick animals. *Neuroscience and Biobehavioral Reviews, 12,* 123–137.

Hart, B. L. (1990). Behavioral adaptations to pathogens and parasites: Five strategies. *Neuroscience and Biobehavioral Reviews, 14,* 273–294.

Hill, G. E. (1991). Plumage coloration is a sexually selected indicator of male quality. *Nature, 350,* 337–339.

Hughes, T. K., Jr., Smith, E. M., Barnett, J. A., Charles, R., & Stefano, G. B. (1991). Lipopolysaccharide and opioids activate distinct populations of Mytilus edulis immunocytes. *Cell Tissue Research, 264,* 317–320.

Hurst, J. L., Payne, C. E., Nevison, C. M., Marie, A. D., Humphries, E., Robertson, D. H. L., Cavaggioni, A., & Beynon, R. J. (2001). Individual recognition in mice by major urinary proteins. *Nature, 414,* 631–634.

Husseini, R. H., Sweet, C., Collie, M. H., Smith, H. (1982). Elevation of nasal viral levels by suppression of fever in ferrets infected with influenza viruses of differing virulence. *Journal of Infectious Diseases, 145,* 520–524.

Johnston, G. R., & Webster, N. R. (2009) Cytokines and the immunomodulatory function of the vagus nerve. *British Journal of Anaesthesia, 102,* 453–462.

Kluger, M. J. (1991). Fever: Role of pyrogens and cryogens. *Physiological Review, 71,* 93–127.

Larson, S. J., & Dunn, A. J. (2005). Behavioral mechanisms for defense against pathogens. In L. Bertok & D. A. Chow (Eds.), *Neuroimmune biology vol 5: Natural immunity* (pp. 351–368). Amsterdam, The Netherlands: Elsevier Science.

Lorenz, K. (1963). *Das sogenannte Böse. Zur Naturgeschichte der Aggression (On aggression).* Vienna: Borotha-Schoeler.

Lucki, I. (1997). The forced swimming test as a model for core and component behavioral effects of antidepressant drugs. *Behavioral Pharmacology, 8,* 523–532.

MacCorquodale, K., & Meehl, P. E. (1948). On a distinction between hypothetical constructs and intervening variables. *Psychological Review, 55,* 95–107.

Maier, S. F., & Watkins, L. R. (1998). The role of the vagus nerve in cytokine-to-brain communication. *Annals of the New York Academy of Sciences, 840,* 1004–1017.

McMurray, G. A. (1955). Congenital insensitivity to pain and its implications for motivation theory. *Canadian Journal of Psychology, 9,* 121–131.

Miller, N. E. (1964). Some psychophysiological studies of motivation and of the behavioural effects of illness. *Bulletin of the Psychological Society, 17,* 1–20.

Murray, M. J., & Murray, A. B. (1979). Anorexia infection as a mechanism of host defense. *American Journal of Clinical Nutrition, 32,* 593–596.

Nahas, G. G., Tannieres, M. L., & Lennon, J. F. (1971). Direct measurement of leukocyte motility: Effects of pH and temperature. *Proceedings of the Society of Experimental Biology and Medicine, 138,* 350.

Ottaviani, E., & Franceschi, C. (1996). The neuroimmunology of stress from invertebrates to man. *Progress in Neurobiology, 48,* 421–440.

Penn, D., & Potts, W. K. (1998). Untrained mice discriminate MHC-determined odors. *Physiology and Behavior, 64,* 235–243.

Porsolt, R. D., Le Pichon, M., & Jalfre, M. (1977). Depression: A new animal model sensitive to antidepressant treatments. *Nature, 266,* 730–732.

Renault, J., & Aubert, A. (2006). Immunity and emotions: Lipopolysaccharide increases defensive behaviours and potentiates despair in mice. *Brain, Behavior and Immunity, 20,* 517–526.

Renault, J., & Aubert, A. (2007). Endotoxin-induced sickness in "demonstrator" mice disrupts the social transmission of food preference in "healthy" conspecifics. *Brain, Behavior and Immunity, 21,* e33.

Renault, J., Gheusi, G., & Aubert, A. (2008). Changes in social exploration of a lipopolysaccharides-treated conspecific in mice: Role of environmental cues. *Brain, Behavior and Immunity, 22,* 1201–1207.

Riley, A. L., & Freeman, K. B. (2004). Conditioned taste aversion: A database. *Pharmacology, Biochemistry and Behavior, 77,* 655–656.

Riviere, S., Challet, L., Fluegge, D., Spehr, M., & Rodriquez, I. (2009). Formyl peptide receptor-like proteins are a novel family of vomeronasal chemosensors. *Nature, 459,* 574–577.

Sherman, J. E., & Liebeskind, J. C. (1979). An endorphinergic, centrifugal substrate of pain modulation: Recent findings, current concepts and complexities. *Proceedings of the Association for Research in Nervous and Mental Diseases.* New York: Raven Press.

Singh, P. B., Brown, R. E., Roser, B. (1987). MHC antigens in urine as olfactory recognition cues. *Nature, 327,* 161–164.

Singh, P. B. (2001). Chemosensation and genetic individuality. *Reproduction,* 121, 529–539.

Suzumura, A. (2008) Immune response in the brain: Glial response and cytokine production. In C. Phelps & E. Korneva (Eds.), *NeuroImmune biology vol. 6: Cytokines and the brain* (pp. 289–306). Amsterdam, The Netherlands: Elsevier Science..

Tinbergen, N. (1963). *On aims and methods of ethology. Zeitschrift für Tierpsychologie, 20,* 410–433.

Traniello, J. F. A., Rosengaus, R. B., & Savoie, K. (2002). The development of immunity in a social insect: Evidence for the group facilitation of disease resistance. *Proceedings of the National Academy of Science USA, 99,* 6838–6842.

Trivers, R. L. (1972). Parental investment and sexual selection. In Campbell, B. (Ed.), *Sexual selection and the descent of man* (pp. 136–179). Chicago: Aldine Publishing Company.

Valsecchi, P., & Galef, B. G., Jr. (1989). Social influences on the food preferences of house mice (Mus musculus). *International Journal of Comparative Psychology, 2,* 245–256.

Vaughn, L. K., Bernheim, H. A., & Kluger, M. J. (1974). Fever in the lizard *Dipsosaurus dorsalis. Nature, 252,* 473–474.

Vaughn, L. K., Veale, W. L., & Cooper, K. E. (1980). Response of rabbits to pyrogen in a helox environment. *Journal of Thermal Biology, 5,* 203–206.

Weinberg, E. D. (1984). Iron withholding: A defense against infection and neoplasia. *Physiological Review, 64,* 65–102.

Whishaw, I. Q., & Kornelson, R. A. (1993). Two types of motivation revealed by ibotenic acid nucleus accumbens lesions: Dissociation of food carrying and hoarding and the role of primary and incentive motivation. *Behavioral Brain Research, 55,* 283–295.

Wing, E. J., & Young, J. B. (1980) Acute starvation protects mice against Listeria monocytogenes. *Infectious Immunology, 28,* 771–776.

Yirmiya, R., Avitsur, R., Donchin, O., & Cohen, E. (1995). Interleukin-1 inhibits sexual behavior in female but not in male rats. *Brain, Behavior and Immunity, 9,* 220–233.

Zillman, D. (1983). Transfer of excitation in emotional behaviour. In T. J. Cacciopo & R. E. Petty (Eds.), *Social psychophysiology: A sourcebook* (pp. 215–240). New York: Guilford Press.

Zillman, D., Johnson, R. C., & Day, K. D. (1974). Attribution of apparent arousal and proficiency of recovery from sympathetic activation affecting excitation transfer to aggressive behavior. *Journal of Experimental Social Psychology, 10,* 503–515.

PART 6

Clinical Methods and Models (Jain to Segerstrom)

Psychoneuroimmunology of Fatigue and Sleep Disturbance: The Role of Pro-inflammatory Cytokines

Shamini Jain, Julienne Bower, *and* Michael R. Irwin

Abstract

Fatigue and sleep disturbance are rampant in today's society and bear significant costs in terms of health-care dollars, productivity, social relationships, and individual quality of life. Fatigue and sleep disturbance often co-occur in relatively healthy populations as well as in several clinical populations. This chapter discusses the psychoneuroimmunological underpinnings of fatigue and sleep disturbance, focusing specifically on the role of pro-inflammatory cytokines as contributors to both fatigue and sleep problems. The chapter provides a basic review of fatigue and sleep, as well as neuro-immune processes underlying these behaviors. Perpetuating factors, treatment approaches, and future research directions are also discussed.

Key Words: fatigue, sleep, sleepiness, sickness behavior, inflammation, HPA

Introduction

Fatigue and sleep disturbance are rampant in today's society, with notable costs in terms of health care dollars, work productivity, and quality of life. Insomnia and daytime sleepiness are thought to affect 30–40% of the general U.S. population (Hossain & Shapiro, 2002), with 10% meeting criteria for chronic syndromal insomnia (Ohayon, 2002). The prevalence of insomnia has been noted to be even higher in younger adults at over 16% (Breslau, Roth, Rosenthal, & Andreski, 1996), likely reflecting statistics that as a nation, the United States is getting less sleep (Jean-Louis, Kripke, Ancoli-Israel, Klauber, & Sepulveda, 2000). Total direct health costs, accidents, and lost productivity for insomnia alone are estimated as $92.5–107.5 billion in the United States (Stoller, 1994). Several epidemiological studies point to increased cardiovascular and noncardiovascular risk of mortality for those suffering from chronic insomnia, particularly in older adults (Bryant, Trinder, & Curtis, 2004; Foley et al., 1995; Gangwisch et al., 2008; Kripke, Garfinkel,

Wingard, Klauber, & Marler, 2002; Mallon, Broman, & Hetta, 2002). Longitudinal studies also support the linkage between sleep loss and mortality: For example, a study utilizing objective measures (i.e., electroencephalography or EEG) of sleep quality and duration in healthy adults indicated that increased sleep latency (i.e., difficulty falling asleep) was predictive of a near two-fold increase in all-cause mortality, independent of socio-demographic and medical factors (Dew et al., 2003).

Fatigue is also a modern plague on society in terms of prevalence and productivity costs (McCrone, Darbishire, Ridsdale, & Seed, 2003; Rosekind et al., 2010). Recent estimates indicate that up to 38% of community dwelling individuals and 43% of primary care patients experience significant fatigue (Fuhrer & Wessely, 1995; Lewis & Wessely, 1992; Pawlikowska et al., 1994). Fatigue can be a co-morbid symptom for many major medical and psychiatric disorders, including HIV/AIDS, cancer, multiple sclerosis, chronic fatigue syndrome, major depression, and schizophrenia, but it also occurs independently, in otherwise healthy individuals, and can lead to substantial disability and cost for society. In the United States, workers with fatigue cost employers $136.4 billion annually in lost productivity (Ricci et al 2007). Fatigue is also considered an additional risk factor for mortality in cardiovascular, cancer, and aging populations (Melamed, Shirom, Toker, Berliner, & Shapira, 2006; Montazeri, 2009; Moreh, Jacobs, & Stessman, 2010).

Sleep disturbance and fatigue frequently co-occur, and both are also associated with depression, leading some to speculate about potential common mechanisms associated with these behavioral disorders. The clustering of sleep disturbance and fatigue has been noted in otherwise healthy populations (Addington, Gallo, Ford, & Eaton, 2001; Fuhrer & Wessely, 1995; Maes, 2009; Taylor, Lichstein, Durrence, Reidel, & Bush, 2005) as well as in various clinical populations, including individuals with depression, cancer, multiple sclerosis, heart failure, fibromyalgia, and chronic fatigue syndrome (Kirkova, Walsh, Aktas, & Davis, 2010; Motl, Suh, & Weikert, 2010; Nisenbaum, Reyes, Unger, & Reeves, 2004; Rutledge, Mouttapa, & Wood, 2009; Smith, Gidron, Kupper, Winter, & Denollet, 2009). On a behavioral level, dysregulations in sleep may trigger fatigue, and chronic fatigue itself triggers sleep disturbance. Although the co-occurrence of fatigue and sleep disorders is common, it is often difficult if not impossible to trace an exact etiology, as their initial manifestation and perpetuation would likely be heterogeneous between and possibly within populations. Specific precipitating as well as perpetuating factors for fatigue and sleep disturbance would naturally depend, not only on the presence and nature of a particular co-morbid disorder, but also on social and behavioral contexts and responses to initial dysregulation.

Despite challenges in clearly elucidating specific etiologies for fatigue and sleep disturbance in various populations, emerging evidence suggests a potential common psychoneuroimmunologic mechanism that may underlie these and related symptoms, including depression. This phenomenon, termed *sickness behavior*, has been studied in animal and human models for over two decades (Dantzer & Kelley, 2007), with new and exciting developments in the area creating a clearer path to our understanding of neuro-immune and endocrine underpinnings associated with the symptoms and clustering of fatigue and sleep disturbance.

In this chapter, we begin with a general explanation of immune terms and pathways important in understanding sickness behavior. We then describe sickness behavior and the progression of research implicating its usefulness for understanding fatigue and sleep disturbance, with examination of the evidence linking PNI mechanisms with these behavioral symptoms in various populations, and discussion of potential physiological pathways that may be serving to prolong or perpetuate sickness behavior responses in the cases of persistent fatigue and insomnia. Finally, we review evidence for both behavioral and pharmacological treatments for insomnia and fatigue, and we speculate on new directions that may be fruitful in treating these pervasive and debilitating symptoms.

Cytokines: An introduction to the key players in the sickness behavior response

As reviewed in other chapters of this volumes, cytokines are a diverse group of potent, low-molecular-weight proteins and glycoproteins that are secreted by white blood cells (and other cell types), which assist in development and proliferation of immune cell subsets, promotion of inflammatory as well as non-inflammatory processes, and alteration of neurochemical and neuroendocrine processes that affect overall physiology and behavior. Hence, cytokines may be thought to function in a manner similar to neurotransmitters and hormones in mediating specific physiological responses, which rely on receptor-ligand interactions with self (autocrine), local (paracrine) and distal (endocrine) effects.

Because of their notable variability in structure and function, there have been many attempts to classify cytokines. A classification system that has proven useful for stress and behavioral medicine researchers is the classification of cytokines as either *pro-inflammatory* or *anti-inflammatory*. For the purposes of this chapter, we will focus on a group of cytokines categorized primarily as pro-inflammatory cytokines.

Pro-inflammatory cytokines, which include IL-1, IL-2, IL-6, TNF-α, and IFN-γ, promote a variety of cell functions that stimulate and enhance inflammation. In response to infection or tissue injury, pro-inflammatory cytokines released by tissue resident macrophages increase vascular permeability and cellular adhesion, allowing cells to leave the blood vessels and migrate to the site of infection. For example, IL-1 activates the expression of the endothelial adhesion molecule intercellular adhesion molecule-1, (ICAM-1) which, when bound to the properly conformed integrin (e.g., LFA-1) on the surface of immune cells, promotes firm adhesion to endothelial cells for eventual extravasation (migration of cells from the circulation to tissue). TNF-α promotes a similar process for neutrophils by stimulating the production of the adhesion molecule E-selectin on the endothelium, which binds to adhesion molecules on neutrophils. TNF-α, IL-6, and IL-1 also promote the activity of *chemokines*, small polypeptides that may directly assist in the adhesion process as well as subsequently guide cells to their proper destinations in the tissues via chemical diffusion gradients. Finally, some pro-inflammatory cytokines, including IL-6 and TNF-α, mediate systemic inflammatory processes by promoting liver production and release of acute phase proteins such C-reactive protein, an inflammatory mediator and important marker of cardiovascular risk. Pro-inflammatory cytokine response and function is also understood to be a central player in sickness behavior responses, as will be described next.

Cytokines and the Central Nervous System

Cytokines mediate more than local immune responses; cytokines and their receptors are present in many other types of cells besides peripheral immune cells. In the past decade, a growing body of research has demonstrated that cytokines play both direct and indirect active roles within the central nervous system (CNS). For example, it is now known that cytokines are secreted by certain classes of brain cells, including microglial cells and astrocytes (Camacho-Arroyo, Lopez-Griego, & Morales-Montor, 2009; Kronfol & Remick, 2000). The endogenous expression of cytokines and their receptors have been found in the hypothalamus, basal ganglia, cerebellum, circumventricular sites, and brainstem nuclei (Anisman & Merali, 2002). Included in the considerably large list of brain-active cytokines are interferons alpha and gamma, tumor necrosis factors alpha and beta, and interleukins 1, 2, 3, 4, 5, 6, 8, 10, and 12 (Camacho-Arroyo et al., 2009; Kronfol & Remick, 2000). Studies involving systematic administration of cytokines in some of the brain regions mentioned earlier indicate that cytokines promote the release of neurotransmitters, including norepinephrine, dopamine, and serotonin (Anisman & Merali, 2002; Camacho-Arroyo et al., 2009). Thus, cytokines may initiate or modulate neurochemical cascades that directly affect behavior, with further effects on mood in humans.

Cytokines also affect the CNS via peripheral mechanisms. Though cytokines are too large to effectively cross the blood-brain barrier, there are several parallel pathways whereby cytokines affect brain activity (Dantzer, 2009; Kronfol & Remick, 2000). One pathway involves circulating cytokines entering the brain via passive transport in areas where the blood-brain barrier is not present (e.g., circumventricular sites) and stimulating release of cytokines and inflammatory mediators such as prostaglandins of the E2 series (PGE2) from macrophage-like cells that exist in the circumventricular organs. Cytokines may also bind to cerebral vascular endothelium, facilitating the release of active second messengers such as nitric oxide, or be transported across the blood-brain-barrier via carrier-mediated transport. Finally, cytokines affect the CNS indirectly via stimulation of peripheral afferent nerve terminals, such as the vagus nerve (Aronson, Mittleman, & Burger, 2001; Floto & Smith, 2003; Maier & Watkins, 1998). Given the importance of the vagal pathway for facilitating immune-to-brain communication, we briefly summarize research on this pathway below.

Among its many functions, the vagus nerve promotes parasympathetic end-organ activity (such as slowing of the heart beat), primarily via acetylcholine release. Although the vagus nerve has been long appreciated for its efferent innervation of secondary and tertiary lymph organs, such as the spleen, gut, thymus, and lymph nodes, the vagus also receives afferent stimulation from these organs as well. The hypothesis that cytokines might affect brain function via peripheral end-organ stimulation of the vagus has been posited since at least the 1990s (Kapcala, He, Gao, Pieper, & DeTolla, 1996; Maier & Watkins, 1998; Watkins, Maier, & Goehler, 1995). The plausibility of such a hypothesis was partially fueled by the discovery that receptors for IL-1 were found on paraganglia, which surround the terminals of the vagus (Goehler et al., 1997; Wang, Wang, Duan, Liu, & Ju, 2000). Moreover, circulating IL-1β was found to stimulate vagal sensory activity (Ek, Kurosawa, Lundeberg, & Ericsson, 1998). Subsequent studies indicated that direct stimulation of the vagus resulted in inhibition of release of pro-inflammatory cytokines TNF-α, IL-1β, and IL-18 in response to endotoxin, but that this vagal stimulation did not inhibit the release of the anti-inflammatory cytokine IL-10 (Borovikova et al., 2000). Another study (Floto & Smith, 2003) demonstrated that blockade of nicotinic acetylcholine α-receptors on vagal terminals prevents this cytokine antagonism, suggesting that the cholinergic system is indeed an important constituent of this anti-inflammatory process.

The vagus is intimately tied to the effects of cytokines on the CNS in the following manner: macrophages in lymphoid structures may release cytokines (evidence is strongest at this point for IL-1β), which bind to their respective receptors in paraganglia near the vagal terminals. Such stimulation may induce acetylcholine release from paraganglia neurons, activating afferent vagal fibers, which then send signals via neural impulses to the dorsal motor nucleus (DMN) via the nucleus tractus solitarius (NTS), resulting in the production and release of pro-inflammatory cytokines in the brain. Activation of the afferent vagus may also lead to activation of the efferent vagal pathway which serves to dampen inflammation via cholinergic mechanism. This "inflammatory reflex" is relatively fast-acting compared to other peripheral mechanisms that appear to rely on passive transport (Johnston & Webster, 2009). In sum, it is increasingly understood that vagal contributions may play a major role in immune-to-brain communications, and that this interaction appears to be salient for health and disease processes.

Cytokines and Sickness Behavior

After summarizing our current understanding about cytokines and their interactions with the CNS, we now consider the role that cytokines and cytokine-CNS interactions play in the phenomenon of sickness behavior. *Sickness behavior* refers to a constellation of behavioral responses that appear to occur as a result of infection. Observed symptoms in animals have included lethargy and sleepiness, as well as decreased interest in feeding, grooming, and socializing. These behaviors are posited as being evolutionarily adaptive in that they allow the organism to mobilize more efficiently immune defenses against an unwanted pathogen (Hart, 1988). In humans, sickness behavior is characterized by similar symptoms of general lethargy or fatigue, depression or irritability, increased pain sensitivity, sleep disturbance, and concentration difficulties.

Although the phenomenon of sickness behavior had been observed in animals and humans in scientific journals in the earlier part of the twentieth century, the physiological mechanisms manifesting the associated symptomatology remained unclear. Some of the first scientific papers positing the existence of inflammatory mediators (then discussed as "endogenous pyrogens" in reference to their fever-causing effects) as contributing factors to sickness behavior in animals were published in the 1960s (N. E. Miller, 1964). Linkages between inflammation and

sickness behavior were further supported by early animal studies reporting increased sickness behavior symptoms such as decreased activity, hypersomnia, decreased feeding behavior, learning impairment, and social withdrawal, after central or peripheral stimulation with cytokines (IL-1β or TNF-α) or endotoxin (lipopolysaccharide or LPS) (Dinarello, 1988; Gibertini, Newton, Friedman, & Klein, 1995; Krueger, Walter, Dinarello, Wolff, & Chedid, 1984; Shimommura et al., 1990). Further studies confirmed that the effects of peripheral administration of LPS or IL-1β were vagally mediated, as vagotomy attenuated the sickness behavior responses but not plasma levels or cytokine production by peritoneal macrophages (Bluthé, Michaud, Kelley, & Dantzer, 1996a, 1996b; Bluthé et al., 1994; Bret-Dibat, Bluthé, Kent, Kelley, & Dantzer, 1995). Other studies suggested that this vagal pathway was important for the behavioral, but not necessarily for febrile, response to inflammation (Konsman, Luheshi, Bluthé, & Dantzer, 2000; Luheshi et al., 2000).

Regarding cytokine-endocrine interactions, Besedovsky and colleagues (Besedovsky, del Rey, Sorkin, & Dinarello, 1986) provided perhaps the first evidence that administration of the previously described "endogenous pyrogen" (now known as interleukin-1 or IL-1) altered hypothalamic-pituitary-adrenal (HPA) axis function while promoting sickness behavior in the rat. A later study suggested that the effects of IL-1 on the HPA were mediated by the activation of corticotrophin releasing factor (CRF) in the paraventricular nucleus of the hypothalamus (Berkenbosch, van Oers, del Rey, Tilders, & Besedovsky, 1987), providing more evidence for the importance of immune-brain interactions in understanding sickness behavior. Studies also suggested that sickness behavior was, not only an adaptive response to innate immune system stimulation (Tazi, Dantzer, Crestani, & Le Moal, 1988), but also that sickness behavior itself was not static; its manifestation and form depended in part on motivational factors (Aubert, Goodall, Dantzer, & Gheusi, 1997). These and other studies (such as the studies described in the previous section of cytokine-CNS interactions) helped to lay the foundation for our understanding of neural-immune processes associated with inflammation and sickness behavior, and they suggest that although initial sickness behavior is an adaptive process aimed at allowing the individual to mobilize resources in order to fight infection, pathology may occur when sickness behavior is prolonged or occurs in absence of a stimulus.

Despite the advances put forth from animal studies, questions remained regarding the influence of inflammatory cytokine activity and sickness behavior-related symptoms (e.g., fatigue, depression, and insomnia) in humans. Studies with various human populations in the last two decades have helped to establish linkages between inflammatory immune activation and sickness behavior. Some of the first observations about sickness behavior were based on cancer patients treated with IFN-α, a potent inducer of inflammatory activity. IFN-α treatment leads to a range of neurobehavioral changes, including fatigue, loss of appetite, and disturbed sleep, as well as cognitive disturbance and hallmark symptoms of depression, such as anhedonia and feelings of sadness (Capuron et al., 2002; Capuron, Ravaud, & Dantzer, 2000). These symptoms seem directly linked to the presence of the exogenous cytokines, because symptoms remit after cessation of cytokine therapy (Anisman & Merali, 2002).

Similar behavioral changes have been observed in experimental studies conducted with healthy individuals. In particular, administration of endotoxin versus placebo leads to increases in feelings of fatigue, sleep disturbance, and depression, as well as social disconnection in healthy participants (Eisenberger, Berkman, et al., 2010; Eisenberger, Inagaki, Mashal, & Irwin, 2010; Harrison et al., 2009; Reichenberg et al., 2001; Spath-Schwalbe et al., 1998). Further, it appears that inflammation-driven changes in mood are associated with neural changes such as reduced functional connectivity between the subgenual anterior cingulate cortex, the amygdala, and the medial prefrontal cortex (Harrison et al., 2009), as well as reduced ventral striatum activity in response to reward cues (Eisenberger, Berkman et al., 2010). This work builds on basic research conducted in animal models to demonstrate a causal role for pro-inflammatory cytokines in sickness behavior. We turn now to a more focused consideration of links between inflammation, fatigue, and sleep disturbance.

Inflammation and Fatigue

Fatigue is a multifactorial construct and may involve mental, physical, cognitive, and emotional components. Fatigue has also been classified as *peripherally related* (e.g., fatigue associated with an inability for the musculature to transmit CNS signals; this type of fatigue is experienced more on a somatic level), or *centrally related* (e.g., fatigue that results in an inability to engage in or maintain voluntary activities; this would include cognitive, motor,

emotional, and social aspects of fatigue) (Ryan et al., 2007). Fatigue may be acute (for example, in response to an acute illness or transient insomnia), or chronic (as in the case of particular disorders or syndromes such as chronic fatigue syndrome or persistent cancer-related fatigue). Although fatigue is a pervasive problem among many different populations, there has been no clear defining instrument for fatigue, nor a defining etiology of fatigue. Fatigue is inherently a subjective phenomenon, and many self-report instruments have been developed to measure fatigue both in the general population (for example, the SF-36 Vitality subscale) as well as within specific clinical populations (for example, the Functional Assessment of Cancer Therapy Fatigue Scale, and Functional Assessment of Chronic Illness Fatigue Scale). Measures and cutoffs for these scales naturally depend on the populations assessed; however, there are efforts to create a more systematic, categorical measurement of fatigue within and across populations (Barsevick et al., 2010; Jhamb, Weisbord, Steel, & Unruh, 2008).

Perhaps the most prevalent area of research examining the relationship between inflammation and fatigue is within cancer populations. Fatigue is one of the most common and distressing side effects of cancer diagnosis and treatment. Prevalence estimates of fatigue during treatment range from 25% to 99% depending on the study sample and method of assessment; in the majority of studies, 30% to 60% of patients report moderate or severe fatigue symptoms (Lawrence, Kupelnick, Miller, Devine, & Lau, 2004, Servaes, Verhagen, & Bleijenberg, 2002). Cancer provides a compelling model for the investigation of cytokine effects on the brain and behavior, because there is a specific triggering event (i.e., the cancer and its treatment) that precipitates increases in fatigue (and other behavioral symptoms) as well as changes in immune and inflammatory markers. Studies have examined the association between pro-inflammatory cytokines and fatigue in cancer patients before, during, and after treatment, and they have generally shown a positive association between inflammation and fatigue (Schubert et al 2007).

Tumors can secrete pro-inflammatory cytokines, and elevations in IL-6 in plasma and ascites are associated with symptoms of fatigue (and other vegetative symptoms of depression) in patients with invasive ovarian cancer prior to surgery (Lutgendorf et al 2008). Cancer treatments, including radiation and chemotherapy, also have pronounced effects on the immune system. The general immunosuppressive side effects of these therapies are well known; for example, chemotherapy generally causes leukopenia, erythropenia, neutropenia, and thrombocytopenia, often due to myelosuppression and sometimes myeloablation (Wijayahadi, Haron, Stanslas, & Yusuf, 2007). However, it is only recently that studies have begun to examine the effects of these treatments on inflammatory processes. A few studies suggest that chemotherapy for breast cancer patients alters levels of inflammatory immune mediators such as interleukin-8, vascular endothelial growth factor (VEGF), and soluble intercellular adhesion molecule-1 (sICAM-1) throughout the course of chemotherapy, with the net effect of chemotherapy being to increase overall activity in these and other inflammatory markers related to chemotaxis and endothelial and platelet activation (Mills et al., 2008; Mills et al., 2004; Pusztai et al., 2004).

Chemotherapy-related alterations in pro-inflammatory cytokines have been linked to fatigue in some reports. For example, a recent study reported increases in serum levels of IL-6 and soluble TNF receptor type I (sTNF-R1) among non-small-cell lung cancer patients treated with chemoradiation treatment that were associated with increases in symptom severity, including fatigue (Wang et al., 2010). Increases in VEGF and sICAM-1 have been found to significantly co-vary with fatigue and quality of life ratings among breast cancer patients undergoing chemotherapy (Mills, Parker, Dimsdale, Sadler, & Ancoli-Israel, 2005). Interestingly, one study has reported that pharmacological blockade of the inflammatory cytokine TNF-alpha during chemotherapy treatment with docetaxel resulted in decreased reports of fatigue in patients (Monk et al., 2006), further suggesting linkages between increases of inflammation and fatigue during chemotherapy.

Increases in inflammation and fatigue have also been associated with radiation therapy in cancer patients. An early study reported concomitant increases in interleukin-1-beta (IL-1β) and fatigue for prostate cancer patients undergoing radiotherapy (Greenberg, Gray, Mannix, Eisenthal, & Carey, 1993). A few studies have also reported significant correlations between increases of interleukin-6 and fatigue levels during radiotherapy (Ahlberg, Ekman, & Gaston-Johansson, 2004), although this result has not always been replicated (Bower et al., 2009; Geinitz et al., 2001). More recent work has shown an association between increases in downstream markers of pro-inflammatory cytokine activity (i.e., interleukin-1 receptor antagonist [IL-1Ra],

C-reactive protein [CRP]) and fatigue in breast and prostate cancer patients undergoing radiation therapy (Bower et al., 2009).

Even after chemotherapy and/or radiation treatments are over, fatigue lingers in about one-third of survivors, with symptoms persisting for up to 10 years (Bower et al., 2006). Findings from several studies suggest that cancer survivors who suffer from persistent posttreatment fatigue have increased plasma levels of inflammatory markers, such as IL-6 and its soluble receptor (sIL-6r), IL-1Ra, CRP, soluble tumor necrosis factor receptor type II (TNF-RII), and neopterin (Alexander, Minton, Andrews, & Stone, 2009; Bower, Ganz, Aziz, & Fahey, 2002; Collado-Hidalgo, Bower, Ganz, Cole, & Irwin, 2006; Inagaki et al., 2008). These findings have been supported by ex vivo studies as well: Comparative increases in IL-6 and TNF-alpha production by LPS-stimulated monocytes have also been found for fatigued versus nonfatigued breast cancer survivors (Collado-Hidalgo, Bower, Ganz, Cole, & Irwin, 2006). Our group has also examined the molecular underpinnings of cancer-related fatigue and found that fatigued survivors show up-regulation of the pro-inflammatory transcription factor nuclear-factor kappa-B (NF-κB) relative to nonfatigued survivors (Bower, Ganz, Irwin, Arevalo, & Cole, 2011), further supporting the hypothesis that increases in inflammation-related cell signaling may contribute to fatigue symptoms. Of note, many of these studies controlled for depressive symptoms (which are typically elevated in fatigued patients), suggesting that the association between inflammation and fatigue is not driven by co-morbid depression.

The mechanisms underlying elevations in cytokine levels during and, particularly, after cancer treatment have not been determined, but they may be due to cellular damage caused by cancer itself or by its treatment (Kurzrock, 2001), by alterations in immune regulatory systems, such as the HPA axis (Bower, Ganz, & Aziz, 2005; Bower et al., 2005; Bower, Ganz, Irwin, Arevalo, & Cole, 2011)), or by preexisting vulnerability factors, including polymorphisms in inflammation-related genes (Aouizerat, et al., 2009; Collado-Hidalgo, Bower, Ganz, Irwin, & Cole, 2008; Miaskowski et al., 2010b). Overall, this growing literature implicates inflammation as potentially causative and, at the very least, associative with fatigue in cancer.

Fatigue is a common symptom of many other medical conditions, and there is some evidence linking inflammation to fatigue among individuals with multiple sclerosis (Heesen et al., 2006),

Sjogren's syndrome (Harboe et al., 2009), and rheumatoid arthritis (Davis et al., 2008), among others. Moreover, TNF antagonists have been associated with reductions in fatigue among individuals with inflammatory conditions such as psoriasis (Tyring et al., 2006). However, results in these populations are inconsistent (Giovannoni, Thompson, Miller, & Thompson, 2001). Similarly, studies examining the association between inflammatory markers and chronic fatigue syndrome have yielded mixed results (Natelson et al., 2002). This likely reflects the heterogeneous nature of these conditions and variability in time of onset, treatment exposure, and other factors. More compelling evidence for an association between inflammation and fatigue outside the cancer context comes from longitudinal studies conducted with healthy individuals, where plasma levels of the pro-inflammatory marker CRP have been shown to predict the development of fatigue (Cho, Seeman, Bower, Kiefe, & Irwin, 2009).

Inflammation and Sleep
Sleep Characteristics

Sleep is currently thought to consist of two major phases, REM sleep and nonrapid eye movement (NREM) sleep. Most investigators conducting preclinical studies using laboratory animals find it sufficient to define only these two phases of sleep. However, in sleep research using human subjects, and in sleep disorders medicine, the phase of NREM sleep is further subdivided into four *stages*—stages 1, 2, 3, and 4—and these stages are determined via electroencephalogram (EEG) analysis of sleep waveforms. The four stages of NREM sleep may generally be considered to parallel a continuum of sleep depth with stage 2 being lighter sleep than stage 4. Stage 1 is the transition between wakefulness and sleep, whereas sleep onset is generally considered to occur when two EEG features characteristic of stage 2 appear, namely, spindles and K-complexes. Spindles are bursts of sinusoidal waves of about 12–14 cycles/second (Hz), whereas K-complexes are transient high-voltage biphasic waves. Sleep spindles and K-complexes are superimposed on a background of low voltage EEG. Human stages 3 and 4 NREM sleep are referred to as slow-wave sleep (SWS) due to the preponderance of high-amplitude, low-frequency components characteristic of the EEG. Differentiating between stages of human sleep is done on the basis of arbitrary criteria. If, during human SWS, the slow waves predominate for less than half of a 30-second period, that period is defined as stage 3. If slow waves predominate for more than half of a 30-second period, the period is considered stage 4.

The arbitrary criteria that are used to define phases and stages of sleep give the impression that sleep consists of discrete units that are quantal in nature. This is not the case. In healthy humans and laboratory animals there is an orderly progression from wakefulness to NREM sleep and REM sleep. Healthy animals and humans enter NREM sleep from wakefulness. From NREM sleep there is a transition to REM sleep. After a period of REM sleep, there may or may not be a brief arousal or awakening and this progression will repeat. These progressions from wakefulness through stages of sleep repeat to form cycles. The number and duration of cycles that occur during a period of sleep are species-specific; the NREM–REM cycle lasts about 8–10 minutes in rats and about 80–110 minutes in humans.

Cytokine Activation and Sleep

The seminal work of Drs. Ishimori and Pieron (Ishimori, 1909; Kubota, 1989) provided the first recent scientific evidence of humoral regulation of sleep. In these studies, cerebrospinal fluid obtained from sleep-deprived animals induced a sleep resembling narcosis when transferred into healthy, well-rested animals (Kornmüller, Lux, Winkel, & Klee, 1961; Monnier & Hoesli, 1964; Nagasaki, Iriki, Inoue, & Uchizono, 1974). This substance, termed Factor S, was identified 15 years later as muramyl peptide, and was recognized as a potent instigator of IL-1 synthesis and secretion (Fontana, Kristensen, Dubs, Gemsa, & Weber, 1982). Further studies demonstrated that injection of IL-1 into rabbits and rats increased non-rapid-eye-movement (NREM) sleep time, suppressed rapid-eye-movement (REM) sleep, and altered the properties of the electroencephalogram (EEG) (Krueger et al., 1984; Tobler, Borbely, Schwyzer, & Fontana, 1984).

As noted earlier, a hallmark sign of sickness behavior in animals and humans is changes in sleep. The past few decades have yielded a notable body of research examining the effects of infections on sleep in animal models. Briefly, mouse models of viral infections (generally with influenza) report increases in NREM sleep during times of usually high activity (Fang, Sanborn, Majde, & Krueger, 1994; Toth & Verhulst, 2003). Evidence suggests that changes in NREM sleep during infection may be mediated by individual differences in interferon (IFN) production, such that animals with genetic alleles that produce high levels of Type 1 IFN-α and

IFN-β also show comparative increases in NREM sleep compared to animals with alleles associated with decreased production of IFN (Toth, 1996).

With respect to bacterial infections, rabbit models have indicated that infection with *Staphylococcus aureus* or *Escherichia coli* result in an initial increase followed by a reduction in NREM sleep, with delta power bands paralleling changes in NREM sleep during the course of infection, suggesting changes in both power and intensity of NREM sleep during infection. The initial increase in NREM sleep is roughly associated with the increase in fever response; however, febrile responses also continue during NREM suppression, suggesting that there is not a one-to-one correspondence with NREM sleep and fever responses to infection. In contrast to the biphasic change in NREM, REM sleep remains suppressed during bacterial infection (Toth & Opp, 2001).

What about the literature supporting relationships with cytokines and sleep, independent of infection? There are basic criteria that Krueger and others have suggested for presuming a substance to be a regulatory sleep factor. (Krueger, Obal, & Fang, 1999). These criteria are: (a) The substance should induce physiological sleep; (b) The substance and its receptors should be present in the animal; (c) The concentration or turnover of the substance or its receptor should vary with the sleep-wake cycle; (d) Induction of the substance should induce sleep; (e) Inactivation of the substance or its receptor should reduce spontaneous sleep; (f) Inactivation of the substance should reduce sleep induced by somnogenic stimuli; and (g) Other biological actions of the substance should be separable, in part, from its sleep-promoting actions.

Current evidence from biochemical, molecular genetics, and electrophysiological studies in animals studies suggest that pro-inflammatory cytokines IL-1β and TNF-α meet all the criteria just noted. These cytokines appear to play a pivotal role in regulating spontaneous NREM sleep, such that NREM sleep is enhanced and REM sleep is suppressed (Krueger & Majde, 2003; Krueger, Obal, Fang, Kubota, & Taishi, 2001; Opp, 2005; Opp & Toth, 2003). Anti-inflammatory cytokines, in particular interleukin-10 (IL-10) and interleukin-4 (IL-4), appear to reduce NREM sleep in mouse and rabbit models, presumably by their suppression of pro-inflammatory cytokine activity (Kushikata, Fang, & Krueger, 1999; Kushikata, Fang, Wang, & Krueger, 1998; Opp, Smith, & Hughes, 1995).

Although the precise mechanisms of these cytokines on somnolence and wakefulness are not yet fully clear, potential known mediators include growth-hormone- releasing hormone, corticotrophin-releasing hormone, prostaglandins, nitric oxide synthase, and activation of NFκβ (Krueger & Majde, 2003).

In humans, studies linking cytokines and sleep are less clear with respect to mechanisms. Administration of endotoxin (*Salmonella abortus*, a lipopolysaccharide that stimulates pro-inflammatory cytokine production by macrophages) has been found to increase NREM stage-2 sleep, whereas slow-wave sleep (SWS) at stages 3 and 4 are relatively unaffected (Hermann et al., 1998; Korth, Mullington, Schreiber, & Pollmacher, 1996; Mullington et al., 2000; Pollmacher, Mullington, Korth, & Hinze-Selch, 1995; Pollmacher et al., 1993). However, because this endotoxin stimulates a variety of cytokines (i.e., TNF-α, IL-6, IL-1ra), as well as results in release of stress hormones such as ACTH and cortisol, the mechanisms by which endotoxin affects sleep in humans are not known. To address this limitation, other studies have examined the effects of subcutaneous injection of IL-6 and IFN-α on sleep; both cytokines induced a reduction of SWS, as well as REM sleep (Spath-Schwalbe et al., 1998; Spath-Schwalbe, Lange, Perras, Fehm, & Born, 2000). Interestingly, the reduced SWS was preceded by reports of increased fatigue measured before sleep, similar in pattern to depressed patients who complain of fatigue and show reduced SWS (Born & Späth-Schwalbe, 1999).

A recent study examined the effects of chronic IFN-α administration in patients with hepatitis C, who had no prior sleep disorder (Raison et al., 2010). IFN-α administration was associated with increases in wake after sleep onset (WASO), as well as decreases in SWS and sleep efficiency. Similar to the studies reported earlier, decreases in SWS resultant from cytokine administration were also associated with increased reports of fatigue, whereas increases in WASO were associated with increases in evening cortisol levels.

Finally, our group (Irwin, Olmstead, Valladares, Breen, & Ehlers, 2009) demonstrated in a randomized, placebo-controlled study that neutralization of TNF α activity was associated with a significant reduction of REM sleep in abstinent alcohol-dependent patients, who had elevated amounts of REM sleep. The reduction in percentage of REM sleep was robust, in which levels of REM sleep approached those typically seen in healthy volunteers without a history of alcohol dependence. Moreover, individual biologic variability in the degree of TNF antagonism, as reflected by circulating levels of sTNFRII, correlated with declines in REM sleep. Taken together, these data further support the hypothesis that circulating levels of TNF α may have a physiologic role in the regulation of REM sleep amounts in humans, and that elevated levels of TNF α contribute to abnormal increases of REM sleep observed in certain clinical populations such as those with alcohol dependence.

Sleep Deprivation and Inflammation

So far we have reviewed evidence suggesting that acute infections and injections with inflammatory agents or antagonists of inflammation alter sleep as well as fatigue levels. Not surprisingly, there is also evidence supporting the notion that acute and chronic sleep disturbance is associated with immune alterations, consistent with the theory that communication between sleep and immunity is bidirectional. Studies examining prolonged sleep deprivation have repeatedly shown disruptions in innate immunity, as reflected by decreases in the NK cells number and activity, as well as decreases in the number of the major lymphocyte subpopulations (Boyum et al., 1996; Dinges et al., 1994; Ozturk et al., 1999). Short-term sleep deprivation experiments have reported increases in inflammatory markers such as IL-6, TNF-α, and C-reactive protein (CRP) after sleep deprivation (Meier-Ewert et al., 2004; Shearer et al., 2001; Vgontzas et al., 2004).

Partial-sleep-deprivation studies on immunity are of particular interest because these studies model more of the type of sleep loss in general and clinical populations and, therefore, may more accurately reflect effects of sleep deprivation on immune function in everyday life. Our group's studies with partial sleep deprivation also point to changes in innate immunity, marked by reductions in natural killer cell activity as well as reductions in stimulated IL-2 production (Irwin et al., 1994; M. Irwin et al., 1996). Further studies by our group (Irwin, Wang, Campomayor, Collado-Hidalgo, & Cole, 2006) indicated that partial sleep deprivation was also associated with increased subsequent morning monocyte production of IL-6 and TNF-α, as well as a greater than threefold increase in IL-6 messenger RNA and a twofold increase in TNF-α messenger RNA. Production of these cytokines in the early and late evening interacted with gender, such that females showed increases in monocytes production of IL-6 and TNF-α, compared to males, who showed a decrease (Irwin, Carrillo, & Olmstead, 2010).

To further understand potential mediating pathways of sleep deprivation's effects on inflammation responses, we examined transcription factor signaling using bioinformatics analyses. These analyses implicated the pro-inflammatory NF-κB/Rel family as well as the CREB/activating transcription factor family, protein kinase C–induced AP-1 family, and mitogen-activated protein kinase–inducible E-26 transformation–specific transcription factor family typified by E-26-like protein 1 (Irwin, Wang, et al., 2006). The potential mediating effects of the NF-κB signaling pathway were also noted in a separate study in which, in both males and females, mononuclear cell NF-κB activation was significantly greater following a night of partial sleep deprivation as compared to uninterrupted baseline or recovery sleep, although the findings were more robust in females (Irwin et al., 2008).

Thus, experimental studies with both prolonged and partial sleep deprivation point to alterations in innate immune function consistent with an inflammatory response. Although further study is certainly warranted with respect to moderating effects of gender, studies generally support the notion that sleep deprivation leads to relatively immediate inflammation-related changes that, if experienced chronically, may lead to further dysregulation and disease.

There is also evidence suggesting that insomnia and sleep disturbance are associated with increases in inflammation. For example, cytokines IL-6 and TNF-α have been found to be elevated during the day in disorders characterized by daytime sleepiness, such as obesity, sleep apnea, and narcolepsy (Alberti et al., 2003; Okun et al., 2004; Vgontzas et al., 1997). Shifts in cytokines IL-6 and TNF-α from daytime to nighttime have also been found in chronic insomniacs; importantly, cytokine shifts associated with chronic insomnia have been associated with a 24-hour cortisol hypersecretion. This may help to explain why insomniacs, who suffer from daytime fatigue, have trouble falling asleep even when provided opportunities for sleep (Vgontzas et al., 2002). With respect to sleep disturbance in the population, increased time in bed, greater variability in bedtime, and later wake times have been found to be associated with elevated TNF-α in older adults (>60), regardless of diagnosed insomnia or caregiving status (Okun et al., 2010).

Fatigue, Sleep Disturbance, and Daytime Sleepiness—Common Mechanisms or Parallel Processes?

The growing literature on inflammation and sickness behavior, as reviewed here and elsewhere, points to a clear linkage between fatigue, sleep, and inflammation. As mentioned earlier, the clustering of fatigue and sleep problems has been noted in various populations, including persons suffering from cardiovascular disease, chronic fatigue syndrome, and cancer-related fatigue (Ancoli-Israel, Moore, & Jones, 2001; Lee et al., 2010; Nisenbaum et al., 2004). The animal literature on sickness behavior supports the clustering of fatigue and sleep disturbance, and recent human research from different laboratories has shown that inflammatory processes are associated with correlated changes in sleep and fatigue. Two independent studies have reported that IFN-α administration leads to decreases in SWS that are associated with self-reports of fatigue (Raison et al., 2010; Spath-Schwalbe et al., 2000). Further, in a sample of healthy adults, Thomas et al. (2011) found that elevated LPS-stimulated production of IL-6 by monocytes in the evening was associated with decreases in SWS that night and with fatigue the following day.

Based on this evidence, it may be tempting to conclude that inflammation is a common mechanism underlying the co-occurring symptoms of fatigue and sleep disturbance in clinical and healthy populations. However, it is important to note that few studies have specifically examined the inter-relationships among these processes; instead, researchers have typically focused on a single symptom of interest (e.g., cancer-related fatigue, insomnia) and examined inflammatory processes in that context. A handful of investigators have examined temporal associations between inflammation, sleep, and fatigue, but more research on the complex dynamics of these symptoms is clearly needed It may also be tempting to suppose that daytime sleepiness and fatigue are interchangeable, such that perceptions of fatigue are actually representative of daytime sleepiness caused by sleep disturbance. However, unlike daytime sleepiness, fatigue is not characterized by a propensity to fall asleep (Vgontzas et al., 2002). It has been proposed, based on data from several studies, that the main difference between disorders characterized by excessive daytime sleepiness (such as sleep apnea and narcolepsy) versus those disorders with chronic fatigue (such as insomnia, fibromyalgia, and chronic fatigue syndrome) may be related to changes in HPA axis functioning, such that increased HPA axis activation combined with increases in inflammation levels or shifts in phase may be more associated with fatigue, whereas increases in inflammation not associated with HPA axis hyperactivation are more associated with daytime sleepiness (Vgontzas et al., 2002). HPA axis dysregulation has been noted in various sleep disorders characterized by fatigue, and HPA axis dysregulation has also been found in fatigue-related disorders associated with sleep disturbance but not necessarily daytime sleepiness (Macedo et al., 2008; Rajeevan et al., 2007; Van Den Eede, Moorkens, Van Houdenhove, Cosyns, & Claes, 2007).

Perpetuating Mechanisms of Sickness Behavior

If sickness behavior is viewed as a natural and adaptive response to acute infection or inflammation, the question remains about what perpetuates this symptomatology in absence of a direct stimulus. For example, why is it that some, but not all, people experience ongoing fatigue after cancer treatment? Why might chronic sleep dysregulation persist in patients with primarily fatigue-related disorders? Perhaps most importantly, what might be done clinically to help patients overcome these debilitating, quality-of-life interfering, and disease-promoting symptoms?

There are a few evidence-based theories on physiological mechanisms that may serve to perpetuate fatigue and sleep disturbance in clinical populations, particularly with respect to continued modulation of inflammatory responses via dysregulated HPA axis functioning, autonomic contributions, and genetic susceptibilities toward increased inflammation (Collado-Hidalgo et al., 2008; Johnston & Webster, 2009; Klimas & Koneru, 2007; Miaskowski et al., 2010a; Miller, Ancoli-Israel, Bower, Capuron, & Irwin, 2008; Vgontzas, Bixler, & Chrousos, 2006). The influence of these factors, along with psychosocial and biobehavioral factors, are depicted in Figure 18.1. However, to date, studies are relatively in their infancy with respect to clearly understanding the causal molecular and systems mechanisms that perpetuate ongoing sickness behavior such as fatigue and sleep disturbance.

It is important to note that these symptoms also may be both a cause and consequence of psychosocial and behavioral responses, and that modulation of these responses may also serve to either perpetuate or mitigate the symptomatology. For example, it is well understood from the sleep-treatment literature that ongoing sleep dysregulation, particularly insomnia, is often largely driven by behavioral conditioning. In cognitive-behavioral models for

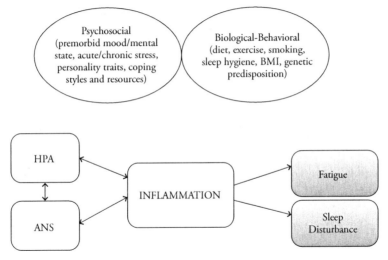

Figure 18.1 Graphical depiction of contributions to fatigue and sleep disturbance. Psychosocial and biobehavioral factors are depicted as latent constructs (ovals) that influence all manifest variables (squares) that contribute to and continue to modulate the experience of fatigue and sleep disturbance. Reciprocal relationships are noted between hypothalamic-adrenal-axis (HPA) functioning, autonomic nervous system (ANS) activity, and inflammation. These physiological systems, as influenced and partially regulated by psychosocial and biobehavioral factors, contribute to the experience of both acute and chronic fatigue and sleep disturbance.

insomnia, for example, it is understood that perpetuating factors (those behaviors that serve to perpetuate insomnia in the absence of the initial precipitating factor) play a large role in maintaining insomnia. These behaviors include things like staying in bed for significant amounts of time while awake, engaging in wakefulness-producing behaviors while in bed (e.g., watching TV or reading), and imbibing caffeine or other stimulants too close to bedtime. Likewise, patients with persistent fatigue report a decrease in activity engagement that is, in part, due to cognitive misperceptions regarding activity level and fatigue (Knoop, Prins, Moss-Morris, & Bleijenberg, 2010); paradoxically, the behavioral withdrawal often leads to increased perceptions of fatigue. Catastrophizing, or expecting negative outcomes with respect to one's fatigue, is also a key predictor of fatigue during and after cancer treatment (Donovan, Small, Andrykowski, Munster, & Jacobsen, 2007, Jacobsen, Andrykowski, & Thors, 2004). It is not unreasonable to suppose that persistent sleep-disrupting or fatigue-perpetuating cognitions and behaviors are associated with consistent dysregulations in neuroimmune and neuroendocrine responses, and that the interaction of both the physiological dysregulation in combination with a maladaptive cognitive-behavioral set of responses serves to maintain the debilitating symptomatology. Evidence from the animal sickness behavior literature has already established that sickness behavior is

behaviorally conditioned and significantly depends on motivational factors (Dantzer & Kelley, 2007).

Chronic stress may well also be a factor that contributes to the persistence of fatigue and sleep disturbance in clinical and other populations, and may be mediated through sickness behavior responses. Vital exhaustion, for example, is a syndrome marked by persistent fatigue often stemming from an inability to cope with one or more chronic stressors, and has been implicated as an independent risk factor for negative cardiovascular events. Vital exhaustion has also been linked in several studies with sleep disturbance (Grossi, Perski, Evengard, Blomkvist, & Orth-Gomer, 2003; Soderstrom, Ekstedt, Akerstedt, Nilsson, & Axelsson, 2004; van Diest & Appels, 1994). In women, vital exhaustion has been linked to elevated circulating TNF-α levels (Grossi et al., 2003), as well as increased C-reactive protein and IL-6 in women with coronary heart disease (Janszky, Lekander, Blom, Georgiades, & Ahnve, 2005). A study comparing vitally exhausted middle-aged males with controls indicated that vital exhaustion was associated with increased IL-6, IL-1ra, and IL-10 levels, as well as increased procoagulant activity (van der Ven et al., 2003). Similarly, a study examining vital versus nonvital exhaustion in male industrial workers (Wirtz et al., 2003) showed decreased glucocorticoid sensitivity for highly exhausted men. In addition, vitally exhausted workers showed significantly increased resting levels of C-reactive protein. Together, these and other findings (Melamed et al., 2006) suggest that continued chronic stress is associated with HPA dysregulations and increased inflammatory activity, and may be associated with prolonged fatigue and sleep disturbance. This points to a need to both assess and provide treatment strategies for chronic stress in populations with persistent fatigue and sleep disturbance.

Treatment of Fatigue and Sleep Disturbance—a PNI Perspective
Psychosocial approaches

There is a large literature on psychosocial intervention effects on sleep disturbance and fatigue, including studies utilizing behavioral, cognitive-behavioral, and mind-body therapies. There is compelling evidence that these treatments have moderate to large beneficial effects on subjective sleep outcomes (Irwin, Cole, & Nicassio, 2006), with more modest effects seen on fatigue (Jacobsen, Donovan, Vadparampil, & Small, 2007), perhaps because fatigue is often not the primary target in these trials. If these symptoms are in part driven by activation of pro-inflammatory cytokines, then treatment-related symptom reduction might be attributable to reductions in pro-inflammatory cytokine activity. However, although there is evidence for psychosocial intervention effects on some immune outcomes (for review, see (McGregor & Antoni, 2009), few studies have specifically examined markers of inflammation or investigated alterations in inflammatory processes as mediators of intervention effects on fatigue and sleep disturbance. For example, a recent randomized controlled trial reported on decreased fatigue and inflammation (as indexed by serum CRP levels) as well as improved quality of life for cancer patients randomized to a Medical QiGong group, as compared to a wait-list control group (Oh et al., 2010), but the mediating role of CRP was not assessed. Even exercise interventions, which have shown beneficial effects on both fatigue and inflammatory markers (Fairey et al., 2005, Milne et al., 2008), have not examined whether decreases in inflammation mediate changes in fatigue outcomes. There is a critical need for studies examining mechanistic PNI processes that may underlie intervention effects on sickness behaviors and other outcomes.

Pharmacological approaches

Pharmacologic therapies have also been examined as potential treatments for fatigue and sleep disturbance. Modafinil (also known as Provigil), is a nonamphetamine based stimulant and a schedule IV drug currently approved for treatment of daytime sleepiness disorders such as narcolepsy, obstructive sleep apnea, and shift-work related sleep disorders. Its precise mechanism of action remains unclear, although it is known to affect histaminergic as well as cholinergic systems, while having relatively small impact on dopaminergic systems, as compared to amphetamine-based stimulants (Ballon & Feifel, 2006). Modafinil has been recently examined for its effects on fatigue as well as treatment-resistant depression. A recent review notes that three of the four studies to date examining the effects of modafinil on cancer-related fatigue have been small, open-label studies, and that more evidence is needed to determine whether modafinil is efficacious for fatigue in cancer patients (Cooper, Bird, & Steinberg, 2009). A recent large, placebo-controlled Phase 3 randomized control trial (RCT) of modafinil for cancer related fatigue found no significant effects of modafinil for the entire group, but modafinil was significantly more effective than placebo in reducing fatigue symptoms for patients who had severe fatigue (Jean-Pierre et al., 2010). A similar review for fatigue in multiple sclerosis noted the initial promise of modafinil in open-label studies; however, more rigorous RCTs have yielded conflicting results (Brown, Howard, & Kemp, 2010). A recent blinded RCT examining the effects of modafinil on fatigue in HIV+ patients reported significant decreases in fatigue for modafinil versus placebo (Rabkin, McElhiney, Rabkin, & McGrath, 2010). None of these studies have reported on effects of modafinil on inflammation markers.

Given the reviewed linkages of inflammation with fatigue and sleep, another reasonable direction for pharmacological interventions has been to examine the effects of anti-inflammatory agents on sickness behavior in samples with inflammation-related medical conditions. As mentioned earlier, a large RCT conducted with psoriasis patients found that treatment with etanercept (an agent that binds to and inhibits the effects of TNF-α) led to clinically meaningful improvements in fatigue, as well as decreases in depressed mood (Tyring et al., 2006). A small, uncontrolled study examined the effects of anakinra (an agent that binds to the IL-1 receptor and, therefore, acts as an antagonist to interleukin-1) on fatigue and disease activity in rheumatoid arthritis (RA) and reported significant reductions in both (Omdal & Gunnarsson, 2005). Another recent, multisite RCT study examined adalimumab (another TNF-α antagonist that binds to TNF-α, preventing its binding with TNF receptors) versus placebo as an adjunct treatment for RA patients. The authors reported significant decreases in fatigue compared to placebo for those with moderate to severe RA (Yount et al., 2007).

A recent pilot study examining infliximab (an antibody against TNF-α) on symptoms and fatigue in lupus patients reported significant improvements in disease activity, nonsignificant decrease in fatigue, and, interestingly, no changes in serum levels of TNF-α or its soluble receptors, sTNFR1 and sTNFR2 (Uppal, Hayat, & Raghupathy, 2009). This agent was also reported to improve sleep disturbance in a small number rheumatoid arthritis patients (Zamarron, Maceiras, Mera, & Gomez-Reino, 2004), although a larger study with the same population reported no significant effect (Wolfe, Michaud, & Li, 2006). There is preliminary evidence that anti-cytokine therapies may also have beneficial effects on fatigue in cancer populations (Monk et al 2006), although increases in fatigue have also been observed in certain groups (Madhusudan et al 2005, Jatoi et al 2010).

Infliximab and some other anti-inflammatory agents' mechanism of action may be due, in part, to their abilities to block the p38 mitogen-activated protein kinase (p38MAPk) pathway. This pathway is a common signaling pathway in inflammation and may have particular relevance in understanding disease progression in certain types of cancer. There has been a considerable amount of research activity examining the effects of p38MAPk blockade in cancer treatment; a recent review suggests that Phase 1 trials examining safety and tolerability, particularly for cardiovascular, gastrointestinal, and neurological symptoms are warranted (Noel et al., 2008). Importantly, p38MAPk pathway activation also influences glucocorticoid receptor function, and influences reuptake mechanisms for dopamine and serotonin, all of which are altered in depression (Pace & Miller, 2009). Future studies will most certainly examine the effects of p38MAPk pathway blockade on sickness behavior as well as inflammation.

Implications for Future Treatment

Although the literature on both psychosocial and pharmacological approaches for the treatment of fatigue and sleep disturbance is arguably in its infancy, the preliminary studies reviewed here suggest promise in mitigating these troubling symptoms. As the literature mentioned earlier suggests,

there does not appear to be a particular "silver bullet" at this time that addresses all concerns for those experiencing sickness behavior. Interestingly, results from a recent work group on sleep treatments in cancer patients concluded that there is little evidence that behavioral treatments for sleep impact fatigue in cancer patients (Zee & Ancoli-Israel, 2009). This, combined with evidence from other behavioral interventions for fatigue that do not impact sleep, and pharmacological studies that are, to date, mixed in terms of impact on fatigue and sleep in patients, suggest once again that while fatigue and sleep disturbance share common variance in terms of physiological pathways, treatment of one symptom does not translate into treatment of another. The data suggest the need for a multimodal or "whole-systems" approach. Such an approach would likely be most effective if personalized to the patient based on several factors—for example, genetic vulnerabilities, disease status and progression, nutritional status, mental health complaints, and sociodemographic resources. This combining of pharmacological, social-behavioral, nutritional, and mind-body restorative practices in treating sickness behavior would aid in addressing both the physiological, psychological, and quality-of-life interfering aspects of these all-too-prevalent symptoms.

Conclusion

Fatigue and sleep disturbance are two the most prevalent complaints among those with disease and those who are otherwise healthy, and they often co-occur along with depression. The growing body of research on these symptoms notes the high costs to society in terms of the effects of prolonged fatigue and sleep disturbance on disease progression, work productivity, and medical costs. Basic research on neuro-immune interactions indicates that pro-inflammatory cytokines can signal the CNS to trigger fatigue, sleep disturbance, and other behavioral symptoms, and science is progressing toward understanding the role of inflammatory processes in the fatigue and sleep problems that occur in healthy and clinical populations. Biobehavioral and psychosocial influences may play a significant role in the perpetuation of the fatigue/sleep disturbance symptom cluster, and, therefore, integrative approaches, for both possible prevention as well as treatment for the fatigue-sleep disturbance cluster, may be warranted.

Future Directions

Although the underlying evidence supporting the influence of inflammatory immune processes on fatigue and sleep disturbance is impressive, much more research is needed to understand the etiology and co-occurrence of these symptoms. Future studies should examine more closely the role of hypothalamic and autonomic system dysregulation as it relates to inflammation and its influence on fatigue and sleep disturbance. Longitudinal studies that examine changes in both molecular and biobehavioral factors from symptom onset through persistence will be useful in terms of identifying precise mechanisms that might underlie the transition from acute to chronic fatigue and sleep disturbance. Finally, effective treatment approaches for these symptoms are highly needed; although some pharmacological and psychosocial treatments have shown promise, no treatment has been shown to be a "gold-standard" approach for ameliorating both fatigue and sleep disturbance. Studies of multimodal or integrative approaches are highly warranted and should include the tracking of relevant biomarkers (including resting and functional immune, EEG, HPA, and ANS markers, with precise biomarkers determined in part by population characteristics) that may indicate mechanisms of improvement of fatigue and sleep disturbance.

References

Addington, A. M., Gallo, J. J., Ford, D. E., & Eaton, W. W. (2001). Epidemiology of unexplained fatigue and major depression in the community: The Baltimore ECA follow-up, 1981–1994. *Psychological Medicine, 31*(6), 1037–1044.

Ahlberg, K., Ekman, T., & Gaston-Johansson, F. (2004). Levels of fatigue compared to levels of cytokines and hemoglobin during pelvic radiotherapy: a pilot study. *Biological Research for Nursing, 5*(3), 203–210.

Alberti, A., Sarchielli, P., Gallinella, E., Floridi, A., Mazzotta, G., & Gallai, V. (2003). Plasma cytokine levels in patients with obstructive sleep apnea syndrome: A preliminary study. *Journal of Sleep Research, 12*(4), 305–311.

Alexander, S., Minton, O., Andrews, P., & Stone, P. (2009). A comparison of the characteristics of disease-free breast cancer survivors with or without cancer-related fatigue syndrome. *European Journal of Cancer, 45*(3), 384–392.

Ancoli-Israel, S., Moore, P., & Jones, V. (2001). The relationship between fatigue and sleep in cancer patients: A review. *European Journal of Cancer Care, 10*, 245–255.

Anisman, H., & Merali, Z. (2002). Cytokines, stress, and depressive illness. *Brain, Behavior, and Immunity, 16*(5), 513–524.

Aouizerat, B. E., Dodd, M., Lee, K., West, C., Paul, S. M., Cooper, B. A., et al. (2009). Preliminary evidence of a genetic association between tumor necrosis factor alpha and the severity of sleep disturbance and morning fatigue. *Biological Research for Nursing, 11*(1), 27–41.

Aronson, D., Mittleman, M. A., & Burger, A. J. (2001). Interleukin-6 levels are inversely correlated with heart rate variability in patients with decompensated heart failure. *Journal of Cardiovascular Electrophysiology, 12*(3), 294–300.

Aubert, A., Goodall, G., Dantzer, R., & Gheusi, G. (1997). Differential effects of lipopolysaccharide on pup retrieving and nest building in lactating mice. *Brain, Behavior, and Immunity, 11*(2), 107–118.

Ballon, J. S., & Feifel, D. (2006). A systematic review of modafinil: Potential clinical uses and mechanisms of action. *Journal of Clinical Psychiatry, 67*(4), 554–566.

Barsevick, A. M., Cleeland, C. S., Manning, D. C., O'Mara, A. M., Reeve, B. B., Scott, J. A., et al. (2010). ASCPRO recommendations for the assessment of fatigue as an outcome in clinical trials. *Journal of Pain and Symptom Management, 39*(6), 1086–1099.

Berkenbosch, F., van Oers, J., del Rey, A., Tilders, F., & Besedovsky, H. (1987). Corticotropin-releasing factor-producing neurons in the rat activated by interleukin-1. *Science, 238*(4826), 524–526.

Besedovsky, H., del Rey, A., Sorkin, E., & Dinarello, C. A. (1986). Immunoregulatory feedback between interleukin-1 and glucocorticoid hormones. *Science, 233*(4764), 652–654.

Bluthé, R. M., Michaud, B., Kelley, K. W., & Dantzer, R. (1996a). Vagotomy attenuates behavioural effects of interleukin-1 injected peripherally but not centrally. *Neuroreport, 7*(9), 1485–1488.

Bluthé, R. M., Michaud, B., Kelley, K. W., & Dantzer, R. (1996b). Vagotomy blocks behavioural effects of interleukin-1 injected via the intraperitoneal route but not via other systemic routes. *Neuroreport, 7*(15–17), 2823–2827.

Bluthé, R. M., Walter, V., Parnet, P., Laye, S., Lestage, J., Verrier, D., et al. (1994). Lipopolysaccharide induces sickness behaviour in rats by a vagal mediated mechanism. *Comptes Rendus de l Academie des Sciences. Serie III, 317*(6), 499–503.

Born, J., & Späth-Schwalbe, E. (1999). The role of interferon-alpha in the regulation of sleep. In N. Müller (Ed.), *Psychiatry, psychoimmunology, and viruses* (pp. 131–144). Vienna: Springer-Verlag.

Borovikova, L. V., Ivanova, S., Zhang, M., Yang, H., Botchkina, G. I., Watkins, L. R., et al. (2000). Vagus nerve stimulation attenuates the systemic inflammatory response to endotoxin. *Nature, 405*(6785), 458–462.

Bower, J. E., Ganz, P. A., Aziz, N., & Fahey, J. L. (2002). Fatigue and pro-inflammatory cytokine activity in breast cancer survivors. *Psychosomatic Medicine, 64*(4), 604–611.

Bower, J. E., Ganz, P. A., & Aziz, N. (2005). Altered cortisol response to psychologic stress in breast cancer survivors with persistent fatigue. *Psychosomatic Medicine, 67*(2), 277–280. doi: 67/2/277 [pii] 10.1097/01.psy.0000155666.55034.c6

Bower, J. E., Ganz, P. A., Desmond, K. A., Bernaards, C., Rowland, J. H., Meyerowitz, B. E., et al. (2006). Fatigue in long-term breast carcinoma survivors: A longitudinal investigation. *Cancer, 106*(4), 751–758.

Bower, J. E., Ganz, P. A., Dickerson, S. S., Petersen, L., Aziz, N., & Fahey, J. L. (2005). Diurnal cortisol rhythm and fatigue in breast cancer survivors. *Psychoneuroendocrinology, 30*(1), 92–100. doi: 10.1016/j.psyneuen.2004.06.003 S0306-4530(04)00112-X [pii]

Bower, J. E., Ganz, P. A., Irwin, M. R., Arevalo, J. M., & Cole, S. W. (2011). Fatigue and gene expression in human leukocytes: increased NF-kappaB and decreased glucocorticoid signaling in breast cancer survivors with persistent fatigue. *Brain, Behavior, and Immunity, 25*(1), 147–150. doi: S0889-1591(10)00468-X [pii] 10.1016/j.bbi.2010.09.010

Bower, J. E., Ganz, P. A., Tao, M. L., Hu, W., Belin, T. R., Sepah, S., et al. (2009). Inflammatory biomarkers and fatigue during radiation therapy for breast and prostate cancer. *Clinical Cancer Research, 15*(17), 5534–5540.

Boyum, A., Wiik, P., Gustavsson, E., Veiby, O. P., Reseland, J., Haugen, A. H., et al. (1996). The effect of strenuous exercise, calorie deficiency and sleep deprivation on white blood cells, plasma immunoglobulins and cytokines. *Scandanavian Journal of Immunology, 43*(2), 228–235.

Breslau, N., Roth, T., Rosenthal, L., & Andreski, P. (1996). Sleep disturbance and psychiatric disorders: A longitudinal epidemiological study of young adults. *Biological Psychiatry, 39*(6), 411–418.

Bret-Dibat, J. L., Bluthé, R. M., Kent, S., Kelley, K. W., & Dantzer, R. (1995). Lipopolysaccharide and interleukin-1 depress food-motivated behavior in mice by a vagal-mediated mechanism. *Brain, Behavior, and Immunity, 9*(3), 242–246.

Brown, J. N., Howard, C. A., & Kemp, D. W. (2010). Modafinil for the treatment of multiple sclerosis-related fatigue. *Annals of Pharmacotherapy, 44*(6), 1098–1103.

Bryant, P. A., Trinder, J., & Curtis, N. (2004). Sick and tired: Does sleep have a vital role in the immune system? *Nature Reviews Immunology, 4*(6), 457–467.

Camacho-Arroyo, I., Lopez-Griego, L., & Morales-Montor, J. (2009). The role of cytokines in the regulation of neurotransmission. *Neuroimmunomodulation, 16*(1), 1–12.

Capuron, L., Gumnick, J. F., Musselman, D. L., Lawson, D. H., Reemsnyder, A., Nemeroff, C. B., et al. (2002). Neurobehavioral effects of interferon-[alpha] in cancer patients*1: Phenomenology and paroxetine responsiveness of symptom dimensions. *Neuropsychopharmacology, 26*(5), 643–652.

Capuron, L., Ravaud, A., & Dantzer, R. (2000). Early depressive symptoms in cancer patients receiving interleukin 2 and/or interferon alfa-2b therapy. *Journal Of Clinical Oncology: Official Journal Of The American Society Of Clinical Oncology, 18*(10), 2143–2151.

Cho, H. J., Seeman, T. E., Bower, J. E., Kiefe, C. I., & Irwin, M. R. (2009). Prospective association between C-reactive protein and fatigue in the coronary artery risk development in young adults study. *Biological Psychiatry, 66*(9), 871–878.

Collado-Hidalgo, A., Bower, J. E., Ganz, P. A., Cole, S. W., & Irwin, M. R. (2006). Inflammatory biomarkers for persistent fatigue in breast cancer survivors. *Clinical Cancer Research, 12*(9), 2759–2766.

Collado-Hidalgo, A., Bower, J. E., Ganz, P. A., Irwin, M. R., & Cole, S. W. (2008). Cytokine gene polymorphisms and fatigue in breast cancer survivors: Early findings. *Brain, Behavior, and Immunology, 22*(8), 1197–1200.

Cooper, M. R., Bird, H. M., & Steinberg, M. (2009). Efficacy and safety of modafinil in the treatment of cancer-related fatigue. *Annals of Pharmacotherapy, 43*(4), 721–725.

Dantzer, R. (2009). Cytokine, sickness behavior, and depression. *Immunology and Allergy Clinics of North America, 29*(2), 247–264.

Dantzer, R., & Kelley, K. W. (2007). Twenty years of research on cytokine-induced sickness behavior. *Brain, Behavior, and Immunity, 21*(2), 153–160.

Davis, M. C., Zautra, A. J., Younger, J., Motivala, S. J., Attrep, J., & Irwin, M. R. (2008). Chronic stress and regulation of cellular markers of inflammation in rheumatoid arthritis: Implications for fatigue. *Brain, Behavior, and Immunity, 22*(1), 24–32

Dew, M. A., Hoch, C. C., Buysse, D. J., Monk, T. H., Begley, A. E., Houck, P. R., et al. (2003). Healthy older adults' sleep predicts all-cause mortality at 4 to 19 years of follow-up. *Psychosomatic Medicine, 65*(1), 63–73.

Dinarello, C. A. (1988). Biology of interleukin 1. *FASEB J, 2*(2), 108–115.

Dinges, D. F., Douglas, S. D., Zaugg, L., Campbell, D. E., McMann, J. M., Whitehouse, W. G., et al. (1994). Leukocytosis and natural killer cell function parallel neurobehavioral fatigue induced by 64 hours of sleep deprivation. *Journal of Clinical Investigation, 93*(5), 1930–1939.

Donovan, K. A., Small, B. J., Andrykowski, M. A., Munster, P., & Jacobsen, P. B. (2007). Utility of a cognitive-behavioral model to predict fatigue following breast cancer treatment. *Health Psychology, 26*(4), 464–72

Eisenberger, N. I., Berkman, E. T., Inagaki, T. K., Rameson, L. T., Mashal, N. M., & Irwin, M. R. (2010). Inflammation-induced anhedonia: Endotoxin reduces ventral striatum responses to reward. *Biological Psychiatry 68*(8), 748–754.

Eisenberger, N. I., Inagaki, T. K., Mashal, N. M., & Irwin, M. R. (2010). Inflammation and social experience: An inflammatory challenge induces feelings of social disconnection in addition to depressed mood. *Brain, Behavior, and Immunity, 24*(4), 558–563.

Ek, M., Kurosawa, M., Lundeberg, T., & Ericsson, A. (1998). Activation of vagal afferents after intravenous injection of interleukin-1beta: Role of endogenous prostaglandins. *Journal of Neuroscience, 18*(22), 9471–9479.

Fairey, A. S., Courneya, K. S., Field, C. J., Bell, G. J., Jones, L. W., Martin, B. S., & Mackey, J. R. (2005). Effect of exercise training on C-reactive protein in postmenopausal breast cancer survivors: A randomized controlled trial. *Brain, Behavior, and Immunity, 19*(5), 381–388.

Fang, J., Sanborn, C. K., Majde, J. A., & Krueger, J. M. (1994). Sleep changes induced by influenza virus infection in mice. *Sleep Research, 23,* 358.

Floto, R. A., & Smith, K. G. (2003). The vagus nerve, macrophages, and nicotine. *Lancet, 361*(9363), 1069–1070.

Foley, D. J., Monjan, A. A., Brown, S. L., Simonsick, E. M., Wallace, R. B., & Blazer, D. G. (1995). Sleep complaints among elderly persons: An epidemiologic study of three communities. *Sleep, 18*(6), 425–432.

Fontana, A., Kristensen, F., Dubs, R., Gemsa, D., & Weber, E. (1982). Production of prostaglandin E and an interleukin-1 like factor by cultured astrocytes and C6 glioma cells. *Journal of Immunology, 129*(6), 2413–2419.

Fuhrer, R., & Wessely, S. (1995). The epidemiology of fatigue and depression: A French primary-care study. *Psychological Medicine, 25*(5), 895–905.

Gangwisch, J. E., Heymsfield, S. B., Boden-Albala, B., Buijs, R. M., Kreier, F., Opler, M. G., et al. (2008). Sleep duration associated with mortality in elderly, but not middle-aged, adults in a large US sample. *Sleep, 31*(8), 1087–1096.

Geinitz, H., Zimmermann, F. B., Stoll, P., Thamm, R., Kaffenberger, W., Ansorg, K., et al. (2001). Fatigue, serum cytokine levels, and blood cell counts during radiotherapy of patients with breast cancer. *International Journal of Radiation Oncology—Biology - Physics, 51*(3), 691–698.

Gibertini, M., Newton, C., Friedman, H., & Klein, T. W. (1995). Spatial learning impairment in mice infected with Legionella pneumophila or administered exogenous interleukin-1-beta. *Brain, Behavior, and Immunity, 9*(2), 113–128.

Giovannoni, G., Thompson, A. J., Miller, D. H., & Thompson, E. J. (2001). Fatigue is not associated with raised inflammatory markers in multiple sclerosis. *Neurology, 57*(4), 676–81.

Goehler, L. E., Relton, J. K., Dripps, D., Kiechle, R., Tartaglia, N., Maier, S. F., et al. (1997). Vagal paraganglia bind biotinylated interleukin-1 receptor antagonist: A possible mechanism for immune-to-brain communication. *Brain Research Bulletin, 43*(3), 357–364.

Greenberg, D. B., Gray, J. L., Mannix, C. M., Eisenthal, S., & Carey, M. (1993). Treatment-related fatigue and serum interleukin-1 levels in patients during external beam irradiation for prostate cancer. *Journal of Pain and Symptom Management, 8*(4), 196–200.

Grossi, G., Perski, A., Evengard, B., Blomkvist, V., & Orth-Gomer, K. (2003). Physiological correlates of burnout among women. *Journal of Psychosomatic Research, 55*(4), 309–316.

Harboe, E., Tjensvoll, A. B., Vefring, H. K., Goransson, L. G., Kvaloy, J. T., & Omdal, R. (2009). Fatigue in primary Sjogren's syndrome: A link to sickness behaviour in animals? *Brain, Behavior, and Immunity, 23*(8), 1104–1108.

Harrison, N. A., Brydon, L., Walker, C., Gray, M. A., Steptoe, A., & Critchley, H. D. (2009). Inflammation causes mood changes through alterations in subgenual cingulate activity and mesolimbic connectivity. *Biological Psychiatry, 66*(5), 407–414.

Hart, B. L. (1988). Biological basis of the behavior of sick animals. *Neuroscience and Biobehavioral Reviews, 12*(2), 123–137.

Heesen, C., Nawrath, L., Reich, C., Bauer, N., Schulz, K. H., & Gold, S. M. (2006). Fatigue in multiple sclerosis: An example of cytokine mediated sickness behaviour? *Journal of Neurology, Neurosurgery, and Psychiatry, 77*(1), 34–39.

Hermann, D. M., Mullington, J., Hinze-Selch, D., Schreiber, W., Galanos, C., & Pollmacher, T. (1998). Endotoxin-induced changes in sleep and sleepiness during the day. *Psychoneuroendocrinology, 23*(5), 427–437.

Hossain, J. L., & Shapiro, C. M. (2002). The prevalence, cost implications, and management of sleep disorders: An overview. *Sleep and Breathing, 6*(2), 85–102.

Inagaki, M., Isono, M., Okuyama, T., Sugawara, Y., Akechi, T., Akizuki, N., et al. (2008). Plasma interleukin-6 and fatigue in terminally ill cancer patients. *Journal of Pain and Symptom Management, 35*(2), 153–161.

Irwin, M., Mascovich, A., Gillin, J. C., Willoughby, R., Pike, J., & Smith, T. L. (1994). Partial sleep deprivation reduces natural killer cell activity in humans. *Psychosomatic Medicine, 56*(6), 493–498.

Irwin, M. R., Carrillo, C., & Olmstead, R. (2010). Sleep loss activates cellular markers of inflammation: Sex differences. *Brain, Behavior, and Immunity, 24*(1), 54–57.

Irwin, M. R., Cole, J. C., & Nicassio, P. M. (2006). Comparative meta-analysis of behavioral interventions for insomnia and their efficacy in middle-aged adults and in older adults 55+ years of age. [Comparative Study Meta-Analysis Research Support, N.I.H., Extramural Research Support, Non-U.S. Gov't Review]. *Health Psychology : Official Journal of the Division of Health Psychology, American Psychological Association, 25*(1), 3–14. doi: 10.1037/0278-6133.25.1.3

Irwin, M. R., Olmstead, R., & Oxman, M. N. (2007). Augmenting immune responses to varicella zoster virus in older adults: A randomized, controlled trial of Tai Chi. *Journal of the American Geriatric Society, 55*(4), 511–517.

Irwin, M. R., Olmstead, R., Valladares, E. M., Breen, E. C., & Ehlers, C. L. (2009). Tumor necrosis factor antagonism normalizes rapid eye movement sleep in alcohol dependence. [Randomized Controlled Trial Research Support, N.I.H., Extramural Research Support, Non-U.S. Gov't].

Biological psychiatry, 66(2), 191-195. doi: 10.1016/j.biopsych.2008.12.004

Irwin, M. R., Valladares, E. M., Motivala, S., Thayer, J. F., & Ehlers, C. L. (2006). Association between nocturnal vagal tone and sleep depth, sleep quality, and fatigue in alcohol dependence. *Psychosomatic Medicine, 68*(1), 159–166.

Irwin, M. R., Wang, M., Campomayor, C. O., Collado-Hidalgo, A., & Cole, S. (2006). Sleep deprivation and activation of morning levels of cellular and genomic markers of inflammation. *Archives of Internal Medicine, 166*(16), 1756–1762.

Irwin, M. R., Wang, M., Ribeiro, D., Cho, H. J., Olmstead, R., Breen, E. C., et al. (2008). Sleep loss activates cellular inflammatory signaling. *Biological Psychiatry, 64*(6), 538–540.

Ishimori, K. (1909). True cause of sleep: A hypnogenic substance as evidenced in the brain of sleep-deprived animals. *Tokyo Igakkai Zasshi, 23,*(429–459).

Jacobsen, P. B., Andrykowski, M. A., & Thors, C. L. (2004). Relationship of catastrophizing to fatigue among women receiving treatment for breast cancer. *Journal of Consulting and Clinical Psychology, 72*(2), 355–361.

Jacobsen, P. B., Donovan, K. A., Vadaparampil, S. T., & Small, B. J. (2007). Systematic review and meta-analysis of psychological and activity-based interventions for cancer-related fatigue. *Health Psychology, 26*(6), 660–667.

Janszky, I., Lekander, M., Blom, M., Georgiades, A., & Ahnve, S. (2005). Self-rated health and vital exhaustion, but not depression, is related to inflammation in women with coronary heart disease. *Brain, Behavior, and Immunity, 19*(6), 555–563.

Jatoi, A., Ritter, H. L., Dueck, A., Nguyen, P. L., Nikcevich, D. A., Luyun, R. F., et al. (2010). A placebo-controlled, double-blind trial of infliximab for cancer-associated weight loss in elderly and/or poor performance non-small cell lung cancer patients (N01C9). *Lung Cancer, 68*(2), 234–239.

Jean-Louis, G., Kripke, D. F., Ancoli-Israel, S., Klauber, M. R., & Sepulveda, R. S. (2000). Sleep duration, illumination, and activity patterns in a population sample: Effects of gender and ethnicity. *Biological Psychiatry, 47*(10), 921–927.

Jean-Pierre, P., Morrow, G. R., Roscoe, J. A., Heckler, C., Mohile, S., Janelsins, M., et al. (2010). A phase 3 randomized, placebo-controlled, double-blind, clinical trial of the effect of modafinil on cancer-related fatigue among 631 patients receiving chemotherapy: A University of Rochester Cancer Center Community Clinical Oncology Program Research base study. *Cancer, 116*(14), 3513–20.

Jhamb, M., Weisbord, S. D., Steel, J. L., & Unruh, M. (2008). Fatigue in patients receiving maintenance dialysis: A review of definitions, measures, and contributing factors. *American Journal of Kidney Disease, 52*(2), 353–365.

Johnston, G. R., & Webster, N. R. (2009). Cytokines and the immunomodulatory function of the vagus nerve. *British Journal of Anaesthia, 102*(4), 453–462.

Kapcala, L. P., He, J. R., Gao, Y., Pieper, J. O., & DeTolla, L. J. (1996). Subdiaphragmatic vagotomy inhibits intra-abdominal interleukin-1 beta stimulation of adrenocorticotropin secretion. *Brain Research, 728*(2), 247–254.

Kirkova, J., Walsh, D., Aktas, A., & Davis, M. P. (2010). Cancer symptom clusters: Old concept but new data. *American Journal of Hospice and Palliative Care, 27*(4), 282–288.

Klimas, N. G., & Koneru, A. O. (2007). Chronic fatigue syndrome: Inflammation, immune function, and neuroendocrine interactions. *Current Rheumatology Reports, 9*(6), 482–487.

Knoop, H., Prins, J. B., Moss-Morris, R., & Bleijenberg, G. (2010). The central role of cognitive processes in the perpetuation of chronic fatigue syndrome. *Journal of Psychosomatic Research, 68*(5), 489–494.

Konsman, J. P., Luheshi, G. N., Bluthé, R. M., & Dantzer, R. (2000). The vagus nerve mediates behavioural depression, but not fever, in response to peripheral immune signals; a functional anatomical analysis. *European Journal of Neuroscience, 12*(12), 4434–4446.

Kornmüller, A., Lux, H., Winkel, K., & Klee, M. (1961). Neurohumoral ausgelöste schlafzustände an tieren mit gekreuztem kreislfau unter kontrolle von EEG-Ableitiungen. *Naturwissenschaften, 14,*(503–505).

Korth, C., Mullington, J., Schreiber, W., & Pollmacher, T. (1996). Influence of endotoxin on daytime sleep in humans. *Infection and Immunity, 64*(4), 1110–1115.

Kripke, D. F., Garfinkel, L., Wingard, D. L., Klauber, M. R., & Marler, M. R. (2002). Mortality associated with sleep duration and insomnia. *Archives of General Psychiatry, 59*(2), 131–136.

Kronfol, Z., & Remick, D. G. (2000). Cytokines and the brain: Implications for clinical psychiatry. *American Journal of Psychiatry, 157*(5), 683–694.

Krueger, J. M., & Majde, J. A. (2003). Humoral links between sleep and the immune system: Research issues. *Annals of the New York Academy of Science, 992,* 9–20.

Krueger, J. M., Obal, F., Jr., & Fang, J. (1999). Humoral regulation of physiological sleep: Cytokines and GHRH. *Journal of Sleep Research, 8*(1), 53–59.

Krueger, J. M., Obal, F. J., Fang, J., Kubota, T., & Taishi, P. (2001). The role of cytokines in physiological sleep regulation. *Annals of the New York Academy of Science, 933,* 211–221.

Krueger, J. M., Walter, J., Dinarello, C. A., Wolff, S. M., & Chedid, L. (1984). Sleep-promoting effects of endogenous pyrogen (interleukin-1). *American Journal of Physiology, 246*(6 Pt 2), R994–999.

Kubota, K. (1989). Kuniomi Ishimori and the first discovery of sleep-inducing substances in the brain. *Neuroscience Research, 6*(6), 497–518.

Kurzrock, R. (2001). The role of cytokines in cancer-related fatigue. *Cancer, 92*(6 Suppl), 1684–1688.

Kushikata, T., Fang, J., & Krueger, J. M. (1999). Interleukin-10 inhibits spontaneous sleep in rabbits. *Journal of Interferon Cytokine Research, 19*(9), 1025–1030.

Kushikata, T., Fang, J., Wang, Y., & Krueger, J. M. (1998). Interleukin-4 inhibits spontaneous sleep in rabbits. *American Journal of Physiology, 275*(4 Pt 2), R1185–1191.

Lawrence, D. P., Kupelnick, B., Miller, K., Devine D., Lau, J. (2004). Evidence report on the occurrence, assessment, and treatment of fatigue in cancer patients. *Journal of the National Cancer Institute: Monographs, 32,* 40–50.

Lee, K. S., Song, E. K., Lennie, T. A., Frazier, S. K., Chung, M. L., Heo, S., et al. (2010). Symptom clusters in men and women with heart failure and their impact on cardiac event-free survival. *Journal of Cardiovascular Nursing, 25*(4), 263–272.

Lewis, G., & Wessely, S. (1992). The epidemiology of fatigue: More questions than answers. *Journal of Epidemiology and Community Health, 46*(2), 92–97.

Luheshi, G. N., Bluthé, R. M., Rushforth, D., Mulcahy, N., Konsman, J. P., Goldbach, M., et al. (2000). Vagotomy attenuates the behavioural but not the pyrogenic effects of interleukin-1 in rats. *Autonomic Neuroscience, 85*(1–3), 127–132.

Lutgendorf, S. K., Weinrib, A. Z., Penedo, F., Russell, D., DeGeest, K., Costanzo, E. S., et al. (2008). Interleukin-6, cortisol, and depressive symptoms in ovarian cancer patients. *Journal of Clinical Oncology, 26*(29), 4820–4827.

Macedo, J. A., Hesse, J., Turner, J. D., Meyer, J., Hellhammer, D. H., & Muller, C. P. (2008). Glucocorticoid sensitivity in fibromyalgia patients: Decreased expression of corticosteroid receptors and glucocorticoid-induced leucine zipper. *Psychoneuroendocrinology, 33*(6), 799–809.

Madhusudan, S., Muthuramalingam, S. R., Braybrooke, J. P., Wilner, S., Kaur, K., Han, C., et al. (2005). Study of etanercept, a tumor necrosis factor-alpha inhibitor, in recurrent ovarian cancer. *Journal of Clinical Oncology, 23*(25), 5950–5959.

Maes, M. (2009). "Functional" or "psychosomatic" symptoms, e.g. a flu-like malaise, aches and pain and fatigue, are major features of major and in particular of melancholic depression. *Neuro Endocrinology Letters, 30*(5), 564–573.

Maier, S. F., & Watkins, L. R. (1998). Cytokines for psychologists: Implications of bidirectional immune-to-brain communication for understanding behavior, mood, and cognition. [Review]. *Psychological Review, 105*(1), 83–105.

Mallon, L., Broman, J. E., & Hetta, J. (2002). Sleep complaints predict coronary artery disease mortality in males: A 12-year follow-up study of a middle-aged Swedish population. *Journal of Internal Medicine, 251*(3), 207–216.

McCrone, P., Darbishire, L., Ridsdale, L., & Seed, P. (2003). The economic cost of chronic fatigue and chronic fatigue syndrome in UK primary care. *Psychological Medicine, 33*(2), 253–261.

McGregor, B. A., & Antoni, M. H. (2009). Psychological intervention and health outcomes among women treated for breast cancer: a review of stress pathways and biological mediators. [Research Support, N.I.H., Extramural Review]. *Brain, Behavior, and Immunity, 23*(2), 159–166. doi: 10.1016/j.bbi.2008.08.002

Meier-Ewert, H. K., Ridker, P. M., Rifai, N., Regan, M. M., Price, N. J., Dinges, D. F., et al. (2004). Effect of sleep loss on C-reactive protein, an inflammatory marker of cardiovascular risk. *Journal of the American College of Cardiology, 43*(4), 678–683.

Melamed, S., Shirom, A., Toker, S., Berliner, S., & Shapira, I. (2006). Burnout and risk of cardiovascular disease: Evidence, possible causal paths, and promising research directions. *Psychological Bulletin, 132*(3), 327–353.

Miaskowski, C., Dodd, M., Lee, K., West, C., Paul, S. M., Cooper, B. A., et al. (2010). Preliminary evidence of an association between a functional interleukin-6 polymorphism and fatigue and sleep disturbance in oncology patients and their family caregivers. *Journal of Pain and Symptom Management, 40*(4), 531–544.

Miller, A. H., Ancoli-Israel, S., Bower, J. E., Capuron, L., & Irwin, M. R. (2008). Neuroendocrine-immune mechanisms of behavioral co-morbidities in patients with cancer. *Journal of Clinical Oncology, 26*(6), 971–982.

Miller, N. E. (1964). Some psychophysiological studies of the motivation and of the behavioral effects of illness. *Bulletin of British Psychology, 17,* 1–20.

Mills, P. J., Ancoli-Israel, S., Parker, B., Natarajan, L., Hong, S., Jain, S., et al. (2008). Predictors of inflammation in response to anthracycline-based chemotherapy for breast cancer. *Brain, Behavior, and Immunity, 22*(1), 98–104.

Mills, P. J., Parker, B., Dimsdale, J. E., Sadler, G. R., & Ancoli-Israel, S. (2005). The relationship between fatigue and quality of life and inflammation during anthracycline-based chemotherapy in breast cancer. *Biological Psychology, 69*(1), 85–96.

Mills, P. J., Parker, B., Jones, V., Adler, K. A., Perez, C. J., Johnson, S., et al. (2004). The effects of standard anthracycline-based chemotherapy on soluble ICAM-1 and vascular endothelial growth factor levels in breast cancer. *Clinical Cancer Research, 10*(15), 4998–5003.

Milne, H. M., Wallman, K. E., Gordon, S., & Courneya, K. S. (2008). Effects of a combined aerobic and resistance exercise program in breast cancer survivors: A randomized controlled trial. *Breast Cancer Research and Treatment, 108*(2), 279–288.

Monk, J. P., Phillips, G., Waite, R., Kuhn, J., Schaaf, L. J., Otterson, G. A., et al. (2006). Assessment of tumor necrosis factor alpha blockade as an intervention to improve tolerability of dose-intensive chemotherapy in cancer patients. *Journal of Clinical Oncology, 24*(12), 1852–1859.

Monnier, M., & Hoesli, L. (1964). Dialysis of sleep and waking factors in blood of the rabbit. *Science, 146*, 796–798.

Montazeri, A. (2009). Quality of life data as prognostic indicators of survival in cancer patients: An overview of the literature from 1982 to 2008. *Health and Quality of Life Outcomes, 7*, 102.

Moreh, E., Jacobs, J. M., & Stessman, J. (2010). Fatigue, function, and mortality in older adults. *Journals of Gerontology Series A: Biological Sciences and Medical Sciences, 65*(8), 887–895.

Motl, R. W., Suh, Y., & Weikert, M. (2010). Symptom cluster and quality of life in multiple sclerosis. *Journal of Pain and Symptom Management, 39*(6), 1025–1032.

Mullington, J., Korth, C., Hermann, D. M., Orth, A., Galanos, C., Holsboer, F., et al. (2000). Dose-dependent effects of endotoxin on human sleep. *American Journal of Physiology: Regulatory, Integrative, and Comparative Physiology, 278*(4), R947–955.

Nagasaki, H., Iriki, M., Inoue, S., & Uchizono, K. (1974). Proceedings: Sleep promoting substances in the brain stem of rats. *Nippon Seirigaku Zasshi, 36*(8–9), 293.

Natelson, B. H., Haghighi, M. H., & Ponzio, N. M. (2002). Evidence for the presence of immune dysfunction in chronic fatigue syndrome. *Clinical and Diagnostic Labratory Immunology, 9*(4), 747–752.

Nisenbaum, R., Reyes, M., Unger, E. R., & Reeves, W. C. (2004). Factor analysis of symptoms among subjects with unexplained chronic fatigue: What can we learn about chronic fatigue syndrome? *Journal of Psychosomatic Research, 56*(2), 171–178.

Noel, J. K., Crean, S., Claflin, J. E., Ranganathan, G., Linz, H., & Lahn, M. (2008). Systematic review to establish the safety profiles for direct and indirect inhibitors of p38 Mitogen-activated protein kinases for treatment of cancer: A systematic review of the literature. *Medical Oncology, 25*(3), 323–330.

Oh, B., Butow, P., Mullan, B., Clarke, S., Beale, P., Pavlakis, N., et al. (2010). Impact of medical Qigong on quality of life, fatigue, mood and inflammation in cancer patients: A randomized controlled trial. *Annals of Oncology, 21*(3), 608–614.

Ohayon, M. M. (2002). Epidemiology of insomnia: What we know and what we still need to learn. *Sleep Medicine Reviews, 6*(2), 97–111.

Okun, M. L., Giese, S., Lin, L., Einen, M., Mignot, E., & Coussons-Read, M. E. (2004). Exploring the cytokine and endocrine involvement in narcolepsy. *Brain, Behavior, and Immunity, 18*(4), 326–332.

Okun, M. L., Reynolds, C. F., III, Buysse, D. J., Monk, T. H., Mazumdar, S., Begley, A., et al. (2010). Sleep variability, health-related practices, and inflammatory markers in a community dwelling sample of older adults. *Psychosomatic Medicine, 73*(2), 142–150.

Omdal, R., & Gunnarsson, R. (2005). The effect of interleukin-1 blockade on fatigue in rheumatoid arthritis: A pilot study. *Rheumatology International, 25*(6), 481–484.

Opp, M. R. (2005). Cytokines and sleep. *Sleep Medicine Reviews, 9*(5), 355–364.

Opp, M. R., Smith, E. M., & Hughes, T. K., Jr. (1995). Interleukin-10 (cytokine synthesis inhibitory factor) acts in the central nervous system of rats to reduce sleep. *Journal of Neuroimmunology, 60*(1–2), 165–168.

Opp, M. R., & Toth, L. A. (2003). Neural-immune interactions in the regulation of sleep. *Frontiers in Bioscience, 8*, d768–779.

Ozturk, L., Pelin, Z., Karadeniz, D., Kaynak, H., Cakar, L., & Gozukirmizi, E. (1999). Effects of 48 hours sleep deprivation on human immune profile. *Sleep Research Online, 2*(4), 107–111.

Pace, T. W., & Miller, A. H. (2009). Cytokines and glucocorticoid receptor signaling: Relevance to major depression. *Annals of the New York Academy of Science, 1179*, 86–105.

Pollmacher, T., Mullington, J., Korth, C., & Hinze-Selch, D. (1995). Influence of host defense activation on sleep in humans. *Advanced Neuroimmunology, 5*(2), 155–169.

Pollmacher, T., Schreiber, W., Gudewill, S., Vedder, H., Fassbender, K., Wiedemann, K., et al. (1993). Influence of endotoxin on nocturnal sleep in humans. *American Journal of Physiology, 264*(6 Pt 2), R1077–1083.

Pawlikowska, T., Chalder, T., Hirsch, S. R., Wallace, P., Wright, D. J., & Wessely, S. C. (1994). Population based study of fatigue and psychological distress. *BMJ, 308*(6931), 763–766.

Pusztai, L., Mendoza, T. R., Reuben, J. M., Martinez, M. M., Willey, J. S., Lara, J., et al. (2004). Changes in plasma levels of inflammatory cytokines in response to paclitaxel chemotherapy. *Cytokine, 25*(3), 94–102.

Rabkin, J. G., McElhiney, M. C., Rabkin, R., & McGrath, P. J. (2010). Modafinil treatment for fatigue in HIV/AIDS: A randomized placebo-controlled study. *Journal of Clinical Psychiatry, 71*(6), 707–715.

Raison, C. L., Rye, D. B., Woolwine, B. J., Vogt, G. J., Bautista, B. M., Spivey, J. R., et al. (2010). Chronic interferon-alpha administration disrupts sleep continuity and depth in patients with hepatitis C: Association with fatigue, motor slowing, and increased evening cortisol. *Biological Psychiatry, 68*(10), 942–949.

Rajeevan, M. S., Smith, A. K., Dimulescu, I., Unger, E. R., Vernon, S. D., Heim, C., et al. (2007). Glucocorticoid receptor polymorphisms and haplotypes associated with chronic fatigue syndrome. *Genes, Brain, and Behavior, 6*(2), 167–176.

Reichenberg, A., Yirmiya, R., Schuld, A., Kraus, T., Haack, M., Morag, A., & Pollmacher, T. (2001). Cytokine-associated emotional and cognitive disturbances in humans. *Archives of General Psychiatry, 58*(5), 445–452.

Ricci, J. A., Chee, E., Lorandeau, A. L., & Berger, J. (2007). Fatigue in the U.S. workforce: Prevalence and implications for lost productive work time. *Journal of Occupational and Environmental Medicine, 49*(1), 1–10.

Rosekind, M. R., Gregory, K. B., Mallis, M. M., Brandt, S. L., Seal, B., & Lerner, D. (2010). The cost of poor sleep: Workplace productivity loss and associated costs. *Journal of Occupational and Environmental Medicine, 52*(1), 91–98.

Rutledge, D. N., Mouttapa, M., & Wood, P. B. (2009). Symptom clusters in fibromyalgia: Potential utility in patient assessment and treatment evaluation. *Nursing Research, 58*(5), 359–367.

Ryan, J. L., Carroll, J. K., Ryan, E. P., Mustian, K. M., Fiscella, K., & Morrow, G. (2007). Mechanisms of cancer-related fatigue. *Oncologist, 12,* 22–34.

Schubert, C., Hong, S., Natarajan, L., Mills, P. J., & Dimsdale, J. E. (2007). The association between fatigue and inflammatory marker levels in cancer patients: A quantitative review. *Brain, Behavior, and Immunity,21*(4), 413–427.

Servaes, P., Verhagen, C., & Bleijenberg, G. (2002). Fatigue in cancer patients during and after treatment: Prevalence, correlates and interventions. *European Journal of Cancer, 38*(1), 27–43.

Shearer, W. T., Reuben, J. M., Mullington, J. M., Price, N. J., Lee, B. N., Smith, E. O., et al. (2001). Soluble TNF-alpha receptor 1 and IL-6 plasma levels in humans subjected to the sleep deprivation model of spaceflight. *Journal of Allergy and Clinical Immunology, 107*(1), 165–170.

Shimommura, Y., Shimizu, H., Takahashi, M., Uehara, Y., Negishi, M., Sato, N., et al. (1990). Effects of peripheral administration of recombinant human interleukin-1 beta on feeding behavior of the rat. *Life Sciences, 47*(24), 2185–2192.

Smith, O. R., Gidron, Y., Kupper, N., Winter, J. B., & Denollet, J. (2009). Vital exhaustion in chronic heart failure: Symptom profiles and clinical outcome. *Journal of Psychosomatic Research, 66*(3), 195–201.

Soderstrom, M., Ekstedt, M., Akerstedt, T., Nilsson, J., & Axelsson, J. (2004). Sleep and sleepiness in young individuals with high burnout scores. *Sleep, 27*(7), 1369–1377.

Spath-Schwalbe, E., Hansen, K., Schmidt, F., Schrezenmeier, H., Marshall, L., Burger, K., et al. (1998). Acute effects of recombinant human interleukin-6 on endocrine and central nervous sleep functions in healthy men. *Journal of Clinicl Endocrinology and Metabolism, 83*(5), 1573–1579.

Spath-Schwalbe, E., Lange, T., Perras, B., Fehm, H. L., & Born, J. (2000). Interferon-alpha acutely impairs sleep in healthy humans. *Cytokine, 12*(5), 518–521.

Stoller, M. K. (1994). Economic effects of insomnia. *Clinical Therepuetics, 16*(5), 873–897; discussion 854.

Taylor, D. J., Lichstein, K. L., Durrence, H. H., Riedel, B. W., & Bush, A. J. (2005). Epidemiology of insomnia, depression, and anxiety. *Sleep, 28*(11), 1457–1464.

Tazi, A., Dantzer, R., Crestani, F., & Le Moal, M. (1988). Interleukin-1 induces conditioned taste aversion in rats: A possible explanation for its pituitary-adrenal stimulating activity. *Brain Research, 473*(2), 369–371.

Tobler, I., Borbely, A. A., Schwyzer, M., & Fontana, A. (1984). Interleukin-1 derived from astrocytes enhances slow wave activity in sleep EEG of the rat. *Eurpean Journal of Pharmacology, 104*(1–2), 191–192.

Toth, L. A. (1996). Strain differences in the somnogenic effects of interferon inducers in mice. *Journal of Interferon and Cytokine Research, 16*(12), 1065–1072.

Toth, L. A., & Opp, M. R. (2001). Cytokine- and microbially induced sleep responses of interleukin-10 deficient mice.

American Journal of Physiology: Regulatory, Integrative, and Comparative Physiology, 280(6), R1806–1814.

Toth, L. A., & Verhulst, S. J. (2003). Strain differences in sleep patterns of healthy and influenza-infected inbred mice. *Behavior Genetics, 33*(3), 325–336.

Tyring, S., Gottlieb, A., Papp, K., Gordon, K., Leonardi, C., Wang, A., et al. (2006). Etanercept and clinical outcomes, fatigue, and depression in psoriasis: double-blind placebo-controlled randomised phase III trial. [Multicenter Study Randomized Controlled Trial Research Support, Non-U.S. Gov't]. *Lancet, 367*(9504), 29–35. doi: 10.1016/S0140-6736(05)67763-X

Uppal, S. S., Hayat, S. J., & Raghupathy, R. (2009). Efficacy and safety of infliximab in active SLE: A pilot study. *Lupus, 18*(8), 690–697.

Van Den Eede, F., Moorkens, G., Van Houdenhove, B., Cosyns, P., & Claes, S. J. (2007). Hypothalamic-pituitary-adrenal axis function in chronic fatigue syndrome. *Neuropsychobiology, 55*(2), 112–120.

van der Ven, A., van Diest, R., Hamulyak, K., Maes, M., Bruggeman, C., & Appels, A. (2003). Herpes viruses, cytokines, and altered hemostasis in vital exhaustion. *Psychosomatic Medicine, 65*(2), 194–200.

van Diest, R., & Appels, W. P. (1994). Sleep physiological characteristics of exhausted men. *Psychosomatic Medicine, 56*(1), 28–35.

Vgontzas, A. N., Bixler, E. O., & Chrousos, G. P. (2006). Obesity-related sleepiness and fatigue: The role of the stress system and cytokines. *Annals of the New York Academy of Science, 1083,* 329–344.

Vgontzas, A. N., Papanicolaou, D. A., Bixler, E. O., Kales, A., Tyson, K., & Chrousos, G. P. (1997). Elevation of plasma cytokines in disorders of excessive daytime sleepiness: Role of sleep disturbance and obesity. *Journal of Clinical Endocrinology and Metabolism, 82*(5), 1313–1316.

Vgontzas, A. N., Zoumakis, E., Bixler, E. O., Lin, H. M., Follett, H., Kales, A., et al. (2004). Adverse effects of modest sleep restriction on sleepiness, performance, and inflammatory cytokines. *Journal of Clinical Endocrinology and Metabolism, 89*(5), 2119–2126.

Vgontzas, A. N., Zoumakis, M., Papanicolaou, D. A., Bixler, E. O., Prolo, P., Lin, H. M., et al. (2002). Chronic insomnia is associated with a shift of interleukin-6 and tumor necrosis factor secretion from nighttime to daytime. *Metabolism, 51*(7), 887–892.

Wang, X., Wang, B., Duan, X., Liu, H., & Ju, G. (2000). The expression of IL-1 receptor type I in nodose ganglion and vagal paraganglion in the rat. *Chinese Journal of Neuroscience, 16,* 90–93.

Wang, X. S., Shi, Q., Williams, L. A., Mao, L., Cleeland, C. S., Komaki, R. R., et al. (2010). Inflammatory cytokines are associated with the development of symptom burden in patients with NSCLC undergoing concurrent chemoradiation therapy. *Brain, Behavior, and Immunity, 24*(6), 968–974.

Watkins, L. R., Maier, S. F., & Goehler, L. E. (1995). Cytokine-to-brain communication: A review & analysis of alternative mechanisms. *Life Sciences, 57*(11), 1011–1026.

Wijayahadi, N., Haron, M. R., Stanslas, J., & Yusuf, Z. (2007). Changes in cellular immunity during chemotherapy for primary breast cancer with anthracycline regimens. *Journal of Chemotherapy, 19*(6), 716–723.

Wirtz, P. H., von Kanel, R., Schnorpfeil, P., Ehlert, U., Frey, K., & Fischer, J. E. (2003). Reduced glucocorticoid sensitivity of monocyte interleukin-6 production in male industrial employees who are vitally exhausted. *Psychosomatic Medicine, 65*(4), 672–678.

Wolfe, F., Michaud, K., & Li, T. (2006). Sleep disturbance in patients with rheumatoid arthritis: Evaluation by medical outcomes study and visual analog sleep scales. *Journal of Rheumatology, 33*(10), 1942–1951.

Yount, S., Sorensen, M. V., Cella, D., Sengupta, N., Grober, J., & Chartash, E. K. (2007). Adalimumab plus methotrexate or standard therapy is more effective than methotrexate or standard therapies alone in the treatment of fatigue in patients with active, inadequately treated rheumatoid arthritis. *Clinical and Experimental Rheumatology, 25*(6), 838–846.

Zamarron, C., Maceiras, F., Mera, A., & Gomez-Reino, J. J. (2004). Effect of the first infliximab infusion on sleep and alertness in patients with active rheumatoid arthritis. *Annals of the Rheumatic Diseases, 63*(1), 88–90.

Zee, P., & Ancoli-Israel, S.(2009). Does effective management of sleep disorders reduce cancer-related fatigue? *Drugs, 69*(2), 29–41.

Psychoneuroimmunology and Cancer: Biobehavioral Influences on Tumor Progression

Susan K. Lutgendorf, Erin S. Costanzo, *and* Anil K. Sood

Abstract

This chapter examines the role of psychosocial factors and stress-related neuroendocrine hormones in cancer progression. The neuroendocrine stress response appears to play a key role in modulating physiological pathways relevant to cancer progression. These include tumor angiogenesis, invasion, anoikis, inflammation, the cellular immune response, and various cell-signaling pathways. These stress-response pathways also potentially interact with cancer treatments. Bidirectional influences of tumor-derived cytokines and other molecules on the hypothalamic pituitary adrenal (HPA) axis and CNS processes are also discussed along with implications for disease progression and survival. These mechanisms point to emerging possibilities for psychosocial, pharmacological, and integrative medicine interventions that have the potential to alter stress-response signaling pathways in cancer.

Key Words: cancer, stress, depression, immunity, inflammation, angiogenesis, invasion, psychoneuroimmunology

Introduction

The extent to which psychological factors can place healthy individuals at risk for developing cancer (cancer incidence) has been highly controversial, and evidence supporting this relationship is equivocal (Chen et al., 1995; Protheroe et al., 1999). In contrast, evidence is much stronger supporting a role for psychosocial factors in cancer progression (the further growth of cancer once a tumor is already present). In this chapter, we will summarize the epidemiological evidence examining the role of psychosocial factors in cancer incidence and progression, and then examine mechanisms by which psychosocial risk factors and stress-related neuroendocrine hormones both directly and indirectly modulate pathways that affect tumor growth. Influences of tumor-derived cytokines and other molecules on the hypothalamic-pituitary-adrenal (HPA) axis and central nervous system (CNS) processes and implications for interventions will be discussed.

Biobehavioral Factors and Cancer Incidence

Although there is some evidence that severe stress, such as that stemming from the death of a spouse or child, may increase cancer risk (Duijts, Zeegers, & Borne, 2003; Geyer, 1991, 1993; Lillberg et al., 2003), most studies have not shown a convincing link between stressful life events and the occurrence of cancer (Brown, Butow, Culjak, Coates, & Dunn, 2000; Duijts et al., 2003; Petticrew, Fraser, & Regan, 1999), and a handful of studies have even reported a reduced risk of breast and gynecologic cancers with increased stress (Kroenke et al., 2004; Nielsen et al., 2007; Nielsen et al., 2005). A recent meta-analysis did not find a significant effect for exposure to stressors on cancer incidence, but findings did suggest that certain personality and coping styles were associated with increased cancer risk (Chida, Hamer, Wardle, & Steptoe, 2008). It may be that long-standing personality traits or approaches to stress play a more salient role in the development of disease than do acute life events. However, other studies have not found links between personality or coping and the development of cancer (Bleiker, Hendriks, Otten, Verbeek, & van der Ploeg, 2008; Nakaya et al., 2010; Persky, Kempthorne-Rawson, & Shekelle, 1987; Price et al., 2001).

The contribution of psychosocial factors to cancer initiation may be more complex than previously thought. There is preliminary evidence that interactions of multiple psychosocial factors may increase risk for cancer development, and that psychosocial factors might moderate other risk factors. For example, among participants in the Women's Health Initiative study (N = 84,335), women who experienced one stressful life event (e.g., death, divorce, major financial trouble) showed a 14% increase in risk for developing breast cancer as compared to women who did not experience any stressful life events (occurrence of additional stressful events did not increase risk). The inclusion of social support in the analyses clarified that this association was most pronounced for women with limited support; there was no significant association between the occurrence of life events and development of breast cancer for women with high levels of social support (Michael et al., 2009). The interaction of life stress and lack of support has also been shown to increase risk for breast cancer in other studies (Price et al., 2001). Psychosocial factors may also interact with other host factors known to increase cancer risk, such as aging, familial cancer risk, or poor health practices. For example, although most studies have not found a relationship between depression and cancer incidence (Butow et al., 2000; McGee, Williams, & Elwood, 1994), a large prospective study found that older adults who reported experiencing chronic depressive symptoms over the course of several years were at greater risk for developing cancer, after controlling for a variety of other risk factors (Penninx et al., 1998). Other studies have documented interactions between depression and smoking status such that when both risk factors are present, the risk for lung and other smoking-related cancers are greater than when either risk factor was present alone (Knekt et al., 1996; Linkins & Comstock, 1990).

Biobehavioral Factors and Progression of Cancer

There is more compelling evidence that psychosocial factors can affect clinical outcomes, particularly mortality, following a cancer diagnosis. Although there have been many contradictory findings, studies with more sophisticated methodology are more likely to find these types of effects (Chida et al., 2008). The most commonly examined factors include markers of emotional distress, such as anxiety and depression, along with coping responses of cancer patients.

DISTRESS AND CANCER PROGRESSION

A cancer diagnosis is generally experienced as a major life stressor (Andersen et al., 1998; Andersen, Kiecolt-Glaser, & Glaser, 1994; Meyerowitz, 1980). Not surprisingly, depression is common among individuals diagnosed cancer, with about one-third of cancer patients reporting depressive symptoms at the time of diagnosis and up to one-fourth suffering from symptoms sufficient to meet criteria for a clinical diagnosis of major depression (Massie, 2004; Spoletini et al., 2008). The extent to which patients experience depression, anxiety, or other emotional distress in the face of a cancer diagnosis can certainly affect quality of life. Additionally, depression is a well-documented risk factor for mortality, particularly for elderly individuals and those with a history of cardiovascular disease (e.g., Blumenthal et al., 2003; Carney, Freedland, Miller, & Jaffe, 2002; Murray & Lopez, 1997; Schulz, Drayer, & Rollman, 2002). Similarly, there is evidence that depression is associated with poorer survival in a number of cancer populations, including patients with breast and lung cancers and those undergoing bone marrow or stem cell transplantation (Buccheri, 1998; Rodrigue, Pearman, & Moreb, 1999; Watson, Haviland, Greer, Davidson, & Bliss, 1999). Anxiety has also been associated with poorer survival in breast cancer patients (Cousson-Gelie, Bruchon-Schweitzer, Dilhuydy, & Jutand, 2007; Groenvold et al., 2007). However, several other studies have failed to replicate these associations (Andrykowski, Brady, & Henslee-Downey, 1994; Faller, Bulzebruck, Drings, & Lang, 1999; Goodwin et al., 2004; Osborne et al., 2004; Tross et al., 1996).

Cancer patients participating in large clinical trials or epidemiological studies often complete standardized measures of quality of life that include indices of emotional well-being or distress. Researchers have taken advantage of these datasets to determine the extent to which quality of life dimensions may serve as prognostic indicators for patients with cancers of various sites. Of those that report on the role of emotional well-being or distress, results are mixed, with both positive (Ashing-Giwa, Lim, & Tang, 2010; Carey et al., 2008; Grande, Farquhar, Barclay, & Todd, 2009; Groenvold et al., 2007) and null findings (e.g., Coyne et al., 2007; Fielding & Wong, 2007; Karvonen-Gutierrez et al., 2008;

McKernan, McMillan, Anderson, Angerson, & Stuart, 2008; Mehanna, De Boer, & Morton, 2008; Meyer et al., 2009). Studies of women with breast or gynecologic cancer appear to be more likely than those of other disease sites to find emotional well-being to be prognostically significant. It may be that hormonally mediated cancers are more sensitive to emotional status, as suggested by Andersen and colleagues (1994).

Given that depression and emotional distress are not uncommon in the context of a cancer diagnosis and treatment, and the duration of depression can be quite variable, it may be that only certain subsets of patients are at greater risk for adverse outcomes. For example, those who suffer severe or chronic depression or those who are depressed prior to their diagnosis may differ from individuals who become acutely depressed following diagnosis. Consistent with this idea, a large epidemiologic study reported that newly diagnosed cancer patients with a prior history of depression were at greater risk for mortality than patients with no history of depression, whereas those experiencing depression for the first time after diagnosis had no decline in survival compared to those without depression (Stommel, Given, & Given, 2002). The type of depression may also be important. For example, Gold and Chrousos (Gold & Chrousos, 2002) have distinguished between hyperactive and hypoactive HPA and autonomic changes associated with depressive symptoms. The downstream effects on tumor progression and mortality would, therefore, also be likely to differ.

COPING STRATEGIES AND CANCER PROGRESSION

The role of cognitive and behavioral coping responses to the stress of a cancer diagnosis and treatment has been an area of interest, particularly given the high potential for translational relevance. Early work focused on the role of approaching cancer with a "fighting spirit." Although this approach was associated with more optimal outcomes in a number of early studies (Greer, Morris, & Pettingale, 1979; Greer, Morris, Pettingale, & Haybittle, 1990; Osborne et al., 2004; Pettingale, 1984; Pettingale, Morris, Greer, & Haybittle, 1985; Tschuschke et al., 2001), much of this research has been criticized for small sample sizes and other methodological issues, and findings have not been replicated in similar patient samples (Akechi et al., 2009; Andrykowski et al., 1994; Giraldi, Rodani, Cartei, & Grassi, 1997; Murphy, Jenkins, & Whittaker, 1996; Phillips et al., 2008; Watson et al., 1999). In contrast, having a pessimistic or hopeless outlook or coping style has been more consistently associated with poorer clinical outcomes, including greater likelihood of relapse and poorer survival among breast cancer patients (Greer et al., 1979; Watson et al., 1999), and shorter survival following a bone marrow transplant (Molassiotis, Van den Akker, Milligan, & Goldman, 1997).

Avoidant coping strategies, including suppressing or avoiding unwanted emotions or thoughts, disengagement, denial, and minimizing the impact of the diagnosis, are typically considered to be maladaptive approaches for managing stress, at least for long-term adjustment (Suls & Fletcher, 1985). Indeed, there is evidence that measures of avoidance are related to poorer survival, particularly when indices of emotional suppression are considered (Brown et al., 2000; Epping-Jordan, Compas, & Howell, 1994; Jensen, 1987; Lehto, Ojanen, Dyba, Aromaa, & Kellokumpu-Lehtinen, 2006; Morris, Pettingale, & Haybittle, 1992; Reynolds et al., 2000; Temoshok et al., 1985; Weihs, Enright, Simmens, & Reiss, 2000). Somewhat surprisingly, however, it appears that denying or minimizing the impact of cancer may have a positive effect, with those who employ this approach showing more optimal outcomes (Butow, Coates, & Dunn, 1999; Butow et al., 2000; Greer et al., 1979; Greer et al., 1990; Lehto et al., 2006; Lehto, Ojanen, Dyba, Aromaa, & Kellokumpu-Lehtinen, 2007; Pettingale, 1984; Pettingale et al., 1985). Although the distinction may be subtle, "wearing rose-colored lenses" and appraising one's disease as less threatening than may objectively be the case appears to have a salubrious influence, but failing to express and acknowledge strong emotions when they do arise can be detrimental. Not all findings are consistent with respect to optimism, however. For example, in one study, patients with non-small-cell lung carcinoma reporting higher levels of optimism showed no differences in survival time than their less optimistic counterparts (Schofield et al., 2004).

SOCIAL SUPPORT/ISOLATION AND CANCER PROGRESSION

The positive influence of social support on health has been well characterized, with epidemiological studies showing robust links between social support and diminished risk for morbidity and mortality (House, Landis, & Umberson, 1988). In addition, social support is thought to moderate the effects of stress (Cohen, 2004). Although some studies of cancer patients have not found a link between social support and survival (Butow et al., 1999; Butow et al., 2000; Giraldi et al., 1997), several large prospective studies have found that social support is related to longer survival among women diagnosed with breast cancer (Funch & Marshall, 1983; Marshall & Funch, 1983; Maunsell, Brisson, & Deschenes, 1995; Reynolds et al., 1994; Reynolds et al., 2000). For example, a comprehensive social network assessment was conducted among Nurses' Health Study participants who were diagnosed with breast cancer (N = 1,753) (Kroenke, Kubzansky, Schernhammer, Holmes, & Kawachi, 2006). After adjusting for a number of biomedical factors and health practices, women who were socially isolated prior to diagnosis had an increased risk of all-cause mortality and were twice as likely to die from breast-cancer related causes than were women considered to be socially integrated.

Other studies have shown links between survival and both quantitative/structural (number of supports, number of sources of emotional support, contact with friends or family) and qualitative/functional (e.g., perceived emotional support, social functioning) indices of breast cancer patients' support networks. In general, better support has been associated with a longer time to recurrence and reduced mortality following diagnosis (Cousson-Gelie et al., 2007; Efficace et al., 2006; Efficace et al., 2008; Levy, 1991; Maunsell et al., 1995; Park, Lechner, Antoni, & Stanton, 2008; Reynolds et al., 1994; Soler-Vila, Kasi, & Jones, 2003; Waxler-Morrison, Hislop, Mears, & Kan, 1991; Weihs et al., 2005). A recent review of prospective, longitudinal studies concluded that there is solid evidence for a relationship between social support and breast cancer progression, although the role of social support for individuals with other types of cancers was inconclusive (Nausheen, Gidron, Peveler, & Moss-Morris, 2009). The authors further noted that although indices of both structural and functional support were associated with reduced risk of mortality, findings for structural support were more robust.

There is evidence for similar links between social support and mortality for individuals with hematologic malignancies undergoing a bone marrow transplant (Colon, Callies, Popkin, & McGlave, 1991; Frick, Motzke, Fischer, Busch, & Bumeder, 2005; Pinquart, Hoffken, Silbereisen, & Wedding, 2007; Rodrigue et al., 1999). Studies assessing links between social support and clinical outcomes for lung cancer (Herndon et al., 1999; Naughton et al., 2002; Saito-Nakaya et al., 2006) and melanoma

(Butow et al., 1999; Lehto et al., 2007) have been less likely to find these relationships. It may be that social support can have a more helpful influence on patients with tumors that are sensitive to hormonal or immune influences, as noted previously (Andersen et al., 1994).

SUMMARY

Although the literature has been mixed, the pattern of findings point to psychosocial profiles of cancer patients who may be more vulnerable to the effects of stress. Those who are chronically depressed and/or socially isolated, as well as those who respond to their diagnosis with a hopeless and pessimistic outlook may be at risk for a poorer clinical course. In contrast, experiencing acute distress or depression after a cancer diagnosis, particularly if the emotions that arise are acknowledged and expressed, does not appear to be problematic. Cancer patients who take a more positive view of their illness appear to do better, as do those with particularly good social support networks, although not all findings are consistent. The majority of studies account for known biomedical risk factors, suggesting findings are not simply reflective of patients' responses to the severity of the prognosis (i.e., those with poorer prognosis are also more depressed). Although the mediating mechanisms are not clear, possibilities include the influence of psychosocial factors on health practices and treatment adherence, as well as on physiological pathways affecting tumor progression. Many studies also accounted for health practices (e.g., Kroenke et al., 2006; Michael et al., 2009; Nielsen et al., 2007; Penninx et al., 1998; Reynolds et al., 2000), with stress-related psychosocial factors remaining significant when these factors are included, suggesting that alternate pathways may be important. The remainder of the chapter will focus on the potential role of stress physiology in tumor development and progression.

Biobehavioral and Neuroendocrine Modulation of Tumor Growth and Progression

Growing evidence indicates that psychosocial factors such as chronic stress, lack of social support, and depression are able to modulate many of the physiological pathways relevant to the growth and metastasis of cancer (e.g., Andersen et al., 1998a; Armaiz-Pena, Lutgendorf, Cole, & Sood, 2009; Reiche, Nunes, & Morimoto, 2004; Thornton, Andersen, Crespin, & Carson, 2007; Antoni et al., 2006; Lutgendorf, Sood, & Antoni, 2010). These effects are mediated in part by the sympathetic nervous system (SNS) (Madden, 2003), the HPA axis (Chrousos, 1992), and a variety of hormones and peptides (McCusker et al., 2007). These pathways are discussed here in brief and are illustrated in Figure 19.1.

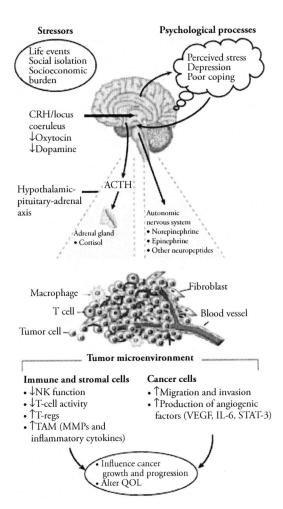

Figure 19.1 Effects of stress and psychological processes on the tumor microenvironment. The stress response results in activation of the autonomic nervous system and the HPA axis. Factors released from these pathways can have direct effects on the tumor microenvironment, resulting in a favorable environment for tumor growth and progression. These dynamics can also adversely affect patient quality of life. Corticotropin-releasing hormone (CRH); adrenocorticotrophic hormone (ACTH); natural killer (NK); regulatory T cells (T-regs) ; tumor-associated macrophages (TAM); matrix metalloprotinease (MMP); VEGF, vascular endothelial growth factor (VEGF); interleukin, (IL); signal transducer and activator of transcription factor-3 (STAT-3); quality of life (QOL). Reprinted with permission © 2008 American Society of Clinical Oncology. All rights reserved. Lutgendorf, S. K. et al. Host Factors and Cancer Progression: Biobehavioral Signaling Pathways and Interventions, *Journal of Clinical Oncology, 28*(26) 2010 (4094–4099).

Stress-related behavioral information is processed via cortical and limbic structures of the central nervous system and ultimately results in modulation of the SNS and the HPA axis (Weiner, 1992). The SNS and HPA affect multiple bodily organs as well as immune cells and tumor tissues. Elevated catecholamine levels have been observed in depressed individuals, those who are socially isolated (Esler et al., 1982; Hamer, Tanaka, Okamura, Tsuda, & Steptoe, 2007; Hughes, Watkins, Blumenthal, Kuhn, & Sherwood, 2004; Light, Kothandapani, & Allen, 1998; Miller, Cohen, Rabin, Skoner, & Doyle, 1999; Seeman & McEwen, 1996; Seeman, Singer, Rowe, Horwitz, & McEwen, 1997; Veith et al., 1994), and individuals experiencing acute or chronic stress (Chrousos, 1992). Both primary and secondary lymphoid organs are directly innervated by fibers of the SNS, which release the catecholamine norepinephrine (NE), which regulates various aspects of leukocyte function (Felten & Felten, 1991). Norepinephrine has been shown to regulate immune cells by stimulating beta-adrenergic receptors (ADRB1 and ADRB2) expressed by leukocytes (Hellstrand, Hermodsson, & Strannegard, 1985; Van Miert, 2002; VanTits et al., 1990). Glucocorticoids such as cortisol are secreted as part of the body's natural adaptation to stress (Chrousos, 1992) and are tightly regulated via the HPA axis (Sapolsky, Krey, & McEwen, 1986). Physiologic levels of glucocorticoids suppress many aspects of the immune response and downregulate inflammation (Gatti et al., 1987; Holbrook, Cox, & Horner, 1983; Ramirez, 1998; Zhou et al., 1997). Glucocorticoids can also act synergistically with adrenergic mechanisms to potentiate adrenergic effects (Nakane et al., 1990).

In addition to effects on cellular immunity and inflammation (which will be discussed later in this chapter), stress-related behavioral factors can influence cancer progression through direct effects on tumor growth mechanisms such as angiogenesis, invasion, and anoikis. These processes are described next.

Mechanisms of Tumor Growth and Progression

THE HALLMARKS OF MALIGNANT TRANSFORMATION

The process by which a normal cell transforms into a tumor cell involves multiple steps, including genetic and epigenetic alterations. (Epigenetic refers to changes in gene expression not caused by alterations in the underlying DNA sequence—but often involving changes in accessibility of DNA with downstream effects on the activity of a gene.) In the process of malignant transformation, cells must overcome the traditional host defense mechanisms limiting their growth and movement. Hanahan and Weinberg (2011) outlined six sequential changes in cell physiology that are essential for the development of cancer. These include (1) self-sufficiency in growth signaling (or the ability to shift from a quiescent state into an active proliferative state without stimulatory signals from outside the cell that are required for normal cells); (2) lack of responsiveness to signals for growth inhibition; (3) ability to avoid programmed cell death (apoptosis); (4) limitless ability to replicate; (5) sustained angiogenesis (growth of tumor vasculature); and (6) ability to invade tissue and metastasize to other parts of the body (Hanahan & Weinberg, 2011). In addition to these six changes, persistent cancer-related inflammation appears to induce genetic instability leading to accumulation of genetic alterations in cancer cells, and this process has been proposed as the seventh hallmark of cancer (Colotta, Allavena, Sica, Garlanda, & Mantovani, 2009; Hanahan & Weinberg, 2011). This series of transformations results in a somatic cell that has enhanced ability to grow and replicate.

TUMORIGENESIS, ANGIOGENESIS, AND METASTASIS

After cells have been transformed and begin to proliferate, vascularization is required for growth and metastatic spread of the tumor (Folkman, 1990, 1995). The process of vascularization, known as *angiogenesis*, is normally under tight control of both positive and negative factors secreted by tumor and host cells (Folkman, 1990; Folkman & Klagsbrun, 1987). Molecules supporting angiogenesis include vascular endothelial growth factor (VEGF), interleukin-6 (IL-6), interleukin 8 (IL-8), and others. When tumors reach approximately 1–2 mm, an "angiogenic switch" is triggered; at this point activities of pro-angiogenic molecules start to predominate, and angiogenesis proceeds (Hanahan & Weinberg, 2011). Following vascularization, tumor cells secrete factors enabling them to more easily **invade** host tissues through the basement membrane and enter peripheral circulation (Fidler, 1997). The process of metastasis involves detachment of tumor cells from the basement membrane. Normally, cells that become detached from a basement membrane undergo apoptosis or programmed cell death, in a process known as *anoikis*. However, tumor cells are able to survive even when not attached to the cellular cytoskeleton, thus evading apoptosis, and then they travel through circulation and arrest in the capillary beds of specific organs, ultimately establishing a microenvironment at a new site (Fidler, 1997). In the next sections, we describe effects of biobehavioral factors and neuroendocrine modulation on these key processes of angiogenesis, invasion, and anoikis.

BIDIRECTIONAL SIGNALING IN THE TUMOR MICROENVIRONMENT

Many of the steps involved in tumorigenesis and metastasis involve bidirectional signaling interactions with surrounding cells of the microenvironment. Stromal cells (which make up the support structures of tissues) can be induced by tumor cells to secrete molecules supporting malignant transformation, proliferation, and angiogenesis (Coussens & Werb, 2002; Fidler, 1995a, 1995b; Hanahan & Weinberg, 2011; Langley & Fidler, 2007; Skobe & Fusenig, 1998; Szlosarek, Charles, & Balkwill, 2006). Increasing evidence has demonstrated that the local microenvironment is influenced by systemic factors, and that behavioral and neuroendocrine factors modulate tumor growth both directly and indirectly (Lutgendorf, Lamkin, Jennings, et al., 2008; Nilsson et al., 2007; Sood, Lutgendorf, & Cole, 2007; Sood et al., 2010; Sood et al., 2006; Sood et al., 2004; Thaker et al., 2006; Yang et al., 2009; Yang et al., 2006). Tumors are also able to induce changes in local as well as distant cells (Aaronson, 1991), including cells of the immune and central nervous systems (Darnell & Posner, 2006). Next, we address effects of behavioral and neuroendocrine factors in the "macroenvironment" on tumor growth, as well as effects of cancer on the systemic environment.

Biobehavioral Factors and Angiogenesis
CLINICAL FINDINGS

Women with ovarian carcinoma who reported higher levels of social support demonstrated lower levels of VEGF perisurgically, both in serum (Lutgendorf et al., 2002) and in tumor tissue (Lutgendorf, Lamkin, Jennings et al., 2008). Among 104 patients with colorectal cancer, higher levels of preoperative depression were associated with higher levels of serum VEGF, both pre-operatively and 6–8 weeks following surgery (Sharma, Greenman, Sharp, Walker, & Monson, 2008). Similarly, more pronounced expression of tumor VEGF was found among 51 patients with newly diagnosed colorectal tumors reporting high levels of loneliness compared to those who were more socially integrated (Nauseen et al., 2010). All these studies controlled for disease stage. Thus, a body of consistent clinical evidence is emerging, demonstrating associations of psychological distress such as depression and loneliness with measures of angiogenesis.

IL-6 is another pro-angiogenic factor (Nilsson, Langley, & Fidler, 2005) that additionally stimulates proliferation of tumor cells (Eustace et al., 1993; Obata, Tamakoshi, Shibata, Kikkawa, & Tomoda, 1997), enhances tumor-cell migration and attachment (Obata et al., 1997), promotes invasion of vascular endothelial cells by tumor (Kitamura, Morita, Nihel, Mishima, & Murota, 1997), and is associated with tumor progression (Berek et al., 1991; Chopra, Dinh, & Hannigan, 1998), shorter disease-free intervals, and poorer overall survival (Scambia et al., 1995). Moreover, IL-6 is responsive to psychosocial factors; it is known to increase with both acute (Zhou, Kusnecov, Shurin, dePaoli, & Rabin, 1993) and chronic stress (Kiecolt-Glaser et al., 2003; Lutgendorf et al., 1999), PTSD, and depression, and to decrease following successful treatment of depression (Dentino et al., 1999; Frommberger et al., 1997; Maes et al., 1999). In vitro, NE induces IL-6 mRNA and protein expression in ovarian cancer cells via a beta-adrenergic pathway (Nilsson et al., 2007). Clinically, women with advanced ovarian cancer who reported poorer perceived social support also were found to have higher levels of IL-6 both in plasma and in ascites, thus demonstrating links between a psychosocial factor and a pro-angiogenic cytokine in the vicinity of the tumor as well in the periphery (Costanzo et al., 2005). Moreover, ovarian cancer patients with higher levels of social isolation had higher levels of tumor NE (Lutgendorf, DeGeest, Dahmoush et al., 2010). These findings suggest a relationship between social support/isolation/loneliness as a measure of distress and important mediators of angiogenesis in the vicinity of the tumor.

NEUROENDOCRINE STRESS HORMONES AND ANGIOGENESIS

Animal and in vivo findings parallel data from the clinical models described earlier. Emerging data has demonstrated that neuroendocrine stress hormones such as NE, epinephrine (E), and the nonspecific beta adrenergic agonist isoproterenol can induce production of angiogenic molecules from a variety of tumor cells, including ovarian, nasopharyngeal, melanoma, and multiple myeloma cells (Lutgendorf et al., 2003; Park et al., 2010; Yang et al., 2009; Yang et al., 2006). Stimulation by catecholamines is effectively blocked by the nonspecific beta-blocker propranolol, and beta adrenergic receptors have been identified on the majority of ovarian cancer cell lines (Thaker et al., 2006) as well as on a variety of other cancer cell lines (Vandewalle, Revillion, & Lefebvre, 1990). Activation of beta adrenergic receptors is linked to accelerated tumor growth in cellular and animal models of breast cancer (Badino, Novelli, & Girardi, 1996; Marchetti, Spinola, Pelletier, & Labrie, 1991; Vandewalle et al., 1990). Extending these in vitro results to an orthotopic mouse model of ovarian cancer, chronic restraint stress resulted in greater tumor burden and a more invasive pattern of metastatic tumor growth with increases in VEGF, angiogenesis, and vascularization. These effects were completely blocked by propranolol, indicating a key role for beta-adrenergic signaling in these stress-induced effects on tumor progression. Moreover, the stress-induced tumor vasculature contained indications suggestive of a more immature vasculature, as compared to tumor vasculature in nonstressed controls (Thaker et al., 2006).

Neuroendocrine stress pathways have also been shown to directly activate angiogenesis-promoting molecules. One such molecule is signal transducer and activator of transcription factor-3 (STAT-3), a key intracellular transcription factor that activates downstream targets to promote tumor cell proliferation and inhibit apoptosis. STAT-3 is thus involved in many pathways supporting tumor progression and can be activated by a variety of cytokines such as VEGF and IL-6. Recent findings in an ovarian carcinoma model have shown that STAT-3 can be directly activated by stress hormones such as NE and E, independent of IL-6. This activation ultimately promotes transcription of genes associated with cell survival, angiogenesis, and cell growth (Landen et al., 2007). The direct activation of STAT-3 by catecholamines thus represents an independent direct pathway by which stress factors can promote tumor progression.

ENRICHED ENVIRONMENT, ANGIOGENESIS, AND TUMOR GROWTH

Cao and colleagues (2010) conducted a series of experiments to determine whether social and physical environments could impact tumor growth. Mice were placed in an enriched (including sensory, cognitive, motor, and social stimulation) versus standard housing environment; those in the enriched environment demonstrated blunted growth of syngeneic melanoma and colon tumors as well as inhibited growth of a spontaneous colon tumor. Serum obtained from "enriched" animals was able to suppress growth of established tumors in vitro as well. The enriched environment enhanced hypothalamic brain-derived neurotropic factor (BDNF), which in turn downregulated leptin production in adipocytes via beta-adrenergic pathways. Decreased leptin directly inhibited cellular proliferation as well as indirectly inhibited inflammation and angiogenesis (Cao et al., 2010). This model is intriguing because of the involvement of leptin in metabolic pathways related to adiposity, the known relationships of adiposity with inflammation and cancer, and the modulation of leptin production in the enriched environment. Possible translational implications of an "enriched" environment need to be explored.

Biobehavioral Effects on Migration, Invasion, and Metastases

As noted earlier, invasion and migration of tumor cells are key components of the metastatic cascade. Matrix metalloproteineases (MMPs) are enzymes that degrade extracellular matrix proteins and thus serve as key promoters of angiogenesis and invasion (Hagemann et al., 2004; Sood et al., 2004). Matrix metalloproteineases are produced by tumor cells, as well as by stromal cells such as macrophages. MMP-2 and -9 are particularly important in ovarian cancer, and have been associated with disease progression (Huang et al., 2002; Kamat et al., 2006; Torng, Mao, Chan, Huang, & Lin, 2004). Incubation with either NE or E induces significant increases in MMP-2 and MMP-9 production by ovarian cancer cells, a process that can be completely blocked by propranolol, indicating beta-adrenergic mediation (Sood et al., 2006). Similar catecholamine-induced MMP increases have been observed in colon and in head and neck cancers (Drell et al., 2003; Masur, Niggemann, Zanker, & Entschladen, 2001; Yang et al., 2002; Yang et al., 2006).

Neuroendocrine stress hormones have also demonstrated direct effects on the invasive potential of ovarian cancer cell lines using the membrane-invasion-culture system, which tests the ability of cells to invade across a collagen matrix. Levels of NE approximating those observed in the stress response increased the in vitro invasive potential of ovarian cancer cells by 89% to 198% in this setting. Similar increases in invasion were induced by E, although they were less pronounced. These catecholamine-induced effects could be completely blocked by either propranolol or by an MMP antagonist, CMT-3 (Sood et al., 2006). In other investigations, the beta agonist isoproterenol has been shown to enhance metastasis-promoting activities such as invasion and adhesion in ovarian cancer cells (Enserink et al., 2004; Rangarajan et al., 2003). Taken together, these findings demonstrate upregulation of the invasive capacity of ovarian cancer cells via β–adrenergic modulation of MMPs and other molecules such as integrins.

Whereas many MMPs are secreted by tumor cells, tumor associated macrophages (TAM) are the principal source of MMPs in ovarian cancer (Huang et al., 2002), and TAM may also be sensitive to stress-related behavioral factors. To examine this potential pathway, Lutgendorf and colleagues analyzed samples of ovarian tumor tissue for TAM and tumor cell expression of MMP-2 and -9. Among 56 women who completed presurgical behavioral assessments, those who reported higher levels of either depression or life stress showed higher levels of MMP-9 expression by TAM, whereas those with greater social support had lower levels of MMP-9 expression by TAM. In contrast, behavioral factors were not associated with MMP-2 expression (Lutgendorf, Lamkin, Jennings et al., 2008). A related in vitro experiment demonstrated that physiologic doses of both NE and cortisol significantly enhanced the production of MMP-9 from monocyte-derived human macrophages, providing further evidence for the ability of neuroendocrine stress hormones to act on macrophages to promote invasion (Lutgendorf, Lamkin, Jennings et al., 2008). In addition to their role in MMP production, TAM are a key source of pro-inflammatory and protumor molecules. This may be another pathway by which stress-related behavioral factors could influence tumor development.

STRESS MODULATION OF ANOIKIS

As mentioned earlier, anoikis is the normal process of cell death that occurs when cells are separated from the extracellular matrix. In the course of malignant transformation, cells develop resistance to anoikis, thereby enhancing their ability to migrate and metastasize to other sites. Recently, Sood and colleagues demonstrated that beta-adrenergic signaling inhibits anoikis through activation of focal adhesion kinase (FAK), a protein involved in cell migration and in regulating the tumor suppressor gene, p53. This ultimately promotes survival of ovarian cancer cells (Sood et al., 2010). This phenomenon was seen both in vitro and in an orthotopic mouse model of ovarian cancer. In this study, ovarian cancer patients reporting higher levels of depression demonstrated higher levels of activated FAK (pFAK^{Y397}) as compared to those who were less depressed, suggesting a greater potential for inhibition of anoikis in the depressed patients. Parallel findings were seen in patients with high versus low tumor NE. Additionally, pFAK^{Y397} was linked to poorer overall survival (Sood et al., 2010). Taken together, these findings suggest that depression- or stress-related modulation of this important protein may contribute to cancer cell survival during the process of metastasis.

Depression, Social Isolation and Patterns of Tumor Gene Activation

Genome-wide transcriptional analysis and promoter-based bioinformatics analyses have now been used to examine differential gene expression patterns of cancer patients according to their behavioral profiles. Lutgendorf and colleagues compared tumors from ovarian cancer patients with high depression and low social support (considered to be the "high risk" group) with tumors from patients with low levels of depression and high social support (deemed "low risk") after being matched for age, grade, stage, and tumor histology. Tumors from high-risk patients showed over 200 upregulated gene transcripts and increased activity of signaling pathways known to be involved in tumor growth and progression (e.g., CREB/ATF, NFKB/Rel, STAT, and ETS-family transcription factors) compared to profiles of low-risk patients. These findings suggest that biobehavioral processes may contribute to regulation of gene expression within solid tumors. Moreover, high-risk patients also showed increased levels of tumor NE (Lutgendorf et al., 2009), suggesting that beta-adrenergic transcription control pathways likely play a key mediating role in these effects. Similar relationships have been identified in animal models of breast cancer, in which social isolation has been related to upregulated mammary gland expression of several important metabolic genes implicated in human carcinogenesis, as well as to increased tumor growth (Williams et al., 2009). Thus, collectively, emerging evidence has shown stress and psychosocial factors to be associated with key elements of the metastatic cascade in vitro, animal and clinical models.

Summary

Findings reviewed in this section demonstrate that stress-response signaling directly induces many of the biological activities that support cancer growth, including angiogenesis, invasion, inhibition of anoikis, apoptosis, and metastases. Mechanisms illustrated in Figure 19.1. Many of these pathways operate simultaneously or work synergistically. Thus, it is reasonable to assume that effects of stress-response pathways are simultaneously occurring via multiple mechanisms to support tumor progression.

Biobehavioral Factors and the Cellular Immune Response in Cancer
The Cellular Immune Response in the Context of Cancer

The role of the immune response in the context of cancer includes immunosurveillance, lysis and destruction of tumor cells, and inflammation. Natural killer (NK) cells and cytotoxic T lymphocytes are two of the primary effector cells involved in the cellular immune response against tumors (Arreygue-Garcia et al., 2008; Smyth et al., 2005). NK cells can lyse tumor or virus-infected cells without prior sensitization, independent of major histocompatability complex (MHC) expression. Natural-killer-cell activation is based on signaling from a variety of stimulatory and inhibitory NK receptors that interact with specific tumor markers and are triggered by cytokines and other cellular signals (Moretta, Biassoni, Bottino, & Moretta, 2000). Natural-killer-cell activity has been associated with clinically significant endpoints including recurrence, treatment response, and progression-free survival in a number of cancers including breast, colorectal, head and neck, and cervical (Beano et al., 2008; Garner, Minton, James, & Hoffman, 1983; Ménard et al., 2009; Pillai, Balaram, Chidambaram, Padmanabhan, & Nair, 1990; Schantz & Goephert, 1987; Textor et al., 2008; Vaquer et al., 1990; Whiteside & Herberman, 1989).

Cytotoxic T lymphocytes (CTL) can recognize tumor cell antigens and target these cells for destruction by lysis (Goedegebuure et al., 1997; Melief & Kast, 1991). CTLs are the predominant effector T cell population involved in tumor surveillance and destruction in murine models (Hamaoka & Fujiwara, 1987; Melief, 1992), and are also known to be important in a variety of human malignancies (Heo, Whiteside, Kanbour, & Herberman, 1988; Ioannides, Freedman, Platsoucas, Rashed, & Kim, 1991). Extent of tumor infiltration of NK, CTL, or dendritic cells has been associated with length of survival for individuals with melanomas as well as cancers of the breast, ovary, bladder, colon, rectum, and prostate (Dunn, Bruce, Ikeda, Old, & Schreiber, 2002). Higher CTL counts have further been associated with longer survival and better performance status among women with metastatic or recurrent breast cancer (Blake-Mortimer, Sephton, Carlson, Stites, & Spiegel, 2004).

Tumors are composed of cells with differing phenotypes that may have heterogeneous morphology, surface antigens, hormone receptors, chemotherapy sensitivity, and metastatic potential (Fidler, 1997). These characteristics influence the ability of immune cells to detect and lyse particular tumor cells—a quality known as *immunogenic potential*. Tumor cells with high immunogenic potential can be readily recognized and destroyed by the immune system, whereas cells with low immunogenic potential may go unrecognized by the immune system. Eradication of more highly immunogenic cells by the immune system actually selects for tumor cells that are resistant to destruction by the immune system, a process known as *immunoselection*. Thus, surviving tumor cells acquire the ability to escape immunosurveillance, a process known as *"immune escape"* (Khong & Restifo, 2002). Tumors often downregulate tumor-associated antigens and Class I major histocompatibility complex (MHC I), thus evading T cell recognition (Garcia-Lora, Algarra, & Garrido, 2003). Tumor cells can also interfere with co-stimulatory signaling, a process that makes it difficult for T-cells and other lymphocytes to eliminate tumor cells (Kowalczyk, 2002; Matzinger, 1994). In addition, tumor cells and other cells in the tumor microenvironment produce an inflammatory milieu that can suppress antitumor physiological responses (Coussens & Werb, 2002).

Stress-Related Immunosuppression Model

Although several biobehavioral pathways linked to tumor progression have now been characterized, as reviewed earlier, links between psychosocial factors and clinical outcomes have been historically thought to be mediated by stress-induced compromise of the cellular immune response (Irwin, 2002; Kiecolt-Glaser et al., 1987; Reiche, Nunes, & Morimoto, 2004; Zorrilla, Luborsky, & McKay, 2001). These relationships were thought to be mediated in large part via adrenergic and glucocorticoid signaling pathways. The underlying assumption of the immunosuppression model is that stress or negative emotions can modulate cancer initiation and development by suppressing elements of the immune response important in tumor surveillance and containment (Andersen et al., 1994; Antoni

et al., 2006; Heffner, Loving, Robles, & Kiecolt-Glaser, 2003; Kiecolt-Glaser, Robles, Heffner, Loving, & Glaser, 2002; Reiche et al., 2004).

PRECLINICAL STUDIES

In animal models, chronic stress, as well as significant but briefer stress (e.g., surgical stress), can promote tumor progression by suppressing cytotoxic activities of T and NK cells, shifting from a Th1 to a Th2 cytokine response, blunting antigen presentation, and enhancing activities of regulatory T-cells (Ben-Eliyahu, Page, Yimira, & Shakhar, 1999; Ben-Eliyahu, Yirmiya, Liebeskind, Taylor, & Gale, 1991; Greenfeld et al., 2007; Saul et al., 2005; Lee et al., 2009). A series of studies by Ben-Eliyahu and colleagues demonstrated that stress-induced release of catecholamines and prostaglandins during the perisurgical period can suppress NK cell activity and other components of the cellular immune response, and this suppression can enhance tumor development and metastasis (Ben-Eliyahu, 2003; Ben-Eliyahu et al., 1999; Ben-Eliyahu, Shakhar, Page, Stefanski, & Shakhar, 2000; Ben-Eliyahu et al., 1991; Page & Ben-Eliyahu, 1999). Natural killer cell activity and NK cell expression of Fas ligand and CD11a were particularly diminished by surgical stress, and corticosterone levels were increased. These effects appear to be mediated by beta-adrenergic processes and can be reversed by combined administration of a beta-adrenergic antagonist and a cyclooxygenase-2 inhibitor (Benish et al., 2008; Glasner et al., 2010). This peri-operative cocktail has been successful in improving survival rates in two models of spontaneous metastasis after surgery in mice (Lewis lung carcinoma or B16F10.9 melanoma) (Glasner et al., 2010). Surgical stress has also been shown to increase angiogenesis and tumor growth in an orthotopic model of ovarian cancer. These effects were blocked by propranolol and were not observed in mice lacking the B-adrenergic receptor (Lee et al., 2009). For a more thorough history of PNI animal models in cancer, readers are referred to a recent review paper (Ben-Eliyahu, Page, & Schleifer, 2007).

CLINICAL STUDIES

The immunosuppression model has been examined in a number of studies of early-stage breast cancer patients. An early series of studies documented that women with breast cancer who felt supported by their partner or physician had greater NK cell activity than women who felt less supported. In contrast, patients reporting more fatigue and depressive symptoms had lower NK cell activity (Levy, Herberman, Lippman, & d'Angelo, 1987; Levy, Heberman, Maluish, Schlein, & Lippman, 1985; Levy, Heberman, Lee, et al., 1990; Levy, Heberman, Whiteside, et al., 1990). The studies accounted for known prognostic factors, and results were replicated at multiple time-points and in more than one patient sample. Psychosocial factors were also associated with time to recurrence; however, NK cell activity was not found to mediate the links between psychosocial factors and recurrence (Levy, Herberman, Lippman, D'Angelo, & Lee, 1991).

Andersen and colleagues have now extended this work in a large sample of breast cancer patients participating in a psychosocial intervention trial. Following breast cancer surgery, women reporting greater distress showed a diminished cellular immune response across a variety of measures including lower NK cell activity, poorer response of NK cells to recombinant IFNγ, and a decreased lymphoproliferative response (Andersen et al., 1998). In a follow-up study of a small subset of these patients (n = 17), women who both reported high levels of stress and had low NK cell cytotoxicity also showed alterations in the expression of both inhibitory (CD158b) and activating (CD94) NK cell receptors (Varker et al., 2007). Among those women who were subsequently randomized to the control group of the intervention trial, the pattern of cellular immune changes during the months following surgery paralleled changes in distress (Thornton, Andersen, Crespin, & Carson, 2007). Specifically, women who showed an early decline in their level of perceived stress also had the most rapid recovery of NK cell activity postsurgery.

The psychosocial intervention conducted by Anderson and colleagues was provided in a supportive group format and targeted coping skills, stress management, health practices, and adherence to treatment, and appeared to have a protective effect on immune functioning. T-cell proliferative responses remained stable or increased during the 4-month intervention period for participants randomized to the intervention, and they declined during the same time frame for women in the control group. This effect was maintained at the 12-month follow-up (Andersen et al., 2007; Andersen et al., 2004). Women who reported clinically significant depressive symptoms were especially likely to benefit (Thornton, Andersen, Schuler, & Carson, 2009). The intervention also improved clinical outcomes. In addition to initial benefits in performance status, functional status, and overall health

status (Andersen et al., 2007), women randomized to the psychosocial intervention showed a reduced risk of breast cancer recurrence and mortality after a median of 11 years of follow-up (Andersen et al., 2008). Furthermore, of the patients who did experience a recurrence, those who had participated in the intervention group showed improved survival, enhanced mood, and improved immune function following the recurrence (Andersen et al., 2010).

Other psychosocial interventions have shown similar protective effects on cellular immunity. For example, breast cancer patients randomized to a 10-session group cognitive-behavioral stress management program showed better lymphoproliferative responses at 3-months, more robust Th1 responses at 6-months, and reduced cortisol over a 12-month follow-up period (Antoni et al., 2009; McGregor et al., 2004; Phillips et al., 2008). A full discussion of psychosocial interventions and cancer is treated in another chapter of this book.

Other recent studies provide further evidence for links between psychosocial factors and alteration of markers of cellular immunity, including NK cell count and activity, lymphoproliferative responses, and B and T cell subsets in breast cancer patients (e.g. Blomberg et al., 2009; Garland et al., 2004; McGregor et al., 2004; Tjemsland, Soreide, Matre, & Malt, 1997; Von Ah, Kang, & Carpenter, 2007). For example, Von Ah and colleagues reported findings that perceived stress was associated with lower NK cell activity and lower IFNγ among breast cancer patients (Von Ah et al., 2007). Similar relationships have also been found among patients with other cancers, including gynecologic, prostate, gastrointestinal, digestive, and liver malignancies (Dunigan, Carr, & Steel, 2007; Lutgendorf et al., 2005; Nan et al., 2004; Penedo et al., 2006; Zhou et al., 2005). For example, Chinese patients with digestive tract cancers who were depressed also had lower lymphocyte and CD56 counts than nondepressed patients, although there was no difference between groups in the CD4:CD8 ratio (Nan et al., 2004).

PROTECTIVE PSYCHOSOCIAL FACTORS

Most research has focused on markers of stress and maladjustment and downregulation of cellular immunity. However, there has been growing attention to processes of resilience that may optimize immune function. For example, in a study of ovarian cancer patients, psychosocial resilience factors such as positive reframing, social support, and positive affect were related to a higher percentage of

NKT cells (a cell subset known to have antitumor activity); however, these positive factors were not associated with NK or T cell percentages or counts (Lamkin et al., 2008). Similarly, positive affect was associated with more robust Th1 cytokine responses (greater IL-12 and IFNγ levels) to stimulation of peripheral mononuclear cells in a group of 134 women who had recently completed breast cancer surgery. In contrast, anxiety was associated with a poorer Th1 response (lower IL-2) (Blomberg et al., 2009). There is evidence that patients who perceive some benefit or find meaning in their illness may have better outcomes. Specifically, women with early-stage breast cancer who were able to find benefit in their experience had a stronger lymphoproliferative response (McGregor et al., 2004). Similarly, patients with hepatocellular carcinoma who scored above the median on a measure of psychological growth showed higher lymphocyte and white blood cell counts both pre- and postchemotherapy (Dunigan et al., 2007). An optimistic outlook also appears to have a positive influence. Among newly diagnosed breast cancer patients, distressed women reporting greater optimism demonstrated better NK cell cytotoxicity than distressed women with low optimism (Von Ah et al., 2007). Similarly, men with localized prostate cancer who were more optimistic and were able to express anger in an adaptive way also showed better NK cell cytotoxicity (Penedo et al., 2006). Continued attention to these directions will be helpful in identifying profiles of resilient cancer patients.

IMMUNE MARKERS IN THE TUMOR MICROENVIRONMENT

Whereas most PNI and cancer research has focused on immune cells and cytokines in peripheral circulation, recent research among ovarian cancer patients has examined cellular immune functioning in the vicinity of the tumor. These studies address the question of whether relationships between psychosocial factors and the immune response exist in the tumor microenvironment. In this work, NK and T cells were derived from tumor-infiltrating lymphocytes (TIL). Psychological distress was associated with poorer NK cell activity and lower TH_1/TH_2 cell ratios both in circulation and in TIL. Conversely, social support was associated with greater NK cell activity in TIL (Lutgendorf Lamkin, DeGeest, et al., 2008; Lutgendorf et al., 2005). These findings indicate that relationships between psychosocial factors and immune cells are

present in the tumor microenvironment, suggesting that even though immune cells are downregulated in the tumor microenvironment, they may still respond more or less optimally depending on the neuroendocrine milieu and mediating psychosocial factors. Interpretation of these results is limited by the fact that functional immune assays were, of necessity, done in vitro, and the immune response to standardized target cells may not fully represent their function within the patient.

Biobehavioral Factors and Inflammation in the Context of Cancer
Inflammation and Cancer: The Role of Macrophages

Many epithelial cancers, including ovarian cancer, are characterized by underlying inflammation, which functions as a tumor initiator and promoter (Szlosarek et al., 2006). Inflammation in the tumor microenvironment is mediated by tumor cells, as well as by stromal and immune cells, particularly macrophages. Tumor associated macrophages (TAM) comprise a large part of most tumor microenvironments (Balkwill & Mantovani, 2001). Tumor-derived chemotactic factors recruit blood monocytes to the tumor, where they differentiate to macrophages and migrate to hypoxic regions. Macrophages were classically thought of as cells that attack tumor cells and promote an antitumor cellular immune response (Pollard, 2004). However, a proinflammatory tumor microenvironment can induce macrophages to switch from a more phagocytic phenotype to a tumor-promoting phenotype (Pollard, 2004; Sica, Schioppa, Mantovani, & Allavena, 2006). Growth-promoting TAM support tumor development in a number of ways, including contributing to the angiogenic switch; directly stimulating proliferation of tumor cells, invasion, and metastases; supporting degradation and remodeling of the surrounding cellular architecture (Huang et al., 2002; Pollard, 2004); and downregulating the adaptive immune response (Hagemann et al., 2004; Huang et al., 2002; Pollard, 2004; Sica, Allavena, & Mantovani, 2008). TAM recruitment is thought to be a requirement for metastatic growth (Nowicki et al., 1996), and presence of TAM is associated with poor clinical outcomes (An et al., 1987; Balkwill, Charles, & Mantovani, 2005; Bingle, Brown, & Lewis, 2002; Tsutsui et al., 2005). Moreover, TAM suppress the adaptive immune response by increasing production of immunosuppressive cytokines, including IL-10 and TGFβ, and suppress production of immunostimulatory cytokines such as IL-12. TAM also produce VEGF and IL-6; downregulate dendritic cells; suppress antigen presentation; inhibit T cell proliferation (Mantovani, Sozzani, Locati, Allavena, & Sica, 2002); and produce chemokines that attract naïve T cell subsets, Th2 cells, and T-regulatory cells (Sica et al., 2008). The net result is anergy and cellular immune suppression, accompanied by conditions that favor tumor promotion.

Behavioral and Neuroendocrine Modulation of Macrophage Activation

Both alpha (Szelenyi, Kiss, Puskas, Szelenyi, & Vizi, 2000) and beta-adrenergic receptors (Van Miert, 2002) have been observed on macrophages. Catecholamines are known to stimulate macrophage production of pro-inflammatory cytokines such as IL-1β and TNFα (Black, 2002; Elenkov & Chrousos, 2002). As noted earlier, Lutgendorf and colleagues have observed that both NE and cortisol enhance MMP-9 production by human monocyte-derived macrophages (Lutgendorf, Lamkin, Jennings, et al., 2008). Moreover, a variety of negative psychosocial factors, including chronic stress, depression, and social isolation are associated with TAM production of MMP-9 (Lutgendorf, Lamkin, Jennings, et al., 2008). These findings suggest that psychosocial factors, via effects on TAM, are able to modulate the tumor microenvironment to supports invasion and tumor progression. Continuing research is investigating the effects of psychosocial factors on TAM.

Sloan and colleagues (2010) examined effects of stress on macrophage-induced tumor growth in an animal model of mammary cancer. Whereas stress-induced neuroendocrine activation had a minimal effect on progression of the primary tumor, it induced a marked (30-fold) enhancement of metastatic spread to distant sites. These effects were mediated by beta-adrenergic stimulation of macrophage infiltration into the tumor microenvironment, where macrophages differentiated into an M-2 (tumor-promoting) phenotype with prometastatic characteristics. Both beta-adrenergic blockers and suppressors of macrophage stimulation abrogated these effects, suggesting that beta-adrenergic stimulation of macrophages is a key component in these metastatic processes.

In sum, these findings demonstrate that macrophages, along with other immune cells and malignant cells are sensitive to neuroendocrine stress hormones, with resultant effects promoting inflammation, tumor growth, and decreasing immunocompetence.

Bidirectional Pathways: Effects of Tumor-Derived Inflammation on Sickness Behaviors and Neuroendocrine Function
Behavioral Effects of Inflammation

Thus far, we have focused on how behavioral factors can modulate inflammatory processes relevant to cancer control. However, it is also known that substantial concentrations of peripheral pro-inflammatory cytokines are produced by certain tumors and by cancer treatment (Herskind, Bamberg, & Rodemann, 1998; Rodemann & Bamberg, 1995; Scambia et al., 1995; Tempfer, Zeisler, Sliutz, Haeusler, & Kainz, 1997). These cytokines can cross into the central nervous system (CNS) by pathways including the vagus nerve and other routes, and evoke a syndrome of behavioral and affective responses known as "sickness behaviors" (Maier & Watkins, 1998; Raison, Capuron, & Miller, 2006; Raison & Miller, 2003). Cardinal sickness-behavior symptoms mimic flu-like vegetative symptoms and include depressed mood, fatigue, anorexia, impaired concentration, sleep disturbance, enhanced pain sensitivity, and reduced activity (Capuron & Dantzer, 2003; Maier & Watkins, 1998; Miller et al., 2008).

As noted earlier, elevated levels of depression have been seen in cancer patients (Massie, 2004; Spoletini et al., 2008), and associations between elevated pro-inflammatory cytokines and depression have been documented in cancer patients (Jehn et al., 2006; Lutgendorf, Weinrib, et al., 2008; Musselman et al., 2001; Rich et al., 2005; Weinrib et al., 2010). The high prevalence of depression among cancer patients has been generally thought to be a reaction to the stress of receiving potentially life-threatening diagnoses and cancer treatment (Spiegel & Giese-Davis, 2003). However, inflammation arising secondary to treatment or tumor growth may also contribute to the pathogenesis of depression, as well as to debilitating fatigue in cancer patients (Lutgendorf, Weinrib, et al., 2008; Musselman et al., 2001; Bower, Ganz, Aziz, & Fahey, 2002; Bower et al., 2005; Collado-Hidalgo, Bower, Ganz, Cole, & Irwin, 2006). For example, elevated levels of plasma IL-6 have been found in depressed cancer patients compared to nondepressed cancer patients and healthy controls (Musselman et al., 2001). Similarly, among ovarian cancer patients, higher levels of vegetative symptoms of depression were related to elevated IL-6 in both plasma and ascites; however, affective symptoms of depression were not related to IL-6 (Lutgendorf, Weinrib, et al., 2008). There is a substantial literature regarding associations between inflammation and fatigue in cancer patients, which is covered in another chapter in this volume. Taken together, these results suggest the possibility that elevated levels of tumor- and inflammation-derived IL-6 contribute to the development of "sickness behaviors" that correspond with indicators of vegetative depression.

PRECLINICAL MODELS

The potential contribution of tumor-derived cytokines to sickness behaviors has been further explicated in animal models, with two studies documenting that depressive behaviors can be induced by the presence of tumors. Pyter and colleagues found that rats with N-nitroso-N-methylurea (NMU)-induced mammary tumors had elevated levels of pro-inflammatory cytokines in mammary tissue (IL-1β) and in the hippocampus (IL-1β, IL-6, TNFα) as compared to controls. Elevations in the anti-inflammatory cytokine IL-10 were also seen in the hippocampus. As compared to non-tumor-bearing controls, these animals demonstrated higher levels of depression-like behaviors including more time floating in the Porsolt forced-swim test, a greater number of floating episodes, and less ingestion of a sucrose solution. Tumor-bearing animals also showed greater burying behaviors (an indicator of obsessive-compulsive anxiety-like behavior). The depression-like behaviors were not observed in NMU-treated animals before the development of tumors, and were not seen before NMU treatment, indicating that the development of tumors was necessary for the expression of these depression-like behaviors. Moreover, blunted corticosterone responses to stress were noted, suggesting a potential breakdown in the negative feedback regulation of cytokine signaling by the HPA axis following tumor development, resulting in an impaired ability to control inflammation in tumor- bearing animals (Pyter, Pineros, Glalang, McClintock, & Prendergast, 2010).

Lamkin and colleagues, using a syngeneic ID8 ovarian cancer model in C57BL/6 mice, found that presence of tumor enhanced depressive-like behaviors including inhibition of sucrose consumption and reduced locomotion while increasing inflammatory cytokines (Lamkin et al., 2011). These two studies provide experimental evidence that presence of tumor can cause depressive-like behavior in animals. Together with the clinical

data, these findings provide emerging support for the hypothesis that tumor-induced inflammation may underlie some of the depression reported by cancer patients.

Neuroendocrine Dysregulation in Cancer

Profound disturbances in circadian rhythms in endocrine hormones such as cortisol have been observed in tumor-bearing animals as well as in human cancer patients (Sephton & Spiegel, 2003; Touitou, Bogdan, Levi, Benavides, & Auzeby, 1996). For example, ovarian cancer patients have shown marked disruption of cortisol rhythms, including erratic peaks and troughs, flattened diurnal slopes, and overall high levels over a 24-hour period (Touitou et al., 1996). Weinrib and colleagues (2010) also documented elevations in nocturnal cortisol among women with ovarian cancer as compared to women with benign gynecologic disease and healthy controls (Weinrib et al., 2010). Similarly, metastatic breast cancer patients have been shown to have flatter diurnal cortisol profiles than healthy women (Abercrombie et al., 2004).

This dysregulation of the diurnal rhythm of the HPA axis may be secondary to tumor-induced inflammation. IL-6 and other pro-inflammatory cytokines (such as IL-1 and TNF-α), acting independently or synergistically, have such potent effects on the HPA axis that they have been collectively called "tissue corticotrophin-releasing factor" (Chrousos, 1995). It is known that chronic stress impairs the negative-feedback system of the HPA axis, leading to chronically elevated cortisol, particularly at night when negative feedback is thought to be at its height (Sapolsky, Alberts, & Altmann, 1997). In a similar fashion, it has been hypothesized that the tumor-induced inflammatory cascade may stimulate the HPA axis to such an extent that its regulatory mechanisms cannot contain cortisol levels within normal limits, and negative feedback may be disrupted (Weinrib et al., 2010). Lutgendorf and colleagues have reported high correlations between IL-6 and nocturnal cortisol, rather than the inverse relationship that one would expect in a functional, well-regulated feedback loop (Lutgendorf, Weinrib, et al., 2008).

BIOBEHAVIORAL CORRELATES OF NEUROENDOCRINE DYSREGULATION

Among ovarian cancer patients, higher levels of nocturnal cortisol and lower cortisol variability were related to fatigue, disability, and vegetative depression (Weinrib et al., 2010). In a similar fashion, among breast cancer survivors, alterations in the diurnal cortisol rhythm, particularly flattening of the diurnal slope, have been associated with poorer performance status, greater functional disability (Sephton & Spiegel, 2003; Touitou et al., 1995), and greater fatigue, with the highest fatigue seen in survivors with the flattest cortisol slopes (Bower et al., 2005). The association between cortisol dysregulation and fatigue may be understood in light of the fact that one of the main functions of cortisol in the body is energy production and regulation (Maier & Watkins, 1998).

It is also possible that disrupted cortisol dynamics may contribute to depression in cancer patients. Depression has been linked with hypercortisolemia, downregulation of cortisol receptors, and dysregulation of the HPA axis (Raison & Miller, 2003) Individuals with diseases of the adrenal gland that lead to greater cortisol secretion are vulnerable to depression at higher rates than the general population (Fava, Sonino, & Morphy, 1987). Thus, the elevations in nocturnal cortisol may directly lead to depression in cancer patients, independent of effects on inflammatory cytokines. Consistent with this interpretation are data from patients with renal cell cancer and metastatic melanoma indicating that higher cortisol levels at the start of cancer treatment predict greater distress two months later (Cohen, de Moor, Devine, Baum, & Amato, 2001).

STRESS AND NEUROENDOCRINE DYSREGULATION

Whereas stress is often implicated in dysregulation of diurnal cortisol in healthy adults, investigations of stress and diurnal cortisol in cancer patients have yielded inconsistent findings (Sephton & Spiegel, 2003). Links between diurnal cortisol alterations and depression, social support, and repressive coping style have been reported (Giese-Davis, Sephton, Abercrombie, Duran, & Spiegel, 2004; Jehn et al., 2006; Turner-Cobb, Sephton, Koopman, Blake-Mortimer, & Spiegel, 2000). However, Weinrib and colleagues (2010) found no association of life stress with cortisol levels among ovarian cancer patients, although greater overall depression as well as vegetative depression were related to blunted cortisol variability. Similarly, no association between cortisol slope and stress was observed among breast cancer patients, whereas, in healthy women, flatter cortisol slope was associated with greater perceived stress (Abercrombie et al., 2004). In a sample of 99 metastatic breast cancer patients, flatter diurnal cortisol slopes were significantly associated with escape

from dexamethasone suppression; however, there was no evidence of an association between cortisol slope and acute stress reactivity. The authors of this study suggested that the flattening of cortisol slopes among cancer patients may be more related to disrupted inhibition of feedback to the HPA axis rather than to hypersensitivity of cancer patients to stress (Spiegel, Giese-Davis, Taylor, & Kraemer, 2006). It is possible that among cancer patients, inflammation-driven dynamics of the HPA axis may interact differently with the stress response than in healthy individuals.

NEUROENDOCRINE DYSREGULATION AND TUMOR GROWTH

Elevated glucocorticoid levels have been directly related to tumor growth. Glucocorticoids directly enhance a survival pathway and inhibit apoptosis (Moran, Gray, Mikosz, & Conzen, 2000); downregulate expression of DNA repair genes, including BRCA1 (Antonova & Mueller, 2008); and decrease paclitaxel chemotherapy-induced apoptosis in vitro (Pang, Kocherginsky, Krausz, Kim, & Conzen, 2006). Glucocorticoids are known to inhibit the cellular immune response (Gatti et al., 1987; Holbrook et al., 1983). Advanced breast cancer patients with higher mean diurnal cortisol demonstrate suppressed cellular immunity to a number of antigens (Sephton et al., 2009). Collectively, these studies suggest that disruptions of diurnal cortisol rhythms and feedback systems may have profound implications for tumor growth, response to treatment, immunosurveillance, and ultimately for survival. Moreover, a flatter diurnal cortisol slope has been linked to poorer survival among women with metastatic breast cancer (Sephton, Sapolsky, Kraemer, & Speigel, 2000).

Conclusions and Future Directions

Converging evidence from clinical, animal, and in vitro models now supports the presence of both direct and indirect links between psychosocial risk factors, related neuroendocrine hormones, and a number of mechanisms that promote cancer growth, modulate immunocompetence, or both. Stress-related factors have been related to impairment of the cellular immune response and upregulation of pathways supporting inflammation, angiogenesis, invasion, and metastases. In some cases, stress may induce various pathways simultaneously. For example, stress can promote tumor angiogenesis via stimulation of VEGF, which itself is capable of downregulating antigen presentation by dendritic cells. Stress effects on TAM support angiogenesis and invasion while increasing the production of IL-10 and downregulating the cellular immune response (Sica et al., 2008). Protective psychosocial factors such as social support can attenuate these effects or even enhance immunocompetence in a cancer setting, and they have also been related to lower levels of pro-angiogenic molecules such as VEGF or IL-6 in systemic circulation and/or in the vicinity of the tumor. These findings suggest that treatments targeting stress-related behavioral factors may modulate physiological pathways relevant to tumor progression.

Translating the findings reviewed here into effective and clinically relevant therapeutic interventions will require continuing research focusing on physiological markers relevant to the clinical population in question, attention to psychosocial profiles likely to influence physiological pathways relevant to cancer control, identification of subsets of patients who are most sensitive to biobehavioral influences, and clarification of the clinical significance of these PNI relationships. Most prior research has focused on women with breast cancer and, more recently, women with ovarian cancer. It will be important to determine whether the biobehavioral relationships documented in these populations are relevant to other cancer sites.

Examination of Clinically Relevant Physiological Pathways

As reviewed in this chapter, biobehavioral research initially focused on the investigation of immune-cell subsets thought to be relevant to immunosurveillance and tumor containment. It is well known that cancers are heterogeneous in their physiology, course, prognosis, and treatment approach. Taking this diversity into account by tailoring the selection of biomarkers to those that delineate pathophysiological processes most relevant to the population in question will be critical in continuing to move the field forward. For example, a focus on biobehavioral mechanisms relevant to viral containment would be highly relevant to HPV-associated cervical cancers that are often identified prior to malignant transformation, whereas a focus on psychosocial influences on angiogenesis is of greater relevance to carcinomas typically diagnosed in later stages, such as ovarian cancer. Examination of how psychosocial factors interact with specific tumor biomarkers and receptors will be important in clarifying these relationships. For example, do neuroendocrine hormones interact differently with Her2neu+ versus

Her2neu- or estrogen receptor positive (ER+) vs. ER- breast cancers? In a recent report of a psychosocial intervention in breast cancer, beneficial effects of the intervention were noted in ER- patients, but not in ER+ patients (Spiegel et al., 2007).

Studies of how biobehavioral factors interact with the efficacy of medical treatments such as cancer vaccines (e.g., the HPV vaccine), chemotherapy, hematopoietic stem-cell transplantation, or monoclonal antibodies are also critical. For example, in breast cancer patients treated with trastuzamab (a drug that blocks the Her2neu receptor), NK cell activity was related to progression-free survival (Beano et al., 2008), but the extent to which psychosocial factors might affect NK activity in this context is an empirical question.

Translational Applications: Hematopoietic Stem-Cell Transplantation and Immunotherapy

The setting of hematopoietic stem-cell transplantation (HSCT) provides an illustrative example of some of the issues already described. HSCT is a potentially curative but rigorous therapy with a significant risk of morbidity and mortality. Patients with hematologic malignancies undergoing this treatment frequently experience physical and psychological sequelae that impair their quality of life and undermine recovery. In addition, 40–70% of patients relapse following autologous stem-cell transplantation (Porrata, Litzow, & Markovic, 2001), and graft-versus-host disease is a common and potentially lethal complication of allogeneic transplantation and a cause of significant long-term disability. Thus, it is not surprising that many patients report significant emotional distress (Neitzert et al., 1998).

Depressed mood and low levels of hope prior to HSCT have predicted poorer survival posttransplant (Colon et al., 1991; Hoodin, Kalbfleisch, Thornton, & Ratanatharathorn, 2004; Molassiotis et al., 1997; Rodrigue et al., 1999). Psychosocial effects on cellular immune responses important to the control of hematologic malignancies and transplant complications could play a critical mediating role in this setting. Specifically, immune reconstitution following transplant is directly associated with reduced relapse risk and overall and progression-free survival (Auletta & Lazarus, 2005; Peggs & Mackinnon, 2004; Porrata et al., 2001; Porrata & Markovic, 2004). In addition to the potential effects on residual disease, recovery of immune competence is also critical for minimizing tissue damage and providing protection against bacterial and viral pathogens

(Auletta & Lazarus, 2005). Psychosocial-immune interactions may be of particular significance for HSCT patients because any modulatory influence on immune processes could have a salient effect on relapse and survival.

Adoptive immunotherapy is another novel cancer treatment involving cultivation of the patient's leukocytes with IL-2 to expand a population of lymphokine-activated killer (LAK) cells known to have antitumor activity. This treatment has been employed in melanoma and renal-cell carcinoma, as well as after HSCT to boost activity against minimal residual disease (MRD). The central role of the cellular immune response in the success of both HSCT and adoptive immunotherapy provides an opportunity to examine how biobehavioral factors influence treatment outcomes.

Preliminary data indicate that psychosocial factors can indeed affect the immune recovery following HSCT. In an initial study, a slower recovery of white blood cell count (WBC) posttransplant was found among transplant recipients reporting higher levels of depression prior to transplant, as well as for those with distress scores that were either very high or very low (McGregor, Langer, & Syrjala, 2005). Similarly, patients reporting higher levels of posttraumatic growth at the time of transplant had a better lymphocyte recovery during the first six months posttransplant (Costanzo, Juckett, Coe, Nelson, & Bourne, 2010). Ongoing research is exploring the extent to which stress-related psychosocial factors are associated with the reconstitution of specific leukocyte subpopulations as well as the impact of these relationships on the clinical course posttransplant.

Identifying At-Risk Patient Populations

Emotional distress, including depressed and anxious mood, are normative responses in the face of a cancer diagnosis and treatment. Attempting to prevent a normal emotional response, especially when acute or already appropriately managed by a patient, may be neither realistic nor adaptive. Moreover, these types of responses may be less likely to be relevant physiologically than more severe or chronic psychological symptoms or maladaptive coping patterns. Consistent with this idea, we have reviewed evidence suggesting that chronically depressed patients were at risk for poorer clinical outcomes, whereas those who developed acute depression following diagnosis were at no greater risk (Stommel et al., 2002). It is also likely that combinations of psychosocial factors are key to identifying vulnerable individuals. A number of studies reviewed in this chapter suggest that the effects of stress on immune functioning and cancer outcomes are stronger for patients who also lack social support or have low levels of optimism (Michael et al., 2009; Price et al., 2001; Von Ah et al., 2007), as well as for those who avoid or suppress their emotions (Epping-Jordan et al., 1994; Lehto et al., 2006; Reynolds et al., 2000; Weihs et al., 2000). Finally, as discussed earlier, there has also been growing attention to positive psychosocial factors that may confer resilience, such as the ability to find meaning or some benefit in one's cancer experience. Emerging data suggest the importance of attending to these influences to gain a fuller picture of patients likely to be vulnerable versus resilient (Dunigan et al., 2007; McGregor et al., 2004; Penedo et al., 2006).

Focusing on populations with psychosocial or disease profiles that confer greater vulnerability to the effects of stress-related behavioral factors is likely to yield the most clinically meaningful results. Psychosocial interventions may be more likely to have a salubrious physiological effect for individuals most at risk. For example, Andersen and colleagues recently tested an intervention combining biobehavioral and cognitive behavioral elements among cancer survivors (largely breast and gynecologic patients) diagnosed with major depressive disorder. The intervention was individually administered. Those who received the intervention showed significant improvements in depressive symptoms, fatigue, and quality of life, and clinical remission of the depression in 19 of 21 study completers (Brothers, Yang, Strunk, & Andersen, 2011). Although effects on physiology were not reported in this study, another study from the same group reported reduced markers of inflammation following a psychosocial intervention, particularly among the subset of early-stage breast cancer patient participants with clinically significant symptoms of depression (Thornton et al., 2009). These studies illustrate the relevance of directing interventions toward at-risk populations.

With respect to the disease context, hormone-sensitive cancers, such as prostate and endometrial cancer, are good targets to consider. Although most prior work has focused on solid tumors, malignancies arising from the bone marrow and lymphatic systems including leukemias, lymphomas, and myelomas are also likely to be sensitive to the types of effects reviewed in this chapter, because the bone marrow and other organs of the lymph system are innervated by SNS fibers. Future work might also take advantages of advances in genomics to identify risk conferring polymorphisms. Specific polymorphisms have been identified that may lead to greater likelihood of inflammation and fatigue in breast cancer survivors (Collado-Hidalgo, Bower, Ganz, Irwin, & Cole, 2008). It may be that individuals with polymorphisms that confer greater sensitivity to stress, such as those with alterations of the serotonin transporter gene (Caspi, Hariri, Holmes, Uher, & Moffitt, 2010; Way & Taylor, 2010), may be more susceptible to stress-related physiological changes promoting tumor growth.

Sensitive Periods for Biobehavioral Influences

Focusing on periods during the disease and treatment trajectory that may be most sensitive to biobehavioral influences is likely to yield the most meaningful effects. Psychosocial factors may be most likely to influence immune functioning in a clinically significant way early in the development of the tumor, rather than after the tumor is well-established, and sophisticated tumor escape mechanisms have developed. The peri-operative period has been proposed to be another critical time period due to the simultaneous occurrence of several risk factors for progression and metastasis, including changes in the balance between pro- and anti-angiogenic factors, secretion of growth factors, shedding of tumor cells, and suppression of cellular immunity (Ben-Eliyahu, 2003; Ben-Eliyahu et al., 2007; Shakhar & Ben-Eliyahu, 2003). During recovery from surgery, as well as from adjuvant therapy, a small number of circulating cancer cells termed minimal residual disease (MRD) can remain and cause disease recurrence. Following immunosuppressive treatment, the immune system must recover sufficiently to both recognize and destroy remaining malignant cells and to protect against secondary infections (Ben-Eliyahu et al., 2007; Mccoy, Rucker, & Petros, 2000; Uchida et al., 1990), making this another window during which psychosocial factors may be more likely to have an effect on the clinical course. Consistent with this notion, the level of pre-surgery depression among breast cancer patients was associated with lower lymphocyte counts one week postsurgery, with particularly pronounced effects on CD4 cells, adjusting for clinical and health practice variables (Tjemsland et al., 1997).

Clinical Significance of Biobehavioral Influences

Whereas relationships reviewed in this chapter are compelling, to date there is limited information regarding the extent to which these relationships are clinically meaningful. In one of the few studies to incorporate both immune markers and clinical outcomes and test the full immunosuppressive model, patients with hepatobiliary carcinoma reporting clinically significant depressive symptomatology died sooner than patients who were not depressed, and a low NK cell count was found to mediate the relationship between depression and survival (Steel, Geller, Gamblin, Olek, & Carr, 2007). However, survival effects of links between psychosocial factors and immune markers have been minimally examined, and findings in those studies that exist have been inconsistent. Incorporating clinical outcomes into research designs will be critical in determining the translational relevance of this body of work. In addition to the traditional focus on mortality, other clinical endpoints relevant to morbidity and quality of life, response to therapy, as well as intermediate markers of disease processes may yield useful results. For example, development of opportunistic infections following immunosuppressive therapy is a complication with relevance to quality of life, health-care utilization, and survival. Tumor markers used as an index of disease processes or treatment response, such as CA125 in ovarian cancer, can easily be assessed. In this light, an initial study suggested that dispositional optimism was associated with lower CA125 after chemotherapy in ovarian cancer patients (de Moor et al., 2006).

Examination of these factors will guide our emerging understanding of who is most vulnerable to stress-related factors in the context of cancer and what types of treatments will be most effective in addressing these issues. Potential interventions to be tested include psychological (stress-management; mindfulness) as well as pharmacological (e.g., beta-blockers, antidepressants, anti-inflammatory agents) and integrative interventions (e.g., yoga, Tai Chi, Qi Gong, Healing Touch, curcumin, and others). The effects of psychosocial intervention are reviewed more thoroughly in another chapter of this volume. To the extent that stress-related factors can modulate physiological processes relevant to cancer progression, these interactions offer a promising avenue for novel interventions to improve survival and quality of life of individuals with cancer.

Acknowledgment

This work was supported in part by grants R01 CA140933 and R01 CA104825 from the National Cancer Institute to SKL, KL2 RR0205012 from the Clinical and Translational Science Award (CTSA) program of the National Center for Research Resources and R21 CA133343 from the National Cancer Institute to ESC, and R01 CA110793, R01 CA109298, and P50 CA083693 (M.D. Anderson Cancer Center SPORE in Ovarian Cancer) from the National Cancer Institute and a Program Project Development Grant from the Ovarian Cancer Research Fund, Inc. to AKS.

Related Chapters

For more information on concepts introduced in this chapter, see also Cole; Antoni; Bower; and Segerstrom and Smith, this volume.

References

Aaronson, S. A. (1991). Growth factors and cancer. *Science, 254,* 1146–1153.

Abercrombie, H. C., Giese-Davis, J., Sephton, S., Epel, E. S., Turner-Cobb, J. M., & Spiegel, D. (2004). Flattened cortisol rhythms in metastatic breast cancer patients. *Psychoneuroendocrinology, 29,* 1082–1092.

Akechi, T., Okamura, H., Okuuyama, T., Furukawa, T. A., Nishiwaki, Y., & Uchitomi, Y. (2009). Psychosocial factors and survival after diagnosis of inoperable non-small cell lung cancer. *Psychooncology, 18,* 23–29.

An, T., Sood, U., Pietruk, T., Cummings, G., Hashimoto, K., & Crissman, J. D. (1987). In situ quantitation of inflammatory mononuclear cells in ductal infiltrating breast carcinoma. Relation to prognostic parameters. *American Journal of Pathology, 128,* 52–60.

Andersen, B., Farrar, W. B., Golden-Kreutz, D., Kutz, L. A., MacCallum, R., Courtney, M. E., et al. (1998). Stress and immune responses after surgical treatment for regional breast cancer. *Journal of the National Cancer Institute, 90,* 30–36.

Andersen, B. L., Farrar, W. B., Golden-Kreutz, D., Emery, C. F., Glaser, R., Crespin, T., et al. (2007). Distress reduction from a psychological intervention contributes to improved health for cancer patients. *Brain, Behavior, & Immunity, 21,* 953–961.

Andersen, B. L., Farrar, W. B., Golden-Kreutz, D. M., Glaser, R., Emery, C. F., Crespin, T. R., et al. (2004). Psychological, behavioral, and immune changes after a psychological intervention: A clinical trial. *Journal of Clinical Oncology, 22,* 3570–3580.

Andersen, B., Kiecolt-Glaser, J., & Glaser, R. (1994). A biobehavioral model of cancer stress and disease course. *American Psychologist, 49,* 389–404.

Andersen, B. L., Thornton, L. M., Shapiro, C. L., Farrar, W. B., Mundy, B. L., Yang, et al. (2010). Biobehavioral, immune, and health benefits following recurrence for psychological intervention participants. *Clinical Cancer Research, 16,* 3270–3278.

Andersen, B. L., Yang, H. C., Farrar, W. B., Golden-Kreutz, D. M., Emery, C. F., Thornton, L. M., et al. (2008). Psychologic intervention improves survival for breast cancer patients: A randomized clinical trial. *Cancer, 113,* 3450–3458.

Andrykowski, M. A., Brady, M. J., & Henslee-Downey, P. J. (1994). Psychosocial factors predictive of survival after allogeneic bone marrow transplantation for leukemia. *Psychosomatic Medicine, 56,* 432–439.

Antoni, M. H., Lechner, S., Diaz, A., Vargas, S., Holley, H., Phillips, K., et al. (2009). Cognitive behavioral stress management effects on psychosocial and physiological adaptation in women undergoing treatment for breast cancer. *Brain, Behavior, & Immunity, 23,* 580–591.

Antoni, M., Lutgendorf, S., Cole, S., Dhabar, F., Sephton, S., Green McDonald, P., et al. (2006). The influence of biobehavioural factors on tumor biology: Pathways and mechanisms. *Nature Reviews, Cancer, 6,* 240–248.

Antoni, M. H., Wimberly, S. R., Lechner, S. C., Kazi, A., Sifre, T., Urcuyo, K. R., et al. (2006). Reduction of cancer-specific thought intrusions and anxiety symptoms with a stress managment intervention among women undergoing treatment for breast cancer. *American Journal of Psychiatry, 163,* 1791–1797.

Antonova, L., & Mueller, C. R. (2008). Hydrocortisone downregulates the tumor suppressor gene BRCA1 in mammary cells: A possible molecular link between stress and breast cancer. *Genes Chromosomes and Cancer, 47,* 341–352.

Armaiz-Pena, G. N., Lutgendorf, S. K., Cole, S. W., & Sood, A. K. (2009). Neuroendocrine modulation of cancer progression. *Brain, Behavior, & Immunity, 23,* 10–15.

Arreygue-Garcia, N. A., Daneri-Navarro, A., del Toro-Arreola, A., Cid-Arregui, A., Gonzalez-Ramella, O., Jave-Suarez, L. F., et al. (2008). Augmented serum level of major histocompatibility complex class I-related chain A (MICA) protein and reduced NKG2D expression on NK and T cells in patients with cervical cancer and precursor lesions. *BMC Cancer, 8,* 16–26.

Ashing-Giwa, K. T., Lim, J. W., & Tang, J. (2010). Surviving cervical cancer: Does health-related quality of life influence survival? *Gynecologic oncology, 118,* 35–42.

Auletta, J. J., & Lazarus, H. M. (2005). Immune restoration following hematopoietic stem cell transplantation: An evolving target. *Bone Marrow Transplantation, 35,* 835–837.

Badino, G. R., Novelli, A., & Girardi, C. E. A. (1996). Evidence for functional beta-adrenoceptor subtypes in CG-5 breast cancer cell. *Pharmacological Research, 33,* 255–260.

Balkwill, F., Charles, K. A., & Mantovani, A. (2005). Smoldering and polarized inflammation in the initiation and promotion of malignant disease. *Cancer Cell, 7,* 211–217.

Balkwill, F., & Mantovani, A. (2001). Inflammation and cancer: Back to Virchow? *Lancet, 357,* 539–545.

Beano, A., Signorino, E., Evangelista, A., Brusa, D., Mistrangelo, M., Polimeni, M. A., et al. (2008). Correlation between NK function and response to trastuzumab in metastatic breast cancer patients. *Journal of Translational Medicine, 16,* 25.

Ben-Eliyahu, S. (2003). The promotion of tumor metastasis by surgery and stress: Immunological basis and implications for psychoneuroimmunology. *Brain, Behavior, & Immunity, 17,* 27–36.

Ben-Eliyahu, S., Page, G. G., & Schleifer, S. J. (2007). Stress, NK cells, and cancer: Still a promissory note. *Brain, Behavior, & Immunity, 21,* 881–887.

Ben-Eliyahu, S., Page, G. G., Yimira, R., & Shakhar, G. (1999). Evidence that stress and surgical interventions promote tumor development by suppressing natural killer cell activity. *International Journal of Cancer, 80,* 880–888.

Ben-Eliyahu, S., Shakhar, G., Page, G. G., Stefanski, V., & Shakhar, K. (2000). Suppression of NK cell activity and of resistance to metastasis by stress: A role for adrenal catecholamines and beta-adrenoceptors. *Neuroimmunomodulation, 8,* 154–164.

Ben-Eliyahu, S., Yirmiya, R., Liebeskind, J. C., Taylor, A. N., & Gale, R. P. (1991). Stress increases metastatic spread of a mammary tumor in rats: Evidence for mediation by the immune system. *Brain, Behavior, & Immunity, 5*, 193–205.

Benish, M., Bartal, I., Goldfarb, Y., Levi, B., Avraham, R., Raz, A., et al. (2008). Perioperative use of beta-blockers and COX-2 inhibitors may improve immune competence and reduce the risk of tumor metastasis. *Annals of Surgical Oncology, 15*, 2042–2052.

Berek, J. S., Chung, C., Kaldi, K., Watson, J. M., Knox, R. M., & Martionez-Maza, O. (1991). Serum interleukin-6 levels correlate with disease status in patients with epithelial ovarian cancer. *American Journal of Obstetrics and Gynecology, 164*, 1038–1043.

Bingle, L., Brown, N. J., & Lewis, C. E. (2002). The role of tumour-associated macrophages in tumour progression: Implications for new anticancer therapies. *Journal of Pathology, 196*, 254–265.

Black, P. H. (2002). Stress and the inflammatory response: A review of neurogenic inflammation. *Brain, Behavior & Immunity, 16*, 622–653.

Blake-Mortimer, J. S., Sephton, S. E., Carlson, R. W., Stites, D., & Spiegel, D. (2004). Cytotoxic T lymphocyte count and survival time in women with metastatic breast cancer. *Breast Journal, 10*, 195–199.

Bleiker, E. M., Hendriks, J. H., Otten, J. D., Verbeek, A. L., & van der Ploeg, H. M. (2008). Personality factors and breast cancer risk: A 13-year follow-up. *Journal of the National Cancer Institute, 100*, 213–218.

Blomberg, B. B., Alvarez, J. P., Diaz, A., Romero, M. G., Lechner, S. C., Carver, C. S., et al. (2009). Psychosocial adaptation and cellular immunity in breast cancer patients in the weeks after surgery: An exploratory study. *Journal of Psychosomatic Research, 67*, 369–376.

Blumenthal, J. A., Lett, H. S., Babyak, M. A., White, W., Smith, P. K., Mark, D. B., et al. (2003). Depression as a risk factor for mortality after coronary artery bypass surgery. *Lancet, 362*, 604–609.

Bower, J. E., Ganz, P. A., Aziz, N., & Fahey, J. L. (2002). Fatigue and proinflammatory cytokine activity in breast cancer survivors. *Psychosomatic Medicine, 64*, 604–611.

Bower, J. E., Ganz, P. A., Dickerson, S. S., Petersen, L., Aziz, N., & Fahey, J. L. (2005). Diurnal cortisol rhythm and fatigue in breast cancer survivors. *Psychoneuroendocrinology, 30*, 92–100.

Brown, J. E., Butow, P. N., Culjak, G., Coates, A. S., & Dunn, S. M. (2000). Psychosocial predictors of outcome: Time to relapse and survival in patients with early stage melanoma. *British Journal of Cancer, 83*, 1448–1453.

Brothers, B. M., Yang, H.-C., Strunk, D. R., Andersen, B. L.(2011). Cancer patients with major depressive disorder: Testing a biobehavioral cognitive behavior intervention. *Journal of Consulting and Clinical Psychology, 79*, 253–260.

Buccheri, G. (1998). Depressive reactions to lung cancer are common and often followed by a poor outcome. *The European respiratory journal, 11*, 173–178.

Butow, P. N., Coates, A. S., & Dunn, S. M. (1999). Psychosocial predictors of survival in metastatic melanoma. *Journal of Clinical Oncology, 17*, 2256–2263.

Butow, P. N., Hiller, J. E., Price, M. A., Thackway, S. V., Kricker, A., & Tennant, C. C. (2000). Epidemiological evidence for a relationship between life events, coping style, and personality factors in the development of breast cancer. *Journal of Psychosomatic Research, 49*, 169–181.

Cao, L., Liu, X., Lin, E. J., Wang, C., Choi, E. Y., Riban, V., et al. (2010). Environmental and genetic activation of a brain-adipocyte BDNF/leptin axis causes cancer remission and inhibition. *Cell, 142*, 52–64.

Ca
puron, L., & Dantzer, R. (2003). Cytokines and depression: The need for a new paradigm. *Brain, Behavior, & Immunity, 17*, S119–S124.

Carey, M. S., Bacon, M., Tu, D., Butler, L., Bezjak, A., & Stuart, G. C. (2008). The prognostic effects of performance status and quality of life scores on progression-free survival in advanced ovarian cancer. *Gynecologic oncology, 108*, 100–105.

Carney, R. M., Freedland, K. E., Miller, G. E., & Jaffe, A. S. (2002). Depression as a risk factor for cardiac mortality and morbidity: A review of potential mechanisms. *Journal of psychosomatic research, 53*, 897–902.

Caspi, A., Hariri, A. R., Holmes, A., Uher, R., & Moffitt, T. E. (2010). Genetic sensitivity to the environment: The case of the serotonin transporter gene and its implications for studying complex diseases and traits. *American Journal of Psychiatry, 167*, 509–527.

Chen, C. C., David, A. S., Nunnerley, H., Michell, M., Dawson, J. L., Berry, H., et al. (1995). Adverse life events and breast cancer: Case-control study. *British Medical Journal, 311*, 1527–1530.

Chida, Y., Hamer, M., Wardle, J., & Steptoe, A. (2008). Do stress-related psychosocial factors contribute to cancer incidence and survival? *Nature clinical practice: Oncology, 5*, 466–475.

Chopra, V., Dinh, T. V., & Hannigan, E. (1998). Circulating serum levels of cytokines and angiogenic factors in patients with cervical cancer. *Cancer Investigation, 16*, 152–159.

Chrousos, G. (1992). The concepts of stress and stress system disorders. *Journal of the American Medical Association, 267*, 1244–1252.

Chrousos, G. P. (1995). The hypothalamic-pituitary-adrenal axis and immune-mediated inflammation. *New England Journal of Medicine, 332*, 1351–1362.

Cohen, L., de Moor, C., Devine, D., Baum, A., & Amato, R. (2001). Endocrine levels at the start of treatment are associated with subsequent psychological adjustment in cancer patients with metastatic disease. *Psychosomatic Medicine, 63*, 951–958.

Cohen, S. (2004). Social relationships and health. *American Psychologist, 59*, 676–684.

Cole, S. W., Hawkley, L. C., Arevalo, J. M., Sung, C. Y., Rose, R. M., & Cacioppo, J. T. (2007). Social regulation of gene expression in human leukocytes. *Genome Biology, 8*, R189.

Collado-Hidalgo, A., Bower, J. E., Ganz, P. A., Irwin, M. R., & Cole, S. W. (2008). Cytokine gene polymorphisms and fatigue in breast cancer survivors: Early findings. *Brain Behavior, & Immunity, 22*, 1197–1200.

Collado-Hidalgo, A., Bower, M. E., Ganz, P. A., Cole, S. W., & Irwin, M. R. (2006). Inflammatory biomarkers for persistent fatigue in breast cancer survivors. *Clinical Cancer Research, 12*, 2759–2766.

Colon, E. A., Callies, A. L., Popkin, M. K., & McGlave, P. B. (1991). Depressed mood and other variables related to bone marrow transplantation survival in acute leukemia. *Psychosomatics, 32*, 420–425.

Colotta, F., Allavena, P., Sica, A., Garlanda, C., & Mantovani, A. (2009). Cancer-related inflammation, the seventh hallmark of cancer: Links to genetic instability. *Carcinogenesis, 30,* 1073–1081.

Costanzo, E. S., Juckett, M. B., Coe, C. L., Nelson, A. M., & Bourne, M. (2010). Posttraumatic growth during recovery from hematopoietic stem cell transplantation. *Psychosomatic Medicine, 72,* A24 [Published abstract].

Costanzo, E. S., Lutgendorf, S. K., Sood, A. K., Anderson, B., Sorosky, J., & Lubaroff, D. M. (2005). Psychosocial factors and interleukin-6 among women with advanced ovarian cancer. *Cancer, 104,* 305–313.

Coussens, L. M., & Werb, Z. (2002). Inflammation and cancer. *Nature, 420,* 860–867.

Cousson-Gelie, F., Bruchon-Schweitzer, M., Dilhuydy, J. M., & Jutand, M. A. (2007). Do anxiety, body image, social support and coping strategies predict survival in breast cancer? A ten-year follow-up study. *Psychosomatics, 48,* 211–216.

Coyne, J. C., Pajak, T. F., Harris, J., Konski, A., Movsas, B., Ang, K., et al. (2007). Emotional well-being does not predict survival in head and neck cancer patients: A radiation therapy oncology group study. *Cancer, 110,* 2568–2575.

Darnell, R. B., & Posner, J. B. (2006). Paraneoplastic syndromes affecting the nervous system. *Seminars in Oncology, 33,* 270–298.

de Moor, J. S., de Moor, C. A., Basen-Engquist, K., Kudelka, A., Bevers, M. W., & Cohen, L. (2006). Optimism, distress, health-related quality of life, and change in cancer antigen 125 among patients with ovarian cancer undergoing chemotherapy. *Psychosomatic Medicine, 68,* 555–562.

Dentino, A. N., Pieper, C. F., Rao, M. K., Currie, M. S., Harris, T., Blazer, D. G., et al. (1999). Association of interleukin-6 and other biologic variables with depression in older people living in the community. *Journal of the American Geriatrics Society, 47,* 6–11.

Drell, T. L., Joseph, J., Lang, K., Niggemann, B., Zaenker, K. S., & Entschladen, F. (2003). Effects of neurotransmitters on the chemokinesis and chemotaxis of MDA-MB-468 human breast carcinoma cells. *Breast Cancer Research and Treatment, 80,* 63–70.

Duijts, S. F. A., Zeegers, M. P. A., & Borne, B. V. (2003). The association between stressful life events and breast cancer risk: A meta-analysis. *International Journal of Cancer, 107,* 1023–1029.

Dunigan, J. T., Carr, B. I., & Steel, J. L. (2007). Posttraumatic growth, immunity and survival in patients with hepatoma. *Digestive Diseases and Sciences, 52,* 2452–2459.

Dunn, G. P., Bruce, A. T., Ikeda, H., Old, L. J., & Schreiber, R. D. (2002). Cancer immunoediting: From immunosurveillance to tumor escape. *Nature Immunology, 3,* 991–998.

Efficace, F., Bottomley, A., Coens, C., Van Steen, K., Conroy, T., Schoffski, P., et al. (2006). Does a patient's self-reported health-related quality of life predict survival beyond key biomedical data in advanced colorectal cancer? *European Journal of Cancer, 42,* 42–49.

Efficace, F., Innominato, P. F., Bjarnason, G., Coens, C., Humblet, Y., Tumolo, S., et al. (2008). Validation of patient's self-reported social functioning as an independent prognostic factor for survival in metastatic colorectal cancer patients: Results of an international study by the Chronotherapy Group of the European Organisation for Research and Treatment of Cancer. *Journal of Clinical Oncology, 26,* 2020–2026.

Elenkov, I. J., & Chrousos, G. P. (2002). Stress hormones, proinflammatory and antiinflammatory cytokines, and autoimmunity. *Annals of New York Academy of Science, 966,* 290–303.

Enserink, J. M., Price, L. S., Methi, T., Mahic, M., Sonnenberg, A., Bos, J. L., et al. (2004). The cAMP-Epac-Rap1 pathway regulates cell spreading and cell adhesion to laminin-5 through the a3b1 integrin but not the a6b4 integrin. *Journal of Biological Chemistry, 279,* 44889–44896.

Epping-Jordan, J., Compas, B., & Howell, D. (1994). Predictors of cancer progression in young adult men and women: Avoidance, intrusive thoughts, and psychological symptoms. *Health Psychology, 13,* 539–547.

Esler, M., Turbott, J., Schwarz, R., Leonard, P., Bobik, A., Skews, H., et al. (1982). The peripheral kinetics of norepinephrine in depressive illness. *Archives of General Psychiatry, 39,* 295–300.

Eustace, D., Han, X., Gooding, R., Rowbottom, A., Riches, P., & Heyderman, E. (1993). Interleukin 6 (IL-6) functions as an autocrine growth factor in cervical carcinomas in vitro. *Gynecologic Oncology, 50,* 15–19.

Faller, H., Bulzebruck, H., Drings, P., & Lang, H. (1999). Coping, distress, and survival among patients with lung cancer. *Archives of General Psychiatry, 56,* 756–762.

Fava, G. A., Sonino, N., & Morphy, M. A. (1987). Major depression associated with endocrine disease. *Psychiatric Developments, 5,* 321–348.

Felten, S., & Felten, D. (1991). Innervation of lymphoid tissue. In R. Ader, D. Felten, & N. Cohen (Eds.), *Psychoneuroimmunology* (2nd ed., pp. 27–71). San Diego, CA: Academic Press.

Fidler, I. J. (1995a). Critical factors in the biology of human cancer metastasis. *American Surgeon, 61,* 1065–1066.

Fidler, I. J. (1995b). Modulation of the organ microenvironment for treatment of cancer metastasis. *Journal of the National Cancer Institute, 87,* 1588–1592.

Fidler, I. J. (1997). *Molecular biology of cancer: Invasion and metastasis.* Philadelphia: Lippincott-Raven Publishers.

Fielding, R., & Wong, W. S. (2007). Quality of life as a predictor of cancer survival among Chinese liver and lung cancer patients. *European Journal of Cancer, 43,* 1723–1730.

Folkman, J. (1990). What is the evidence that tumors are angiogenesis dependant? *Journal of the National Cancer Institute, 82,* 4–6.

Folkman, J. (1995). Tumor angiogenesis. In J. Mendelsohn, P. M. Howley, M. A. Israel, & L. A. Liotta (Eds.), *The molecular basis of cancer* (pp. 206–232). Philadelphia: WB Saunders.

Folkman, J., & Klagsbrun, M. (1987). Angiogenic factors. *Science, 235,* 442–447.

Frick, E., Motzke, C., Fischer, N., Busch, R., & Bumeder, I. (2005). Is perceived social support a predictor of survival for patients undergoing autologous peripheral blood stem cell transplantation? *Psycho-oncology, 14,* 759–770.

Frommberger, U. H., Bauer, J., Haselbauer, P., Fraulin, A., Rieman, D., & Berger, M. (1997). Interleukin-6 plasma levels in depression and schizophrenia: Comparison between the acute state and after remission. *European Archives of Psychiatry & Clinical Neuroscience, 247,* 228–233.

Funch, D. P., & Marshall, J. (1983). The role of stress, social support and age in survival from breast cancer. *Journal of Psychosomatic Research, 27,* 77–83.

Garcia-Lora, A., Algarra, I., & Garrido, F. (2003). MHC class I antigens, immune surveillance, and tumor escape. *Journal of Cell Physiology, 195,* 346–355.

Garland, M. R., Lavelle, E., Doherty, D., Golden-Mason, L., Fitzpatrick, P., Hill, A., et al. (2004). Cortisol does not mediate the suppressive effects of psychiatric morbidity on natural killer cell activity: A cross-sectional study of patients with early breast cancer. *Psychological Medicine, 34,* 481–490.

Garner, W., Minton, J., James, A., & Hoffman, C. (1983). Human breast cancer and impaired NK cell function. *Journal of Surgical Oncology, 24,* 64–66.

Gatti, G., Cavallo, R., Sartori, M., Delponte, D., Masera, R., Salvadori, A., et al. (1987). Inhibition of human natural killer cell activity by cortisol. *Journal of Steroid Biochemistry, 265,* 29–58.

Geyer, S. (1991). Life events prior to manifestation of breast cancer: A limited prospective study covering eight years before diagnosis. *Journal of psychosomatic research, 35,* 355–363.

Geyer, S. (1993). Life events, chronic difficulties and vulnerability factors preceding breast cancer. *Social science & medicine, 37,* 1545–1555.

Giese-Davis, J., Sephton, S., Abercrombie, H., Duran, R., & Spiegel, D. (2004). Repression and high anxiety are associated with aberrant diurnal cortisol rhythms in women with metastatic breast cancer. *Health Psychology, 23,* 645–650.

Giraldi, T., Rodani, M. G., Cartei, G., & Grassi, L. (1997). Psychosocial factors and breast cancer: A 6-year Italian follow-up study. *Psychotherapy and Psychosomatics, 66,* 229–236.

Glasner, A., Avraham, R., Rosenne, E., Benish, M., Zmora, O., Shemer, S., et al. (2010). Improving survival rates in two models of spontaneous postoperative metastasis in mice by combined administration of a beta-adrenergic antagonist and a cyclooxygenase-2 inhibitor. *Journal of Immunology, 184,* 2449–2457.

Goedegebuure, P., Douville, C. C., Doherty, J. M., Linehan, D. C., Lee, K. Y., Ganguly, E. K., et al. (1997). Simultaneous production of T helper-1-like cytokines and cytolytic activity by tumor-specific T cells in ovarian and breast cancer. *Cellular Immunology, 175,* 150–156.

Gold, P. W., & Chrousos, G. P. (2002). Organization of the stress system and its dysregulation in melancholic and atypical depression: High vs low CRH/NE states. *Molecular Psychiatry, 7,* 254–275.

Goodwin, P. J., Ennis, M., Bordeleau, L. J., Pritchard, K. I., Trudeau, M. E., Koo, J., et al. (2004). Health-related quality of life and psychosocial status in breast cancer prognosis: Analysis of multiple variables. *Journal of Clinical Oncology, 22,* 4184–4192.

Grande, G. E., Farquhar, M. C., Barclay, S. I., & Todd, C. J. (2009). Quality of life measures (EORTC QLQ-C30 and SF-36) as predictors of survival in palliative colorectal and lung cancer patients. *Palliative Support Care, 7,* 289–297.

Greenfeld, K., Avraham, R., Benish, M., Goldfarb, Y., Rosenne, E., Shapira, Y., et al. (2007). Immune suppression while awaiting surgery and following it: Dissociations between plasma cytokine levels, their induced production, and NK cell cytotoxicity. *Brain, Behavior, & Immunity, 21,* 503–513.

Greer, S., Morris, T., & Pettingale, K. W. (1979). Psychological response to breast cancer: Effect on outcome. *Lancet, 2,* 785–787.

Greer, S., Morris, T., Pettingale, K. W., & Haybittle, J. L. (1990). Psychological response to breast cancer and 15-year outcome. *Lancet, 335,* 49–50.

Hagemann, T., Robinson, S. C., Schulz, M., Trümper, L., Balkwill, F. R., & Binder, C. (2004). Enhanced invasiveness of breast cancer cell lines upon co-cultivation with mac-rophages is due to TNF-alpha dependent up-regulation of matrix metalloproteases. *Carcinogenesis, 25,* 1543–1549.

Hamaoka, T., & Fujiwara, H. (1987). Phenotypically and functionally distinct T-cell subsets in anti-tumor responses. *Immunology Today, 8,* 267–269.

Hamer, M., Tanaka, G., Okamura, H., Tsuda, A., & Steptoe, A. (2007). The effects of depressive symptoms on cardiovascular and catecholamine responses to the induction of depressive mood. *Biological Psychology, 74,* 20–25.

Hanahan, D., & Weinberg, R. A. (2011). Hallmarks of cancer: The next generation. *Cell, 144,* 646–674.

Heffner, K. L., Loving, T. J., Robles, T. F., & Kiecolt-Glaser, J. K. (2003). Examining psychosocial factors related to cancer incidence and progression: In search of the silver lining. *Brain, Behavior, & Immunity, 17*(1), S109–111.

Hellstrand, K., Hermodsson, S., & Strannegard, O. (1985). Evidence for B-adrenoceptor mediated regulation of human natural killer cells. *Journal of Immunology, 134,* 4095–4099.

Heo, D., Whiteside, T., Kanbour, A., & Herberman, R. (1988). Lymphocytes infiltrating human ovarian tumors I: Role of Leu-19 (NKH1)-positive recombinant IL-2-activated cultures of lymphocytes infiltrating human ovarian tumors. *Journal of Immunology, 140,* 4042–4049.

Herndon, J. N., Fleishman, S., Kornblith, A. B., Kosty, M., Green, M. R., & Holland, J. C. (1999). Is quality of life predictive of the survival of patients with advanced nonsmall cell lung carcinoma? *Cancer, 85,* 333–340.

Herskind, C., Bamberg, M., & Rodemann, H. (1998). The role of cytokines in the development of normal tissue reactions after radiotherapy. Suppliment 3. *Strahlentherapie und Onkologie, 174,* 12–15.

Holbrook, N., Cox, W., & Horner, H. (1983). Direct suppression of natural killer activity in human peripheral blood leukocyte cultures by glucocorticoids and its modulation by interferon. *Cancer Research, 43,* 4019–4025.

Hoodin, F., Kalbfleisch, K. R., Thornton, J., & Ratanatharathorn, V. (2004). Psychosocial influences on 305 adults' survival after bone marrow transplantation: Depression, smoking, and behavioral self-regulation. *Journal of Psychosomatic Research, 57,* 145–154.

House, J. S., Landis, K. R., & Umberson, D. (1988). Social relationships and health. *Science, 241,* 540–545.

Huang, S., Van Arsdall, M., Tedjarati, S., McCarty, M., Wu, W., Langley, R., et al. (2002). Contributions of Stromal Metalloproteinase-9 to angiogenesis and growth of human ovarian carcinoma in mice. *Journal of the National Cancer Institute, 94,* 1134–1142.

Hughes, J. W., Watkins, L., Blumenthal, J. A., Kuhn, C., & Sherwood, A. (2004). Depression and anxiety symptoms are related to increased 24-hour urinary norepinephrine excretion among healthy middle-aged women. *Journal of Psychosomatic Research, 57,* 353–358.

Ioannides, C., Freedman, R., Platsoucas, C., Rashed, S., & Kim, Y. (1991). Cytotoxic T cell clones isolated from ovarian tumor-infiltrating lymphocytes recognize multiple antigenic epitopes on autologous tumor cells. *Journal of Immunology, 146,* 1700–1707.

Irwin, M. (2002). Psychoneuroimmunology of depression: Clinical implications. *Brain Behavior & Immunity, 16,* 1–16.

Jehn, C. F., Kuehnhardt, D., Bartholomae, A., Pfeiffer, S., Krebs, M., Regierer, A. C., et al. (2006). Biomarkers of depression in cancer patients. *Cancer, 107,* 2723–2729.

Jensen, M. R. (1987). Psychobiological factors predicting the course of breast cancer. *Journal of Personality, 55,* 317–342.

Kamat, A. A., Fletcher, M. S., Gruman, L., Mueller, P., Lopez, A., Landen, C. N., et al. (2006). The clinical relevance of stromal matrix metalloprotinease (MMP) expression in ovarian cancer. *Clinical Cancer Research, 12,* 1707–1714.

Karvonen-Gutierrez, C. A., Ronis, D. L., Fowler, K. E., Terrell, J. E., Gruber, S. B., & Duffy, S. A. (2008). Quality of life scores predict survival among patients with head and neck cancer. *Journal of Clinical Oncology, 26,* 2754–2760.

Khong, H. T., & Restifo, N. P. (2002). Natural selection of tumor variants in the generation of "tumor escape" phenotypes. *Nature Immunology, 3,* 999–1005.

Kiecolt-Glaser, J., Fisher, L., Ogrocki, P., Stout, J., Speicher, C., & Glaser, R. (1987). Marital quality, marital disruption, and immune function. *Psychosomatic Medicine, 49,* 13–34.

Kiecolt-Glaser, J. K., Preacher, K. J., MacCallum, R. C., Atkinson, C., Malarkey, W. B., & Glaser, R. (2003). Chronic stress and age-related increases in the proinflammatory cytokine IL-6. *Proceedings of the National Academy of Sciences of the United States of America, 100,* 9090–9095.

Kiecolt-Glaser, J. K., Robles, T. F., Heffner, K. L., Loving, T. J., & Glaser, R. (2002). Psycho-oncology and cancer: Psychoneuroimmunology and cancer. *Annals of Oncology, 13,* 165–169.

Kitamura, Y., Morita, I., Nihei, Z., Mishima, Y., & Murota, S. (1997). Effects of IL-6 on tumor cells invasion of vascular endothelial monolayers. *Japanese Journal of Surgery, 27,* 534–541.

Knekt, P., Raitasalo, R., Hellovaara, M., Lehtinen, V., Pukkala, E., Teppo, L., et al. (1996). Elevated lung cancer risk among persons with depressed mood. *American journal of epidemiology, 144,* 1096–1103.

Kowalczyk, D. W. (2002). Tumors and the danger model. *Acta Biochimica Polonica, 49,* 295–302.

Kroenke, C. H., Hankinson, S. E., Schernhammer, E. S., Colditz, G. A., Kawachi, I., & Holmes, M. D. (2004). Caregiving stress, endogenous sex hormone levels, and breast cancer incidence. *American journal of epidemiology, 59,* 1019–1027.

Kroenke, C. H., Kubzansky, L. D., Schernhammer, E. S., Holmes, M. D., & Kawachi, I. (2006). Social networks, social support, and survival after breast cancer diagnosis. *Journal of Clinical Oncology, 24,* 1105–1111.

Lamkin, D. M., Lutgendorf, S. K., Lubaroff, D. M., Sood, A. K., Beltz, T. G., & Johnson, A. K. (2011). Cancer induces inflammation and depressive-like behavior in the mouse: Modulation by social housing. *Brain, Behavior, and Immunity, 25,* 555–564.

Lamkin, D. M., Lutgendorf, S. K., McGinn, S., Dao, M., Maiseri, H., DeGeest, K., et al. (2008). Positive psychosocial factors and NKT cells in ovarian cancer patients. *Brain, Behavior, and Immunity, 22,* 65–73.

Landen, C. N., Lin, Y. G., Armaiz-Pena, G. N., Das, P. D., Arevalo, J. M., Kamat, A. A., et al. (2007). Neuroendocrine modulation of signal transducer and activator of transcription-3 in ovarian cancer. *Cancer Research, 67,* 10389–10396.

Langley, R. R., & Fidler, I. J. (2007). Tumor cell-organ microenvironment interactions in the pathogenesis of cancer metastasis. *Endocrine Reviews, 28,* 297–321.

Lee, J. W., Shahzad, M., Lin, Y., Armaiz-Pena, G., Mangala, S., Han, H.-D., et al. (2009). Surgical stress promotes tumor growth in ovarian carcinoma. *Clinical Cancer Research, 15,* 2695–2702.

Lehto, U. S., Ojanen, M., Dyba, T., Aromaa, A., & Kellokumpu-Lehtinen, P. (2006). Baseline psychosocial predictors of survival in localised breast cancer. *British Journal of Cancer, 94,* 1245–1252.

Lehto, U. S., Ojanen, M., Dyba, T., Aromaa, A., & Kellokumpu-Lehtinen, P. (2007). Baseline psychosocial predictors of survival in localized melanoma. *Psychosomatic research, 63,* 9–15.

Levy, S., Herberman, R., Lippman, M., & d'Angelo, T. (1987). Correlation of stress factors with sustained depression of natural killer cell activity and predicted pronosis in patients with breast cancer. *Journal of Clinical Oncology, 5,* 348–353.

Levy, S., Herberman, R., Lippman, M., D'Angelo, T., & Lee, J. (1991). Immunological and psychosocial predictors of disease recurrence in patients with early-stage breast cancer. *Behavioral Medicine, 17,* 67–75.

Levy, S. M. (Ed.). (1991). *Behavioral and immunological host factors in cancer risk.* Hillsdale, NJ: Erlbaum.

Levy, S. M., Herberman, R. B., Lee, J., Whiteside, T., Kirkwood, J., & McFeeley, S. (1990). Estrogen receptor concentration and social factors as predictors of natural killer cell acitivity in early-stage breast cancer patients: Confirmation of a model. *Natural immunity and cell growth regulation, 9,* 313–324.

Levy, S. M., Heberman, R. B., Maluish, A. M., Schlein, B., & Lippman, M. (1985). Prognostic risk assessment in primary breast cancer by behavioral and immunological parameters. *Health Psychology, 4,* 99–113.

Levy, S. M., Heberman, R. B., Whiteside, T., Sanzo, K., Lee, J., & Kirkwood, J. (1990). Perceived social support and tumor estrogen/progesterone receptor status as predictors of natural killer cell activity in breast cancer patients. *Psychosomatic Medicine, 52,* 73–85.

Light, K. C., Kothandapani, R. V., & Allen, M. T. (1998). Enhanced cardiovascular and catecholamine responses in women with depressive symptoms. *International Journal of Psychophysiology, 28,* 157–166.

Lillberg, K., Verkasalo, P. K., Kaprio, J., Teppo, L., Helenius, H., & Koskenvuo, M. (2003). Stressful life events and risk of breast cancer in 10,808 women: A cohort study. *American journal of epidemiology, 157,* 415–423.

Linkins, R. W., & Comstock, G. W. (1990). Depressed mood and development of cancer. *American journal of epidemiology, 132,* 962–972.

Lutgendorf, S. K., Cole, S., Costanzo, E., Bradley, S., Coffin, J., Jabbari, S., et al. (2003). Stress-related mediators stimulate vascular endothelial growth factor secretion by two ovarian cancer cell lines. *Clinical Cancer Research, 9,* 4514–4521.

Lutgendorf, S. K., DeGeest, K., Sung, C. Y., Arevalo, J. M. G., Penedo, F., Lucci, J. A. I., et al. (2009). Depression, social support, and beta-adrenergic transcription control in human ovarian cancer. *Brain, Behavior, & Immunity, 23,* 176–183.

Lutgendorf, S., Garand, L., Buckwalter, K., Tripp-Reimer, T., Hong, S., & Lubaroff, D. (1999). Life stress, mood disturbance, and elevated IL-6 in healthy older women. *Journals of Gerontology. Series A, Biological Sciences & Medical Sciences, 54,* M434–439.

Lutgendorf, S. K., Johnsen, E. L., Cooper, B., Anderson, B., Sorosky, J. I., Butler, R. E., et al. (2002). Vascular endothelial growth factor and social support in patients with ovarian carcinoma. *Cancer, 95,* 808–815.

Lutgendorf, S. K., Lamkin, D. M., DeGeest, K., Anderson, B., Dao, M., McGinn, S., et al. (2008). Depressed and anxious mood and T-cell cytokine expressing populations in ovarian cancer patients. *Brain, Behavior, &Immunity, 22,* 890–900.

Lutgendorf, S. K., Lamkin, D. M., Jennings, N. B., Arevalo, J. M. G., Penedo, F., DeGeest, K., et al. (2008). Biobehavioral influences on matrix metalloproteinase expression in ovarian carcinoma. *Clinical Cancer Research, 14,* 6839–6846.

Lutgendorf, S. K., Sood, A. K., Andersen, B., McGinn, S., Maiseri, H., Dao, M., et al. (2005). Social support, psychological distress, and natural killer cell activity in ovarian cancer. *Journal of Clinical Oncology, 23,* 7105–7113.

Lutgendorf, S., Sood, A., & Antoni, M. H. (2010). Host factors and cancer progression: Biobehavioral signaling pathways and interventions. *Journal of Clinical Oncology, 28,* 4094–4099.

Lutgendorf, S. K., Weinrib, A. Z., Penedo, F., Russell, D., DeGeest, K., Costanzo, E. S., et al. (2008). Interleukin-6, Cortisol, and depressive symptoms in ovarian cancer patients. *Journal of Clinical Oncology, 26,* 4820–4827.

Madden, K. (2003). Catcholamines, sympathetic innervation, and immunity. *Brain, Behavior & Immunity, 17,* S5–S10.

Maes, M., Lin, A. H., Delmire, L., Van Gastel, A., Kenis, G., De Jongh, R., et al. (1999). Elevated serum interleukin-6 (IL-6) and IL-6 receptor concentrations in posttraumatic stress disorder following accidental man-made traumatic events. *Biological Psychiatry, 45,* 833–839.

Maier, S., & Watkins, L. (1998). Cytokines for psychologists: Implications of bidirectional immune to brain communication for understanding behavior, mood, and cognition. *Psychological Review, 105,* 83–107.

Mantovani, A., Sozzani, S., Locati, M., Allavena, P., & Sica, A. (2002). Macrophage polarization: Tumor-associated macrophages as a paradigm for polarized M2 mononuclear phagocytes. *Trends in Immunology, 23,* 549–555.

Marchetti, B., Spinola, P. G., Pelletier, G., & Labrie, F. (1991). A potential role for catecholamines in the development and progression of carcinogen-induced mammary tumors: Hormonal control of beta-adrenergic receptors and correlation with tumor growth. *Journal of Steroid Biochemistry and Molecular Biology, 38,* 307–320.

Marshall, J., & Funch, D. P. (1983). Social environment and breast cancer: A cohort analysis of patient survival. *Cancer, 52,* 1546–1550.

Massie, M. J. (2004). Prevalence of depression in patients with cancer. *Journal of the National Cancer Institute: Monographs, 32,* 57–71.

Masur, K., Niggemann, B., Zanker, K. S., & Entschladen, F. (2001). Norepinephrine-induced migration of SW 480 colon carcinoma cells is inhibited by beta-blockers. *Cancer Research, 61,* 2866–2869.

Matzinger, P. (1994). Tolerance, danger, and the extended family. *Annual Review of Immunology, 12,* 991–1045.

Maunsell, E., Brisson, J., & Deschenes, L. (1995). Social support and survival among women with breast cancer. *Cancer, 76,* 631–637.

Mccoy, J. L., Rucker, R., & Petros, J. A. (2000). Cell-mediated immunity to tumor-associated antigens is a better predictor of survival in early stage breast cancer than stage, grade or lymph node status. *Breast Cancer Research and Treatment, 60,* 227–234.

McCusker, R. H., Strle, K., Broussard, S. R., Dantzer, R., Bluthé, R. M., & Kelley, K. W. (2007). Crosstalk between insulin-like growth factors and pro-inflammatory cytokines. In R. Ader, D. Felten, & N. Cohen (Eds.),

Psychoneuroimmunology (4th ed., Vol. 1, pp. 171–192). San Diego, CA: Elsevier.

McGee, R., Williams, S., & Elwood, M. (1994). Depression and the development of cancer: A meta-analysis. *Social science & medicine, 38,* 187–192.

McGregor, B., Langer, S. L., & Syrjala, K. L. (2005). The effect of pre-transplant distress on immune reconstitution among adult hematopoietic cell transplant patients. *Psychosomatic Medicine, 67,* A24 [Published abstract].

McGregor, B. A., Antoni, M. H., Boyers, A., Alferi, S. M., Blomberg, B. B., & Carver, C. S. (2004). Cognitive-behavioral stress management increased benefit finding and immune function among women with early-stage breast cancer. *Journal of Psychosomatic Research, 56,* 1–8.

McKernan, M., McMillan, D. C., Anderson, J. R., Angerson, W. J., & Stuart, R. C. (2008). The relationship between quality of life (EORTC QLQ-C30) and survival in patients with gastro-oesophageal cancer. *British Journal of Cancer, 98,* 888–893.

Mehanna, H. M., De Boer, M. F., & Morton, R. P. (2008). The association of psycho-social factors and survival in head and neck cancer. *Clinical Otolaryngology, 33,* 83–89.

Melief, C. (1992). Tumor eradication by adoptive transfer of cytotoxic T lymphocytes. *Advances in Cancer Research, 58,* 143–175.

Melief, C., & Kast, W. (1991). Cytotoxic T lymphocyte therapy of cancer and tumor escape mechanisms. *Cancer Biology and Therapy, 2,* 347–353.

Ménard, C., Blay, J. Y., Borg, C., Michiels, S., Ghiringhelli, F., Robert, C., et al. (2009). Natural killer cell IFN-gamma levels predict long-term survival with imatinib mesylate therapy in gastrointestinal stromal tumor-bearing patients. *Cancer Research, 69,* 3563–3569.

Meyer, F., Fortin, A., Gelinas, M., Nabid, A., Brochet, F., Tetu, B., et al. (2009). Health-related quality of life as a survival predictor for patients with localized head and neck cancer treated with radiation therapy. *Journal of Clinical Oncology, 27,* 2970–2976.

Meyerowitz, B. (1980). Psychosocial correlates of breast cancer and its treatments. *Psychological Bulletin, 87,* 108–131.

Michael, Y. L., Carlson, N. E., Chlebowski, R. T., Aickin, M., Weihs, K. L., Ockene, J. K., et al. (2009). Influence of stressors on breast cancer incidence in the Women's Health Initiative. *Health Psychology, 28,* 137–146.

Miller, G. E., Chen, E., Sze, J., Marin, T., Arevalo, J. M., Doll, R., et al. (2008). A functional genomic fingerprint of chronic stress in humans: Blunted glucocorticoid and increased NF-kappaB signaling. *Biological Psychiatry, 64,* 266–272.

Miller, G. E., Cohen, S., Rabin, B. S., Skoner, D. P., & Doyle, W. J. (1999). Personality and tonic cardiovascular, neuroendocrine, and immune parameters. *Brain, Behavior, & Immunity, 13,* 109–123.

Molassiotis, A., Van den Akker, O. B. A., Milligan, D. W., & Goldman, J. M. (1997). Symptom distress, coping style and biological variables as predictors of survival after bone marrow transplantation. *Journal of Psychosomatic Research, 42,* 275–285.

Moran, T. J., Gray, S., Mikosz, C. A., & Conzen, S. D. (2000). The glucocorticoid receptor mediates a survival signal in human mammary epithelial cells. *Cancer Research, 60,* 867–872.

Moretta, A., Biassoni, R., Bottino, C., & Moretta, L. (2000). Surface receptors delivering opposite signals regulate the function of human NK cells. *Seminars in Immunology, 12,* 129–138.

Morris, T., Pettingale, K. W., & Haybittle, J. L. (1992). Psychological response to cancer diagnosis and disease outcome in patients with breast cancer and lymphoma. *Psychooncology, 1,* 105–114.

Murphy, K. C., Jenkins, P. L., & Whittaker, J. A. (1996). Psychosocial morbidity and survival in adult bone marrow transplant recipients: A follow-up study. *Bone Marrow Transplantation, 18,* 199–201.

Murray, C. J., & Lopez, A. D. (1997). Global mortality, disability, and the contribution of risk factors: Global burden of disease study. *Lancet, 349,* 1436–1442.

Musselman, D. L., Miller, A. H., Porter, M. R., Manatunga, A., Gao, F., Penna, S., et al. (2001). Higher than normal plasma interleukin-6 concentrations in cancer patients with depression: Preliminary findings. *American Journal of Psychiatry, 158,* 1252–1257.

Nakane, T., Szentendrei, T., Stern, L., Virmani, M., Seely, J., & Kunos, G. (1990). Effects of IL-1 and cortisol on beta-adrenergic receptors, cell proliferation, and differentiation in cultured human A549 lung tumor cells. *Journal of Immunology, 145,* 260–266.

Nakaya, N., Bidstrup, P. E., Saito-Nakaya, K., Frederiksen, K., Koskenvuo, M., Pukkala, E., et al. (2010). Personality traits and cancer risk and survival based on Finnish and Swedish registry data. *American Journal of Epidemiology, 172,* 377–385.

Nan, K., Wei, Y., Zhou, F. L., Li, C. L., Sui, C. G., Hui, L. Y., et al. (2004). Effects of depression on parameters of cell-mediated immunity in patients with digestive tract cancers. *World Journal of Gastroenterology, 10,* 268–272.

Naughton, M. J., Herndon, J. N., Shumaker, S. A., Miller, A. A., Kornblith, A. B., Chao, D., et al. (2002). The health-related quality of life and survival of small-cell lung cancer patients: Results of a companion study to CALGB 9033. *Quality of life research, 11,* 235–248.

Nauseen, B., Carr, N. J., Peveler, R. C., Moss-Morris, R., Verrill, C., Robbins, E., et al. (2010). The relationships between loneliness and proangiogenic cytokines in newly diagnosed tumors of colon and rectum. *Psychosomatic Medicine, 72,* 912–916.

Nausheen, B., Gidron, Y., Peveler, R., & Moss-Morris, R. (2009). Social support and cancer progression: A systematic review. *Journal of Psychosomatic Research, 67,* 403–415.

Neitzert, C. S., Ritvo, P., Dancey, J., Weiser, K., Murray, C., & Avery, J. (1998). The psychosocial impact of bone marrow transplantation: A review of the literature. *Bone Marrow Transplantation, 22,* 409–422.

Nielsen, N. R., Strandberg-Larsen, K., Gronbaek, M., Kristensen, T. S., Schnohr, P., & Zhang, Z. F. (2007). Self-reported stress and risk of endometrial cancer: A prospective cohort study. *Psychosomatic Medicine, 69,* 383–389.

Nielsen, N. R., Zhang, Z. F., Kristensen, T. S., Netterstrom, B., Schnohr, P., & Gronbaek, M. (2005). Self reported stress and risk of breast cancer: A prospective cohort study. *BMJ, 331,* 548.

Nilsson, M. B., Armaiz-Pena, G., Takahashi, R., Lin, Y. G., Trevino, J., Li, Y., et al. (2007). Stress hormones regulate IL-6 expression by human ovarian carcinoma cells through a SRC-dependent mechanism. *Journal of Biological Chemistry, 282,* 29919–29926.

Nilsson, M. B., Langley, R. R., & Fidler, I. J. (2005). Interleukin-6, secreted by human ovarian carcinoma cells, is a potent proangiogenic cytokine. *Cancer Research, 65,* 10794–10800.

Nowicki, A., Szenajch, J., Ostrowska, G., Wojtowicz, A., Wojtowicz, K., Kruszewski, A. A., et al. (1996). Impaired tumor growth in colony-stimulating factor 1 (CSF-1)-deficient, macrophage-deficient op/op mouse: Evidence for a role of CSF-1-dependent macrophages in formation of tumor stroma. *International Journal of Cancer, 65,* 112–119.

Obata, N. H., Tamakoshi, K., Shibata, K., Kikkawa, F., & Tomoda, Y. (1997). Effects of interleukin-6 on in vitro cell attachment, migration, and invasion of human ovarian carcinoma. *Anticancer Research, 17,* 337–342.

Osborne, R. H., Sali, A., Aaronson, N. K., Elsworth, G. R., Mdzewski, B., & Sinclair, A. J. (2004). Immune function and adjustment style: Do they predict survival in breast cancer? *Psychooncology, 13,* 199–210.

Page, G. G., & Ben-Eliyahu, S. (1999). A role for NK cells in greater susceptibility of young rats to metastatic formation. *Developmental and Comparative Immunology, 23,* 87–96.

Pang, D., Kocherginsky, M., Krausz, T., Kim, S. Y., & Conzen, S. D. (2006). Dexamethasone decreases xenograft response to Paclitaxel through inhibition of tumor cell apoptosis. *Cancer Biology & Therapy, 5,* 933–940.

Park, C. L., Lechner, S. C., Antoni, M. H., & Stanton, A. L. (2008). *Medical illness and positive life change: Can crisis lead to personal transformation?* Washington, DC: American Psychological Association.

Park, S. Y., Kang, J. H., Jeong, K. J., Lee, J., Han, J. W., Choi, W. S., et al. (2010). Norepinephrine induces VEGF expression and angiogenesis by a hypoxia-inducible factor-1alpha protein-dependent mechanism. *International Journal of Cancer, 128,* 2306–2316.

Peggs, K. S., & Mackinnon, S. (2004). Immune reconstitution following haematopoietic stem cell transplantation. *British Journal of Haematology, 124,* 407–420.

Penedo, F. J., Dahn, J. R., Kinsinger, D., Antoni, M. H., Molton, I., Gonzalez, J. S., et al. (2006). Anger suppression mediates the relationship between optimism and natural killer cell cytotoxicity in men treated for localized prostate cancer. *Journal of Psychosomatic Research, 60,* 423–427.

Penninx, B. W., Guralnik, J. M., Pahor, M., Ferrucci, L., Cerhan, J. R., Wallace, R. B., et al. (1998). Chronically depressed mood and cancer risk in older persons. *Journal of the National Cancer Institute, 90,* 1888–1893.

Persky, V. W., Kempthorne-Rawson, J., & Shekelle, R. B. (1987). Personality and risk of cancer: 20-year follow-up of the Western Electric Study. *Psychosomatic medicine, 49,* 435–449.

Petticrew, M., Fraser, J. M., & Regan, M. F. (1999). Adverse life-events and risk of breast cancer: A meta-analysis. *British Journal of Health Psychology, 4,* 1–17.

Pettingale, K. W. (1984). Coping and cancer prognosis. *Journal of psychosomatic research, 28,* 363–364.

Pettingale, K. W., Morris, T., Greer, S., & Haybittle, J. (1985). Mental attitudes to cancer: An additional prognostic factor. *Lancet, 1,* 750.

Phillips, K. M., Antoni, M. H., Lechner, S. C., Blomberg, B. B., Llabre, M. M., Avisar, E., et al. (2008). Stress management intervention reduces serum cortisol and increases relaxation during treatment for nonmetastatic breast cancer. *Psychosomatic Medicine, 70,* 1044–1049.

Pillai, M., Balaram, P., Chidambaram, S., Padmanabhan, T., & Nair, M. (1990). Development of an immunological staging system to prognosticate disease course in malignant cervical neoplasia. *Gynecologic Oncology, 37*, 200–205.

Pinquart, M., Hoffken, K., Silbereisen, R. K., & Wedding, U. (2007). Social support and survival in patients with acute myeloid leukaemia. *Supportive Care in Cancer, 15*, 81–87.

Pollard, J. W. (2004). Tumour-educated macrophages promote tumour progression and metastasis. *Nature Reviews: Cancer, 4*, 71–78.

Porrata, L. F., Litzow, M., & Markovic, S. N. (2001). Immune reconstitution after autologous hematopoietic stem cell transplantation. *Mayo Clinic Proceedings, 76*, 407–412.

Porrata, L. F., & Markovic, S. N. (2004). Timely reconstitution of immune competence affects clinical outcome following autologous stem cell transplantation. *Clinical and Experimental Medicine, 4*, 78–85.

Price, M., Tennant, C., Smith, R., Butow, P., Kennedy, S., Kossoff, M., et al. (2001). The role of psychosocial factors in the development of breast carcinoma part 1: The cancer prone personality. *Cancer, 91*, 679–685.

Protheroe, D., Turvey, K., Horgan, K., Benson, E., Bowers, D., & House, A. (1999). Stressful life events and difficulties and onset of breast cancer: Case-control study. *British Medical Journal, 319*, 1027–1030.

Pyter, L. M., Pineros, V., Glalang, J. A., McClintock, M. K., & Prendergast, B. J. (2010). Peripheral tumors induce depressive-like behaviors and cytokine production and alter hypothalamic-pituitary-adrenal axis regulation. *Proceedings of the National Academy of Sciences, 106*, 9069–9074.

Raison, C. L., Capuron, L., & Miller, A. H. (2006). Cytokines sing the blues: Inflammation and the pathogenesis of depression. *TRENDS in Immunology, 27*, 24–31.

Raison, C. L., & Miller, A. H. (2003). When not enough is too much: The role of insufficient glucocoticoid signaling in the pathophysiology of stress-related disorders. *American Journal of Psychiatry, 160*, 1554–1565.

Ramirez, F. (1998). Glucocorticoids induce a Th2 response in vitro. *Developmental Immunology, 6*, 233–243.

Rangarajan, S., Enserink, J. M., Kuiperij, H. B., de Rooij, J., Price, L. S., Schwede, F., et al. (2003). Cyclic AMP induces integrin-mediated cell adhesion through Epac and Rap1 upon stimulation of the β 2-adrenergic receptor. *Journal of Cell Biology, 160*, 487–493.

Reiche, E. M., Nunes, S. O., & Morimoto, H. K. (2004). Stress, depression, the immune system, and cancer. *Lancet Oncology, 5*, 617–625.

Reynolds, P., Boyd, P. T., Blacklow, R. S., Jackson, J. S., Greenberg, R. S., Austin, D. F., et al. (1994). The relationship between social ties and survival among black and white breast cancer patients: National Cancer Institute Black/White Cancer Survival Study Group. *Cancer Epidemiology, Biomarkers and Prevention, 3*, 253–259.

Reynolds, P., Hurley, S., Torres, M., Jackson, J., Boyd, P. T., Chen, V. W., et al. (2000). Use of coping strategies and breast cancer survival: Results from the Black/White Cancer Survival Study. *American Journal of Epidemiology, 152*, 940–949.

Rich, T., Innominato, P. F., Boerner, J., Mormont, M. C., Iacobelli, S., Baron, B., et al. (2005). Elevated serum cytokines correlated with altered behavior, serum cortisol rhythm, and dampened 24-hour rest-activity patterns in patients

with metastic colorectal cancer. *Clinical Cancer Research, 11*, 1757–1764.

Rodemann, H. P., & Bamberg, M. (1995). Cellular basis of radiation-induced fibrosis. *Radiotherapy and Oncology, 35*, 83–90.

Rodrigue, J. R., Pearman, T. P., & Moreb, J. (1999). Morbidity and mortality following bone marrow transplantation: Predictive utility of pre-BMT affective functioning, compliance, and social support stability. *International Journal of Behavioral Medicine, 6*, 241–254.

Saito-Nakaya, K., Nakaya, N., Fujimori, M., Akizuki, N., Yoshikawa, E., Kobayakawa, M., et al. (2006). Marital status, social support and survival after curative resection in non-small-cell lung cancer. *Cancer Science, 97*, 206–213.

Sapolsky, R. M., Alberts, S. C., & Altmann, J. (1997). Hypercortisolism associated with social subordinance or social isolation among wild baboons. *Archives of General Psychiatry, 54*, 1137–1143.

Sapolsky, R., Krey, L., & McEwen, B. (1986). The neuroendocrinology of stress and aging: the glucocorticoid cascade hypothesis. *Endocrinology Review, 7*, 284–301.

Saul, A. N., Oberyszyn, T. M., Daugherty, C., Kusewitt, D., Jones, S., Jewell, S., et al. (2005). Chronic stress and susceptibility to skin cancer. *Journal of the National Cancer Institute, 97*, 1760–1767.

Scambia, G., Testa, U., Benedetti, P., Foti, E., Nartucci, R., Gadducci, A., et al. (1995). Prognostic significance of IL-6 serum levels in patients with ovarian cancer. *British Journal of Cancer, 71*, 352–356.

Schantz, S., & Goephert, H. (1987). Multimodal therapy and distant metastasis: The impact of NK cell activity. *Archives Otolaryngology Head and Neck Surgery, 113*, 1207–1213.

Schofield, P., Ball, D., Smith, J. G., Borland, R., O'Brien, P., Davis, S., et al. (2004). *Cancer, 100*, 1276–1282.

Schulz, R., Drayer, R. A., & Rollman, B. L. (2002). Depression as a risk factor for non-suicide mortality in the elderly. *Biological Psychiatry, 52*, 205–225.

Seeman, T., & McEwen, B. (1996). Impact of social environment characterisitics on neuroendocrine regulation. *Psychosomatic Medicine, 58*, 459–471.

Seeman, T. E., Singer, B. H., Rowe, J. W., Horwitz, R. I., & McEwen, B. (1997). Price of adaptation: Allostatic load and its health consequences. *Archives of Internal Medicine, 157*, 2259–2268.

Sephton, S. E., Dhabhar, F. S., Keuroghlian, A. S., Giese-Davis, J., McEwen, B. S., Ionan, A. C., et al. (2009). Depression, cortisol, and suppressed cell-mediated immunity in metastatic breast cancer. *Brain, Behavior, & Immunity, 23*, 1148–1155.

Sephton, S., Sapolsky, R. M., Kraemer, H. C., & Speigel, D. (2000). Early mortality in metastatic breast cancer patients with absent of abnormal diurnal cortisol rhythms. *Journal of the National Cancer Institute, 92*, 994–1000.

Sephton, S., & Spiegel, D. (2003). Circadian disruption in cancer: A neuroendocrine-immune pathway from stress to disease? *Brain, Behavior, and Immunity, 17*, 321–328.

Shakhar, G., & Ben-Eliyahu, S. (2003). Potential prophylactic measures against postoperative immunosuppression: Could they reduce recurrence rates in oncological patients? *Annals of Clinical Oncology, 10*, 972–992.

Sharma, A., Greenman, J., Sharp, D. M., Walker, L. G., & Monson, J. R. (2008). Vascular endothelial growth factor and psychosocial factors in colorectal cancer. *Psychooncology, 17,* 66–73.

Sica, A., Allavena, P., & Mantovani, A. (2008). Cancer related inflammation: The macrophage connection. *Cancer Letters, 267,* 204–215.

Sica, A., Schioppa, T., Mantovani, A., & Allavena, P. (2006). Tumour-associated macrophages are a distinct M2 polarised population promoting tumour. *European Journal of Cancer, 42,* 717–727.

Skobe, M., & Fusenig, N. E. (1998). Tumorigenic conversion of immortal human keratinocytres through stromal cell activation. *Proceedings of the National Academy of Sciences of the United States of America, 95,* 1050–1055.

Sloan, E. K., Priceman, S. J., Cox, B. F., Yu, S., Pimentel, M. A., Tangkanangnukul, V., et al. (2010). The sympathetic nervous system induces a metastatic switch in primary breast cancer. *Cancer Research, 70,* 7042–7052.

Smyth, M. J., Cretney, E., Kelly, J. M., Westwood, J. A., Street, S. E., Yagita, H., et al. (2005). Activation of NK cell cytotoxicity. *Molecular Immunology, 42,* 501–510.

Soler-Vila, H., Kasi, S. V., & Jones, B. A. (2003). Prognostic significance of psychosocial factors in African-American and white breast cancer patients: A population-based study. *Cancer, 98,* 1299–1308.

Sood, A. K., Armaiz-Pena, G., Halder, J., Nick, A., Stone, R., Hu, W., et al. (2010). Adrenergic modulation of focal adhesion kinase protects human ovarian cancer cells from anoikis. *Journal of Clinical Investigation, 120,* 1515–1523.

Sood, A. K., Bhatty, R., Kamat, A. A., Landen, C. N., Han, L., Thaker, P. H., et al. (2006). Stress hormone mediated invasion of ovarian cancer cells. *Clinical Cancer Research, 12,* 369–375.

Sood, A. K., Coffin, J. E., Schneider, G. B., Fletcher, M. S., DeYoung, B. R., Gruman, L. M., et al. (2004). Biological significance of focal adhesion kinase in ovarian cancer: Role in migration and invasion. *American Journal of Pathology, 165,* 1087–1095.

Sood, A. K., Fletcher, M. S., Coffin, J. E., Yang, M., Seftor, E. A., Gruman, L. M., et al. (2004). Functional role of matrix metalloprotineases in ovarian tumor cell plasticity. *American Journal of Obstetrics and Gynecology, 190,* 899–909.

Sood, A., Lutgendorf, S., & Cole, S. (2007). Neuroendocrine regulation of cancer progression I: Biological mechanisms and clinical relevance. In N. C. R. Ader & D., Felten (Eds.), *Psychoneuroimmunology* (Vol. IV, pp. 233–250). San Diego, CA: Elsevier.

Spiegel, D., Butler, L. D., Giese-Davis, J., Koopman, C., Miller, E., DiMiceli, S., et al. (2007). Effects of supportive-expressive group therapy on survival of patients with metastatic breast cancer: A randomized prospective trial. *Cancer, 110,* 1130–1138.

Spiegel, D., & Giese-Davis, J. (2003). Depression and cancer: Mechanisms and disease progression. *Biological Psychiatry, 54,* 269–282.

Spiegel, D., Giese-Davis, J., Taylor, C. B., & Kraemer, H. (2006). Stress sensitivity in metastic breast cancer: Analysis of hypothalamic-pituitary-adrenal axis function. *Psychoneuroendocrinology, 31,* 1231–1244.

Spoletini, I., Gianni, W., Repetto, L., Bria, P., Caltagirone, C., Bossù, P., et al. (2008). Depression and cancer: An unexplored and unresolved emergent issue in elderly patients. *Critical Reviews in Oncology/Hematology, 65,* 143–155.

Steel, J. L., Geller, D. A., Gamblin, T. C., Olek, M. C., & Carr, B. I. (2007). Depression, immunity, and survival in patients with hepatobiliary carcinoma. *Journal of Clinical Oncology, 25,* 2397–2405.

Stommel, M., Given, B. A., & Given, C. W. (2002). Depression and functional status as predictors of death among cancer patients. *Cancer, 94,* 2719–2727.

Suls, J., & Fletcher, B. (1985). The relative efficacy of avoidant and nonavoidant coping strategies: A meta-analysis. *Health Psychology, 4,* 249–288.

Szelenyi, J., Kiss, J. P., Puskas, E., Szelenyi, M., & Vizi, E. S. (2000). Contribution of differently localized alpha 2- and beta-adrenoceptors in the modulation of TNF-alpha and IL-10 production in endotoxemic mice. *Annals of the New York Academy of Sciences, 917,* 145–153.

Szlosarek, P., Charles, K. A., & Balkwill, F. R. (2006). Tumour necrosis factor-a as a tumour promoter. *European Journal of Cancer, 42,* 745–750.

Temoshok, L., Heller, B., Sagebiel, R. W., Blois, M. S., Sweet, D. M., DiClemente, R. J., et al. (1985). The relationship of psychosocial factors to prognostic indicators in cutaneous malignant melanoma. *Journal of Psychosomatic Research, 29,* 139–153.

Tempfer, C., Zeisler, H., Sliutz, G., Haeusler, G., E., H., & Kainz, C. (1997). Serum evaluation of interleukin 6 in ovarian cancer patients. *Gynecologic Oncology, 66,* 27–30.

Textor, S., Dürst, M., Jansen, L., Accardi, R., Tommasino, M., Trunk, M. J., et al. (2008). Activating NK cell receptor ligands are differentially expressed during progression to cervical cancer. *International Journal of Cancer, 123,* 2343–2353.

Thaker, P., Han, L. Y., Kamat, A. A., Arevalo, J. M., Takahashi, R., Lu C., et al. (2006). Chronic stress promotes tumor growth and metastasis in ovarian carcinoma. *Nature Medicine, 12,* 939–944.

Thornton, L. M., Andersen, B. L., Crespin, T. R., & Carson, W. E. (2007). Individual trajectories in stress covary with immunity during recovery from cancer diagnosis and treatments. *Brain, Behavior, and Immunity, 21,* 185–194.

Thornton, L. M., Andersen, B. L., Schuler, T. A., & Carson, W. E. (2009). A psychological intervention reduces inflammatory markers by alleviating depressive symptoms: Secondary analysis of a randomized controlled trial. *Psychosomatic Medicine, 71,* 715–724.

Tjemsland, T., Soreide, J. A., Matre, R., & Malt, U. F. (1997). Preoperative psychological variables predict immunological status in patients with operable breast cancer. *Psycho-Oncology, 6,* 311–320.

Torng, P. L., Mao, T. L., Chan, W. Y., Huang, S. C., & Lin, C. T. (2004). Prognostic significance of stromal metalloproteinase-2 in ovarian adenocarcinoma and its relation to carcinoma progression. *Gynecologic Oncology, 92,* 559–567.

Touitou, Y., Bogdan, A., Levi, F., Benavides, M., & Auzeby, A. (1996). Disruption of the circadian patterns of serum cortisol in breast and ovarian cancer patients: Relationships with tumour marker antigens. *British Journal of Cancer, 74,* 1248–1252.

Touitou, Y., Levi, F., Bogdan, A., Benavides, M., Bailleul, F., & Misser, J.-L. (1995). Rhythm alteration in patients with metastatic breast cancer and poor prognostic factors. *Journal of Cancer Research and Clinical Oncology, 121,* 181–188.

Tross, S., Herndon, J. N., Korzun, A., Kornblith, A. B., Cella, D. F., Holland, J. F., et al. (1996). Psychological symptoms and disease-free and overall survival in women with stage II breast cancer: Cancer and leukemia Group B. *Journal of the National Cancer Institute, 88,* 661–667.

Tschuschke, V., Hertenstein, B., Arnold, R., Bunjes, D., Denzinger, R., & Kaechele, H. (2001). Associations between coping and survival time of adults leukemia patients receiving allogeneic bone marrow transplantation: Results of a prospective study. *Journal of Psychosomatic research, 50,* 277–285.

Tsutsui, S., Yasuda, K., Suzuki, K., Tahara, K., Higashi, H., & Era, S. (2005). Macrophage infiltration and its prognostic implications in breast cancer: The relationship with VEGF expression and microvessel density. *Oncology Reports, 14,* 425–431.

Turner-Cobb, J., Sephton, S., Koopman, C., Blake-Mortimer, J., & Spiegel, D. (2000). Social support and salivary cortisol in women with metastatic breast cancer. *Psychosomatic Medicine, 62,* 337–345.

Uchida, A., Kariya, Y., Okamoto, N., Sugie, K., Fujimoto, T., & Yagita, M. (1990). Prediction of postoperative clinical course by autologous tumor-killing activity in lung cancer patients. *Journal of the National Cancer Institute, 82,* 1697–1701.

Van Miert, A. (2002). Present concepts on the inflammatory modulators with special reference to cytokines. *Veterinary Research Communications, 26,* 111–126.

Vandewalle, B., Revillion, F., & Lefebvre, J. (1990). Functional beta-adrenergic receptors in breast cancer cells. *Journal of Cancer Research and Clinical Oncology, 116,* 303–306.

VanTits, L., Michel, M., Grosse-Wilde, H., Happel, M., Eigler, F., Solimam, A., et al. (1990). Catecholamines increase lymphocyte beta-2-adrenergic receptors via a beta-2-adrenergic, spleen dependent process. *American Journal of Physiology, 258,* E191–E202.

Vaquer, S., Jordá, J., López de la Osa, E., Alvarez de los Heros, J., López-García, N., & Alvarez de Mon, M. (1990). Clinical implications of natural killer (NK) cytotoxicity in patients with squamous cell carcinoma of the uterine cervix. *Gynecologic Oncology, 36,* 90–92.

Varker, K. A., Terrell, C. E., Welt, M., Suleiman, S., Thornton, L., Andersen, B., et al. (2007). Impaired natural killer cell lysis in breast cancer patients with high levels of psycholigcal stress is associated with altered expression of killer immunoglobin-like receptors. *Journal of Surgical Research, 139,* 36–44.

Veith, R. C., Lewis, N., Linares, O. A., Barnes, R. F., Raskind, M. A., Villacres, E. C., et al. (1994). Sympathetic nervous system activity in major depression: Basal and desipramine-induced alterations in plasma norepinephrine kinetics. *Archives of General Psychiatry, 51,* 411–422.

Von Ah, D., Kang, D., & Carpenter, J. (2007). Stress, optimism, and social support: Impact on immune responses in breast cancer. *Research in Nursing & Health, 30,* 72–83.

Watson, M., Haviland, J. S., Greer, S., Davidson, J., & Bliss, J. M. (1999). Influence of psychological response on survival in breast cancer: A population-based cohort study. *Lancet, 354,* 1331–1336.

Waxler-Morrison, N., Hislop, T. G., Mears, B., & Kan, L. (1991). Effects of social relationships on survival for women with breast cancer: A prospective study. *Social Science & Medicine, 33,* 177–183.

Way, B. M., & Taylor, S. E. (2010). Social influences on health: Is serotonin a critical mediator? *Psychosomatic Medicine, 72,* 107–112.

Weihs, K. L., Enright, T. M., Simmens, S. J., & Reiss, D. (2000). Negative affectivity, restriction of emotions, and site of metastases predict mortality in recurrent breast cancer. *Journal of Psychosomatic Research, 49,* 59–68.

Weihs, K. L., Simmens, S. J., Mizrahi, J., Enright, T. M., Hunt, M. E., & Siegel, R. S. (2005). Dependable social relationships predict overall survival in Stages II and III breast carcinoma patients. *Journal of psychosomatic research, 59,* 299–306.

Weiner, H. (1992). *Perturbing the organism: The biology of stressful experience.* Chicago: University of Chicago Press.

Weinrib, A., Sephton, S. E., DeGeest, K., Penedo, F., Bender, D., Zimmerman, B., et al. (2010). Diurnal cortisol dysregulation, functional disability, and depression in women with ovarian cancer. *Cancer, 116,* 4410–4419.

Whiteside, T., & Herberman, R. (1989). The role of natural killer cells in human disease. *Clinical Immunology Immunopathology, 53,* 1–23.

Williams, J. B., Pang, D., Delgado, B., Kocherginsky, M., Tretiakova, M., Krausz, T., et al. (2009). A model of gene-environment interaction reveals altered mammary gland gene expression and increased tumor growth following social isolation. *Cancer Preventative Research, 2,* 850–61.

Yang, E., Bane, C. M., MacCallum, R. C., Kiecolt-Glaser, J. K., Malarkey, W. B., & Glaser, R. (2002). Stress-related modulation of matrix metalloproteinase expression. *Journal of Neuroimmunology, 133,* 144–150.

Yang, E. V., Kim, S. J., Donovan, E. L., Chen, M., Gross, A. C., Webster Marketon, J. I., et al. (2009). Norepinephrine upregulates VEGF, IL-8, and IL-6 expression in human melanoma tumor cell lines: implications for stress-related enhancement of tumor progression. *Brain, Behavior, & Immunity, 23,* 267–275.

Yang, E. V., Sood, A. K., Chen, M., Li, Y., Eubank, T. D., Marsh, C. B., et al. (2006). Norepinephrine up-regulates the expression of vascular endothelial growth factor, matrix metalloproteinase (MMP)-2, and MMP-9 in nasopharyngeal carcinoma tumor cells. *Cancer Research, 66,* 10357–10364.

Zhou, D., Kusnecov, A., Shurin, M., dePaoli, M., & Rabin, B. (1993). Exposure to physical and psychological stressors elevates plasma interleukin-6: Relationship to the activation of hypothalamic-pituitary-adrenal axis. *Endocrinology, 133,* 2523–2530.

Zhou, F. L., Zhang, W. G., Wei, Y. C., Xu, L. Y., Wang, X. S., & Li, M. Z. (2005). Impact of comorbid anxiety and depression on quality of life and cellular immunity changes in patients with digestive tract cancers. *World Journal of Gastroenterology, 11,* 2313–18.

Zhou, J., Olsen, S., Moldovan, J., Fu, X., Sarkar, F., Moudgil, V., et al. (1997). Glucocorticoid regulation of natural cytotoxicity: Effects of cortisol on the phenotype and function of a cloned human natural killer cell line. *Cellular Immunology, 178,* 108–116.

Zorrilla, E. P., Luborsky, L., & McKay, J. R. (2001). The relationship of depression and stressors to immunological assays: A meta-analytic review. *Brain, Behavior, and Immunity, 15,* 199–226.

Regulation of Target System Sensitivity in Neuroinflammation: Role of GRK2 in Chronic Pain

Annemieke Kavelaars, Anibal Garza Carbajal, *and* Cobi J. Heijnen

Abstract

Scientists and clinicians have long used the *level* of hormones or the *level* of inflammatory mediators as an important parameter of functional activity of the neuro-endocrine or immune system. However, not much focus has been given to the role of the *sensitivity* of the target tissue, such as receptors or components of the intracellular signalosome. This is important because, as recent literature has shown, the sensitivity of the target tissue may change during pathological processes such as inflammation or chronic stress. This chapter focuses on changes in sensitivity of target tissue by focussing on a kinase known as G protein receptor kinase 2 (GRK2), which appears to be an important regulator of the severity and duration of inflammatory pain. GRK2 regulates the sensitivity of target systems, including immune and nervous systems, for signals given by G protein-coupled receptors via regulating receptor desensitization. In addition, GRK2 regulates intracellular signaling via direct effects on elements of the signalosome of the cell. The contribution of GRK2 to chronic pain is discussed in the context of the idea that regulation of the sensitivity of target systems is an important process during neuro-inflammation and should be taken into account when investigating neuro-immune communication in inflammatory pathologies.

Key Words: hyperalgesia, cellular signaling, neuro-inflammation, cellular signaling; Cre-Lox technology, G protein-coupled receptors, central sensitization, chronic pain

Introduction

It is now well established that bidirectional neuro-immune communication contributes to regulation of the immune response as well as to regulation of the behavioral response to infection, tissue damage, and inflammation (Dantzer & Kelley 2007). Cells of the immune system express receptors for hormones and neurotransmitters and, conversely, cells in the central nervous system are capable of responding to signals given by inflammatory mediators via expression of their cognate receptors (Blalock & Smith 1985). When examining neuro-immune interactions, the focus has long been on determining changes in the level of hormones and neurotransmitters in an attempt to relate these changes to changes in the activity of the immune system. Conversely, many studies measure circulating levels of cytokines or chemokines to determine the relation between these mediators of inflammation and specific behavioral characteristics. Although such studies have provided important information on the possible functional relations between immune system and nervous system, a major aspect of neuro-immune communication may well be missed by focusing on soluble mediator production when describing and investigating this interaction. We propose that, in fact, the receivers of these communication signals, that is, specific receptors for hormones, neurotransmitters, cytokines, chemokines, and so forth, are as important in determining the functional consequences of neuro-immune communication (Heijnen & Kavelaars 1999). This chapter describes a specific molecular mechanism by which neuro-immune communication is regulated at the level of the sensitivity of the target system. The focus is on the effect of inflammatory processes on the regulation of the sensitivity of receptors for hormones, neurotransmitters, and inflammatory mediators with a special emphasis on inflammatory pain.

In the first part of this chapter, we will describe some general mechanisms involved in regulation of receptor function on target cells. We zoom in on a specific class of receptors, that is, the class of G protein-coupled receptors (GPCR) and describe how inflammatory disorders can change the functioning of receptors of the GPCR class. GPCR functioning is regulated by a kinase known as G protein coupled receptor kinase 2 (GRK2). We will describe how the expression of this key regulator of signaling is modulated in the context of chronic inflammation and how changes in the level of expression of GRK2 affect the course of inflammatory disorders. Finally, we will summarize recent evidence from our work showing that GRK2 is an important regulator of inflammatory pain.

Interindividual Differences in Sensitivity of the Target System

There are multiple examples of interindividual differences in sensitivity of the target system to signals provided by hormones and neurotransmitters. These interindividual differences in the response of target systems to signals provided by hormones and neurotransmitters can sometimes be related to genetic factors. Multiple studies have presented evidence for the relation between specific single nucleotide polymorphisms in genes encoding receptors that determine how patients will respond to medication (Mellen & Herrington 2005; Polanczyk, Bigarella, Hutz, & Rohde, 2010; Tsikouris & Peeters 2007). For example, there is evidence that common genetic polymorphism in the angiotensin receptor or in angiotensin converting enzyme can predict the response to treatment with antihypertensive medication. These and similar findings have evoked the idea that the efficacy of pharmacological intervention can be markedly increased by the design of tailored treatments that take these genetic differences in receptor reactivity into account.

Interindividual differences in the response to hormones and neurotransmitters can also be associated with developmental aspects or with environmental factors such as exposure to stress, prolonged treatment with agonists, or chronic inflammation. For example, by comparing the effect of the glucocorticoid agonist dexamethasone on lymphocyte proliferation at various stages during human development we showed that the sensitivity of these cells to regulation by dexamethasone is lower in adulthood than in newborns. At birth, lymphocytes from cord blood are much more sensitive to the inhibitory effects of dexamethasone on cell proliferation than lymphocytes from peripheral blood obtained from adults. During the first year of life, sensitivity to glucocorticoids gradually decreases to reach adult levels at an age of 1–2 years (Kavelaars et al. 1995; Kavelaars et al. 1996).

There is also evidence that exposure to traumatic events can modify the response of cells from the immune system to regulation by dexamethasone. We have shown that lymphocytes from veterans, who had been exposed to a traumatic event during military deployment and developed posttraumatic stress disorder, are relatively resistant to inhibition by dexamethasone of mitogen-induced T lymphocyte proliferation (de Kloet et al. 2007).

Interestingly, our most recent studies have shown that glucocorticoid binding characteristics of peripheral blood mononuclear cells before exposure to a traumatic event may even predict the likelihood of developing posttraumatic stress disorder (van Zuiden et al. 2011). Apparently, the status of intracellular glucocorticoid receptors in peripheral blood leukocytes reflects a certain capacity of the individual to deal with trauma at the psychological level. Whether there is a causal relation between GR and trauma sensitivity or whether it can only be classified as a possible biomarker for vulnerability to develop posttraumatic stress symptoms remains to be evaluated in experimental mechanistic studies.

Other well-known examples of pathological conditions that are associated with changes in the sensitivity of target systems to signals provided by the neuroendocrine system include insulin resistance in patients with type II diabetes. In this case, there is direct evidence that the resistance of insulin receptors on target cells (e.g., adipose cells and skeletal muscle) to insulin is responsible for the pathology associated with type II diabetes (Eckardt, Taube, & Eckel, 2011).

Prolonged exposure to certain agonists, such as occurs in patients receiving morphine-treatment for prolonged pain, can cause desensitization of the target system via a cellular mechanism that involves uncoupling of receptors from the intracellular signaling pathways and subsequent internalization of a specific receptor, in this case the μ-opioid receptor, in a process called desensitization (Mao,

Price, & Mayer, 1995). Similarly, chronic treatment of asthma patients with beta-adrenergic receptor agonists may lead to desensitization of the receptor and, consequently, therapy resistance (Black, Oliver, & Roth, 2009).

Collectively, the findings just summarized underline the need to take the possibility into account that the *reactivity* of the relevant target system is a major player in neuro-immune interactions and subsequent pathology. In this chapter, we will focus on the contribution of a kinase known as G protein-coupled receptor kinase 2 (GRK2) which regulates the sensitivity of the target tissues (Premont & Gainetdinov 2007), to the regulation of neuro-immune interactions in the context of inflammatory pain.

Mechanisms Regulating Target System Sensitivity for G Protein-coupled Receptors

G protein-coupled receptors or 7-trans membrane domain receptors form the largest family of membrane receptors. They play a key role in multiple physiological processes as is attested by the notion that more than 50% of all drugs that are currently on the market target a G protein-coupled receptor or its immediate signaling routes (Brink, Harvey, Bodenstein, Venter, & Oliver, 2004; Gudermann, Nurnberg, & Schultz, 1995). There is a wide array of GPCRs involved in neuro-immune interactions. For example, inflammatory mediators including chemokines, prostaglandins, and leukotrienes as well as a myriad of neuropeptides and neurotransmitters such as substance P, serotonin, epinephrine (EPI), norepinephrine (NE), calcitonin gene-related protein (CGRP), and vasoactive intestinal protein (VIP) signal via GPCRs (Lombardi et al. 2002). Interestingly, GPCR signaling is regulated at multiple levels, and chronic inflammation as well as chronic stress has been implicated in the regulation of GPCR function.

In our laboratory, we have long been interested in the effect of chronic inflammation on the sensitivity of the immune system to regulation by signals from the sympathetic nervous system. In our initial studies, we showed that chronic inflammatory disorders are associated with changes in the subtype of adrenergic receptor expressed on leukocytes. All adrenergic receptors belong to the family of GPCR and can be divided into three main classes: $\alpha 1$, $\alpha 2$, and β-adrenergic receptors, of which each subclass contains multiple subtypes. In a first set of experiments, we analyzed peripheral blood mononuclear cells of patients with juvenile idiopathic arthritis (JIA).

Juvenile idiopathic arthritis is a chronic inflammatory disorder of childhood, and the main characteristic of the disease is chronic inflammation of one or more joints. The disease is considered to be a chronic autoimmune disease and, especially in those children in whom multiple joints are affected, treatment can be difficult. Commonly, steroids are used, and if steroid treatment is not effective, cytostatic treatment is often applied. Although the disease can resolve after adolescence, permanent damage to the joints has often occurred and this is a frequent cause of pain and disability. We described that JIA is associated with marked changes in the way cells from the immune system respond to signals given by the catecholamines norepinephrine (NE) and epinephrine (EPI). Lymphocytes from normal, healthy individuals express $\beta 2$-adrenergic receptors ($\beta 2$-AR) on their surface to respond to signals given by NE and EPI (Sanders & Straub 2002). There is some evidence in the literature that macrophages also express $\alpha 2$-AR, but most studies to date show that the other subtypes of adrenergic receptors are not expressed on leukocytes from healthy individuals (Spengler, Chensue, Giacherio, Blenk, & Kunkel, 1994). However, when examining expression of mRNA encoding $\alpha 1$-AR subtypes in peripheral blood mononuclear cells from children with JIA, we observed that cells from most patients contained detectable levels of mRNA encoding one or more subtypes of the α-1 adrenergic receptor subtype. In contrast, samples from 19 out of 20 healthy controls did not express this subtype of adrenergic receptor (Heijnen et al. 1996; Kavelaars, Rouppe van der Voort, & Heijnen, 1999). Functionally, the presence of $\alpha 1$-AR on cells from JIA patients was associated with increased IL-6 production after in vitro stimulation of peripheral blood samples with a specific $\alpha 1$-AR agonist. The in vivo relevance of the presence of these receptors was highlighted by the observation that exposure of patients with JIA to a short-lasting noradrenergic stressor (cold pressor test; 2-minute immersion of one hand in ice water, leading to vasoconstriction and secretion of (nor) epinephrine) induced an increase in IL-6 production (Rouppe van der Voort, Heijnen, Wulffraat, Kuis, & Kavelaars, 2000). In contrast, we did not observe any effect of this acute stressor on IL-6 production in healthy controls. Notably, the increase in plasma NE in response to the stressor did not differ between JIA patients and controls. These findings indicate that the chronic inflammatory process in patients with JIA is associated with the appearance of a specific subtype of receptor on leukocytes that is normally not expressed or functional in these cells, and expression of this receptor subtype leads to pro-inflammatory cytokine production by the target tissue, which may contribute to the pathology of this debilitating chronic arthritis in children.

In adults with rheumatoid arthritis, signaling via adrenergic receptors is also different from healthy individuals, but the underlying mechanism in adults is not the same as in children with JIA. Rheumatoid arthritis is a chronic inflammatory disease in which mainly synovial joints are affected. As a result of the ongoing inflammatory activity in these joints, the articular cartilage of the joints is damaged. At present there is no curative intervention, and treatment focuses on the use of disease-modifying medication, including anti-inflammatory drugs, and steroid and anticytokine interventions. It is known that β2-AR agonists inhibit the LPS-induced production of the pro-inflammatory cytokine TNFα. Comparing the dose-response curves for inhibition of TNFα production in samples from healthy individuals and patients with rheumatoid arthritis revealed that the inhibitory effect of the β2-AR agonist is more profound in the patients than in controls (Lombardi et al. 1999). However, the number of receptors per cell did not differ between cells from rheumatoid arthritis patients and controls. Moreover, the first cellular response to stimulation with a βAR agonist (that is, the increase in intracellular cAMP) was increased in patients compared to controls as well. Based on these findings, we proposed that the chronic inflammatory process in patients with rheumatoid arthritis sensitizes the immune system to catecholaminergic stimulation by affecting the regulation of GPCR signaling and, thereby, the response of cells to catecholamines. If the sensitivity of leukocytes to β-adrenergic signaling could be translated to other target tissues, such as the sympathetic nervous system or the spleen, we can envisage that receptor regulation by (chronic) inflammation may contribute to the pathology of a disease such as rheumatoid arthritis.

G Protein-coupled Receptor Signaling and Desensitization

Signaling via GPCRs involves a rapid and transient change in the level of so-called second messengers—for example, calcium, cAMP, inositol-triphosphate (IP3), and cGMP—in the target cell (Figure 20.1). These second messengers serve to activate further downstream signaling molecules including a myriad of kinases that ultimately regulate the cellular response to the GPCR ligand. An important feature of GPCR signaling is that the response is rapid and transient. Moreover, it is well known that, upon stimulation with a GPCR ligand, cells become temporarily refractory to restimulation with the same agonist. This process is known as homologous receptor desensitization, and members of the G protein-coupled receptor kinase (GRK) family play a central role in this process (Premont & Gainetdinov 2007; Vroon, Heijnen, & Kavelaars, 2006).

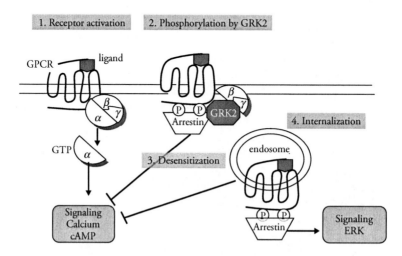

Figure 20.1 G protein-coupled receptor signaling and desensitization by GRK2. Ligand binding induces activation of a heterotrimeric G protein, leading to the activation of second messenger signaling. Receptor activation also leads to recruitment of GRK2 and phosphorylation of the intracellular domain of the receptor. The phosphorylation of the GPCR facilitates binding of arrestins, which promotes internalization of the receptor. Upon internalization, the GPCR can be targeted to degradation, re-expression, and/or further activation of signaling via the GPCR/arrrestin complex.

GRK2 is the most widely studied member of the GRK family. GRK2 is a ubiquitously expressed kinase that restrains GPCR-signaling by interfering at various levels of the transduction cascade. The classical, first described pathway that GRK2 uses to protect cells against overstimulation takes place at the level of the G protein coupled receptor (Figure 20.1). When a GPCR is activated by its ligand, conformational changes in the receptor unmask phosphorylation sites for GRKs in the intracellular domains of the receptor. The phosphorylated residues, in turn, act as binding sites for proteins from the β-arrestin family, which are recruited to the activated receptor. Binding of these β-arrestin proteins to the receptor uncouples the receptor from its interaction with heterotrimeric G-proteins, thereby terminating this phase of the response to the ligand. Via this mechanism GRK2 regulates termination of receptor signaling and protects cells against overstimulation by GPCR ligands. This mechanism constitutes not only the main desensitization mechanism for many GPCRs, but also a necessary step for the endocytosis and recycling of the receptor to the membrane (Pitcher, Freedman, & Lefkowitz, 1998).

Increasing evidence suggests that the regulatory function of GRK2 extends well beyond this first identified action of this serine kinase. GRK2 also phosphorylates and inhibits activity of receptors that do not belong to the GPCR class of receptors, such as the receptors for the growth factor PDGF that signals via a tyrosine kinase receptor (Hildreth et al. 2004). In addition, GRK2 directly binds and phosphorylates proteins that are associated with the cytoskeleton including tubulin, synuclein, and ezrin, as well as the transcription factor DREAM (Lombardi, Kavelaars, & Heijnen, 2002; Vroon et al. 2006; Jurado-Pueyo, Campos, Mayor, & Murga, 2008). Even more excitingly, it has recently become clear that GRK2 also directly regulates the activity of a variety of nonreceptor signaling proteins including members of the MAP kinase family, PI3kinase, and Smad (Jimenez-Sainz et al. 2006). As this mode of action of GRK2 depends on direct interaction of GRK2 with intracellular kinases or other regulators of cellular activity, it does not require GPCR activation, but it can regulate cellular responses to other stimuli that act via receptors that do not belong to the GPCR class of receptors. Interestingly, there is a large body of evidence linking activity of the MAPkinase p38 to cytokine-induced pain and depression (Bruchas et al. 2007; Ji & Suter 2007). Therefore, the recent finding that GRK2 is an endogenous inhibitor of p38 deserves further attention in the study on neuroinflammation and cytokine-induced sickness behavior and depression (see section on The Role of GRK2 in Pain).

(Neuro)inflammatory Processes are Associated with Changes in GRK2 Level

In view of the wide variety of functions of GRK2 in terminating signaling and preventing overstimulation of cells, it is not surprising that its intracellular level is tightly regulated and that a number of pathological conditions are associated with alterations in GRK2 expression.

Our initial studies have shown that peripheral blood mononuclear cells from patients with the chronic inflammatory disease rheumatoid arthritis express a reduced level of GRK2 (Lombardi et al. 1999). A similar observation was made when comparing GRK2 levels in peripheral blood mononuclear cells from patients with multiple sclerosis and healthy individuals (Vroon et al. 2005). Multiple sclerosis is a relapsing remitting disorder associated with chronic inflammation in which the myelin sheets around neurons becomes damaged. As a consequence, patients suffer from a variety of neurological problems including motor deficits and sensory impairments. Further studies indicated that this decrease in GRK2 protein expression may well be due to the ongoing inflammatory response in these individuals. First of all, induction of adjuvant arthritis in rats, an animal model of rheumatoid arthritis in humans, induces a reduction in splenocyte GRK2 protein that restores to baseline levels after remission of the disease (Lombardi et al., 2001). Similarly, experimental autoimmune encephalomyelitis (EAE), a rat model for multiple sclerosis in humans, induces a marked reduction in splenocyte GRK2 that also normalizes after resolution of EAE (Vroon, Lombardi, Kavelaars, & Heijnen, 2003). Inflammatory processes in the central nervous system have also been reported to be associated with a reduction in GRK2. For example, exposure of neonatal rats or mice to hypoxic-ischemic brain damage induces a reduction in neuronal GRK2 (Lombardi et al. 2004). Interestingly, this reduction in GRK2 protein precedes the loss of neurons, and more recent studies showed that low neuronal GRK2 increases glutamate-induced neuronal death (Nijboer et al. 2008).

The neuro-inflammatory response that develops in response to intracerebroventricular (i.c.v.) infusion of beta amyloid peptide to model Alzheimer disease also induces a decrease in neuronal GRK2 expression, particularly in the temporal cortex. Inhibition of cerebral inflammatory activity by administration of minocycline to inhibit microglia prevents this reduction in GRK2 (Suo, Wu, Citron, Wong, & Festoff, 2004). Similarly, lesioning of the dopaminergic system to model Parkinson disease reduces GRK2 expression in specific areas in the lesioned hemisphere (Ahmed, Bychkov, Gurevich, Benovic, & Gurevich, 2008).

The hypothesis that the reduction in cellular GRK2 level in these models that involve neuroinflammation is mediated by the inflammatory response is supported by results from in vitro studies. Culturing of peripheral blood mononuclear cells, astroglia, or aortic smooth muscle cells with inflammatory mediators like oxygen radicals and pro-inflammatory cytokines reduces the cellular level of GRK2 protein (Cobelens et al. 2007; Lombardi et al. 1999; Penela, Ribas, & Mayor, 2003). More specifically, IL-1β, TNFα, and IFN-γ all inhibit GRK2 promoter activity in aortic smooth muscle cells (Ramos-Ruiz, Penela, Penn, Mayor, 2000). Exposure of peripheral blood mononuclear cells to oxygen radicals down-regulates GRK2 protein level by increasing the calpain-mediated degradation of the protein (Cobelens et al. 2007; Lombardi et al. 2007). Finally, LPS-induced signaling through the TLR4 pathway down-regulates chemokine-induced expression of GRK2 in polymorphonuclear neutrophils (PMN) (Fan & Malik, 2003). In summary, both in vivo and in vitro inflammatory activity can induce a reduction in the level of GRK2 protein in multiple cell types.

Pathophysiological Consequences of GRK2 Deficiency

Down-regulation of GRK2 levels in immune cells during inflammatory disease may represent an *adaptive* mechanism of cells responding to a disease state, but it may also become *maladaptive,* thereby contributing to disease progression. For example, in the cardiac system, there is evidence that the increased level of GRK2 protein that occurs in patients with hypertension or cardiac failure is maladaptive (Choi, Koch, Hunter, & Rockman, 1997; Rockman et al. 1998). Studies in animal models showed that targeted overexpression of GRK2 in vascular smooth muscle results in development of hypertension and cardiac hypertrophy (Eckhart, Ozaki, Tevaearai, Rockman, & Koch, 2002). These findings clearly show that maintaining "normal" GRK2 levels is required for adequate vascular control. Additional evidence of the importance of

normal GRK2 protein levels for physiology comes from gene-deletion models in vivo.

Total knock-out models for GRK2 are not available, because this manipulation causes the death of the organism before birth (Jaber et al. 1996). The lethality of homozygous GRK2 deletion is related to defective formation/function of the heart in the absence of GRK2. Instead, partial deletions of GRK2 as heterozygous GRK2$^{+/-}$ mice have been obtained. Interestingly, the hemizygous deletion of the GRK2 gene in these model systems is sufficient to induce a 40–60% reduction in GRK2 protein, depending on the tissue examined (Vroon et al. 2004; Kleibeuker et al. 2007; Nijboer et al. 2010). As a similar reduction in GRK2 proteins was observed in humans and animals with chronic inflammatory disorders, these mice with a partial GRK2 deficiency represent an excellent model to study the pathophysiological consequences of reduced GRK2.

The more recent development of a mouse transgenic for GRK2 flanked by LoxP sites (GRK2-fLoxP mouse) provides an excellent tool for investigation of the contribution of cell-specific reductions in GRK2 to pathology and physiology by using Cre-Lox technology. This technology uses the capacity of the enzyme Cre (Causes recombination) to remove DNA sequences between two LoxP sites. A LoxP site is a specific short DNA sequence that can be artificially inserted into the DNA at required sites to allow excision of the gene that is flanked by two LoxP sites. Thus, if a certain cell contains two alleles of GRK2 flanked by LoxP sites and at the same time expresses the Cre enzyme, then the GRK2 gene will be removed from the DNA and that cell will not express GRK2. Thus, depending on where or when Cre is expressed, GRK2 deficiency can be induced in specific cells (conditional knockout) or at a specific time (inducible knockout). A widely used application of this technique is the induction of a specific deletion by breeding mice transgenic for a gene of interest flanked by LoxP sites with mice transgenic for Cre under the control of a tamoxifen-inducible promoter. Only when expression of the Cre enzyme is induced by treating offspring with tamoxifen will the gene of interest be removed. Similarly, cell- or tissue-specific deletion can be obtained by crossing mice transgenic for the gene of interest flanked by LoxP sites with mice transgenic for Cre under the control of a cell-specific promoter. Thus, GRK2-fLoxP mice can be used to generate mice with reduced GRK2 only in microglia/macrophages/granulocytes by crossing them with mice transgenic for Cre under the control of the lysozyme M promoter that is only active in microglia/macrophages/granulocytes (LysM-GRK2$^{+/-}$ mice). Similarly, GFAP-Cre mice can be used to generate mice with astrocyte-specific deletion of GRK2, and Calmodulin kinase 2A-Cre mice can serve to generate mice with targeted reduction of GRK2 in forebrain neurons.

Using mice with reduced GRK2 in all cells or in specific cells, we and others have been able to elucidate the contribution of GRK2 to multiple pathophysiological processes. For example, the 40–60% reduction in GRK2 protein in all cells that is present in GRK2$^{+/-}$ mice has important consequences for the course of chronic relapsing, MOG-induced EAE. This rodent model for the human disease multiple sclerosis is based on the induction of a T cell response against myelin oligodendrocyte glycoprotein, an important component of the myelin sheet around neurons. This autoimmune T cell response causes damage to the myelin sheet similar to the damage observed in patients with multiple sclerosis. The extent of paralysis that results from the damage of the myelin is scored as a readout of disease severity. The onset of the disease is significantly advanced in GRK2$^{+/-}$ mice in association with increased early infiltration of T cells into the central nervous system (Vroon et al. 2005). Hypoxic-ischemic brain damage is also increased in these GRK2$^{+/-}$ mice as compared to wild type littermates (Nijboer et al. 2008). Interestingly, this increased sensitivity to hypoxic-ischemic brain damage was also observed in mice with low GRK2 only in CaM-kinase 2a positive neurons (Nijboer et al. 2010). These findings indicate that a low level of GRK2 in forebrain neurons is sufficient to cause increased brain damage. In specific situations, low cellular levels of GRK2 can also have protective effects. For example, GRK2$^{+/-}$ mice are protected against development of type II diabetes in response to aging or high fat diets (Garcia-Guerra et al., 2010).

The first evidence that GRK2 was linked to pain processing came after the observation that the level of GRK2 is decreased in the dorsal horn of the spinal cord in rodent models of chronic pain (Kleibeuker et al., 2007). Before we go further into the role of GRK2 in chronic pain, we will first give some background on chronic pain and the underlying mechanisms.

Chronic Pain as a Health Problem

"Pain" is defined as the perception of an unpleasant sensation originating from a particular region of the body. This definition, which may seem too vague and ambiguous for such a tangible feeling (a toothache can be associated with many adjectives, but ambiguous is rarely one of them), speaks to the subjective nature of pain. Resulting from a combination of the peripheral signals conveyed by sensory neurons specialized in the detection of noxious stimuli and the central processing of these signals, pain arises, not as a direct result of the simple detection of the noxious signal, but as a result of the interpretation by signal processing in the central nervous system.

Pain perception has evolved as a self-protective system for the organism. Tissue damage or stimuli with the potential to cause tissue damage are perceived as painful. This provides the organism with a system to detect and react to the presence of a potential damaging condition, and in this way, the organism can protect its own integrity. Due to the particular noxious nature of the stimulus that elicits nociceptive signals, these signals have a priority status in the constant influx of sensory information to the central nervous system. This priority processing ensures immediate attention and development of a protective reaction from the organism aimed at preventing further damage. The importance of pain as an organism's warning system is evident when we consider the consequences of impaired pain perception, as observed in uncommon disorders as the congenital insensitivity to pain. These individuals do not receive the warning signals, and burns or other serious tissue damage are frequent consequences of the inability to respond to pain signals.

Unfortunately, the opposite condition—a pathological increased pain perception—is by far more common within the population, and has become an important health problem in many countries. Contrary to normal pain perception, most forms of pathological pain do not arise from the presence of noxious stimuli, but from an *abnormal activation* of the pain-sensing systems in response to non-noxious stimulation (Gold & Gebhart 2010). Because these signals are indistinguishable to the nervous system from a true noxious signal, they still call the complete attention of the system and tend to elicit a response. However, in this pathological situation, attempts to elicit an adequate response are utterly pointless and ineffective in terminating the cause of the signal. The abnormal and sustained activity of pain-sensing circuits and associated systems may have another side effect. In a process that has many points in common with certain types of memory, the increased activity of the system can self-consolidate through its neuronal and non-neuronal components, becoming a chronic condition that may be present for decades. The physical, psychological, and social consequences of this condition may affect the quality of life of the patient permanently.

If this scenario was not negative enough for the patient with chronic pain, most of the treatments currently available for this condition are only targeting the pain symptoms and do not correct the cause of the increased pain perception. The latter situation forces the ·patient to keep for years under constant and—in many cases—ineffective medication and palliative treatments.

Chronic pain-related disorders are a widespread pathology. The National Center for Health Statistics in the United States reported that more than 25% of Americans age >20 years (or 76.5 milion) report that they have had a problem with persisting pain of some sort (http://www.cdc.gov/nchs/data/hus/hus06.pdf). The lack of effective treatments for chronic pain is partially a consequence of a lack of understanding of the mechanisms involved in pain perception and its modulation in the organism. Although impressive advances have been achieved in the last years, the understanding of the mechanisms responsible for increased and chronic pain perception is still insufficient. Identification of the processes and components behind the pathophysiology of pain is essential to design new and more successful approaches and tools to treat the causes of pain pathologies.

Normal Pain Signaling

As any sensory information, nociception depends on the transduction of physical forces into electrical currents by the peripheral terminal of the sensory neuron. The difference in potential generated by this process will, in turn, be reflected in the patterns of electrical activity conveyed by the neuron into the spinal cord. Noxious stimuli are perceived as a sensory modality by itself, and its detection is achieved by a specific subset of sensory neurons, denominated nociceptors, that are specialized in the detection of stimuli whose intensity or chemical identity relate to tissue damage. Although many nociceptor sensory terminals constitute simple nude nerve endings, the presence of specialized transduction components on these nerve terminals grants its activation only by a specific subset of stimuli. The transduction components are only partially known, and they include ion channels sensitive to mechanical stress, chemical agents, and temperature. In general, nociceptive neurons are medium- or small-sized neurons with axons belonging to the Aδ or C subtypes. Noxious

modalities include heat, cold, mechanical stress, and certain chemical agents. To which of these modalities a particular nociceptor reacts depends on the transducer combinations expressed in its peripheral terminal. Although most nociceptors are able to react to more than one specific modality, unimodal nociceptors show a marked preference to a certain kind of stimulus. In contrast, polymodal nociceptors are equally stimulated by different types of stimulation. The stimulus preference, conduction characteristics (based on axon diameter, myelinization, and ion channel expression), and particular input area at the dorsal horn of the spinal cord are correlated, showing the functional organization of the nociceptive system. Although the physical forces acting on the nociceptor transduction systems are the same as in other sensory modalities (e.g., pressure or temperature), the particular architecture of the nociceptor terminal and the operational parameters of the transducer apparatus warrant its activation only when the stimulation intensity reaches noxious levels. In this way, low intensity stimuli (innocuous) and high intensity stimuli (noxious) are detected by separate sensory systems and processed in separate ways.

Inflammatory Pain and Peripheral Sensitization

Inflammation constitutes an important indicator of tissue damage, and nociceptors are highly reactive to chemical agents released under inflammatory conditions. Agents such as prostaglandin E2 (PGE_2), substance P, or Interleukin-1β (IL-1β) modify nociceptor function by increasing its sensitivity (peripheral sensitization; Figure 20.2) and reactivity to stimulation, thus creating the phenomenon of hyperalgesia (increased pain sensitivity; Gold and Gebhart 2010). Posttranslational modifications of the signaling components expressed in the nociceptor constitute the basis of these alterations, and, consequently, they are short lived. In the absence of persistent stimulation, these signals fade away as the intracellular machinery of the nociceptor reverts the modifications made in the different components involved. If, on the contrary, the stimulation is sustained, the short-term modifications of the nociceptor initiate second-order modifications, which include changes in protein expression and reorganization of the intracellular components of the cell. These modifications, although functionally similar to the short-term modifications, constitute a much more permanent and profound alteration in the operation of the nociceptor. In a mechanism

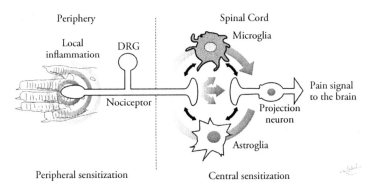

Figure 20.2 Cells involved in pain signaling in the context of inflammation or tissue damage. Exposure of peripheral nociceptors to inflammatory mediators induces an increase in the reactivity of these pain sensing neurons known as peripheral sensitization. When inflammation is ongoing or when nerve damage is occurring, microglia and astroglia in the spinal cord are activated. Local production of inflammatory mediators further enhances pain signaling via a mechanism known as central sensitization.

analogous to the events taking place in the nociceptor, the increased input from the nociceptor induces modifications in ion channels and membrane receptors that increase the gain of the second order neuron to stimulation. In an activity-dependent way, these changes lead to more permanent changes in protein expression and subcellular structures that tend to sustain the increased activity of the neuron. If this activity is sustained long enough, this will finally lead to the modification of the neuronal circuits at the level of the spinal cord and higher areas, in a process involving neuroplastic mechanisms analogous to memory formation and known as central sensitization (Figure 20.2).

Glia and Central Sensitization

Contrary to early interpretations, it is now known that the phenomena related to pain are not purely neurogenic. Glial cells in the CNS have a decisive role in defining pain intensity and duration, although their exact role is still only partially understood (Milligan & Watkins 2009; Ren & Dubner 2010; Romero-Sandoval, Horvath, & DeLeo, 2008). The central nervous system has a neuron:glia proportion of nearly 1:1, and instead of mere bystanders of the neuronal activity, it is now known that glial cells contribute to neuronal signal processing at multiple levels. In the particular context of pain processing, microglia, the inflammatory cells of the CNS, seem to have an important role in the transition from acute to chronic pain in many rodent pain models (Ji & Suter 2007; Milligan & Watkins 2009; Watkins et al. 2007).

Microglia represent more than 10% of the total number of cells in the nervous system. Originating from the mononuclear phagocyte lineage, they constitute the CNS resident macrophages, and are the only immune cells belonging to the CNS. Although their functions –as those of other macrophage populations– include support, defense, and debris-cleaning, several characteristics of microglial cells distinguish them from other monocyte-macrophage subtypes (Graeber 2010). Among these functional characteristics, probably the most important one is the neuromodulatory role that these microglia can exert based on their reciprocal communication with neurons. Microglial cells can express a vast repertoire of ligand-, ion-, and voltage-gated channels; membrane receptors; and an impressive arsenal of signaling molecules, including peptides, cytokines, and neurotransmitters (Colton & Wilcock 2010). This enables microglia to modulate neuronal activity and to be modulated by neuronal signals. Although equipped with the potential to express any of these molecules, microglia express (combinations of) these markers in a function-specific way. This allows macrophages/microglia to exhibit a broad gamut of responses depending on the particular stimulus and the context in which it takes place. Although microglial cells constitute a resident self-renewing population in the nervous system, peripheral macrophages can also access the CNS and can acquire microglial characteristics under certain pathologic conditions. An opposite conversion has been observed in vitro when isolated microglia could be stimulated to acquire a macrophage phenotype. The latter underlines the importance of the (neuronal) environment as a key factor defining the microglial phenotype (Ponomarev, Veremeyko, Barteneva, Krichevsky, & Weiner, 2011).

The CNS is an immunosuppressive environment, and resting microglia resemble in several ways an immunosupressed macrophage. Isolated from the rest of the organism by the blood-brain barrier, neurons and astroglia actively keep microglia in an inhibited state by the expression of soluble factors and surface molecules that act as suppressive factors. The expression of these factors is a direct reflection of the normal operation of the neuronal networks and tissue integrity in the CNS. These signals keep the microglia in a "resting" phenotype, which functionally implies the active surveillance of the neural environment (Ransohoff & Perry 2009). Enabled with multiple philopodial processes radiating from the cell body and a low secretory profile, resting microglia constantly patrol the CNS by sampling and sensing the neural environment. The high motility of microglial cells allows them to cover large areas in a short time and to efficiently migrate toward the source of any distress signal (according to some estimates, a complete brain scan can be achieved in only a few hours by the resident microglia) (Nimmerjahn, Kirchhoff, & Helmchen, 2005).

ATP, glutamate, certain neuropeptides or the presence of foreign molecules are activating signals for the resting microglia (Basbaum, Bautista, Scherrer, & Julius, 2009a). The presence of and the balance between these factors and the inhibitory signals released by the CNS environment will define the activation status of microglial cells. A loss of inhibitory signals and/or an increase in activating signals—such as, for example, occurs in conditions of nerve damage—induces microglial activation and the restructuring of their phenotype (Ransohoff & Perry 2009; Basbaum, Bautista, Scherrer, & Julius, 2009b). Similar to what happens with other macrophage populations, the phenotype of active microglia is shaped by the context and identity of the incoming signals, ensuring a response appropriate to the stimulation. In an oversimplified way, microglia/macrophage phenotype can be classified as defensive-pro-inflammatory (M1) or healing-anti-inflammatory (M2), with multiple intermediate or combined states in between (Martinez, Sica, Mantovani, & Locati, 2008). The M1 phenotype is characterized by the production of pro-inflammatory factors as TNFα, IL-1β, IL-12 and NO. The M2 phenotype is characterized by the inhibited production of pro-inflammatory factors and the production of anti-inflammatory cytokines, like IL-10 and TGFβ. Although macrophage/microglial activation does not follow a linear path,

a progression from M1→M2 is common, because many of the released factors in the M1 phenotype induce the transition to the M2 phenotype, as part of a negative feedback loop. In either state of activation (M1 or M2), the factors released by active microglia can have a large effect on the operation of the CNS. Neurons express receptors for many of the pro-inflammatory factors released in M1, such as TNFα, IL-1β or PGE2 that increase neuronal excitability, and are linked to hyperalgesia observed in inflammatory conditions.

Pain-related neurogenic activation of microglia may arise from changes in the patterns of activity at the level of the nociceptive circuits. The presence of abnormal activity in the dorsal horn terminals from nociceptive afferents has been suggested as a primary cause of microglial activation in several neuropathic pain models (Biggs, Lu, Stebbing, Balasubramanyon, & Smith, 2010). The existing evidence suggests that increases in glutamate and the release of factors such as ATP or substance P (to which microglia are highly reactive) contribute to microglial activation (Gosselin, Suter, Ji, & Decosterd, 2010). Activated microglia in turn releases a second wave of signaling molecules that increase the excitability of the second order neurons and/or provide a positive feedback loop for microglial and astroglial activation. Among these factors is brain-derived neurotropic factor (BDNF), which is important in removing the synaptic inhibition over the second order neuron (Biggs et al. 2010). This, in turn, increases the neuronal input to microglia. Although this process has the potential of developing into an ongoing positive feedback loop, the transition of microglia/macrophages to the M2 phenotype prevents this from happening. In the absence of further external stimulation, the microglial initial response should decrease and disappear as the cells progress to the anti-inflammatory phenotype, allowing the nervous system to return to its normal levels of activity. Recent evidence suggests that IL-10, a powerful immunosuppressive cytokine, seems to be important in the deactivation process (Shechter et al., 2009). Recently, microglial activation has gained increasing interest, as several neuropathologies—Alzheimer and persistent pain included—are associated with persistent microglial activation (Graeber 2010; Lue, Kuo, Beach, & Walker, 2010; Milligan & Watkins 2009; Walker, Sing-Hernandez, Campbell, & Lue, 2009). In the case of chronic pain, in several models, agents suppressing microglial activity (e.g., minocycline) have been shown to have a therapeutic potential

(Ledeboer et al., 2005). Consequently, microglia have been considered as a key element for the establishment of chronic pain via termination of central sensitization.

The Role of GRK2 in Pain

As described in the earlier section, Mechanisms Regulating Target System Sensitivity for G Protein-Coupled Receptors, the kinase GRK2 has the potential to regulate sensitivity of target tissues at the level of GPCRs as well as at the level of intracellular signaling cascades. Chronic pain is a condition in which the sensitivity of target systems has undergone marked changes. Moreover, there is evidence that GPCR ligands play a major role in pain signaling in conditions of chronic pain. Inflammatory activity in the periphery or in the spinal cord has marked consequences for pain signaling and can also lead to reduction of cellular GRK2 protein levels. Based on these findings, we came up with a model for the possible involvement of GRK2 in chronic pain that is depicted in Figure 20.3 We hypothesized that, in response to ongoing inflammatory activity (elevation of cytokines) either in the periphery or in the spinal cord, GRK2 levels in specific cells will be reduced leading to increased and/or prolonged activation of these cells and thereby to an altered sensitivity to painful stimuli.

This hypothesis was tested using a stepwise approach. First, we examined whether chronic neuropathic pain or chronic inflammatory pain were

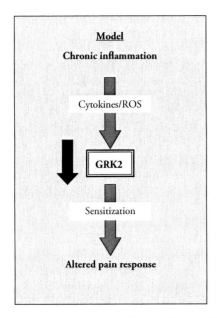

Figure 20.3 Hypothetical model of the contribution of GRK2 to pain. For details see text.

associated with changes in GRK2 protein expression levels in cells that are involved in regulation of the pain response, that is, microglia in the spinal cord and nociceptors.

As predicted, in response to chronic inflammation of the hind paw, the level of GRK2 in nociceptors was decreased (Eijkelkamp, Wang et al. 2010). Interestingly, this decrease in GRK2 protein was limited to a subtype of nociceptors, i.e., the IB4+ nociceptors that are thought to be the main class of nociceptors responsible for the transmission of inflammatory pain signals (Eijkelkamp, Wang, et al. 2010; Wang et al. 2011). In this respect it is of interest that it has now been shown that culturing dorsal root ganglion neurons with the pro-inflammatory cytokine IL-1β reduces GRK2 levels in these cells. In addition, neuropathic pain induced by spinal nerve transection induces also a reduction in GRK2 protein in microglia isolated from the lumbar spinal cord (Eijkelkamp, Heijnen, et al. 2010).

The findings just summarized support the upper part of the hypothesis depicted in Figure 20.3. The next question that needs to be addressed is: Does reduced GRK2 have consequences for the pain response as we hypothesize in the lower part of the scheme Figure 20.3? First of all, we showed that, under baseline conditions, there was no difference in heat withdrawal latency or mechanical sensitivity between WT and GRK2[+/-] mice (Eijkelkamp, Heijnen, et al. 2010; Eijkelkamp, Wang, et al. 2010; Willemen et al. 2010). These findings indicate that low GRK2 does not alter normal pain sensitivity. However, a totally different picture emerges when examining the pain response in WT and GRK2[+/-] mice under inflammatory conditions. It has been known for a long time that induction of a transient inflammatory response in the paw increases pain sensitivity as measured by determining the reduction in the latency to withdraw from a heat source (thermal hyperalgesia) or the reduction in mechanical force needed to induce a withdrawal response (mechanical hyperalgesia). This hyperalgesic response to peripheral inflammation is rapidly induced upon injection of an inflammatory stimulus, for example, carrageenan, pro-inflammatory cytokines, chemokines, or other inflammatory mediators. In wild-type animals, the hyperalgesic response fades away as inflammation resolves. For example, in response to intraplantar injection of a low dose of carrageenan, an extract of seaweed that induces activation of innate immunity via Toll-like receptor 4, thermal hyperalgesia rapidly develops and thermal sensitivity normalizes within approximately 3 days (Figure 20.4; Eijkelkamp,

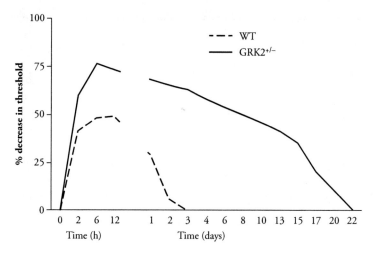

Figure 20.4 Carrageenan induced inflammatory hyperalgesia. Cartoon of the course of carrageenan-induced thermal hyperalgesia in WT and GRK2-deficient mice. X-axis depicts time, Y-axis depicts the decrease in time to withdraw from a heat stimulus after injection of carrageenan into the hind paw. Heat withdrawal latency at baseline was approximately 8 seconds. Based on data presented in Eijkelkamp, Heijnen, et al. 2010.

Heijnen, et al., 2010). However, if the same dose of carrageenan is applied in GRK2[+/−] mice, hyperalgesia lasts up to three weeks. Notably, we did not observe any difference in heat withdrawal latency or mechanical sensitivity at baseline when comparing GRK2[+/−] and WT mice.

Interestingly, the marked prolongation of hyperalgesia in GRK2[+/−] mice was not associated with increased or prolonged inflammatory activity in the paw. Also in response to a single injection of an inflammatory mediator into the hind paw, GRK2[+/−] mice develop markedly prolonged hyperalgesia. For example, CCL3-induced hyperalgesia lasts less than one day in WT mice, but up to 10 days in GRK2[+/−] mice. Similarly, hyperalgesia induced by a single intraplantar injection of IL-1β, epinephrine, and PGE$_2$ lasts markedly longer in GRK2-deficient mice (Eijkelkamp, Heijnen, et al. 2010; Eijkelkamp, Wang, et al. 2010; Willemen et al. 2010).

GRK2-deficiency does not only prolong inflammatory hyperalgesia, it also increases the hyperalgesic response to some but not all stimuli. In fact, existing evidence indicates that in GRK2[+/−] mice, the acute hyperalgesic response to the GPCR ligands CCL3, PGE$_2$, and EPI is increased, whereas the response to IL-1β that signals via another class of receptors is not affected. In vitro studies provided evidence for a possible underlying mechanism. Primary neurons from GRK2[+/−] mice show a more pronounced calcium response to the GPCR ligand CCL3. CCL3 is known to signal via CCR1

or CCR5, which are two receptors from the GPCR class that are expressed on dorsal root ganglion neurons and that are known to be regulated by GRK2. It is likely that the more pronounced hyperalgesic response to CCL3 is mediated via increased GPCR signaling due to inefficient desensitization in GRK2-deficient mice.

Contribution of GRK2 in Specific Cell Types to Pain

As mentioned earlier, there are multiple cell types involved in regulating pain signaling. Figure 20.2 provides a schematic overview of the cells involved, focusing on spinal cord and peripheral nervous system. In addition, signal processing in the brain and descending modulatory signals contribute to the pain response, but we will not discuss these in the context of this chapter. To get more insight into the contribution of low GRK2 in specific cell types, we used mice with a cell specific decrease in GRK2 that were generated as described earlier in the section Chronic Pain as a Health Problem.

In line with our hypothesis that increased CCL3-induced GPCR signaling underlies the enhanced acute hyperalgesic response in GRK2[+/−] mice, we also observed that in mice with a selective decrease in GRK2 only in nociceptors (SNS-GRK2[+/−] mice), CCL3 hyperalgesia is increased. In contrast, hyperalgesia induced by the non-GPCR ligand IL-1β was not affected by a decrease in GRK2 expression in nociceptors. Moreover, we also observed that the reduction of GRK2 in nociceptors only was not sufficient to prolong CCL3 or IL-1β hyperalgesia, indicating that GRK2 levels in other cells contribute to the regulation of duration of hyperalgesia (Eijkelkamp, Heijnen, et al. 2010; Willemen et al. 2010).

As described earlier, microglia and astrocytes are thought to be important for the regulation of chronic pain. Indeed, the prolonged carrageenan hyperalgesia in GRK2+/− mice was associated with ongoing microglial activation in the spinal cord. Moreover, inhibition of microglial activation by minocycline prevents the transition to chronic carrageenan or IL-1β hyperalgesia in GRK2+/− mice (Willemen et al., 2010). These findings strongly indicate that the prolongation of hyperalgesia in GRK2-deficient mice is mediated via prolonged activation of spinal cord microglia. The next question is whether this prolonged microglial activation is dependent on low microglial GRK2. LysM-GRK2+/− mice have low GRK2 in microglia as well as in macrophages and granulocytes. The hyperalgesic response to carrageenan lasts approximately 3 weeks in these mice, whereas it lasts only 2–3 days in littermate controls with normal GRK2 in all cells. Thus, low GRK2 in microglia/macrophages appears to be sufficient for marked prolongation of carrageenan hyperalgesia. Moreover, also Il-1β hyperalgesia and CCL3 hyperalgesia were markedly prolonged in mice deficient for GRK2 in microglia/macrophages/granulocytes. We now also know that, even in LysM-GRK2+/− mice depleted from granulocytes, hyperalgesia is prolonged. These findings tell us that microglia and/or macrophages with low GRK2 mediate the transition to chronic hyperalgesia.

Mechanism of Prolonged Microglial Activation in GRK2-deficient Mice

Further investigation of the mechanism involved in the ongoing hyperalgesia in GRK2-deficient mice revealed that, during the chronic phase of hyperalgesia, spinal cord microglial activation is maintained via a fractalkine-dependent pathway. Fractalkine is known to signal via the GPCR CX3CR1 and is known to contribute to chronic pain (Clark, Yip, & Malcangio, 2009). Therefore, it is possible that reduced GRK2 in microglia/macrophages leads to increased fractalkine signaling and thereby to the prolongation of hyperalgesia in GRK2-deficient mice. Although this is an interesting possibility, it is probably not the whole story, because only late, but not early, inhibition of fractalkine signaling attenuates chronic hyperalgesia in GRK2-deficient mice.

These findings indicate that ongoing fractalkine signaling in GRK2-deficient mice is required for maintaining ongoing microglial activity and prolongation of chronic pain (Willemen et al., 2010). To further investigate the contribution of spinal cord microglia to the ongoing pain response in these mice, we used the tetracycline-derivative minocycline. This antibiotic does not only have bactericidal properties, but also is well-known for its capacity to inhibit cytokine release by microglia and macropahges. Based on this capacity, minocycline is frequently used to assess the contribution of microglial/macrophage activity to (patho-) physiological processes. Interestingly, early inhibition of spinal cord microglial activity by intrathecal administration of minocycline, as well as by intrathecal treatment with an inhibitor of p38 clearly prevents transition to chronic hyperalgesia in GRK2-deficient mice. This is an interesting observation because it is known that the p38 MAPK pathway is regulated directly by GRK2 in a receptor-independent manner. Co-immunoprecipitation studies using cellular extracts show that GRK2 and the MAPkinase p38 are found in the same protein complex (Jurado-Pueyo et al. 2008; Mayor, Jurado-Pueyo, Campos, & Murga, 2007; Peregrin et al. 2006). In vitro assays in which purified GRK2 was added to purified p38 MAPkinase have confirmed that GRK2 directly binds p38 MAPkinase. Upon binding to p38, GRK2 phosphorylates p38 at Thr 123, a residue that is located at the entrance of the docking groove of p38 (Peregrin et al. 2006). This is important because this phosphorylation event severely impairs binding of MKK6, the upstream activator of p38, and thereby inhibits activation of p38 resulting in decreased phosphorylation of downstream substrates such as MEF2, MK2 and ATF2.

The functional importance of the direct interaction between GRK2 and p38 has been demonstrated in three different assays. (a) overexpression of GRK2 dose dependently reduces activation of p38 by MKK6; (b) overexpression of GRK2 inhibits differentiation of pre-adipocytic cells into adipocytes, a process that is known to be p38 dependent; (c) the LPS-induced production of the pro-inflammatory cytokine TNFα by macrophages or microglia deficient for GRK2 is significantly increased and this effect is p38 dependent (Eijkelkamp, Heijnen, et al. 2010; Nijboer et al. 2010; Peregrin et al. 2006).

Thus, we propose that the transition from acute to chronic hyperalgesia in response to peripheral inflammation that develops in mice deficient for GRK2 in microglia mice is mediated via a pathway involving increased microglial p38 activation and pro-inflammatory cytokine production. Indeed, not only inhibition of p38, but also intrathecal administration of the TNF-inhibitor Etanercept prevents transition to chronic hyperalgesia in GRK2-deficient mice.

Conclusion

In conclusion, we propose that chronic peripheral inflammation as well as peripheral nerve damage evokes a decrease in the level of GRK2 in spinal cord microglia. This reduction in microglial GRK2 protein level is sufficient to mediate transition from acute to chronic hyperalgesia in response to an inflammatory stimulus, such as the cytokine response that will be present in the periphery and/or at the level of the spinal cord.

Future directions

1. Future research should focus on studying in depth the sensitivity of receptors and possible changes in the behavior of intracellular signaling cascades in the context of prolonged or chronic inflammation, chronic stress, or depression, and chronic pain.

2. In the context of the important role GRK2 may play in neuroinflammation, the research in this field should focus on ways to up-regulate GRK2 during inflammation in order to therapeutically prevent the increase in sensitivity of receptors or signaling cascades that are responsible for the transition of acute to chronic pain.

3. Using this strategy, a problem may arise by the possibility that GRK2 is also increased in tissues that do not benefit from the increase in GRK2, such as in cardiac myocytes, that function less well when GRK2 is increased.

4. Future research should, therefore, concentrate on finding novel ways to prevent the inflammation-mediated *breakdown* of GRK2.

5. Since the response of the receptor for the stress hormone epinephrine (β-adrenergic receptor) is also tightly regulated by GRK2, future studies may concentrate on the role of chronic stress and catecholamine secretion on the reactivity of various target tissues. Investigating GRK2 in response to chronic stress may, therefore, contribute to elucidation of the mechanism of various stress-mediated pathologies.

Acknowledgments

This work has been supported in part by NIH grants RO1- NS073939 and RO1-NS074999 to A.K.

References

Ahmed M. R., Bychkov E., Gurevich, V. V., Benovic, J. L., Gurevich, E. V. (2008). Altered expression and subcellular distribution of GRK subtypes in the dopamine-depleted rat basal ganglia is not normalized by l-DOPA treatment. *Journal of Neurochemistry, 104,* 1622–1636.

Basbaum, A. I., Bautista, D. M., Scherrer, G., & Julius, D. (2009a) Cellular and molecular mechanisms of pain. *Cell, 139,,267–284.*

Basbaum, A. I., Bautista, D. M., Scherrer, G., & Julius, D. (2009b) Cellular and molecular mechanisms of pain. *Cell, 139,* 267–284.

Biggs, J. E., Lu, V. B., Stebbing, M. J., Balasubramanyan, S., & Smith, P. A. (2010). Is BDNF sufficient for information transfer between microglia and dorsal horn neurons during the onset of central sensitization? *Molecular Pain, 6,* 44.

Black, J. L., Oliver, B. G., Roth, M. (2009). Molecular mechanisms of combination therapy with inhaled corticosteroids and long-acting beta-agonists. *Chest, 136,*1095–1100.

Blalock, J. E., Smith, E. M. (1985). A complete regulatory loop between the immune and neuroendocrine systems. *Federation Proceedings, 44,*108–112.

Brink, C. B., Harvey, B. H., Bodenstein, J., Venter, D. P., & Oliver, D. W. (2004). Recent advances in drug action and therapeutics: Relevance of novel concepts in G-protein-coupled receptor and signal transduction pharmacology. *British Journal of Clinical Pharmacology, 57,* 373–387.

Bruchas, M. R., Land, B. B., Aita, M., Xu, M., Barot, S. K., Li, S., et al. (2007). Stress-induced p38 mitogen-activated protein kinase activation mediates kappa-opioid-dependent dysphoria. *Journal of Neuroscience,27,* 11614–11623.

Choi, D. J., Koch, W. J., Hunter, J. J., & Rockman, H. A. (1997). Mechanism of beta-adrenergic receptor desensitization in cardiac hypertrophy is increased beta-adrenergic receptor kinase. *Journal of Biological Chemistry, 272,* 17223–17229.

Clark, A. K., Yip, P. K., Malcangio, M. (2009). The liberation of fractalkine in the dorsal horn requires microglial cathepsin S. *Journal of Neuroscience 29,* 6945–6954.

Cobelens, P. M., Kavelaars, A., Heijnen, C. J., Ribas, C., Mayor, F., Jr., Penela, P. (2007). Hydrogen peroxide impairs GRK2 translation via a calpain-dependent and cdk1-mediated pathway. *Cell Signal, 19,* 269–277.

Colton, C. A., & Wilcock, D. M. (2010). Assessing activation states in microglia. *CNS Neurological Disorders Drug—Targets, 9,*174–191.

Dantzer, R., Kelley, K. W. (2007). Twenty years of research on cytokine-induced sickness behavior. *Brain, Behavior and Immunity, 21,* 153–160.

de Kloet, C. S., Vermetten, E., Bikker, A., Meulman, E., Geuze, E., Kavelaars, A., et al. (2007). Leukocyte glucocorticoid receptor expression and immunoregulation in veterans with and without post-traumatic stress disorder. *Molecular Psychiatry, 12,* 443–453.

Eckardt, K., Taube, A., Eckel, J. (2011). Obesity-associated insulin resistance in skeletal muscle: Role of lipid accumulation and physical inactivity. *Reviews in Endocrine and Metabolic Disorders, 12,* 163–172.

Eckhart, A. D., Ozaki, T., Tevaearai, H., Rockman, H. A., Koch, W. J. (2002). Vascular-targeted overexpression of G protein-coupled receptor kinase-2 in transgenic mice attenuates beta-adrenergic receptor signaling and increases resting blood pressure. *Molecular Pharmacology, 61,* 749–758.

Eijkelkamp, N., Heijnen, C. J., Willemen, H. L., Deumens, R., Joosten, E. A., Kleibeuker, W., et al. (2010). GRK2: A novel cell-specific regulator of severity and duration of inflammatory pain. *Journal of Neuroscience, 30,* 2138–2149.

Eijkelkamp, N., Wang, H., Garza Carbajal, A., Willemen, H. L., Zwartkruis, F. J., Wood, J. N., et al. (2010). Low nociceptor GRK2 prolongs PGE_2 hyperalgesia via biased cAMP signaling to Epac/Rap1, PKCε and MEK/ERK. *Journal of Neuroscience, 30,* 12806–12815.

Fan, J., Malik, A. B. (2003). Toll-like receptor-4 (TLR4) signaling augments chemokine-induced neutrophil migration by modulating cell surface expression of chemokine receptors. *Nature Medicine, 9,* 315–321.

Garcia-Guerra, L., Nieto-Vazquez, I., Vila-Bedmar, R., Jurado-Pueyo, M., Zalba, G., Diez, J., et al. (2010). G protein-coupled receptor kinase 2 plays a relevant role in insulin resistance and obesity. *Diabetes, 59,* 2407–2417.

Gold, M. S., & Gebhart, G. F. (2010). Nociceptor sensitization in pain pathogenesis. *Nature Medicine, 16,* 1248–1257.

Gosselin, R. D., Suter, M. R., Ji, R. R., & Decosterd, I. (2010). Glial cells and chronic pain. *Neuroscientist, 16,* 519–531.

Graeber, M. B. (2010). Changing face of microglia. *Science, 330,* 783–788.

Gudermann, T., Nurnberg, B., & Schultz, G. (1995). Receptors and G proteins as primary components of transmembrane signal transduction. Part 1. G-protein-coupled receptors: structure and function. *Journal of Molecular Medicine, 73,* 51–63.

Heijnen, C. J., Kavelaars, A. (1999). The importance of being receptive. *Journal of Neuroimmunology, 100,*197–202.

Heijnen, C. J., Rouppe van der Voort, C., Wulffraat, N., van der Net, J., Kuis, W., & Kavelaars, A. (1996). Functional α1-adrenergic receptors on leukocytes of patients with polyarticular juvenile rheumatoid arthritis. *Journal of Neuroimmunology, 71,* 223–226.

Hildreth, K. L., Wu, J. H., Barak, L. S., Exum, S. T., Kim, L. K., Peppel, K., et al. (2004). Phosphorylation of the platelet-derived growth factor receptor-beta by G protein-coupled receptor kinase-2 reduces receptor signaling and interaction with the Na(+)/H(+) exchanger regulatory factor. *Journal of Biological Chemistry, 279,* 41775–41782.

Jaber, M., Koch, W. J., Rockman, H., Smith, B., Bond, R. A., Sulik, K. K., et al. (1996). Essential role of beta-adrenergic receptor kinase 1 in cardiac development and function. *Proceedings of the National Academy of Science USA, 93,* 12974–12979.

Ji, R. R., & Suter, M. R. (2007). p38 MAPK, microglial signaling, and neuropathic pain. *Molecular Pain, 3,* 33.

Jimenez-Sainz, M. C., Murga, C., Kavelaars, A., Jurado-Pueyo, M., Krakstad, B. F., Heijnen, C. J., et al. (2006). G protein-coupled receptor kinase 2 negatively regulates chemokine signaling at a level downstream from G protein subunits. *Molecular Biology of the Cell, 17,* 25–31.

Jurado-Pueyo, M., Campos, P. M., Mayor, F., Murga, C. (2008). GRK2-dependent desensitization downstream of G proteins. *Journal of Receptors and Signal Transductors Research, 28,* 59–70.

Kavelaars, A., Cats, B., Visser, G. H. A., Zegers, B. J. M., Bakker, J. M., Van Rees, E. P., et al. (1996). Ontogeny of the response of human peripheral blood T cells to glucocorticoids. *Brain, Behavior and Immunity, 10,* 288–297.

Kavelaars, A., Rouppe van der Voort, C., & Heijnen, C. J. (1999). α1-adrenergic receptor subtypes in human peripheral blood lymphocytes. *Hypertension, 34,* e5.

Kavelaars, A., Zijlstra, J., Bakker, J. M., Van Rees, E. P., Visser, G. H. A., Zegers, B. J. M., et al. (1995). Increased dexamethasone sensitivity of neonatal leukocytes: Different mechanisms of glucocorticoid inhibition of T cell proliferation in adult and neonatal cells. *European Journal of Immunology, 25,* 1346–1351.

Kleibeuker, W., Ledeboer, A., Eijkelkamp, N., Watkins, L. R., Maier, S. F., Zijlstra, J., et al. (2007). A role for G protein-coupled receptor kinase 2 in mechanical allodynia. *European Journal of Neuroscience, 2,* 1696–1704.

Ledeboer, A., Sloane, E. M., Milligan, E. D., Frank, M. G., Mahony, J. H., Maier, S. F., et al. (2005). Minocycline attenuates mechanical allodynia and proinflammatory cytokine expression in rat models of pain facilitation. *Pain, 115,* 71–83.

Lombardi, M. S., Kavelaars, A., Cobelens, P., Schmidt, R. E., Schedlowski, M., & Heijnen, C. J. (2001). Adjuvant arthritis induces downregulation of G-protein-coupled receptor kinases in the immune system. *Journal of Immunology, 166,* 1635–1640.

Lombardi, M. S., Kavelaars, A., & Heijnen, C. J. (2002). Role and modulation of G protein-coupled receptor signaling in inflammatory processes. *Critical Reviews in Immunology, 22,* 141–163.

Lombardi, M. S., Kavelaars, A., Schedlowski, M., Bijlsma, J. W., Okihara, K. L., van de P. M., et al. (1999). Decreased expression and activity of G-protein-coupled receptor kinases in peripheral blood mononuclear cells of patients with rheumatoid arthritis. *FASEB Journal, 13,* 715–725.

Lombardi, M. S., van den Tweel, E. R., Kavelaars, A., Groenendaal, F., Van Bel, F., & Heijnen, C. J. (2004). Hypoxia-ischemia modulates G protein-coupled receptor kinase 2 and arrestin1 levels in the neonatal rat brain. *Stroke, 35,* 981–986.

Lombardi, M. S., Vroon, A., Sodaar, P., van Muiswinkel, F. L., Heijnen, C. J., & Kavelaars, A. (2007). Down-regulation of GRK2 after oxygen and glucose deprivation in rat hippocampal slices: role of the PI3-kinase pathway. *Journal of Neurochemistry,102,* 731–740.

Lue, L. F., Kuo, Y. M., Beach, T., & Walker, D. G. (2010). Microglia activation and anti-inflammatory regulation in Alzheimer's disease. *Molecular Neurobiology, 41,* 115–128.

Mao, J., Price, D. D., & Mayer, D. J. (1995). Mechanisms of hyperalgesia and morphine tolerance: A current view of their possible interactions. *Pain, 62,* 259–274.

Martinez, F. O., Sica, A., Mantovani, A., & Locati, M. (2008). Macrophage activation and polarization. *Frontiers in Bioscience, 13,* 453–461.

Mayor, F., Jr., Jurado-Pueyo, M., Campos, P. M., & Murga, C. (2007). Interfering with MAP kinase docking interactions: implications and perspective for the p38 route. *Cell Cycle, 6,* 528–533.

Mellen, P. B., & Herrington, D. M. (2005). Pharmacogenomics of blood pressure response to antihypertensive treatment. *Journal of Hypertension, 23,* 1311–1325.

Milligan, E. D., & Watkins, L. R. (2009). Pathological and protective roles of glia in chronic pain. *National Review of Neuroscience, 10,* 23–36.

Nijboer, C. H., Heijnen, C. J., Willemen, H. L., Groenendaal, F., Dorn, G. W., Van Bel, F., et al. (2010). Cell-specific roles of GRK2 in onset and severity of hypoxic-ischemic brain damage in neonatal mice. *Brain, Behavior and Immunity, 24,* 420–426.

Nijboer, C. H., Kavelaars, A., Vroon, A., Groenendaal, F., Van Bel, F., & Heijnen, C. J. (2008). Low endogenous G-protein-coupled receptor kinase 2 sensitizes the immature brain to hypoxia-ischemia-induced gray and white matter damage. *Journal of Neuroscience, 28,* 3324–3332.

Nimmerjahn, A., Kirchhoff, F., & Helmchen, F. (2005). Resting microglial cells are highly dynamic surveillants of brain parenchyma in vivo. *Science, 308,*1314–1318.

Penela, P., Ribas, C., & Mayor, F., Jr. (2003). Mechanisms of regulation of the expression and function of G protein-coupled receptor kinases. *Cell Signal, 15,* 973–981.

Peregrin, S., Jurado-Pueyo, M., Campos, P. M., Sanz-Moreno, V., Ruiz-Gomez, A., Crespo, P., et al. (2006). Phosphorylation of p38 by GRK2 at the docking groove unveils a novel mechanism for inactivating p38MAPK. *Current Biology, 16,* 2042–2047.

Pitcher, J. A., Freedman, N. J., & Lefkowitz, R. J. (1998). G protein-coupled receptor kinases. *Annual Review of Biochemistry, 67,* 653–692.

Polanczyk, G., Bigarella, M. P., Hutz, M. H., & Rohde, L. A. (2010). Pharmacogenetic approach for a better drug treatment in children. *Current Pharmaceutical Design, 16,* 2462–2473.

Ponomarev, E. D., Veremeyko, T., Barteneva, N., Krichevsky, A. M., & Weiner, H. L. (2011). MicroRNA-124 promotes microglia quiescence and suppresses EAE by deactivating macrophages via the C/EBP-alpha-PU.1 pathway. *Nature Medicine, 17,* 64–70.

Premont, R. T., & Gainetdinov, R. R. (2007). Physiological roles of G protein-coupled receptor kinases and arrestins. *Annual Review of Physiology,69,* 511–534.

Ramos-Ruiz, R., Penela, P., Penn, R. B., & Mayor, F., Jr. (2000). Analysis of the human G protein-coupled receptor kinase 2 (GRK2) gene promoter: regulation by signal transduction systems in aortic smooth muscle cells. *Circulation, 101,* 2083–2089.

Ransohoff, R. M., & Perry, V. H. (2009). Microglial physiology: unique stimuli, specialized responses. *Annual Review of Immunology, 27,* 119–145.

Ren, K., & Dubner, R. (2010). Interactions between the immune and nervous system in pain. *Nature Medicine, 16,* 1267–1276.

Rockman, H. A., Choi, D. J., Akhter, S. A., Jaber, M., Giros, B., Lefkowitz, R. J., et al. (1998). Control of myocardial contractile function by the level of beta-adrenergic receptor kinase 1 in gene-targeted mice. *Journal of Biological Chemistry, 27,* 18180–18184.

Romero-Sandoval, E. A., Horvath, R. J., & DeLeo, J. A. (2008). Neuroimmune interactions and pain: Focus on glial-modulating targets. *Current Opinions in Investigational Drugs, 9,* 726–734.

Rouppe van der Voort, C., Heijnen, C. J., Wulffraat, N., Kuis, W., & Kavelaars, A. (2000). Stress-induced increase in IL-6 production by leukocytes of patients with the chronic inflammatory disease juvenile rheumatoid arthritis:a putative role for α1-adrenergic receptors. *Journal of Neuroimmunology, 110,* 223–229.

Sanders, V. M., & Straub, R. H. (2002). Norepinephrine, the beta-adrenergic receptor, and immunity. *Brain, Behavior and Immunity, 16,* 290–332.

Shechter, R., London, A., Varol, C., Raposo, C., Cusimano, M., Yovel, et al. (2009). Infiltrating blood-derived macrophages are vital cells playing an anti-inflammatory role in recovery from spinal cord injury in mice. PLoS Med 2009;6: e1000113.

Spengler, R. N., Chensue, S. W., Giacherio, G. A., Blenk, N., & Kunkel, S. L. (1994). Endogenous norepinephrine regulates tumor necrosis factor-α production from macrophages in vitro. *Journal of Immunology, 152,* 3024–3031.

Suo, Z., Wu, M., Citron, B. A., Wong, G. T., & Festoff, B. W. (2004). Abnormality of G-protein-coupled receptor kinases at prodromal and early stages of Alzheimer's disease: an association with early beta-amyloid accumulation. *Journal of Neuroscience, 24,* 3444–3452.

Tsikouris, J. P., & Peeters, M. J. (2007). Pharmacogenomics of renin angiotensin system inhibitors in coronary artery disease. *Cardiovascular Drugs and Therapy, 21,* 121–132.

van Zuiden, M., Geuze, E., Willemen, H. L., Vermetten, E., Maas, M., Heijnen, C. J., et al. (2011). Pre-existing high glucocorticoid receptor number predicting development of posttraumatic stress symptoms after military deployment. *American Journal of Psychiatry, 168,* 89–96.

Vroon, A., Heijnen, C., Lombardi, M. S., Cobelens, P., Mayor, F., Caron, M. G., et al. (2004). Reduced GRK2 level in T cells potentiates chemotaxis and signaling in response to CCL4. *Journal of Leukocyte Biology, 75,* 901–909.

Vroon, A., Heijnen, C. J., & Kavelaars, A. (2006). GRKs and arrestins: regulators of migration and inflammation. *Journal of Leukocyte Biology, 80,*1214–1221.

Vroon, A., Kavelaars, A., Limmroth, V., Lombardi, M. S., Goebel, M. U., Van Dam, A. M., et al. (2005). G protein-coupled receptor kinase 2 in multiple sclerosis and experimental autoimmune encephalomyelitis. *Journal of Immunology, 174,* 4400–4406.

Vroon, A., Lombardi, M. S., Kavelaars, A., & Heijnen, C. J. (2003). Changes in the G protein coupled receptor desensitization machinery during relapsing progressive experimental autoimmune encephalomyelitis. *Journal of Neuroimmunology, 137,* 79–86.

Walker, D. G., Sing-Hernandez, J. E., Campbell, N. A., & Lue, L. F. (2009). Decreased expression of CD200 and CD200 receptor in Alzheimer's disease: a potential mechanism leading to chronic inflammation. *Experimental Neurology, 215,* 5–19.

Wang, H., Heijnen, C. J., Eijkelkamp, N., Garza Carbacal, A., Schedlowsky, M., Kelley, K. W., Dantzer, R.,Kavelaars, A., (2011). GRK2 in sensory neurons regulates epinephrine-induced signaling and duration of mechanical hyperalgesia. *Pain, 152,* 1649–1658.

Watkins, L. R., Hutchinson, M. R., Ledeboer, A., Wieseler-Frank, J., Milligan, E. D., & Maier, S. F. (2007). Norman Cousins Lecture. Glia as the "bad guys": Implications for improving clinical pain control and the clinical utility of opioids. *Brain, Behavior and Immunity, 21,* 131–146.

Willemen, H. L., Eijkelkamp, N,. Wang, H., Dantzer, R., Dorn, G. W., Kelley, K. W., et al. (2010). Microglial/macrophage GRK2 determines duration of peripheral IL-1beta-induced hyperalgesia: Contribution of spinal cord CX3CR1, p38 and IL-1 signaling. *Pain, 150,* 550–560.

Stress Management, PNI, and Disease

Michael H. Antoni

Abstract

As our understanding of the immunologic processes that underlie the vulnerability to certain infectious, neoplastic, and inflammatory diseases and other immunoregulatory conditions has grown so too has the empirical basis relating psychosocial processes and stress physiology to these same immunologic processes. This provides a rationale for first examining the influence of stress processes on disease risk and disease course, and second for the development of interventions to mitigate stress processes in persons at risk for, or managing a wide range of diseases where the immune system plays some role in health outcomes. This chapter will summarize the state of the field of research examining the effects of stress management-based interventions on psychoneuroimmunologic (PNI) processes and health outcomes using a few examples of diseases involving some type of immune system alteration.

Key Words: HIV/AIDS, breast cancer, infectious, neoplastic, inflammatory, immunoregulatory, chronic fatigue syndrome, cardiovascular disease

Overview

Many of the chapters in this book have carefully reviewed the psychoneuroimmunologic (PNI) literature relating immune system components to personality, affect, and social processes and have demonstrated how these associations may be affected during normal development as well as during the development of diseases. Most of the research used to establish these relationships has involved observational and experimental animal models that were used as a prelude to human models of personality traits such as optimism, stress and coping processes, persistant distress states, and interpersonal relationships. This work has nicely set the stage for the development and testing of interventions that can be used to modify some of these psychosocial processes in order to reduce the risk of disease, speed recovery after medical treatments such as surgery and drug/

chemotherapy, promote optimal disease management, and decrease morbidity and mortality. This chapter summarizes research examining the effects of stress-management-based interventions on PNI processes and health outcomes using a few examples of diseases involving some type of immune system alteration.

This chapter will first characterize some widely studied, highly prevalent diseases according to their relationship to the functioning of the immune system. These will be designated as infectious, neoplastic, inflammatory, and immunoregulatory diseases or disorders. Although many different behavioral interventions have been tested in PNI studies targeting one disease or another, the most widely tested intervention approaches in PNI research have used relaxation-based or cognitive-behavioral techniques to reduce or manage stress responses. In fact, it is now possible to review the effects of "stress-management" interventions across the classifications of disease already noted. Because of this, I shall focus on PNI studies of stress-management interventions in clinical populations that represent one example for each of these disease classes noted previously. Accordingly, I shall present the rationale for stress management in each of four examples of these disease types: human immunodeficiency virus infection and acquired immune deficiency syndrome (HIV/AIDS) as an infectious disease; breast cancer (BCa) as a neoplastic disease; cardiovascular disease (CVD) as an inflammatory disease; and chronic fatigue syndrome (CFS) as an immunoregulatory condition.

I summarize the evidence for stress and psychosocial influences on clinical disease outcomes in each of these four diseases or syndromes. I note the immune processes relevant to the pathogenesis or pathophysiology of these conditions, which have also been related to stress and psychosocial factors. Next, I describe the evidence from randomized controlled trials that stress management affects PNI processes and clinical outcomes in samples of patients with these conditions. I will then review issues germane to testing the effects of interventions such as stress management in clinical-trial designs, noting the advantages and limitations of this research line. I end with suggestions for future directions in this field by (a) addressing the needs for innovations in the "who, what, when and how" of optimal stress-management approaches; (b) describing emerging analytic approaches that are sensitive to the nonlinear patterns of change that occur in the psychotherapeutic process as well as in the evolution of changes in biologic systems once perturbed by intervention-associated changes in stress processing; (c) discussing emerging measurement tools for capturing how such biological changes can be characterized in immune cells and disease-affected tissue; and (d) suggesting ways to use community-based methods and telecommunication technology to enhance the reach of stress management and PNI research to understudied disease populations who have been poorly represented in the PNI literature to date. The hope is that this summary will help future investigators who wish to take the building blocks established in PNI-based intervention research over the past to develop stress-management interventions to reduce disease risk, hasten recovery after diagnosis and medical treatment, and better manage diseases that are influenced by the interactions of psychosocial and biobehavioral processes.

Overview of PNI Processes in Different Diseases

Classes of Diseases Putatively Affected by PNI Processes

Although many of the disease classes used in this chapter are certainly multiply determined and are characterized by concurrent alterations in several physiological systems and disruptions in multiple organs, one way to characterize their association with the immune system is to "force" each of them into one of four groups as noted in Table 21.1. Using two columns designating the nonself versus self categories commonly used in immunology, and two rows indicating the direction of proposed disruption in the immune system (up- versus down-regulation) one can create four artificial classes of disease or disorder as follows: *Down-regulated or deficient responses to nonself pathogens* such as viruses or bacteria often characterize infectious diseases such as HIV/AIDS; *down-regulated immune responses to self-initiated cellular mutations* may permit the promotion and progression of neoplastic disease of which cancer is the most prevalent example. On the other hand disruptions in the immune system in other diseases or syndromes may be the result of an *up-regulation of inflammatory reactions to specific tissue (self) changes* or may involve a *systemic up-regulation of specific aspects of the immune system to extrinsic (nonself) factors* that are more likely due to a breakdown in immunoregulatory signaling resulting in systemic effects. For example, diseases such as cardiovascular disease (CVD) is now understood to be caused, in part, by inflammatory reactions to tissue changes (self) in the walls (lumen) of the coronary arteries. Alternatively, some poorly understood syndromes such as chronic fatigue syndrome (CFS) may feature problems with immunoregulation wherein sudden exposure to extrinsic nonself factors such as allergens, toxins, vaccines, or drugs may trigger a

Table 21.1 Organization of Medical Conditions in Relation to Immune System Disruption

Disruption	Non-Self	Self
Down-regulated	Infectious: HIV/AIDS	Neoplastic: Cancer
Up-regulated	Immunoregulatory: CFS	Inflammatory: CVD

HIV/AIDS: Human Immunodeficiency Virus/Acquired Immune Deficiency Syndrome
CFS: Chronic Fatigue Syndrome
CVD: Cardiovascular Disease

cascade of immunologic reactions that are closely tied to the chronic and repeating flu-like symptom flares of this condition.

As noted previously I will organize the bulk of this chapter around each of these classes of disease/disorder using as examples, HIV/AIDS, breast cancer, CVD, and CFS. I will summarize the evidence for the influence of stress and psychosocial factors on the development and clinical course of each condition, and I will present a model for the role of the immune system as a potential mediator of the effects of stress and psychosocial factors on health outcomes. I also present evidence for the effects of stress-modulating behavioral and psychosocial interventions on symptoms and disease endpoints as well as PNI changes that occur during these interventions and that may explain their effects on health outcomes.

Stress Management in PNI Research: Rationale and Relevant Mechanisms to Target and Measure

Before beginning a detailed review of the role of stress-management interventions in each of these four areas ,it is helpful to review the rationale for expecting that such interventions can affect PNI processes. Behavioral interventions have been used for decades to help patients with various medical conditions better adapt to the stress of diagnosis and treatment to better their quality of life (QOL). Over the past 25 years, there has been emerging interest in the question of whether these interventions may provide physical health benefits including optimal disease management and minimization of symptoms, decreased risk of recurrence, slowed disease progression, and increased survival time. Over this period of time, a small but gradually expanding empirical base has accumulated demonstrating that behavioral interventions may also modulate immune system functioning by modifying stress responses, building personal and interpersonal resources, reducing negative mood states, and improving positive psychological states. Many of the behavioral interventions comprising this empirical base include elements designed to reduce anxiety, depressed and negative affect, and other aspects of distress. These elements target bodily relaxation, modify extreme cognitive appraisals about stress and disease, teach new behavioral and interpersonal coping skills, and provide social support, especially when they are delivered in a group format. For this chapter, these intervention approaches will be collectively referred to as "stress management" interventions.

HOW DOES MODIFYING BEHAVIORAL AND PSYCHOSOCIAL PROCESSES THROUGH STRESS MANAGEMENT AFFECT THE IMMUNE SYSTEM AND, IN TURN, THE COURSE OF PHYSICAL DISEASE?

Although empirical support for the biobehavioral mechanisms underlying stress- management interventions are still incomplete, the extensive body of PNI research documenting interactions of behavioral, neural, endocrine, and immune systems across a wide variety of species and situations—much of which is described in this volume—is often used to explain their effects on disease outcomes. The PNI research that can be used to explain the effect of stress-management interventions on health outcomes derives from animal models of central nervous system and endocrine-mediated activation of immune cellular pathways, and from observational studies relating immune parameters to acute laboratory-induced behavioral challenges, chronic and acute "field" stressors, negative mood states, and a variety of stress moderating variables describing personality (e.g., optimism) and interpersonal (e.g., social-support) processes. Although it is beyond the scope of this chapter to review each of these lines of evidence in any detail, I shall review the basic and clinical human PNI evidence supporting the use of stress-management interventions to modify psychosocial and physiological processes relevant to the pathological processes underlying the four disease conditions noted previously.

PNI Associations in Human Studies

PNI studies conducted during the 1980s and 1990s related associated field stressors and negative mood states to various immunologic indices including lymphocyte proliferative responses to mitogens, natural killer (NK) cell cytotoxicity (NKCC), antibody titers to herpes viruses, production of cytokines such as interferon (IFN), and changes in the numbers of circulating leukocytes. Stressors examined ranged from common daily experiences such as medical-school exams and sleep deprivation, to intense short-term events like splashdown after space travel, to more major events reflecting protracted periods of burden such as divorce, family caregiving, spousal bereavement, and natural disasters (see for example Herbert & Cohen, 1993a; Ironson et al., 1997; Kiecolt-Glaser et al. 1987). Most of the parallel body of work examining immunologic correlates of negative mood states has focused on clinical depression (Herbert & Cohen, 1993b), though there is an emerging interest in the effects of positive affect and positive attitudes and states of mind (Moskowitz, 2003; McGregor et al., 2004).

Across the human PNI literature up to the early 1990s the most consistent immune correlates of psychological variables were those reflecting cellular immune processes as indexed by lymphoproliferative responses to mitogens, NKCC, immunoglobulin levels, and herpes virus antibody titers (Herbert & Cohen, 1993a). Importantly, these associations may be accounted for by neuroendocrine-cytokine interactions. For instance, production of interleukin-2 (IL-2), a cytokine that mediates both lymphocyte proliferation and NKCC, and which is suppressed in the face of stressors (Glaser, Kenedy, Lafuse, & Kiecolt-Glaser, 1990), is down-regulated by both catecholamines and corticosteroids, neuroendocrines that have been associated with both chronic stress and negative mood states (McEwen, 1998). Decrements in cellular immunity can have implications for increased susceptibility to viral infections in particular. Lymphocyte proliferative responses to specific viral antigens (e.g., herpes simplex virus [HSV]) and elevated HSV antibody titers (reflecting re-infection or latent virus reactivation) are suppressed among persons dealing with interpersonal stressors such as family caregiving (Glaser & Kiecolt-Glaser, 1997), and marital separation and divorce (Kiecolt-Glaser et al., 1987), and demonstrate some of the highest stress-immune effect sizes in humans (Herbert & Cohen, 1993a). This supports the possibility that stressors may relate to indicators of immune responses to pathogens that may contribute directly to disease. Meta-analytic reviews of studies relating depression and immunity reveal reliable relationships between depression and decrements in a variety of measures of cell-mediated immunity including lymphocyte proliferation and NKCC (Herbert & Cohen, 1993b). This suggests that depression may relate to compromised cellular immunity via similar pathways to those implicated for stressors.

Because neuroendocrine responses to stress may vary based on an individual's *appraisal* (i.e., controllable versus uncontrollable) and *coping response* (i.e., active versus passive) to stressors it is reasonable to consider the role of individual differences in intrapersonal factors in PNI research (e.g., personality factors such as optimism and self-efficacy; Segerstrom, 2000). Similarly because elevations in adrenocortical hormones have also been observed in those reporting increased loneliness and marital strife (Kiecolt-Glaser et al., 1984; Kiecolt-Glaser

et al., 1987) we also know that interpersonal factors such as social support may significantly influence the impact of stressors on immune parameters. Taken together, this work suggests that many PNI relationships might be mediated, in part, by disruptions in neuroendocrine processes linked to an individual's appraisals of, coping responses to, and resources available for dealing with environmental stimuli (Antoni, Schneiderman & Penedo, 2006). These intrapersonal and interpersonal processes can moderate the nature, degree, and duration of neuroendocrine responses as well as neuro-anatomical changes involving structures critical for hypothalamic pituitary adrenal (HPA) (McEwen, 1998) and sympathoadrenomedullary (SAM) (Felten, 1996) hormonal regulation and efficient neuroimmune interactions that are relevant for understanding the negative health consequences of chronic and repeated stressor exposure and persisting negative mood states.

Endocrine-immune Interactions

Much of the work aiming to explain PNI associations in humans has focused on adrenal hormonal substances such as cortisol and catecholamines such as epinephrine (E) and norepinephrine (NE), which are liberated into the circulation where they are free to interact with cells in the bloodstream, lymphatic fluid, and lymphoid organs (e.g., spleen and lymph nodes). It is well established that corticosteroids, such as cortisol, directly impair or modify several cellular immune functions and modulate production of cytokines that direct them. Elevations in peripheral NE and other β-adrenergic agonists relate to decreased cellular immune indices such as NKCC and T lymphocyte proliferation, and promote a predominance of T-helper cell Type 2 (Th2) over Th1 cytokines, which tends to down-regulate these cellular immune functions. In humans, these changes may compound the pathogenic processes already established in diseases such as HIV/AIDS by dampening cellular immune function (Cole, Kemeny, Naliboff, Fahey, & Zack, 2001), and in certain types of cancer, by promoting tumor growth and metastasis (Lutgendorf, Cole & Costanza, 2003).

Thus, at least two stress-related pathways are capable of orchestrating behavioral-immune interactions: the HPA axis by way of corticosteroids, and the sympathetic nervous system (SNS), by way of peripheral catecholamine production (Chrousos & Gold, 1992, McEwen, 1998). Consequently, chronic stress or psychological distress and negative affect states (e.g., depression) that are characterized by disruptions in HPA and SNS functioning may have the greatest effects on certain immune-system functions that are relevant in major diseases. Keep in mind that a large research literature demonstrates that other hormones such as testosterone, estrogens and progesterone, met-enkephalin, β-endorphin, and substance P, growth hormone, thyroid hormones, androgens and estrogens, prolactin, arginine vasopressin, and neuropeptide-Y can modulate immune functioning, though a review of this work is beyond the scope of this chapter.

PNI and Disease Processes

Up until recently, most human PNI studies were designed to elucidate mechanisms underlying associations between stressors and affect on the one hand and infectious and neoplastic disease on the other (Antoni et al., 2006). Thus, the effects of stressors and depression on down-regulation of immune parameters received the greatest research attention, especially in conditions such as HIV/AIDS (Antoni & Carrico, 2010) and in some cancers (Antoni, Lutgendorf, Cole et al., 2006). This work has evolved to a consideration of stress-induced neuroendocrine changes on inflammatory as well as immune surveillance processes in each of these sets of diseases (e.g., Lutgendorf, Sood & Antoni, 2010). There is an increasing focus, as well, on examining relations between psychological factors, stress physiology, and inflammatory processes to develop PNI models for other conditions such as cardiovascular disease (CVD) (Steptoe & Brydon, 2005) and rheumatoid arthritis (Heijnen & Kavelaars, 2005). Acute psychological stressors can induce transient endothelial dysfunction, and increases in pro-inflammatory cytokines such as IL-1β, IL-10, IL-6 and tumor necrosis factor-alpha (TNFα), as well as cortisol and NE in healthy individuals (Ghiadoni, Donald, Cropley et al., 2000; Altemus, Rao, Dhabhar, Ding, & Granstein, 2001). There is also an increase in peripheral leukocyte adhesion molecule expression and density after acute psychological laboratory stress (Goebel & Mills, 2000), as well as increased chemotaxis of peripheral blood mononuclear cells (Redwine, Snow, Mills & Irwin, 2003). In the latter study, increases in catecholamine levels paralleled increased lymphocyte expression of Mac-1 and decreased L-selectin expression, suggesting that the expression of these adhesion molecules is mediated by adrenergic receptors (Redwine et al., 2003).

Chronic stress and inflammation have been associated with exacerbations of autoimmune disease (Harbuz, Chover-Gonzalez & Jessop, 2003) and CVD (Appels, Bar, Bar, Bruggeman, & de Bates, 2000). In individuals with autoimmune disease or severe atherosclerosis, prolonged stress related to chronically activated pro-inflammatory cytokine production, possibly exacerbating pathophysiology and symptoms. These changes are believed to be due, in part, to a down-regulation of leukocyte corticosteroid receptors with chronic stress (Miller, Cohen & Ritchey, 2002). With cortisol unable to suppress inflammatory signaling, pro-inflammatory cytokines may be produced in excess, thereby exacerbating disease processes and symptoms. We know that chronic stress is associated with increased swelling and reduced mobility in rheumatoid arthritis (Affleck et al., 1997) and an exacerbation of disease in multiple sclerosis (Mohr, Hart, Julian, Cox, & Pelletier, 2004). In coronary heart disease, elevated levels of inflammatory markers, such as C-reactive protein (CRP) predict myocardial infarction, even beyond cholesterol, blood pressure, and smoking (Morrow & Ridker, 2000).

One other relevant set of conditions for this discussion include medically unexplained conditions such as chronic fatigue syndrome (CFS), which are characterized by overactivation of some immune cell subpopulations (Cruess, Klimas, Helder, Antoni & Fletcher, 2000), elevations in circulating pro-inflammatory cytokines (Patarca, Klimas, Lutgendorf, Antoni, & Fletcher, 1994) and down-regulated cellular immune functions such as NKCC (Klimas & Koneru, 2007). The fact that CFS patients also show down-regulated HPA axis responses to challenge (Demitrack & Dale, 1991) and stress-related exacerbation of symptoms (Lutgendorf et al., 1995) suggests that chronic stress may contribute to symptom flares via neuroendocrine alterations (Antoni & Weiss, 2003).

PNI Rationale for Using Behavioral Interventions to Affect Disease Processes.

Using a PNI rationale one could reason that the most effective behavioral interventions for helping stressed and distressed individuals handle the challenges in their lives, while optimizing physical health, need to consider the role of psychosocial, neuroendocrine and immunologic mechanisms. Much of the promise of human PNI research has lain in the notion that stress-induced immune suppressive processes might be offset by behavioral interventions that change stress responses. This rationale is particularly germane to patients dealing with conditions associated with down-regulated cellular immune functioning like viral infections and cancers. To the extent that stressors also contribute to the course of conditions where the immune system and inflammatory processes are up-regulated, then it is plausible that behavioral interventions that reduce chronic stress and cortisol production in dysregulated systems may lead to an up-regulation of cortisol receptors on immune cells, thereby decreasing inflammation.

It follows that those stress reduction interventions that are of greatest clinical value are the ones that are found to be effective in individuals whose immune systems are down-regulated to external antigens (e.g., HIV/AIDS) or self-associated cellular mutations (e.g., cancer), or up-regulated to internal inflammatory signals (e.g., CVD) or external stimuli (e.g., chronic fatigue syndrome). The following sections focus on examples of work applying stress-management interventions to each of these chronic disease populations.

Stress Management, PNI, and Infectious Diseases: HIV/AIDS

Disease Processes in HIV/AIDS

As an example of the use of stress management in PNI research with an infectious disease I will focus on research on HIV/AIDS. HIV/AIDS is caused by a retrovirus, which works in reverse of typical viral infections by converting viral RNA to DNA in host cells. HIV selectively targets a subpopulation of T lymphocytes referred to as CD4+ T helper cells (Klatzmann et al., 1984; Varmus, 1988). These cells are used as hosts for transcribing HIV RNA and ultimately new HIV virions that can go on to infect other host cells bearing the CD4 receptor. In so doing, the infected person experiences a loss of CD4+ T cells, and HIV virus concentration in the peripheral blood or "viral load" increases (Pantaleo, Graziosi, & Fauci, 1993). Beyond the rapid viral replication, the fact that HIV is constantly mutating diminishes the effectiveness of antiviral immune mechanisms (Gaines et al., 1990).

After an initial period of an acute mononucleosis-like syndrome for about a month after seroconversion, most people remain asymptomatic for a period of years (Tindall & Cooper, 1991). During this period, however, these individuals reveal increasing viral load and decreasing CD4+ cell count. When clinical symptoms do appear, they come in the form of non-life-threatening infections (Candida, hairy cell leukoplakia) that diminish quality of life, but are treatable (Pantaleo et al., 1993). Many individuals go on to develop full-blown AIDS when their CD4+ T cells fall below 200 cell/mm³ or when they are diagnosed with AIDS-defining opportunistic infections such as pneumonia, or neoplasias such as Kaposi's Sarcoma, Burkitt's lymphoma, or invasive cervical cancer (CDC, 1992).

It is unclear what accounts for the variability in the number and severity of manifest clinical symptoms and time course to the development of AIDS among HIV-infected persons. Differences in the course of the disease may be determined by negative health behaviors (e.g., substance use or poor medication adherence) and mood states (e.g., depression), which may facilitate increased virus replication or decrease the individual's ability to preserve certain key immune system components in spite of the HIV infection. Some of these immune components may include CD8+ T cytotoxic lymphocytes and natural killer (NK) cells, which are important for viral and neoplastic surveillance (Ironson et al., 2001). Importantly the PNI literature shows that the functioning of these immune cells (e.g., natural killer cell cytotoxicity, NKCC) are influenced by stressors, negative mood, coping, and decreased social support in persons with HIV (for review see Antoni & Carrico, in press).

Psychological Factors and HIV Disease Progression

Persons dealing with HIV/AIDS are at elevated risk of increased stressful life events as well as affective and anxiety disorders (Carrico, Antoni, Young, & Gorman, 2008; Bing et al., 2001; Ciesla & Roberts, 2001). Our group previously hypothesized that chronic stress, depression, and other mental health challenges may impact disease course in HIV via increased risk of negative health behaviors (increased substance use and poorer HIV medication adherence) and/or via PNI processes secondary to stressors and distress states (Antoni et al., 1990; Antoni & Carrico, in press). Most of the evidence suggesting the latter has come from longitudinal studies of the health sequelae of distress states like depression, and from the burden of accumulating stressful life events. These studies typically track biological and clinical health effects in cohorts of asymptomatic HIV-infected persons and relate psychological factors to disease indicators while controlling for the influence of negative health behaviors.

It is well established that depression is associated with poorer immune status, faster HIV disease progression, and a greater risk of mortality in persons with HIV (Leserman, 2008), though it is plausible that, as the disease progresses, depressive symptoms may increase reactively (Kalichman, Difonzo, Austin, Luke, & Rompa, 2002). However, longitudinal work reveals that depressive symptoms predict reduced CD8+ and NK cell counts (Leserman et al., 1997), and more rapid CD4+ cell count decline over periods of several years in cohorts of HIV+ men (Burack et al., 1993; Vedhara et al., 1997) and women (Ickovics et al., 2001). Cumulative depressive symptoms, hopelessness, and avoidant coping scores over a 2-year period were associated with decreased CD4+ cell counts and higher HIV viral load, even after controlling for antiretroviral therapy (ART) adherence (Ironson et al., 2005). The cumulative burden of depressive symptoms over longer periods have also been related to faster progression to an AIDS diagnosis and shorter survival (Leserman et al., 2002; Mayne, Vittinghoff, Chesney, Barrett, & Coates, 1996; Ickovics et al., 2001). Beyond depressive symptoms, increased anger and anxiety have been associated with faster progression to AIDS (Leserman et al., 2002), and higher HIV viral load (Evans et al., 2002).

Cumulative negative life events have also been associated with reduced NK and CD8+ T cell counts and faster disease progression over a serial set of follow-ups of initially asymptomatic HIV+ men spanning 9 years (Leserman et al., 1997; 1999; 2000; 2002). Importantly for considerations of PNI mechanisms, this team also found that greater serum concentrations of cortisol measured cumulatively were independently associated with faster progression to AIDS, development of an AIDS-related condition, and mortality over a 9-year period (Leserman et al. 2002). More recent work confirms this in showing that cumulative negative life events relate to increases in HIV viral load in cohorts of HIV-infected men and women treated with Highly Active Antiretroviral Therapy (HAART), the treatment of choice for the past decade (Ironson et al., 2005). This work supports the contention that chronic stress may contribute to accelerated HIV disease progression.

Other work has focused on whether individual differences in stressor appraisals, coping strategies, and social support—all key targets of stress-management interventions—can moderate the impact of stressors and distress states on disease progression and related PNI processes in persons with HIV. For instance, "positive" psychological states may relate to slowed HIV disease progression (Ironson & Hayward, 2008). Among both HIV-infected men and women, greater levels of constructs such as positive affect, positive HIV outcome expectancies,

and benefit finding predicted less rapid CD4+ T cell decline and greater survival over time (Ickovics et al., 2006; Moskowitz, 2003). Social support may be beneficial to HIV-infected persons by operating through multiple pathways (Zuckerman & Antoni, 1995). Generally this work has shown that more positive outlook, use of more adaptive coping strategies, and having adequate social support have salutary effects on psychological and immunological status and the course of HIV infection (for review, see Antoni, 2010).

As previously noted, the effects of stressors, mood, and distress states on immune parameters relevant for HIV disease progression may be explained via disruptions in neuroendocrine regulation governed by SNS and HPA processes (Antoni and Carrico, in press). As we shall see, PNI mechanisms have also been proposed to explain the potential health benefits of stress-management interventions in persons with HIV (Antoni, 2003a; Caricco & Antoni, 2008). It should be noted that a separate area of behavioral medicine research has focused on behavioral interventions targeting health behavior pathways (to change substance use, medication adherence, sexual behaviors) to optimize HIV disease management. Though beyond the scope of this chapter, more information on this area of work can be found elsewhere (e.g., Gore-Felton & Koopman, 2008; Safren et al., 2006; Kalichman, 2008; DesJarlais & Semaan, 2008).

Rationale for Stress-Management Intervention in HIV/AIDS

The use of psychosocial interventions to help individuals with HIV cope with their illness and other stressors in their lives has been extensively researched in the past 20 years. One model focused on a specific form of stress management—cognitive-behavioral stress management (CBSM)—has been refined over this period (Antoni, 2003a; Antoni et al., 1990). The rationale for using CBSM intervention in HIV/AIDS is as follows: Because stressors, cognitive appraisals, coping strategies, and interpersonal processes (e.g., social support) may influence psychological adjustment, biobehavioral processes, and physical health status in persons dealing with HIV, a multimodal intervention designed to modify stressor perceptions and responses using cognitive behavioral and relaxation techniques may improve psychological adaptation and possibly physical health.

It was specifically hypothesized that stress-management intervention can improve psychological adaptation by first teaching anxiety-reduction behavioral skills such as relaxation, imagery, deep breathing, and meditation. Second cognitive-behavioral and interpersonal skills training was hypothesized to reduce negative mood and distress states by changing cognitive appraisals to improve outlook and attitudes, teaching new coping strategies to increase a sense of self-efficacy, and providing skills to better evaluate, attract, and maintain positive social support and decrease interpersonal conflict (Antoni, 2003a; Antoni, Ironson, & Schneiderman, 2007). It was hypothesized that subsequent changes in perceived stress, distress, or depression would parallel improved regulation of SNS and HPA axis functioning since: (a) changes in distress and mood states were previously associated with alterations in neuroendocrine regulation (McEwen, 1998; Chrousos & Gold, 1992), and (b) circulating levels of cortisol and catecholamines are altered as a function of an individual's appraisals of and coping responses to stressors (McEwen, 1998; Sapolsky, Romero, & Munck, 2000). If so, then improvements in neuroendocrine regulation after stress-management intervention may produce a partial "normalization" of immune system functions in HIV-infected persons (Antoni & Schneiderman, 1998).

Although most of the links in this chain of hypothesized events had previously been established in healthy organisms, there was reason to suspect that these associations might apply to HIV-infected persons. First, in-vitro studies show that cortisol synergizes with gp120—the major host cell HIV attachment site—to enhance rates of CD4+ T cell decline (Nair et al., 2000) and apoptosis (programmed cell death) (Amendola et al., 1996). Cortisol also enhances in-vitro HIV p24 antigen production in human macrophages (which also bear the CD4 receptor) (Swanson, Zeller, & Spear, 1998). Finally, as noted previously, in-vivo work shows that serum cortisol concentrations in HIV-infected men are associated with progression to AIDS, development of an AIDS-Related Complex (ARC) symptom, and mortality over a 9-year period (Leserman et al., 2002).

There is also convincing evidence that another adrenal hormone, norepinephrine (NE), known to be associated with increased anxiety and distress, can affect immune system functions known to be compromised in HIV disease. Catecholamines such as NE (and epinephrine, E) bind to lymphocyte membrane β_2 adrenergic receptors where they tend to down-regulate cellular immune functions by activating the G protein linked adenyl cyclase-cAMP-protein kinase A, signaling cascade and decreasing protein synthesis

(Kobilka, 1992). This can suppress cellular immune functions, such as lymphocyte proliferation, decrease Th1 cytokines, and increase Th2 cytokines, which normally orchestrate immunologic responses, such as lymphocyte proliferation, and increase CD8+ T-cell and NK-cell mediated killing necessary for antiviral and antitumor responses. Importantly, Th1/Th2 reversal predicts elevations in HIV viral load over time (Cole, Korin, Fahey, & Zack, 1998). In terms of the pathophysiology of HIV/AIDS there is an emerging body of research demonstrating that neuroendocrine factors may mediate stress effects on HIV disease progression through direct effects on dysregulation of Th1 cytokines, chemokines, and HIV transcription factors that favor increased HIV replication rate (Cole, 2008). Increased HIV replication rate predates increased viral load in the circulation and ultimately clinical disease progression. There is, in fact, direct evidence that HIV-infected people with elevated resting autonomic nervous system activity (likely accompanied by increased adrenal production of NE and cortisol) prior to beginning antiretroviral therapy demonstrate poorer suppression of HIV viral load and decreased CD4+ T-cell reconstitution (Cole et al., 2001). Thus, a reasonable case can be made for stress-management interventions targeting stress and mood improvement to effect changes in adrenal hormones that can contribute to biomarkers of HIV disease progression.

In terms of clinical pathways, one can postulate that, if changing stress physiology influences cytokine regulation and other aspects of immune system communication, then HIV-infected persons undergoing stress-reduction interventions such as CBSM might show more efficient surveillance of opportunistic pathogens (e.g., reactivated latent herpesvirus infections). These infections, if poorly controlled, can contribute directly to increased HIV replication through "transactivation" of HIV-infected CD4+ T cells resulting in a rising viral load (for review see Antoni, Esterling, Lutgendorf, Fletcher, & Schneiderman, 1995). Opportunistic oncogenic viral infections that are highly prevalent in HIV-infected persons (e.g., human papillomavirus, HPV; Epstein-Barr virus, EBV) if poorly controlled can produce neoplastic cell changes and result in AIDS-related cancers such as cervical cancer and Burkitt's lymphoma (e.g., Antoni et al., 1995; Jensen, Lehman, Antoni, & Pereira, 2007). Thus, stress management may help normalize immune surveillance, which may, in turn, slow stress-associated increases in viral load and clinical disease progression.

Efficacy of Psychosocial Interventions and Stress Management in HIV/AIDS

A number of reviews have summarized the effects of behavioral interventions on anxiety and depressed mood in HIV-infected men and women (e.g., Carrico Antoni, Young, & Gorman, 2008). Reviews most relevant to this chapter have focused specifically on the effects of these interventions on physiological parameters such as neuroendocrine and immune variables in HIV-infected persons (Antoni, 2003a; Crepaz, et al., 2008; Carrico & Antoni, 2008). Before summarizing this work, I again stress that behavioral interventions have also been shown to modulate sexual risk behaviors (Kalichmen, 2008), drug use (DesJarlais & Semaan, 2008), and HIV medication adherence (Simoni, Pearson, Pantalone, Marks, & Crepaz, 2006), which may, in turn, affect HIV disease progression. However, I focus here on work examining the effects of behavioral interventions on mood and neuroimmune variables that are relevant to HIV disease progression.

One meta-analysis summarized cognitive-behavioral intervention effects on psychological (depression, anxiety, anger, and stress) and immune (CD4+ T cell counts) outcomes in 15 studies of persons with HIV that were published from 1988–2005 (Crepaz et al., 2008). Most of these were group-based interventions, delivered over 3–17 sessions (median = 10), with a focus on cognitive re-appraisal/cognitive restructuring, coping-skills training, stress-management-skills training, and/or social support. Effect sizes for psychological outcomes were mostly significant and ranged from 0.30 to 1.00, but no significant effects were reported on CD4+ T-cells. Interestingly, significant effects on depression and anxiety were only found in studies providing stress management and in those having at least 10 intervention sessions (Crepaz et al., 2008). The absence of intervention effects on overall CD4+ cell counts in this review may be due to the fact that stress-response processes may not relate directly (especially over short follow-up periods) to the numbers of immune cells, but rather to their functions (lymphocyte proliferative response and antiviral mechanisms, including NKCC) and the regulation of cytokines that orchestrate these functions. Why would one expect stress processes, including stress-management interventions, to affect immune functioning in the absence of reliable changes in immune cell counts? It is possible that cell counts (T-cells or NK cells) can remain constant in the face of neuroendocrine changes while the per cell functionality might be altered by way of stimulation of adrenergic membrane receptors or glucocorticoid intracytoplasmic receptor-mediated changes in these cells. Prior reviews of the human PNI have shown much more robust associations between psychological variables (chronic stress, negative mood) and immune functional indices than for immune cell counts (Herbert & Cohen, 1993a,b).

A qualitative review published in 2008 conducted a more fine-grained analysis focused on the effects of psychological interventions on neuroendocrine and immune parameters in 14 randomized controlled trials published from 1987 to 2007 in persons with HIV/AIDS (Carrico & Antoni, 2008). As in the meta-analysis by Crepaz et al. (2008) most of the studies in this review were group-based with a mode of 10 weeks duration. This review, however, included studies that were published after the period covered by the Crepaz et al. analysis, which allowed for the inclusion of some work encompassing the era of highly active antiretroviral therapy (HAART) and which measured changes in HIV viral load. The studies were classified as cognitive behavioral (mixture of cognitive-behavioral therapy and relaxation-related strategies), those using relaxation only or meditation only, and those focused on emotional expression.

Many of the studies showed PNI effects. The majority of the studies showing significant effects on psychological states (anxiety and depressed mood), neuroendocrine hormones (cortisol and catecholamines), and immune and viral parameters (lymphocyte proliferation, herpesvirus antibody titers, HIV viral load) were based on interventions that employed at least 10 weeks of group-based sessions and that focused on stress- management techniques. A second major finding of this review was that those interventions that were most successful in reducing depressed mood, anxiety, and distress were more likely to have significant effects on neuroendocrine measures and immune status. This pattern suggests that, in order for behavioral interventions to modulate health-relevant immune and viral parameters, they must modulate distress or mood states. It is plausible then that the putative health effects of these interventions may be mediated by successful manipulation of stress and coping processes and subsequent changes in stress physiology. A closer look at some of the CBSM intervention research reveals how intervention-associated changes in distress and mood indicators appear to parallel changes in neuroendocrine indicators, which each predate apparently beneficial changes in immunologic and viral biomarkers of disease. However I first summarize some of the features of CBSM intervention, how its specific contents and sequence was developed, and the types of clinical considerations that are relevant when delivering this intervention.

THE COGNITIVE BEHAVIORAL STRESS-MANAGEMENT INTERVENTION

The CBSM intervention was designed to be a group-based training distributed over 10 weekly 2-hour sessions delivered in groups of 4–8 participants led by two co-leaders who had completed a 20-hr training session. Within the first 45 minutes of each session, various relaxation techniques were taught, which progressed from simple 7- and 4-muscle relaxation exercises to muscle relaxation on cue, based on a counting method, and on to deep breathing, autogenic exercises, and mindfulness meditation. This portion of the intervention also included provision of a recording (cassettes or CDs) made in the group leader's voice, which the participants were instructed to listen to on a daily basis. The 45-minute relaxation portion of each session was designed to give participants an immediate experience of relief and anxiety reduction at the beginning of each session, which we hypothesized would make them more focused and suggestible for the remaining 90-minute cognitive behavioral (CB) portion of each session (Antoni, Ironson & Schneiderman, 2007; Antoni, 2003c).

After a 15-minute break from the relaxation exercises, the CB portion of each session commenced. Participants initially learned about stressors and stress responses and participated in exercises designed to raise their awareness of these stress responses and mood changes. This continued for the first 2 weeks of the program, followed in weeks 3 and 4 by a focus on cognitive restructuring and rational thought replacement, techniques designed to increase awareness of the link between cognitive appraisal of stressors and other stimuli, and affective and behavioral responses. In weeks 5 and 6, the focus turned to coping-effectiveness training (Folkman et al., 1991), wherein participants first reviewed their coping repertoire and classified their coping responses into direct and indirect, emotion- and problem-focused strategies. The second part of the coping sessions was focused on teaching participants to separate stressors into changeable and unchangeable aspects and then to match direct, problem-focused strategies with changeable aspects of stressful situations, and direct, emotion-focused strategies with unchangeable aspects of stressful

situations. The remaining modules of the program focused on teaching participants interpersonal skills that could be used to manage stress. These included anger management, assertiveness training, and social-support building. In addition to the weekly CB modules, participants received homework assignments (e.g., diary keeping, mood ratings, recordings of cognitive appraisals used for daily stressors, coping strategies matched to aspects of stressors, assertive responses to interpersonal exchanges, how feelings of anger were expressed, types of social support requested and received in response to specific stressors, etc.) that were designed to reinforce their skills in using the techniques presented in the sessions. Throughout all the weekly CB modules, the protocol was to begin each session with a review of homework, then introduce a new topic and set of techniques through didactics delivered by the group leaders, then a period for role-playing, and finally, a review of the session. A final session served as a review of the prior weekly sessions. Sessions summaries and homework assignments were contained in a participant workbook.

The program was designed to be led by persons with at least a Master's level of training in psychology or related mental-health fields, but it is feasible that this material could be delivered by nurses or other health-care professionals. This intervention was not designed for delivery as a self-help method, though certain aspects of it (e.g., muscle relaxation), are in fact self-administered. All the evidence for the efficacy of CBSM are based on using a live group format, and it is hypothesized that some of its effects are realized through nonspecific group processes. Work is currently underway to see if this group experience can be translated into effective programs delivered remotely via videophone- and web-based technologies.

EFFECTS OF CBSM IN HIV

The effects of CBSM on psychosocial and physiological variables relevant to health outcomes have been evaluated in a series of studies of men who have sex with men (MSM) and lower-income minority women who are, at various points, in the disease experience. We know that CBSM buffers the initial distress and immune changes upon learning of a seropositive diagnosis in MSMs (Antoni, Baggett, Ironson, August et al., 1991; LaPerriere et al., 1990). Men in this trial also showed significant decreases in IgG antibody titers (reflecting better immunologic control) to two herpesviruses, EBV, and human herpes virus Type-6 (HHV-6), over the subsequent

5 weeks. Their IgG values, in fact, moved into the normal range for age-matched healthy-male laboratory control values following the intervention (Esterling et al., 1992). Importantly, the men who revealed less distress at diagnosis, decreased HIV-specific denial coping after diagnosis, attended more CBSM sessions, and practiced their homework more showed lower and slower disease progression to symptoms and AIDS 2 years later (Ironson et al., 1994). Thus, individual differences in the "uptake" of CBSM predicted HIV disease progression over time.

A subsequent trial focused on men with more progressed disease and conducted a more fine-grained analysis of cognitive-behavioral and inter-personal processes. Men with mild non-AIDS symptoms (category B of the 1993 CDC definition) assigned to CBSM showed decreased depressive symptoms, anxiety, and total mood disturbance over the 10-week intervention period (Lutgendorf et al., 1998). In this trial, changes in cognitive coping strategies (acceptance, and positive reinterpretation and growth) and social support (social attachment, guidance) during the intervention, mediated its effects on these mood variables (Lutgendorf et al., 1998). In parallel to these observations, men assigned to CBSM also showed decreases in IgG antibody titers to herpes simplex virus-type 2 (HSV-2) (Lutgendorf et al., 1997). Reductions in HSV-2 titers were proportional to decreases in depressive symptoms (Lutgendorf et al., 1997), and to increases in perceived social support and relaxation-associated distress reduction during home practice over the 10-week period (Cruess, Antoni, Cruess et al., 2000). This was among the first evidence that changes in the targets of CBSM—depression, social support, and relaxation—would happen in parallel with increases in an in-vivo indicator of antiviral immunity specific to an opportunistic herpes virus that is associated with marked pathology in HIV-infected persons.

Were These Changes Accompanied by Changes in Adrenal Stress Hormones Hypothesized to be Affected by Stress Management?

Those men assigned to CBSM did, in fact, show significant decreases in 24-hour urinary free cortisol over this 10-week period (Antoni, Wagner, Cruess, et al., 2000), and these cortisol decreases were associated with decreases in both depressed mood and HSV-2 antibody titers (Cruess, Antoni, McGregor, et al., 2000). These findings support a PNI model wherein changes and mood and cortisol regulation

parallel improved immunologic control over a latent herpes virus—a potential analog for susceptibility to other opportunistic viral infections. When we followed these individuals over a longer period, we found that men assigned to CBSM showed a greater evidence of immune system reconstitution (transitional naïve T-helper cells) at 6–12 month follow-up (Antoni et al., 2002). Importantly, reductions in both depressed mood and urinary free cortisol during the initial 10-week intervention period appeared to "co-mediate" CBSM effects on recovery of these transitional naïve T-cell counts up to 12 months later (Antoni et al., 2005).

Men assigned to CBSM also showed decreases in urinary NE during the 10-week intervention period, which were associated with reductions in anxiety but not depressed mood. When we followed this cohort of men we found that NE reductions during the 10-week intervention period predicted greater preservation of CD8+ T cells at 6–12 months (Antoni, Cruess, et al., 2000). CBSM appeared to decrease anxiety in parallel with NE reductions, which predicted levels of CD8+T cells. Often referred to as cytotoxic or "killer" T-cells, this is an important immune component necessary for responding to viral infections and neoplastic cell changes. It is plausible that the immune changes observed in these two sets of analyses—transitional naïve T cells and CD8+ cytotoxic T cells—may have changed, secondary to other immunologic changes (decreased HIV viral load, better Th1 cytokine regulation), which we now know may be directly tied to neuroendocrine regulation (Cole, 2008). It is plausible that the recovery or preservation of cell populations observed in men receiving CBSM may have been secondary to decreases in circulating HIV virions occurring over the follow-up period. However, measuring viral load in these early studies was not practical due to excessive costs and relative insensitivity of assays available. With the advent of HAART in 1996 and the need for careful monitoring of changes in both medication adherence and HIV RNA levels in the circulation, it became possible to explore the effects of CBSM on viral load while carefully controlling for changes in medication adherence.

We first examined how stress and coping processes related to the evolution of medication adherence and viral load over time in a cohort of men and women recently initiating a HAART regimen (Weaver et al., 2005). We found that avoidant coping, lower social support, and negative mood all related to greater viral load over time. Since our prior work showed that CBSM improved negative mood, coping, and social support (Lutgendorf et al., 1998; Cruess, Wagner, Cruess et al., 2000) in tandem with improved neuroendocrine (Antoni, Wagner, Cruess, et al., 2000) and immunologic status (Antoni, Cruess, et al., 2000; Antoni et al., 2005; Lutgendorf et al., 1997), it seemed plausible that CBSM might also improve the ways people on HAART handled stress in parallel with improvements in health-related outcomes such as viral load. We found that HIV+ men (who had a detectable HIV viral load at baseline) who were assigned to CBSM showed greater than a half-log reduction in HIV viral load over the 15-month investigation period, a clinically meaningful effect that held, even after controlling for HAART medication adherence over this entire period, and the reduction appeared to be mediated by reductions in depressed mood (Antoni, Carrico, et al., 2006). Paralleling earlier work with CBSM (Ironson et al., 1994), we noted that greater attendance at CBSM sessions was associated with lower HIV viral load at follow-up. Future work should investigate whether the influence of depression reductions on viral load were explained by changes in neuroendocrine (urinary cortisol and catecholamines) and/or health behaviors (substance use, sleep). In each of the cohorts of men with HIV who we have studied, the effects of CBSM on mental health and immune and virologic variables appear to be tied to the neuroendocrine changes reflecting changes in stress physiology. Recent longitudinal work in another HAART-treated sample showed that greater urinary NE predicted less effectiveness of a newly initiated HAART regimen in reducing HIV viral load over a 6-month period (Ironson et al., 2008). Investigating whether changes in NE and cortisol during CBSM parallel its effects on HIV viral load in HAART-treated patients seems like a worthwhile effort. Mapping these changes in viral load onto specific clinical outcomes is yet to be done, and doing so would be a key culmination of this research line. Interestingly, we might be closer to identifying such effects in women with HIV.

A separate line of studies has shown that stress processes and CBSM may be associated with specific indicators of clinical disease progression in women dealing with HIV. This work focuses on lower income women with HIV who are at elevated risk for developing an AIDS-defining clinical outcome—cervical cancer—due to being co-infected with a type of carcinogenic virus, human papilloma virus (HPV). Women co-infected with HIV and certain types of HPVs (HIV+HPV+) are at increased risk for developing cervical intraepithelial neoplasia (CIN) as well as invasive cervical carcinoma (Maiman et al., 1997; Jensen et al., 2007). Importantly, CIN and cervical cancer were designated as ARC-defining and AIDS-defining conditions, respectively, by the Centers of Disease Control in 1992 (CDC, 1992).

Prospective studies show that HIV+HPV+ women reporting greater negative life events over the prior year had a greater subsequent risk of CIN (Pereira et al., 2003a) and HSV-2 genital herpes virus outbreaks (Pereira et al., 2003b) one year later. This study was followed by another showing that a separate cohort of HIV+HPV+ women assigned to CBSM showed significant decreases in perceived stress and a decreased risk for persistent CIN at 6-month follow-up (Antoni et al., 2008), effects that held after controlling for HPV type, CD4+ cell counts, HAART medications, and tobacco smoking at study entry. Future work should examine whether these effects can be explained by changes in neuroendocrine (urinary cortisol and NE) and immunologic (NKCC, HIV viral load) variables as well as health-behavior-change variables (e.g., sexual behaviors, smoking, alcohol and drug use, medication adherence). There is strong evidence that stress-associated neuroendocrine factors could affect, not only immune surveillance over latent HPV infection, but also multiple steps in HPV viral oncogenesis (see Antoni, Lutgendorf, et al., 2006; Jensen et al., 2007). Other viral-associated cancers may present plausible PNI models for prevention of AIDS-related cancers. Some of these include HPV-associated anal carcinoma, human herpes virus type 8 (HHV-8), associated Kaposi's sarcoma, and EBV-associated Burkitt's lymphoma (Huang et al., 2001; Suligoi et al., 2003; Killibrew & Shiramizu, 2004). One place to begin this work may be in persons with a background of immunosuppression secondary to HIV infection.

Summary

In summary, stress management and other related interventions can improve psychological variables such as distress and depressive symptoms in men and women with HIV/AIDS. In studies focused specifically on examining PNI outcomes—mostly involving group-based CBSM—there is a strong trend for these psychological changes to parallel neuroendocrine changes that relate to improvements in immunological and viral biomarkers of disease progression (Carrico & Antoni, 2008). More recently published studies suggest that CBSM may also affect specific disease activity processes such as

HIV viral load and cervical neoplasia. Reviewing the effects of CBSM across multiple studies reveals that this form of intervention helps individuals manage the "stress" of HIV infection by improving psychological adjustment and physiological regulation at several points in the HIV disease experience including: serostatus testing and notification, the early symptomatic stage preceding AIDS, and throughout disease management with antiretroviral therapy including HAART regimens. In general, this provides empirical support for a PNI model that changes in stress-related processes, and distress states may relate reliably to neuroendocrine and immune-system indicators that are relevant for this disease (see Table 21.2 for summary of effects of CBSM in HIV/AIDS).

Taken together, these findings make a strong case for the efficacy of CBSM—an intervention designed to modify stress and coping responses as individuals manage HIV infection—for optimizing mental and physical health outcomes. However, not all studies of CBSM have shown improvements in disease status (HIV viral load, CD4 cell counts), even when the interventions produced positive improvements in mental-health variables (Berger et al., 2008; McCain et al., 2003). It is plausible that the specific techniques used across these studies varied in a systematic way. There is also evidence that alternative forms of psychosocial intervention targeting stress and distress states, including Tai Chi, massage, and written emotional expression may produce significant effects on certain immune parameters in persons with HIV (McCain et al., 2008; Diego et al., 2001; Petrie, Fontanilla, Thomas, Booth, & Pennebaker, 2004). These interventions may work on alleviating unexpressed concerns, bodily tension, and physiological activation. Although these approaches have shown short-term effects, it remains unclear how they might improve coping with future HIV-related stressors, and, thus, their effects may be time limited.

Most studies investigating the effects of stress-management interventions in HIV have been focused on distress, depressive symptoms, and other indicators of negative affect. Given that positive affect and an increased sense of meaning have been shown to predict better disease course in HIV (Moskowitz, 2003; Bower, Kemeny, Taylor, & Fahey, 1998), it is worth testing whether approaches such as group-based CBSM and expressive writing can modulate constructs such as positive affect, positive states of mind, and benefit finding in parallel with neuroendocrine and immune parameters such as those studies to date.

It is also arguable that much more work needs to be done to test whether the effects of CBSM and other stress management approaches are generalizable to real-life situations, which is where HIV is taking its greatest tolls. In particular, there is a conspicuous lack of CBSM studies of HIV-infected populations outside of middle class, white MSM. Although some work shows encouraging results with group-based CBSM (Antoni et al., 2008) and CBSM-like (Lechner et al., 2003; Weiss, Tobin,

Table 21.2 Summary of Cognitive-Behavioral Stress-Management (CBSM) Intervention Effects in Persons with HIV/AIDS:

(1) CBSM decreases indicators of distress (anxiety and depressed mood) by increasing the use of adaptive cognitive coping strategies (greater acceptance and positive reframing and less denial and avoidance) and perceived social support (instrumental and emotional).

(2) CBSM decreases distress in parallel with reductions in SNS activity (urinary norepinephrine, NE) and Hypothalamic Pituitary Adrenal (HPA) axis output (urinary cortisol).

(3) CBSM reductions in distress and neuroendocrine output during the 10-week intervention predict more favorable immune status (greater immune system reconstitution and cytotoxic T cell numbers and better control of latent herpesviruses) concurrently and up to 12 months later.

(4) CBSM reductions in depressed mood predict lower disease activity (HIV viral load) and clinical disease progression (cervical intraepithelial neoplasias, CIN) over time.

(5) CBSM intervention gains in psychological, neuroendocrine, immunologic and viral outcomes are proportional to the "dose" of CBSM received (group attendance) or practiced (home practice) suggesting these effects are specific to CBSM.

Antoni et al., 2011) interventions that have been tailored to be acceptable among lower-income women with HIV, little is known about their longer-term effects on disease course or the mechanisms that could explain their effects. Research aiming to modify stress and coping processes in ethnic minority populations requires carefully adapting the intervention material to be culturally sensitive and relevant to the stressors that participants are dealing with (e.g., Pereira, 2002). The role of family processes also needs more attention in this line of work. Intervention directed at the level of the dyad (Fife, Scott, Fineberg, & Zwickil, 2008) and family system (Szapocnik et al., 2004) will ensure optimal carryover to the setting in which newly learned stress coping skills will be enacted.

Stress Management, PNI, and Neoplastic Disease: Cancers
Rationale for Psychological Intervention in Breast Cancer

Many reviews have addressed the possible role of the immune system and PNI processes in the incidence and progression of different types of human cancers (Antoni, Lutgendorf, Cole et al., 2006; Lutgendorf, Sood, & Antoni, 2010; Bovjberg, 1991; Kiecolt-Glaser, Robles, Heffner, Loving, & Glaser, 2002; Antoni, 2003b; Andersen, Kiecolt-Glaser, & Glaser, 1994; Goodkin, Antoni, Fox, & Sevin, 1993). Despite the fact that this area has been of some interest for several decades definitive PNI work linking stress-endocrine-immune processes to cancer outcomes is only now emerging. Another chapter 19 in this volume by Lutgendorf, Costanzo, and Sood has summarized this body of work. Therefore, the present chapter will focus on psychosocial and stress-management intervention studies that have attempted to elucidate PNI and other biobehavioral processes that could explain the effects of psychosocial interventions on health outcomes in persons dealing with neoplastic disease. Because the research in breast cancer has generated the largest body of empirical studies, I shall focus exclusively on this area.

There is growing evidence that psychological distress, and associated alterations in the HPA axis and SNS, can negatively influence biological processes relevant for breast cancer (McGregor & Antoni, 2009). The consensus in the field is that although the evidence linking psychological factors to breast cancer incidence is weak, there is support for an association among distress states, neuroimmune interactions, and the *progression* of breast cancer after it has been diagnosed and initially treated

(Antoni & Lutgendorf, 2007). Since distress states such as anxiety and negative mood are associated with neuroendocrine and immune system components (as reviewed earlier in this chapter and others), then psychological interventions that reduce psychological distress could positively influence the course of breast cancer.

Efficacy of Psychosocial Intervention and Stress Management in Breast Cancer

With evidence for associations between stress, psychosocial processes, and neuroendocrine changes that can promote cancer progression (e.g., Antoni, Lutgendorf, et al., 2006; Lutgendorf, Sood, & Antoni, 2010), it is surprising that there is yet murky evidence for effects of psychological interventions on cancer progression and survival. Over 300 trials of psychological interventions have been conducted in cancer patients over the past 50 years. Many trials have been criticized for flaws and heterogeneity in sampling, design, and reporting (Newell, Sanson-Fisher, & Savolainen, 2002; Coyne, Stefanek, & Palmer, 2007; Spiegel, 2002). However, the consensus has been that different forms of psychosocial intervention that teach relaxation and stress management, help patients ventilate their feelings and anxiety, and provide social support are able to improve quality of life. The effects and sample sizes of these interventions are generally small, and efficacy varies as a function of intervention content and format and the specific intervention targets of interest (Newell et al., 2002). Only a small minority of these studies have even tested for intervention effects on biological measures, and based on these reviews one could also come to the conclusion that the science demonstrating the effects of such interventions on biological and clinical outcomes among breast cancer survivors is quite preliminary.

In 1989, Spiegel et al. published a seminal study showing that women with metastatic breast cancer assigned to an expressive-supportive-group-therapy (ESGT) intervention lived for about 36 months compared to those in a control condition, who survived for about 18 months (Spiegel, Bloom, Kramer, & Gottheil, 1989). Attempts to replicate these effects in women with metastatic breast cancer have been unsuccessful (Goodwin et al., 2001; Kissane et al., 2007; Spiegel et al., 2007). In one of these trials, EGST was associated with survival effects but only in a small subset of women with estrogen-receptor negative tumors (Spiegel et al., 2007). However, a re-analysis of the ER women in Kissane et al.'s trial revealed no survival effects of ESGT. This line of research has not included studies probing biobehavioral mechanisms, and, therefore, inconsistencies among trial results remains a mystery.

One more recently published trial reported on women with nonmetastatic breast cancer assigned to 4 months of weekly and 8 months of monthly sessions of group-based intervention during the course of their treatment (Andersen et al., 2008). The intervention included training in stress management, positive coping skills, problem solving, improving utilization of social support, improving health behaviors, and various relaxation techniques (progressive muscle relaxation and others). Participants also received disease and breast-cancer-treatment education to improve treatment adherence. Women assigned to the intervention showed a significant reduction in overall and breast-cancer-specific mortality rates as well as reduced risk of breast-cancer recurrence at a median of 11 years follow-up (Andersen et al., 2008). Results were not attributable to site of accrual, sociodemographic factors, disease stage, prognostic markers, surgery type, or adjuvant therapies received during the trial nor extratrial psychiatric medications or counseling received. Recall that, in three earlier trials among women with metastatic breast cancer (Kissane et al., 2007; Goodwin et al., 2001; Spiegel et al., 2007), those assigned to a 12-month course of weekly group-based ESGT focused on emotional expression, social-support provision, and encouraging acceptance of mortality and decreasing the anxiety surrounding death showed no overall survival advantage. These recent results, like those of most psychosocial intervention trials of the past, are clearly disparate. How did they differ?

First, Andersen et al. studied women who were undergoing treatment for nonmetastatic disease (Stage 2 and 3 breast cancer), whereas the other three trials involved women with Stage 4 metastatic disease. Although each intervention was group based and 12 months in duration, the intervention content differed among the studies, as it should have. Whereas the Andersen et al. trial used an intervention based mostly on cognitive-behavioral stress reduction and lifestyle change, the Kissane et al., Goodwin et al., and Spiegel et al. interventions focused more on the expression of emotions and transitions in future life expectations. These are reasonable targets for each population, given that women with nonmetastatic disease are planning their return to daily roles and employment, whereas women with metastatic disease may be more focused on processing existential issues. These studies were

similarly powered. Andersen et al.'s study of 227 women (114 in the intervention arm) and Kissane et al.'s study of women with metastatic breast cancer (147 in the intervention arm) are among the largest samples studied for psychological intervention effects on survival in breast cancer. It may be far more difficult to demonstrate a health benefit from psychological interventions in women with metastatic disease versus nonmetastatic disease due to disease- and treatment-related factors. Because of a lack of clear support for a survival benefit of ESGT in women with metastatic breast cancer in these recently published trials, should we place more weight on the evidence for effects of psychosocial (and stress-reduction focused) interventions in women with nonmetastatic disease? Although the Andersen et al. trial has been criticized for its analytic approach (Stefanek, Palmer, Thombs, & Coyne, 2009) it is worthwhile, for this chapter, to place these results in the context of PNI work in the field that has reported possible biobehavioral mechanisms to explain these effects.

Psychosocial Interventions and PNI Processes in Breast Cancer

Previously, Andersen et al. reported that over the initial intensive monthly training period of their intervention women revealed alterations in stress-related immunoregulatory processes that could contribute to improved general health and possibly altered disease course. They showed that women assigned to the intervention showed increases in cellular immunity (lymphocyte proliferative responses, LPR) (Andersen et al., 2004) at 4-month follow-up. These effects were small and should be interpreted in light of other immune measures that did not change in this study. Importantly, women in the intervention also reported more healthy eating habits, reduced smoking rates, and better treatment adherence (Andersen et al., 2004). At the 12-month follow-up, chart reviews and patient interviews revealed that health status was better in the intervention group than in the comparison group. Reductions in distress at the 4-month time point predicted improved health at 12 months among the intervention participants (Andersen et al., 2007). In a subgroup of the depressed women, the investigators reported what they interpreted as decreases in inflammatory markers in those assigned to the psychosocial intervention (Thornton, Anderson, Scholer, & Carson, 2009).

Importantly, women who ultimately showed disease recurrence revealed greater serum cortisol and greater levels of inflammatory markers (e.g., elevated leukocyte counts) 17 months prior to their recurrence compared to those who remained disease free (Thornton, Andersen, & Carson, 2008). Moreover, those women who experienced a local recurrence at this point had stronger cellular immune responses (NKCC, lymphocyte proliferation) yet fewer signs of general inflammation compared to those who experienced a distal recurrence. Thus, one possible explanation for the positive effects of this intervention on recurrence may be the normalization of stress- and treatment-associated neuroendocrine and immunologic regulation during a critical period following treatment and preceding recurrence. In the context of breast cancer, reducing stress following surgery for cancer may reinforce immunologic components (e.g., NKCC) capable of responding to the metastatic spread of cancer cells (see Ben-Eliyahu, 2003; Shakkar & Ben-Eliyahu, 2003). Other work has suggested that inflammation may contribute to cancer progression (for review see Lutgendorf et al., 2010).

The Andersen group is not the first to demonstrate that stress-reducing interventions can modulate neuroendocrine and immune measures in women with breast cancer. Studies conducted between 1990 and 2000 suggested that psychosocial interventions such as relaxation could influence indices of neuroendocrine and immune function among breast-cancer patients (Schedlowski, Jung, Schimanski, Tewes, & Schmoll, 1994; Larson, Duberstein, Talbot, Caldwell, & Moynihan, 2000). However, these studies were conducted on small samples, lacked sufficient controls, and had short follow-up periods. During the past decade, stress-reduction techniques such as CBSM and meditation-based stress reduction (MBSR) have been shown in larger samples to modulate distress states, neuroendocrine and immunologic indicators in recent completed trials in women with nonmetastatic breast cancer who received the interventions in the midst of medical treatment (see McGregor & Antoni, 2009 for review). These effects have included reductions in anxiety, intrusive thoughts, negative mood, and interpersonal disruption and increases in quality of life, positive mood and benefit finding. Women receiving these interventions also show decreases in PM serum cortisol and increases in immune indicators such as lymphocyte proliferation, Th1 cytokine production (interleukin-2 [IL-2] and interferon-gamma [IFN-γ] and Th1/Th2 production ratio (Carlson, Speca, Faris, & Patel, 2007; McGregor et al., 2004; Phillips et al., 2008; Antoni et al.,

2009; Witek-Janisek et al., 2008). Since the MBSR trials were not randomized clinical trials (RCTs) caution is in order when interpreting the validity of these findings (Carlson et al., 2007; Witek-Janisek et al., 2008). The consistency of results across studies however is provocative. I now focus on the work with CBSM.

To date a 10-week group-based CBSM intervention (Antoni, 2003c) has been shown to improve adaptation to the experience of breast cancer in two separate cohorts of approximately 300 total women recruited in the weeks after surgery and followed across the period of adjuvant therapy out to a 12-month follow-up (Antoni et al., 2001; Antoni, Lechner, et al., 2006; Antoni, Wimberly, et al., 2006). This CBSM intervention also decreased late afternoon cortisol levels immediately postintervention (Cruess, Antoni, McGregor et al., 2000) in the first trial and up to 12-month follow-up in the second trial (Phillips et al., 2008). In each case, the cortisol reductions were greatest in the women who showed the largest psychological changes or who perceived greater confidence in using newly learned CBSM skills such as relaxation (e.g., Phillips et al, 2011). Showing reliable reductions in cortisol is important because flatter diurnal cortisol slopes (possibly due to higher P.M. levels) have been associated with decreased survival among women with metastatic breast cancer (Sephton, Sapolsky, Kraemer, & Spiegel, 2000).

Women in CBSM also showed increased lymphocyte proliferative responses (LPR) to stimulation with anti-CD3 (the T cell receptor) (McGregor et al., 2004). These increases in LPR could have clinical significance since mitogen stimulated proliferation of peripheral blood mononuclear cells (PBMCs) derived from patients with breast cancer is a good clinical predictor for disease recurrence (Wiltschke et al., 1995). To explore the cell-signaling processes that may have underlain these changes in cellular immune functioning, a second trial showed that women in CBSM showed increases in anti-CD3 stimulated lymphocyte production of two Th1 cytokines—IL-2 and IFN-γ—as well as increases in the ratio of Th1/Th2 cytokines produced, an effect that was evident at 6-month follow-up (Antoni et al., 2009). Th1 cytokines are important for supporting cellular immune processes that are involved in tumor eradication, such as antigen presenting cells, cytotoxic- T-cells, and T regulatory cells (Disis & Lyerly, 2005).

Some work has targeted CBT-based interventions to address sleep disruptions in breast-cancer patients, a relatively common condition (Vargas et al., 2010). Breast-cancer patients randomized to an 8-week group CBT intervention to treat insomnia (versus those in a control condition) reported better subjective sleep, lower levels of depression and anxiety, and better global quality of life immediately after the intervention and at 12-month follow-up (Savard, Simard, Ivers, & Morin, 2005a). Those in the intervention also had greater in vitro IFN-γ production immediately after the intervention and at 12-month follow-up (Savard, Simard, Ivers, & Morin, 2005b). These findings are remarkably similar to the effects demonstrated for a 10-week CBSM intervention noted previously (Antoni et al., 2009). It is plausible that interventions that use CBT techniques to teach better stress and sleep management in combination may have the greatest impact on psychological adaptation and associated changes in biological processes that could promote optimal health outcomes.

Across the literature in breast cancer, it appears that stress-reducing interventions show effects on physiological indicators such as cortisol and immune function that parallel the size of their psychological effects. Moreover, studies failing to establish psychological effects generally did not show physiological effects (see McGregor & Antoni, 2009). This pattern of PNI effects parallels conclusions of studies of stress management and other psychosocial interventions in HIV-infected persons (Carrico & Antoni, 2008). In fine-grained analyses of CBSM effects, positive psychological changes (decreased distress, anxiety and social disruption; increased quality of life, positive affect and benefit finding) and cortisol decreases were paralleled by increased confidence in using relaxation to manage stress (Antoni et al., 2006; Phillips et al., 2008; Phillips et al., 2011). These findings mirror those of Andersen, Shelby, and Golden-Kruetz (2007) who also showed that many of the psychological effects of their intervention were explained by women's reported improvements in relaxations skills. Reported relaxation-skill improvements may actually "mediate" intervention effects on outcomes, or they may, instead, serve as simply a marker of women's buy-in of the value of the intervention, their enhanced sense of self-efficacy, or numerous other psychosocial processes. "Dismantling" designs will need to be used to compare the relative efficacy of well-controlled experimental conditions focused on the specific elements of multimodal approaches such as CBSM or MBSR (e.g., controlling for the presence/absence of relaxation effects by comparing relaxation only versus CBT-only versus an attention-matched control condition). Such trials are underway.

Although it is yet to be determined whether the women enrolled in these stress reduction-focused interventions (CBSM, MBSR) will demonstrate less disease recurrence and greater survival as reported by Andersen et al. (2008), it seems worthwhile to invest in following these extant cohorts who have already completed the intervention phase, with a priority placed on following samples from RCTs. Given that tests of survival in such intervention studies would be rendered as post hoc secondary analyses, great caution is in order in interpreting their results alongside prior trials that listed survival as an *apriori* primary outcome (Coyne et al., 2007). Here, it would be critical to look for consistency across intervention effects, as well as putative biobehavioral mechanisms, as a guide for which interventions are likely to provide benefits in terms of recurrence and survival in future trials.

It is also important to consider that the Andersen et al. (2008) intervention effects on disease outcomes may have been mediated by other stress-related biologic processes, independent of immune regulation. Several of these have been outlined in another chapter in this volume (see chapter 19) and they include metastasis, angiogenesis, tumor cell migration, and invasion. It would be intriguing if Andersen et al. and other researchers who completed similar trials could analyze archival samples for some of the biomarkers that index these processes. It is essential to also investigate whether the women in these trials successfully changed their health behaviors (more exercise, better nutrition, less alcohol consumption, better adherence to hormonal medications and attendance at follow-up appointments, etc,) and actually got more effective medical treatment and larger doses of adjuvant therapy (e.g., co-intervention effects). Disproportionate changes in medical treatment received across psychosocial intervention study conditions could confer greater protection against disease progression and facilitate better health outcomes independently of or in interaction with stress-reduction processes. Importantly, women assigned to the psychosocial intervention in the Andersen et al. trial were more likely to receive more varied adjuvant therapies than controls (Andersen et al., 2004). These investigators might probe whether their intervention effects on survival or recurrence are more pronounced in those women who ended up receiving more cancer treatment.

In designing future studies examining the effects of psychosocial interventions in women with breast cancer, one must weigh out both the likelihood of specific health outcomes in women recruited at specific cancer stages (and types of tumors) as well as the theoretical basis for expecting effects of psychosocial intervention on these health outcomes. When designing intervention studies in cancer patients, in general, it is also important to consider other stress-related health outcomes beyond survival and disease recurrence such as the incidence of moderate to severe opportunistic infections (OI) during and after the completion of surgical and adjuvant therapy, a period of dampened immunologic functioning. Stress-related changes in upper respiratory infections, reactivation of latent herpes virus infections, and the progression of virally associated neoplastic processes are well established in the literature (Cohen Tyrell, & Smith, 1991; Glaser et al., 1987; Pereira et al., 2003). It has yet to be shown that stress reduction can decrease the risk of OI in cancer patients undergoing active treatment (Lutgendorf et al, 2010).

Summary

Although there is growing evidence that stress-related processes can impact cancer progression, the evidence for the efficacy of psychosocial interventions and stress management in altering the course of cancer remains inconclusive, and the biobehavioral mechanisms that might explain any such effects are yet to be established. Future work in the field should monitor intervention effects on indicators representing putative pathways. Some of these might include a set of psychosocial variables (stress, depression, and social support); health behavior changes including adherence to adjuvant therapy regimen; neuroendocrine regulatory indicators; cytokines reflecting optimal immune regulation (adequate cellular immune responsivity to specific antigenic challenge and lower background inflammation) locally and systemically; and measurements of tissue and molecular changes reflecting alterations in circulating micrometastatic cells, and processes supporting metastasis, angiogenesis, and tumor cell migration and invasion in tumor and stromal (e.g., myeloid cells) (Lutgendorf et al., 2010).

We still know very little about what the best point is in the cancer continuum to begin intervention and how to space the readouts that we take after an intervention is completed. Using statistical procedures like growth modeling techniques might help us understand the architecture of immune (and neuroendocrine) changes across the cancer experience by monitoring blood samples from the point of diagnosis to pre- and postsurgical time points during cancer treatment. This could lay the groundwork for planning the timing of biological assessments for future large-scale intervention studies. Because different trials have incorporated different intervention approaches, it is critical to utilize a standardized and manualized approach to facilitate comparisons across trials. Because most single-site intervention trials involve samples of breast-cancer patients that range from 50–200 collected over multiple years, it is clear that multisite trials are needed to generate the much larger cohort of women who can be used to form a cohort and followed annually for several years. Because the vast majority of psychosocial intervention studies with breast-cancer patients have used white, middle-class samples, there is a real limit to the generalizability of this work. In sum, future stress-management intervention work in breast cancer needs to incorporate multiethnic samples of patients; the use of standardized, manualized, and culturally relevant psychosocial intervention protocols; repeated measurements of relevant psychosocial, biological, and disease activity markers; and the analytic techniques that can model linear as well as nonlinear changes over time (McGregor & Antoni, 2009).

This section has focused on research examining the effects of stress management and other psychosocial interventions in breast-cancer patients. This may serve as a model for other PNI-cancer research that can be conducted using intervention paradigms in other relatively common cancers such as prostate cancer, malignant melanoma, cervical cancer, ovarian cancer, colorectal cancer, head and neck cancers, and leukemias and lymphomas, to name a few. However, it is important to understand that though these conditions are collectively referred to as cancers, and in most cases reflect atypical cell growth that has evaded bodily defense systems, they represent different diseases with different etiologies, promoters, progression rates, treatments regimens, and prognostic courses. Justifying the exploration of stress-reduction effects on health outcomes in each of these different conditions will require linking the most well-validated intervention approaches to improved psychological adaptation in parallel with changes in neuroendocrine, immune, and tumor-growth processes that can be related to the pathophysiology of each of these separate diseases. This requires a systematic program of research beginning with observational basic research moving through various translational stages before clinical trials research can begin. We have a long, long way to go.

Stress Management, PNI, and Inflammatory Conditions: Cardiovascular Disease
Immune Processes in Cardiovascular Disease

Inflammation's role in atherosclerosis and cardiovascular disease (CVD) have been shown in studies involving accumulating low-density lipoprotein (LDL) cholesterol getting lodged in the intima of the coronary artery vessel walls, which in turn triggers an inflammatory response (Libby, Ridker, & Maseri, 2002; Ross. 1999). Endothelial dysfunction, following endothelial injury, is likely promoted by elevated concentrations of LDL-cholesterol, free radicals, homocysteine, vasoactive amines, and hepresviruses such as cytomegalovirus (CMV). Once the endothelium is injured, LDL cholesterol accumulates in the "subendothelial space" beneath the intima, where it can undergo oxidation due to exposure to the products of vascular cells. This produces minimally oxidized LDL species with pro-inflammatory activity, which signal endothelial and smooth muscle cells to secrete chemokines that attract monocytes. Monocytes ultimately squeeze between now dilated endothelial cell spaces and gain access to the intima, where they multiply and mature into active macrophages. Other pro-inflammatory cytokines produced by the endothelium, smooth muscle cells, and leukocytes also facilitate leukocyte recruitment and adhesion. (Scheiderman, Antoni, Penedo & Ironson, 2010).

Monocytes, T lymphocytes and platelet-leukocytes aggregate and migrate into the intima and upregulate pro-inflammatory cytokine signaling that helps form a lesion. Upon entering the intima of the vessel, monocytes transform into macrophages, which ingest oxidized LDL (ox-LDL), contributing to the formation of foam cells, which die, and form the bulk of the necrotic core of the lesion. Activated T cells act to amplify this process by producing inflammatory cytokines that stimulate macrophages and vascular endothelial cells, and induce smooth muscle cells to migrate to the surface of the intima and synthesize components of extracellular matrix that ultimately form a fibrous cap covering a necrotic core together forming an atherosclerotic plaque. Over time, these plaques may push inward causing stenosis, or they may rupture causing a thrombus (blood clot), and a myocardial infarction. Thus, symptomatic CVD follows a long period of chronic, low-grade inflammation.

Psychosocial Factors, Inflammation, and CVD

Based upon the well-established association between depression and CVD in healthy persons and those who have had heart attacks (Rugulies, 2002), some have suggested that depression may exacerbate vascular inflammation (Broadley, Korszun, Jones, & Frenneaux, 2002). Depressed people have higher IL-6 and C-reactive protein (CRP) levels than nondepressed individuals (Miller et al., 2002), and cardiac patients with depressive-like symptoms (vital exhaustion) showed elevated serum IL-1β, TNFα, and IL-6 in one study (Appels et al., 2000), and increases in soluble ICAM-1 and CRP levels in another (Lésperance, Frasure-Smith, Theroux and Irwin, 2004). Appels et al., (2000) have proposed that depression, vital exhaustion, or fatigue may simply be symptoms of underlying inflammation associated with CVD, and those symptoms are akin to the sickness behavior pattern that has been widely studied in PNI research (Dantzer, 2001). Accordingly, pro-inflammatory cytokines initiate behavioral, affective, and motivational changes by binding to receptors in the hypothalamus and other limbic structures (Dantzer, 2001) or accessing brain regions through the afferent limb of the vagus nerve or by diffusing across relatively permeable portions of the blood-brain barrier (Rivest, 2001). The pro-inflammatory cytokines that influence the CNS produce a set of behavioral changes collectively known as "sickness behavior," characterized by a sense of fatigue, weakness, malaise, and listlessness a well as decreased appetite and weight, altered sleeping patterns, loss of interest, and concentration problems. Many of these are also cardinal symptoms of depression (Schneiderman et al., 2010).

Thus, elevations in pro-inflammatory cytokines may be associated with heightened risk for CVD and increased depression, fatigue, and related symptoms, which are also known to occur with CVD. Two studies showed that CVD patients with vital exhaustion (compared to nonexhausted CVD patients) had greater levels of pro-inflammatory cytokines and signs of activated viral infections. One found elevated antibody titers against chlamydia pneumoniae and CMV among exhausted CVD patients (Appels et al., 2000), whereas the other found that exhausted CVD patients had greater number of seropositive tests to herpes simplex virus, varicella-zoster virus, EBV, and CMV than nonexhausted CVD patients (Van Der Ven et al., 2003). If one believes that measures of depression and exhaustion are assessing the same construct (Wojciechowski,

Strik, Falger, Lousberg, & Honig, 2000), then this work may indicate that depression is a correlate of both pathogen burden and inflammatory responses in CVD patients. Depression may also exacerbate inflammation through neuroendocrine dysregulations involving the HPA axis. Some have suggested that persisting negative mood states (and chronic stress) may be accompanied by chronically elevated cortisol levels that induce a downregulation in the number of cortisol receptors in monocytes thereby reducing the "anti-inflammatory" effects of cortisol (Miller et al., 2002). It follows that if cortisol is unable to suppress inflammation, chronic stress or depression may continue to promote proinflammatory cytokines, exacerbating processes such as atherosclerosis (Schneiderman et al., 2010).

Psychosocial Intervention and Stress Management in CVD

If HPA and SAM axes are involved in chronic stress or negative affect states in persons diagnosed with or at risk for developing CVD, then psychosocial (e.g., CBT or CBSM) or pharmacological (selective serotonin reuptake inhibitors: SSRIs) interventions may decrease chronic stress and depression, and possibly decreasing inflammation and slowing atherosclerotic processes in CVD. Despite this exciting evidence relating depression, inflammation, and CVD, it is interesting that there is no current evidence that stress management or other psychosocial interventions capable of modifying PNI processes can affect inflammation markers in persons with CVD. There is, however, strong evidence that stress-reducing interventions may improve disease course in persons with CVD. Four meta-analyses have examined randomized psychosocial-behavioral interventions in patients with coronary heart disease (CHD) (Clark, Hartling, Vandermeer, & McAlister, 2005; Dusseldorp, van Elderen, Maes, Meulman, & Kraaij, 1999; Linden, Phillips, & Leclerc, 2007; Linden, Stossel, & Maurice, 1996). These reviews have found that psychosocial interventions were associated with as much as a 34% reduction in cardiovascular mortality, and a 29% reduction in MI recurrence. The pattern across these meta-analyses was consistent (e.g., Linden et al., 2007).

The Enhancing Recovery in Coronary Heart Disease (ENRICHD) clinical trial enrolled nearly 2500 post-MI patients and showed that those who received a combined pharmacologic regimen and group-based CBT stress management reported decreased depression and social isolation across the sample of men and women (Berkman

et al., 2003), and among white men, being in the intervention was associated with lower cardiac death and decreased nonfatal myocardial infarction (Schneiderman et al., 2004). Two recent Scandinavian reports indicated that women with CVD who were assigned to CBT-based stress-management intervention showed decreases in mortality and recurrence of disease (Burell, Svardsudd, & Gulliksson, 2010; Orth-Gomer et al., 2009). In one of these, the Stockholm Women's Intervention Trial for Coronary Heart Disease (SWITCHD) trial, 273 women with severe CHD were randomized to either 20 group sessions over a 12-month period (focused on health education, relaxation, CBT, and coping skills training) or usual care. Over a mean follow-up period of over 7 years, 20% of women in usual care died versus only 8% in the intervention, effects that held after controlling for baseline medication regimen (Orth-Gomer et al., 2009). This is an exciting area of research that is likely to hasten the adoption of behavioral medicine interventions and stress management into standard postoperative coronary care.

Summary

There is growing evidence that chronic stress and depression may contribute to the pathophysiology of CVD by way of PNI processes, mostly involving regulation of inflammation. There is also evidence that stress-management interventions may decrease the risk of recurrent disease and mortality in patients treated for CVD-associated conditions such as myocardial infarction, and in those with established heart disease. However, because there were no markers of inflammation collected in the intervention trials conducted to date, it is unclear how these stress-management approaches had their effects on survival and disease recurrence. It remains to be seen whether intervention-associated changes in CVD clinical outcomes are mediated via PNI processes. Future work might investigate whether these interventions modulate circulating levels of inflammatory biomarkers such as CRP and IL-6, tissue-associated macrophage activation, and then gene expression of endocrine/SNS interactions with inflammatory signaling pathways in circulating immune cells and in affected tissue.

Stress Management, PNI, and Immunoregulatory Conditions: Chronic Fatigue Syndrome

I now focus on the use of stress management to improve physical symptoms, quality of life, and putative biobehavioral processes in a poorly understood condition known as chronic fatigue syndrome (CFS). For the purposes of this chapter, I have classified CFS as an immunoregulatory disorder wherein the host shows signs of overactivation in some immune parameters as well as deficiencies in others. This may make CFS patients more prone to show exaggerated and protracted flulike symptoms after they are exposed to extrinsic stimuli or when they engage in excessive physical activity.

Immune Processes in CFS

According to the CDC, the overall prevalence of CFS in the United States is 235 per 100,000 persons (Reyes et al., 2003) and about 80% are women (Jason et al., 1999). Individuals with CFS suffer from severe fatigue that impairs daily activity, diminishes quality of life for years, and has no known cure (Bombardier & Buchwald, 1995). Symptoms beyond debilitating fatigue include low-grade fever, lymph-node pain and tenderness, pharyngitis, myalgias, arthralgias, cognitive difficulties, and mood changes (Buchwald, Sullivan, & Komaroff, 1987; Jones & Straus, 1987; Taerk, Toner, Salit, Garfinkel, & Ozersky, 1987). Symptoms may emerge at unpredictable times, one of the features of CFS that makes it particularly stressful. Initiating events for CFS symptom flares include infections, vaccinations, psychiatric trauma, and exposure to toxins, though etiology remains unknown (Prinz, vanderMeer & Bleijenberg, 2006).

Many of the symptoms of CFS resemble a chronic viral infection like influenza, and such symptoms have prompted a theory of infection-induced illness (Klimas, Morgan, Salvado, & Fletcher, 1990; Evengard & Klimas, 2002) that presents with acute or gradual onset of illness, with systemic "flulike" symptoms that do not subside (Evengard, Jonzon, Sandberg, Theorell, & Lindh, 2003). These observations have led to reports of associated microbial infection or reactivation of latent viral infections (Klimas et al., 1990; Straus, et al., 1985; Glaser et al., 2005; Ledina et al., 2007). There is corresponding evidence that CFS patients also show abnormalities on several indices of immune functioning (e.g., elevated IgG, impaired natural killer cell cytotoxicty, NKCC, Klimas, Salvato, Morgan & Fletcher, 1990), elevated levels of circulating mostly pro-inflammatory cytokine peptides and/or mRNA (Fletcher, Zeng, Barnes, Lewis, & Klimas, 2009), and abnormalities in the numbers and activation states of certain lymphocyte subpopulations (Buchwald, Cheney & Peterson, 1992; Caliguri

et al., 1987; Klimas, Ashman & Fletcher, 1988; Klimas et al., 1990; Klimas, Patarca & Fletcher, 1992; Lutgendorf et al., 1993; Patarca, et al. 1994; Salvato, Landay, Jessop, Lenette & Levy, 1991). Recent work in the United States isolating a gamma-retrovirus virus (XMRV) in the etiologic pathway of CFS adds strength to the notion of a chronic immune system activation (Lombardi et al., 2009) though this XMRV finding has failed to replicate in a UK population study (Erlwein et al., 2010).

Psychosocial Factors, PNI Processes, and CFS

Over the past two decades, PNI research in CFS has related the severity of symptoms to immune system impairments, though the mechanisms maintaining and exacerbating these symptoms have been elusive. Our group previously posited that CFS symptoms can be understood through a *neuroimmune model* (Antoni & Weiss, 2003). Our model proposes that CFS involves an immunologic dysregulation (due to extrinsic stimulation) characterized by chronic lymphocyte activation with elevated expression of lymphocyte activation markers, episodic increased expression of inflammatory cytokines, such as tumor necrosis factor (TNF)-α and β peptide and soluble receptor in serum/plasma, and mRNA in circulating lymphocytes, and associated decrements in cellular immune function. Those decrements in cellular immune function, in turn, hamper antiviral immunity and fail to eradicate viral infections, thus promoting further immune activation (Klimas & Koneru, 2007; Antoni & Weiss, 2003). CFS patients are also hypothesized to have an HPA axis dysregulation (Cleare, 2004; Demitrack & Crofford, 1998; Evengard, Jonzon, Sandberg, Theorell & Lindh, 2003; Gaab et al., 2005; Torres-Harding et al., 2009) (which may be aggravated by stress), and altered immunoregulation, which serve to maintain the symptom cluster of CFS such as fatigue, muscle pain, unrefreshing sleep, and weakness.

Patients may experience *distress reactions* that are secondary to the flaring of these flulike symptoms (Kennedy, 1988). As CFS patients' ability to carry out activities of daily living decreases, anxiety, depression, and irritability may increase (Brickman & Fins, 1993). This *distress cascade* may further deplete energy resulting in additional decrements in attention and vigilance, thus worsening the fatigue symptoms. Distress reactions may also further dysregulate the immune system since distress/depressive states are related to several pro-inflammatory cytokines possibly via alterations in HPA axis hormones such as cortisol (Fuite, Vernon, & Broderick, 2008; Miller, Cohen, & Ritchey, 2002).

Because distress reactions appear to be related to the fatigue, HPA axis alterations, and immune dysfunction characterizing this syndrome, we reasoned that effective treatment would need to focus on reducing patients' distress reactions. This makes sense in view of the interdependency among CFS symptom severity, psychological response processes, HPA functioning, and the immune system. This model is the basis for a program of research with a stress-management intervention designed to modulate CFS patients' distress responses in order to influence symptomatology via changes in neuroimmune processes (Antoni & Weiss, 2003; Weiss, Helder, & Antoni, 2003).

WHAT IS THE EVIDENCE THAT IMMUNE DYSREGULATIONS MIGHT CONTRIBUTE TO CFS SYMPTOMS? AND IF SO HOW MIGHT STRESS/DISTRESS BE INVOLVED?

CFS patients with the greatest fatigue severity and lowest vigor reveal lower NKCC and greater signs of lymphocyte activation (increased CD2+CD3+CD26+ T-cells). TNF-α and soluble TNF receptor-type I (sTNF-RI) were greater in the low NKCC group versus the normal NKCC group (Siegel et al., 2006). Thus, elevated pro-inflammatory cytokines such as TNF-α may accompany both decrements in antiviral immunity (via NKCC) and greater CFS symptom expression. TNF-α and β are primary modifiers of the inflammatory response to injury or infection, and are primarily produced by macrophages. Overproduction or inappropriate expression of TNF is associated with fever, slow-wave sleep induction, and appetite suppression (Dinarello, 1992; Dinarello, Cannon & Wolff, 1986; Shohan, Davenne, & Cady, 1987;), which could underlie the fatigue, lassitude, and excessive sleepiness associated with CFS (Moldovsky, 1989). CFS symptoms may be part of a complex referred to as "sickness behavior" wherein fatigue, sleep disturbances, pain, and other CFS-like symptoms are believed secondary to chronically elevated levels of pro-inflammatory cytokines (IL-1, IL-6, TNF) (Capuron & Dantzer, 2003; Dantzer, 2001). This pattern of increased pro-inflammatory cytokine production may be triggered by antigenic stimulation (e.g., viral infection) and maintained by stress/mood-related HPA axis alterations (e.g, flattened diurnal secretion of glucocorticoids, and/or decreased glucocorticoid sensitivity in immune cells that produce pro-inflammatory cytokines)

(Vgontzas & Chrousos, 2002). Sickness behavior symptoms and accompanying elevations in pro-inflammatory cytokines (e.g., TNF) are compatible with the symptom picture and cytokine patterns identified in CFS patients by our group (Patarca-Montero, Antoni, Fletcher & Klimas, 2001).

ARE STRESS PROCESSES RELATED TO CFS SYMPTOMS?

We know that daily life event stress is associated with greater reports of symptom burden in persons with CFS, and these stress effects are moderated by *cognitive appraisals* (more optimism, less frequent cognitive distortions), *coping strategies* (more active coping, planning, and acceptance, and less denial and disengagement), and *social support* (Antoni, et al., 1994). In other work, CFS patients who experienced the stress of Hurricane Andrew showed CFS exacerbations compared to well-matched CFS patients not directly exposed to the hurricane (Lutgendorf et al. 1995). This included increased clinician-rated symptom relapses and increased severity and frequency of sleep disturbances, muscle weakness, and fatigue after modest exercise; worse functional indicators such as work impairment and illness burden; and increased levels of circulating TNF-α. Greater emotional responses to the hurricane (independent of material damages) related to greater risk of symptom relapse. Converesely, perceived social support and an optimistic attitude (cognitive appraisal) were associated with less likelihood of a clinical relapse and lower reports of symptom burden. So, external stressors may exacerbate CFS symptoms and cognitive-behavioral-interpersonal factors such as cognitive appraisals, coping strategies, and social support that affect stress responses may moderate these stress effects. Emotional distress increases may modulate the immune system, possibly exacerbating cytokine dysregulations, which then intensifies physical (e.g., inflammatory) symptoms. There is growing evidence for an association between HPA axis substances, such as cortisol and pro-inflammatory cytokines (Vgontzas, & Chrousos, 2002), and of altered cortisol diurnal pattern and multiple CFS symptoms (Torres-Harding et al., 2009). As such, it is plausible that documented stress-induced exacerbations in CFS physical symptoms (Lutgendorf et al. 1995) are mediated by HPA axis disruption and circulating cytokines. What is the evidence that psychosocial interventions can improve CFS symptomatology?

Efficacy of Psychosocial Intervention and Stress Management in CFS

Most of behavioral intervention studies for CFS are based on a model of activity avoidance and deconditioning as exacerbating factors in CFS, and they use cognitive behavioral therapy (CBT) to change attitudes toward avoidance of exercise and physical activity and to initiate a prescription of titrated reintroduction to exercise and physical activity sometimes referred to as graded exercise therapy (White et al., 2011). Sharpe and colleagues (Sharpe et al., 1996) note that CBT may be effective in breaking the vicious cycle of fatigue, negative cognitions, increased attention to symptoms, distress reactions, physiologic arousal, and other changes, and exacerbation of CFS symptoms, including fatigue. Also, CBT may be preferred over medications by CFS patients reluctant to take drugs or endure their side effects (Sharpe et al., 1996).

Several studies have demonstrated the effectiveness of cognitive-behavioral treatment in the reduction of concomitant emotional factors of CFS (i.e., anxiety, depression), negative cognitions, physical symptoms (particularly fatigue), physiological arousal, and distress reactions in CFS patients (Butler, Chalder, & Ron, 1991; Deale, Chalder, Marks, & Wesley, 1997; Friedberg & Krupp, 1994; Sharpe et al., 1996). Meta-analyses find moderate effects for individual-based CBT interventions focused on physical activity and deconditioning models in CFS, though drop-out rates range up to 42% (Malouff,, Thorsteinsson, Rooks, Bhuliar, & Schutte, 2008). Group-based CBT combined with body awareness and exercise training has also been shown to be effective for CFS in recent work (Stubhaug, Alte, Ursin, & Eriksen, 2008).

More recently, stress-management techniques have been tested as a way to modulate stress physiology processes believed to exacerbate CFS symptomology. In line with a stress-neuroimmune model of CFS symptom exacerbation previously described (Antoni & Weiss, 2003), our work has focused on testing group-based CBSM intervention, which is designed to reduce stress through relaxation, decrease depression by modifying participants' outlook and cognitive appraisals through cognitive restructuring, teach adaptive coping strategies and interpersonal skills such as assertiveness and anger management, and, when conducted in a group format, it may also improve group members' perceptions of social support.

Our conceptual model specifies the ways in which psychological distress, HPA axis functioning, and immunologic abnormalities may act as *mediators* of stress-related exacerbation and/or maintenance of CFS physical symptoms (Antoni & Weiss, 2003). Specifically, CBSM intervention may modulate the presenting physical symptoms of CFS by several pathways: (a) Enhanced psychological status (increased feelings of self-efficacy and sense of control and decreased rumination) may reduce the perceived severity of CFS physical symptoms (e.g., chronic pain perceptions are markedly impacted by cognitive appraisal factors; Turk, Holzman & Kerns,1986). (b) Improved psychological status, if accompanied by reductions in distress and depression may also help to normalize immunologic functioning (Antoni & Schneiderman, 1998). (c) Modulation of immunologic status may also impact physical status by way of increased surveillance of ubiquitous viruses (e.g., rhinoviruses, herpesviruses; Esterling et al, 1992). (d) Enhancing immune surveillance against virally associated infections (e.g., upper respiratory infections) may reduce CFS physical symptoms through lowered virally induced elevations in immunologic activation and production of pro-inflammatory cytokines such as TNF (Glaser et al., 1991). Thus, CBSM intervention may improve physical problems that CFS patients suffer from by modulating neuroimmune processes believed to contribute to the maintenance and exacerbation of CFS symptoms.

We developed a group-based CBSM intervention program specifically for men and women with CFS (Antoni & Weiss, 2003; Weiss, Helder, & Antoni, 2003). The structure and content of each component of the intervention was partially adopted from a similar protocol implemented with HIV-infected patients (Antoni, 2003a; Antoni, Ironson & Scheiderman, 2007), but enhanced with an emphasis on particular symptom exacerbations and associated losses (i.e., job, social activities) that accompany CFS (Weiss, Helder, & Antoni, 2003). It is a closed, structured CBSM group intervention, meeting once weekly for 2 hours in groups of 5–8 members, facilitated by a group leader. Men and women with diagnosed CFS participating within the group-based CBSM intervention showed significant reductions in perceived stress, mood disturbance, and improvements in quality of life (Lopez et al., 2011). Intervention participants also showed decreased severity of CDC-based CFS symptoms.

In pilot work, we have identified neuroimmune associations that might explain these CBSM effects on symptoms by assessing CFS symptoms, HPA axis regulation (di-urnal salivary cortisol output), and circulating pro-inflammatory cytokines among a sample of patients diagnosed with CFS. We found that greater severity of CFS symptoms was associated with greater levels of circulating pro-inflammatory cytokines, and these symptoms and cytokine levels were greater in cases with lower salivary cortisol output and poorer diurnal regulation of cortisol (Antoni, 2009). This suggested that HPA axis dysregulation may be a central target for intervention in this population. Because stress management has been shown to modulate cortisol levels in prior work with other populations, we hypothesized that CBSM would alter salivary cortisol patterns in patients with CFS. This is the basis for ongoing work.

Summary

CFS remains a poorly understood medical condition characterized by disruptions in immune system regulation. Given the lack of knowledge concerning an etiologic agent responsible for the onset of CFS, the chronic nature of this syndrome, and the possibility of a stress-neuroimmune mechanism maintaining its physical and affective presentation, it can be reasoned that interventions designed to reduce psychological distress and alter cognitive appraisals may be effective in interrupting the mechanism(s) maintaining or exacerbating some of the health complaints associated with CFS. However, work evaluating the effects of stress-management interventions in CFS is just beginning. Monitoring changes in the diurnal cycle of salivary cortisol secretion and a comprehensive panel of pro-inflammatory cytokines in association with changes in CFS symptoms before and after a stress-management intervention will provide stronger evidence of a neuroimmune model of CFS than would be possible with a natural history study. Monitoring concomitant changes in stress/distress and psychosocial functioning in patients will allow us to identify the contribution of cognitive, behavioral, and interpersonal processes to neuroimmune and symptom changes so that future interventions can be further refined.

Conclusion

This chapter has provided a rationale for the use of stress management and other psychosocial and behavioral interventions to better manage a number of chronic diseases and other conditions characterized by immune-system abnormalities. This chapter framed this body of work in the context of PNI models to explain the role of stressors and psychosocial factors on disease course and physical health by way of alterations in neuroendocrine and immune system functioning. I summarized the results of several trials testing the effects of psychosocial interventions on health outcomes and biobehavioral processes in medical conditions including infectious, neoplastic, inflammatory, and immunoregulatory disorders. For the purpose of illustration, I have focused most of the work in this chapter on stress-management-based interventions, but I have also noted instances in which other psychosocial intervention approaches might be fruitful. Across many disease conditions there appears to be reasonable evidence that time-limited, manualized stress-management interventions may be efficacious in modulating neuroendocrine and immune-system parameters, and in some cases these interventions have shown to have an impact on biomarkers of subclinical disease progression as well as hard clinical endpoints, such as clinical disease recurrence and mortality. Due to the lack of replication across trials, the lack of standardized intervention protocols, assessment instruments, and analytic procedures, it remains difficult to say how close we are to moving this line of work into clinical practice. This will require large-scale multisite trials with standardized and objective endpoints before medical practitioners and third-party payers will view this work as providing evidence-based validated treatments.

Using an intervention paradigm as a probe to identify as well as intervene on biobehavioral mechanisms relevant to disease processes appears to be a very efficient way to conduct research. Advantages are that one can gain insight into the temporality of changes in PNI processes (e.g., Do psychosocial changes precede neuroendocrine and immunologic changes en route to health and disease changes?). The use of a randomized controlled trial (RCT) design also allows one to entertain causal pathways. However, this work is not without limitations. All RCTs have some degree of flaws that impact their quality, and systems have been developed to rate them for diseases such as cancer (e.g., Newell et al., 2002). To aid in the burdens of proof placed on investigators conducting RCTs, CONSORT reporting guidelines have been developed. One would be then wise to learn these guidelines when designing and consuming intervention research in the field. However, aside from establishing proper guidelines for reporting the results of intervention work, what are the best ways for this field to invest its energies and funding sources in intervention research in the coming decade?

Future Directions

The next steps in the line of research that has been the focus of this chapter might be summarized as addressing the "Who, What, When, and How" of optimal stress-management interventions in different diseases and clinical conditions.

Who?

The *who* questions concern choosing the best target populations to focus on in order to model disease. Should we focus on pure cases that are dealing with only one condition, or should we allow for co-morbidities, age range, different disease types? Often a line of intervention work begins by establishing efficacy within a relatively homogeneous group and then expands outward along the generalizability gradient to increase the external and ecological validity of the findings. Incorporating measures of hypothesized biobehavioral mechanisms at each step in this programmatic line as well as developing agreed upon methods for controlling confounding factors can make this a particularly efficient enterprise.

PNI intervention research needs to increase its reach to populations who have been understudied to date. Much of the human PNI research in the past two decades has focused on white, middle-class, well-educated samples that have been recruited from university campuses and medical centers. Moreover, the studies of medical outpatients have often been restricted to patients that live in metropolitan areas in close proximity to medical centers. It is arguable that the underserved medical populations made up of lower-income minority individuals, persons in rural communities, and those who lack the energy, transportation, and child-care resources to attend structured intervention sessions do not participate in this line of research. Moving beyond the convenience samples that typify PNI stress-management research conducted to date requires outreach in the community using the give and take of community-based participatory research methods. Isolated studies in the field have made use of these methods in conducting psychosocial intervention research among lower income women with HIV/AIDS (Weiss et al., 2011; Lechner et al., 2003), but they still remain the exception. Expanding into minority populations often requires linguistic and cultural translation of interventions and assessments, as well as an understanding of how that culture views the health-care system and the collection of biosamples (e.g., for genetic tests) that could be used for discriminatory practices.

Attracting understudied and "hard-to-reach" populations may involve developing more portable interventions and harnassing telecommunication technology to facilitate outreach, increase efficiency, and capture assessment of intervention adherence in real time. Combining community-based participatory research methods and advances in telephone- and web-based technologies (Heckman et al.,2006; Stein et al., 2007) is likely to be a powerful combination in reaching the most understudied groups. Work using telephone-delivered "groups" to test stress management in the homes of patients with mobility-limiting conditions (e.g., chronic fatigue syndrome; Antoni, 2009) may be one model for adapting our intervention studies to other groups with severe disease and major treatment side effects or significant transportation and child-care barriers. The use of telephone technology (audio and video-phones) allows for the testing of successful interventions in a controlled, private, and high-fidelity venue. Applying telephone technology to the delivery of group stress-management interventions is likely to be only a first step. Web-based technology to increase the scalability and global reach of those approaches may follow from successful efficacy demonstrated using phone-delivered versions.. Using remote collections of biosamples and psychosocial data along with home-delivered interventions may play a great role in expanding the reach of PNI intervention research as well as testing the effects of these interventions in real-world settings. Comprehensive stress-management interventions of the future will be those that use techniques such as CBSM in combination with optimal medical treatments, medication adherence training, and lifestyle change programs that are carefully designed to be relevant, acceptable, scalable, and deliverable to the largest populations.

What?

The *what* questions should specify the optimal content and format that the intervention should take, and it should be informed by psychosocial targets of interventions that are most relevant to the recipients and the plausibility that intervention-associated changes in these stress and psychosocial targets can influence disease-relevant PNI processes. When we consider *content*, we address questions pertaining to whether one should isolate pure elements (e.g., muscle relaxation) versus "molecules" of stress management that present interlocking approaches that may reinforce one another. Another consideration would be work that attempts to test intervention elements that "match" the personality or social environment of the recipient. Although intriguing, this latter approach should be considered a more advanced line of inquiry that can be explored only once a body of intervention research in a given disease has matured. Another aspect of the *what* question concerns the *format* of the intervention. Here considerations arise about whether the intervention is best tested in individual rather than group-based sessions or some combination of both. Also worth considering is whether couples- or family-based approaches might be the best way to ensure carryover of intervention effects into the home environment. This is a reasonable consideration given that social adversity and social support may have stress-buffering effects on biobehavioral processes (e.g., Cole, 2009) and health outcomes (e.g., House, Landis, & Umberson, 1988).

Another *what* question concerns the optimal *length and frequency* of stress- management sessions. This requires a balance of minimal sufficient dose for short- versus longer-term effects, patient burden, and costs of delivery. In PNI research, one would want to design an intervention capable of driving clinically meaningful changes in PNI processes and changes in risk of disease progression or other health outcomes. This raises the question of the value of maintenance/booster sessions after an acute training period. Recall that in the successful intervention work of Andersen et al. (2008) the intervention actually featured a 4-month intensive period during which sessions were conducted weekly, followed by monthly maintenance sessions offered over the subsequent 8 months. However, the use of intensive year-long interventions, as have been used widely in research in cancer and CVD, needs to be offset by considerations of whether the intervention is scalable as a public-health tool.

The final *what* question concerns the choice of the comparison group(s) in RCT research. Clearly, most intervention research involves comparing a comprehensive intervention against some form of "usual care." However, once efficacy has been demonstrated, it is expected that more elaborate control conditions will be used such as attention-matched controls, equivalent but different active intervention (e.g., comparative effectiveness trials), and combination or stepped-care approaches that may or may not blend pharmacologic and behavioral approaches (e.g., ENRICHD trial; Berkman et al., 2003).

When?

The *when* question involves deciding on the optimal timing of the psychosocial intervention within disease phenomenology and the spacing of the outcomes measurements, decisions that are all too often made on the basis of convenience, with little consideration of the translation of the work for clinical practice. To some degree, decisions about the timing of an intervention depend on whether it has a primary, secondary, tertiary, or quaternary prevention goal. Does the intervention seek to prevent disease, hasten and optimize screening, aid adjustment to a new diagnosis, or offer tools for chronic disease management? Beyond clinical application considerations, PNI intervention research adds the additional complexity of needing to work around medical treatments that may confound outcome variables.

Managing the timing of stress-management intervention onset and measurements involves the challenge of dodging confounders of biobehavioral readouts by working around known treatment regimens and monitoring the medical happenstances that can occur during and after treatment is completed. Intervention researchers must often balance the potential clinical yield of peritreatment timing against noisy readouts. Taking the example of cancer patients receiving chemotherapy or radiation treatments, can we get close to the cyclone and deliver our treatments during a patients' stressor apex and still get interpretable neuroendocrine and immune results? One can wait until a "safe window" appears, after the end of treatment, and then begin an intervention, but will patients' distress levels justify the need for stress management and will such delayed intervention affect the trajectory of disease outcomes? Or is it better still to collect pre-intervention baseline data before the storm, intervene during active treatment, and wait for patients to complete the regimen before taking poststorm readouts, and continue to take them over clinically meaningful periods?

This latter approach may minimize some confounders of medical treatments but many powerful medical treatments have unclear posttreatment side-effect kinetics, so it is difficult to plan for "when" the coast is clear. Conservative approaches that enroll patients well after treatment completion will still miss opportunities to see how stress management "buffers" or moderates impact of medical treatment acutely, and they will fail to observe the shape of the recovery curve. Because some have hypothesized that the critical period for stress-mediated immunosuppression increases the risk of breast cancer's metastatic spread in the weeks after surgery (Ben-Eliyahu, 2003), it seems as though some PNI intervention research in cancer patients may have to contend with these timing issues head on.

How?

Before summarizing some of the methods available to probe for PNI mediators underlying the effects of psychosocial interventions on health outcomes it seems worthwhile to highlight a few of the areas of "disconnect" that have plagued our field for the past two decades.

Multiple studies have demonstrated that psychosocial interventions, including stress management, may be associated with changes in neuroendocrine and immunologic parameters that are hypothesized to have potential health effects in specific populations, such as persons with HIV and certain cancers. However, it is quite rare to find that intervention-associated changes in these neuroimmune indicators, often made using single point-in-time blood samples pre- and postintervention, have actually mediated the effects of the intervention on a health outcome, such as disease progression or recurrence, or on survival (Carrico & Antoni, 2008; Lutgendorf et al., 2010). A few exceptions exist in the cancer literature. A study by Fawzy and colleagues reported the effects of a group-based psychosocial intervention in malignant melanoma patients and was one of the few to show intervention effects on mood and immunologic status (NK cell activity) at 6- month follow-up in parallel with improved survival outcomes at 6 years (Fawzy, Kemeny, et al., 1990). However, careful analyses of the nature of these effects revealed that the increases in NK cell activity at 6 months did not mediate the effects of the intervention on survival outcomes (Fawzy et al., 1993). In a more recent series focused on women with nonmetastatic breast cancer, Andersen showed that a psychosocial intervention was associated with decreases in distress and lymphocyte proliferation at 4 months (Andersen et al., 2004) and with decreased mortality and disease recurrence at 7- to 11-year follow-up (Andersen et al., 2008). However these changes in lymphocyte proliferation did not appear to mediate the effects of the intervention on survival and recurrence. The authors have suggested in subsequent reports that women in the intervention group showed decreased indicators of inflammation (e.g., elevated leukocyte counts) several years after the intervention, which were associated, in turn, with a decreased risk of recurrence in the subsequent 17-month period (Thornton, Andersen, & Carson, 2008). Given the post hoc nature of these tests, and the fact that increases in total leukocytes may be a less-than-optimal indicator of chronic inflammation, one must exercise caution in presenting them as evidence that the intervention's effects on disease outcomes was mediated by intervention-associated changes in inflammation.

How can we explain the lack of clear evidence that intervention-associated changes in neuroendocrine and immunologic indicators actually predict or mediate the effects of these interventions on hard clinical endpoints such as recurrence and mortality among cancer patients? One possibility is that intervention-associated changes in immune status, which may be relevant in recovering cancer patients, have little bearing on longer-term disease outcomes. This would of course not rule out that such immune changes are relevant for infectious disease during recovery, an important but rarely studied phenomenon in PNI research in cancer patients. Another possibility is that the use of single point-in-time measures of immune cell counts or cell functions taken from a blood sample does not accurately reflect the lasting effects of stress physiology on the immune system to the extent necessary to impact cancer disease outcomes. Emerging technologies allow us now to investigate stress-related changes in leukocyte transcriptional indicators of neuroendocrine impact on immune-cell signaling pathways, which could represent a better indicator of more long-lasting immune status of a nature that could impact disease promoting processes related to inflammation and angiogenesis (Antoni et al., 2012).

Many potential biobehavioral mechanisms to explain the health effects of psychosocial interventions and stress management have been summarized in this chapter. Future key *how* questions in PNI intervention research seek to understand how best to measure and model the pattern of intervention effects over time as well as their underlying mediators. A typical pattern of change over time with psychosocial interventions might be that effects on mood and related stress physiology are greatest in the 6-month period after the intervention when participants are actively using techniques to deal with ongoing stressors. This might be followed by a leveling off or slight fading of intervention gains thereafter. Analyzing data that does not follow linear patterns of change can present some challenges. Designs that include multiple repeated measures may increase the likelihood of missing data during follow-ups. Standard analysis of variance (ANOVA) procedures and trend analyses offer some options, but most programs are plagued by list-wise deletion of missing data that can compromise power and introduce biases. Using latent-growth modeling, a special case of structural equation modeling, to assess the timing and shape of intervention effects, plateauing, and fading, is powerful and robust against missing data. These procedures offer very practical information. For instance, an latent-growth model analysis could estimate the point at which a specific intervention's effects begins to level off or decline (e.g., Antoni, Wimberly et al., 2006) and thereby guide the judicial use of additional training sessions or posttraining booster sessions to mitigate plateauing or fading of effects in order to "carry" a person through a known period of stress.

Another *how* question pertains to the best ways to operationalize biological and physiological functions that PNI researchers use to identify biobehavioral mechanisms of intervention effects on health outcomes. For years, investigators would track stress-management intervention effects on stress physiology by measuring adrenal hormones in blood or 24-hour urine samples and then relate these changes to immunologic parameters measured in the blood. The widespread availability of salivary measures of cortisol and analogs of SNS activity (alpha amylase) make it now possible to collect serial samples across the diurnal cycle in a noninvasive fashion. However, this new and often large influx of data points creates analytic challenges. Multiple indices of diurnal regulation of hormones have been developed and are now available (e.g., mean level of salivary cortisol or AUC versus slopes; Fekeulegn et al., 2007).

Although these measures provide a window into the diurnal output of specific hormones, they do not inform investigators on how these hormones interact with immune cells and other tissue. One approach to do so is a mathematical one. Using a systems-biology approach, one can gain an understanding into how stress or stress management affects dynamic changes in ways biobehavioral variables intercommunicate over time. For instance ongoing work in systems biology is examining how variability in cortisol, pro-inflammatory cytokines, and fatigue symptoms align over time in persons with chronic fatigue syndrome (Fuite et al., 2008).

A more powerful approach would be examining transcriptional (gene expression) changes in immune cells hypothesized to be impacted by stress physiology, one of the basic tenets of PNI. This involves moving from separate measures of circulating hormones and immune cells that hypothetically interact to studying the genomic "footprints" of such interactions, and inferring their effects on signaling pathways in immune cells and disease-affected tissue that contribute to pathogenesis and pathophysiology through bioinformatics programs (Cole, 2009; Cole et al., 2007). Specifically this work conducts genomic (microarray) analyses of logical and theoretically dictated sets of genes in immune cells (lymphocytes, monocytes) that are expressed/up-regulated and repressed/down-regulated in synchrony with improved or recovered immune surveillance repertoire, SNS activation, glucocorticoid resistance, inflammation, and with oxidative stress, wound healing, and tumor-growth processes like angiogenesis and tissue invasion (e.g., Lutgendorf et al., 2009). Interpreting microarray data of this nature requires bioinformatics software and algorithms to make sense of data on the status of hundreds of harmonizing genes singing at different volumes. Fortunately, such software is available (Cole, Arevalo, Takahashi, et al., 2010). Given that we know that social adversity is associated with transcriptional changes in many of these pathways (Chen et al., 2009; Lutgendorf et al., 2009, Cole et al., 2010), it remains to be seen whether psychosocial interventions and stress management in particular is capable of reversing or modifying some of the genomic changes that may have been brought about by stress and social adversity in specific patient groups, and whether such changes predict clinical health benefits in the types of conditions presented in this chapter. Early work applying this approach in studying stress management effects in breast cancer is encouraging but will require replication (Antoni et al., 2012). It is important that PNI researchers, examining the effects of psychosocial and behavioral interventions on PNI processes and health outcomes, continue to incorporate these and other emerging advances in our understanding of how stress physiology can be impacted in ways that are sufficient for influencing disease processes over longer more clinically meaningful periods.

Acknowledgments

The work described in this chapter was supported by the grants from the National Institutes of Health (CA064710, P50 CA84944, NS055672-01, PO1 MH49548, U01 AI45940) and from the Sylvester Cancer Center at the University of Miami Miller School of Medicine.

References

Affleck, G., Urrows, S., Tennen, H., Higgins, P., Pav, D., Aloisi, R. (1997). A dual pathway model of daily stressor effects on rheumatoid arthritis. *Annals of Behavioral Medicine, 19,* 161–170.

Altemus, M., Rao, B., Dhabhar, F., Ding, W., & Granstein, R.. (2001). Stress-induced changes in skin barrier function in healthy women. *Journal of Investigative Dermatology, 117,* 309–317.

Amendola, A., Gougeon, M. L., Poccia, F., Bondurand, A., Fesus, L., & Piacentini, M. (1996). Induction of tissue transglutaminase in HIV pathogenesis: Evidence for high rate of apoptosis on CD4+ T lymphocytes and accessory cells in lymphoid tissues. *Proclamation of the National Academy of Sciences USA, 93,* 11057–11062.

Andersen, B. L., Farrar, W. B., Golden-Kreutz, D., Emery, C. F., Glaser, R., Crespin, T., et al. (2007). Distress reduction from a psychological intervention contributes to improved health for cancer patients. *Brain, Behavior and Immunity, 21*(7), 953–961.

Andersen, B., Farrar, W., Goolden-Freutz, D., Glaser, R., Emery, C., Crespin, T., et al. (2004). Psychological, behavioral, and immune changes after a psychosocial intervention: A clinical trial. *Journal of Clinical Oncology, 22,* 3570–3580.

Andersen, B., Kiecolt-Glaser, J., & Glaser, R. (1994). A biobehavioral model of cancer stress and disease course. *American Psychologist, 49,* 389–404.

Andersen, B., Shelby, R., Golden-Kreutz, D. (2007). RCT of a psychological intervention for persons with cancer. I. Mechanisms of change. *Journal of Consulting and Clinical Psychology, 75,* 927–938.

Andersen, B., Yang, H., Farrar, W., Golden-Kreutz, D., Emery, C., Thornton, L., et al. (2008). Psychologic intervention improves survival for breast cancer patients. *Cancer, 113,* 3450–3458.

Antoni. M. H. (2003a) Stress management and psychoneuroimmunology in HIV infection. *CNS Spectrums, 8,* 40–51.

Antoni, M. H. (2003b) Stress management effects on psychological, endocrinological and immune function in men with HIV: Empirical support for a psychoneuroimmunological model. *Stress, 6,* 173–188.

Antoni, M. H. (2003c) *Stress management intervention for women with breast cancer.* Washington DC: American Psychological Association Press.

Antoni, M. H. (2009) *Calling in cognitive behavioral stress management for chronic fatigue syndrome.* Presented at International Association of Chronic Fatigue Syndrome/ME Bi-annual meeting. Reno, Nevada.

Antoni, M. H. (2010). Stress, coping and health in HIV/AIDS. In S. Folkman (Ed.), *Oxford handbook of stress, coping and health* (pp 428–452). New York: Oxford University Press.

Antoni, M. H., Baggett, L., Ironson, G., August, S., LaPerriere, A., Klimas, N., et al. (1991). Cognitive–behavioral stress management intervention buffers distress responses and immunologic changes following notification of HIV-1 seropositivity. *Journal of Consulting and Clinical Psychology, 59*(6), 906–915.

Antoni, M. H., Brickman, A., Klimas, N., Finns, A., Lutgendorf, S., Patorca, R., et al. (1994). Psychosocial correlates of Illness burden in chronic fatigue syndrome patients. *Clinical Infectious Diseases, 18,* S73–S78.

Antoni, M. H., & Carrico, A. (in press). Psychological and Bio-Behavioral processes in HIV disease. In A. Baum & T. Revenson (Eds), *Handbook of Clinical Health Psychology.* NY: Psychology Press.

Antoni, M. H., Carrico, A. W., Durán, R. E., Spitzer, S., Penedo, F., Ironson, G., et al. (2006). Randomized clinical trial of cognitive behavioral stress management on human immunodeficiency virus viral load in gay men treated with highly active antiretroviral therapy. *Psychosomatic Medicine, 68,* 143–151.

Antoni, M. H., Cruess, D., Klimas, N., Carrico, A. W., Maher, K., Cruess, S., et al. (2005). Increases in a marker of immune system reconstitution are predated by decreases in 24-hour urinary cortisol output and depressed mood during a 10-week stress management intervention in symptomatic HIV-infected gay men. *Journal of Psychosomatic Research, 58,* 3–13.

Antoni, M. H., Cruess, D., Klimas, N., Maher, K., Cruess, S., Kumar, M., et al. (2002). Stress management and immune system reconstitution in symptomatic HIV-infected gay men over time: Effects on transitional naïve T-cells (CD4+CD45RA+CD29+). *American Journal of Psychiatry, 159,* 143–145.

Antoni, M. H., Cruess, D., Wagner, S., Lutgendorf, S., Kumar, M., Ironson, G., et al. (2000). Cognitive behavioral stress management effects on anxiety, 24-hour urinary catecholamine output, and T-Cytotoxic/suppressor cells over time among symptomatic HIV-infected gay men. *Journal of Consulting and Clinical Psychology, 68,* 31–45.

Antoni, M. H., Esterling, B., Lutgendorf, S., Fletcher, M. A., & Schneiderman, N. (1995). Psychosocial stressors, herpes virus reactivation and HIV-1 infection. In M. Stein & A. Baum (Eds.), *AIDS and oncology: Perspectives in behavioral medicine.* Hillsdale, NJ: Erlbaum.

Antoni, M. H., Ironson, G., & Schneiderman, N. (2007). *Stress management for persons with HIV Infection.* New York: Oxford University Press.

Antoni, M. H., Lechner, S., Diaz, A., Vargas, S., Holley, H., Phillips, K., et al. (2009) Cognitive behavioral stress management effects on psychosocial and physiological adaptation in women undergoing treatment for breast cancer. *Brain, Behavior and Immunity, 23,* 580–591.

Antoni, M. H., Lechner, S. C., Kazi, A., Wimberly, S. R., Sifre, T., Urcuyo, K. R., et al. (2006). How stress management improves quality of life after treatment for breast cancer. *Journal of Consulting and Clinical Psychology, 74*(6), 1143–1152.

Antoni, M. H., Lehman, J. M., Kilbourn, K. M., Boyers, A. E., Culver, J. L., Alferi, S. M., et al. (2001). Cognitive-behavioral stress management intervention decreases the prevalence of depression and enhances benefit finding among women under treatment for early-stage breast cancer. *Health Psychology, 20*(1), 20–32.

Antoni, M. H., Lutgendorf, S. K., Cole, S. W., Dhabhar, F. S., Sephton, S. E., McDonald, P. G., et al. (2006b). The influence of bio-behavioural factors on tumour biology: Pathways and mechanisms. *Nature Review Cancer, 6*(3), 240–248.

Antoni, M. H., & Lutgendorf, S. (2007). Psychosocial factors and disease progression in cancer. *Current Directions in Psychological Science, 16,* 42–46.

Antoni, M. H, Pereira, D. B., Buscher, I., Ennis, N., Peake-Andrasik, M. Rose, R., et al. (2008). Stress management effects on perceived stress and cervical intraepithelial neoplasia in low-income HIV infected women. *Journal of Psychosomatic Research, 65,* 389–401.

Antoni, M. H. & Schneiderman, N. (1998). HIV/AIDS. In A. Bellack & M. Hersen (Eds.), *Comprehensive clinical psychology*. (pp. 237–275). New York: Elsevier Science.

Antoni, M. H., Schneiderman, N., Fletcher, M., Goldstein, D., Laperriere, A., & Ironson, G. (1990). Psychoneuroimmunology and HIV-1. *Journal of Consulting and Clinical Psychology, 58*(1), 38–49.

Antoni, M. H., Schneiderman, N. & Penedo, F. (2006). Behavioral interventions: Immunologic mediators and disease outcomes. In R. Ader, R. Glaser, N. Cohen, & M. Irwin, (Eds.), *Psychoneuroimmunology* (4th ed, pp. 675–703). New York: Academic.

Antoni, M. H., Wagner, S., Cruess, D., Kumar, M., Lutgendorf, S., Ironson, G., et al. (2000). Cognitive behavioral stress management reduces distress and 24-hour urinary free cortisol among symptomatic HIV-infected gay men. *Annals of Behavioral Medicine, 22*, 29–37.

Antoni, M. H. & Weiss, D. (2003) Stress and immunity. In: L. Jason, P. Fenell, & R. Taylor (Eds.), *Handbook of chronic fatigue syndrome and fatiguing illnesses* (pp. 527–545) New York: Wiley.

Antoni, M. H., Wimberly, S. R., Lechner, S. C., Kazi, A., Sifre, T., Urcuyo, K. R., Dettmer, E., Williams, J., Klimas, N., Fletcher, M.A. & Schneiderman, N. (2006). Reduction of cancer-specific thought intrusions and anxiety symptoms with a stress management intervention among women undergoing treatment for breast cancer. *American Journal of Psychiatry, 163*(10), 1791–1797.

Antoni, M. H., Lutgendorf, S., Blomberg, B., Carver, C. S., Lechner, S., Diaz, A., et al. (2012). Cognitive-behavioral stress management reverses anxiety-related leukocyte transcriptional dynamics. *Biological Psychiatry, 71*, 366–372.

Appels, A., Bar, F. W., Bar, J., Bruggeman, C., & de Bates, M. (2000). Inflammation, depressive symptomatology, and coronary artery disease. *Psychosomatic Medicine, 62*, 601–605.

Ben-Eliyahu, S. (2003) The promotion of tumor metastasis by surgery and stress: Immunological basis and implications for Psychoneuroimmunology. *Brain, Behavior and Immunity, 17*, S27–38).

Berger, S., Schad, T., VonWyl, V., Ehlert, U., Zellweger, C., Furrer, H., et al. (2008). Effects of cognitive behavioral stress management on HIV-1 RNA, CD4 cell counts and psychosocial parameters of HIV-infected persons. *AIDS, 22*, 767–775.

Berkman, L. F., Blumenthal, J., Burg, M., Carney, R. M., Catellier, D., et al. (2003). Effects of treating depression and low perceived social support on clinical events after myocardial infarction: The Enhancing Recovery in Coronary Heart Disease Patients (ENRICHD) Randomized Trial. *JAMA, 289*, 3106–3116.

Bing, E. G., Burnam, M. A., Longshore, D., Fleishman, J. A., Sherbourne, C. D., London, A. S., et al. (2001). Psychiatric disorders and drug use among human immunodeficiency virus-infected adults in the United States. *Archives of General Psychiatry, 58*, 721–728.

Bombardier C, & Buchwald D. (1995). Outcome and prognosis of patients with chronic fatigue vs. chronic fatigue syndrome. *Archives of Internal Medicine,155*, 2105–2110. PMID: 7575071.

Bovjberg, D. (1991) Psychoneuroimmunology: Implications for oncology? *Cancer, 67*, 828–832.

Bower, J., Kemeny, M., Taylor, S. & Fahey, J. L. (1998). Cognitive processing, discovery of meaning, CD4 decline and AIDS-related mortality among bereaved HIV-positive seropositive men. *Journal of Consulting and Clinical Psychology, 66*, 979–986.

Brickman, A., & Fins, A. (1993). Psychological and cognitive aspects of chronic fatigue syndrome. In P. Goodnik & N. Klimas (Eds), *Chronic fatigue & related immunodeficiency syndrome* (pp. 67–94). New York: American Psychiatric Press.

Broadley, A. J., Korszun, A., Jones, C. J., Frenneaux, M. P. (2002). Arterial endothelial function is impaired in treated depression. *Heart, 88*, 521–523.

Buchwald, D., Cheney, P., & Peterson, J. (1992). A chronic illness characterized by fatigue, neurologic and immunologic disorders, and active human herpesvirus-type 6 infection, *Annals of Internal Medicine, 116*, 103–113.

Buchwald, D., Sullivan J., & Komaroff, A. (1987). Frequency of chronic active Epstein-Barr virus infection in a general medical practice. *JAMA*, 257, 2303–2307.

Burack, J. H., Barrett, D. C., Stall, R. D., Chesney, M. A., Ekstrand, M. L., & Coates, T. J. (1993). Depressive symptoms and CD4 lymphocyte decline among HIV-infected men. *Journal of the American Medical Association, 270*, 2568–2573.

Burell, G., Svardsudd, K., & Guilliksson, M. (August, 2010). *Stress management prolongs life for CHD patients: A randomized clinical trial assessing the effects of group intervention on all cause mortality, recurrent cardiovascular disease, and quality of life.* Presented at the International Congress of Behavioral Medicine, Washington, DC.

Butler, S., Chalder, T., & Ron, M., (1991). Cognitive behavior therapy in chronic fatigue syndrome. *Journal of Neurology, Neurosurgery, and Psychiatry, 54*, 153–158.

Caliguri, M., Murray, C., Buchwald, C., Levine, H., Cheney, P., Peterson, D., et al. (1987). Phenotypic and functional deficiency of natural killer cells in patients with chronic fatigue syndrome. *Journal of Immunity, 139*, 3306–3313.

Capuron, L., Dantzer, R. (2003). Cytokines and depression: the need for a new paradigm. *Brain, Behavior and Immunity, 17*(1), S119–S124.

Carlson, L. E., Speca, M., Faris, P., & Patel, K. D. (2007). One year pre-post intervention follow-up of psychological, immune, endocrine and blood pressure outcomes of mindfulness-based stress reduction (MBSR) in breast and prostate cancer outpatients. *Brain, Behavior and Immunity, 21*(8), 1038–1049.

Carrico, A. W. & Antoni, M. H. (2008). The effects of psychological interventions on neuroendocrine hormone regulation and immune status in HIV-positive persons: A review of randomized controlled trials. *Psychosomatic Medicine, 70*, 575–584.

Carrico, A. W., Antoni, M. H., Young, L., & Gorman, J. M. (2008). Psychoneuroimmunology and HIV. In M. A. Cohen & J. M. Gorman (Eds.), *Comprehensive Textbook of AIDS Psychiatry* (pp. 27–38). Oxford, England: Oxford University Press.

Centers for Disease Control. (1992). 1993 revised classification system for HIV infection and expanded surveillance case definition for AIDS among adolescents and adults. *Morbidity and Mortality Weekly Report, 41*, RR-171–19.

Chen, E., Miller, G., Walker, H., Arevalo, J., Sung, C. & Cole, S. (2009) Genome-wide transcriptional profiling linked to social class in asthma. *Thorax, 64*, 38–43.

Chrousos, G., & Gold, P. (1992) The concepts of stress and stress system disorders: Overview of physical and behavioral homeostasis. *JAMA, 267*, 1244–1252.

Cielsa, J. A., & Roberts, J. E. (2001). Meta-analysis of the relationship between HIV infection and the risk for depressive disorders. *American Journal of Psychiatry, 158,* 725–730.

Clark, A. M., Hartling, L., Vandermeer, B., & McAlister, F. A. (2005). Secondary prevention program for patients with coronary artery disease: a meta-analysis of randomized control trials. *Annals of Internal Medicine, 143,* 659–672.

Cleare, A. J. (2004). The HPA axis and the genesis of chronic fatigue syndrome. *Trends in Endocrinology and Metabolism,* 15(2), 55–59.

Cohen, S., Tyrrell, D. A., & Smith, A. P. (1991). Psychological stress in humans and susceptibility to the common cold. *New England Journal of Medicine, 325,* 606–612.

Cole, S., Arevalo, J., Takahashi R., et al. (2010). Computational identification of gene-social environment interaction at the human IL6 locus. *Proceedings of the National Academy of Science USA, 107,* 5681–5686.

Cole, S. W. (2008). Psychosocial influences on HIV-1 disease progression: Neural, endocrine, and virologic mechanisms. *Psychosomatic Medicine, 70,* 562–568.

Cole, S. W. (2009). Social regulation of human gene expression. *Current Directions in Psychological Science, 18,* 132–137.

Cole, S. W., Hawkley, L. C., Arevalo, J. M., Sung, C. Y., Rose, R. M., Cacioppo, J. T. (2007). Social regulation of gene expression in human leukocytes. *Genome Biology* 2007;8:R189.

Cole, S., Kemeny, M., Naliboff, B., Fahey, J., & Zack, J. (2001). ANS enhancement of HIV Pathogenesis. *Brain, Behavior and Immunity,15,* 121.

Cole, S. W., Korin, Y. D., Fahey, J. L., & Zack, J. A. (1998). Norepinephrine accelerates HIV replication via protein kinase A-dependent effects on cytokine production. *Journal of Immunology, 161,* 610–616.

Cole, S. W., Naliboff, B. D., Kemeny, M. E., Griswold, M. P., Fahey, J. L., & Zack, J. A. (2001). Impaired response to HAART in HIV-infected individuals with high autonomic nervous system activity. *Proceedings of the National Academy of Sciences USA, 98,* 12695–12700.

Coyne, J., Stefanek, M., & Palmer, S. (2007) Psychotherapy and survival in cancer: The conflict between hope and evidence. *Psychological Bulletin, 133,* 367–394.

Crepaz, N., Passin, W., Herbst, J., Rama, S, Malow, R., Purcell, D, et al. (2008). Meta-analysis of cognitive behavioral interventions on HIV-positive person's mental health and immune functioning. *Health Psychology, 27,* 4–14.

Cruess, D. G., Antoni, M. H., McGregor, B. A., Kilbourn, K. M., Boyers, A. E., Alfieri, S. M., et al. (2000). Cognitive-behavioral stress management reduces serum cortisol by enhancing benefit finding among women being treated for early stage breast cancer. *Psychosomatic Medicine,* 62(3), 304–308.

Cruess, S., Antoni, M. H., Cruess, D., Fletcher, M. A., Ironson, G., Kumar, M., et al. (2000). Reductions in HSV-2 antibody titers after cognitive behavioral stress management and relationships with neuroendocrine function, relaxation skills, and social support in HIV+ gay men. *Psychosomatic Medicine, 62,* 828–837.

Cruess, S., Klimas, N., Helder, L., Antoni, M. H., & Fletcher, M. A. (2000) Immunologic status correlates with severity of physical symptoms and perceived illness burden in Chronic Fatigue Syndrome patients. *Journal of Chronic Fatigue Syndrome,* 7(1), 39–52.

Dantzer, R. (2001). Cytokine-induced sickness behavior: where do we stand? *Brain, Behavior and Immunity, 15,* 7–24.

Deale, A., Chalder, T., Marks, I. & Wessley, S. (1997) Cognitive behavioral therapy for chronic fatigue syndrome: A randomized controlled trial. *American Journal of Psychiatry, 154,* 408–414.

Demitrack, M. & Crofford, L. (1998). Evidence for and pathophysiological implications of hypothalamic pituitary adrenal axis dysregulation in fibromyalgia and chronic fatigue syndrome. *Annals of the New York Academy of Sciences, 840,* 684–697. PMID: 9629295.

Demitrack, M., & Dale, J. (1991). Evidence for impaired activation of the hypothalamic-pituitary-adrenal axis in patients with chronic fatigue syndrome. *Journal of Clinical Endocrinology and Metabolism, 73,* 1224–1234.

DesJarlais, D., & Semaan, S. (2008). HIV prevention and injecting drug users: The first 25 years and counting. *Psychosomatic Medicine, 70,* 606–611.

Diego, M. A., Field, T., Hernandez-Reif, M., Shaw, K., Friedman, L., & Ironson, G.. (2001). HIV adolescents show improved immune function following massage therapy. *International Journal of Neuroscience, 106,* 35–45.

Dinarello, C. (1992). Interleukin-1 and tumor necrosis factor: Effector cytokines in autoimmune diseases. *Seminars in Immunology,* 4(3), 133–145. PMID: 1320950.

Dinarello, C., Cannon, J., & Wolff, S. (1986). Tumor necrosis factor (cachectin) is an endogenous pyrogen and induces production of interleukin-1. *Journal of Experimental Medicine, 63,* 1433–1450. PMID: 3486936.

Disis, M. L., & Lyerly, H. K. (2005). Global role of the immune system in identifying cancer initiation and limiting disease progression. *Journal of Clinical Oncology,* 23(35), 8923–8925.

Dusseldorp, E., vanElderen, T., Maes, S., Meulman, J., & Kraaij, V. (1999). A meta-analysis of psychoeducational programs for coronary heart disease patients. *Health Psychology, 18,* 506–519.

Erlwein, O., Kaye, S., McClure, M., Weber, J., Wills, G., Collier, D., et al. (2010). Failure to detect the novel retrovirus XMRV in chronic fatigue syndrome. *PLoS One,* 6(1): e8519.

Esterling, B., Antoni, M., Schneiderman, N., Ironson, G., LaPerriere, A., Klimas, N., et al. (1992). Psychosocial modulation of antibody to Epstein-Barr viral capsid antigen and herpes virus type-6 in HIV-1 infected and at-risk gay men. *Psychosomatic Medicine, 54,* 354–371.

Evans, D. L., Ten Have, T. R., Douglas, S. D., Gettes, D., Morrison, C. H., Chiappini, M. S., et al. (2002). Association of depression with viral load, CD8 T lymphocytes, and natural killer cells in women with HIV infection. *American Journal of Psychiatry, 159,* 1752–1759.

Evengård, B., Jonzon, E., Sandberg, A., Theorell, T., & Lindh, G. (2003). Differences between patients with chronic fatigue syndrome and with chronic fatigue at an infectious disease clinic in Stockholm, Sweden. *Psychiatry and Clinical Neuroscience, 57,* 361–368.

Evengård, B., & Klimas, N. (2002). Chronic fatigue syndrome: Probable pathogenesis and possible treatments. *Drugs, 62,* 2433–2446.

Fawzy F., Fawzy N., Hyun C., Elashoff, R., Guthrie, D., Fahey, J. L., et al. (1993). Malignant melanoma. Effects of an early structured psychiatric intervention, coping, and affective state on recurrence and survival 6 years later. *Archives of General Psychiatry, 50,* 681–689.

Fawzy, F. I., Kemeny, M. E., Fawzy, N., Elashoff, R. Morton, D., et al. (1990). A structured psychiatric intervention for cancer patients. II. Changes over time in immunological measures. *Archives of General Psychiatry, 47,* 729–735.

Fekeulegn, D., Andrew, M., Burchfiel, C., Violanti, J., Hartley, T., Charles, L., et al. (2007). Area under the curve and other summary indicators of repeated waking cortisol measurements. *Psychosomatic Medicine, 69,* 651–650.

Felten, D. (1996). Changes in the neural innervation of lymphoid tissues with age. In N. Hall, F. Altman, & S. Blumenthal (Eds), *Mind-body interactions and disease and psychoneuroimmunological aspects of health and disease. Proceedings of conference on stress, immunity and health. National Institutes of Health* (pp.157–164) Washington, DC: Heath Dateline Press.

Fife, B., Scott, L., Fineberg, N., & Zwickil, B. (2008). Promoting adaptive coping by persons with HIV disease: Evaluation of a patient/partner intervention model. *Journal of the Association of Nurses in AIDS Care, 19,* 75–84.

Fletcher, M. A., Zeng, X. R., Barnes, Z., Lewis, S., & Klimas, N. G. (2009). Plasma cytokines in women with chronic fatigue syndrome. *Journal of Translational Medicine, 7,* 96. Retrieved at http://www.translational- medicine.com/content/7/1/96

Folkman, S., Chesney, M., McKusick, L., Ironson, G., Johnson, D., & Coates, T. (1991). Translating coping theory into intervention. In J. Eckenrode (Ed.), *The social context of coping* (pp. 239–259). New York: Plenum.

Friedberg, F., & Krupp, L. (1994). A comparison of cognitive behavioral treatment for chronic fatigue syndrome and primary depression. *Clinical Infectious Diseases, 18,* S105–S110.

Fuite, J., Vernon, S.D., & Broderick, G. (2008). Neuroendocrine and immune network re-modeling in chronic fatigue syndrome: an exploratory analysis. *Genomics, 92,* 393–399.

Gaab, J., Rohleder, N., Heitz, V., Engert, V., Schad, T., Schürmeyer, T. H., et al. (2005). Stress-induced changes in LPS-induced pro-inflammatory cytokine production in chronic fatigue syndrome. *Psychoneuroendocrinology, 30(2),* 188–198.

Gaines, H., von Sydow, M. A., von Stedingk, L.V., Biberfeld, G., Bottiger, B., Hansson, L. O. et al. (1990). Immunological changes in primary HIV-1 infection. *AIDS, 4,* 995–999.

Ghiadoni, L., Donald, A.E., Cropley, M., Mullen, M., Oakley, G., Taylor, M., et al. (2000). Mental stress induces transient endothelial dysfunction in humans. *Circulation, 102,* 2473–2478.

Glaser, R., Kennedy, S., Lafuse, W., & Kiecolt-Glaser, J. (1990). Psychological stress-induced modulation of IL-2 receptor gene expression and IL-2 production in peripheral blood leukocytes. *Archives of General Psychiatry, 47,* 729–735.

Glaser, R., & Kiecolt-Glaser, J. (1997). Chronic stress modulates the virus-specifiic immune response to latent herpes simplex virus type 1. *Annals of Behavioral Medicine, 19,* 78–82.

Glaser, R., Padgett, D. A., Litsky, M. L., Baiocchi, R. A., Yang, E. V., Chen, M., et al. (2005). Stress-associated changes in the steady-state expression of latent Epstein-Barr virus: implications for chronic fatigue syndrome and cancer. *Brain, Behavior, and Immunity, 19,* 91–103.

Glaser, R., Pearson, G. R., Jones, J. F., Hillhouse, J., Kennedy, S., Mao, H. Y., et al. (1991). Stress-related activation of Epstein-Barr virus. *Brain, Behavior and Immunity, 5,* 219–232.

Glaser, R., Rice, J., Sheridan, J., Fertel, R., Stout, J., Speicher, C., et al. (1987). Stress-related immune suppresion: Health implications. *Brain, Behavior and Immunity, 1,* 7–20.

Goebel, M. U., & Mills, P. J. (2000). Acute psychological stress and exercise and changes in peripheral leukocyte adhesion molecule expression and density. *Psychosomatic Medicine, 62,* 664–670.

Goodkin, K., Antoni, M. H., Fox, B. H., & Sevin, B. (1993) A partially testable model of psychosocial factors in the etiology of cervical cancer. II. Psychoneuroimmunological aspects, critique and prospective integration. *Psycho-oncology, 2(2):* 99–121.

Goodwin, P. J., Leszcz, M,, Ennis, M., Koopmans, J., Vincent, L., Guther, H., et al. (2001). The effect of group psychosocial support on survival in metastatic breast cancer. *New England Journal of Medicine, 345,* 1719–1726.

Gore-Felton, C. & Koopman, C. (2008). Behavioral mediation of the relationship between psychosocial factors and HIV disease progression. *Psychosomatic Medicine, 70,* 569–574.

Harbuz, M. S., Chover-Gonzalez, A. J., Jessop, D. S. (2003). Hypothalamo-pituitary-adrenal axis and chronic immune activation. *Annals of the New York Academy of Science, 992,* 99–106.

Heckman, T. G., Barcikowski, R., Ogles, B., Suhr, J., Carlson, B., Holroyd, K., et al. (2006). A telephone-delivered coping improvement group intervention for middle-aged and older adults living with HIV/AIDS. *Annals of Behavioral Medicine, 32,* 27–38.

Heijnen, C. & Kavelaars, A. (2005). Psychoneuorimmunology and chronic autoimmune disease: rheumatoid arthritis. In K. Vedhara & M. Irwin (Eds), *Human psychoneuroimmunology* (pp. 195–218). Oxford, England: Oxford University Press.

Herbert, T. & Cohen, S. (1993a) Stress and immunity in humans: A meta-analytic review. *Psychosomatic Medicine, 55,* 364–379.

Herbert, T. & Cohen, S. (1993b) Depression and immunity: A meta-analytic review. *Psychological Bulletin, 113,* 472–486

House, J. S., Landis, K. R., Umberson, D. (1988) Social relationships and health. *Science, 241,* 540–545

Huang, L. M., Chao, M. F., Chen, M. Y., Shih, H. M., Chiang, Y. P., Chuang, C. Y., et al. (2001). Reciprocal regulatory interaction between Human Herpesvirus 8 and Human Immunodeficiency Virus Type 1. *Journal of Biological Chemistry, 276,* 13427–13432.

Ickovics, J.R., Hamburger, M.E., Vlahov, D., Schoenbaum, E.E., Schuman, P., Boland, R.J., et al. (2001). Mortality, CD4 cell count decline, and depressive symptoms among HIV-seropositive women: Longitudinal analysis from the HIV Epidemiology Research Study. *Journal of the American Medical Association, 285,* 1460–1465.

Ickovics, J. R., Milan, S., Boland R., Schoenbaum, E., Schuman, P., Vlahov, D., et al. (2006). Psychological resources protect health: 5-year survival and immune function among HIV-infected women from four U.S. cities. *AIDS, 20,* 1851–1860.

Ironson, G., Balbin, G., Solomon, G., Fahey, J., Klimas, N., Schneiderman, N., et al. (2001). Relative preservation of natural killer cell cytotoxicity and number in healthy AIDS patients with low CD4 cell counts. *AIDS, 15,* 2065–2073.

Ironson, G., Balbin, E., Stieren, E., Detz, K., Fletcher, M.A., Schneiderman, N., et al. (2008) Perceived stress and norepinephrine predict effectiveness of response to protease inhibitors in HIV. *International Journal of Behavioral Medicine, 15,* 221–226.

Ironson, G., Friedman, A., Klimas, N., Antoni, M. H., Fletcher, M. A., LaPerriere, A., et al. (1994). Distress, denial and low adherence to behavioral intervention predict faster disease progression in gay men infected with human immunodeficiency virus. *International Journal of Behavioral Medicine, 1,* 90–105.

Ironson, G. & Hayward, H. (2008). Do positive psychological factors predict disease progression in HIV-1? A review of the evidence. *Psychosomatic Medicine, 70,* 546–554.

Ironson, G., O'Cleirigh, C., Fletcher, M. A., Laurenceau, J. P., Balbin, E., Klimas, N., et al. (2005). Psychosocial factors predict CD4 and viral load change in men and women with human immunodeficiency virus in the era of highly active antiretroviral therapy. *Psychosomatic Medicine, 67,* 1013–1021.

Ironson, G., Wynings, C., Schneiderman, N., Baum, A., Rodriquez, M., Greenwood, D., et al. (1997). Post traumatic stress symptoms, intrusive thoughts, loss and immune function after Hurricane Andrew. *Psychosomatic Medicine, 59,* 128–141.

Jason, L. A., Richman, J. A., Rademaker, A.W., Jordan, K. M., Plioplys, A.V., Taylor, R.R., et al. (1999). A community-based study of chronic fatigue syndrome. *Archives of Internal Medicine,159,* 2129–2137.

Jensen, S., Lehman, B., Antoni, M. H. & Pereira, D. (2007). Psychoneuroimmunologic applications to human papillomavirus mediated cervical neoplasia research among the iatrogenically immunocompromised. *Brain, Behavior and Immunity, 21,* 758–766.

Jones J., & Straus S. (1987). Chronic Epstein-Barr virus infection. *Annual Review of Medicine, 38,* 195–209.

Kalichman, S. (2008). Co-occurrence of treatment nonadherence and continued HIV transmission risk behaviors: Implications for positive prevention interventions. *Psychosomatic Medicine, 5*(70), 593–597.

Kalichman, S. C., Difonzo, K., Austin, J., Luke, W., & Rompa, D. (2002). Prospective study of emotional reactions to changes in HIV viral load. *AIDS Patient Care and STD's, 16*(3), 113–120.

Kennedy, H. G. (1988). Fatigue and fatigability. *British Journal of Psychiatry, 153,* 1–5.

Kiecolt-Glaser, J., Fisher, L., Ogrocki, P., Stout, J., Speicher, C., & Glaser, R. (1987) Marital quality, marital disruption, and immune function. *Psychosomatic Medicine, 49,* 13–34.

Kiecolt-Glaser, J., Ricker, D., George, J., Messick, G., Speicher, C., Garner, W., et al. (1984). Urinary cortisol levels, cellular immunocompetency, and loneliness in psychiatric inpatients. *Psychosomatic Medicine, 46*(1), 15–23.

Kiecolt-Glaser, J. K., Robles, T. F., Heffner, K. Loving, T., & Glaser, R. (2002). Psycho-oncology and cancer: psychoneuroimmunology and cancer. *Annals of Oncology, 13*(4), 165–169.

Killebrew, D. & Shiramizu, B. (2004) Pathogenesis of HIV-associated nonHodgkin lymphoma. *Current HIV Research, 2,* 215–221.

Kissane, D., Grabsch, B., Clarke, D., Smith, G., Love, A., Bloch, S., & Li, Y. (2007). Supportive-expressive group therapy for women with metastatic breast cancer: Survival and psychosocial outcomes from a randomized controlled trial. *Psycho-Oncology, 16,* 277–286.

Klatzmann, D., Champagne, E., Chamaret, S., Gruest, J., Guetard, D., Hercend, T., et al. (1984). T lymphocyte T4 molecule behaves as the receptor for human retrovirus LAV. *Nature, 312,* 767–768.

Klimas, N. G., & Koneru, A. O. (2007) Chronic fatigue syndrome: inflammation, immune function, and neuroendocrine interactions. *Current Rheumatology Reports, 9*(6):482–7.

Klimas, N. G., Morgan, R., Salvado, F., & Fletcher, M. A. (1990). Immunologic abnormalities of chronic fatigue syndrome. *Journal of Clinical Microbiology, 28,*1403–1410.

Klimas, N., Patarca, R., & Fletcher, M. A. (1992). Psychoneuroimmunology and chronic fatigue syndrome. In N. Schneiderman & A. Baum (Eds), *Perspectives in behavioral medicine,* Mahwah,NJ: Erlbaum.

Kobilka, B. (1992). Adrenergic receptors as models for G-protein coupled receptors. *Annual Review of Neuroscience, 15,* 87.

Landay, A. Jessop, C., Lenette, E. & Levy, J. (1991). Chronic fatigue syndrome: clinical condition associated with immune activation. *Lancet, 338,* 707–712. PMID: 1679864.

LaPerriere, A., Antoni, M. H., Ironson, G. Klimas, N., Ingram, F., Fletcher, M. A., & Schneiderman, N. (1990). Exercise training buffers emotional distress and immune decrements in gay males learning of their HIV-1 antibody status. *Biofeedback and Self-Regulation, 15*(3), 229–242.

Larson, M. R., Duberstein, P. R., Talbot, N. L., Caldwell, C., & Moynihan, J. A., 2000. A presurgical psychosocial intervention for breast cancer patients: Psychological distress and the immune response. *Journal of Psychosomatic Research, 48*(2), 187–194.

Lechner, S., Antoni, M. H., Lydston, D., LaPerriere, A., Ishii, M., Stanley, H., et al. (2003). Cognitive-behavioral interventions improve quality of life in women with AIDS. *Journal of Psychosomatic Research, 54,* 253–261.

Ledina, D., Bradari, N., Milas, I., Ivi, I., Brnci, N., & Kuzmici, N. (2007). Chronic fatigue syndrome after Q fever. *Medical Science Monitor, 13,* CS88–92.

Leserman, J. (2008). Role of depression, stress, and trauma in HIV disease progression. *Psychosomatic Medicine, 70,* 539–545.

Leserman, J., Jackson, E. D., Petitto, J. M., Golden, R. N., Silva, S. G., Perkins, D. O., et al. (1999). Progression to AIDS: The effects of stress, depressive symptoms and social support. *Psychosomatic Medicine, 61,* 397–406.

Leserman, J, Petitto, J. M, Golden, R. N, Gaynes, B. N, Gu, H., Perkins, D. O., et al. (2000). Impact of stressful life events, depression, social support, coping, and cortisol on progression to AIDS. *American Journal of Psychiatry, 157,* 1221–1228.

Leserman, J., Petitto, J. M., Gu, H., Gaynes, B. N., Barroso, J., Golden, R. N., et al. (2002). Progression to AIDS, a clinical AIDS condition and mortality: Psychosocial and physiological predictors. *Psychological Medicine, 32,* 1059–1073.

Leserman, J., Petitto, J. M., Perkins, D. O., Folds, J. D., Golden, R. N., & Evans, D. L. (1997). Severe stress and depressive symptoms, and changes in lymphocyte subsets in human immunodeficiency virus infected men. *Archives of General Psychiatry, 54,* 279–285.

Lesperance, F., Frasure-Smith, N., Theroux, P. & Irwin, M. (2004). The association between major depression and levels of soluble intercellular adhesion molecule 1, interleukin-6, and C-reactive protein in patients with recent acute coronary syndromes. *American Journal of Psychiatry, 161*(2), 271–277.

Libby, P., Ridker, P. M., & Maseri, A. (2002). Inflammation and atherosclerosis. *Circulation, 105,* 1135–43.

Linden, W., Phillips, M. J., & Leclerc, J. (2007). Psychological treatment of cardiac patients; a meta-analysis. *European Heart Journal, 28,* 2972–2984.

Linden, W., Stossel, C., & Maurice, J. (1996). Psychosocial interventions for patients with coronary artery disease. *Archives of Internal Medicine, 156,* 745–52.

Lombardi, V., Ruscetti, F., Das Gupta, J., Plost, M., Hagen, K., Peterson, D., et al. (2009). Detection of an infectious retrovirus, XMRV, in blood cells of patients with chronic fatigue syndrome. *Science, 326,* 585–589.

Lopez, C., Antoni, M., Penedo, F., Weiss, D., Cruess, S., Segotas, M. C., et al. (2011). A pilot study of cognitive behavioral stress management effects on stress, quality of life, and symptoms in persons with chronic fatigue syndrome. *Journal of Psychosomatic Research, 70*(4), 328–334.

Lutgendorf, S., Costanzo, E., & Sood, A. (in press). Cancer. In S. Segerstrom (Ed), *Psychoneuroimmuology.* Oxford, England: Oxford University Press.

Lutgendorf, S., Antoni, M. H., Brickman A., Klimas, N., Ironson, G., Patarca, R., et al. (1993). Immunologic correlates of cognitive difficulties in chronic fatigue syndrome. *Psychosomatic Medicine, 55,* 227 (abstract).

Lutgendorf, S., Antoni, M. H., Ironson, G., Fletcher, M. A., Penedo, F., VanRiel, F., et al. (1995) Physical symptoms of chronic fatigue syndrome are exacerbated by the stress of Hurricane Andrew. *Psychosomatic Medicine, 57,* 310–323.

Lutgendorf, S. K., Antoni, M. H., Ironson, G., Klimas, N., Kumar, M., Starr, K., et al. (1997). Cognitive behavioral stress management intervention decreases dysphoria and herpes simplex virus-type 2 titers in symptomatic HIV-seropositive gay men. *Journal of Consulting and Clinical Psychology, 65,* 23–31.

Lutgendorf, S., Antoni, M. H., Ironson, G., Starr, K., Costello, N., Zuckerman, M., et al. (1998) Changes in cognitive coping skills and social support mediate distress outcomes in symptomatic HIV-seropositive gay men during a cognitive behavioral stress-management intervention. *Psychosomatic Medicine, 60,* 204–214.

Lutgendorf, S., Cole, S., Costanzo, E., Bradley, S., Coffin, J., Jabari, S., et al. (2003). Stress-related mediators stimulate vascular endothelial growth factor secretion by two ovarian cancer cell lines. *Clinical Cancer Research, 9,* 4514–4521.

Lutgendorf, S. K., DeGeest, K., Sung, C. Y., Arevalo, J. M. G., Penedo, F., Lucci, J. A. I., et al. (2009) Depression, social support, and beta-adrenergic transcription control in human ovarian cancer. *Brain, Behavior and Immunity, 23,* 176–183.

Lutgendorf, S., Sood, A. & Antoni, M. H. (2010). Host factors and cancer progression: Biobehavioral signaling pathways and interventions. *Journal of Clinical Oncology, 28,* 4094–4099.

Maiman, M., Fruchter, R., Clark, M., Arrastia, C., Matthews, R., & Gates, E. J.(1997). Cervical cancer as an AIDS-defining illness. *Obstetrics and Gynecology, 89,* 76–80.

Malouff, J., Thorsteinsson, E., Rooks, S., Bhuliar, N., & Schutte, N. (2008). Efficacy of cognitive behavioral therapy for chronic fatigue syndrome: A meta-analysis. *Immunology Review, 5,* 736–745.

Mayne, T. J., Vittinghoff, E., Chesney, M. A., Barrett, D. C., & Coates, T. J. (1996). Depressive affect and survival among gay and bisexual men infected with HIV. *Archives of Internal Medicine, 156,* 2233–2238.

McCain, N., Gray, D., Elswick, R., Robins, J., Tuck, I., Walter, J., et al. (2008). A randomized clinical trial of alternative stress management interventions in persons with HIV infection. *Journal of Consulting and Clinical Psychology, 76,* 431–441.

McCain, N. Munjas, B., Munro, C., Elswick, R., Robins, J., Ferreira-Gonzalez, A., et al. (2003). Effects of stress management on PNI-based outcomes in persons with HIV disease. *Research in Nursing and Health, 26,* 102–117.

McEwen, B. (1998). Protective and damaging effects of stress mediators. *New England Journal of Medicine, 338,* 171–179.

McGregor B., & Antoni M. H. (2009). Psychological intervention and health outcomes among women treated for breast cancer: A review of stress pathways and biological mediators. *Brain, Behavior and Immunity, 23,*159–166.

McGregor, B., Antoni, M. H., Boyers, A., Alferi, S., Cruess, D., Blomberg, B., et al. (2004) Effects of cognitive behavioral stress management on immune function and positive contributions in women with early-stage breast cancer. *Journal of Psychosomatic Research, 54,*1–8.

Miller, G. E., Cohen, S., & Ritchey, A. K. (2002). Chronic psychological stress and the regulation of pro-inflammatory cytokines: A glucocorticoid-resistance model. *Health Psychology, 21,* 531–541.

Mohr, D. C., Hart, S. L., Julian, L., Cox, D., & Pelletier, D. (2004). Association between stressful life events and exacerbation in multiple sclerosis: A meta-analysis. *British Medical Journal, 328,* 731.

Moldovsky, H. (1989). Nonrestorative sleep and symptoms after a febrile illness in patients with fibrosis and chronic fatigue syndrome, *Journal of Rheumatology, 16*(19), 150–153.

Morrow, D. A., & Ridker, P. M. (2000). C-reactive protein, inflammation, and coronary disease. *Medical Clinics of North America, 81,* 149–161.

Moskowitz, J. T. (2003). Positive affect predicts lower risk of AIDS mortality. *Psychosomatic Medicine, 65,* 620–626.

Nair, M. P. N., Mahajan, S., Hou, J., Sweet, A. M., Schwartz, S. A. (2000). The stress hormone, cortisol, synergizes with HIV-1 gp120 to induce apoptosis of normal human peripheral blood mononuclear cells. *Cellular and Molecular Biology, 46*(7), 122–1238.

Newell, S., Sanson-Fisher, R, & Savolainen, N. (2002) Systematic review of psychological therapies for cancer patients: Overview and recommendations for future research. *Journal of the National Cancer Institute, 94,* 558–584.

Orth-Gomér, K., Schneiderman, N., Wang, H., Walldin, C., Bloom, M. & Jernberg, T. (2009). Stress reduction prolongs life in women with coronary disease: The Stockholm Women's Intervention Trial for Coronary Heart Disease (SWITCHD). *Circulation: Cardiovascular Quality and Outcomes, 2,* 25–32.

Pantaleo, G., Graziosi, C., & Fauci, A. S. (1993). The immunopathogenesis of human immunodeficiency virus infection. *The New England Journal of Medicine, 328,* 327–335.

Patarca, R., Klimas, N., Lutgendorf, S., Antoni, M. H., & Fletcher, M. A. (1994). Dysregulated expression of tumor necrosis factor (TNF) in the chronic fatigue immune dysfunction syndrome: Interrelationships with cellular sources and soluble immune mediator expression patterns. *Clinical Infectious Diseases, 18,* S147–153.

Patarca-Montero, R., Antoni, M., Fletcher, M. A., & Klimas, N. G. (2001) Cytokine and other immunologic markers in chronic fatigue syndrome and their relation to neuropsychological factors. *Applied Neuropsychology, 8*(1),51–64.

Pereira, D. (2002). Interventions for mothers during pregnancy and postpartum: Behavioral and pharmacological approaches. In M. Chesney & M. H. Antoni (Eds.), *Innovative approaches to health psychology: Prevention and treatment lessons from AIDS* (pp. 141–166). Washington, DC: American Psychological Association Press.

Pereira, D., Antoni, M. H., Simon, T., Efantis-Potter, J., Carver, C. S., Durán, R., et al. (2003a) Stress and squamous intra-epithelial lesions in women with Human Papillomavirus and Human Immunodeficiency Virus. *Psychosomatic Medicine, 65,* 427–434.

Pereira, D., Antoni, M. H., Simon, T., Efantis-Potter, J., Carver, C. S., Durán, R., et al. (2003b). Stress as a predictor of symptomatic genital herpes virus recurrence in women with Human Immunodeficiency Virus. *Journal of Psychosomatic Research, 54,* 237–244.

Petrie, K. J, Fontanilla, I, Thomas, M. G, Booth, R. J., & Pennebaker, J. W. (2004): Effect of written emotional expression on immune function in patients with human immuno-deficiency virus infection: A randomized trial. *Psychosomatic Medicine, 66,* 272–275.

Phillips, K., Antoni, M. H., Lechner, S., Blomberg, B., Llabre, M., Avisar, E., et al. (2008) Stress management intervention reduces serum cortisol and increases relaxation during treatment for non-metastatic breast cancer. *Psychosomatic Medicine, 70,* 1044–1049.

Phillips, K. M., Antoni, M. H., Carver, C. S., Lechner, S. C., Penedo, F. J., McCullough, M. E., et al. (2011). Stress management skills and reductions in serum cortisol across the year after surgery for non-metastatic breast cancer. *Cognitive Therapy and Research, 35,* 595–600.

Prinz, J., Van der Meer, J., & Bleijenberg, G. (2006). Chronic fatigue syndrome. *Lancet, 367,* 346–355.

Redwine, L., Snow, S., Mills, P., & Irwin, M. (2003). Acute psychological stress: Effects on chemotaxis and cellular adhesion molecule expression. *Psychosomatic Medicine, 65,* 598–603.

Reyes, M., Nisenbaum, R., Hoaglin, D. C., Unger, E. R., Emmons, C., Randall, B., et al. (2003). Prevalence and incidence of chronic fatigue syndrome in Wichita, Kansas. *Archives of Internal Medicine, 163,* 1530–1536.

Rivest, S. (2001). How circulating cytokines trigger the neural circuits that control the hypothalamic-pituitary-adrenal axis. *Psychoneuroendocrinology, 26,* 761–788.

Ross, R. (1999). Atherosclerosis—an inflammatory disease. *New England Journal of Medicine, 340,* 115–126.

Rugulies, R. (2002). Depression as a predictor for coronary heart disease. *American Journal of Preventive Medicine, 23,* 51–61.

Safren, S., Knauz, R. O., O'Cleirigh, C., Lerner, J., Greer, J., Harwood, M., et al. (2006). CBT for HIV medication adherence and depression: Process and outcome at post-treatment and three-month cross over. *Annals of Behavioral Medicine, 31,* S006.

Salvato, F., Klimas, N., Ashman, M., & Fletcher, M. (1988). Immune dysfunction among chronic fatigue syndrome patients with evidence of Epstein-Barr virus reactivation. *Journal of Clinical Cancer Research, 7,* 89.

Sapolsky, R. M, Romero, L. M., & Munck, A. U. (2000). How do glucocorticoids influence stress responses? Integrating permissive, suppressive, stimulatory, and preparative actions. *Endocrine Reviews, 21,* 55–89.

Savard, J., Simard, S., Ivers, H., & Morin, C. M. (2005a) Randomized study on the efficacy of cognitive-behavioral therapy for insomnia secondary to breast cancer, part i: Sleep and psychological effects. *Journal of Clinical Oncology, 23*(25), 6083–6096.

Savard, J., Simard, S., Ivers, H., & Morin, C. M. (2005b). Randomized study on the efficacy of cognitive-behavioral therapy for insomnia secondary to breast cancer, part ii: Immunologic effects. *Journal of Clinical Oncology, 23*(25), 6097–6106.

Schedlowski, M., Jung, C., Schimanski, G., Tewes, U., & Schmoll, H. J. (1994). Effects of behavioral intervention on plasma cortisol and lymphocytes in breast cancer patients: An exploratory study. *Psychooncology, 3,* 181–187.

Schneiderman, N., Saab, P. G., Catellier, D., Powell, L. H., DeBusk, L. F., et al. (2004). Psychosocial treatment within sex by ethnicity subgroups in the Enhancing Recovery in Coronary Heart Disease clinical trial. *Psychosomatic Medicine 66,* 475–483.

Schneiderman, N., Antoni, M. H., Penedo, F., & Ironson, G. (2010). Psychosocial and Behavioral Interventions in the Treatment of Physical Illnesses and Disease Processes. In A. Steptoe (Ed.), *Handbook of behavioral medicine: Methods and applications* (pp. 989–1007). NY: Springer.

Segerstrom, S. C. (2000). Personality and the immune system: models, methods, and mechanisms. *Annals of Behavioral Medicine, 22*(3), 180–190.

Sephton, S. E., Sapolsky, R. M., Kraemer, H. C., & Spiegel, D. (2000). Diurnal cortisol rhythm as a predictor of breast cancer survival. *Journal of the National Cancer Institute, 92*(12), 994–1000.

Shakhar, G., & Ben-Eliyahu, S. (2003). Potential prophylactic measures against postoperative immunosuppression: Could they reduce recurrence rates in oncological patients? *Annals of Surgical Oncology,* 10, 972–992.

Sharpe, M., Hawton, K., Simkin, S., Surawy, C., Hackman, A., Klimes, I., et al. (1996) Cognitive behavior therapy for chronic fatigue syndrome: A randomized controlled trial. *British Medical Journal, 312,* 21–26.

Shoham, S., Davenne, D., & Cady, A. (1987). Recombinant tumor necrosis factor and interleukin 1 enhance slow-wave sleep. *American Journal of Physiology, 253,* R142. PMID: 3496800.

Siegel, S., Antoni, M. H., Fletcher, M. A., Maher, K., Segota, M. C. Klimas, N. (2006). Impaired natural immunity, cognitive dysfunction, and physical symptoms in patients with chronic fatigue syndrome: Preliminary evidence for a sub-group? *Journal of Psychosomatic Research, 60,* 559–566.

Simoni, J. M., Pearson, C. R., Pantalone, D. W., Marks, G., & Crepaz, N. (2006). Efficacy of interventions in improving highly active antiretroviral therapy adherence and HIV-1 RNA viral load: A meta-analytic review of randomized controlled trials. *Journal of Acquired Immune Deficiency Syndromes, 43*(1), S23–S35.

Spiegel D. (2002) Effects of psychotherapy on cancer survival. *Nature Reviews Cancer, 2,* 383–389.

Spiegel, D., Bloom, J. R., Kraemer, H. C., & Gottheil, E., (1989). Effect of psychosocial treatment on survival of patients with metastatic breast cancer. *Lancet, 2*(8668), 888–891.

Spiegel, D., Butler, L. D., Giese-Davis, J., Koopman, C., Miller, E., DiMiceli, S., et al. (2007). Effects of supportive-expressive group therapy on survival of patients with meta-static breast cancer: A randomized prospective trial. *Cancer, 110*(5), 1130–1138.

Stefanek, M., Palmer, S., Thombs, B., Coyne, J. (2009). Finding what there is not: Unwarranted claims of an effects of psy-chosocial intervention on recurrence and survival. *Cancer, 115,* 5612–5616.

Stein, M. D, Herman, D. S, Bishop, D., Anderson, B. J,, Trisvan, E., Lopez, R., et al. (2007). A telephone-based intervention for depression in HIV patients: negative results from a randomized clinical trial. *AIDS Behavior, 11*, 15–23.

Steptoe, A., & Brydon, L. (2005). Psychoneuroimmunology and coronary heart disease. In K. Vedhara & M. Irwin (Eds), *Human psychoneuroimmunology* (pp. 107–136). Oxford, England: Oxford University Press.

Straus, S. E., Tosato, G., Armstrong, G., Lawley, T., Preble, O.T., Henle, W., et al. (1985). Persisting illness and fatigue diagnostic instrument in adults with evidence of Epstein-Barr virus infection. *Annals of Internal Medicine, 102*, 7–16. PMID: 2578268.

Stubhaug, B., Atle, S., Ursin, H. & Eriksen, H. (2008). Cognitive-behavioural therapy v. mirtazapine for chronic fatigue and neurasthenia: Randomized placebo-controlled trial. *British Journal of Psychiatry, 192*, 217–223.

Suligoi, B., Dorrucci, M., Uccella, I., Andreoni, M., & Rezza, G. (2003). Effect of multiple herpesvirus infectins on the progression of HIV disease in a cohort of HIV seroconverters. *Journal of Medicial Virology, 69*, 182–187.

Swanson, B., Zeller, J. M., & Spear, G. T. (1998). Cortisol upregulates HIV p24 antigen production in cultured human monocyte-derived macrophages. *Journal of the Association of Nurses in AIDS Care, 9(4)*, 78–84.

Szapocznik, J., Feaster, D. J., Mitrani, V. B., Prado, G., Smith, L., Robinson-Batista, C., et al. (2004). Structural ecosystems therapy for HIV-seropositive African American women: Effects on psychological distress, family hassles, and family support. *Journal of Consulting Clinical Psychology, 72*, 288–303.

Taerk, G., Toner, B. B., Salit, I. E., Garfinkel, P. E., & Ozersky, S. (1987). Depression in patients with neuromyasthenia (benign myalgic encephoalomyelitis) *Intern. J. Psychiatry in Medicine, 17*, 49–56.

Thornton, L., Andersen, B. & Carson, W. (2008). Immune, endocrine, and behavioral precursors to breast cancer recurrence: a case-control analysis. *Cancer Immunology, Immunotherapy, 57*, 1471–1481.

Thornton, L., Andersen, B., Scholer, T & Carson, W. (2009). A psychological intervention reduces inflammatory markers by alleviating depressive symptoms: Secondary analysis of a randomized controlled trial. *Psychosomatic Medicine, 71*, 715–724.

Tindall, B. & Cooper, D.A. (1991). Primary HIV infection: Host responses and intervention strategies. *AIDS, 5*, 1–15.

Torres-Harding, S., Sorenson, M., Jason, L.A., Reynolds, N., Brown, M, Maher, et al. (2009). The associations between basal salivary cortisol levels and illness symptomatology in chronic fatigue syndrome. *Journal of Applied Biobehavioral Research, 13,*157–160.

Turk, D., Holzman, A., & Kerns R., (1986). Chronic pain. In K. Holroyd & I. Creer (Eds), *Self-management of chronic disease: Handbook of clinical interventions and research*. Orlando, FL: Academic.

Van Der Ven, A., Van Diest, R., Hamulyak, K., Maes, M., Bruggeman, C., & Appels, A. (2003). Herpes viruses, cytokines, and altered hemostasis in vital exhaustion. *Psychosomatic Medicine, 65*, 194–200.

Vargas, S., Wohlgemuth, W., Antoni, M. H., Lechner, S., Holley, H. & Carver, C. S. (2010). Brief report: Sleep dysfunction and psychosocial adaptation among women undergoing treatment for non-metastatic breast cancer. *Psycho-Oncology, 19*, 669–673.

Varmus, H. (1988). Retroviruses. *Science, 240*, 1427–1434.

Vedhara, K., Nott, K.H., Bradbeer, C. S., Davidson, E. A. F., Ong, E. L. C., Snow, M. H., et al. (1997). Greater emotional distress is associated with accelerated CD4+ cell decline in HIV infection. *Journal of Psychosomatic Research, 42*, 379–390.

Vgontzas, A. N. & Chrousos, G. P. (2002) Sleep, the hypothalamic-pituitary-adrenal axis, and cytokines: Multiple interactions and disturbances in sleep disorders. *Endocrinology Metabolism Clinics of North America, 31*, 15–36. PMID: 12055986.

Weaver, K. E., Llabre, M. M., Duran, R. E., Antoni, M. H., Ironson, G., Penedo, F. J., et al. (2005). A stress and coping model of medication adherence and viral load in HIV-positive men and women on highly active antiretroviral therapy (HAART). *Health Psychology, 24(4)*, 385–392.

Weiss, D., Helder, L., & Antoni, M. H. (2003). Development of the SMART-ENERGY program. In L. Jason, P. Fenell, & R. Taylor (Eds), *Handbook of chronic fatigue syndrome and fatiguing Illnesses*. (pp. 546–560.) New York: Wiley.

Weiss, S., Tobin, J., Antoni, M. H., Ironson, G., Ishii, M., Vaughn, A., and the SMART/EST Women's Project Team (2011). Empowering women of color living with HIV/AIDS: The SMART/EST Women's Project. *The International Journal of Women's Health, 3*, 63–77.

White, P. D., Goldsmith, K. A., Johnson, A. L., Potts, L., Walwyn, R., DeCesare, J. C., et al. (2011). Comparison of adaptive pacing therapy, cognitive behaviour therapy, graded exercise therapy, and specialist medical care for chronic fatigue syndrome (PACE): A randomised trial. *The Lancet, 377*, 823–836.

Wiltschke, C., Krainer, M., Budinsky, A. C., Berger, A., Muller, C., Zeillinger, R., et al. (1995). Reduced mitogenic stimulation of peripheral blood mononuclear cells as a prognostic parameter for the course of breast cancer: A prospective longitudinal study. *British Journal of Cancer, 71(6)*, 1292–1296.

Witek-Janusek, L., Albuquerque, K., Chroniak, K. R., Chroniak, C., Durazo-Arvizu, R., & Mathews, H. (2008). Effect of mindfulness-based stress reduction on immune function, quality of life and coping in women newly diagnosed with early stage breast cancer. *Brain, Behavior and Immunity, 22*, 969–981.

Wojciechowski, F. L., Strik, J. J. M. H., Falger, P., Lousberg, R., & Honig, A. (2000). The relationship between depressive and vital exhaustion symptomatology post-myocardial infarction. *Acta Psychiatrica Scandinavica, 102*, 359–365.

Zuckerman, M., & Antoni, M.H. (1995). Social support and its relationship to psychological physical and immune variables in HIV infection. *Clinical Psychology and Psychotherapy, 2(4)*, 210–219.

Methods, Variance, and Error in Psychoneuroimmunology Research: The Good, the Bad, and the Ugly

Suzanne C. Segerstrom *and* Gregory T. Smith

Abstract

Every researcher deals with error at some level. In psychoneuroimmunology (PNI) research, there may be error due to substantive fluctuations in immune parameters (e.g., as related to stress, time of day, or activity). This error is significant for some parameters, but it can and should be minimized by taking multiple measurements or converted into "good," substantive variance by measuring variables that can predict the fluctuations. Type I and Type II "bad" errors are of more concern; many PNI studies have far too few subjects for the number of effects they test. Of studies included in a recent meta-analysis of stress and human immunity, several studies actually had fewer subjects than they had statistical tests. Finally, variance due to assay or supply variability contributes to "ugly" error, and it should be addressed by analysis of covariance or partial variance. However, too often, important variance due to factors such as age is designated as "ugly" rather than incorporated into the model. We suggest solutions for addressing "good," "bad," and "ugly" error and look into the future of physiometrics.

Key Words: immune, error, reliability, generalizability, validity, covariance

Psychoneuroimmunology (PNI) research typically requires (a) significant effort to recruit participants who meet stringent inclusion and exclusion criteria or who have particular diseases in particular stages; (b) significant interdisciplinary coordination to effectively assess participants across different psychological and physiological dimensions; and (c) significant financial investment, often of our own taxpayer dollars in the form of federal grant funding. This kind of up-front investment is made in the hope of not only a statistically significant finding, but also a substantively significant finding: one that can be replicated and act as a foundation for further research. Unfortunately, some conventional methods in PNI do not fulfill this promise. The purpose of this chapter is to suggest approaches that could increase the return on investment for PNI scientists—both those who are generating the research and those who rely on it to

inform research hypotheses, clinical applications, or both.

The problem that has to be overcome can generally be described as error. Many kinds of error are inherent to research, not just PNI research, but we will focus here on those that seem to be the biggest threats to the robustness, replicability, and validity of findings in PNI. Some "error" comes from undesired variability in the outcome measure; as we describe later, this error can be mitigated against or even converted into desired variability, and so we characterize that error as "good" error. However, other error is "bad" because it contributes to findings that are difficult if not impossible to replicate and may send PNI down blind alleys. Bad error, however, can and should be addressed a priori through design. Finally, there is error that is "ugly." There is nothing redeeming about ugly error. As we explain later, the biggest problem with ugly error is the tendency to relegate variance to this category that does not deserve the label.

The good
What is Good Error?

It is widely recognized that many biological parameters have phasic changes over minutes, hours, and days. These changes may be related to diurnal rhythms: For example, cortisol and proinflammatory cytokines typically change over the course of the day (e.g., Van Cauter, Leproult, & Kupfer, 1996; Vgontzas, Bixler, Lin, Prolo, Trakada, & Chrousos, 2005). They may also be related to momentary stress, arousal, activity, or pain: For example, the number of natural killer cells in circulation increases in response to sympathetic activation (e.g., Schedlowski et al., 1996). There are many other potential influences.

These changes create error variance for scientists interested in longer-term differences between groups or people or in changes over longer periods such as months or years. The typical approach to addressing this error is adopted from classical test theory. If one adds more randomly sampled observations within the focus of interest (people, months, or years), momentary effects that are not of interest will ultimately cancel each other out.

The question, of course, is how many observations are required to cancel out this error and achieve a reliable assessment of the parameter of interest at the level of interest. This question has received the most attention from researchers who study cortisol. The MacArthur Network includes on its Web page specific recommendations to collect cortisol over 3 to 6 days to reliably characterize stable individual differences in mean cortisol and cortisol slope, respectively (Stewart & Seeman, 2000). Kraemer and colleagues (2006) examined this issue in older adults and found less error variance, resulting in a recommendation that 2 days are sufficient in this sample to reliably characterize individual differences in cortisol slope. Sephton and Segerstrom (2011) examined this issue in young, healthy law students, yielding recommendations more like those from the MacArthur Network: at least 3 days for mean cortisol and 11 days for cortisol slope.

Some studies have also assessed variance in immune parameters (see Table 22.1). Typically these studies focused on the degree to which common immune assays capture stable individual differences between people or animals over a period of days to years. There is an important pattern in these studies that is worth noting. Typically, it is more difficult to capture an individual difference that is stable over a longer period of time than one that is stable over a shorter period of time. If one detects individual differences in the proliferative response, those individual differences are very likely to persist over a period of days (Fletcher et al., 1992). Over a longer period of time, in part due to intervening influences that, in this case, introduce "noise," those individual differences are harder to detect without multiple assessments (Van Rood et al., 1991).

What should be done?

Whereas concerns about the psychometrics of questionnaires or items are commonly raised by grant or manuscript reviewers, it is uncommon for a reviewer to raise this issue of what might be called physiometrics, or the reliability and validity of physiological parameters. However, the consequences of substituting a single assessment for multiple assessments can be serious. If single assessments prove not to be reliable indicators of a person's immunological "trait," one important consequence is that true findings, or findings that characterize the population, may not be detectable. The formula for estimating the maximum correlation between two variables as a function of the reliability of each is given by

$$r_{xy}(\text{max}) = \sqrt{r_{xx} r_{yy}}$$

where r_{xy} refers to the correlation between two variables, x and y, and r_{xx} and r_{yy} refer to reliability/stability estimates of each (Nunnally & Bernstein, 1994). Suppose one correlates an immunological variable, such as serum level of a cytokine, with a measure of personality that has a reliability coefficient of 0.80. If the cytokine is relatively stable over time, and its reliability is also 0.80, then the maximum possible correlation between the two variables is the square root of 0.80 squared, or 0.80. The less-than-perfect reliability constrains the possible correlation to a maximum of 0.80, not the preferred maximum of 1.0. If, in the population, the true variables were perfectly correlated, one would find a correlation of 0.80 or less in one's sample. This level of maximum correlation characterizes research using measures that are considered quite reliable, and it reflects the ubiquity of downward-biasing error in research.

More seriously, now suppose that the cytokine fluctuates over time and, therefore, a single measurement is much less reliable, having a reliability coefficient of 0.50. Consider the impact on the

Table 22.1 Studies assessing the reliability of inflammatory, functional, and enumerative immune parameters

	Method	Parameter	
Study	Reliability	Test-retest	% P variance
Inflammatory markers			
Hamer et al. (2006)	91 adult men studied twice over 4 weeks	CRP	47%
Rao et al. (1994)	12 older adults studied 8 times over 36 days	D-dimer	86%
		IL-6	87%
Cava et al. (2000)	15 adults studied monthly for 6 months	sIL2R	93%
		IL-6	37%
Functional assays			
Fletcher et al. (1992)	7 adults studied twice over 2 weeks	PHA	74%
		PWM	86%
Van Rood et al. (1991)	47 adults studied 5 times over 1 year	PHA	60%
		PWM	53%
		ConA	48–51%
Segerstrom et al. (2006)	6 male rhesus macaques studied 9 times over 7 months	NKCC	31–39%
		ConA	30%
	18 male rhesus macaques studied 13 times over 1 year	NKCC	25%
		ConA	26%
Segerstrom et al. (2009)	43 adolescent bonnet and pigtail monkeys studied 9 times over 2 years	NKCC	44–71%
		Per-cell NKCC	15–53%
Enumerative assays			
Van Rood et al. (1991)	47 adults studied 5 times over 1 year	Basophil	20%
		Eosinophil	50%
		Monocyte	24%
		Lymphocyte	41%
		Neutrophil	45%
		CD3	68%
		CD4	63%
		CD8	80%
		CD16	70%

(*continued*)

Table 22.1 (continued)

Study	Method	Parameter	
	Reliability	Test-retest	% P variance
Segerstrom et al. (2009)	43 adolescent bonnet and pigtail monkeys studied 9 times over 2 years	Basophil	1%
		Eosinophil	37%
		Monocyte	20%
		Lymphocyte	33%
		Neutrophil	28%
		CD2	48%
		CD4	46%
		CD8	69%
		CD16	56%
		CD20	35%

maximum possible correlation. In such a case, the maximum correlation would be given by

$$\sqrt{(0.80)*(0.50)} = \sqrt{0.40} = 0.63$$

Even if the true variables were perfectly correlated in the population and the personality variable were measured with good reliability, the largest correlation one would observe would be 0.63: one would have vastly underestimated the effect size, estimating that personality and the serum cytokine overlapped only by 40% rather than the true 100%. Of course, the variables of interest to PNI researchers are never perfectly correlated. In a more realistic metric, one could obtain a small effect size of $R^2 = 0.04$ due only to unreliability of the cytokine measurement when the true effect size was actually a medium effect size of $R^2 = 0.10$.

To underestimate modest (but important) effect sizes is to run the serious risk of concluding that these effects are negligible (and not statistically significant) when the true relationships in the population are actually quite noteworthy and meaningful. The result is that good theory, and important findings, could be discarded due to a failure to assess immunological variables reliably.

How Do You Know if There is a Problem with Your Physiometry?

We know full well that many variables of interest to PNI researchers vary as a function of stress, arousal, activity, pain, and many other factors. For such variables, there is no reason to assume that single assessments would prove reliable or stable; on the contrary, there is good reason to assume that would not be the case (cf. Stone, Broderick, & Kaell, 2010). Researchers who are studying variables known to fluctuate significantly in these ways have, by definition, a problem with their physiometry if they are relying on single assessments.

There are viable strategies for determining the extent of the problem. For example, to the degree that there are existing data sets that do include multiple assessments, researchers can use techniques such as generalizability theory to determine the amount of variance that lies at the level of interest (usually the person but also potentially other levels such as time point) and use the results in "decision studies" (Fletcher, Klimas, Morgan, & Gjerset, 1992; Segerstrom & Laudenslager, 2009; Segerstrom, Lubach, & Coe, 2006; Shavelson & Webb, 1991). Decision studies estimate the number of observations necessary to achieve a desired reliability and as such can be quite useful in planning future studies. Table 22.1 shows the results of the relatively few studies that have examined variability in immune parameters and, for most parameters, the amount of variance in a single assessment that was due to stable individual differences. These estimates are only available for functional and enumerative immune parameters (no such estimates have been given for cytokines, for example, despite their current popularity) and range from encouraging to alarming when planning a single measurement of that parameter.

Another approach adopted by Segerstrom, Lubach, and Coe (2006) was to conduct a series of prediction comparisons, in which they correlated immune parameters with other individual differences (rearing condition, handedness) using different numbers of immunological observations. In this example, which represents typical assessment of variables of interest to PNI researchers, the change in magnitude of effect and the resulting implications for theory and practice are striking. A "true" unstandardized beta weight between handedness and natural killer cell cytotoxicity (NKCC) and its 95% confidence interval were derived using a reliable (0.84) average of 13 measures of NKCC. One of the measures of NKCC per subject was then randomly sampled 1,000 times and used to obtain new beta weights. Reliability of the single sample was much lower (0.29); as a consequence, a quarter of the 1,000 obtained beta weights were outside the confidence interval for the "true" beta weight, illustrating the problematic results that can arise from the use of unreliable measures.

This approach illustrates empirically the magnitude of influence on a predictive relationship when the physiological variable is measured once, twice, or more often. It can also be illustrated theoretically by examining the inputs to the *standardized* beta weight, which is more commonly reported. If a single assessment is less reliable than multiple assessments, one will find that the standardized beta weight will be smaller in the single assessment case when reliability is at a minimum and increases as one includes more assessments. Consider that the standardized beta weight β is given by the product of the unstandardized beta weight and the ratio of the standard deviation of the predictor x and the standard deviation of the outcome variable y:

$$\beta = B*(SDx/SDy)$$

One can see that as SDy decreases, β will increase accordingly, and the easiest way to decrease SDy is to measure y more reliably. Another approach, which can be employed in the absence of existing data sets with multiple observations, is to conduct Monte Carlo studies. In a Monte Carlo study, one constructs a simulated data set, specifying the magnitude of the "true" effect in the simulated population and including multiple observations of the physiological variable; the multiple observations vary as a function of a standard deviation that is specified in advance. One can then compare a series of predictive equations, each using a measure of the physiological variable derived from a different number of observations. Because the true effect is known, it is a straightforward matter to determine how many observations one needs to estimate the population effect in an accurate, unbiased fashion. Overviews of Monte Carlo methods are provided by Mooney (1997) and Paxton, Curran, Bollen, Kirby, and Chen (2001).

These procedures, two using existing data and the other using simulated datasets, can provide guidance concerning how many observations are necessary to produce an assessment that is reliable enough to make it possible to identify the magnitude of associations among variables with reasonable accuracy. It is, of course, true that financial and other practical considerations often work against a multiple observation methodology, but researchers should be armed with the knowledge of the implications of using too few observations, so they can both make design decisions in an informed way and advocate effectively with funding agencies for the support necessary to do accurate science.

A closely related problem concerns tests of mediational hypotheses. For example, if one believes variation in an immune parameter mediates the relationship between a medical intervention and survival (e.g., Fawzy et al., 1993), one's ability to test that hypothesis depends heavily on the reliability of the assessment of the immune parameter. Statistical tests of mediation involve calculating the product of two beta weights: That between the putative independent variable and the mediator, and that between the mediator and the putative dependent variable (MacKinnon, Fairchild, & Fritz, 2007). Using the logic from the preceding, if the independent and dependent variables are both measured with reliability of 0.80, but the mediator is estimated with reliability of 0.50, each of the two beta weight values will significantly underestimate the true values in the population (i.e., the poor reliability of the mediating variable constrains the magnitude of the relationship between the independent variable and the mediator as well as that between the mediator and the dependent variable). The downward biasing property of the unreliable assessment of the immune parameter is effectively squared when these two relationships (predictor to mediator and mediator to outcome) are multiplied by each other to estimate the magnitude of the mediational pathway. Therefore, poor reliability in the mediator compromises researchers' ability to find mediational processes that actually do operate in the population. Because important models of PNI posit that immune parameters mediate between psychological factors or interventions and health (e.g., Kemeny, Cohen, Zegans, & Conant, 1989), it becomes imperative in testing such models that these parameters be measured reliably.

The error that comes from phasic changes that are not of interest can be characterized as "good" error, not because it can be easily addressed with meticulous research design (although it can), but because, with a change of focus, it can go from being error to being substantive variance. For example, one might be measuring salivary IgA daily in order to test whether there are personality correlates of this immune parameter (individual differences). In that case, it is important to aggregate across enough days to get a reliable measure of individual differences in IgA. However, if daily differences in stress or affect were also measured, it would be possible to link changes in these predictors to daily changes in IgA (Stone, Cox, Valdimarsdottir, Jandorf, & Neale, 1987; Stone, Neale, Cox, Napoli, Valdimarsdottir, & Kennedy-Moore, 1994). Likewise, daily variation in fatigue correlates with daily change in diurnal cortisol slope, turning day-to-day "error" into substantive variance (Adam, Hawkley, Kudielka, & Cacioppo, 2006; Sephton & Segerstrom, 2011; see also Smyth, Ockenfels, Porter, Kirschbaum, Hellhammer, & Stone, 1998).

The Bad
What is Bad Error?

It is the nature of much PNI research to test multiple dependent variables. For example, we may wish to characterize the balance between Th1 and Th2 cytokines by assessing interleukin (IL)-2, interferon-γ, IL-4, and IL-10. In some cases, multiple dependent variables may be reduced to a composite for analysis (e.g., a ratio between pro-inflammatory and anti-inflammatory variables; a mean of delayed-type hypersensitivity responses to different antigens). In other cases, dependent variables are analyzed separately.

The ubiquity of this multivariate approach is illustrated using data from a meta-analysis of stress and immunity in humans (Segerstrom & Miller, 2004). In the process of this meta-analysis, effect sizes were extracted from 332 studies published from 1960 through 2001. The illustration has to do with the number of effect sizes reported per study as well as the ratio of number of subjects to number of effect sizes. The modal study reported only one

effect size (26%), but the median number of effect sizes was 4, and there was a large range of 1 to 38. There was a small secular trend for the number of effect sizes reported to increase over time ($r = .13$, $p < .05$).

The error associated with the performance of many statistical tests, of course, is Type I error: the likelihood that a particular effect was statistically significant by chance. The amount of Type I error associated with a particular study is additive across the number of tests performed. In the absence of correction for Type I error, then, 15% of the studies of stress and immunity had a 50% or better chance of reporting an effect as statistically significant when it was actually obtained by chance because they reported 10 or more effect sizes.

Were these studies published in obscure journals in which a Type I error would be unlikely to affect the progress of the field? No. Many of them were published in the top journals for this kind of work, including *Psychosomatic Medicine*; *Brain, Behavior, and Immunity;* and *Biological Psychiatry*.

Most important, did these studies correct for Type I error? A random sample of 10 of the 54 studies contributing 10 or more effect sizes showed that only 1 made a partial correction for Type I error. Two others acknowledged that Type I error was a potential problem but made no correction in the statistical analysis. In other studies, this failure may have slipped by editors and reviewers because they were not aware of the number of tests being performed on the same sample: One-third of the studies with the largest number of reported effect sizes (10 or more) *split* these reports among two or more publications.

Another way of looking at these data is to compare the number of effect sizes reported to the number of subjects. Ideally, there should be a positive correlation between the number of effects reported and the number of subjects, because each additional test not only compounds the risk of Type I error, but also Type II error. Imagine that a study is adequately powered to detect a medium effect size ($r = 0.30$) with power of 0.80 and tests three correlations (e.g., between stress and three different cytokines, understood to be independent of each other), each of which correlations actually has a population value of 0.30. The odds that the study will miss one of these correlations is 0.60 (Type II error = 1—power = 0.20 * 3 tests = 0.60). If the three correlations were not independent of each other, the risk of Type II error would increase further. Therefore, with an increasing number of tests, an increasing number of subjects is needed to protect against Type II error.

Unfortunately, in the stress and immunity literature reviewed by Segerstrom and Miller (2004), there is a *negative* correlation between number of tests and number of subjects ($r = -0.30$, $p < 0.001$). The largest Ns per effect size were to be found in studies that reported only one effect size. The range of Ns per effect size in those studies was 4–618, with a respectable median of 41. This sample size would have power of 0.80 to detect a single effect with a magnitude of $r = 0.37$.

In studies that reported multiple effect sizes, the situation gets worse. The range of Ns per effect size in these studies was 0.4–308, with a median of only 7. The correlation between number of effects and number of subjects per effect reported was still negative ($r = -.19$, $p < .003$), a large proportion of all studies (30%) had fewer than 5 subjects per effect reported, and seven studies actually had fewer subjects than effects. These seven studies were mostly published in top journals.

What Should be Done?

Rosenthal and DiMatteo (2001) offered this simple, "prose" equation:

$$\text{Significance Test} = \text{Effect Size} \times \text{Sample Size}$$

This equation serves as a reminder that statistical significance is only partly a function of the magnitude of an effect in a sample; it is also very much a function of the size of the sample. Thus, as noted in the Segerstrom and Miller (2004) meta-analysis, the many studies that have a high ratio of effects tested to study participants run the risk of committing Type II error, possibly depriving researchers and practitioners of knowledge of important effects. It is simply inappropriate to confuse statistical significance with magnitude of an effect in a sample or population. One important strategy for PNI researchers is to be aware of this problem and, when conducting research, conduct an appropriate number of tests for the sample size, and, when consuming research, modify conclusions they draw from either the absence or presence of statistical significance in light of the number of effects tested, whether there is a correction for Type I error, and the ratio of effects reported to study participants.

One very useful technique for mitigating the effects of this problem on the field is meta-analysis. One of the important advantages to meta-analysis is its focus on effect size, rather than statistical significance. Meta-analysis can help researchers rely less on the statistical significance or the absence of statistical significance of any one finding and, instead, focus on patterns of effect-size magnitude across studies. As researchers combine both significant and nonsignificant effects using meta-analysis, the pattern and magnitude of effects becomes clearer. Using meta-analytic aggregation techniques, researchers are less vulnerable to the operation of both Type I and Type II error in individual studies.

Of course, researchers should be mindful of the nature of risks for Type I and Type II error as they design individual studies. If one wants to draw inferences about multiple effects in a single study, one should do everything possible to have a sample size large enough to avoid misleading the field by reporting nonsignificant results that could easily be Type II error. When it is necessary to conduct multiple tests within a single study, and those tests are not independent, researchers should note that is the case, so readers can appropriately temper their conclusions. Similarly, when researchers report results from the same sample in multiple papers, they should make readers aware that they have done so, again so readers can draw more accurate conclusions.

The ugly
What is "ugly" error?

There is another error that is simply irredeemable. This "ugly" error arises from sheer noise that occurs in the process of doing research. For example, Segerstrom and Sephton (2010) assessed the delayed-type hypersensitivity response, using a skin-test antigen derived from either mumps or candida, in first year law students, for five consecutive years. The change in antigen was necessary because manufacture of the mumps antigen was discontinued after the first two years of the study. In addition, because the antigen had short expiration dates, multiple batches of each antigen had to be used. There was nothing to be done about error variance related to antigen type and batch. Good design could address only where this variance would lie. The same antigen batch was used for the same person throughout each year, so each person always received the same antigen and batch, although people in different years received different antigens and batches. Surprisingly, batches within the "same" antigen accounted for more variance than "different" antigens. Figure 22.1 shows the mean induration associated with the various antigens in this study. It is important to note that this kind of error is true of both in vivo and in vitro assays. When labs have kept track of variance related to antigen or

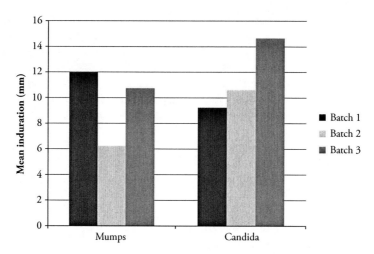

Figure 22.1 Mean induration in a DTH skin test resulting from the use of three different batches of two antigens (Segerstrom & Sephton, 2010). There was a significant effect of batch ($p < 0.0001$), but not antigen type.

reagent batch, this variance has at times been very large (Kiecolt-Glaser & Glaser, 1995).

What Should be Done?

One appropriate step is to attempt to isolate this "ugly" variance from the variance of interest. In a simple, cross-sectional study of differences among people, one should attempt to use the same supplies for all the participants. In longitudinal studies, in which freezing does not seriously compromise the results of assays, it would be ideal to freeze samples and assay them all together using the same supplies. This may not always be possible. In that case, one should try to isolate the effect of interest (differences between people or changes within people) from the error variance by using the same supplies within the appropriate effect. Where between-person differences are of most interest, the same supplies should be used across people; where within-person differences are of most interest, the same supplies should be used within people.

Even this may not be possible. In that case, the remaining strategy is statistical control via analysis of covariance or regression. In fact, the analysis of covariance is most appropriately used for this kind of situation. When a variable contributes to "noise" in the dependent variable but is unrelated to other pieces of the model (experimental groups or predictors), then it can and should be used as a covariate in regression or ANCOVA (Miller & Chapman, 2001)

What Should not be Done?

Covariates, therefore, are best conceptualized as "ugly" error with no redeeming or substantive

value. However, other kinds of variance have been relegated to this category, mostly in the interest of determining whether the predictor of interest is related to the outcome above and beyond the covariate. Unfortunately, covariates can create as many interpretational problems as they solve. Numerous articles have pointed out that "ANCOVA remains a widely misused approach to dealing with substantive group differences on potential covariates" (Miller & Chapman, p. 40), "it is essential to remember that 'statistical control' is nothing more than a highly fallible process" (Christenfeld, Sloan, Carroll, & Greenland, 2004, p. 874), and the overuse of covariates constitutes "threats to psychoneuroimmunology research" (Segerstrom, 2009, p. 885). These threats can be grouped into three broad categories: undercontrol, overcontrol, and perilous partialling.

UNDERCONTROL

There are two types of undercontrol in the use of covariates. In the first, researchers covary out the effects of one or more variables, but they do not actually include those covariates that have the strongest relationship with the dependent variable. This can occur because theory has not yet identified the most important covariates, or simply because the most important covariates were not included in the data set. The second type of undercontrol concerns the reliability of the covariate. Often, less attention is paid to the psychometric properties of covariates than to the properties of target variables (Christenfeld et al., 2004; Zinbarg et al., 2010), even though the magnitude of target variable correlations with covariates plays a key role in any analysis of covariation. As is true of other elements of the model, if the covariate is not measured reliably, it is likely that important true variance associated with the covariate is not removed statistically (because it was not represented in the measure of the covariate): the statistical control will be more apparent than real.

OVERCONTROL

Researchers sometimes use variables as covariates that should actually play an important role in the substantive model (Christenfeld et al., 2004; Meehl, 1971; Segerstrom, 2009). For example, in an attempt to specify a relationship between an individual difference variable and an immune parameter, researchers sometimes covary out age, so they can describe the relationship independent of age. As appealing as this may seem, it may often be the case that theory will be advanced by considering a variable like age as a potential predictor or moderator. If one simply covaries out the influence of age, one will not know whether the relationship between the individual difference variable and the immune parameter is different at different ages. In a similar way, variables that are sometimes handled as covariates might profitably be considered as potential mediators or moderators, or even as potential antecedents to, or consequences of, both variables of interest.

PERILOUS PARTIALLING

Lynam, Hoyle, and Newman (2006) provided a very useful analysis of the process of partialling out variance from one variable in evaluating the relationship between two other variables (as in analysis of covariance). As they note, partialling out, or "covarying out" the influence of one set of variables makes it possible to determine whether an independent variable of interest is related to a dependent variable above and beyond the influence of other variables not of interest to the researcher. The capacity to use multiple regression and ANCOVA to covary out variables makes it possible to test interesting and rigorous hypotheses.

There is, however, an underappreciated but crucial consideration with respect to partialling (Lynam et al., 2006): It is difficult to know what construct is represented by an independent variable once the variance it shares with other variables is removed. That is, there is a core, substantive problem: What is the meaning of that part of the independent variable that is left, once those parts of the variable that overlap with other variables have been removed

(Miller & Chapman, 2001)? It is often the case that, after covarying out "nuisance variables," or variables not of central interest, researchers draw conclusions about the original, "whole" independent variable, even though their analyses applied only to a residual variable (Lynam et al., 2006).

Suppose one studies the relationship between neuroticism and NKCC and wants to draw conclusions about that relationship independent of age. The typical way to do so is to covary out that variance in neuroticism that is associated with age, and then report that neuroticism has such-and-such a relationship with NKCC, holding age constant. But in fact, using this method, one has actually examined the relationship between NKCC and that part of neuroticism that is unrelated to age. One has studied a residual variable, not "whole" neuroticism. The difficulty is that there is not an existing body of theory and empirical evidence describing the meaning of the construct "neuroticism unrelated to age." There are two aspects to this difficulty. The first is that researchers do not always appreciate that their findings pertain to a residual variable, not the target variable of interest, and inappropriately draw conclusions about the original, target variable. The second is that researchers typically do not know the substantive meaning of variation among people in the residual variable: for example, the substantive meaning of that part of neuroticism unrelated to age. Personality is understood to develop from the combination of genetic disposition and experience. Different ages reflect different levels and types of experience that influence personality trait domains and contribute to developmental change in traits such as neuroticism across the lifespan (Roberts, Walton, & Viechtbauer, 2006): What is neuroticism independent of these influences?

Often, the distinction between the "whole" variable and the residual variable matters a great deal. Suppose the independent variable and the covariate are correlated $r = 0.50$. When the covariate is partialled out, 25% of the variance of the independent variable is removed. Often, covariates correlate even more highly with independent variables, resulting, of course, in even more dramatic changes from the original, "whole" variable to the residual variable: When the correlation is $r = 0.70$, virtually half of the variance (49%) in the independent variable is removed through partialling. To add to the difficulty, it is, of course, the case that the variance removed is, by definition, part of the reliable variance of the independent variable (the nonreliable variance is random and so could not correlate with a covariate). One can consider the variance of the independent variable as having three components: reliable variance shared with the covariate, reliable variance independent of the covariate, and random error variance. After partialling, one is left with only some of the original, reliable variance and all of the error variance. Thus, the ratio between "true score" and "noise" is changed, and not for the better. The residual variable is less reliable than the original, "whole" variable. In examples provided by Lynam et al., (2006), beginning with an independent variable with reliability = 0.80, partialling out a covariate correlated 0.50 reduces the reliability of the residual to 0.73, and partialling out a covariate correlated 0.75 reduced the reliability of the residual to 0.54.

An additional, related difficulty is that different researchers covary out different sets of variables from an independent variable. It is often not appreciated that, to the degree this is true, each study is actually investigating a different residual variable. Thus, not only are the problems described earlier present, but those problems are manifest differently in different studies. O'Connor et al. (2009) recommend the following covariates in analysis of proinflammatory markers based on the strength and reliability of the relationships between them and inflammation in the literature: age, sex, socioeconomic status, ethnic and racial differences, body mass index (BMI), alcohol use, sleep quality, sleep habits, and use of four medications (aspirin, statins, antihypertensives, and SSRIs). A study that covariates out some, but not all, of these variables is actually investigating a different variable from one that is studied when all of O'Connor et al.'s (2009) recommendations are followed, from one that is studied without including any such covariates, and from one that is studied using a different subset.

What, then, should researchers do? We recommend the following. First, be judicious in the inclusion of covariates; select covariates because they are a considerable source of "nuisance" variance and are likely to be treated the same way by other researchers. Overuse of idiosyncratic or trivial covariates creates a literature in which it is difficult to compare what is ostensibly the same variable across studies. Second, consider carefully whether a prospective covariate really is a "nuisance" variable or does, in fact, represent an important, substantive source of variance. If the latter is the case, then consider research and analytic designs that recognize the role of the covariate. Moderation and mediation designs are two possibilities. Third, be both clear and careful about interpreting effects when covariates are included, so that readers do not mistakenly

conclude that a given effect applies to the original, "whole" independent variable of interest. Fourth, when appropriate, report results both with and without covariates, thus providing readers with a more complete picture. Fifth, consider the reliability with which prospective covariates are measured, and exclude variables that are not measured reliably. Sixth, consider carefully the implications for the reliability of model tests if covariates are used, particularly when prospective covariates are highly related to the independent variable. Seventh, exercise care in comparing results from different studies that used different covariates.

Future Directions

1. We hope to see the development of the field of physiometrics in the coming years. This will require that the single sample assessment methodology play a lesser and lesser role until the adequacy of such methodology can be assessed for the various parameters that PNI researchers employ. In the meantime, researchers should plan multiple assessments, with the exact number based on the best available data, and compute the physiometrics of these assessments to inform future research design. Archival data can also be mined to answer these questions (Segerstrom et al., 2006; Segerstrom & Laudenslager, 2009).

2. Most of the physiometric analyses that have been performed have been focused on how one assesses reliable differences between individuals (e.g., "person" or "trait" variance). However, new methods for assessing the reliability of measures to capture change over time have been proposed (Cranford et al., 2006). A measure that can reliably capture the difference between *Person* A and *Person* B may not reliably capture the difference between *Time* A and *Time* B. If one wishes to capture reliable change over time (e.g., in an intervention or longitudinal study), this kind of reliability needs to be assessed as well.

3. Likewise, increased accessibility of statistical analyses that can account for variance at different levels (e.g., multilevel models, hierarchical linear modeling) provide the opportunity to predict good "error" variance. If researchers not only take multiple immunological measurements (enough to reliably measure individual differences) but also include multiple assessments of the psychological constructs of interest, it is possible to not only reveal differences *between* people in PNI relationships, but also changes *within* people.

References

Adam, E. K., Hawkley, L. C., Kudielka, B. M., & Cacioppo, J. T. (2006). Day-to-day dynamics of experience-cortisol associations in a population-based sample of older adults. *PNAS, 103*, 17058–17063.

Cava, F., González, C., Pascual, M. J., Navajo, J. A., & González-Buitrago, J. M. (2000). Biological variation of interleukin 6 (IL-6) and soluble interleukin 2 receptor (sIL2R) in serum of healthy individuals. *Cytokine, 12*, 1423–1425.

Christenfeld, N. J. S., Sloan, R. P., Carroll, D., & Greenland, S. (2004). Risk factors, confounding, and the illusion of statistical control. *Psychosomatic Medicine, 66*, 868–875.

Cranford, J. A., Shrout, P. E., Iida, M., Rafaeli, E., Yip, T., & Bolger, N. (2006). A procedure for evaluating sensitivity to within-person change: Can mood measures in diary studies detect change reliably? *Personality and Social Psychology Bulletin, 32*, 917–929.

Fawzy, F. I., Fawzy, N. W., Hyun, C. S., Elashoff, R., Guthrie, D., Fahey, J.L.et al. (1993). Malignant melanoma: Effects of an early structured psychiatric intervention, coping, and affective state on recurrence and survival 6 years later. *Archives of General Psychiatry, 50*, 681–689.

Fletcher, M. A., Klimas, N. G., Morgan, R., & Gjerset, G. (1992). Lymphocyte proliferation. In N. R. Rose, E. Conway de Macario, J. L. Fahey, H. Friedman, & G. M. Penn (Eds.), *Manual of clinical laboratory immunology (3rd ed.*, pp. 213–219). Washington, DC: American Society for Microbiology.

Hamer, M., Gibson, E. L., Vuononvirta, R., Williams, E., & Steptoe, A. (2006). Inflammatory and hemostatic responses to repeated mental stress: Individual stability and habituation over time. *Brain, Behavior, and Immunity, 20*, 456–459.

Kemeny, M. E., Cohen, F., Zegans, L. S., & Conant, M. A. (1989). Psychological and immunological predictors of genital herpes recurrence. *Psychosomatic Medicine, 51*, 195–208.

Kiecolt-Glaser, J. K., & Glaser, R. (1995). Measurement of immune response. In S. Cohen, R. C. Kessler, & L. U. Gordon (Eds.), *Measuring stress: A guide for health and social scientists* (pp. 213–229). New York: Oxford University Press.

Kraemer, H. C., Giese-Davis, J., Yutsis, M., Neri, E., Gallagher-Thompson, D., Taylor, C. B., et al. (2006). Design decisions to optimize reliability of daytime cortisol slopes in an older population. *American Journal of Geriatric Psychiatry, 14*, 325–333.

Lynam, D. R., Hoyle, R. H., & Newman, J. P. (2006). The perils of partialling: Cautionary tales from aggression and psychopathy. *Assessment, 13*, 328–341.

MacKinnon, D. P., Fairchild, A. J., & Fritz, M. S. (2007). Mediation analysis. *Annual Review of Psychology, 58*, 593–614.

Meehl, P. E. (1971). High school yearbooks: A reply to Schwarz. *Journal of Abnormal Psychology, 77*, 143–148.

Miller, G. A., & Chapman, J. P. (2001). Misunderstanding analysis of covariance. *Journal of Abnormal Psychology, 100*, 40–48.

Mooney, C. Z. (1997). *Monte Carlo simulation.* Thousand Oaks, CA: Sage.

Nunnally, J. C., & Bernstein, I. H. (1994). *Psychometric Theory.* New York, NY: McGraw-Hill.

O'Connor, M. F., Bower, J. E., Cho, H. J., Creswell, J. D., Dimitrov, S.,… Irwin, M. R. (2009). To assess, to control, to exclude: Effects of biobehavioral factors on circulating inflammatory markers. *Brain, Behavior, and Immunity, 23*, 887–897.

Paxton, P., Curran, P. J., Bollen, K. A., Kirby, J., & Chen, F. (2001). Monte Carlo experiments: Design and implementation. *Structural Equation Modeling, 8*, 287–312.

Rao, K. M. K., Pieper, C. S., Currie, M. S., & Cohen, H. J. (1994). Variability of plasma IL-6 and crosslinked fibrin dimers over time in community dwelling elderly subjects. *Coagulation and Transfusion Medicine, 102*, 802–805.

Roberts, B. W., Walton, K. E., & Viechtbauer, W. (2006). Patterns of mean-level change in personality traits across the life course: A meta-analysis of longitudinal studies. *Psychological Bulletin, 132*, 1–25.

Rosenthal, R., & DiMatteo, M. R. (2001). Meta-analysis: Recent developments in quantitative methods for literature reviews. *Annual Review of Psychology, 52*, 59–82.

Schedlowski, M., Hosch, W., Oberbeck, R., Benschop, R. J., Jacobs, R., Raab, H. R., & Schmidt, R. E. (1996). Catecholamines modulate human NK cell circulation and function via spleen-independent β2-adrenergic mechanisms. *Journal of Immunology, 156*, 93–99.

Segerstrom, S. C. (2009). Biobehavioral controls: Threats to psychoneuroimmunology research? *Brain, Behavior, and Immunity, 23*, 885–886.

Segerstrom, S. C., & Laudenslager, M. L. (2009). When is enough, enough? Generalizability of primate immunity over time. *Brain, Behavior, and Immunity, 23*, 986–992.

Segerstrom, S. C., Lubach, G. R., & Coe, C. L. (2006). Identifying immune traits and biobehavioral correlates: Generalizability and reliability of immune responses in rhesus macaques. *Brain, Behavior, and Immunity, 20*, 349–358.

Segerstrom, S. C., & Miller, G. E. (2004). Psychological stress and the human immune system: A meta-analytic study of 30 years of inquiry. *Psychological Bulletin, 130*, 601–630.

Segerstrom, S. C., & Sephton, S. E. (2010). Optimistic expectancies and cell-mediated immunity: The role of positive affect. *Psychological Science, 21*, 448–455.

Sephton, S. E., & Segerstrom, S. C. (2011). *Reliability and generalizability of diurnal cortisol parameters.* Manuscript in preparation.

Shavelson, R. J., & Webb, N. M. (1991). *Generalizability theory: A primer.* Newbury Park, CA: Sage.

Smyth, J., Ockenfels, M. C., Porter, L., Kirschbaum, Hellhammer, D. H., & Stone, A. A. (1998). Stressors and mood measured on a momentary basis are associated with salivary cortisol secretion. *Psychoneuroendocrinology, 23*, 353–370.

Stewart, J., & Seeman, T. (2000). Salivary cortisol measurement. *MacArthur Research Network on SES and Health.* Retrieved May 13, 2011, from http://www.macses.ucsf.edu/research/allostatic/salivarycort.php

Stone, A. A., Broderick, J. E., & Kaell, A. (2010). Single momentary assessments are not reliable outcomes for clinical trials. *Contemporary Clinical Trials, 31*, 466–472.

Stone, A. A., Cox, D. S., Valdimarsdottir, H., Jandorf, L., & Neale, J. M. (1987). Evidence that secretory IgA antibody is associated with daily mood. *Journal of Personality and Social Psychology, 52*, 988–993.

Stone, A. A., Neale, J.M., Cox, D. S., Napoli, A., Valdimarsdottir, H., & Kennedy-Moore, E. (1994). Daily events are associated with a secretory immune response to an oral antigen in men. *Health Psychology, 13*, 440–446.

Van Cauter, E., Leproult, R., & Kupfer, D. J. (1996). Effects of gender and age on the levels and circadian rhythmicity of plasma cortisol. *Journal of Clinical Endocrinology and Metabolism, 81*, 2468–2473.

Van Rood, Y., Goulmy, E., Blokland, E., Pool, J., Van Rood, J., & Van Houwelingen, H. (1991). Month-related variability in immunological test results; implications for immunological follow-up studies. *Clinical and Experimental Immunology, 86*, 349–354.

Vgontzas, A. N., Bixler, E. O., Lin, H. M., Prolo, P., Trakada, G., & Chrousos, G. P. (2005). IL-6 and its circadian secretion in humans. *Neuroimmunomodulation, 12*, 131–140.

Zinbarg, R. E., Suzuki, S., Uliszek, A. A., & Lewis, A. R. (2010). Biased parameter estimates and inflated type I error rates in analysis of covariance (and analysis of partial variance) arising from unreliability: Alternatives and remedial strategies. *Journal of Abnormal Psychology, 119*, 307–319.

PART 7

Conclusion

Looking into the Future: Conclusion to the Oxford Handbook of Psychoneuroimmunology

Suzanne C. Segerstrom

Abstract

All authors in this volume forecast the most important work to be done in their areas, and synthesizing these forecasts reveals some old and new themes for the future of psychoneuroimmunology research. The desire to understand mechanisms of PNI relationships is a long-standing one, but new methods will advance progress toward satisfaction of this desire. The desire to understand causality and to effect meaningful clinical change underlies the calls for intervention research. This research will be advanced when more kinds of intervention become available. Good, longitudinal methodology and large samples will be required to demonstrate that immune changes mediate between psychological factors and health. Finally, forward-looking research will be examining how the many intraindividual, interpersonal, social, and developmental factors influencing immunity interact with each other.

Key Words: psychoneuroimmunology, mechanisms, behavior, interventions, causality, clinical significance, development

It is an interesting exercise to read all the final sections of the chapters in this volume, in which the authors forecast the most important work to be done in their areas. This look forward reveals some perennial questions and goals of psychoneuroimmunology (PNI) and also some new ways of addressing the complexity of psychological influences on immunity.

Everything Old is New Again

Three themes emerge that have long been of interest in PNI research. First, almost every chapter mentions mechanisms as a direction for future research and locates these mechanisms at every stage in the pathway from the brain to the immune system and vice versa. For example, what immune parameters most strongly influence health outcomes? What brain regions are active when it is modulating the immune system, and what brain regions are active

when it is being modulated by the immune system? Are there common pathways from specific psychological states to immunological change, or is there specificity in the way that states influence immunity? What is happening at the molecular level in immune cells when they are signaled by the brain?

The answers to some of these questions can be answered better now than ever due to advances in neuroscience and molecular biology. The hardware available to scan the brain and the expertise and software to extract meaningful data are improving all the time. One critique of scanning approaches is that they can be atheoretical and capitalize on chance findings in small samples (Vul, Harris, Winkielman, & Pashler, 2009). Fortunately, PNI approaches are increasingly theoretically driven, and these theories often point to brain regions of interest (ROI). With a priori hypotheses about how neural activity in these ROI mediates between psychological states and immunological outcomes (and vice versa), theoretically and methodologically sound studies based on PNI hypotheses can and will continue to be designed. Likewise, molecular biology offers a closer look at the cellular level of PNI by using genomic and proteomic approaches. PNI has a long history of examining (e.g., through pharmacological approaches) the gateways to the cell: receptors. Now we can look inside the cell to see the consequences of those signals.

Another new look at mechanisms has to do with behavior. Health behavior has had a limited role in much of PNI research, except where it was the explicit focus (e.g., exercise intervention trials; Kohut et al., 2004). In nonhuman animal research, health behaviors such as diet are controlled by the experimenter. In human research, health behaviors, when not the explicit focus of the study, have often been relegated to the list of covariates and controlled for as if they contributed only noise variance. In contrast, many of the present chapters bring health behavior back into the spotlight. As Smith and I note in chapter 22, covariates should be related to the outcome or dependent variable but not the predictor, thereby reducing extraneous variance in the outcome variable while not interfering with the predictive power of the predictor. Many health behaviors, however, are related to predictors of interest, such as personality, depression, social relationships, and social status, and, as such, they should have a substantive role in understanding how these factors are related to immunity. Several chapters call for the examination of health behaviors as mediators and moderators in PNI models.

The second theme that has a long history in PNI is the desire to use interventions to either improve causal inference or improve health. The importance of interventions and particularly randomized clinical trials for health research can be traced, at least in part, back to Sir Austin Bradford Hill (Hill, 1965). Hill, an epidemiologist, laid out several criteria for making causal inference regarding relationships between the environment and disease. Hill wrote,

> ...with the aims of occupational, and almost synonymous preventive, medicine in mind the decisive question is where the frequency of the undesirable event B will be influenced by a change in the environmental feature A. *How* such a change exerts that influence may call for a great deal of research, However, before deducing "causation" and taking action we shall not invariably have to

sit around awaiting the results of the research. The whole chain may have to be unraveled or a few links may suffice. It will depend upon circumstances. (p. 295)

Of Hill's pieces of evidence that imply causation, one could argue that PNI has generated evidence for *strength* of association and its *plausibility*, as well as *gradient*, that is, continuous or dose-response relationships, and meta-analyses are providing evidence for the *consistency* of these effects. A future direction already mentioned is *specificity* in PNI relationships. The desire to see more intervention research in PNI addresses two more: *temporality* and *experiment*.

Temporality, as Hill put it, asks "which is the cart and which is the horse?" (p. 297). Importantly, this question cannot be answered with cross-sectional research. Cross-sectional research informs all the other pieces mentioned earlier: strength, plausibility, gradient, consistency, and specificity. All those pieces being established, however, only longitudinal and experimental research can establish whether psychosocial factors or behavior *precede* their immunological correlates. An illustrative example is the relationship between depression and immunity. Early, cross-sectional investigations showed that there was a substantial, gradiated, consistent relationship between depression and immunity, and the causal conclusion was that depression suppressed immunity (Herbert & Cohen, 1993). However, later it has come to be understood that changes in immunity, particularly inflammation, can also affect levels of depression.

This understanding came in part from a natural *experiment* in which the level of inflammatory activity is manipulated in a treatment context (Raison, Capuron, & Miller, 2006). This research is just one example of the understanding that experimental manipulation can provide. Behaviors such as physical activity can be manipulated directly and their effects measured in terms of both manipulation checks (e.g., increases in cardiovascular fitness or strength) and immunological consequences. However, when it comes to psychological states, we must rely on manipulations with varying amounts of ecological validity that are intended to change internal states (e.g., shame, stress, support), but we cannot manipulate those states directly. Nonetheless, such interventions—whether they are short-term attempts to manipulate affect, such as film clips, or long-term attempts to manipulate coping patterns—provide an important piece of evidence for causality.

One problem to be overcome is the paucity of validated interventions for changing the psychological constructs that PNI researchers are interested in. For example, in my experience, findings that the personality trait of optimism can have healthy consequences (e.g., Kim, Park, & Peterson, 2011) often lead to a flurry of questions from the press about how to become more optimistic. The fact is, although we know something about the correlates of optimism's natural change (e.g., Segerstrom, 2007), there is almost nothing in the literature that would indicate a valid or reliable method for changing optimism intentionally. (Also in my experience, this is not a very satisfactory answer if you are a reporter.) In general, where the P in PNI is recognized as a clinical problem (e.g., psychopathology or marital conflict), effective and valid interventions have been developed, but where it is not so recognized (e.g., well-being or marital satisfaction), interventions cannot be applied to PNI questions until they have been better developed and validated. One then needs to address the question of tailoring the intervention to the population of interest and its unique needs, interests, and abilities (Antoni, chapter 21, this volume).

Finally, it is obvious that PNI researchers are still working to fulfill the promise of establishing the clinical significance of their work. This work is taking the form of increased focus on diseases and developmental stages in which the immune system is involved or vulnerable, respectively. As Coussons-Read (chapter 1, this volume) notes, it is important to establish the magnitude of change or difference in the immune system necessary to result in clinical outcomes. One challenge in this work is that studies that link immune parameters to morbidity and mortality are often epidemiological studies that report small effect sizes. These effects, in addition to being clinically significant (and see Rosenthal & Rubin, 1982, for a nice demonstration of the potential importance of small effect sizes), are statistically significant in the large samples characteristic of these studies. However, much PNI research is based on smaller sample sizes, which make it more difficult to reliably replicate such findings. Furthermore, the mediational test in which psychological or behavioral factors lead to immunologic differences, which lead to disease outcomes, is power-hungry and particularly prone to being missed in small-sample research. Of course, the long-term public health significance of PNI research relies on making continual progress toward the goal of demonstrating its relevance for disease.

Future Directions, Future Dimensions

Figure 23.1 is an attempt to distill some of the emerging complexity in how psychological influences on the immune system are conceptualized, particularly with regard to three dimensions that revisit themes in the Introduction: development, level of analysis, and finally positive versus negative content. The figure shows development over time, from the prenatal period to old age, and the embedding of the individual in close individual

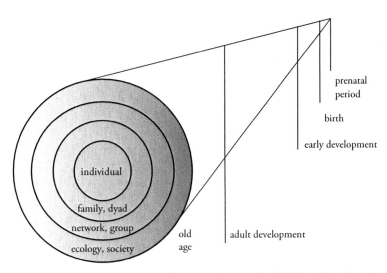

Figure 23.1 Levels of analysis in PNI: Development (conical projection), context (embedded circles), and positive or negative valence (shading)

relationships, such as those with parents, romantic partners, and family; these relationships exist within larger social groups such as networks; and the individual, his or her relationships, and his or her social network exist in a larger ecological and societal context. In addition, within each of these levels and across development, it is important to recognize that there are positive, functional, adaptive qualities as well as negative, dysfunctional, maladaptive qualities, represented by the shading of the circles. For example, an individual can by happy or hostile; a dyad can be securely attached or conflicted; a social network can provide support or criticism; and a society can afford opportunity or oppression.

The future directions identified by the chapters in this volume point to the importance of interactions within and among these levels. The objective then moves from identifying those who are vulnerable due to a single "hit" to biobehavioral health, for example, from stress, to identifying those combinations of "hits" that confer the greatest vulnerability. These combinations can occur within a level. In fact, several recent reports indicate that the relationship of low psychosocial well-being or high ill-being to high basal pro-inflammatory cytokines such as IL-6 is strongest when combined with other individual factors, including older age, lack of physical activity, poor sleep, and low education (Friedman et al., 2005; Morozink, Friedman, Coe, & Ryff, 2010; Morris et al., 2011; Rethorst, Moynihan, Lyness, Heffner, & Chapman, 2011; Steptoe, O'Donnell, Badrick, Kumari, & Marmot, 2008). As noted in the earlier discussion of mechanisms, these factors have often been treated as covariates or noise, but these tests of interactions are also bringing health behavior back into the substantive model. Interactions can also occur across dimensions, as noted in several of the chapters. Do self-conscious emotions depend on the social group context (Dickerson, chapter 5, this volume)? Does the fit between a nonhuman animal's personality and its ecology determine its immunocompetence (Adamo, chapter 15, Michael and Cavigelli chapter 8, this volume)? The way that "hits" interact may account for the effectiveness of multimodel therapies such as cognitive behavioral stress management (Antoni, chapter 21, this volume). Because risks may be synergistic, a synergistic approach to intervention may not be effective when dismantled.

Finally, the temporal dimension depicted in the figure represents macro influences of change and development. Those influences might in turn affect how the levels—alone and in combination—interact

with the immune system. At this macro level, developmental stage can itself act as a factor that affects the influence of stress or psychological health. It can also indicate the presence of a critical period, in which PNI relationships set the stage for later resilience or vulnerability. Not shown in the figure but also of importance are micro influences of change. Weil and Nelson (chapter 16, this volume) review the effects of seasonal variation on immunity, and this is another source of immunological change within development. Ram and Gerstorf (2009) provide a useful taxonomy of change in which *intraindividual variability* is "conceptualized as fluctuations, inconsistency, instability, oscillations, or "noise" that manifests on microtime scales (e.g., minutes, hours, days, weeks)" and is embedded in *intraindividual change*, which is "directional changes resulting from long-term processes such as development, maturation, aging or senescence that manifest on a macrotime scale" (p. 779). Studying change over time not only allows for tests of how time affects the immune system per se (e.g., senescence or seasonal change) and how psychosocial factors' effects on the immune system may depend on time, but with appropriate design, can help establish *temporality* (see earlier) in PNI relationships.

The research represented in this volume samples from the best and most sophisticated applications of psychology to PNI, whether those applications arise from affective science, development, behavioral neuroscience, or clinical psychology. In both the old and new directions in PNI, this kind of work shall continue to make a significant impact on the field.

References

Friedman, E. M., Hayney, M. S., Love, G. D., Urry, H. L., Rosenkranz, M. A., Davidson, et al. (2005). Social relationships, sleep quality, and interleukin-6 in aging women. *Proceedings of the National Academy of Sciences, 102,* 18757–18762.

Herbert, T. B., & Cohen, S. (1993). Depression and immunity: A meta-analytic review. *Psychological Bulletin, 113,* 472–486.

Hill, A. B. (1965). The environment and disease: Association or causation? *Proceedings of the Royal Society of Medicine, 58,* 295–300.

Kim, E. S., Park, N., & Peterson, C. (2011). Dispositional optimism protects older adults from stroke: The Health and Retirement Study. *Stroke.* Published online before print, July 21, 2011. doi: 10.1161/STROKEAHA.111.613448

Kohut, M. L., Arntson, B. A., Lee, W., Rozeboom, K., Yoon, K. J., Cunnick, J. E., et al.. (2004). Moderate exercise improves antibody response to influenza vaccination in older adults. *Vaccine, 22,* 2298–2306.

Morozink, J. A., Friedman, E. M., Coe, C. L., & Ryff, C. D. (2010). Socioeconomic and psychosocial predictors of interleukin-6 in the MIDUS national sample. *Health Psychology, 29*, 626–635.

Morris, A. A., Zhao, L., Ahmed, Y., Stoyanova, N., De Staercke, C., Hooper, W. C., et al. (2011). Association between depression and inflammation—differences by race and sex: The META-Health Study. *Psychosomatic Medicine, 73*, 462–468.

Raison, C. L., Capuron, L., & Miller, A. H. (2006). Cytokines sing the blues: Inflammation and the pathogenesis of depression. *Trends in Immunology, 27*, 24–31.

Ram, N., & Gerstorf, D. (2009). Time-structured and net intraindividual variability: Tools for examining the development of dynamic characteristics and processes. *Psychology and Aging, 24*, 778–791.

Rethorst, C. D., Moynihan, J., Lyness, J. M., Heffner, K. L., & Chapman, B. P. (2011). Moderating effects of moderate-intensity physical activity in the relationship between

depressive symptoms and interleukin-6 in primary care patients. *Psychosomatic Medicine, 73*, 265–269.

Rosenthal, R., & Rubin, D. B. (1982). A simple, general purpose display of magnitude of experimental effect. *Journal of Educational Psychology, 74*, 166–169.

Segerstrom, S. C. (2007). Optimism and resources: Effects on each other and on health over 10 years. *Journal of Research in Personality, 41*, 772–786.

Steptoe, A., O'Donnell, K., Badrick, E., Kumari, M., & Marmot, M. (2008). Neuroendocrine and inflammatory factors associated with positive affect in healthy men and women: The Whitehall II Study. *American Journal of Epidemiology, 167*, 96–102.

Vul, E., Harris, C., Winkielman, P., & Pashler, H. (2009). Puzzlingly high correlations in fMRI studies of emotion, personality, and social cognition. *Perspectives on Psychological Science, 4*, 274–290.

AUTHOR INDEX

A

Aag, S., 30
Aalto, A-M., 179
Aaronson, N. K., 342, 343
Aaronson, S. A., 346
Abbas, A. K., 214–215
Abbey, S., 405
Abbott, D. H., 135
Abel, K. M., 12–13, 133–134, 261–262
Abeni, D., 115–116
Abercrombie, H. C., 354, 355
Abizaid, A., 80–81, 82, 88
Abo, T., 296–297
Abraham, J., 44–45
Abramson, J. L., 186
Abramson, L. Y., 155–156
Abril, I., 12
Abrous, D. N., 24
Accardi, R., 349
Achanzar, K., 171
Ackerman, J. M., 131–132
Ackerman, K. D., 225
Ackland-Berglund, C. E., 265–267
Adam, E. K., 204, 426
Adame, D. D., 98
Adamo, S. A., 277, 278, 279, 279–280, 280–281, 282, 285–286, 312
Adamopoulos, E., 109
Adams, D. O., 171–172
Adams, J. S., 71
Adams, S., 135
Addington, A. M., 322
Addy, C., 23
Adegnika, A. A., 22
Adelson, J. D., 295–296
Ader, H. J., 292
Ader, R., xvii, 19, 38, 217–218, 277, 306

Adinolfi, M., 21–22
Adler, K. A., 325–326
Adler, N., 52, 93
Adler, N. E., 71–72, 234–235, 235–236, 237
Adler, U. C., 178
Adyiga, O., 20
Affleck, G., 389
Agarwal, S., 39–40
Agerbo, E., 23–24
Aggarwal, B. B., 44–45
Agnji, S. T., 22
Ahlberg, K., 326
Ahleman, S., 96, 107–108
Ahluwalia, B., 20
Ahmadzadeh, M., 67
Ahmed, M. R., 373–374
Ahmed, Y., 438
Ahnve, S., 331–332
Ahrens, A. H., 155–156
Aicher, A., 67–68
Aickin, M., 342, 344, 357
Aiello, A. E., 238–241, 241–242, 247
Aita, M., 373
Akbar, A. N., 66–67, 71
Akechi, T., 326, 343
Akello, M., 22
Akerstedt, T., 331–332
Akhter, S. A., 374
Akinbami, M., 292, 297
Akizuki, N., 326, 344
Aknin, L. B., 83
Aktas, A., 322
Akurut, H., 22
Al'Absi, M., 94
Albers, K. M., 259
Albert, M. A., 243–244
Alberti, A., 329
Alberts, S. C., 354–355
Albuquerque, K., 50–51, 98, 400

Alderman, B. W., 7
Alexander, G. J., 265–267
Alexander, M., 314
Alexander, R. W., 175
Alexander, S., 326
Alferi, S. M., 220–221, 351–352, 357, 387–388, 389–390, 395, 400
Algarra, I., 350
Alghamdi, A., 279
Alho, O-P., 25–26
Aljada, A., 173
Alkon, A., 135
Allaire, J. C., 51–52
Allan, T. M., 291, 297
Allavena, P., 345–346, 352–353, 355–356
Allcock, R., 188
Allen, J., 177
Allen, K. A., 85, 135
Allen, M. T., 345
Alleva, E., 313–314
Alley, D. E., 46, 238, 239–241t, 247
Alley, P. G., 115
Alleyne, S., 197–198
Allsopp, R., 66, 67–68
Almawi, W., 94
Almeida, D. M., 226
Almeida, N. D., 236–237, 241–242, 242–243t
Almeida, O. P., 188
Almeida-Oliveira, A., 40
Aloisi, R., 389
Alonso, A., 133, 138
Alper, C. M., 43, 93, 94, 134, 149, 151, 153–154, 160
Alpert, A., 29
Alt, J. M., 263
Altemus, M., 389
Altincicek, B., 285
Altmann, J., 354–355

Backer, V., 298–299
Backlund, E., 197
Bacon, M., 342–343
Bacon, S. L., 94
Badino, G. R., 347
Badrick, E., 44–45, 438
Baeza, I., 136
Baggett, L., 394–395, 407
Bagley, C., 93
Bagni, R., 405
Bagnoli, F., 24–25
Bagot, R., 256–257, 260–261
Bailey, M. T., 27–28
Bailleul, F., 355
Baillie, S. R., 294, 295
Bain, V. G., 265–267
Baines, D., 285
Baiocchi, R. A., 405
Baithun, S., 297
Baker, A. M., 344, 346–347
Baker, I. A., 176
Baker, K. H., 96
Bakker, J. M., 6–7, 26–27, 370
Bakker, T. C. M., 133
Balaban, J., 6
Balaram, P., 349
Balasubramanyan, S., 378–379
Balbin, E., 108, 112–113, 390–391,
    395–396
Balbin, G., 390
Baldaro, B., 94
Baldwin, M. W., 135, 224
Baliko, B., 397
Baljet, M., 217–218
Balkwill, F. R., 333, 346, 348, 352–353
Ball, D., 343
Ball, G. F., 292–293
Ballantyne, C. M., 177
Ballard, T. J., 23
Ballas, Z. K., 67–68
Ballon, J. S., 332
Bamberg, M., 353
Bamberger, C. M., 258–259
Banaschewski, T., 133
Bandura, A., 130
Bane, C. M., 348
Banich, M. T., 227
Banjevic, M., 135
Banks, J., 236
Banks, L., 265–267
Banks, W. A., 108–109, 161, 162,
    182–183, 187, 306–307
Bannuru, R., 49
Bar, F. W., 403
Bar, J., 403
Barak, L. S., 373

Barakat, B., 3–4, 4–5
Barcikowski, R., 409
Barclay, C. J., 235
Barclay, S. I., 342–343
Bard, J. M., 177
Barefoot, J. C., 161, 173–174, 187,
    246–247
Barengolts, E. I., 68
Bargellini, A., 153
Bargmann, C. I., 279
Barkan, S. E., 23
Barker, D. J., 20, 29, 299
Barker, J. P., 296–297
Barker, R. N., 24–25
Barkhof, F., 292
Barkin, A., 149, 152, 154, 155,
    217–218, 221–222, 225, 255
Barlow, D. H., 80
Barnes, G. T., 248
Barnes, L. L., 42
Barnes, R. F., 345
Barnes, Z., 405
Barnett, J. A., 312
Baron, A. E., 7
Baron, B., 353–354
Baron, K. G., 201–202
Baron, R. M., 223–224
Baron, R. S., 222–223
Baroncelli, S., 264–265
Barot, S. K., 373
Barrera, M., 222, 227–228
Barrett, C. E., 130, 136–137
Barrett, D. C., 390–391
Barrett, D. J., 20
Barroso, J., 390–391, 392
Barry, P. A., 21–22
Barsevick, A. M., 325
Bartal, I., 350
Barteneva, N., 377
Bartfai, T., 306–307
Barth, J., 214–215
Bartholomae, A., 353–354, 355
Bartholomew, J. S., 265–267
Bartlett, A., 280–281
Bartmann, P., 10, 24–25
Bartness, T. J., 296
Barton, B. E., 216–217
Barton, S., 150, 153
Bartrop, R. W., 38
Barve, S. S., 3–4, 5–6, 9
Basbaum, A. I., 378
Basen-Engquist, K., 358
Bates, M. P., 171
Bateson, P., 20
Battegay, M., 397

Batten, S. V., 110
Batty, G. D., 236, 246–247
Baucom, D. H., 115, 209–210
Bauer, J., 347
Bauer, M. E., 51
Bauer, N., 326–327
Bauknecht, T., 265–267
Baum, A., xvii–xviii, 94–95, 114, 224,
    355, 387–388, 389–390, 406
Baum, M. K., 220
Baumann, H., 179
Baumgartner, T., 224–225
Bautista, B. M., 330
Bautista, D. M., 378
Baxter, M. R., 130–131
Bayer, B. M., 225
Beach, S. R. H., 202–203, 313
Beach, T., 378–379
Beaglehole, R., 171
Beal, W. E., 107, 110
Beale, P., 332
Beall, S. K., 105–106, 106–107, 116
Beano, A., 349, 356
Beaseley, R., 20
Beck, A. T., 152, 172–173, 179
Beck, G., 265–267
Beck, M. H., 286, 402
Becker, D. V., 131–132
Becker, K. A., 139–140
Becker, R. C., 162, 297
Becker, T., 280–281
Beckerman, K. P., 20
Beddoe, A. E., 13
Bedoui, S., 19
Begley, A. E., 321
Behrens, M., 306–307
Beilin, B., 225
Beiting, D. J., 259
Beksinska, M., 239–241t, 241–242,
    242–243t
Belaise, C., 53–54
Belin, T. R., 326
Bell, A., 129–130, 131, 137
Bell, G. J., 332
Bell, I. R., 134, 136–137
Bellinger, D. L., 94
Bellingrath, S., 180
Beltz, T. G., 179–180, 354
Belwood, J., 282–284
Ben-Eliyahu, S., 225, 350, 358,
    399–400, 410–411
Ben-Shlomo, Y., 236–237
Benach, J., 236
Benavides, M., 354, 355
Benca, R. M., 52–53
Bendayan, P., 68

Brummett, B. H., 162
Brunet, A., 29
Brunner, E., 239–241t, , 241–242242–243t
Brunner, E. J., 180, 181–182, 245–246
Brunton, P. J., 11
Brusa, D., 349, 356
Bruscke, A. P., 136–137

Bryant, F. B., 96, 97
Bryant, P. A., 321
Brydon, L., 158, 245, 325, 389
Bryer, H. P., 68
Buccheri, G., 342
Buchanan, T. W., 94
Buchinsky, F. J., 68
Buchman, A. S., 42, 45
Buchwald, C., 405
Buchwald, D., 405
Buck, G. M., 7
Buckwalter, K., 347
Budaev, S. V., 130–131
Budinsky, A. C., 400
Buekers, T. E., 347
Buhrfeind, E. D., 106–107, 107
Buijs, R. M., 321
Bukusuba, J., 22
Buller, R., 216–217, 218, 221–222, 222–223, 223, 225
Bulpitt, C. J., 238
Bulzebruck, H., 342
Bumeder, I., 344
Bunde, J., 173, 174, 187–188
Bunjes, D., 343
Bunn, D. K., 234–235
Bunney, W. E., 256
Buonocore, G., 24–25
Burack, J. H., 390–391
Burchfiel, C., 412
Burdick, N., 100–101
Burell, G., 404
Burg, M., 410
Burger, A. J., 323
Burger, K., 325, 328
Burger, M., 19–20
Burgess, J. A., 3–4
Buring, J., 171, 186
Burk, R. D., 265–267
Burke, A. P., 176
Burke, P. A., 108
Burke, P. J., 215–216
Burleson, M. H., 225
Burman, B., 198
Burnam, M. A., 390
Burnett, F. M., 218–219
Burns, V. E., 96, 151, 153–154, 201, 206–207, 217–218, 221–222

Burrows, G., 151, 160
Burt, D. J., 265–267
Burt, T. D., 20
Burton, R., 152, 152–153, 153–154
Busch, F. N., 173
Busch, M. P., 20
Busch, R., 344
Buscher, I., 396, 397–398
Bush, A. J., 322
Bushnell, P. J., 139–140
Buss, A. H., 161
Buss, C., 6, 11
Busse, P. J., 39–40, 40
Buswell, B. N., 80, 81
Butler, J. J., 70
Butler, L., 342–343
Butler, L. D., 356, 398–399
Butler, R., 67–68
Butler, R. E., 346–347
Butler, S., 407
Butow, P. N., 332, 341–342, 343–344, 344, 357
Butterfield, R. M., 201–202
Buttgereit, F., xviii–xix
Buysse, D. J., 52–53, 53, 202, 321
Bychkov, E., 373–374
Byrne, M., 23–24
Byrne-Davis, L., 109

C

Cabanac, M., 309
Caccavari, R., 94
Cacioppo, J. T., 38–39, 53, 110–111, 134, 199–200, 200–201, 204, 205, 206, 216, 216–217, 220, 221, 223, 225, 227, 255, 258, 264, 265–267, 269, 412, 426
Cady, A., 406
Cai, Q., 6
Cakar, L., 329
Calatroni, A., 6–7, 19–20
Caldji, C., 256, 256–257, 260–261
Caldwell, C., 400
Caldwell, D., 111–112
Calhoun, K. S., 110
Caligiuri, M., 81, 405
Calil, H. M., 178
Callahan, R., 9
Callies, A. L., 344, 356–357
Caltagirone, C., 342, 353–354
Calver, B. L., 66
Camacho, T. C., 171
Camacho-Arroyo, I., 323
Cameron, C. L., 114
Cameron, J. L., 223, 227
Cameron, L. D., 114–115, 117–118
Campbell, C. Y., 44–45

Campbell, D. E., 329
Campbell, N. A., 378–379
Campbell, R. S., 108
Campisi, J., 65
Campomayor, C. O., 256, 329
Campos, B., 209
Campos, P. M., 373, 381
Canner, R., 239–241t, 241–242, 242–243t
Cannon, C. P., 297
Cannon, J., 406
Cannon, J. G., 4
Cannon, J. T., 310–311
Cano, A., 208
Cano, J., 133
Cantell, K., 298
Cao, L., 347–348
Cao, W., 66
Capitanio, J. P., 119, 129, 130, 130–131, 133–134, 134, 135, 256, 258–259, 259, 261–262, 263–264, 264–265
Capri, M., 44–45
Capuron, L., 140, 178, 325, 330, 353, 406, 436
Caramaschi, D., 133
Carceller, R., 12
Cardinal, J., 10
Carey, J. C., 22
Carey, M. S., 326, 342–343
Carey, P., 164–165
Carlos Letelier, J., 120
Carlson, B., 409
Carlson, L. E., 95, 98, 400
Carlson, N. E., 342, 344, 357
Carlson, R. W., 349–350, 398–399
Carlson, S. L., 94, 259
Carlson, W., 399, 411
Carmichael, S. L., 4–5
Carney, D. R., 83
Carney, R. M., 108–109, 161, 162, 182–183, 187, 342, 410
Carobrez, A. P., 135–136
Caron, M. G., 373, 374
Carpenter, C. J., 298
Carpenter, J. S., 216–217, 219, 351, 351–352, 357
Carr, B. I., 351, 351–352, 357
Carr, N. J., 344, 346–347
Carrera, P., 280–281
Carrico, A. W., 389, 390, 391, 393, 395, 395–396, 396–397, 401, 411
Carrillo, C., 329
Carroll, D., 46, 80–81, 82, 85, 96, 97, 151, 153–154, 201, 206–207, 217–218, 221–222, 428

Hamer, M., 86, 179, 180–181, 181–182, 204, 224–225, 244, 341–342, 342, 345, 423–424t
Hamilton, J. G. Lobel, M., 6
Hamilton, W. D., 263, 314
Hammock, B. D., 71
Hamovitch, M., 215
Hamrick, N., 219, 263
Hamsten, A., 238–241
Hamulyak, K., 331–332, 403–404
Han, C., 333
Han, H.-D., 350
Han, J. W., 347
Han, L. Y., 256, 298, 346, 347, 348
Han, X., 347
Han, Y., 67
Hanahan, D., 345–346, 346
Hanewald, G., 106–107
Hanita, T., 21–22
Hankins, M., 206
Hankinson, S. E., 341–342
Hanlon, R. T., 138
Hannan, P. J., 297–298
Hannestad, J., 178
Hannigan, E., 347
Hansel, A., 44–45
Hansen, A. V., 19
Hansen, D., 6
Hansen, K., 8, 325, 328
Hansen, R., 22–23
Hanson, B. S., 220
Hanson, M. A., 299
Hanson, M. D., 83, 246
Hansson, G. K., 170, 176, 177
Hansson, L. O., 390
Hantsoo, L., 40, 69
Hao, L-Y., 23–24
Hao, X-Q., 23–24
Happel, M., 345
Haratani, T., 216–217, 217
Harbeck, R. J., 28
Harboe, E., 326–327
Harbuz, M. S., 247, 389
Harding, R., 21–22
Hariri, A. R., 88, 357–358
Harker, L., 176, 175
Harley, C. B., 66, 67–68
Harlow, H. F., 130–131
Harman, J. E., 114–115
Harmon-Jones, E., 85
Haron, M. R., 325–326
Harralson, T. L., 171
Harrington, H., 255
Harris, C. R., 85, 435–436
Harris, J. W., 23, 342–343
Harris, M. H., 65
Harris, S. D., 400

Harris, T. B., 238, 239–241t, 347
Harrison, C. M., 96
Harrison, D. G., 207
Harrison, L. K., 96
Harrison, M. J., 234–235
Harrison, N. A., 325
Hart, B. L., 278, 280, 294–295, 314–315, 324
Hart, C. L., 246–247
Hart, D. J., 68
Hart, S. L., 51, 389
Hartley, T., 412
Hartling, L., 404
Hartwig, A., 100
Harvey, J. H., 99–100
Harwood, M., 391
Haselbauer, P., 347
Hashimoto, K., 352–353
Hashimoto, T., 108–109
Haskett, R. F., 173
Hasselquist, D, 282–284
Hatch, M. C., 30
Hathcock, K. S., 66–67
Haugen, A. H., 329
Haughie, P., 177
Hauser, P. M., 234
Haussy, C., 294–295
Haverkamp, A. D., 7
Haviland, J. S., 342, 343
Hawk, D. M., 200
Hawken, S., 174
Hawkins, M., 4–5, 6
Hawkley, L. C., 46–47, 53, 134, 216–217, 225, 255, 258, 264, 269, 412, 426
Hawton, K., 407
Hay, F. C., 46, 238–241, 244–245
Hayano, J., 94
Hayat, S. J., 333
Haybittle, J. L., 343
Hayden, M. J., 187
Hayes, L. J., 238, 238–241
Haynes, E. N., 248
Haynes, L., 216, 217–218, 219
Haynes, M. T., 224–225
Hayney, M. S., 46, 216–217, 221–222, 438
Hays, Q. R., 278–279
Hayward, H., 48, 219–220, 220
Hazan, C., 203
He, J. R., 323
He, L., 81, 292–293, 294
Head, J., 245–246
Head, K., 6
Heaney, J. L., 51
Heatherton, T., 223, 227
Heberman, R. B., 350–351

Heckler, C., 332
Heckman, J. J., 256, 261, 264, 412
Heckman, T. G., 409
Hector, M., 4–5
Hedblad, B., 245–246
Hedegaard, M., 30
Hedrick, A. V., 282–284
Heemskerk, B., 67
Heeren, T. C., 94, 97, 107–108
Heesen, C., 326–327
Heffner, K. L., 350, 398, 438
Hegeman, I. M., 164–165
Heijnen, C. J., 6–7, 26–27, 138, 183–184, 369–370, 371, 372, 373, 374, 375, 379, 379–380, 380–381, 381, 389
Heilman, M. J., 263
Heim, C., 256, 330
Heimberg, R. G., 110
Heinrichs, M., 224–225
Heise, E. R., 155
Heiss, G., 242–243t
Heitz, V., 405
Helder, L., 405–406, 407
Helenius, H., 341–342
Heller, A. R., 280–281
Heller, B., 343
Heller, W., 227
Hellhammer, D. H., 6–7, 84, 94, 203, 330, 426
Hellovaara, M., 342
Hellstrand, K., 345
Helmchen, F., 378
Helmerhorst, E. J., 80–81, 82, 85
Helps, S. C., 139–140
Hemingway, H., 245–246
Henderson, B. N., 114, 247
Henderson, P. J., 325–326
Hendriks, J. H., 341–342
Hendrix, S. W., 12
Henle, W., 405
Henley, S. J., 234
Hennekens, C. H., 177, 179–180, 186, 216–217
Henriksen, T. B., 30
Henry, J. P., 258, 261, 263–264, 264
Henslee-Downey, P. J., 342, 343
Heo, D., 349–350
Heo, S., 330
Her, S., 256
Herberman, R. B., 49–50, 218, 349–350, 349, 350–351, 405
Herbert, A., 67–68
Herbert, T. B., 92, 177–178, 222, 387–388, 388, 393
Herbst, J., 393
Hercend, T., 390

Herd, P., 46, 238, 239–241t
Herderick, E. E., xix
Herman, D. S., 409
Hermann, D. M., 328
Hermodsson, S., 345
Hernandez, J., 67
Hernandez-Reif, M., 397
Hernanz, A., 136
Herndon, J. N., 342, 344
Hernez, M., 225
Hernez-Reif, M., 11
Heron, M., 37
Herrald, M. M., 85–86
Herrell, R., 298
Herrera, A. J., 133
Herrington, D. M., 370
Herrington, J. D., 227
Hershfield, M. S., 69–70
Herskind, C., 353
Hertenstein, B., 343
Hertz-Picciotto, I., 22–23
Hertzog, C., 99
Hesse, F. W., 95
Hesse, J., 330
Hessing, M. J., 138
Het, S., 82
Hetta, J., 321
Hewison, M., 71
Heyderman, E., 347
Heymsfield, S. B., 321
Hicklin, D., 222–223
Hickman, H. D., 264–265
Hida, S., 68
Higashi, H., 352–353
Higgins, J. P., 216–217, 238
Higgins, P., 389
Hik, D., 282–284
Hildreth, K. L., 373
Hill, A. M., 263, 351
Hill, G. E., 314
Hill, J. A., 8
Hill, J. M., 265–267
Hiller, J. E., 342, 343–344
Hiller, S. L., 22
Hillhouse, J., 407
Hillier, S. L., 9
Hillis, S. L., 99–100
Hilmert, C. J., 203, 223, 227
Hilner, J. E., 238
Hinderliter, A. L., 94
Hinze-Selch, D., 328
Hirji, K., 66, 67–68
Hirokawa, K., 291–292
Hirsch, S. R., 321–322
Hirte, H. W., 70–71
Hislop, T. G., 344
Hjalmarsson, L., 108

Ho, B., 280
Ho, J., 67
Ho, J. Z. S., 280
Ho, M. R., 227
Hoaglin, D. C., 405
Hoare, S., 333
Hoath, S. B., 12
Hobbins, J. C., 9
Hoch, C. C., 321
Hock, J. M., 68
Hodes, R., 66–67
Hodgson, D. M., 19
Hoekstra, R., 298
Hoesli, L., 327
Hoffken, K., 344
Hoffman, C., 349
Hoffman, G., 131–132
Hoffman, J. M., 197–198, 201,
    203–204, 208
Hoffman, T., 19
Hoffmann, J., 67–68
Hoffmann, J. A., 255
Hoffmeister, A., 247
Hofmann, S. G., 85
Hogan, V., 3–4, 5–6, 9
Hohm, E., 133
Holahan, C. J., 221
Holbrook, N., 345, 355
Holbrook, N. J., 224–225
Holdorf, A. D., 65
Hole, D. J., 246–247
Holland, J. C., 344
Holland, J. F., 342
Holley, H., 50, 351, 400–401
Holliday, J., xvii–xviii, 200–201
Holloway, J. A., 20
Holm, J., 176
Holmang, A., 12
Holmes, A., 357–358
Holmes, M. D., 341–342, 343–344, 344
Holroyd, K., 409
Holsboer, F., 10, 328
Holstad, M., 48
Holt-Lunstad, J., 207, 214–215. 216,
    221, 227–228
Holtmann, M., 133
Holzman, A., 407
Holzman, I. R., 23
Homish, G. G., 201–202
Hong, D. S., 217
Hong, S. Y., 44–45, 99–100, 325,
    325–326, 347
Honig, A., 403–404
Hoodin, F., 356–357
Hooper, W. C., 438
Hooton, J. W., 63
Hoppitt, L., 109

Höppler, S., 29
Hoppmann, C., 203–204
Hopster, H., 129, 129–130, 131, 137
Horbury, S. R., 294–295
Horgan, K., 65, 341
Horgan, M., 115–116
Horn, M. C., 226
Horner, H., 345, 355
Hornig, M., 21–22, 22
Horsten, M., 197–198, 238–241
Horvath, J., 41–42
Horvath, R. J., 377
Horwitz, R. I., 345
Horwood, L. J., 20
Hosch, W., 422
Hoshino, A., 131–132
Hoshino, K., 294
Hoskin, D. W., 69–70, 70
Hossain, J. L., 321
Hotchkiss, A. K., 291–292, 293, 294
Hou, J., 392
Hou, W., 208–209
Houck, P. R., 321
Hougaard, K. S., 6
Houldin, A., 202–203
House, A., 341
House, J. S., 45, 214–215, 215, 220,
    222–223, 226–227, 343–344,
    409–410
Houts, C., 200
Howard, B. V., 238
Howe, R., 7
Howell, D., 343, 357
Howley, P. M., 262–263, 265
Howren, M. B., 44–45, 179, 180
Hoyle, R. H., 429, 429–430
Hu, F., 258
Hu, P., 238, 239–241t
Hu, W., 326, 346, 348–349
Huang, B., 235
Huang, C. L., 117–118
Huang, H., 23, 387–388
Huang, J., 70
Huang, S., 348, 352–353
Huang, S. C., 67, 348
Huang, S. P., 117–118
Hubbard, B., 131
Hubbard, G. B., 292–293
Hubbard, R. E., 66
Hubbard, R. W., 94
Hucklebridge, F., 97, 99, 238–241
Huehn, J., 29
Hughes, C. F., 107
Hughes, G. A., 265–267
Hughes, J., 217–218
Hughes, J. W., 345
Hughes, T. K., 312, 328

Klock, S. C., 4–5
Kloner, R. A., 297
Klug, L., 296–297
Kluger, M. J., 225, 279, 308
Klumb, P., 203–204
Knackstedt, M. K., 3–4, 10
Knapp, P. H., 94, 97, 107–108
Knauz, R. O., 391
Knekt, P., 342
Knickmeyer, R. C., 6, 23
Knipe, D. M., 262–263, 265
Knoll, M. D., 171
Knoop, H., 330–331
Knorr, E., 285
Knox, R. M., 347
Knox, S. S., 225
Knudsen, T. B., 298–299
Knudson, M., 67–68
Knutsson, A., 53
Kobayakawa, M., 344
Kobayashi, F., 216–217, 217
Kobayashi, K., 21–22
Kobayashi, Y., 21–22
Kobilka, B., 392
Kobor, M. S., 19–20, 255–256, 258
Kobrosly, R., 179
Koç, C., 134
Kocelak, P., 187
Koch, W. J., 374
Kocherginsky, M., 349, 355
Koehl, M., 23–24, 24
Koenig, W., 187, 247
Kohda, M., 96–97
Kohm, A. P., 224
Kohut, M. L., 49, 52, 156, 436
Koivu, M., 25–26
Koizumi, M., 45
Kolodgie, F. D., 176
Komaki, R. R., 323, 326
Komaroff, A., 405
Komarow, H., 131–132
Konarzewski, M., 291–292
Koneru, A. O., 330, 389–390, 405
Kong, Y. Y., 68
Konno, A., 291–292
Konski, A., 342–343
Konsman, J. P., 324
Koo, J., 342
Koolhaas, J. M., 129, 129–130, 131, 132, 132–133, 137
Koopman, C., 218, 219, 222, 224–225, 355, 356, 391, 398–399
Kop, W. J., 178–179, 179
Kopp, H., 247
Korczykowski, M., 223, 227
Korin, Y. D., 264–265, 265–267, 392
Kornblith, A. B., 342, 344

Kornelson, R. A., 310
Kornmüller, A., 327
Korszun, A., 403
Korte, S. M., 129, 129–130, 131, 137
Korth, C., 328
Korzan, W., 138
Korzun, A., 342
Koskenvuo, M., 341–342
Kossoff, M., 341–342, 342, 357
Kostaki, A., 6
Koster, A., 238, 239–241t
Kosty, M., 344
Kothandapani, R. V., 345
Kotrschal, K., 130
Kotur, M., 402
Koukoulas, I., 29–30
Kouro, T., 24–25
Kouznetsova, T., 68
Kovacsics, C. E., 130, 131–132, 136–137
Kowalczyk, D. W., 350
Kozak, L. J., 247
Kozak, M. J., 223, 227
Kozak, W., 279
Kozanian, T. A., 82
Kraal, G., 9
Kraemer, H. C., 355, 355, 398–399, 400, 422
Kraenzlin, M. E., 68
Kraft, C. A., 109–110
Kraft, J. K., 19
Krainer, M., 400
Krakowiak, P., 22–23
Krakstad, B. F., 373
Kralj-Fiser, S., 130
Kramer, J., 353–354
Kraus, T., 325
Krause, N., 45
Krause, P. R., 265–267
Krausz, T., 349, 355
Krebs, M., 353–354, 355
Kreibig, S. D., 85–86
Kreier, F., 321
Kremsner, P. G., 22
Krey, L. C., 295–296, 345
Krichevsky, A. M., 377
Kricker, A., 342, 343–344
Krieger, N., 236
Kriegsfeld, L. J., 291, 292, 293–294
Kriegsman, D. M. W., 221
Kripke, D. F., 321
Krishnan, R. R., 161, 176–177, 179–180, 182, 183–184, 186, 187, 326–327, 332–333
Kristensen, F., 327
Kristensen, T. S., 341–342, 344
Kristenson, M., 185

Kristiansen, O. P., 216–217
Kritchevsky, S. B., 238, 239–241t
Kroenke, C. H., 67, 341–342, 343–344
Kroes, H., 6–7
Krohn, M. A., 22
Kronfol, Z., 323
Krueger, G., 347
Krueger, J. M., 324, 327–328
Krueger, P. M., 53
Kruk, M. R., 133
Krupp, L., 407
Kruschinski, C., 19
Kruse, N., 8–9
Kruszewski, A. A., 352–353
Ksiek, A., 291–292
Kubista, E., 400
Kubota, K., 327
Kubota, T., 328
Kubzansky, L. D., 172–173, 174, 343–344, 344
Kudelka, A., 358
Kudielka, B. M., 180, 426
Kuehnhardt, D., 353–354, 355
Kuh, D., 236–237
Kuhlwein, E., 297
Kuhn, C., 11, 161, 172, 174, 182, 183, 345
Kuhn, I. N., 296–297
Kuhn, J., 326, 333
Kuhns, D. B., 200
Kuiperij, H. B., 348
Kuis, W., 371
Kukreja, S. C., 68
Kulik, J. A., 206, 207
Kulkarni, S., 67–68
Kuller, L. H., 176, 207
Kumagai, K., 296–297
Kumar, M., 113, 152, 220, 389–390, 395, 395–396, 400, 409
Kumari, M., 44–45, 51, 96–97, 241–242, 242–243t, 438
Kumsta, R., 6–7
Kunkel, S. L., 371
Kunos, G., 345
Kunst, A. E., 234–235
Kunz-Ebrecht, S. R., 179, 238–241, 244–245
Kunze, M., 247
Kunzmann, U., 41
Kuo, Y. M., 378–379
Kupelnick, B., 325
Kupfer, D. J., 422
Kupfer, S. R., 265–267
Kupper, N., 322
Kurashima, C., 291–292
Kuratsune, H., 96
Kurian, J. R., 204–205

Manolagas, S. C., 216–217, 217
Mantell, J., 215
Mantero-Atienza, E., 220
Mantovani, A., 263, 345–346, 352–353, 355–356
Manuck, S. B., 44, 98–99, 135, 151, 153, 153–154, 155, 160, 160–161, 162, 163–164, 171, 179–180, 179, 187, 203–204, 216–217, 217, 219, 221–222, 222–223, 224, 225–226, 235, 241–242, 246, 239–241t, 242–243t
Mao, H. Y., 199–200, 200–201, 205, 407
Mao, J., 370–371
Mao, L., 323, 326
Mao, T. L., 348
Maple, T. J., 130–131
Maras, A., 133
Marchetti, B., 347
Marco, E. M., 136
Marcus, S. M., 29–30
Marder, V. J., 174–175
Margolin, G., 198
Margolin, K. A., 96–97
Margulies, S., 113
Marin, T., 255, 258–259, 264
Mark, D. B., 342
Markides, K., 171
Markovic, S. N., 356–357
Markowe, H. L., 238
Markowitz, N., 153, 153–154, 158
Marks, G., 99–100, 157–158, 393
Marks, I., 407
Marks, J. S., 23
Marler, M. R., 321
Marmot, M. G., 44–45, 94, 197–198, 227–228, 234, 235, 237, 238, 241–242, 244, 245–246, 247, 248, 438
Marniemi, J., 239–241t, 242–243t
Marques, A. H., 178
Marsden, A. K., 297
Marsh, C. B., 346, 347, 348
Marshall, G. D., 405
Marshall, J., 343–344
Marshall, L., 325, 328
Marsland, A. L., 44, 98–99, 151, 153, 153–154, 160, 160–161, 162, 163–164, 179–180, 179, 187, 203–204, 216–217, 219, 221–222, 222–223, 224, 225–226, 239–241t, 242–243t
Marten-Mittag, B., 187
Martin, B. S., 332
Martin, D. H., 22

Martin, L. B., 278, 285, 292–293, 295–296
Martin, M. A., 149–150, 150, 152, 153–154, 262–263, 265
Martin, R., 172
Martin, R. B., 96, 107–108
Martin, R. P., 12
Martinez, E., 21–22
Martinez, F. O., 263
Martinez, M. M., 325–326
Martino, G., 378–379
Martionez-Maza, O., 347
Marucha, P. T., 4, 12, 46, 81, 115, 204, 206, 216–217, 217, 222
Marx, B. P., 107, 110, 116–117
Marx, F., 69
Marx, K., 235–236
Marx, L., 8–9
Masaki, K. H., 221
Masaki, Y., 8
Mascovich, A., 329
Masera, R., 345
Maseri, A., 403
Mashal, N. M., 325
Mashoodh, R., 255–256, 256–257, 260–261
Mason, J. W., 84
Mason, W. A., 133–134, 134, 256, 259, 263–264, 264–265
Massie, M. J., 342, 353–354
Massing, M., 237
Masson, M., 24–25
Masterman, D., 67–68, 68–69
Masters, A. M., 297
Mastorakos, G., 9–10
Masur, K., 348
Masurel, N., 217–218
Matera, L., 137–138
Matheson, K., 80–81, 82, 82–83, 83–84, 88
Mathews, H. L., 98, 285, 286, 400
Mathias, C. J., 227
Matis, J., 30
Matre, R., 351, 358
Matsuda, T., 21–22
Matsumoto, T., 285–286
Matsunaga, M., 97
Matt, K. S., 197–198, 201, 203–204, 208
Mattar, B. I., 333
Matthews, K. A., 161, 172, 180–181, 207, 227–228, 235, 247, 248
Matthews, R., 396
Matthews, S. G., 6
Matthiesen, L., 8
Maturana, H., 120
Maturana, H. R., 120

Matzinger, P., 350
Maue, A. C., 216, 217–218, 219
Mauer, M. H., 397–398
Maunsell, E., 343–344
Mauricas, M., 67
Maurice, J., 404
Mawa, P. A., 22
Maxwell, A. E., 184–185
May, J. C., 223, 227
May, R. M., 265
Mayanagi, T., 6
Mayer, D. J., 370–371
Mayer, K. H., 391
Mayne, T. J., 108, 200–201, 205, 390–391
Mayor, F., 373, 374, 375, 381
Mayr, M., 247
Mazor, M., 9
Mazuc, J., 294–295
Mazzanti, C., 115–116
Mazzotta, G., 329
McAlister, F. A., 404
McAuley, E., 52
McCain, N., 397
McCalla, J., 396, 397–398
McCann, J., 96
McCarthy, D. O., 219
McCarty, M., 176, 348, 352–353
McChesney, M. B., 133–134, 261–262
McClelland, D. C., 96
McClintick, J., 329
McClintock, M. K., 130, 136–137, 354
McConnachie, A., 239–241t
McCormick, M. C., 23
Mccoy, J. L., 358
McCrady, B., 200–201, 205
McCrae, R. R., 130–131, 146, 148, 150–151, 172
McCraty, R., 98
McCrone, P., 321–322
McCune, J. M., 20
McCusker, R. H., 344–345
McCutchan, A. J., 157–158
McCutchan, J. A., 219–220
McDade, T. W., 216–217, 269
McDonald, P. G., 44, 254–255, 256, 265–267, 396, 398
McDougall, P. T., 129–130
McElhaney, J. E., 37, 39–40, 63, 436
McElhiney, M. C., 332
McEwen, B. S., 87, 129, 198–199, 207, 235, 282–284, 284–285, 295–296, 345, 355, 388–389, 391–392
McFeeley, S., 350–351
McFree, J., 20–21
McGee, R., 130–131, 342

Mills, P. J., 162–163, 164, 171–172, 204, 325, 325–326, 326, 389
Mills, R. S. L., 83
Milne, B. J., 248, 255
Milne, H. M., 332
Milne, K., 67
Min, Y. K., 285–286
Minchoff, B., 96
Minden, S., 405
Mingam, R., 278–279
Minton, J., 349
Minton, O., 326
Minville, V., 21–22
Miquel, J., 136
Miranda, N., 109–110
Mirowsky, J., 236
Mischel, W., xviii
Mishima, Y., 347
Misiti, S., 70–71
Misser, J.-L., 355
Mistrangelo, M., 349, 356
Mitchell, M. D., 9
Mitrani, V. B., 397–398
Mitsuyasu, R. T., 70
Mittal, R., 265–267
Mittleman, M. A., 197–198, 323
Mittwoch-Jaffe, T., 96–97, 107–108
Miwa, H., 21–22
Miyakoshi, M., 97
Miyazaki, T., 216–217, 217
Mizrahi, J., 215, 344
Mletzko, T., 256
Mocchegiani, E., 40
Modlin, R. L., 71
Moestl, E., 130
Moestrup, T., 220
Moffitt, T. E., 132–133, 133, 244, 248, 255, 357–358
Mohamed-Ali, V., 46, 96–97, 238–241, 244–245, 245
Mohanty, A., 227
Mohanty, P., 173
Mohideen, N., 265–267
Mohile, S., 332
Mohr, D. C., 389
Mokyr, M. B., 264–265
Molassiotis, A., 343, 356–357
Mold, J. E., 20
Moldovan, J., 345
Moldovsky, H., 406
Molloy, G. J., 129, 180–181, 181–182
Molton, I., 351, 351–352, 357
Mommersteeg, P. M. C., 183–184
Monjan, A. A., 321
Monk, J. P., 326, 333
Monk, T. H., 321
Monnier, M., 327

Monroe, S. M., 203–204
Monson, J. R., 346–347
Montazeri, A., 321–322
Montebarocci, O., 94
Montecino-Rodriguez, E., 52
Montella, F., 112
Montross, L. P., 42
Mooney, C. Z., 425
Moons, W. G., 82, 88
Moore, A. N., 82
Moore, D. D., 265–267
Moore, J., 280
Moore, M. C., 284
Moore, P., 330
Moore, S. E., 299
Moorkens, G., 330
Moos, R. H., xvii, 92, 221
Morag, A., 152, 153–154, 325
Morag, M., 152, 153–154
Morales-Montor, J., 323
Moran, T. J., 355
Moranis, A., 278–279
Morcos, M., 87
Moreau, J. L., 265–267
Moreb, J., 342, 344, 356–357
Moreh, E., 321–322
Moretta, A., 349
Moretta, L., 349
Morgan, D. L., 227–228
Morgan, R., 405, 422, 423–424t, 424–425
Morgan, T. M., 81
Mori, S., 23
Moriabadi, N. F., 8–9
Morimoto, H. K., 344–345, 350
Morin, C. M., 400–401
Morison, L. A., 22
Morita, I., 347
Morita, K., 256
Morita, T., 6
Moritz, K., 29–30
Morizono, K., 353
Mormède, P., 137–138
Mormont, M. C., 353–354
Morosini, M., 67
Morozink, J. A., 46, 438
Morphy, M. A., 355
Morris, A. A., 438
Morris, C., 23–24, 29
Morris, R. M., 115–116
Morris, R. W., 238–241
Morris, T., 343
Morrison, C. H., 391
Morrison, D. C., 139
Morrissey, P. J., 29
Morrow, D. A., 186, 389
Morrow, G. R., 325, 332
Morrow, J. D., 71–72

Mortensen, C. R., 131–132
Mortensen, L. H., 246–247
Mortensen, P., 23–24
Morton, C., 114–115
Morton, D. L., 411
Morton, R. P., 342–343
Morton, S. M., 299
Moschen, A. R., 238
Moschos, N., 297
Moscovitch, D. A., 85
Moser, B., 115
Moses, R. G., 3–4
Moses, S., 4–5
Moskowitz, J. T., 71–72, 93, 387–388, 391, 397
Moss, A. J., 174–175, 186
Moss, H. B., 99–100
Moss, J., 258
Moss, N. E., 236
Moss, R. B., 99–100
Moss-Morris, R., 215, 330–331, 344, 346–347
Motivala, S. J., 185, 326–327, 328–329
Motl, R. W., 52, 322
Motzke, C., 344
Mou, D., 70
Moudgil, V., 345
Moul, D. E., 299–300
Mouridsen, H. T., 342, 342–343
Moussa, M., 108
Moussavi, S., 129
Mouttapa, M., 171, 322
Movsas, B., 342–343
Moynihan, J. A., 46, 217–218, 400, 438
Mpairwe, H., 22
Mpodozis, J., 120
Mrekar, P., 248
Mroczek, D. K., 41
Mrup-Poulsen, T., 216–217
Muche, R., 247
Mueller, C. R., 355
Mueller, P., 348
Muench, M. O., 20
Muennig, P., 238, 239–241t
Mueser, K. T., 209–210
Muftuler, L. T., 6
Muggeo, M., 247
Muhangi, L., 22
Mujahid, M. S., 237, 243–244
Muldoon, M. F., 44, 98–99, 160–161, 162, 163–164, 173, 179–180, 180, 181–182, 182, 187, 216–217, 219, 221–222, 222–223, 224, 225–226, 241–242, 246, 242–243t
Mullan, B., 332
Mullen, L., 282

Muller, C., 400
Muller, C. P., 330
Muller, D., 98
Muller, J., 297
Mullington, J. M., 328, 329
Muluk, N. B., 134
Munck, A., 224–225
Munck, A. U., 224–225, 282–284, 284, 391–392
Munjas, B., 397
Munoz, H., 9
Munro, C., 397
Munster, P., 330–331
Muntaner, C., 236
Murabito, J. M., 236–237, 241–242, 242–243t
Murakami, H., 97
Murata, C., 53
Murata, S., 68
Murga, C., 373, 375, 381
Murgia, F., 112
Murota, S., 347
Murphy, J. R., 22
Murphy, K. C., 343
Murphy, V. E., 29–30
Murray, A. B., 294–295, 308–309
Murray, C. J., 342, 356, 405
Murray, E. J., 106–107
Murray, J. C., 29–30
Murray, M. A., 238–241
Murray, M. J., 294–295, 308–309
Murray, T. E., 234
Musaad, S., 248
Musselman, D. L., 172–173, 325, 353–354
Mustian, K. M., 325
Muthuramalingam, S. R., 333
Muwanga, M., 22
Mycek, P. M., 80, 80–81, 82, 83, 88
Myers, H. F., 71–72, 110–111, 163, 199–200, 205

N

Nabi, H., 174
Nabid, A., 342–343
Nabulime, J., 22
Naeim, F., 65
Nagarathna, R., 13
Nagasaki, H., 327
Nagashima, M., 108
Nagendra, H. R., 13
Nahas, G. G., 308
Nail, L. M., 106–107
Nair, C., 297
Nair, M., 349
Nair, M. P. N., 392
Naitza, S., 153, 154, 155

Nakajima, A., 108
Nakane, T., 345
Nakashima, Y., 175–176
Nakata, A., 216–217, 217
Nakaya, N., 341–342, 344
Nakshatri, H., 265–267
Naliboff, B. D., 119, 134, 164–165, 255, 264–265, 265–267, 388, 392
Nalini, M., 282
Nam, E. J., 350
Namatovu, A., 22
Nampijja, M., 22
Namujju, P. B., 22
Nan, K., 351
Nance, D. M., 282
Nanni, S., 70–71
Nannis, E., 219–220
Nanteza, B., 22
Napier, B. J., 94
Napoli, A., 426
Napolitano, P. G., 20
Naqvi, S. S. A., 186
Naqvi, T. Z., 186
Nar, H., 298
Narendran, S., 13
Narendran, V., 12
Nartucci, R., 347, 353
Nascimbene, C., 67
Nassar, M. A., 379, 379–380, 380–381
Nast-Kolb, D., 137–138
Natarajan, D., 133
Natarajan, L., 325, 325–326
Natelson, B. H., 265–267, 326–327
Nater, U. M., 256
Nation, J. L., 281
Naughton, M. J., 344
Naumann, E., 133
Nauseen, B., 344, 346–347
Nausheen, B., 215
Navara, K. J., 294
Nawrath, L., 326–327
Nawroth, P. P., 87
Naylor, R. J., 135–136
Nazmi, A., 241, 241–242, 242–243t
Nazroo, J. Y., 237
Ndibazza, J., 22
Neale, J. M., 96, 99, 426
Nealey, J. B., 85
Negi, L. T., 98
Negishi, M., 324
Nehlsen-Cannarella, S. L., 292–293, 293–294, 295
Nehrenberg, D. L., 133
Neidenthal, P. M., 80
Neigh, G. N., 293
Neitzert, C. S., 356
Nelesen, R. A., 162–163, 164

Nelson, A. M., 357
Nelson, E. L., 6–7
Nelson, L. D., 180–181
Nelson, P., 96
Nelson, R. J., 285, 291–292, 292–293, 293–294, 294–295, 295–296, 296–297
Nemeroff, C. B., 172–173, 325
Nepper-Christensen, S., 298–299
Neri, E., 422
Nesbitt, C., 256, 256–257, 260–261
Nestel, A. R., 65
Netterstrom, B., 341–342
Nettles, C. D., 5–6, 12–13, 216–217
Neuberg, S. L., 131–132
Neuhaus, J. M., 158
Neumann, S. A., 94
Newberger, E. H., 23
Newbern, E. C., 235
Newell, S., 398, 408
Newman, A. B., 238, 239–241t
Newman, J. P., 429, 429–430
Newman, M. A., 65
Newman, R. D., 22
Newman, W., 65
Newsom, J. T., 227–228
Newton, C., 324
Newton, T., 198, 199–200, 200–201, 205, 205–206, 208–209
Ng, D. M., 220–221
Ng, E., 236
Ng, H. L., 66, 70
Ng, R., 221
Nguyen, H. C., 71–72, 295
Nguyen, P. L., 333
Ni, H., 238, 239–241t
Niaura, R., 171
Nicassio, P. M., 332
Nicholls, E. F., 255, 258–259, 258, 260–261
Nicholls, G., 114–115, 117–118
Nichols, A., 248
Nick, A., 346, 348–349, 350
Nicklas, J. M., 197–198
Nickolaus, M. S., 156
Niederhoffer, K. G., 105–106
Nielsen, J. S., 67
Nielsen, N. M., 19
Nielsen, N. R., 341–342, 344
Nieman, D. C., 282
Nieto, F. J., 237
Nieto-Vazquez, I., 375
Niggemann, B., 348
Nihel, Z., 347
Nijagal, A., 20
Nijboer, C. H., 373, 374, 375, 379, 379–380, 380–381, 381

Peterson, R. A., 197–198
Petitto, J. M., 133, 134, 391, 390–391, 392
Peto, T., 407
Petraitis, T., 67
Petrie, K. J., 105–106, 107, 107–108, 108, 112, 113–114, 115, 397
Petronis, V. M., 400
Petros, J. A., 358
Petrov, D., 87
Petrow-Sadowski, C., 405
Pettersson, K., 171
Petticrew, M., 341–342
Pettingale, K. W., 343
Peveler, R. C., 215, 344, 346–347
Pezeshki, G., 247
Pfeifer, D., 23
Pfeiffer, S., 353–354, 355
Pfister, G., 39–40
Pham, L. N., 278
Philippot, P., 105–106, 234–235
Phillips, A. C., 46, 51, 151, 153–154, 201, 206–207, 217–218, 221–222
Phillips, D. I., 29–30
Phillips, G., 326, 333
Phillips, J. E., 241–242, 242–243t
Phillips, K. M., 50, 343, 351, 389, 400, 401
Phillips, M. J., 404
Phillis, A., 279
Phillpotts, J., 148–149
Phillpotts, R. J., 134, 264–265
Piacentini, M., 392
Piccini, A., 265–267
Piccinni, M. P., 8–9, 24–25
Pichler, J., 20, 24–25
Pickering, T. G., 85, 135
Pieper, C. F., 85, 135, 347
Pieper, J. O., 323
Pieraccini, F., 291
Pierce, G. R., 227–228
Pierson, D. L., 69
Pietruk, T., 352–353
Pietschmann, P., 68
Pike, J., 329
Pillai, M., 349
Pilote, L., 46, 236–237, 241–242, 242–243t
Pimentel, M. A., 353
Pinal, C. S., 299
Pinelli, M., 153
Pineros, V., 354
Pinner, R., 296–297
Pinquart, M., 344
Pinsky, D., 402
Pintado, P., 24
Pirke, K. M., 84

Pitcher, J. A., 373
Pitsavos, C., 179, 186, 238, 239–241t
Pitts, C. G., 107–108
Plas, D. R., 65
Platsoucas, C., 349–350
Pletnikov, M., 23–24, 29
Plost, M., 405
Ploutz-Snyder, R., 201–202
Pluchino, S., 378–379
Plummer, M., 297–298
Plump, A. S., 175–176
Poccia, F., 392
Poehlmann, K. M., 204, 225, 265–267
Poellinger, L., 265–267
Poewe, W., 247
Polanczyk, G., 370
Poland, G. A., 69
Polimeni, M. A., 349, 356
Polinsky, P., 175–176
Polk, D. E., 94
Pollak, S. D., 19, 30, 204–205
Pollard, J. W., 352–353
Pollard, M., 23–24, 29
Pollitt, R. A., 235, 242–243t
Pollmacher, T., 325, 328
Pollock, B. G., 188
Polonsky, W., 97, 107–108
Poltorak, A., 294
Polychronopoulos, E., 238, 239–241t
Pongratz, G., xviii–xix
Ponomarev, E. D., 377
Ponti, C., 44
Ponzio, N. M., 326–327
Poole, W. K., 297
Poon, L. W., 42
Pope, R. M., 8
Popkin, M. K., 344, 356–357
Porrata, L. F., 356–357, 356
Porsolt, R. D., 312–313
Porter, L., 94, 426
Porter, L. S., 115
Porter, M. R., 353–354
Porter, V. R., 65, 67–68, 68–69
Portier, C., 285
Porto, M., 3–4, 12, 29–30
Poskitt, E. M., 299
Posner, J. B., 346
Posner, M. I., 98
Post, A., 402
Postolache, T. T., 131–132, 298
Potter, P. T., 197–198, 201, 203–204, 208
Pottinger, T. G., 138
Pouilles, J. M., 68
Poulton, R., 19, 244, 248, 255
Poulton, T., 46, 238–241, 244–245
Pournajafi-Nazarloo, H., 204–205, 206
Pouslen, G., 29–30

Poustka, L., 133
Powell, L. H., 161, 404
Power, A., 217–218
Power, C., 241–242, 242–243t
Prado, G., 397–398
Prasad, A., 247
Prather, A. A., 44, 153, 160–161, 162, 163–164
Preacher, K. J., 38, 180–181, 180, 238, 347
Preble, O. T., 405
Preisinger, E., 68
Preisler, H. K., 286
Premont, R. T., 371, 372
Prendergast, B. J., 206, 291–292, 292, 293, 293–294, 295–296, 354
Prentice, A. M., 299
Pressman, S. D., 38–39, 53, 92, 93, 94, 94–95, 100, 149, 152, 154, 155, 203–204, 206, 217–218, 221–222, 225, 255
Pretorius, C. J., 10
Price, A. A., 400
Price, D. D., 370–371
Price, L. S., 348
Price, M. A., 341–342, 342, 343–344, 344, 357
Price, N. J., 329
Price, T., 131
Priceman, S. J., 353
Primeau, F., 298
Prins, J. B., 71, 330–331
Prinz, J., 405
Pritchard, K. I., 342
Prolo, P., 329, 330, 422
Protheroe, D., 341
Proud, K., 278
Provenzano, K. M., 107
Pruessner, J. C., 135
Pruett, S. B., 285
Pryds, O., 6
Pudrovska, T., 45
Pugliatti, M., 299
Pukkala, E., 341–342, 342
Pulkki-Råback, L., 182, 185, 239–241t, 242–243t
Pulman, K. G., 138
Pupkin, M., 3–4, 4–5
Purcell, D., 393
Purdom, C. L., 7
Puskas, E., 353
Pusztai, L., 325–326
Pyter, L. M., 292–293, 293, 294, 295–296, 354

Q
Qamhieh, H. T., 238
Quan, F. S., 285–286

Richard, H., 236–237, 241–242, 242–243t
Richards, C., 227–228
Richards, J. M., 107, 110
Richardson, H. N., 6
Richardson, J. L., 157–158
Riches, P., 347
Richman, J. A., 226–227
Ricker, D., 388
Riddell, C. E., 279
Ridker, P. M., 44–45, 170, 171, 177, 179–180, 186, 207, 216–217, 329, 389, 403
Ridsdale, L., 321–322
Rieckmann, N., 174
Rieckmann, P., 8–9
Rieder, M., 94
Riedl, M., 225
Rieman, D., 347
Rifai, N., 171, 179–180, 186, 216–217, 329
Riggs, B. L., 67–68
Riggs, T., 24–25
Rigo, J. J. R., 21
Riley, A. L., 315
Riley, J. L., 65
Rimé, B., 105–106
Rimon, R., 298
Riney, S., 84
Ring, C., 96, 97, 201, 206–207, 217–218, 221–222
Rippin, G., 247
Riquelme, E., 69
Ritchey, A. K., 389, 403, 405–406
Ritchie, J., 218
Ritter, H. L., 333
Ritvo, P., 356
Ritz, I., 405
Rivest, S., 403
Rivier, C. L., 6
Riviere, S., 315
Rivkin, I. D., 112–113
Rixon, L., 206
Robbins, E., 344, 346–347
Robbins, M. S., 397–398
Robert, A., 234–235
Robert, C., 349
Roberts, B. W., 429
Roberts, D., 298
Roberts, F., xviii
Roberts, J. L., 280–281, 282
Roberts, J. E., 390
Roberts, R. E., 171
Roberts, S. B., 299
Robertson, A. L., 176
Robertson, J. L., 286
Robertson, M., 239–241t

Robertson, R. M., 285
Robins, J., 397
Robins, L., 197
Robins, R. W., 79, 80
Robinson, C., 163
Robinson, F. P., 98, 285, 286
Robinson, S. C., 348, 352–353
Robinson-Batista, C., 397–398
Robles, T. F., 100, 182, 198–199, 200, 202, 202–203, 203–204, 204, 206, 209, 217, 350, 398
Rocha, V. Z., 170, 177
Rockman, H., 374
Rockman, H. A., 374
Rodani, M. G., 343, 343–344
Rodemann, H., 353
Rodin, J., 156
Rodrigue, J. R., 342, 344, 356–357
Rodriguez, B. L., 221
Rodriguez, C. H., 109–110
Rodriguez, M. S., 219, 263
Rodriguiz, R., 134
Rodriguiz, R. M., 133
Rodriquez, M., 387–388
Roeder, T., 280, 281
Roenneberg, T., 296
Rogge, R. D., 208–209
Rohde, L. A., 370
Rohleder, N., 82, 84, 85, 86, 87–88, 88, 325–326, 405
Rohrbaugh, M. J., 197–198, 207
Roitman-Johnson, B., 177
Roitt, I., 8–9
Roizman, B., 262–263, 265
Rojas, I., 9
Rollman, B. L., 342
Rolls, A., 378–379
Romagnani, S., 8–9, 24–25
Romanos, M., 265–267
Romero, D. F., 68
Romero, L. M., 282–284, 284–285, 391–392
Romero, M. G., 224–225, 351, 351–352
Romero, R., 9, 25
Romero-Sandoval, E. A., 377
Romo, A., 12
Rompa, D., 390–391
Ron, M., 407
Ronchi, E., 295–296
Ronis, D. L., 342–343
Rook, G. A., 10
Rook, K. S., 220–221, 221, 222, 227–228
Rooks, R. N., 238, 239–241t
Rooks, S., 407
Rosahn, P. D., 297

Rosas-Ballina, M., 69
Rosato, E., 279
Roscoe, J. A., 332
Rose, G., 234
Rose, K. M., 235, 242–243t
Rose, L., 171
Rose, R., 396, 397–398
Rose, R. M., 134, 255, 258, 264, 412
Rosekind, M. R., 321–322
Rosen, D., 29
Rosenberg, H. J., 114
Rosenberg, L., 96
Rosenberg, L. T., 28
Rosenberg, R., 6
Rosenberg, S. D., 114
Rosenblatt, H. M., 298
Rosenfeld, M. E., 175–176
Rosengaus, R. B., 314–315
Rosengren, A., 174
Rosenkranz, M. A., 44, 98, 216–217, 221–222, 298, 438
Rosenne, E., 350
Rosenthal, G. E., 197
Rosenthal, G. J., 285
Rosenthal, L., 321
Rosenthal, N. E., 298
Rosenthal, R., 202–203, 427, 437
Roskam, A. J., 234–235
Ross, C. E., 236
Ross, J. S., 248, 374
Ross, N. W., 280–281, 282
Ross, R., xix, 161, 170, 171, 175–176, 177, 179–180, 214–215
Rostron, B. L., 37
Rosvall, M., 245–246
Roth, T., 321
Roth, W. T., 85
Rothenbacher, D., 247
Rother, E., 8
Rotheram-Borus, M. J., 215
Rothman, A. D., 208–209
Rothstein, G., 26–27
Rouppe van der Voort, C., 371
Rovesti, S., 153
Rowbottom, A., 347
Rowe, J. W., 41–42, 221, 225, 345
Rowland-Jones, S., 71–72
Rowley, D. L., 23
Roy, B., 48, 156–157
Rozanski, A., 170–171, 172–173, 173, 174
Rozeboom, K., 436
Rozlog, L. A., 204, 265–267
Rubin, D. B., 437
Rubin, S. M., 238, 239–241t
Rucinski, B., 68
Rucker, R., 358

Smith, P. A., 378–379

Smith, P. K., 342

Smith, R. G., 10, 29–30, 177–178, 178, 179–180, 341–342, 342, 357, 400

Smith, R. S., 177–178, 178, 179–180, 298

Smith, T. B., 214–215. 215, 216, 221

Smith, T. L., xvii–xviii, 329

Smith, T. W., 85, 161, 172, 173–174, 174, 201–202, 224

Smith, V. J., 280, 281

Smith-Carvalho, M., 40

Smyth, J., 94, 426

Smyth, J. M., 105–106, 106–107, 111, 116–117, 349

Snidman, N., 255, 264–265

Snow, M. H., 390–391

Snow, S., 389

Snowdon, C. T., 135

Snowdon, D. A., 55

Snydersmith, M., 110–111, 204, 205

Soares, M. V., 66–67

Sodaar, P., 374

Soderstrom, M., 331–332

Sohler, N., 238, 239–241t

Sohr, R., 23

Sol, D., 129–130

Solano, L., 112

Solari, N., 67

Sole, J., 248

Soler-Vila, H., 344

Solfrini, V., 153

Solimam, A., 345

Solomayer, E. F., 67

Solomon, G. F., xvii, 19, 92, 133, 390

Somers, D. E., 292

Sompayrac, L., 64

Sondergaard, C., 235

Sondik, E. J., 30

Song, C., 5–6, 298

Song, E. K., 330

Song, X. Y., 223–224

Sonino, N., 355

Sonko, B. J., 299

Sonnega, J. S., 197–198

Sonnenberg, A., 348

Sood, A. K., 216–217, 218, 222, 259, 261, 264, 325–326, 344–345, 346, 347, 348, 348–349, 350, 351, 352, 353, 354, 389, 396, 398, 402, 411

Sood, U., 352–353

Sorbi, M. J., 111–112

Soreide, J. A., 351, 358

Sørensen, C., 138

Sorensen, H. T., 235

Sorenson, M. V., 332–333, 405, 406

Soriano, J. J., 298

Sorkin, E., 324

Sorlie, P., 237

Sorlie, P. D., 197

Sorosky, J. I., 216–217, 218, 221–222, 222–223, 223, 225, 346–347, 347

Sorrells, S. F., 133

Sorri, M., 25–26

Soszynski, D., 225, 279

Sotgiu, M. A., 299

Sotgiu, S., 299

Soulimani, R., 136

Southwick, S. M., 84

Sozzani, S., 352–353

Spahr, A., 247

Sparks, C. E., 174–175, 186

Spath-Schwalbe, E., 325, 328, 330

Spaulding, C. C., 65, 66, 70–71

Spaulding, C. S., 66

Spear, G. T., 392

Speca, M., 98, 400

Spector, T. D., 68

Spehr, M. Rodriquez, I., 315

Speicher, C. E., xvii–xviii, 200–201, 206, 219, 222–223, 226, 350, 387–388, 388, 402

Speigel, D., 355

Speiser, P., 400

Spencer, F. A., 297

Spencer, N., 280–281

Spencer, R. L., 295–296

Spengler, R. N., 371

Spera, S. P., 106–107, 107

Spiegel, D., 49–50, 218, 219, 222, 224–225, 349–350, 353–354, 354, 355, 356, 398–399, 400, 422

Spielberger, C. D., 172

Spies, K., 95

Spinola, P. G., 347

Spiro, A., 41

Spitz, A. M., 23

Spitzer, S., 395–396

Spivey, J. R., 330

Spoletini, I., 342, 353–354

Springer, K. W., 45

Spyridopoulos, I., 67–68

Srendi, B., 96–97, 107–108

Srinivasan, S., 20

McMurry, S. T., 293–294

Stahl, G., 95

Stainbrook, D., 111–112

Stall, R. D., 390–391

Stallings, J. D., 20

Stamatelou, F., 10

Stamler, J., 171

Stampfer, M. J., 177, 179–180, 216–217

Stanley, H., 397–398, 409

Stanley, M. A., 265–267

Stanslas, J., 325–326

Stanton, A. L., 109, 114, 344

Staras, S. A., 39–40

Stark, J. L., 81, 86, 87–88, 133, 258–259

Starr, J. M., 246–247

Starr, K., 395, 395–396

Stary, H. C., 176

Stebbing, M. J., 378–379

Steel, J. L., 325, 351, 351–352, 357

Steer, R. A., 152, 172–173, 179

Stefanadis, C., 238, 239–241t

Stefanek, M. E., 396, 398–399, 401

Stefanski, V., 350

Steimer, T., 137–138

Stein, D. J., 164–165

Stein, M., 315

Stein, M. D., 409

Stein, P. K., 178–179

Steinberg, M., 332

Steiner, I., 265–267

Steiner, M., 139–140

Steiner, S. C., 203–204

Steinfeld, S., 6

Steinhauer, S. R., 94

Stenman, U-H., 30

Stephan, M., 19

Stephens, P. M., 258, 261, 263–264, 264

Stephenson, T., 23

Steptoe, A., 38–39, 44–45, 46–47, 51–52, 52–53, 86, 93, 94, 129, 158, 173, 179, 187, 204, 224–225, 235, 238–241, 244, 244–245, 247, 248, 325, 341–342, 342, 345, 389, 423–424t, 438

Sterling, P., 263–264

Stern, L., 345

Sternberg, E. M., 281, 285

Sterner, J., 114, 118

Stessman, J., 321–322

Stetler, C. A., 108–109, 113–114, 161, 162, 182, 182–183, 187

Stevens, J. G., 265–267

Stevens, S. Y., 110–111, 163, 199–200, 205

Stevens, W. J., 108

Stevenson-Hinde, J., 130–131

Stewart, J., 234, 237

Stewart, J. A., 405

Webb, A. G., 227
Webb, D., 299–300
Webb, E. L., 22
Webb, J. R., 67
Webb, N. M., 424–425
Webb, R. T., 12–13
Weber, E., 327
Weber, K., 40–41
Weber, M., 235–236
Weber, R., 397
Webster Marketon, J. I., 346, 347
Webster, J. I., 281
Webster, N. R., 306–307, 324, 330
Wedding, U., 344
Weers, P. M. M., 282
Wegener, G., 6
Wegner, D. M., 107
Wegorzewska, M., 20
Wehr, T. A., 298, 299–300
Wei, L., 65–66, 67–68
Wei, Y.-L., 23–24
Wei, Y., 351
Wei, Y. C., 351
Weidenfeld, J., 10
Weidner, G., 264
Weigent, D. A., 52
Weihs, K. L., 197–198, 215, 342, 343,
    344, 357
Weikert, M., 322
Weil, G. J., 29
Weil, Z. M., 285, 292–293, 295–296
Weiler, H. A., 83
Weimann, E., 137–138
Weinberg, E. D., 308–309
Weinberg, R. A., 345–346, 346
Weinberg, V., 264
Weinberger, B., 39–40
Weiner, H. L., xvii–xviii, 219–220,
    257–258, 261, 264, 345, 377
Weingarten, I., 112–113
Weinman, J., 115, 206
Weinrib, A. Z., 325–326, 353–354,
    355
Weins, S., 85
Weinstock, M., 6, 23–24
Weinstock, R. S., 201–202
Weisbord, S. D., 325
Weiser, K., 356
Weiskopf, D., 39–40
Weiss, A., 150, 153, 154, 155, 157
Weiss, D., 389–390, 405–406, 407
Weiss, J. W., 171
Weiss, S. J., 13, 220–221, 397–398,
    409
Weisse, C. S., xvii–xviii
Weissing, F. J., 132–133
Weitzman, O. B., 164, 264–265

Welberg, L. A., 23–24
Wells, K. A., 400
Welsh, T., 100–101
Welt, M., 351
Wen, J., 70–71
Wen, J. C., 294, 295
Wendel, M., 280–281
Wendt, T., 87
Weng, N. P., 66–67
Wensley, F., 216–217, 238
Werb, Z., 346, 350
Wesley, B., 20
Wesseling, G., 248
Wessley, S. C., 321–322, 407
West, C., 326, 330
Westel, W. C., 133
Westenberg, H. G., 370
Westengard, J., 96–97
Wester, A. E., 84
Westermann, R., 95
Westwood, J. A., 349
Wetherell, M. A., 111, 285
Wetmore, G. S., 223, 227
Weyand, C. M., 63–64, 65, 69
Whaley, F. S., 297–298
Whalley, L. J., 246–247
Wheatley, S. C., 265–267
Whincup, P. H., 216–217, 238,
    238–241
Whishaw, I. Q., 310
Whistler, T., 256
White, D. E., 67
White, J., 329
White, W., 342
White, W. L., 26–27
Whitehead, R. G., 299
Whitehouse, W. G., 329
Whiteside, T., 218, 349–350, 350–351,
    405
Whittaker, J. A., 343
Whitworth, J. A., 22
Whorwood, C. B., 29–30
Wick, D. A., 67
Wick, G., 247
Wickrama, K. A. S., 197–198
Wiebe, J. S., 108–109, 163
Wieczorek, G., 29
Wiedemann, K., 328
Wiedermann, C. J., 247
Wieg, S. J., 225
Wiegant, V. M., 138
Wiegers, G. J., 10
Wielgosz, A., 234–235
Wieseler-Frank, J., 377
Wigdahl, B., 265–267
Wigger, A., 136
Wiik, P., 329

Wijayahadi, N., 325–326
Wikby, A., 66–67, 67, 71
Wikelski, M., 293
Wilcock, D. M., 377
Wilcock, G. K., 69, 201, 225
Wilder, R. L., 216–217, 217
Wildman, D. E., 25
Wilfley, D. E., 82
Wilhelm, F. H., 85
Willeit, J., 247
Willemen, H. L., 370, 374, 375, 379,
    379–380, 380–381
Willemsen, G., 97
Willette, A. A., 279
Willey, J. S., 325–326
Willheim, M., 68
Williams, B. J., 85
Williams, D. R., 236, 243–244
Williams, J. B., 349
Williams, K. L., 70
Williams, L. A., 323, 326
Williams, M. V., 405
Williams, R., 265–267
Williams, R. B., 129, 161, 162,
    171–172, 187
Williams, S. G., 20, 24, 130–131, 178,
    342
Williamson, H. A., 4–5
Willoughby, R. R., 152, 329
Wills, T. A., 214–215, 216, 219, 222,
    225–226, 226–227
Wilner, S., 333
Wilsenack, K., 137–138
Wilson, D. H., 298
Wilson, D. S., 129–130
Wilson, J., 224–225
Wilson, T. W., 221, 238
Wilson, V., 246–247
Wiltschke, C., 400
Wimberly, S. R., 344–345, 350, 389,
    400, 401
Windle, R. J., 247
Wing, E. J., 308–309
Wingard, D. L., 321
Wingfield, J. C., 129, 278, 278–279,
    282–284, 284–285, 285
Winkel, K., 327
Winkielman, P., 435–436
Winter, C., 23
Winter, J. B., 322
Wintour, E. M., 29–30
Wirtz, P. H., 180, 181, 331–332
Wisenbaker, J. M., 12
Witek-Janusek, L., 50–51, 98, 285,
    286, 400
Witter, F. R., 19–20
Wittert, G., 298

SUBJECT INDEX

comparative psychoneuroimmunology, 277, 278–279

emotional expression and disclosure, 107–108, 108, 110–111, 111, 111–112, 119

imbalance in hostility, 185

in immunity, 20, 20–21, 21, 29, 30

influences on motivation, 306–307, 312

in personality, human, 153, 154, 156–157, 160–161, 162, 163–164, 166

positive affect and, 96–97, 98, 100

pregnancy and stress, 4, 8–9, 11–12

reliability formulae, 422–424

social support, 216–217, 221–222, 224, 225

stress management interventions, 387–388, 389–390, 400, 403–404, 406

Cytokines (proinflammatory). *See also specific cytokines*

aging and well-being, 38, 40, 43–45, 45–47, 48, 50

aging of immune system, 66, 68, 69–70

fatigue and sleep disturbance
activation, sleep and, 327–329
CNS mediation by, 323–324
overview, 322–323
sickness behavior and, 324–325
sleep-inducing criteria, 328

GRK2 and, 372, 374, 378, 379–380, 381

inflammation role generally, 171, 178

marriage effects on, 200, 204–205

in personality, animal, 133, 135, 137–138, 138, 139–140

in seasonality, 294, 296–297, 298

in self-conscious emotions, 79–80, 81, 86, 86–87

Cytomegalovirus
aging and well-being, 39–40
aging of immune system, 63–64, 66–67, 69, 71
socioeconomic status, 238–241, 247

D

Daytime sleepiness, 321, 329, 330. *See also* Fatigue and sleep disturbance

Death rate patterns, 19

Dehydroepiandrosterone sulfate (DHEAS), 69

Delayed-type hypersensitivity. *See also* Allergies
emotional expression and disclosure, 119

personality, human, 159, 164

seasonality, 293, 298

social support, 218, 219

Depression
adiposity, obesity effects, 187

causal pathways, 178–179

C-reactive protein, 178–179, 179–180, 180–181, 183

cross-sectional relationships, 179–180

directionality (prospective) studies, 180–181

dose-response association, 179

fatigue and sleep disturbance, 322

fibrinogen, 180–181

gender effects, 186–187

interferon-α, 178

interleukin-2, 178

interleukin-6, 178–179, 179–180, 180–181

interleukin-8, 179–180

interleukin-10, 181

interleukin-1 species, 179–180, 181

leptin, 187

macrophage-T-lymphocyte hypothesis, 177–178, 179–180

marriage effects on, 202–203, 203–204

measures of, 172–173

meta-analysis of studies, 179

overview, 174

personality, animal, 138–140

social support, 224

stress management interventions, 387–388, 390–391, 403–404

studies of generally, 177–178, 181–182

temporal relationships, 181

TNF-α, 182–185, 187

Development, 19

Diabetes type 2, 67–68

Disclosure. *See* Emotional expression and disclosure

Docetaxel, 326

Dopamine, 323

DTH response. *See* Delayed-type hypersensitivity

Dyskeratosis congenita, 67–68

E

Emotional expression and disclosure
adaptive immunity, 119

anger, 109–110, 115

arteriosclerosis, 108–109

asthma, 111

attentional bias, 109

autonomic nervous system effects, 107, 118–119

B cells, 113–114

best possible self, 109, 117–118

cancer, 114–115

cardiovascular reactivity, 107, 108–109

CD4 cells, 108, 112–113

CD8 cells, 107–108

cognitive processing, 108, 109, 111–112, 115, 117

coping strategies, 109, 114–115, 131

C-reactive protein, 111

cytokines, 107–108, 108, 110–111, 111–112, 119

delayed-type hypersensitivity response, 119

disinhibition, 117

emotional effects, 107, 117–118

Epstein-Barr virus, 113

expressive writing studies, 106–107

future research directions, 120

goals, 109, 115

headaches, 109–110

health benefits of, 105–106, 106–107, 116–117

heart disease, 107, 108–109

HIV/AIDS, 108, 112–113

hostility, 108–109, 109, 115

HPA axis, 118–119

immune system effects, 107–108

inflammation, 108–109, 111, 115–116

interferon-γ, 111, 111–112, 119

interleukins, 107–108, 108, 110–111, 111–112, 119

marital conflict, 110–111

meaning-making, 117

meta-analyses, 116–117

migraines, 109–110

moderators of, 108–109

natural killer cells, 107–108, 108–109

neuroimmune mechanisms, 118–119, 120

overview, 105–106, 116, 120

pain alleviation, 109–110

psoriasis, 115–116

psychological processes, theories, 117–118

psychosis, posttraumatic stress, 110, 117–118

racism, 113–114

reflection, narrative reconstruction, 120

repressor (type D) personalities, 108

rheumatoid arthritis, 108, 111–112

secure attachment style personalities, 108

Hormones. *See also specific hormones* (cont.)
overview, 278
in positive emotions (positive affect), 94
in pregnancy and stress, 9–10
in seasonality, 299–300
stress (*See* Stress hormones)

Hostility
adiposity, obesity effects, 187
chemokines, 184–185
CMHO scale measurement, 183–185
C-reactive protein, 182–185, 185–186, 187
cross-sectional studies, 182–185
cytokine imbalance in, 185
directionality (prospective) studies, 185
emotional expression and disclosure, 108–109, 109, 115
factor interaction findings, 185–186
gender effects, 186–187
high density lipoprotein (HDL), 185, 185–186
instinctive theory of aggression, 307–308
interferon-γ, 183–185
interleukin-2, 183–185
interleukin-4, 183–185
interleukin-5, 183–185
interleukin-6, 182–185, 185–186, 187
interleukin-10, 183–185, 185
marriage effects on, 199–200, 206
personality, human, 161–164
TNF-α, 182–185

HPA axis
activity in self-conscious emotions, 81, 83, 84
aging and well-being, 51–52
emotional expression and disclosure, 118–119
fatigue and sleep disturbance, 324, 326, 330
marriage effects on, 204
modulation of cancer by, 344–345, 345f, 354–355
motivation, 306–307, 312, 313
personality, animal, 132–134, 137–138
personality, animal, 151
positive affect and, 94, 94–95
pregnancy and stress, 6–7, 9–10, 11
seasonality, 295–296, 299–300
in social regulation of gene expression, 257–258, 258

social support, 224–225
socioeconomic status, function and, 247
stress management interventions, 388, 388–389, 389–390, 405–406
HPG axis, 295
HTERT, 70

I

ICAM-1
fatigue and sleep disturbance, 322–323
sICAM-1, 183, 325–326
socioeconomic status, 238–241, 242–243t
stress management interventions, 403–404
IL6 gene, 261–262, 266f
Illness-induced anorexia, 278, 278–279, 279–281

Immunity
adaptive, 18–19, 28
aging in (*See* Aging of immune system)
allergies, 19–20, 20, 24–25
antenatal corticosteroids, 24–25, 26–27
antibodies, 19, 25–26, 26f
asthma, 19–20
bacterial vaginosis, 22
Bifidobacteria, 27–28
cytokines, 20, 20–21, 21, 29, 30
dexamethasone, 26
evolutionary processes, natural selection, 24–25, 29–30
fetal brain development, 21f, 22–23, 29
fetal immunomodulation, 21–24, 29
fetal outcomes, 23–24, 29–30
fetal programming, 20, 24
fetus, 19–20
future research directions, 31
immunomodulation, 20, 20–21, 21f, 29
infections, 21–22, 22, 22–23, 27–28, 29
influenza, 22–23
innate, 18–19, 28
interferon, 20
interleukin-1β, 20–21
interleukin-5, 20
interleukin-6, 20–21, 22–23, 30
interleukin-8, 20–21
interleukin-12, 20
intestinal disease, 27–28
Lactobacilli, 27–28

as learning system, 19
lymphocyte responses, 19
microbiota, 19, 27–28
MNCs, 25, 26–27
monoamine neurotransmitters, 23–24
neurodevelopmental disorders, 22–23
overview, 18–20, 30–31
passive immunity, 19, 25–26, 26f, 30
placenta, 19, 20, 21–22, 24–25, 29
pregnancy, 19–20, 20–21, 21f, 29(*See also* Pregnancy and stress)
prenatal processes in, 20
progenitor cells, 24–25
proinflammatory cytokines, 21, 22f, 23
protective factors, resiliency, 24, 30
psychological processes, 22–24, 29–30
rearing environment in, 19, 24–25, 26–27, 27f, 27t, 28–29, 29f, 30
separation anxiety, stress, 28, 28t
small molecular weight proteins, 24–25
suppressor T cells, 26–27, 27f, 27t
T cell memory, 19, 25
thymus, 20, 24–25, 29
TNF-α, 21, 22f
tolerance, 20, 20–21, 21f, 29
trauma, violence, 23, 29–30
weaning cytokines, 28, 28t
worms, parasites, 22

Immunoglobulins
personality, animal, 134, 135, 136, 139–140
personality, animal, 156
positive emotions (positive affect), 96
salivary immunoglobulin A (sIgA), 238–241
secretory immunoglobulin A (sIgA), 96, 99
socioeconomic status, 238–241

Infections
bacterial
in fatigue, sleep disturbance, 328
in social regulation of gene expression, 262–264
in socioeconomic status, 238–241, 247
cytomegalovirus (*See* Cytomegalovirus)
early life exposure to, 236–237, 246, 247
Epstein-Barr (*See* Epstein-Barr virus)
immunity generally, 21–22, 22–23, 27–28, 29
intimate social, 262–264

NGF gene, 256
NGF/IFNB/SIV system remodeling, 259–261
Norepinephrine
    cancer, 344–345, 347, 348, 353
    in comparative psychoneuroimmunology, 278
    in fatigue, sleep disturbance, 323
    GRK2 and, 371–372
    marriage, 198–199
    positive emotions (positive affect), 94
    seasonality, 296
    social regulation of gene expression, 259–261
    social support, 225
    stress management interventions, 388–389, 392, 395–396
NUPDQ assessment, 6
Nurses' Health Study, 343–344

O

Obstructive sleep apnea, 201–202
Octopamine, 280, 281–282, 283f, 285
Opiates, 94
M-opioid receptor, 370–371
Osteoporosis, 68
Oxidative stress, 64, 65–66, 68

P

Parkinson's disease, 373–374
personality, animal
    affiliation, sociability, 131–132, 134–135, 137
    aggression, 132–134, 137
    animal models generally, 129–130, 134–135
    arthritis, 138
    autonomic nervous system function, 135
    behavioral inhibition, 130–131
    behavioral syndrome, 131
    cancer, 138, 139
    CD4 cells, 134, 136
    CD8 cells, 136
    coping strategies, 109, 114–115, 131, 137–138
    corticosterone, 133, 136, 138, 139
    cortisol, 133–134, 138
    definitions, 130–131
    depression, 138–140
    disease, 131–132
    exploration, 130–131, 136–137
    extraversion, 130–131
    fear/anxiety, 130–131, 133, 135–136, 137–138
    Five-Factor model, 130–131
    Flinders rats, 139–140

forced-swim test, 139
future research directions, 140
genetic linkages, 134
glucocorticoids, 133
health, 131–132
HIV/AIDS, 134
HPA axis, 132–134, 137–138
immune function, 131–132, 134–135
immunoglobulins, 134, 135, 136, 139–140
infection, 139
interferon-α, 139
interferon-γ, 133, 137–138, 138, 139–140
interleukins, 133, 136, 137–138, 138, 139–140
keyhole limpet hemocyanin (KLH), 138
learned helplessness, 138–139
life spans, 136
lymph node innervation, 135
natural killer cells, 133, 136
novelty-seeking, 130–131, 136–137
overview, 129–130, 140
proactive coping, 130–131, 132–133, 135, 137–138
pro-inflammatory cytokines, 133, 135, 137–138, 138, 139–140
prolactin, 137–138
reactive coping, 130–131, 132–133, 137–138
sensation-seeking, 130–131, 136–137
short vs. long attack latency, 133
simian immunodeficiency disorder (SIV), 133–134
sleep patterns, 139–140
SNS reactivity, 133
sucrose-preference test, 139
T cells, 134, 137–138
terminology, 130
tetanus, 134, 135
TNF-α, 136–137
type-health status relationships, 129
vaccination, 134, 135
personality, human
    agreeableness, 155
    assessment of personality, 147
    Big Five traits, 146, 148, 166
    cardiovascular disease, 161
    causal inferences, 148
    CD species cells, 149–150, 152–153, 153, 154, 156, 158, 162–163
    conscientiousness, 154–155, 165–166
    coping strategies, 158–159

C-reactive protein, 153, 154, 156–157, 162
delayed-type hypersensitivity, 159, 164
environmental alterations, 146–147
Epstein-Barr virus, 152
extraversion, 148–150
future research directions, 165–166
herpes recurrence, 150, 153
HIV/AIDS, 150, 153, 154, 157–158, 164–165
hostility, 161–164
HPA axis, 151
immune altering behaviors, 146–147
immunoglobulins, 156
infectious disease, 147, 148–149, 151, 154, 160
inflammation markers, 153, 154, 156–157, 160–161, 162, 163–164, 166
influence of traits, 146–147
interferon-γ, 161–162
interleukin-6, 152–153, 154, 156–157, 158, 160–161, 162, 163–164
interleukins, 152–153, 153, 156, 160–161, 161–162
introversion, 148–150
lymphocytes, lymphocyte subsets, 149–150, 152–153, 156
main vs. stress-modulating effects, 147
measures of immunity, 147
natural killer cells, 149–150, 152–153, 153, 158–159, 162–163, 164
NEO scale, 148
neuroticism, 150–154
openness to experience, 155
optimism, 155–159
overview, 146, 165
phytohemagglutinin (PHA), 149–150, 152–153, 156
positive affect, 160–161
social inhibition, 164–165
stress effect moderation, 150, 151, 153, 158–159, 162–163, 166
subtraits, 166
T cells, 149–150
telomere length, 157
TNF-α, 152–153, 160–161, 161–162
vaccination, 149, 151–152, 152, 154, 156, 158, 160
Photoperiodism. See also Seasonality
    immune response to, 292–293, 293
    inflammation response, 293, 295–296

cytokines, 387–388, 389–390, 400, 403–404, 406

depression, 387–388, 390–391, 403–404

disease classes, 386–387

ENRICHD trial, 404

epinephrine, 388–389, 392

HAART, 391, 395–396

HIV/AIDS

classification of, 386–387

cognitive behavioral stress management (CBSM) (*See* Cognitive-behavioral stress management (CBSM), above)

disease processes in, 389, 390

endocrine-immune interactions, 388–389

opportunistic infections in, 392

psychological factors in disease progression, 390–391

HPA axis, 388, 388–389, 389–390, 405–406

HPV, 396

ICAM-1, 403–404

inflammatory processes, 389–390

interferon-γ, 400

interleukin-1, 406

interleukin-1β, 389, 403–404

interleukin-2, 387–388, 400

interleukin-6, 389, 403–404, 406

interleukin-10, 389

leukocyte adhesion molecules, 389

lymphocyte proliferative response, 400

Mac-1, 389

multiple sclerosis, 389

natural killer cells, 387–388, 389–390

negative life events, cumulative, 391

neuroendocrine response, 387–388

norepinephrine, 388–389, 389, 392, 395–396

opportunistic infections, 392, 402

optimization

content, format, 409–410

methodology, 411–412

target populations, 409

timing, 410–411

overview, 385–386, 408

peripheral blood mononuclear cells, 389, 400

rationale, relevant mechanisms

disease processes, PNI and, 389–390

endocrine-immune interactions, 388–389

human studies, 387–388

overview, 387

PNI rationale, 390

rheumatoid arthritis, 389

L-selectin, 389

sickness behaviors, 403–404, 406

sleep disruptions, 400–401

SNS activation, 388, 388–389

social support, isolation, 388, 391, 406

stress hormones, 388–389, 395–396

SWITCHD trial, 404

TNFα, 389, 403–404, 406

vaccination, 387–388

Substance P, 376–377, 378–379

Sympathetic nervous system. *See* SNS activation

T

T'ai chi, 49, 71

T cells

aging of immune system, 63–64, 65–66, 66–67

chronically stimulated in immune system aging, 65–66

cytotoxic in immune system aging, 64–65

emotional expression and disclosure, 107–108, 112–113

in inflammation, 176

memory, 19, 25

personality, human, 149–150

seasonality, 293, 296–297

social support, 219, 220

socioeconomic status, 238–241, 244–245

suppressor, 26–27, 27f, 27t

Telomerase targeting, 70–71

Telomere length

aging of immune system, 65–66, 67–69, 69

personality, human, 157

Temperament. *See* personality, human; personality, human

Testosterone, 282–284

Third National Health and Nutrition Examination Survey, 186–187

THROMBO study, 174–175

TLR4 pathway, 374

TNF-α

aging and well-being, 46

aging of immune system, 66, 68, 70–71

anger, 182–185

in depression, 182–185, 187

emotional expression and disclosure, 108, 110–111

fatigue and sleep disturbance, 322–323, 323, 324, 326, 328–329, 329, 331–332

GRK2 and, 372, 374, 378, 381

hostility, 182–185

in immunity, 21, 22f

marriage effects on, 200, 204–205

personality, human, 152–153, 160–161, 161–162

positive emotions (positive affect), 96–97

pregnancy and stress, 9, 11–12

self-conscious emotions, 81, 86, 86–87

social support, 217

socioeconomic status, 244–245, 239–241t

Tumor associated macrophages (TAMs)

behavioral, neuroendocrine modulation of, 353

role of, 348, 352–353

stress effects on, 345f, 355–356

V

Vaccination

aging and well-being, 49

aging of immune system, 63, 69, 71

emotional expression and disclosure, 113–114, 119

personality, human, 149, 151–152, 152, 154, 156, 158, 160

response in seasonality, 296–297

social support, 217–218

VEGF

cancer, 345f, 346, 346–347, 352–353, 355–356

fatigue and sleep disturbance, 325–326

Viral infections. *See* Infections

W

Well-being and aging. *See* Aging and well-being

Whitehall Psychobiology Study, 244–245

WLS study, 46

Women's Health Initiative study, 342

Wound healing

comparative psychoneuroimmunology, 284

emotional expression and disclosure, 115

marriage effects on, 206

positive emotions (positive affect), 100

Wound infection, 282